Trease and Evans

Pharmacognosy

For Elsevier
Commissioning Editor: Pauline Graham
Development Editor: Janice Urquhart, Fiona Conn
Project Manager: Gail Wright
Design Direction: George Ajayi

Trease and Evans
Pharmacognosy

William Charles Evans BPharm BSc PhD DSc FIBiol FLS FRPharmS

Revised with the assistance of
Daphne Evans BA MA

SIXTEENTH EDITION

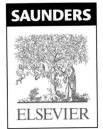

SAUNDERS

ELSEVIER

Edinburgh London New York Philadelphia St Louis Sydney Toronto 2009

SAUNDERS
ELSEVIER

© 2009, Elsevier Limited. All rights reserved.
First published 1934
Sixteenth edition 2009
Fifteenth edition 2002
Fourteenth edition 1996
Thirteenth edition 1989
Twelfth edition 1983

ISBN 978-0-7020-2933-2
International Edition ISBN 978-0-7020-2934-9

British Library Cataloguing in Publication Data
A catalogue record for this book is available from the British Library

Library of Congress Cataloging in Publication Data
A catalog record for this book is available from the Library of Congress

Notice

Knowledge and best practice in this field are constantly changing. As new research and experience
broaden our knowledge, changes in practice, treatment and drug therapy may become necessary or
appropriate. Readers are advised to check the most current information provided (i) on procedures
featured or (ii) by the manufacturer of each product to be administered, to verify the recommended
dose or formula, the method and duration of administration, and contraindications. It is the
responsibility of the practitioner, relying on their own experience and knowledge of the patient, to
make diagnoses, to determine dosages and the best treatment for each individual patient, and to take
all appropriate safety precautions. To the fullest extent of the law, neither the Publisher nor the Editor
assumes any liability for any injury and/or damage to persons or property arising out of or related to
any use of the material contained in this book.

The Publisher

Working together to grow
libraries in developing countries

www.elsevier.com | www.bookaid.org | www.sabre.org

ELSEVIER   BOOK AID International   Sabre Foundation

The
publisher's
policy is to use
**paper manufactured
from sustainable forests**

Printed in China

Contents

Preface

Pharmacognosy embraces a number of scientific and other disciplines providing a unified and comprehensive treatment of medicinal plants. There are constant advances and changes affecting all areas of the subject and, as in the past, this 16th edition addresses these new developments while at the same time maintaining the fundamental concepts required for the teaching of all aspects of the subject. It should continue to be of value not only to those of a pharmaceutical and medical persuasion but also to scholars of other disciplines who have an interest in natural products.

Over 60 crude drugs, recently included in editions of the European and British pharmacopoeias, have now been given separate entries in Part 3. Cognizance has been taken of the shift away from material collected in the wild, which results in the endangerment of species, towards cultivation under controlled conditions. The implementation of legal requirements for the quality control of herbal drugs and medicines has given an even greater significance to the development of additional standardization and analytical procedures; similarly for traditional Asian and Chinese medicines.

Subsequent to the publication of the 15th edition of this book, many new phytochemicals, their structures and pharmacological activities, have been reported, especially from those plant materials having current interest. In this respect, a new chapter covering plant nutraceuticals gives emphasis to the attention now being given to this diverse group of pharmacologically active food constituents. Genetic fingerprinting, now widely used by plant taxonomists, is becoming increasingly important for the characterization of closely related species of medicinal plants and for the recognition of chemical races with variable pharmacological properties; a number of examples will be found throughout the text.

As previously, I am much indebted to the contributors, who have given of their time and expertise to provide new or revised chapters on topics of current interest. It is with much regret that I record the death of my former colleague Dr Mohammed Aslam, who with characteristic enthusiasm had initiated and continued to update the chapter on Asian medicine, Thanks are due to Dr R. Hardman, Dr K. Helliwell, Dr L. W. Levy and Prof. J. D. Phillipson for aspects concerning current developments, and to Seven Seas Limited, Marfleet, for kindly updating entries on fish oils. Library facilities were made available by the Universities of Bath, Bristol, Exeter and Reading, the Royal Pharmaceutical Society of Great Britain, the Secretariat of the European Scientific Cooperative for Phytotherapy and the Taunton Public Library.

Daphne, my wife, has assisted me throughout by providing miscellaneous contributions to the text, carrying out literature searches and helping with the organization of the manuscript; without her dedicated help, this edition would not have been possible. Miscellaneous practical support afforded by other family members is also much appreciated.

I am grateful to the publishers in Edinburgh for their usual helpful assistance and understanding.

W. C. E.
2009

Contributors

Robin Baker
RoA Services Ltd, Harwich, UK

Peter J. Houghton BPharm PhD FRPharmS CChem FRSC
Department of Pharmacy, King's College London, London, UK

Jane A. Lewis BSc PhD
Medicines Research Centre, GlaxoSmithKline, Stevenage, UK

G. Brian Lockwood BPharm PhD MRPharmS
School of Pharmacy and Pharmaceutical Sciences, University of Manchester, Manchester, UK

Simon Y. Mills MA FNIMH MCCP
Centre for Complementary Health Studies, University of Exeter, Exeter, UK

Melanie J. O'Neill BPharm PhD MRPharmS
Medicines Research Centre, GlaxoSmithKline, Stevenage, UK

Abayomi Sofowora BPharm PhD
Faculty of Pharmacy, Obafemi Awolowo University, Ife-Ife, Nigeria

Samantha E. Weston BPharm MBA MRPharmS
School of Pharmacy, University of Reading, Reading, UK

Elizabeth M. Williamson BSc PhD MRPharmS FLS
School of Pharmacy, University of Reading, Reading, UK

Colin W. Wright BPharm MSc PhD MRPharmS
School of Pharmacy, University of Bradford, Bradford, UK

PART

1 | Introduction

1

Plants in medicine: the origins of pharmacognosy

The universal role of plants in the treatment of disease is exemplified by their employment in all the major systems of medicine irrespective of the underlying philosophical premise. As examples, we have Western medicine with origins in Mesopotamia and Egypt, the Unani (Islamic) and Ayurvedic (Hindu) systems centred in western Asia and the Indian subcontinent and those of the Orient (China, Japan, Tibet, etc.). How and when such medicinal plants were first used is, in many cases, lost in pre-history, indeed animals, other than man, appear to have their own materia medica. Following the oral transmission of medical information came the use of writing (e.g. the Egyptian *Papyrus Ebers c.* 1600 BC), baked clay tablets (some 660 cuneiform tablets *c.* 650 BC from Ashurbanipal's library at Nineveh, now in the British Museum, refer to drugs well-known today), parchments and manuscript herbals, printed herbals (invention of printing 1440 AD), pharmacopoeias and other works of reference (first *London Pharmacopoeia*, 1618; first *British Pharmacopoeia*, 1864), and most recently electronic storage of data. Similar records exist for Chinese medicinal plants (texts from the 4th century BC), Ayurvedic medicine (Ayurveda 2500–600 BC) and Unani medicine (*Kitab-Al-Shifa*, the Magnum Opus of Avicenna, 980–1037 AD).

In addition to the above recorded information there is a great wealth of knowledge concerning the medicinal, narcotic and other properties of plants that is still transmitted orally from generation to generation by tribal societies, particularly those of tropical Africa, North and South America and the Pacific countries. These are areas containing the world's greatest number of plant species, not found elsewhere, and with the westernization of so many of the peoples of these zones there is a pressing need to record local knowledge before it is lost forever. In addition, with the extermination of plant species progressing at an alarming rate in certain regions, even before plants have been botanically recorded, much less studied chemically and pharmacologically, the need arises for increased efforts directed towards the conservation of gene pools.

A complete understanding of medicinal plants involves a number of disciplines including commerce, botany, horticulture, chemistry, enzymology, genetics, quality control and pharmacology. Pharmacognosy is not any one of these per se but seeks to embrace them in a unified whole for the better understanding and utilization of medicinal plants. A perusal of the monographs on crude drugs in a modern pharmacopoeia at once illustrates the necessity for a multidisciplinary approach. Unlike those who laid the foundations of pharmacognosy, no one person can now expect to be an expert in all areas and, as is illustrated in the next chapter, pharmacognosy can be independently approached from a number of viewpoints.

The word 'pharmacognosy' had its debut in the early 19th century to designate the discipline related to medicinal plants; it is derived from the Greek pharmakon, 'a drug', and gignosco, 'to acquire a knowledge of' and, as recorded by Dr K. Ganzinger (*Sci. Pharm.*, 1982, **50**, 351), the terms 'pharmacognosy' and 'pharmacodynamics' were probably first coined by Johann Adam Schmidt (1759–1809) in his hand-written manuscript *Lehrbuch der Materia Medica*, which was posthumously published in Vienna in 1811. Schmidt was, until his death, professor at the medico-surgical Joseph Academy in Vienna; interestingly he was also Beethoven's physician. Shortly after the above publication, 'pharmacognosy' appears again in 1815 in a small work by Chr. Aenotheus Seydler entitled *Analecta Pharmacognostica*.

Pharmacognosy is closely related to botany and plant chemistry and, indeed, both originated from the earlier scientific studies on medicinal plants. As late as the beginning of the 20th century, the subject had developed mainly on the botanical side, being concerned with the description and identification of drugs, both in the whole state and in powder, and with their history, commerce, collection, preparation and storage. In his series *A History of British Pharmacognosy (1842–1980)*, E. J. Shellard (*Pharm. J.*, 1980, **225**, 680) wrote:

> It is a recognised fact that in the historical development of any subject the role of certain individuals is of considerable importance. This is true in pharmacognosy. The first British pharmacognosist was Jonathan Pereira (1804–1853), who as the first teacher of the subject gave it its pharmaceutical basis. He may be considered as the founder of British pharmacognosy. Daniel Hanbury (1825–1875) was the most outstanding applied pharmacognosist while the contribution made by E. M. Holmes (1843–1930) as an applied pharmacognosist stands out both in quality and quantity. H. G. Greenish (1855–1933), and T. E. Wallis (1876–1973) transformed the old academic pharmacognosy by their contribution to the elimination of adulteration from powdered drugs. Their exploitation of the microscope in pharmacognosy ensures their position as the pillars of the halcyon days (of pharmacognosy).

Such branches of pharmacognosy are still of fundamental importance, particularly for pharmacopoeial identification and quality control purposes, but rapid developments in other areas have enormously expanded the subject.

The use of modern isolation techniques and pharmacological testing procedures means that new plant drugs may find their way into medicine as purified substances rather than in the form of galenical preparations which, for various reasons, would be unsatisfactory. Preparation is usually confined to one or a few companies who process all the raw material; thus, few pharmacists have occasion to handle dried *Catharanthus roseus* although they are familiar with formulations of the isolated alkaloids vinblastine and vincristine. For these new drugs it is important that the pharmacist is cognisant of the physical, chemical and chromatographic standards applicable to the identification, purity, etc. of such products. Similar remarks apply to other anticancer drugs derived from *Taxus, Podophyllum* and *Ochrosia* spp.

When specific plants, including those used in traditional medicine, suddenly become of interest to the world at large, the local wild sources soon become exhausted. This necessitates, as in the case of *Catharanthus roseus, Coleus forskohlii, Ginkgo biloba, Arnica montana* and *Taxus brevifolia*, research into the cultivation or artificial propagation by cell culture, etc., of such species. In order to avert the type of supply crisis that arose at the clinical trial stage with the anticancer drug taxol, isolated from *T. brevifolia*, the US National Cancer Institute initiated plans for future action should a similar situation again arise (see G. M. Cragg *et al., J. Nat. Prod.*, 1993, **56**, 1657). However, it was reported that as a result of the original demand for the drug galanthamine (q.v.) for the treatment of Alzheimer's disease, the native source of *Leucojum aestivum* was endangered. The situation was partially resolved following the commercial synthesis of galanthamine.

The use of single pure compounds, including synthetic drugs, is not without its limitations, and in recent years there has been an immense revival in interest in the herbal and homoeopathic systems of medicine, both of which rely heavily on plant sources. At the 9th Congress of the Italian Society of Pharmacognosy (1998) it was stated that the current return of phytotherapy was clearly reflected by the increased market of such products. In 1995 the latter, for Europe, reached a figure of $6 billion, with consumption for Germany $2.5 billion, France $1.6 billion and Italy 600 million. In the US, where the use of herbal products has never been as strong as in continental Europe, the increase in recent years has also been unprecedented with the market for all herb sales reaching a peak in 1998 approaching $700 million. Again, illustrating the same trend, the editor of *Journal of Natural Products*, 1999, wrote that in response to the increasing prominence of herbal remedies, additional contributions describing scientific investigations of a rigorous nature would be welcomed, a suggestion that appears to have been fully endorsed!

Undoubtedly, the plant kingdom still holds many species of plants containing substances of medicinal value which have yet to be discovered; large numbers of plants are constantly being screened for their possible pharmacological value (particularly for their anti-inflammatory, hypotensive, hypoglycaemic, amoebicidal, antifertility, cytotoxic, antibiotic and anti-Parkinsonism properties). Pharmacognosists with a multidisciplinary background are able to make valuable contributions to these rapidly developing fields of study and pharmacists in general need to have a knowledge of, and to give professional advice on, the many herbal preparations available to the public.

2

The scope and practice of pharmacognosy

Until relatively recently pharmacognosy was regarded, almost exclusively, as a subject in the pharmaceutical curriculum focused on those natural products employed in the allopathic system of medicine. Coincident with the increasing attractiveness of alternative (complementary) therapies and the tremendous range of herbal products now generally available to the public, regulatory requirements covering medicinal herbs have been put in place by many countries in order to control the quality of these products. Monographs are now available on a large number of such drugs giving descriptions, tests for identity and purity and assays of active constituents. These monographs are being compiled by a number of bodies (see below). In this respect recognition should be given to the pioneering production of the *British Herbal Pharmacopoeia*, first produced in 1974 with the latest volume in 1996. Pharmacognosy is also important in those countries having their own systems of medicine in which plants are important components.

Many crude drugs once generally categorized as herbal remedies are now, in accordance with Continental European practice, described in the *British Pharmacopoeia* (*BP*). Chromatographic, chemical and physical tests, together with assay procedures, are given for many drugs for which previously there was no quantitative evaluation of the chemical constituents available. The importance of quality control is paramount, as the demand and the possibility of substitution has increased. The upsurge in the marketing of Chinese and Asian traditional medicines worldwide, for which there is a need for adequate control, adds a further dimension to pharmacognosy; pharmacopoeial monographs now include Liquorice for use in Chinese medicine, Chinese angelica root and Astragalus root. It is understood that further monographs on Chinese and Indian drugs for use in traditional medicine are to be included in the *BP* 2009.

Although pharmacognosy is principally concerned with plant materials, there are a small number of animal products which are traditionally encompassed within the subject; these include such items as beeswax, gelatin, woolfat, vitamins, etc. Other natural products such as the antibiotics, hormones and others may or may not be involved, depending on the teaching practice of a particular institution. Marine organisms, both plant and animal, with potent pharmacological actions are receiving increasing attention in the search for new drugs. Materials having no pharmacological action which are of interest to pharmacognosists are natural fibres, flavouring and suspending agents, colourants, disintegrants, stabilizers and filtering and support media. Other areas that have natural associations with the subject are poisonous and hallucinogenic plants, allergens, herbicides, insecticides and molluscicides.

Vegetable drugs can be arranged for study under the following headings.

1. *Alphabetical.* Either Latin or vernacular names may be used. This arrangement is employed for dictionaries, pharmacopoeias, etc. Although suitable for quick reference it gives no indication of interrelationships between drugs.
2. *Taxonomic.* On the basis of an accepted system of botanical classification (Chapter 3), the drugs are arranged according to the plants from which they are obtained, in classes, orders, families, genera and species. It allows for a precise and ordered arrangement and accommodates any drug without ambiguity. As the basic botanical knowledge of pharmacy students decreases over the years this system is becoming less popular for teaching purposes.
3. *Morphological.* The drugs are divided into groups such as the following: leaves, flowers, fruits, seeds, herbs and entire organisms, woods, barks, rhizomes and roots (known as organized drugs), and dried latices, extracts, gums, resins, oils, fats and waxes (unorganized drugs).

These groupings have some advantages for the practical study of crude drugs; the identification of powdered drugs (see Chapter 43) is often based on micro-morphological characters.

4. *Pharmacological or Therapeutic*. This classification involves the grouping of drugs according to the pharmacological action of their most important constituent or their therapeutic use. R. Pratt and H. W. Youngken Jr. were, in 1956, the first to use this approach for an English language textbook and now, with so many plant materials being screened for specific pharmacological activity, this type of listing is found increasingly in the literature. Its use is illustrated in Chapters 27–32. However, it is important to appreciate that the constituents of any one drug may fall into different pharmacological groups.

5. *Chemical or Biogenetic*. The important constituents, e.g. alkaloids, glycosides, volatile oils, etc., or their biosynthetic pathways, form the basis of classification of the drugs. This is a popular approach when the teaching of pharmacognosy is phytochemically biased. Ambiguities arise when particular drugs possess a number of active principles belonging to different phytochemical groups, as illustrated by liquorice, ginseng, valerian, etc. The scheme is employed in Chapters 19–26 for arranging the established pharmacopoeial drugs.

The following list of works, arranged in the above five groups, will serve as examples and also provide a useful list of textbooks and works of reference; those no longer in print may be found in established pharmaceutical libraries.

1. Alphabetical

Barnes J, Anderson LA, Phillipson JD 2007 Herbal medicines, 3rd edn. Pharmaceutical Press, London
Bisset NG (ed), Wichtl M 1996 Herbal drugs, a handbook for practice on a scientific basis. Medpharm Scientific Publishers, Stuttgart
Bradley PR 1992, 2006 British herbal compendium, Vols I, II. British Herbal Medicine Association, Bournemouth, UK
British Pharmacopoeia 2008 and preceding edns
British Herbal Pharmacopoeia 1996. British Herbal Medicine Association, Exeter, UK
Duke JA 2002 Handbook of medicinal herbs, 2nd edn. CRC Press, New York
Martindale: the Complete Drug Reference, 35th edn 2007. Pharmaceutical Press, London
United States Pharmacopoeia 29/National Formulary 24 and Supplement 2006
Williamson EM 2002 Potter's herbal cyclopaedia. CW Daniel Co, Saffron Walden

The national pharmacopoeias of many countries and the European Pharmacopoeia; *the relevant crude drug monographs of the latter are included in the British Pharmacopoeia*

2. Taxonomic

Paris RR, Moyse H 1965, 1967, 1971 Matière médicale. Masson, Paris, 3 vols
Thoms H 1929 Handbuch der Pharmacie. Urban and Schwarzenberg, Berlin, Band V, 2 vols, Pharmacognosy
Trease GE, Evans WC 1972 Pharmacognosy, 10th edn. Baillière Tindall and Cassell, London

3. Morphological

Berger F Handbuch der Drogenkunde. Maudrich, Vienna, Vol I, Barks and flowers, 1949; Vol II, Leaves, 1950; Vol III, Fruits and woods, 1952; Vol IV, Herbs, 1954; Vol V, Roots, 1960; Vol VI, Resins etc and seeds, 1964; Vol VII, Index, 1967
Jackson BP, Snowdon DW 1990 Atlas of microscopy of medicinal plants, culinary herbs and spices. Belhaven Press, London
Wallis TE, 1967 Textbook of pharmacognosy, 5th edn. Churchill Livingstone, London

4. Pharmacological or Therapeutic

Der Marderosian A, Liberti LE 1988 Natural product medicine. GF Stickley, Philadelphia, PA, USA
Heinrich M, Barnes J, Gibbons S, Williamson EM 2004 Pharmacognosy and phytotherapy. Churchill Livingstone, Edinburgh
Pratt R, Youngken HW, Jr 1956 Pharmacognosy, 2nd edn. Lippincott, Philadelphia, PA, USA
Ross MSF, Brain KR 1977 An introduction to phytopharmacy. Pitman Medical, Tunbridge Wells

5. Chemical

Bruneton J 1999 Pharmacognosy, phytochemistry, medicinal plants. Intercept Scientific, Medical and Technical Publications
Dewick PM 2002 Medicinal natural products, a biosynthetic approach, 2nd edn. John Wiley, Chichester
Hänsel R, Sticher O, Steinegger E 1999 Pharmakognosie-Phytopharmazie, 6th edn. Springer, Berlin (*in German*)
Robbers JE, Speedie MK, Tyler VE 1996 Pharmacognosy and pharmacobiotechnology. Williams & Wilkins, Baltimore
Tschirch A Handbuch der Pharmakognosie. Tauchnitz, Leipzig (*two editions and numerous volumes up to 1933*)

With the increase in interest in medicinal plants world-wide there are now many publications covering regional areas of the globe. Treatment of the plants in these works may be on any of the above lines. Some examples are given following the Introduction to Part VI.

As mentioned previously, a number of bodies have implemented research and published monographs on medicinal herbs. The aim has been to set standards for quality, efficacy and safety in order that the many traditional herbs meet legal requirements. The following are of note:

German Commission E monographs. These were developed for the German Federal Health Authority between 1978–1994 and involve 324 herbs used in German traditional medicine. The monographs give sources, constituents and considerable pharmacological and clinical information. They have now been translated into English and published by the American Botanical Council in 1999 as a single work followed by expanded monographs in 2000.

ESCOP monographs. ESCOP (European Scientific Cooperative for Phytotherapy) is an affiliation of European associations which has produced 60 monographs on herbal drugs, published in loose-leaf form in six fascicules, harmonizing the standards for these drugs throughout the European Union. Information is given on approved therapeutic uses, and unlike the Commission E monographs, provides references. The second edition of *ESCOP Monographs* was published in 2003, and a third edition is in the course of preparation.

AHP monographs. The *American Herbal Pharmacopoeia* (1997–2005) has monographs on a selection of traditional indigenous herbs with some overlap with the European monographs. Treatment of individual drugs can be extensive, for example, the St John's wort monograph published in *HerbalGram* 1997, No 4 extends to 32 pages with over 150 references, colour photographs and chemical formulae.

WHO monographs. The World Health Organization published Volume 1 of its *Monographs on Selected Medicinal Plants* in 1999. It contains standards for quality of drugs together with a therapeutic section; 31 plant species, the majority of which are also included in the above lists, are considered. Volume 2 was published in 2002.

USP monographs. The United States Pharmacopoeia is also producing herbal monographs. Eleven have been published, all involving drugs treated above, and twelve more were expected during 2000.

Current awareness. Students wishing to read original research will find many references in this book and should learn how to find similar ones for themselves. As no one can hope to read all the scientific literature that is published, special journals are devoted to the publication of brief abstracts from the original papers. Such abstracts give the author's name, the subject of the research, the reference necessary to locate the paper in the original journal and usually a brief outline of the work it contains. Most pharmacy department libraries contain *Chemical Abstracts* and *Biological Abstracts*, which in the appropriate sections cover all areas of pharmacognosy. Even so, the systematic searching of the abstracts to cover a broad field of interests can itself be most time-consuming, and publications such as *Chemical Titles* and *Current Contents* can be used to give a more rapid indication of recent publications. *Phytotherapy Research* regularly includes a selected bibliography relating to plant drugs. Information storage and retrieval is now itself a science, and a glance at the shelf-space occupied by succeeding years of *Chemical Abstracts* is sufficient to indicate that before long, if not already, manual searches of the literature will become impossibly long procedures. In many libraries, hard copies of these publications and of the journals mentioned below are no longer available, but they can be accessed on-line. Inevitably it will be necessary to rely on databases for literature scanning. *Pharmacognosy Titles* is a computer abstract coverage of phytochemical research publications up to 1974 (10 vols) produced under the direction of Professor N. Farnsworth, University of Illinois. Subsequently, Farnsworth introduced NAPRALERT, a Natural Product Database which is mainly, but not entirely, post-1975 and is viewed by many as a logical and indispensable collection of pharmacognostic information. The NAPRALERT database is available on a scheduled-fee basis to scientists, industrial firms, government agencies and academic institutions. Among other useful databases having a relevance to pharmacognosy and published on the Web are MEDLINE, compiled by the US National Library of Medicine and EMBASE, produced by Excerpta Medica.

Some journals—for example, *Planta Medica, Journal of Ethnopharmacology, Phytochemistry* and *Journal of Natural Products*—periodically contain reviews on some aspect of medicinal plants. Other journals containing research papers of pharmacognostical interest are *Natural Product Research* and *Natural Product Sciences*. Periodical publications appearing in bound form and devoted to reviews on certain aspects of plant constituents are useful for updating; often the reviews cover only the advances in a particular field since the previous volume. Examples are *Natural Product Reports* (six issues per year) and *Alkaloids* (Academic Press).

A series of multi-author books *Medicinal and Aromatic Plants – Industrial Profiles* (R. Hardman, series editor, CRC Press, Boca Raton, FL) provides an in-depth coverage of major medicinal and aromatic plants for specific genera; to date (2007) forty-five volumes have been published. Individual books for appropriate drugs are cited in Part 5 under 'Further reading'. Books that are not part of a series but, like the above, multi-author and dealing with certain specialized areas (e.g. alkaloids, flavonoids, isoprenoids), continually appear and generally give up-to-date information (in so far as any book can). Symposia which cover various aspects of pharmacognosy are frequently held in various parts of the world and scientists can easily become acquainted with others having like interests. Often the informal discussions which invariably arise at such meetings can be an extremely useful means of disseminating information. In addition, the lectures presented at such meetings are often subsequently published in book form. Modern communication systems make world-wide contact between researchers much simpler.

Now available to Western scientists interested in oriental medicine is the quarterly journal *Abstracts of Chinese Medicine*, published by the Chinese University of Hong Kong. This gives abstracts in English of significant Chinese research papers from more than one hundred scientific journals not readily available outside China.

Useful dictionaries to be found in most University libraries include *Dictionary of Organic Compounds* consisting of 7 volumes and 10 supplements (to 1992), *Dictionary of Alkaloids* (2 volumes) (1989), *Dictionary of Terpenoids* (1991) and *Dictionary of Natural Products* (1994) all published by Chapman and Hall and also *Phytochemical Dictionary: A Handbook of Bioactive Compounds from Plants* (1993), published by Taylor and Francis. Some of these more expensive volumes are available on CD-ROM.

3

Plant nomenclature and taxonomy

BOTANICAL NOMENCLATURE

Before the time of Linnaeus (1707–1778) many plants were known by a double Latin title; however, it is to this great Swedish biologist that we owe the general adoption of the present binomial system, in which the first name denotes the genus, while the second (specific) name denotes the species. All specific names may be written with small initial letters although formerly capitals were used where species were named after persons. Thus the species of *Cinchona* named after Charles Ledger, who brought its seeds from Brazil in 1865, is now written *Cinchona ledgeriana* rather than *Cinchona Ledgeriana*.

The specific name is usually chosen to indicate some striking characteristic of the plant—for example, the hemlock with the spotted stem is named *Conium maculatum* (*maculatus, -a, -um*, spotted). Sometimes the reason for the name is not as obvious as in the example just mentioned, but once it is discovered it will serve as a reminder of a characteristic of the plant—for example, *Strychnos potatorum* (*potator, -oris*, a drinker) bears a name which is only intelligible when it is known that the seeds of this species are used in India for clearing water. A particular species can also exhibit a number of varieties; these are especially evident with cultivated plants but are also found in the wild. For a medicinal example, see *Mentha piperita* below.

The modern rules governing the terminology of plant taxonomy are laid down in the *International Code of Botanical Nomenclature*.

Unlike the names of chemical substances, which are subject to changes which conform to evolving systems of nomenclature, systematic plant names are strictly controlled by rules which give precedence to that name used by the botanist who first described the species. Nevertheless, this seemingly straightforward approach can give rise to various quirks in spelling. The following are three examples involving medicinal plants: *Rauvolfia* vis à vis *Rauwolfia*; the former name was given to this Apocynaceous genus by Plumier in 1703, honouring the botanist Leonard Rauwolf. This spelling oversight caused much contention over the years centring on whether Plumier's obvious intention should be adopted in the name *Rauwolfia*. Both spellings are commonly found but the rules dictate that *Rauvolfia* has priority. In another example the downy thornapple may be encountered as either *Datura innoxia* or *Datura inoxia*. The former, as *Datura innoxia* Miller, was used in 1768 (*Gard. Dict.*, edn. 8, *Datura* no. 5) and this spelling was invariably employed for some 200 years; however in Miller's original description, the plant was characterized as: 'Datura (*Inoxia*) pericarpiis spinosis inoxiis ovatis propendentibus foliis cordatis pubescentibus' (W. E. Safford, *J. Wash. Acad. Sci.*, 1921, **11**, 173) and taxonomists now consider *D. inoxia* Miller to have priority. Both versions are still commonly encountered. A third example concerns the genus of the coca plant which may appear as *Erythroxylum*, or in older literature as *Erythroxylon*. Uppsala Monitoring Centre (a WHO collaborating centre for International Drug Monitoring) has published 'Accepted scientific names of therapeutic plants and their synonyms'.

SUBDIVISIONS OF THE PHYLA

The branches of the genealogical tree differ so much in size that it is not easy to decide which are of equal systematic importance, and what one biologist may consider as a family another may regard as a subfamily. Similarly, the species of one botanist may be the subspecies or variety of another. The main hierarchical subdivisions of a division, arranged according to Engler's scheme, may be illustrated by the following example showing the systematic position of peppermint.

Division	Angiospermae
Class	Dicotyledoneae
Subclass	Sympetalae
Order	Tubiflorae
Suborder	Verbenineae
Family	Labiatae (Lamiaceae)
Subfamily	Stachydoideae
Tribe	Satureieae
Genus	*Mentha*
Species	*Mentha piperita* Linnaeus (Peppermint)
Varieties	*Mentha piperita* var. *officinalis* Sole (White Peppermint)
	Mentha piperita var. *vulgaris* Sole (Black Peppermint)

It will be noted that in pharmacopoeias and in research publications botanical names are followed by the names of persons or their accepted abbreviations (e.g. Linnaeus and Sole in the case of peppermint given above). These refer to the botanist who first described the species or variety. Students need not attempt to memorize these names, and in the following pages they are usually omitted except in cases where different botanical names have at different times been applied to the same plant and there is possibility of confusion. The source of cloves, for example, is now usually given as *Syzygium aromaticum* (L.) Merr. et Perry; prior to 1980 the *BP* used the name *Eugenia caryophyllus* (Spreng.) Sprague; other synonyms which may be found in the older literature are *E. caryophyllata* Thunb. and *E. aromatica* (L.) Baill. Worldwide, not all authors of research papers use the currently accepted name so caution is necessary and botanical sources should be checked.

The letters s.l. following the botanist's name refers to collective species and varieties and imply 'in the widest sense' (*sensu latiore*), e.g. *Thymus serpyllum* L.s.l.

BOTANICAL SYSTEMS OF CLASSIFICATION

Before the widespread acceptance of the principle of evolution, biologists, being convinced of the fixity of species and lacking much of the information available today, confined themselves to more or less artificial methods of classification, their systems being frequently based on one or a few characters instead of upon the organism as a whole. These earlier systems are now mainly of historic interest, but certain of their features—for example, the large division of seed plants into monocotyledons and dicotyledons as used by John Ray (1628–1705)—survive today. Linnaeus' *Species Plantarum* of 1753 is the starting point for the modern nomenclature of plants, although his actual system of classification is entirely artificial and of little significance today. The *Prodromus*, started by A. P. de Candolle (1778–1841) and completed under the editorship of his son Alphonse (1806–93), was a massive work of 17 volumes which professed to be an account of every flowering plant then known. The system of classification employed was a modification and extension of that introduced earlier by De Jussieu (1748–1836) and further demonstrated the inadequacies of the Linnaean system which were then becoming apparent. Bentham and Hooker's *Genera Plantarum* (1862–1883) was patterned on the de Candolles' work, each genus being redescribed from herbarium specimens and not consisting of a restatement of earlier literature. Although largely artificial, it was convenient to retain this system as a basis for collections such as the herbaria of Kew and the British Museum, with continuous revision based on molecular systematics.

During the last 100 years a considerable number of phylogenetic systems of classification have been propounded; these systems arrange taxa (any groups used for classification such as orders, families, genera, etc.) to indicate the possible relationship of one taxon to another. Such systems are clearly susceptible to change with increasing knowledge, and no final system acceptable to all taxonomists is in sight; indeed, for some practical purposes a stable, workable phenetic system is often preferable. A close examination of the phylogenetic systems reveals that certain taxa form precise groups, others have less well-defined boundaries and other groups are difficult to accommodate phylogenetically. The work of Engler (1844–1930) in association with other German systematists is still adhered to in this connection. Engler's scheme of classification largely embodied the fundamental concepts of Eichler (1839–87) and was exemplified in the 20-volume work (1887–89) *Die natürlichen Pflanzenfamilien*, by Engler and Prantl. Subsequent to this, there appeared many editions of Engler's *Syllabus der Pflanzenfamilien*, the eleventh by Engler and Diels in 1936. The last version of the *Syllabus*, produced by Melchoir as two volumes, was published in 1964; the plant families in Chapter 5 of this textbook are arranged in this order. The immediate popularity of Engler's works was due to their applicability to plants of the whole world; they afforded a means of identifying all known genera.

Obviously, large works such as the above are not easily compiled and many taxonomists have produced phylogenetic schemes directed at various levels of classification without the complete systematics of the Engler series. Of the schemes, those of Cronquist (1981) and Takhtajan (1959) are generally similar whereas that of Hutchinson (1992) differs in that the dicotyledons are divided into two large groups—those characteristically and primitively woody (Lignosae) and those characteristically and primitively herbaceous (Herbaceae). These schemes incorporate data often not accessible to the earlier taxonomists; thus Cronquist, while emphasizing classical morphological characters and following the strobilar theory of Angiosperm evolution also takes account of micromorphological data (e.g. embryology and pollen structure), chemical data (e.g. secondary metabolites and serology) and the fossil record.

Dahlgren's proposals (1983), which involve a taxonomic method termed cladistics, demonstrate the distribution of characters and his cladograms of the orders of Angiosperms can be conveniently used for illustrating the occurrence of secondary metabolites throughout the higher plants. In this method (cladistics), clade is a group of plants at any level sharing a common ancestor and formed by a splitting to give two new species, which themselves in the course of time may split again. Clades may be very large or small, with clades within clades; as they comprise hypothetical relationships, they are subject to change as new knowledge becomes available. Evolutionary changes as envisaged in cladistics are sudden and widespread vis à vis the continuous gradual evolution taking place by small changes over a long period of time, as postulated by Darwin. Cladistics are now widely employed by modern taxonomists.

A modern replacement for Engler's classical work, now in the course of compilation, is *The families and genera of vascular plants* [K. Kubitzki *et al.* (eds)]. So far (2007), nine volumes have been published.

TAXONOMIC CHARACTERS

All plants possess hundreds of characters of a morphological, histological, embryological, serological, chemical and genetic nature which are potentially available for building up a classification of the plant kingdom. In the artificial schemes the characters employed were those that experience had shown could be used to produce suitable groups or taxa. The eventual scheme, into which could be inserted new plants as they were discovered or in which any plant could easily be traced, resembled a catalogue with a 'telephone directory' arrangement of plants in which the groups of individuals listed together did not necessarily have any phylogenetic relationship, but merely possessed certain common features.

Phylogenetic classifications, which endeavour to indicate the relationship of one taxon to another, imply the use of characters that are capable of showing such relationships. Because some groups of plants are more primitive than others on the evolutionary scale, certain characters will also be primitive, whereas other characters will have evolved from them. Thus, woody plants are generally regarded as more primitive than herbaceous ones and flowers with few parts more advanced than those with many parts.

The difficulties facing the taxonomist are appreciable. The appearance of a particular character in certain plants does not necessarily imply a relationship between these plants, because at some time in the past, under favourable conditions, whole groups of unrelated plants could have undergone this change (e.g. the development of fused corollas from polypetalous flowers; this is known as *convergence*). Alternatively, related plants may, in some point of time, have started to diverge in their characteristics so that the modern phenotypes appear very dissimilar—this is *divergence*. *Parallelism* refers to the similar evolution of characters in related plants or related groups of plants. Having decided which characters are of value and how many can be used, the taxonomist then has to consider whether each character should be given equal value or whether a 'weighting' system should be employed. Computers have an obvious role in dealing with large numbers of characters applied to thousands of plants, not only from the aspect of storage and retrieval of information, but also for the science of *numerical taxonomy*, which will probably play an increasing role in the development of systematics. For a fuller discussion of this subject the reader is referred to Heywood's *Plant Taxonomy*.

CHEMICAL PLANT TAXONOMY

This subject has recently attracted much attention and has, after many years, brought the plant chemist back to systematic botany. The concept that plants can be classified on the basis of their chemical constituents is not new; for example, early workers classified the algae into green, brown and red forms, but it is only during the last 40 years that modern techniques of isolation and characterization have led to the chemical screening of many thousands of plant samples. Compared with morphological characters, chemical constituents are often more precisely definable and can be of more fundamental significance for classification purposes. Plant taxonomists, in general, hold the view that chemical characters are yet another type of character to be considered alongside those used traditionally, but it does not necessarily follow that taxa constructed on a purely chemical basis, if such were possible on the data at present available, would necessarily coincide with those arrived at by classical methods.

The characters employed in chemical taxonomy need to be those of intermediate distribution in the plant kingdom. The presence of such ubiquitous compounds as the essential amino acids and common sugars is of little diagnostic value and, at the other extreme, the occurrence of coniine in the single species *Conium maculatum* of the large family Umbelliferae is also of little taxonomic significance. Characters most studied in this connection are therefore secondary metabolites (alkaloids, isoprenoids, flavonoids, characteristic glycosides, etc.), many of which are of established pharmaceutical interest.

However, as discussed later, secondary metabolites may be subject to considerable variation in the living plant, depending on environmental and ontogenetic factors, and more stable chemical characteristics are offered by those closely associated with DNA composition of the species. Increasingly, it is becoming possible to use DNA hybridization, serotaxonomy and amino acid sequencing techniques for taxonomic purposes. One pharmacognostical application (Y. Mino *et al.*, *Phytochemistry*, 1993, **33**, 601) has been the determination of the complete amino acid sequence of one of the iron sulphur ferredoxins present in varieties of *Datura stramonium*. The results support the view that the white and purple forms are varieties of a single species and that the tree daturas (e.g. *D. arborea*) are best regarded as constituting one section of the genus *Datura* and not a separate genus (*Idem.*, *ibid.*, 1994, **37**, 429; 1995, **43**, 1186); work with *D. quercifolia* and *D. fastuosa* also suggests that the amino acid sequence depends not on the species, but on the section. Similar studies were subsequently applied to *Physalis* (Y. Mino and K. Yasuda *Phytochemistry*, 1998, **49**, 1631).

A second example (H. Mizukami *et al.*, *Biol. Pharm. Bull.*, 1993, **16**, 388) shows that restriction fragment length polymorphisms (RFLPs) can be used as a simple and efficient method for distinguishing between *Duboisia leichhardtii*, *D. myoporoides* and the hybrid of the two species (RFLPs are produced by digestion of DNA with restriction endonucleases and vary in number and size according to genus, species etc.) However, the same group found (*ibid.*, 1993, **16**, 611) that the technique did not distinguish between the various geographical strains of the traditional Chinese drug *Glehnia littoralis* (Umbelliferae) containing different furanocoumarin compositions but did so with *Bupleurum falcatum* (*ibid.*, p. 279).

The differentiation between samples of *Panax ginseng* (Oriental ginseng), *P. quinquefolium* (American ginseng) and adulterants can be difficult by conventional means and F. Ngan *et al.* (*Phytochemistry*, 1999, **50**, 787) have reported on the authentication and differentiation, one from another, of six species of *Panax* and also their adulterants, using RFLPs involving the DNA sequences in a selected ribosomal region; see also J. Wang *et al.*, *Planta Medica*, 2001, **67**, 781 and Z. Zhao *et al.*, *Planta Medica*, 2006, **72**, 865 for the authentication of Chinese herbal medicines. *Salvia divinorum*, which contains the hallucinogenic diterpenoid salvinorin A not present in other species of *Salvia* (e.g. the sage plant), can be identified unequivocally by the combined use of analytical chemistry (HPLC-MS) and molecular DNA fingerprinting (C. M. Bertea *et al.*, *Phytochemistry*, 2006, **67**, 371).

Random amplified polymorphic DNA analysis has been used to distinguish between the various subspecies of *Melissa officinalis* common on the pharmaceutical market and now included in the *BP/EP*. Previously, samples have been classified according to the distribution pattern of compounds present in the lemon balm oil (H.-T. Wolf *et al.*, *Planta Medica*, 1999, **65**, 83).

Recent examples of the correspondence of genetic profiles and chemical constituents for the delineation of closely related plant species and chemotypes is illustrated by research on *Withania somnifera* (R. S. Dhar *et al.*, *Phytochemistry*, 2006, **67**, 2269), *Zingiber officinalis* and related species (H. L. Jiang *et al.*, *Phytochemistry*, 2006, **67**, 1673), and *Hypericum* spp. (A. Smelcerovic *et al.*, *Phytochemistry*, 2006, **67**, 171).

Serotaxonomic studies of *Acacia* gum exudates have demonstrated the value of such immunological tests in the chemotaxonomic analyses of these economically important products (T. C. Baldwin *et al.*, *Phytochemistry*, 1990, **50**, 599).

A standard work on chemotaxonomy (in German) is that of Hegnauer (see 'Further reading'); it comprises 11 volumes published over nearly 40 years. A four-volume work in English is that of Darnley Gibbs, published in 1974; unfortunately, it does not appear to have been updated.

Further reading
Plant nomenclature
Gledhill D 2008 The names of plants, 4th edn. Cambridge University Press, Cambridge, UK

Spencer R, Cross R, Lumley P 2007 Plant names, a guide to botanical nomenclature, 3rd edn. Cabi, Wallingford, UK

General taxonomy
Cronquist A 1981 An integrated system of classification of flowering plants. Columbia University Press, New York, USA

Engler A, Melchoir H, Werdermann E 1954, 1964 Syllabus der Pflanzenfamilien. Gebrüder Borntraeger, Berlin, Germany, 2 vols

Heywood VH 1987 Plant taxonomy, 3rd edn. Edward Arnold, London, UK

Holmes S 1986 Outline of plant classification. Longman, Harlow, Essex, UK

Jeffrey C 1989 Biological nomenclature, 3rd edn. Edward Arnold, London, UK

Judd WS, Campbell CS, Kellogg EA et al 2002 Plant systematics: a phylogenetic approach. Sinauer Associates Inc., US

Minelli A 1993 Biological systematics. Chapman and Hall, London, UK

Sivarajan VV 1991 Introduction to the principles of plant taxonomy (ed Robson NKP), 2nd edn. Cambridge University Press, Cambridge, UK

Stace CA 1991 Plant taxonomy and biosystematics, 2nd edn. Cambridge University Press, Cambridge, UK

Chemical taxonomy
Gibbs R Darnley 1974 Chemotaxonomy of flowering plants. McGill University Press, Montreal, Canada, 4 vols

Harborne JB, Turner BL 1984 Plant chemosystematics. Academic Press, London, UK

Harborne JB, Williams CA 1994 Recent advances in the chemosystematics of the Monocotyledons. Phytochemistry 37(1): 3–18

Hawkes JG (ed) 1968 Chemotaxonomy and serotaxonomy. Academic Press, London, UK

Hegnauer R 1962–1992 Chemotaxonomie der Pflanzen. Birkhäuser, Basle, Switzerland, Vols I–X

Hegnauer R, Hegnauer MH 1994, 1996 Chemotaxonomie der Pflanzen. Birkhäuser, Basle, Switzerland, XIa and XIb, Leguminosae parts 1 and 2

PART

2 | The plant and animal kingdoms as sources of drugs

4

Biological and geographical sources of drugs

Current estimates of the number of species of flowering plants range between 200 000 and 250 000 in some 300 families and 10 500 genera. Despite a rapidly expanding literature on phytochemistry, only a small percentage of the total species has been examined chemically, and there is a large field for future research.

However, man did not require the modern methods of investigation to collect for himself a materia medica of plants which he often used in conjunction with magical and other ritual practices. Such folk medicines naturally varied according to the plants available in a particular climatic area and can be studied today in those more or less undisturbed primitive societies which still exist. It is interesting to reflect that such collections of herbal medicines compiled over centuries by trial and error, and presumably using the patient as the experimental animal throughout, must surely contain some material worthy of further investigation and should not be too readily discarded. Is it not also possible that those materials producing adverse reactions, one of the principal problems in the introduction of new drugs, might also have been eliminated by such a system of development?

In the current search for new drugs having, for example, antitumour or hypotensive activity the plants involved, unlike many of the more traditional medicaments, very often show no immediate indications of pharmacological activity. Investigators are thus faced with the problem of making a systematic investigation from among the thousands of species still unexamined. One obvious line of approach is to start with folk medicines of the world on the assumption that these materials have already been subjected to some human screening, however crude, and found acceptable to those cultures that use them. For many areas of the world, the plants used in folklore have been adequately recorded; but for other regions—for example, in South America, with its vast flora of potentially useful plants—the art of folk medicine in aboriginal societies is in rapid decline owing to a changing mode of life of the people. Ethnobotanists are currently fighting a battle against time to record such information before, within a generation or so, it is lost and with it a possible short cut to some medicinally useful plant. However, the urgency is well-recognized and as described in Chapter 8, the biological and geographical sources of many traditional plant remedies are being actively researched and documented. Often, successful research on a particular drug prompts the investigation of related species indigenous elsewhere, as evidenced with *Hypericum* and *Taxus*; the same is now happening with the bee product propolis. Much recorded information still requires sifting. An example of the employment of a combination of literature surveys and data from other sources in the search for new drugs is the US National Cancer Institute's screening of thousands of plant extracts for antineoplastic and cytotoxic activity. This undertaking involves the team-work of botanists, phytochemists, pharmacologists and clinicians. In the absence of such sophisticated collaboration, much useful research by one discipline fails to be followed through to a utilitarian conclusion.

An inspection of the plant or plant-derived drugs included in western pharmacopoeias shows them to be composed of those which have survived from Greek and Roman eras, including some spices, those more characteristic of our own flora (e.g. digitalis) and introduced at a later date, other pharmacologically active drugs (e.g. cinchona—quinine—and ipecacuanha) added as a result of increased travel and colonial expansion, drugs (e.g. rauwolfia—reserpine) long used in other systems of medicine but of more recent introduction into Western medicine, and finally, recently discovered plant constituents of therapeutic value (e.g. vinblastine and vincristine from *Catharanthus roseus*) and those semisynthetic products (e.g. steroidal hormones) which depend on plant sources for starting material.

4

A perusal of the current literature soon reveals that, with the general availability of sophisticated methods of phytochemical analysis and pharmacological screening, together with the establishment of research centres, many traditional remedies not previously considered by Western scientists are being investigated in their countries of origin.

An examination of the list of drugs derived from natural sources, as included in any pharmacopoeia, indicates that the majority are derived from the Spermatophyta—the dominant seedbearing plants of the land. Within the Spermatophyta the number of species and the number of useful medicinal plants is divided unevenly between the phyla Gymnospermae, which yields some useful oils, resins and the alkaloid ephedrine, and the Angiospermae, which is divided into Monocotyledons and Dicotyledons (both of these provide many useful drugs but especially the Dicotyledons). Of the other divisions of the plant kingdom, the fungi provide a number of useful drugs, especially antibiotics, and are important in pharmacy in a number of other ways. The algae are a source of a limited number of drugs (e.g. agar and alginic acid), but the full pharmacological importance of this large group of aquatic plants has still to be realized. At the moment, lichens and mosses contribute little to medicine and the Pteridophytes are pharmaceutically best-known for the taenicidal ferns and lycopodium. Land animals provide such traditional pharmaceutical materials as gelatin, wool fat, beeswax and cochineal, and are a source of hormones, vitamins and sera. Among the many important pharmaceutical aspects of the Bacteriophyta are the production of antibiotics, their use in effecting various chemical conversions of added substrates and their employment in genetic engineering as, for example, in the production of human insulin and the transformation of higher plant cells by incorporation of part of the DNA of a bacterial plastid into the plant genome.

Researchers in the US have genetically engineered microbes to produce a precursor of the antimalarial artemisinin, which is then chemically manipulated to give the bioequivalent drug. It is hoped to have the product available for distribution by 2010 (report by K. Purcell, *HerbalGram*, 2006, **69**, 24). This would alleviate the shortage, and high cost, of natural artemesinin, which is currently derived from the Chinese *Artemisia annua* (Chenopodiaceae).

GEOGRAPHICAL SOURCES

Two factors which determine the commercial geographical sources of a drug are the suitability of the plant to a particular environment and the economic factors associated with the production of a drug in a particular area.

Many plants grow equally well in numerous localities having similar climates; and as economic conditions change in one area, so the collection or cultivation of a drug plant may move in accordance. Developing countries may also start the cultivation of medicinal plants, and in this respect South America, India and S.E. Asian countries have been particularly active. Cinnamon, traditionally produced in Sri Lanka, has been introduced to the Seychelles as a commercial crop, with so much success that the plant has now become a weed! Cinnamon also grows well in West Africa but is not commercially utilized there. It must be remembered, however, that a plant may grow well in different situations but fail to produce the same constituents (e.g. cinchonas growing at altitude and in the plains). The commercial cultivation of belladonna, stramonium, hyoscyamus and valerian in England has long been uneconomic and material is now imported from Eastern Europe, largely via Germany. Similarly, the USA, which at one time utilized domestic supplies of the solanaceous drugs, now obtains such raw materials from Eastern Europe; the production of labiate oils has been largely transferred to China. During and after World War II, agar production was initiated around New Zealand, Australia and South Africa, but with the re-emergence of the Japanese industry these sources became less important. Scarcity of acacia from the Sudan prompted the exploitation of the Nigerian gum. Pharmacopoeial ginger once came exclusively from Jamaica; a decline in production in Jamaica and a vast improvement in the quality of some African gingers has led to the use of these and Chinese ginger on a large scale. Official storax was once derived only from the Turkish *Liquidambar orientalis* (e.g. *USP* from 1851) but limited supplies led to the admission into many pharmacopoeias of American storax, *L. styraciflua* (e.g. *USP* from 1936). Similarly, a lasting shortage of Rio (Brazilian) ipecacuanha root has led to the widespread use of the Cartagena, Nicaragua and Panama varieties, which are obtainable from a much wider area of South and Central America. With the exception of India, attempts to cultivate the drug in other areas (e.g. Malaya) met with only limited success. In contrast, the cinchonas, indigenous to the Andes of South America, were most successfully introduced to Indonesia (particularly Java) and India. These became the principal geographical sources for the bark and its alkaloids. Java fell to the Japanese in 1942 and, as India normally consumes most of its own quinine production, there was a great shortage of this vital alkaloid at a time when large armies were fighting in malarial areas. Expeditions searched the original South American habitats and wild trees supplied useful but inadequate quantities. Fortunately, very successful synthetic antimalarials were discovered at this time and put into large-scale production. However, 50 years on the malarial parasite became extremely resistant to these drugs and the use of quinine was again invoked. There is also a steady demand for other cinchona alkaloids, and Zaire and other African states, together with Guatemala, produce most of the world's bark.

China has now emerged as a major producer of a number of quality medicinal plant products including coumarin, menthol and oils of eucalyptus, peppermint, spearmint, sassafras and valerian in addition to its established listings. Other changes evident from market reports include the acceptance by the European market of expensive high-quality Australian coriander, Guatemala as the principal producer of cardamons and *Podophyllum emodi* from China.

Many countries produce limited quantities of medicinal plants and spices for domestic consumption and these are not listed on the international market.

Governmental policies on the export of raw materials may affect geographical sources, as when the Indian government limited the export of crude rauwolfia root, selling only the more highly priced extract. Supplies of the root were subsequently obtained from Thailand. Changes in the legal cultivation of medicinal opium in Turkey must eventually affect the geographical source of the drug; thus, the opium poppy has been cultivated in Tasmania on a large scale in recent years but political factors are militating against the continuation of this source. Political considerations have also led to changes in the starting materials for corticosteroids. Up to 1970 the sole intermediate source material for the manufacture of contraceptive steroids was diosgenin derived from the Mexican yam. Then the Mexican government nationalized diosgenin production and increased prices to above those for total synthesis; as a result, in subsequent years manufacturers have turned to other starting materials such as hecogenin (from sisal), solasodine (from *Solanum* spp.), microbiological products from cholesterol, stigmasterol, sitosterol and squalene, and petroleum products. The more recent emergence of China as a producer of high-quality, low-priced diosgenin has again changed the situation.

National and international restrictions on the collection of wild plants have also affected the sources of some drugs; the Washington Convention on International Trade in Endangered Species (CITES) placed all species of *Aloe* except *A. vera* on the protected list without warning; this caused problems in the marketing of aloes produced from the usual species. Other medicinal plants which have recently been given CITES listing include *Hydrastis canadensis* (1997) and *Prunus africana* (1998).

A number of the above factors have given added impetus to research on the application of cloning techniques in cultivation and to the artificial culture of plant cells and organs (see Chapter 13).

Further reading

Journal of Ethnopharmacology, special issue 1996 51(1–3). Intellectual property rights, naturally-derived bioactive compounds and resource conservation

4

5

A taxonomic approach to the study of medicinal plants and animal-derived drugs

For classification purposes the plant and animal kingdoms are each divided into a number of phyla and in addition to the phyla, the classification includes groupings of gradually diminishing size, namely divisions, classes, orders, suborders and families. According to the system used, these groupings may, or may not, indicate phylogenetic relationships.

In this chapter the principal plant families of pharmaceutical interest are arranged according to the botanical scheme of Engler (q.v.). The chapter is divided into six parts: Thallophytes; Bryophytes and Pteridophytes; Gymnosperms; Angiosperms (Dicotyledons); Angiosperms (Monocotyledons); Animal Products. At the beginning of each large taxon of plants a table is given to clarify the orders and families involved. Following the listed genera for each family, notes on the uses and constituents of specific plants not included in Part 5 are given. According to the botanical system of classification considered, schemes vary, as do the numbers of families, genera and species cited within an order.

THALLOPHYTES

The old term 'thallophyte' includes those plants which are not differentiated into root, stem and leaves. Engler divides them into 13 phyla. They include bacteria, algae, fungi and lichens. The positions of the main families of pharmaceutical interest are indicated below.

Phyla	Orders	Families
Bacteriophyta	Eubacteriales	Rhizobiaceae, Micrococcaceae
Chrysophyta (Diatomeae)	Discales	Actinodiscaceae
	Pennatales	Fragilariaceae, Naviculariaceae
Phaeophyta (Brown Algae)	Laminariales	Laminariaceae
	Fucales	Fucaceae, Sargassaceae
Rhodophyta (Red Algae)	Gelidiales	Gelidiaceae
	Gigartinales	Gracilariaceae, Gigartinaceae

BACTERIA AND ALGAE

BACTERIOPHYTA

The bacteria are unicellular organisms, the great majority of which range in size from 0.75 to 8 μm. They reproduce by binary fission. Most species of bacteria contain no chlorophyll, although there is one group whose members contain a chlorophyll-like pigment and photosynthesize. Recent research has revealed much more of the details of cellular structure and it has been possible to distinguish in certain species, in no small detail, the various components of the cell. For example, in *Escherichia coli* the cell wall consists of a four-layer structure, the inner one being rigid, the three outer ones non-rigid. Within the three-layer wall structure lies a protoplast membrane enclosing the cytoplasm. The protoplast membrane acts as a permeability barrier to all but very large molecules and contains enzymes concerned with respiration and the active transport of metabolites.

Bacteria exist in a number of characteristic shapes, namely:

1. Rod-shaped or bacillary forms (e.g. *Clostridium welchii*, *Escherichia coli* and *Bacillus subtilis*).

2. Spherical or coccal forms, which can occur singly but are usually found in characteristic aggregates—i.e. in chains (streptococci), in groups of two (diplococci), four (tetracocci) or eight (sarcinae). Aggregates of irregular pattern are said to be of staphylococcal form.
3. Twisted or spirillar forms which, if having a single twist, belong to the genus *Vibrio*, while those with more than one twist belong to the genus *Spirillum*.
4. Branched forms which sometimes occur in the genus *Mycobacterium*.

Other important morphological features which are of value in classifying bacteria are: (1) The possession of flagella, thread-like processes whose number and position are often of diagnostic importance. (2) The formation of capsules consisting of polysaccharide material which is of great importance in relation to the immunological properties of the organism. (3) The possession of endospores, which are highly refractive bodies formed by certain species under what appear to be adverse environmental conditions. The position of the spore in relation to the rest of the cell is of diagnostic importance. (4) Pigmentation; many bacteria are capable of elaborating complex colouring matters.

Bacteria are able to carry out a very wide range of chemical reactions, some of which are used for identification and differentiation, in addition to forming the basis of many important industrial processes. Bacterial action is used, for example, in the production of vinegar, acetone, butyl alcohol, lactic acid and L-sorbose. Notable examples of reactions which are useful for characterizing bacteria are the ability to ferment carbohydrates with the formation of acidic and gaseous products; the ability to digest protein, as shown by gelatin liquefaction; the production of hydrogen sulphide from organic sulphur compounds.

Bacteria are most important in medicine and pharmacy in the following respects: as disease-producing organisms (about 10% of bacteria are probably pathogenic); for producing antibiotics (Chapter 30); for effecting biochemical conversions; as agents in the deterioration of crude drugs and medicaments (Chapter 15); the production of transformed root cultures and transgenic medicinal plants by *Agrobacterium* spp. (Chapters 11 and 12); in genetic engineering involving recombinant DNA (e.g. the production of human insulin). Bacteria also play a vital role in nature—for example, in the nitrogen cycle atmospheric nitrogen is fixed by *Azotobacter* or, symbiotically, by various species of *Rhizobium*. *Nitrosomonas* is able to oxidize ammonia to nitrite, while *Nitrobacter* can oxidize nitrite to nitrate. Bacteria are important in sewage purification, in the retting of fibres such as jute and flax, and in the ripening of cheese.

CHRYSOPHYTA: DISCALES

Actinodiscaceae
The Chrysophyta has three classes, one of which is the Bacillariophyceae (Diatomeae), containing some 10 000 species of diatom. They are unicellular algae, have a silica skeleton, and show infinite variety in shape and in the sculpturing of the cell wall. There are two main types: the subclass Centricae (in which Discales is one of the orders) and subclass Pennatae (which includes the order Pennatales). The Centricae are centric or discoid in shape and generally marine, while the Pennatae are pennate or naviculoid and more often occur in fresh water.

An example of the family Actinodiscaceae is *Arachnoidiscus*, found in Japanese agar (q.v.) and other genera are found in the fossil deposits of diatomite or kieselguhr (q.v.).

CHRYSOPHYTA: PENNATALES

Fragilariaceae and Naviculariaceae
Species of these two families occur in diatomite and are illustrated in Fig. 34.1.

PHAEOPHYTA: LAMINARIALES

Laminariaceae
The brown algae are mainly marine and vary from microscopic branched filaments to leathery frond-like forms up to 60 m in length. They owe their brown colour to the carotenoid pigment fucoxanthin, which masks the other pigments.

Many of the 30 species of *Laminaria* are used in coastal districts for agricultural purposes. They are used for the manufacture of alginic acid (q.v.), mannitol and iodine.

PHAEOPHYTA: FUCALES

Fucaceae and Sargassaceae
Examples of the Fucaceae are *Fucus* (about 30 spp.) and *Pelvetia*; and of the Sargassaceae about 250 species of *Sargassum*. These are collected on a large scale in many parts of the world for the production of alginic acid and its derivatives. The species have been much investigated for biologically active properties; *F. vesiculosus*, for example, gives water-soluble extracts that inhibit the activity of the HIV reverse-transcriptase enzyme.

RHODOPHYTA: GELIDIALES

Gelidiaceae
The red algae are divided into 11 orders. The 3000 species are mainly marine and are particularly abundant in the tropics and subtropics. Most are relatively small. Their plastids contain chlorophyll, the red pigment phycoerythrin (usually in sufficient quantity to mask the other pigments), and sometimes the blue pigment phycocyanin.

Important genera of the Gelidiaceae are *Gelidium* (about 40 spp.) and *Pterocladia* (5 spp.). Many of these are used in the preparation of agars (q.v.).

RHODOPHYTA: GIGARTINALES

Gracilariaceae and Gigartinaceae
Gracilaria (100 spp.) is a source of agar, particularly *G. lichenoides*, found in the Indian Ocean. In the Gigartinaceae *Chondrus crispus* yields carageen or Irish moss (q.v.); *Gigartina stellata* has been investigated as a source of British agar.

FUNGI

The fungi are saprophytic or parasitic members of the Thallophyta, entirely devoid of chlorophyll. The plant body is made up of filaments or hyphae, which together constitute the mycelium. The hyphae may be aseptate and coenocytic, but are often septate, the individual segments being uni-, bi- or multinucleate. In the formation of fruiting bodies the hyphae may become woven into dense masses of pseudoparenchyma (e.g. the sclerotium of ergot).

The protoplast of fungal cells consists of granular or reticulate cytoplasm, which in older cells is often vacuolated. The nucleus may show a delicate reticulum and one or more nucleoli or its contents may be condensed into a chromatin body. The cell wall in many Archimycetes and some Phycomycetes (Oomycetes) and in the yeasts consists mainly of cellulose, but in other fungi cellulose is replaced by the nitrogenous substance chitin.

Sexual and asexual reproduction occur. The characteristic spores of the sporophyte generation are known as oospores (produced endogenously) or basidiospores (produced exogenously). In the Fungi Imperfecti the sporophyte generation is missing. The fungi also produce spores having no significance in the alternation of the generations; they are borne on the gametophyte (Phycomycetes and Ascomycetes) or on the sporophyte (rusts and some Autobasidiomycetes). These accessory spores often take the form of conidia, non-motile spores, borne externally on conidiophores.

The Archimycetes are the simplest fungi, in which the mycelium is absent or rudimentary. A member of this group causes wart disease in potatoes. The following groups and families are of pharmaceutical interest.

Class	Order	Families
Phycomycetes	Mucorales	Mucoraceae
Ascomycetes	Protoascales	Saccharomycetaceae
	Plectascales	Aspergillaceae
	Sphaeriales	Hypocreaceae
	Clavicipitales	Clavicipitaceae
Basidiomycetes	Polyporinales	Polyporaceae
	Agaricales	Tricholometaceae
		Amanitaceae
		Agaricaceae
	Phallinales	Phallinaceae
Fungi Imperfecti	Moniliales	Dematiaceae

PHYCOMYCETES: MUCORALES

Mucoraceae

These fungi have an aseptate mycelium; members include *Phytophthora infestans*, which causes potato blight. In the Mucoraceae we have *Mucor* (40 spp.) and *Rhizopus* (8 spp.), which are among the moulds associated with badly stored food products. Some *Rhizopus* species are used industrially for the saccharification of starchy material and for producing D-lactic acid from glucose; they are important in the microbiological conversions of steroids (q.v.).

ASCOMYCETES: PROTOASCALES

Saccharomycetaceae

This group includes the yeasts, some 30 species of *Saccharomyces*. Dried yeast (q.v.) is prepared from a strain of *S. cerevisiae*. A member of the related family Cryptococcaceae is *Candida utilis*, which produces torula yeast, a rich source of proteins and vitamins.

PLECTASCALES

Aspergillaceae

In this order the conidial stage is more prominent than the ascal stage. *Penicillium* (over 100 spp.) yields important antibiotics (q.v.) such as penicillin and griseofulvin; also the immunosuppressant mycophenolic acid. *P. islandicum* forms emodin. Among the 60 species of *Aspergillus* may be noted *A. oryzae*, used in the manufacture of soya sauce; *A. fumigatus*, producing the antibiotic fumagillin; and *A. flavus* producing aflatoxin in poorly stored feeding materials.

SPHAERIALES

Hypocreaceae

Gibberella (10 spp.) produces the plant growth regulators known as gibberellins, first isolated from *G. fugikuroi*, see Chapter 12.

CLAVICIPITALES

Clavicipitaceae

Like other Ascomycetes, the ascospores are produced in a sac or ascus. *Claviceps* (10 spp.) includes ergot, the sclerotium of *C. purpurea*; *Cordyceps* (100 spp.) includes *C. sinensis*, one of the most valued species in Chinese traditional medicine but limited in use by a shortage of supply. *C. militaris* has similar properties and efforts are devoted to its artificial culture; R. Yu *et al.*, have purified and identified four polysaccharides from cultured material (*Fitoterapia*, 2004, **75**, 662).

BASIDIOMYCETES: POLYPORINALES

The Basidiomycetes produce basidiospores, borne externally on the spore mothercell or basidium. They have septate mycelia which produce elaborate fruiting bodies (e.g. mushrooms). Some members are edible, others poisonous.

Polyporaceae

The Polyporaceae includes *Polyporus*, *Polystichus*, *Fomes*, *Ganoderma* and *Boletus* (200 spp.). *Polyporus officinalis* (white agaric) and *P. fomentarius* were formerly used in medicine. *Ganoderma lucida* has long been used in Chinese medicine and its biologically active triterpenoids have attracted attention. *Boletus edulis* is edible.

AGARICALES

An order of several families.

Tricholometaceae

The Tricholometaceae contains *Clitocybe* (80 spp.), species of which produce muscarine (q.v.). Other families of the order contain *Stropharia*, *Psilocybe* and *Conocybe*, which produce hallucinogenic substances (q.v.) such as psilosin and psilocybin.

Amanitaceae

The family includes *Amanita* (50–60 spp.) and *Pluteus*; *Amanita muscaria* (fly agaric) and *A. pantherina* contain muscarine (q.v.).

Agaricaceae

This family includes the common mushroom, *Agaricus campestris*. The genus *Agaricus* (*Psalliota*) contains about 30 species.

PHALLINALES

The order contains two families.

Phallinaceae

The Phallinaceae takes its name from *Phallus* (10 spp.). *Phallus impudicus* is the stinkhorn.

FUNGI IMPERFECTI: MONILIALES

The Fungi Imperfecti is a group in which sexual spores have not been demonstrated. Some members may be Ascomycetes which have completely lost the ascus stage.

Dematiaceae

The family Dematiaceae contains *Helminthosporium* (150–200 spp.), a species of which, *H. graminium*, produces helminthosporin (q.v.). Another family of the group, the Tuberculariaceae, contains *Fusarium* (65 spp.). *Fusarium lini* will transform digitoxigenin into digoxigenin.

Fungal spores are a common source of allergens.

LICHENS

A lichen is a symbiotic association of an alga and a fungal partner. Some, particularly in arctic regions, are used as food. The desert species *Lecanora esculenta* is regarded as the biblical manna. The 'oak moss' used as a fixative in perfumery is the lichen *Evernia prunastri*. Many lichens contain derivatives of orcinol, orcellic acid and lecanoric acid; these compounds are termed depsides and are phenolic acids formed by the interaction of the carboxyl group of one molecule with the hydroxyl group of another. A class of these acids termed depsidones (e.g. norstictic and psoromic acids) complex with metals and are probably responsible for the ability of lichens to flourish on mineral-rich soils including mine tailings and to accumulate large quantities of metals, such as copper, zinc etc.

Lichen dyes were formerly much used in the textile industry. Litmus, produced from certain lichens (e.g. *Lecanora*, *Roccella* spp.) by fermentation, is used as an indicator.

Iceland moss, *Cetraria islandica*, has been used for disguising the taste of nauseous medicines and with other species (e.g. *Cladonia* spp.) for the treatment of cough. It contains the very bitter depsidone, cetraric acid. Many lichens have antibiotic properties as illustrated by usnic acid, found in *Cladonia* and *Usnea* spp. (see E. R. Correché *et al.* 1998, *Fitoterapia*, **69**, 493; V. Marcano *et al.*, *J. Ethnopharmacology*, 1999, **66**, 343); 29 species of Icelandic lichens have recently been investigated for their cancer chemopreventive and cytotoxic activity (K. Ingólfsdóttir *et al.*, *Pharm. Biol.*, 2000, **38**, 313).

It is possible to isolate and grow the algae from lichens as suspension cultures (see P. Härmälä *et al.*, *Fitoterapia*, 1992, **63**, 217).

The accompanying list indicates some of the families and genera of recent interest.

Order	Family	Genera
Roccellales	Roccellaceae	*Roccella* (31 spp.)
Lecanorales	Pertusariaceae	*Pertusaria* (608 spp.)
	Lecanoraceae	*Lecanora* (1100 spp.)
	Parmeliaceae	*Parmelia* (800 spp.)
		Cetraria (62 spp.)
	Usneaceae	*Usnea* (500 spp.)
		Evernia (8 spp.)
		Alectoria (48 spp.)
Caloplacales	Caloplacaceae	*Caloplaca* (480 spp.)
	Teloschistaceae	*Xanthoria* (21 spp.)

BRYOPHYTES AND PTERIDOPHYTES

These two phyla are of relatively small pharmaceutical importance, but have some phytochemical interest.

BRYOPHYTA

The phylum is divided into two classes, Hepaticae (liverworts) and Musci (mosses). Both show alternation of generations. The more conspicuous gametophyte generation is a leaf-like thallus in the liverworts and a leafy plant with a stem in the mosses. On the latter is borne the sporophyte generation with sporangium.

Of the many bryophyte orders, families and genera, a few which have been subjects of recent research are listed below.

Class	Order	Genera
Hepaticae	Jungermaniinales	*Bazzania, Solenostoma, Gymnomitrion, Diplophyllum*
	Jubulineales	*Lunularia*
Musci	Sphagnales	*Sphagnum* (336 spp.)
	Dicranales	*Dicranum* (52 spp.)
	Funariales	*Funaria* (117 spp.)

Peat, long used as a domestic fuel, consists of partly decayed mosses and other plants. In some areas (e.g. parts of Ireland) deposits of bog moss (largely species of *Sphagnum*) are many feet thick, and after the surface has been skimmed off, soil may be excavated in a very pure form. Sphagnum moss, consisting of a mixture of various species of *Sphagnum*, can be collected in many parts of Britain. It may be used (enclosed in muslin bags) as an absorbent dressing or compressed into sheets, making absorbent mattresses. Large quantities were used in this way in World War I.

The pharmacologically active terpenoids (sesquiterpenes, diterpenes) and aromatic compounds of the bryophytes have been well studied. (For a review see Y. Asakawa, *Proc. Phytochem. Soc. Eur.*, 1990, **29**, 369. This volume (eds. H. D. Zinsmeister and R. Mues), published by Clarendon Press, Oxford, also includes a further 28 review articles covering the chemistry and chemical taxonomy of the Bryophytes.)

PTERIDOPHYTA

The Pteridophyta includes the Filices (ferns), Articulatae (horsetails) and Lycopsida (club mosses). They show an alternation of generations, the sporophyte being the larger. A few are of medical importance.

Of the many families, subfamilies and genera the following may be noted.

Class	Order	Family	Genera
Filices	Filicales	Polypodiaceae (divided into many subfamilies)	*Polypodium* (about 50 spp.)
			Dryopteris (about 150 spp.)
			Pteris (280 spp.)
			Pteridium (1 sp.)
			Onychium (6 spp.)
			Dennstaedtia (70 spp.)
			Adiantum (about 200 spp.)
			Athyrium (180 spp.)
			Asplenium (about 700 spp.)
Articulatae	Equisetales	Equisetaceae	*Equisetum* (32 spp.)
Lycopsida	Lycopodiales	Lycopodiaceae	*Lycopodium* (about 450 spp.)

5

Male fern rhizome (q.v.) derived from *Dryopteris filix-mas* is one of many ferns containing phloroglucinol derivatives. The insect-moulding hormones or pterosins are widely distributed in ferns and attract considerable research.

Various species of *Adiantum* (the maiden hair ferns) are recorded as used in traditional medicine in Europe, Saudi Arabia, Africa and the Indian subcontinent. They contain hopane triterpenoids, a group of squalane-derived compounds more commonly associated with bacterial membranes. G. Brahmachari and D. Chatterjee record the isolation of a new one-such constituent from *A. lunulactum* (syn. *A. philippense*) (*Fitoterapia*, 2002, **73**, 363).

The dried sterile stems of the horsetail, *Equisetum arvense* are used in herbal medicine and are listed in the *BHP* (1996) and the *BP/EP*. There are apparently two chemotypes of the species with different flavonoid compositions. Horsetails give a high mineral ash containing considerable amounts of silica. Correct identification of the herb is important because the related species *E. palustre* is poisonous.

The spores of lycopodium (*Lycopodium clavatum*) are used in quantitative microscopy (q.v.) and to a limited extent in medicated snuffs, dusting powders and lubricants. As a dusting powder for rubber gloves it has been known to give rise to dermatitis and mild caution has been expressed regarding its use as a lubricant non-stick agent for condoms relative to a possible cause of granulomas. The lycopodium alkaloids have been extensively studied (for a review see W. A. Ayer and L. S. Trifonov, *Alkaloids*, 1994, **45**, 233). *Huperzia serrata* (a club moss), now assigned to *Lycopodium*, contains the unusual alkaloid huperzine A and has been long-used in Chinese medicine for the treatment Alzheimer's and related conditions (see also Chapter 8).

Bracken (*Pteridium aquilinum*) has been a recent cause of concern owing to its carcinogenic properties and known bovine poisoning. The use of the young shoots for culinary purposes is discouraged and avoidance of bracken spores in the atmosphere suggested. The toxic constituent is ptaquiloside, an unstable glycoside of an illudane-type norsesquiterpene. Other similar compounds are widely distributed in the genus *Pteridium*.

GYMNOSPERMS

The division Gymnospermae contains many fossil members. Of the 11 orders in the Engler classification, it is only necessary to mention five orders and 10 families:

Orders	Families
Cycadales	Cycadaceae
Ginkgoales	Ginkgoaceae
Coniferae	Pinaceae, Taxodiaceae, Cupressaceae, Araucariaceae, Podocarpaceae, Cephalotaxaceae
Taxales	Taxaceae
Gnetales	Ephedraceae

The gymnosperms are one of the two great divisions of the seed-bearing plants or spermaphyta. They differ from the angiosperms in having ovules which are not enclosed in an ovary. A perianth is absent except in the Gnetales. The seeds usually contain one mature embryo with from two to 15 cotyledons embedded in endosperm. The wood is composed largely of tracheids, vessels being absent.

CYCADALES

Cycadaceae

The order contains only 10 genera and about 100 species. The family Cycadaceae contains the single genus *Cycas*, with 20 species. A sago (not to be confused with that from certain palms) is obtained from the pith of *Cycas circinalis* and *C. revolula*.

GINKGOALES

Ginkgoaceae

With the exception of *Ginkgo biloba*, the maidenhair-tree, the plants of this order are found only as fossils. In recent years, owing to their increasing use for the treatment of various diseases associated with the ageing process, the leaves of the ginkgo tree have been extensively investigated. For further details see 'Diterpenoids'.

CONIFERAE (OR CONIFERALES)

Pinaceae

All members of the order are trees or shrubs; mostly evergreen with needle-like leaves; monoecious or dioecious. Sporophylls usually in cones. Resin ducts occur in all parts.

The Pinaceae are trees, rarely shrubs. Important genera are: *Abies* (50 spp.), *Pseudotsuga* (7 spp.), *Tsuga* (15 spp.), *Picea* (50 spp.), *Larix* (11 spp.), *Cedrus* (4 spp.), and *Pinus* (70–100 spp.). They are abundant in the northern hemisphere and extend southwards to Indonesia and Central America. Apart from their great value as timber and paper-making material, many species (e.g. *Pinus*) yield oleoresin (see 'Colophony Resin and Crude Turpentine'). Other species are *Abies balsamea*, yielding Canada balsam; *Pseudotsuga taxifolia* (Douglas fir); *Picea abies* (Norway spruce); and *Larix europaeus* (larch). The barks of larch and hemlock spruce are tanning materials. *Pinus pinea* (the umbrella pine) produces large edible seeds (pignons). An extract of the bark of *P. pinaster* (*P. maritima*) var. *atlantica* containing bioflavonoids, particularly procyanidins (q.v.), is marketed as a food supplement (Pycnogenol®) having antioxidant properties. Some members of the family are a potential source of shikimic acid (q.v.).

Taxodiaceae

A small family of 10 genera, including *Sequoia*, *Taxodium*, *Cryptomeria*, *Tetraclinis*, *Taiwania* and *Cunninghamia*; 16 species.

The resin sandarac is produced in North Africa and Spain from *Tetraclinis articulata*. Some of the family contain antifungal diterpenes, others alkaloids.

Cupressaceae

A family of 19 genera and 130 species of trees and shrubs.

Members differ from the Pinaceae in that the leaves and cone-scales are usually opposite or whorled and the ovules erect. The genera include *Callitris* (16 spp., Australasia), *Thuja* (5 spp., China, Japan and North America), *Cupressus* (15–20 spp.), *Chamaecyparis* (7 spp.), *Juniperus* (60 spp., northern hemisphere). *Juniperus communis* yields juniper berries and volatile oil (q.v.); *J. virginiana*, the red cedar wood used for pencils; and *J. sabina*, volatile oil of savin; *J. oxycedrus*, by destructive distillation, yields oil of cade, which was formerly much used in veterinary work. This tar-like oil contains cadinene and phenols. Various diterpenes and flavonoids of the family have been studied.

Araucariaceae

Two genera and 38 species of trees, which sometimes have pungent leaves.

Araucaria (18 spp.) provides useful timbers; and *Agathis* (20 spp.), the resins known as copals or animes, which are used for varnish. Manila copal is obtained from the Malaysian *Agathis alba*; and kauri copal from *A. australis*, the kauri pine, in Australia and New Zealand. The best copals are usually those found in the ground long after the trees are dead.

Podocarpaceae
Six genera and 125 species of trees and shrubs. The largest genus, *Podocarpus* (100 spp.), extends from tropical to temperate zones and yields valuable timbers. A characteristic chemical feature of this genus is the widespread occurrence of norditerpene and bisnorditerpene dilactones; these compounds exhibit a variety of biological activities (see I. Kubo *et al.*, *Phytochemistry*, 1992, **31**, 1545).

Cephalotaxaceae
A family of one genus (*Cephalotaxus*) and seven species of trees and shrubs (plum yews) found from the eastern Himalayas to Japan. They have been intensively studied for their antitumour constituents in particular, the alkaloids harringtonine and homoharringtonine from *C. harringtonia*.

TAXALES

Taxaceae
An order of only one family, which includes the genera *Taxus* (10 spp.), *Pseudotaxus*, *Torreya*, *Austrotaxus* and *Amentotaxus*.

The common yew, *Taxus baccata*, produces valuable wood. The fruit has a fleshy red aril. All parts of the plant are very poisonous, and cattle and horses can die very rapidly after eating the leaves and stems. In addition to alkaloids, a cyanogenetic glycoside and anti-tumour agent have been reported in the genus.

Taxus brevifolia (the Pacific yew). The bark of this species yields the anticancer drug taxol, a nitrogenous diterpene. Low yields from the bark and the scarcity of raw material leading to damage to forests by, often illegal, over-collection hampered the development of the drug. The investigation of alternative sources led to tissue culture procedures for the production of taxol but the yields are still low. A development involving a renewable source has been the isolation of 10-deacetylbaccatin from the fresh needles of *T. baccata* in up to 0.1% yield and its chemical conversion to taxol. *T. media*, *T. cuspidata* and *T. chinensis* are other species investigated for taxane alkaloids.

GNETALES

Ephedraceae
The order consists of three families (Gnetaceae, Ephedraceae and Welwitchiaceae), three genera and about 70–75 species.

The Ephedraceae contains the single genus *Ephedra* (q.v.), about 40 species of shrubs. They occur in arid regions of the subtropics and tropics. Their seed, with two cotyledons, is enclosed in a perianth which becomes woody. Various species yield the drug ephedra (q.v.) and the alkaloid ephedrine.

ANGIOSPERMS: DICOTYLEDONS

The angiosperms or flowering plants include more than 250 000 species of herbs, shrubs and trees. The sporophylls (stamens and carpels) are usually arranged with other leaves (the perianth) to form a 'flower'. The ovules are enclosed in a chamber (the ovary) formed from the carpels, and a stigma is provided for the reception and germination of the pollen. The embryo plant contained in the seed has one or two seed leaves or cotyledons. The wood almost invariably contains true vessels. The phylum is divided into monocotyledons and dicotyledons.

The dicotyledons are herbs, shrubs or trees, the seeds of which have two cotyledons. The leaves are usually reticulately veined and the typical stem structure is a ring of open vascular bundles. Unlike the monocotyledons, which typically have their floral parts in threes, dicotyledonous flowers are usually pentamerous or tetramerous. The flowers may be unisexual (e.g. Salicaceae), but are more usually bisexual. The perianth may or may not be differentiated into sepals and petals, and the latter may be free from one another or fused.

The classification adopted in the following pages is that of Engler, who divides the dicotyledons into two groups, the Archichlamydeae and Sympetalae. The Archichlamydeae are further divided into 37 orders and about 226 families and the Sympetalae into 11 orders and about 63 families.

The names of the orders terminate in '-ales', suborders in '-neae', families usually in '-aceae' (Compositae, Gramineae and Labiatae are exceptions), and sometimes into subfamilies ending in '-oideae'.

The Archichlamydeae contain those families that in early editions were grouped under Monochlamydeae and Dialypetalae. The flowers have either no perianth or a perianth that is differentiated into sepals and petals, the latter being free. Engler's classification of the Dicotyledons is given in a somewhat abbreviated form below.

Order	Family
Subclass Archichlamydeae	
Juglandales	Myricaceae, Juglandaceae
Salicales	Salicaceae
Fagales	Betulaceae, Fagaceae
Urticales	Ulmaceae, Moraceae (including Cannabinaceae) and Urticaceae
Proteales	Proteaceae
Santalales	Olacaceae, Santalaceae, Loranthaceae
Polygonales	Polygonaceae
Centrospermae	Phytolaccaceae, Caryophyllaceae, Chenopodiaceae
Cactales	Cactaceae
Magnoliales	Magnoliaceae, Winteraceae, Annonaceae, Eupomatiaceae, Myristicaceae, Canellaceae, Schisandraceae, Illiciaceae, Monimiaceae, Calycanthaceae, Lauraceae, Hernandiaceae
Ranunculales	Ranunculaceae, Berberidaceae, Menispermaceae, Nymphaeaceae
Piperales	Piperaceae
Aristolochiales	Aristolochiaceae
Guttiferales	Paeoniaceae, Dipterocarpaceae, Theaceae, Guttiferae
Sarraceniales	Sarraceniaceae, Nepenthaceae, Droseraceae
Papaverales	Papaveraceae (including Fumariaceae), Capparaceae, Cruciferae
Rosales	Hamamelidaceae, Crassulaceae, Saxifragaceae, Rosaceae, Leguminosae, Krameriaceae
Geraniales	Geraniaceae, Zygophyllaceae, Linaceae, Erythroxylaceae, Euphorbiaceae

(Continued)

5

Order	Family
Subclass Archichlamydeae (continued)	
Rutales	Rutaceae, Simaroubaceae, Burseraceae, Meliaceae, Malpighiaceae, Polygalaceae
Sapindales	Anacardiaceae, Aceraceae, Sapindaceae, Hippocastanaceae
Celastrales	Aquifoliaceae, Celastraceae, Buxaceae
Rhamnales	Rhamnaceae, Vitaceae
Malvales	Elaeocarpaceae, Tiliaceae, Malvaceae, Bombacaceae, Sterculiaceae
Thymelaeales	Thymelaeaceae, Elaeagnaceae
Violales	Flacourtiaceae, Violaceae, Turneraceae, Passifloraceae, Cistaceae, Bixaceae, Tamaricaceae, Caricaceae
Cucurbitales	Cucurbitaceae
Myrtiflorae	Lythraceae, Myrtaceae, Punicaceae, Rhizophoraceae, Combretaceae, Onagraceae
Umbelliflorae	Alangiaceae, Cornaceae, Garryaceae, Araliaceae, Umbelliferae
Subclass Sympetalae	
Ericales	Ericaceae
Primulales	Myrsinaceae, Primulaceae
Plumbaginales	Plumbaginaceae
Ebenales	Sapotaceae, Ebenaceae, Styracaceae
Oleales	Oleaceae
Gentianales	Loganiaceae, Gentianaceae, Menyanthaceae, Apocynaceae, Asclepiadaceae, Rubiaceae
Tubiflorae	Polemoniaceae, Convolvulaceae, Boraginaceae, Verbenaceae, Labiatae, Solanaceae, Buddlejaceae, Scrophulariaceae, Bignoniaceae, Acanthaceae, Pedaliaceae, Gesneriaceae, Myoporaceae
Plantaginales	Plantaginaceae
Dipsacales	Caprifoliaceae, Valerianaceae, Dipsacaceae
Campanulales	Campanulaceae (including Lobeliaceae), Compositae

SUBCLASS ARCHICHLAMYDEAE

JUGLANDALES

Myricaceae and Juglandaceae
The order contains only these two small families.

The Myricaceae has three or four genera of trees and shrubs with unisexual flowers. Some members contain volatile oil (e.g. *Myrica gale*, the bog myrtle).

The Juglandaceae has seven or eight genera and the best-known species is the walnut, *Juglans regia*, which produces timber and edible nuts. *Juglans* contains the naphthoquinone juglone, the sugars raffinose and stachyose, flavonoids and phenolic acids.

The leaves and pericarp of *J. regia* have long been used as extracts in traditional medicine and pharmacologically demonstrated to be antihelmintic, antidiarrhoeal, antifungal, astringent, hypoglycaemic and, more recently, sedative; see M. Girzu *et al.*, *Pharm. Biol.*, 1998, **36**, 280.

SALICALES

Salicaceae
The single family of the order contains only two genera, *Salix* (500 spp.) and *Populus* (35 spp.). The dioecious flowers are in catkins.

Both genera contain phenolic glycosides such as fragilin, salicin and populin. Salicin, formerly used in medicine, has been replaced by other drugs. Willow charcoal is the chief kind of wood charcoal used in Britain. Osiers (*Salix purpurea* and *S. viminalis*) are used for basket-making, and *S. alba* var. *caerulea* is used for cricket-bats. Species of *Populus* contain raffinose and stachyose. The dried winter buds of various species of poplar (*P. nigra*, *P. candicans*, *P. tacamahaca*) constitute Balm of Gilead Bud *BHP* 1996, *BHC* Vol 1, 1992. It is used as an expectorant and contains flavonoids, phenolic esters and free acids (caffeic acid, etc.). The hive product propolis may be derived from poplar bud exudates.

FAGALES

Betulaceae and Fagaceae
These families consist of monoecious trees and shrubs. Their classification together is confirmed by similarities in constituents.

The Betulaceae has two genera, *Alnus* (35 spp.) and *Betula* (60 spp.). Constituents include many phenolic substances such as myricetin, delphinidin and ellagic acid; also terpenoids such as lupeol and betulin. The wood of *Betula alba* is used for charcoal.

The Fagaceae has eight genera and about 900 species. *Fagus* (10 spp.) includes the beech, *F. sylvatica*, the nuts of which are expressed to yield oil; *Castanea* (12 spp.) includes the sweet chestnut, *C. sativa*, which yields timber and a bark used for tanning. The edible nut serves as a component of a gluten-free diet in cases of coeliac disease and in paediatrics for the treatment of gastroenteritis. For the isolation of a pyrrole alkaloid from the seeds, see A. Hiermann *et al.*, *Fitoterapia*, 2002, **73**, 22. *Quercus* (450 spp.) provides valuable timber. Different *Quercus* spp. contain shikimic acid (a cyclitol), methyl salicylate and terpenoids. The cupules and unripe acorns of *Q. aegelops* (valonia) are used in tanning. *Q. ilex* and *Q. robur* yield tanning barks and *Q. tinctoria*, a yellow dye. *Q. suber* affords the commonly used cork, in an industry worth (1987) some £120 million p.a. to Portugal's economy; because there was no planned re-afforestation the industry now faces a decline. An extract of *Q. stenophylla* has been marketed for the acceleration of the elimination of renal and urethral calculi. Turkish galls (q.v.), an important source of tannic acid, are vegetable growths formed on the young twigs of the dyer's oak, *Q. infectoria*, as a result of the activity of a gall-wasp. Similar galls are produced on the English oak, *Q. robur*.

URTICALES

Ulmaceae, Moraceae, Cannabinaceae, Urticaceae
The Cannabinaceae, originally included in the Moraceae, is now regarded as a separate family.

1. The Ulmaceae contains 15 genera and 200 species of tropical or temperate shrubs and trees. Genera include *Ulmus* (45 spp.), *Celtis* (80 spp.) and *Trema* (30 spp.). Members contain no latex (distinction from Moraceae). Mucilage is abundant in the barks of *Ulmus rubra* (see 'Slippery Elm Bark') and *U. campestris*; raffinose and stachyose occur in *Ulmus*, an indole alkaloid occurs in *Celtis*.
2. The Moraceae has about 53 genera and 1400 species. They are mainly tropical or subtropical shrubs or trees containing latex. The fruit is often multiple, as in *Ficus*, the fig. The large genus *Ficus* (about 800 spp.) includes trees and shrubs of very varied habit.

These include *F. benghalensis* (banyan), *F. elastica* (indiarubber tree) and *F. carica* (common fig). The latex is often anthelmintic, owing to the proteolytic enzyme ficin. Another genus *Castilloa* (10 spp.), yields, from *C. elastica*, Panama rubber or caoutchouc. Among other constituents reported in the family are cardenolides (in five genera) and pyridine alkaloids (in two genera). Species of *Morus* are used in oriental medicine.

3. The Cannabinaceae or Cannabidaceae consists of the two genera *Cannabis* and *Humulus* comprising *C. sativa* (hemp), *H. lupulus* (common hop) (q.v.) and *H. japonica* (Japanese hop). The chemistry of these plants is a justification for their separation from the Moraceae. *Cannabis* produces the best hemp when grown in a temperate climate, whilst the more active samples of Indian hemp (q.v.) are usually associated with warmer climates.

4. The Urticaceae has 45 genera and 550 species; tropical or temperate herbs or undershrubs without latex. Some genera have stinging hairs (e.g. *Urtica*, 50 species of stinging nettle), others lack such-hairs (e.g. *Pilea*, *Boehmeria* and *Parietaria*). Root and leaf extracts of the common stinging nettle (q.v.) are used in herbal medicine, often in combination with other species, for the treatment of benign prostate hyperplasia. For a review with 78 references see E. Bombardelli and P. Morazzoni, *Fitoterapia*, 1997, **68**, 387.

PROTEALES

Proteaceae

The single family of the order, the Proteaceae, contains 62 genera and 1050 species. Shrubs and trees are particularly abundant in Australia, New Zealand and South Africa. Many species have been examined chemically, and the constituents reported include cyanogenetic compounds, alkaloids, tannins, leucoanthocyanins, arbutin and the sugar alcohol polygalitol. Genera include *Protea* (130 spp.), *Grevillea*, *Persoonia*, *Hakea* and *Knightia*.

SANTALALES

Olacaceae, Santalaceae, Loranthaceae

The order contains seven families of which only four need be mentioned.

The Olacaceae has about 27 genera and 250 species. Few have been examined chemically. Acetylenic acids occur in *Olax stricta*.

The Santalaceae contains about 30 genera and 400 species. Of the genera, *Santalum* contains 25 species and *Thesium* about 325 species. Monoterpenes and sesquiterpenes occur in several genera. The plants are hemiparasitic herbs, shrubs and small trees. *Santalum album* yields sandalwood and sandalwood oil (q.v.) and is rich in sesquiterpene alcohols. Australian sandalwood and its oil are obtained from another member of the family, *Eucarya spicata*.

The Loranthaceae is a fairly large family of 36 genera and 1300 species. The genus *Viscum* consists of about 60 species of parasitic evergreen shrubs, which often contain cyclitols. The dried aerial parts of the common mistletoe, *Viscum album*, which grows on apple and other trees are included in the *BHP* 1996 and are used for various circulatory conditions. It contains glycoproteins (the mistletoe lectins), polypeptides (viscotoxins), lignans, flavonoids, etc. The flavonoid glycosides involve glucose, apiose and *trans*-cinnamic acid; for glycoside isolations from *V. album* ssp. *atlantica* grown on apricot (*Armeniaca vulgaris*) in Turkey, see D. Deliorman Orhan *et al.*, *Pharm. Biol.*, 2002, **40**, 380.

POLYGONALES

Polygonaceae

This one-family order occupies an isolated position. It has about 40 genera and 800 species, mostly herbs. About 29 species are indigenous to Britain. Genera include *Rheum* (50 spp.), *Rumex* (about 180 spp.), *Fagopyrum* (15 spp.), *Coccoloba* (150 spp.) and *Polygonum*. The fruit is a one-seeded, usually three-winged nut (e.g. dock and buckwheat). Anthocyanin pigments are common; also flavones and flavonols—for example, buckwheat, *Fagopyrum esculentum*, is a commercial source of rutin. Quinones (anthraquinones, phenanthraquinones, anthrones and dianthrones) are found in many species of *Rheum* (q.v.), *Rumex* and *Polygonum*. The root of *Rumex crispus* (yellow dock, curled dock), *BHP* 1983, contains hydroxyanthraquinone derivatives; it is indicated for the treatment of chronic skin diseases, obstructive jaundice and psoriasis.

CENTROSPERMAE

Phytolaccaceae, Caryophyllaceae, Chenopodiaceae

The order contains 13 families which show a passage from the monochlamydeous type of flower (e.g. Phytolaccaceae and Chenopodiaceae) to the dichlamydeous type of flower (e.g. Caryophyllaceae). Most families of the order, except the Caryophyllaceae, produce characteristic betacyanin and betaxanthin pigments, which indicate affinity with the Cactales (the next order, below).

The Phytolaccaceae is a family of 12 genera and 100 species; herbs, shrubs and trees, found particularly in tropical America and South Africa. *Phytolacca* (35 spp.) includes *Phytolacca americana* (Poke root), the leaves and roots of which have been found as an adulterant of belladonna: its berries contain a dyestuff. The roots which contain saponins are included in the *BHP* (1996) for the treatment of rheumatic diseases; however, arising from its toxicity the drug is not strongly recommended and excessive use should be avoided. The toxicity is primarily due to mitogenic proteins (lectins) and triterpene saponins. Other species have been shown to have molluscicidal activity.

The Caryophyllaceae has 70 genera and about 1750 species, mostly herbs, and is wide-spread. Genera include *Saponaria*, *Stellaria*, *Arenaria*, *Spergularia*, *Herniaria*, *Silene*, *Lychnis*, *Gypsophila* (125 spp.) and *Dianthus* (300 spp.). Many of these plants are rich in saponins. The root of *Saponaria officinalis* has been included in many pharmacopoeias. It contains about 5% of saponins and is widely used as a domestic detergent.

The Chenopodiaceae contains 102 genera and 1400 species; most grow naturally in soils containing much salt (halophytes). Genera include *Beta* (6 spp.), *Chenopodium* (100–150 spp.), *Salicornia*, *Atriplex* and *Anabasis*. From the wild *Beta vulgaris* (sea-beet) have been derived garden beetroot, sugar-beet and the mangold-wurzel. *Chenopodium anthelminticum* yields the anthelmintic Mexican tea or 'wormseed' and its oil of chenopodium (q.v.).

CACTALES

Cactaceae

The Cactaceae is the only family of the order and contains from 50 to 150 genera and about 2000 species. The plants are xerophytes and, with possibly one exception, are all native to the Americas. They will not grow where there is virtually no rainfall, but thrive in deserts where there is a reasonable rainfall even if rain occurs very infrequently. Some cacti occur in rain forests, where they are often epiphytes (e.g. *Epiphyllum*). The majority are succulent and store water in their stems. The plant body is usually globular or cylindrical and bears wool, spines and flowers, but in *Epiphyllum* the stems are flattened and consist of jointed segments, which are often mistaken for leaves. Among the genera are *Epiphyllum* (21 spp.), *Opuntia* (250 spp.), *Cephalocereus* (48 spp.), *Cereus* (50 spp.) and *Echinocereus* (75 spp.). The leaves of *Opuntia* and *Nopolea* provide food for cochineal insects (q.v.). *Opuntia ficus-indica*, the prickly-pear, is sometimes grown as a hedge but can become a troublesome weed. Dried cactus flowers (*Opuntia* spp.) are used as an astringent herbal remedy. *O. dillenii* finds various medicinal uses in India. *Lophophora williamsii* is the plant producing peyote, anhalonium or 'mescal buttons'; it contains mescaline (q.v.). Several genera contain simple isoquinoline alkaloids; cyanogenetic glycosides are very rare or absent; most species contain abundant mucilage.

MAGNOLIALES

Magnoliaceae, Winteraceae, Annonaceae, Myristicaceae, Canellaceae, Schisandraceae, Illiciaceae, Monimiaceae, Lauraceae and Hernandiaceae

This order contains 22 families.

1. The Magnoliaceae contains 12 genera and about 230 species, which occur in both temperate and tropical regions. They are trees or shrubs with oil cells in the parenchyma. Genera include *Magnolia* (180 spp.), *Michelia* (50 spp.) and *Liriodendron* (1 sp.), tulip tree. The remedial properties of *L. tulipifera*, which is reported to contain alkaloids (e.g. dihydroglaucine) and sesquiterpenes, have been assessed (Crellin, J. K. *Pharm. J.*, 1988, **240**, 29).

2. The Winteraceae comprises 7 genera and 120 species. *Drimys winteri* (Winter's bark) has been much used for its stimulant and tonic properties and a number of pharmacological investigations have been reported in the literature. The bark contains volatile oil, sesquiterpenes, lactones, flavonoids and polygodial derivatives (V. C. Filho *et al.*, *J. Ethnopharmacology*, 1998, **62**, 223).

3. The Annonaceae contains 120 genera and about 2100 species, which are found mainly in the tropical regions of the Old World. Genera include *Uvaria* (150 spp.), *Xylopia* (100–150 spp.), *Monodora* (20 spp.) and *Annona* (120 spp.). The seeds of *Monodora myristica* are used like nutmegs. Many members of the family contain alkaloids mainly of the isoquinoline type. The family is of importance in folk medicine.

4. The Myristicaceae is a family of 18 genera and 300 species, which are mainly found in tropical Asia. Genera include *Myristica* (120 spp.), *Virola* (60 spp.), *Horsfieldia* (80 spp.) and *Knema* (37 spp.). The flowers are dioecious and consist of an inconspicuous three-lobed perianth with 3–18 monadelphous stamens or a solitary carpel containing a basal anatropous ovule. The fruit is a fleshy drupe, which splits along both dorsal and ventral sutures. The single seed is more or less completely enveloped in a lobed aril. The chemistry of the family has not been thoroughly investigated. Some species (see 'Nutmeg' and 'Mace') contain volatile oil and hallucinogenic substances.

5. The Canellaceae is a small family of five genera and 16 species; trees with gland-dotted leaves. Fruit is a berry. Genera include *Canella*, *Cinnamodendron* and *Warburgia*. Canella bark, a spice, is obtained from *Canella alba*, grown in the Bahamas and Florida.

6. The Schisandraceae comprises two genera and 47 species of climbing shrubs. *Schisandra* has 25 species; lignans are common constituents. *S. chinensis* produces antihepatoxic constituents (q.v.).

7. The Illiciaceae, sometimes classified under Magnoliaceae, has the single genus *Illicium* (42 spp.), found in Asia, Atlantic North America and the West Indies. See 'Star-anise Fruit and Oil'.

8. The Monimiaceae includes 20 genera and 150 species of trees and shrubs, which often contain volatile oil and resin. In South America there are many traditional uses of plants of this family; G. G. Leitao *et al.* (*J. Ethnopharmacology*, 1999, **65**, 87), have reviewed the pharmacology and chemistry. The genera include *Hedycarya* (25 spp.) and *Peumus* (one sp.). *Peumus boldus* (q.v.) has a hard wood, its bark yields a dye and its leaves contain the alkaloid boldine.

9. The Lauraceae has 32 genera and about 2000–2500 species. These are tropical or subtropical trees and shrubs with leathery, evergreen leaves; the flowers are usually bisexual (e.g. *Cinnamomum*), rarely unisexual (e.g. *Laurus*). The fruit is a berry or drupe. Alkaloids, volatile oils and fixed oils occur in many species. Volatile oil cells occur in the leaves and cortex. Genera include *Persea* (150 spp.), *Ocotea* (300–400 spp.), *Cinnamomum* (250 spp.), *Aniba* (40 spp.), *Litsea* (400 spp.), *Neolitsea* (80 spp.), *Lindera* (100 spp.), *Laurus* (2 spp.) and *Cryptocarya* (200–250 spp.). A number of Taiwanese species of the above genera have been tested for bioactivity (C. T. Lin *et al.*, *Pharm. Biol.*, 2007, **45**, 638).

   The bark of *Cryptocarya massoia* yields an essential oil that has a coconut-like aroma and is used as a cosmetic additive, e.g. in shampoos; *C. moschata* gives the mace of Brazilian nutmeg. The bay laurel, *Laurus nobilis*, is the only European representative of the family; 45 constituents of the essential oil have been identified, the principal one being 1,8-cineole. Other constituents of the leaves are glycosylated flavonoids, (−)-epicatechin, (+)-catechin, (+)-epigallocatechin and procyanidins. For research and other references, see C. Fiorini *et al.*, *Phytochemistry*, 1998, **47**, 1821; M. Simić *et al.*, *Fitoterapia*, 2003, **74**, 613; S. D. Acqua *et al.*, *Chem. Pharm. Bull.*, 2006, **54**, 1187. For drugs see 'Cinnamon bark', 'Cassia bark' and 'Camphor'.

10. The Hernandiaceae has three genera and 54 species. Members are tropical trees, shrubs or lianes with oil cells. Species of *Hernandia* (24 spp.) contain tumour-inhibiting alkaloids and lignans including podophyllotoxin; they have been used in traditional Samoan medicine. About 128 alkaloids belonging to 17 structural types are known for the family, see L. M. Conserva *et al.*, *The Alkaloids*, 2005, **62**, 175.

RANUNCULALES:

Ranunculaceae, Berberidaceae, Menispermaceae and Nymphaeaceae

Of the seven families in this order the above four are of medicinal interest. The families show a considerable variety of plant constituents and alkaloids are very common. In the four named families the alkaloids are often based on benzylisoquinoline, bisbenzylisoquinoline or aporphine.

1. The Ranunculaceae comprises 59 genera and about 1900 species. The plants are mostly perennial herbs with a rhizome or rootstock. They are well represented in Britain. Many members are poisonous. The flowers are bisexual, regular (e.g. *Ranunculus*) or zygomorphic (e.g. *Aconitum*). The perianth is simple or differentiated into calyx and corolla. The stamens are numerous and free. The carpels are usually numerous in the regular flowers or fewer in the zygomorphic ones. The fruit is an etaerio of achenes or follicles, or a berry. Genera include *Helleborus* (20 spp.), *Aconitum* (300 spp.), *Thalictrum* (150 spp.), *Clematis* (250 spp.), *Actaea* (10 spp.), *Ranunculus* (400 spp.), *Anemone* (150 spp.), *Delphinium* (250 spp.), *Adonis* (20 spp.) and *Hepatica* (10 spp.). The family has diverse chemical constituents and is of considerable phytochemical and chemotaxonomic interest. For example, the chromosomes, based

on size and shape, fall into two distinct groups, the *Ranunculus* type (R-type) and the *Thalictrum* type (T-type). The glycoside ranunculin has been found only in plants of the R-type. This glycoside hydrolyses to protoanemonin, which is vesicant and accounts for this property in many species. Isoquinoline-derived alkaloids occur in *Thalictrum*, *Aquilegia* and *Hydrastis*; diterpene-derived alkaloids in *Delphinium* and *Aconitum*. Saponins, mainly triterpenoid, occur in *Ranunculus*, *Trollius*, *Clematis*, *Anemone* and *Thalictrum*, cyanogenetic glycosides in *Ranunculus* and *Clematis*; cardenolides in *Adonis*, bufodienolides in *Helleborus*. Black hellebore rhizome, from *Helleborus niger*, contains very powerful cardiac glycosides but is now little used in medicine. Various aconite roots, containing highly toxic alkaloids (q.v.) have also lost much of their former popularity. Black Cohosh BHP 1996 is the dried rhizome of *Cimicifuga racemosa*; it contains triterpenoid glycosides structurally related to cycloartenol, also isoflavones including formononetin. The drug contains substances with endocrine activity and is used in herbal medicine to treat menopausal and other female disorders, and also various rheumatic conditions. A number of other species e.g. *C. simplex*, are used in Chinese medicine (see, for example, A. Kussano *et al.*, *Chem. Pharm. Bull.*, 1999, **47**, 1175). The European *C. foetida* (bugbane) is a traditional vermin preventative.

2. The Berberidaceae has 14 genera and about 575 species, they are perennial shrubs usually with spiny leaves. The flowers are hermaphrodite, regular and hypogynous. The perianth is differentiated into calyx and corolla. The stamens are generally in two whorls and the ovary is composed of one carpel. The fruit is a berry with one to numerous seeds. Genera include *Berberis* (450 spp.), *Mahonia* (70 spp.), *Epimedium*, *Vancouveria* and *Leontice*.
   The Berberidaceae contains alkaloids of the benzylisoquinoline, bisbenzylisoquinoline and aporphine types. *Leontice* contains an alkaloidal amine and quinolizidine. Lignans such as dehydropodophyllotoxin occur; also triterpenoid saponins. The root tubers of *Leontice leontopetalum* contain saponin and alkaloids and have been used for the treatment of epilepsy. For other drugs see under 'Hydrastis', 'Podophyllum' and 'Indian Podophyllum'.
   In some members of the family there is a close resemblance to the Ranunculaceae. *Hydrastis*, for example, is sometimes placed in the Ranunculaceae in the same tribe as the peony. There are also relationships with the Papaveraceae, narcotine being found in both families.

3. The Menispermaceae is a family of 65 genera and 350 species; mainly tropical twining shrubs, herbs or trees. The plants usually have palmately lobed leaves and dioecious flowers. Anomalous stem structure is frequently found and abnormal secondary growth often takes place in the roots (e.g. of *Chondodendron tomentosum*), successive cambia being produced to give concentric rings of wood. The broad primary medullary rays found in the stem of *Coscinium* are a family characteristic. The fruit is a drupe the dorsal side of which develops more rapidly than the ventral, as in the fish berry *Anamirta cocculus*. These contain the highly toxic substance picrotoxin. For drugs see 'Calumba' and 'Curare'.
   The genera include *Chondodendron* (8 spp.), *Tiliacora* (25 spp.), *Triclisia* (25 spp.), *Anamirta* (1 sp.), *Coscinium* (8 spp.), *Tinospora* (40 spp.), *Jateorhiza* (2 spp.), *Abuta* (35 spp.), *Cocculus* (11 spp.), *Menispermum* (3 spp.), *Stephania* (40 spp.), *Cissampelos* (30 spp.) and *Cyclea* (30 spp.).
   Alkaloids are important constituents of the family and have been reviewed (J. M. Barbosa-Filho *et al.*, *The Alkaloids*, 2000, **54**, 1). Saponins are present in many species. *Coscinium fenestratum* ('false calumba', 'tree turmeric') stems are widely used in SE Asia and India for the treatment of a variety of ailments. The principal

alkaloid constituents are berberine and jatrorrhizine, the former being responsible for its antibacterial activity (G. M. Nair *et al.*, *Fitoterapia*, 2005, **76**, 285); for an investigation of the hypotensive and toxicological properties of an extract, see T. Wongcome *et al.*, *J. Ethnopharm.*, 2007, **111**, 468. *Stephania pierrii* (*S. erecta*) contains bisbenzylisoquinoline alkaloids and is used in Thai folk medicine as a muscle relaxant. *Tinospora cordifolia* is used in Ayurvedic medicine and a considerable number of pharmacological actions, including immunomodulatory, have been demonstrated for the drug. For other drugs see 'Calumba' and 'Curare'.

4. The Nymphaeaceae is a small family of about six genera and 70 species. Species of *Nymphaea* (water-lilies) are widely cultivated. The genera include *Nymphaea* (50 spp.), *Nuphar* (25 spp.), *Nelumbo* (2 spp.) and *Ondinea*. Alkaloids occur which resemble those of other families of the order but the chemistry of the family requires further research. *Nuphar variegatum* rhizomes contain antibacterial tannins and have long been used in folk medicine, similarly *Nymphaea* spp.. *Nelumbo nucifera* (the sacred lotus) and *Nymphaea lotus* (the white lotus) were revered in the ancient civilizations of India, China, Tibet and Egypt. *Nymphaea stellata* has been traditionally used in Indian medicine.

PIPERALES

Piperaceae

Four families are included in the Piperales; only the Piperaceae is considered here.

The Piperaceae (excluding the Peperomiaceae) consists of four genera and about 2000 species. The plants are tropical, mostly climbing shrubs or lianes, with swollen nodes and fleshy spikes of flowers. The leaves contain oil cells. The one-celled ovary has a single basal ovule and develops into a berry. The seeds contain endosperm and abundant perisperm. The four genera are *Piper* (about 2000 spp.), *Trianaeopiper* (18 spp.), *Ottonia* (70 spp.) and *Pothomorphe* (10 spp.). In addition to the above, Engler includes in the Piperaceae the Peperomiaceae with its four genera and about 1000 species of succulent herbs and subshrubs. All but 5 of its species belong to the genus *Peperomia*. The Piperaceae contains phenolic esters and ethers; pyrrolidine alkaloids; volatile oils and lignans. The peppers (q.v.) are widely used as condiments. Cubebs, *Piper cubeba*, was formerly used in medicine but is now obsolescent. In the South Pacific islands an aqueous extract of the roots of *P. methysticum* (kava-kava) is consumed as a ritual stimulant; large doses cause intoxication. In herbal medicine the root is used as a diuretic, stimulant and tonic. the active principles are pyrone derivatives (kava lactones); a number of piperidine alkaloids, including pipermethysticine, have also been isolated (K. Dragull *et al.*, *Phytochemistry*, 2003, **63**, 193).

ARISTOLOCHIALES

Aristolochiaceae

The order comprises three families, of which only the Aristolochiaceae is of importance.

The Aristolochiaceae has seven genera and about 500 species. Members occur in the tropics and warm temperate zones, excluding Australia. Most are herbs or climbing shrubs. Oil-secreting cells occur throughout the family, often forming transparent dots on the leaves. The principal genera are *Aristolochia* (350 spp.) and *Asarum* (70 spp.). Constituents of the family include alkaloids (aporphine and protoberberine), aristolochic acid, phenolic esters and ethers, volatile oils and flavonoids. Some species show tumour-inhibiting properties. *Asarum europaeum*, asarabacca root, was formerly used in European medicine.

5

GUTTIFERALES

Paeoniaceae, Dipterocarpaceae, Theaceae, Guttiferae

Of the 16 families in the order, only the four above need be noted.

1. The Paeoniaceae contains the single genus *Paeonia* with 33 species which are perennial rhizomatous herbs, occasionally shrubby. *Paeonia mascula* is one of Britain's rarest wild plants; it grows on the island of Steep Holme, in the Bristol Channel, having been introduced there by monks in the 14th century for medicinal purposes. Peony root is important in Chinese medicine and the species used, *P. lactiflora*, has been extensively investigated. It is a constituent of a herbal tea which, in the UK, has come into prominence for the treatment of children's eczema. The active anti-inflammatory ingredient appears to be paeonol, 2'-hydroxy-4'-methoxyacetophenone; other constituents of the rhizome are monoterpenoid glycosides one of which, paeoniflorin, is used as a basis for the quality control of the drug by HPLC. New glycosidic paeoniflorin derivatives have recently been reported (A. Braca *et al.*, *Fitoterapia*, 2008, **79**, 117).

2. The Dipterocarpaceae has 15 genera and about 580 species. Many are large trees yielding useful timbers. Oleoresins are a character of the family. Genera include *Dipterocarpus* (76 spp.), *Shorea* (180 spp.), *Dryobalanops* (9 spp.) and *Hopea* (90 spp.). Products include: gurjun balsam from *Dipterocarpus turbinatus*; varnish resins from species of *Shorea*, *Hopea* and *Balanocarpus*; an edible fat which can be used instead of cocoa butter in chocolate manufacture, from the nuts of *Shorea macrophylla*; and Borneo camphor, from *Dryobalanops aromatica*.

3. The Theaceae or Ternstroemiaceae consists of 16 genera and about 500 species of tropical and subtropical trees and shrubs. Genera include *Camellia* (82 spp.) and *Ternstroemia* (100 spp.). Among the constituents are purine bases in *Camellia*, saponins, tannins and fixed oils. By far the most important plant commercially is *Camellia sinensis*, which yields tea and caffeine. The so-called 'tea seed oil' is an edible oil which is a possible adulterant of the more expensive olive oil and is obtained from *Camellia sasanqa*.

4. The Guttiferae contains about 40 genera and 1000 species. They are trees, shrubs or lianes, except *Hypericum*, which is often treated as a separate family, the Hypericaceae. The main genera are *Hypericum* (400 spp.), *Kielmeyera* (20 spp.), *Clusia* (145 spp.), *Garcinia* (400 spp.) and *Calophyllum* (112 spp.). Constituents of the family include resins, volatile oils, alkaloids, xanthones and seed oils. Products include resin from *Calophyllum* and gamboge, a coloured gum resin, from *Garcinia*. The edible fruit mangosteen is obtained from *Garcinia mangostana*.

SARRACENIALES

Sarraceniaceae, Nepenthaceae, Droseraceae

The three small families of insectivorous plants forming this order are of minor pharmaceutical interest.

The Sarraceniaceae consists of three genera and 17 species of pitcher-plants. The Nepenthaceae has two genera and 68 species, of which 67 belong to *Nepenthes*. In these plants, which occur mainly in tropical Asia, the leaves are modified into pitchers, which attract insects by their colour and honey-like secretion. The Droseraceae has four genera and 105 species. Of these, 100 belong to *Drosera*, which is represented in Britain by three sundews. The European sundew, *Drosera rotundifolia*, has long been employed in folk medicine and has been included in some pharmacopoeias (*BHP* 1983). In Italy it is an ingredient of a liqueur. It contains the naphthoquinone plumbagone, which has antimicrobial activity.

PAPAVERALES

Papaveraceae, Fumariaceae, Capparaceae, Cruciferae

An order of seven families, if the Fumariaceae is separated from the Papaveraceae. The Papaveraceae belongs to the suborder Papaverineae and the Capparaceae and Cruciferae to the Capparineae. Some workers regard the Papaveraceae as related to the Ranunculales and the Capparineae as derived from the Cistales. Chemical support for this view is that alkaloids of the Papaveraceae are related to those of the Ranunculaceae, and that thiogluconates are absent from the Papaveraceae but present in the other two families.

1. The Papaveraceae is a family of 26 genera and about 300 species. The plants are usually herbs with solitary, showy flowers of the floral formula K 2 – 3, C 2 + 2 or 2 + 4, A ∞, G (2 – ∞). The fruit is generally a capsule, with numerous seeds, each containing a small embryo in an oily endosperm. Genera include *Platystemon* (about 60 spp.), *Romneya* (2 spp.), *Eschscholtzia* (10 spp.), *Sanguinaria* (1 sp.), *Chelidonium* (1 sp.), *Bocconia* (10 spp.), *Glaucium* (25 spp.), *Meconopsis* (43 spp.), *Argemone* (10 spp.) and *Papaver* (100 spp.). All members contain latex tissue. The latex is sometimes in vessels which accompany the vascular system (e.g. in *Papaver*); sometimes in latex sacs (e.g. *Sanguinaria*). The family is rich in alkaloids. Some, such as the opium alkaloids (q.v.), are of great medical and economic importance. *Eschscholtzia californica*, used by the Californian Indians as a sedative and now similarly prescribed in Europe, has been validated experimentally. The aerial parts of *Glaucium grandiflorum* are used in Iranian medicine for the treatment of dermatitis (K. Morteza-Semnani *et al.*, *Fitoterapia*, 2004, **75**, 123). Mustard oil glycosides appear to be absent from the family (compare Capparaceae and Cruciferae).

2. Fumariaceae. Included in the Papaveraceae by Engler but now generally regarded as a separate family. It contains 16 genera and about 55 species: they contain a watery, not milky, juice. Isoquinoline alkaloids are a feature of the family. Fumitory is used for liver disorders, see Chapter 29.

3. Capparaceae. A family of 30 genera and 650 species; usually trees or shrubs, often xerophytic. The genus *Capparis* (250 spp.) includes *Capparis spinosa*, the buds of which (capers) are used in flavouring. Like the Cruciferae, the family has myrosin cells and mustard-oil glycosides such as glucocapparin. The only alkaloid reported is pyrrolidine in two genera. Cardenolides, which occur in some Cruciferae, have not been found in the Capparaceae.

4. Cruciferae. A family of 375 genera and about 3200 species; herbs and a few undershrubs. The inflorescence is typically a raceme without bracts. The flowers are of the type, K 2 + 2, C 2 + 2, A 2 + 4, G(2). The stamens are tetradynamous and the ovary is divided into two loculi by a replum uniting the two parietal placentas. The fruit is called a siliqua when elongated, as in the wallflower and mustards; or silicula when almost as broad as long, as in shepherd's purse and horseradish. The testas of the seeds often contain mucilage. Genera include *Brassica* (about 30 spp.), *Sinapis* (10 spp.), *Nasturtium* (6 spp.), *Lepidium* (150 spp.), *Hesperis* (30 spp.), *Cheiranthus* (10 spp.), *Isatis* (45 spp.), *Erysimum* (100 spp.), *Crambe* (25 spp.) and *Lunaria* (3 spp.). Cultivated *Brassica* species include: *B. nigra* (black mustard); *B. oleracea* (cabbage, cauliflower, broccoli, etc.); *B. campestris*, turnip; and *B. napus*, rape or colza oil. *Sinapis alba* yields white mustard; *Nasturtium officinale*, water cress; *Lepidium sativum*, garden cress; *Crambe maritima*, the sea kale. The ancient dyestuff woad was made by grinding and fermenting the leaves of *Isatis tinctoria* to produce deep blue indigo, isatin A being the major indoxyl glycoside precursor of the dye. For the significance

of indoxyl derivatives in this connection and further studies, see T. Kokubun *et al.*, *Phytochemistry*, 1998, **49**, 79; C. Oberthur *et al.*, *Phytochemistry*, 2004, **65**, 3261 and 'Colourants', Chapter 33. Many members of the Cruciferae contain mustard-oil glycosides and in special myrosin cells contain the enzymes necessary for their hydrolysis. Cardiac glycosides occur in some genera and the seeds usually contain mucilage and fixed oil.

ROSALES

Hamamelidaceae, Crassulaceae, Saxifragaceae, Rosaceae, Leguminosae, Krameriaceae

The order Rosales consists of 19 families divided into four suborders. The families to be considered fall into the suborders as follows: Hamamelidineae (Hamamelidaceae); Saxifragineae (Crassulaceae, Saxifragaceae and Pittosporaceae); Rosineae (Rosaceae); Leguminosineae (Leguminosae and Krameriaceae). The flowers are usually hermaphrodite (rarely bisexual by abortion: e.g. kousso flowers from *Brayera*); hypogynous, perigynous or epigynous. The sepals and petals are usually free; stamens and carpels free or united.

1. Hamamelidaceae. A family of 26 genera and 106 species of trees and shrubs, chiefly subtropical. Genera include *Hamamelis* (6 spp.) and *Liquidambar* (6 spp.). Drugs (q.v.) include hamamelis leaves (*Hamamelis virginiana*), Levant storax (*Liquidambar orientalis*) and American storax or sweet gum (*L. styraciflua*). The family contains tannins, balsamic resins, phenolic acids and cyclitols; alkaloids are absent.

2. Crassulaceae. A family of 35 genera and 1500 species; many perennial xerophytes. Genera include *Sedum* (about 600 spp.), *Sempervivum* (25 spp.), (*Rhodiola*) and *Crassula* (about 300 spp.). An interesting chemical character of the family is the presence, often in large amounts, of isocitric acid; it was in this xerophytic family that a distinctive build-up of malic acid during the hours of darkness was first noticed and the term crassulacean acid metabolism (CAM) given to this particular adaptation of the photosynthetic cycle (see Chapter 18). The carbohydrate sedoheptulose occurs in both the Crassulaceae and the Saxifragaceae. Cyanogenetic glycosides and cardiac glycosides occur in some species; tannins are common but alkaloids rare. Species of *Sedum* have been used medicinally as antihepatotoxics. The roots and rhizomes of *Rhodiola rosea* (arctic root), indigenous to Northern Europe and Northern Asia, have been used in traditional medicine for centuries. Recently, the drug has attracted considerable attention in the West, principally as an adaptogen for the treatment of stress. It has been extensively investigated, pharmacologically and chemically. Constituents include flavonoids, proanthocyanidin glycosides, e.g. rosavin, monoterpenoid glycosides, lotaustralin, etc. For further information, see R. P. Brown and G. Gerberg with B. Graham 2004, *The Rhodiola Revolution*, 260 pp., Rodale, New York; G. Ma *et al.*, *Chem. Pharm. Bull.*, 2006, **54**, 1229.

3. The Saxifragaceae is a family of 30 genera and about 580 species; chiefly north temperate herbs. Genera include *Saxifrage* (370 spp.), *Astilbe* and *Ribes*. The latter, sometimes separated as the family Grossulariaceae, includes such well-known fruits as the blackcurrant, redcurrant and gooseberry. These are rich in citric and malic acids and in ascorbic acid. Black Currant Syrup is used medicinally. Some members of the Saxifragaceae contain tannins and saponins, but alkaloids are rare.

4. Rosaceae. A family which includes about 100 genera and 2000 species of herbs, shrubs and trees. The leaves are simple (e.g. *Prunus*) or compound (e.g. *Rosa*). Considerable variety exists in the flowers and fruits. There are no anatomical features characteristic of the family as a whole, and the various subfamilies frequently show differences in stomatal arrangement, origin of cork, etc. Genera include *Spiraea* (100 spp.), *Quillaja* (3 spp.), *Pyrus* (3 spp.), *Malus* (35 spp.), *Sorbus* (100 spp.), *Kerria* (1 sp.), Rubus (250 spp.), *Potentilla* (500 spp.), *Geum* (40 spp.), *Alchemilla* (250 spp.), *Agrimonia* (15 spp.), *Poterium* (25 spp.), *Rosa* (250 spp.), *Prunus*, including *Laurocerasus* (430 spp.) and *Crataegus* (200 spp.). Constituents of the Rosaceae include cyanogenetic glycosides, saponins, tannins, seed fats, sugar alcohols, cyclitols, terpenoids and mucilage; alkaloids and coumarins are rare. The secondary metabolites of the family have been the basis for a number of chemosystematic studies (for such studies involving hydrolysable tannins see T. Okuda *et al.*, *Phytochemistry*, 1992, **31**, 3091). Important products (q.v.) are oil of rose (*Rosa damascena*), rose hips (*R. canina*), wild cherry bark (*Prunus serotina*), almond oil (*Prunus amygdalus*), quillaia bark (*Quillaia saponaria*), hawthorn (*Crataegus oxycanthoides*). Other products are cherry-laurel leaves (*Prunus laurocerasus*), quince seeds (*Pyrus cydonia*), prunes (*Prunus domestica*), raspberry fruits and leaves (*Rubus idaeus*) and morello cherries (*Prunus cerasus*). Comparative studies on the antibacterial and free-radical scavenging activities of extracts of *Prunus padus* (bird cherry) and *P. spinosa* (blackthorn, sloe) have been reported (Y. Kumarasamy *et al.*, *Fitoterapia*, 2004, **75**, 77).

5. Leguminosae. This is the second-largest family of flowering plants and contains 600 genera and about 12000 species. It includes more important drugs than any other family. It is divided into three subfamilies—the Papilionaceae, the Mimosoideae and the Caesalpinoideae, containing, respectively, about 377, 40 and 133 genera. Important characters and genera in each subfamily are:

   (1) Papilionaceae: Herbs, shrubs or trees; leaves simple or compound; flowers zygomorphic and papilionaceous (e.g. in broom); stamens 10, monadelphous or diadelphous; fruit a legume. Genera include *Myroxylon* (2 spp.), *Sophora* (50 spp.), *Crotalaria* (550 spp.), *Lupinus* (200 spp.), *Cytisus* (25–30 spp.), *Ononis* (75 spp.), *Medicago* (100 spp.), *Melilotus* (25 spp.), *Trifolium* (300 spp.), *Psoralea* (130 spp.), *Indigofera* (700 spp.), *Astragalus* (2000 spp.), *Vicia* (150 spp.), *Lens* (10 spp.), *Lathyrus* (130 spp.), *Pisum* (6 spp.), *Abrus* (12 spp.), *Glycine* (10 spp.), *Erythrina* (100 spp.), *Mucuna* (120 spp.), *Phaseolus* (200–240 spp.), *Arachis* (15 spp.), *Trigonella* (about 100 spp.), *Butea* (30 spp.), *Derris* (80 spp.), *Lonchocarpus* (150 spp.), *Copaifera* (25 spp.) and *Erythrophleum* (17 spp.). Drugs (q.v.) from this subfamily are fenugreek seeds, calabar bean, tonco seed, liquorice root, derris, lonchocarpus, Tolu balsam, Peru balsam, arachis oil and tragacanth gum. Common British plants with poisonous properties include broom (*Cytisus scoparius*), laburnum (*Cytisus laburnum*) and many species of *Lupinus*. Among economic products other than drugs may be mentioned sunn hemp (*Crotalaria juncea*), lentils (*Lens esculents*), peas (*Pisum sativum*), soya bean (*Glycine hispida*), scarlet runner, French and Lima beans (*Phaseolus* spp.), groundnut (*Arachis hypogaea*) and copaiba oleoresin and copals (*Copaifera* spp.). Species of *Indigofera*, including *I. tinctoria*, are a source of indigo (for biosynthesis of indigo see Z.-Q. Xia and M. H. Zenk, *Phytochemistry*, 1992, **31**, 2695).

   (2) Mimosoideae: Most members of this subfamily are trees or shrubs; leaves usually bipinnate; flowers regular; calyx usually gamosepalous; stamens equal in number to the petals or twice as numerous; fruit a legume. Important genera are *Mimosa* (450–500 spp.) and *Acacia* (750–800 spp.). Products include acacia gums from *Acacia* spp., wattle barks used in tanning from

5

Acacia spp. and volatile oil such as oil of cassie (*A. farnesiana*), which are used in perfumery.

(3) Caesalpinoideae: Members are trees or shrubs; leaves pinnate or bipinnate; flowers zygomorphic; typical floral formula K5, C5, A 5 + 5, G1. Drugs derived from this subfamily are senna leaves and pods, cassia pods and tamarinds. Other products are the redwoods logwood, from *Haematoxylon*, and sappan wood, from *Caesalpinia*; sassy bark, from *Erythrophleum guineense*, and carob beans from *Ceratonia siliqua*. *Caesalpina bonducella* seeds are traditionally used in Indian medicine for a variety of conditions.

Of the three subfamilies, the Mimosoideae and Caesalpinoideae are mostly tropical plants, while the Papilionaceae occur in both tropical and temperate regions. Tannin sacs are common, particularly in the Mimosoideae and Caesalpinoideae. The constituents of the Leguminosae show many similarities to those of the Rosaceae. Both contain cyanogenetic glycosides, saponins, tannins, mucilage and anthocyanins. Alkaloids, however, are common in the Leguminosae but rare in the Rosaceae. For a discussion of the chemotaxonomic relevance of seed polysaccharides and flavonoids in the family see R. Hegnauer and R. J. Grayer-Barkmeijer, *Phytochem.*, 1993, **34**, 3. An important work of reference for the family is *Phytochemical Dictionary of the Leguminosae*, Vols 1 and 2 (1994), compiled by I. W. Southon and published by Chapman and Hall, London.

(4) Krameriaceae: This, often included in the Leguminosae (q.v.), is a family of one genus, *Krameria*, and 20 species. They are shrubs or herbs found from the southern USA to the Argentine. The flowers resemble the Caesalpinoideae, but two of the petals are modified into glands and there are only three stamens. They contain phlobatannins; see 'Rhatany'.

GERANIALES

Geraniaceae, Zygophyllaceae, Linaceae, Erythroxylaceae, Euphorbiaceae

The order Geraniales consists of nine families.

1. The Geraniaceae consists of five genera and 750 species; mostly herbs. Members of the two large genera, *Geranium* (400 spp.) and *Pelargonium* (250 spp.) are popularly called 'geraniums' and the commercial rose geranium oil is obtained from a *Pelargonium*. The family contains volatile oils which are widely used in perfumery; more research is needed on other constituents.

2. The Zygophyllaceae is a family of 25 genera and 240 species; mostly woody perennials, tropical and subtropical. Genera include *Zygophyllum* (100 spp.), *Tribulus* (20 spp.), *Guaiacum* (6 spp.), *Peganum* (5 or 6 spp.) and *Balanites* (25 spp.). *Peganum harmala* and *Tribulus terrestris* are used in Indian medicine; the alkaloids of the former (harmine, harmaline and derivatives) have been produced in hairy root cultures and the saponins of the latter have been extensively studied (see Y.-X. Xu *et al.*, *Phytochemistry*, 1998, **49**, 199; J. Conrad *et al.*, *Fitoterapia*, 2004, **75**, 117). Some members contain alkaloids, steroidal saponins or lignans. For drugs see 'Guaiacum Resin'.

3. The Linaceae is a family of 19 genera and about 290 species; mostly herbs or shrubs. About 230 of the species belong to *Linum*. Constituents of the family include cyanogenetic glycosides, fixed oils, mucilages, diterpenes and triterpenes. Flax and linseed and its oil (q.v.) are obtained from *Linum usitatissimum*.

4. The Erythroxylaceae is closely related to the Linaceae and comprises some three to four genera with *Erythroxylum* pre-eminent (about 200 spp). The other small genera including *Nectaropetalum*

are represented by about 10 species. *Erythroxylum* spp. are distributed widely throughout tropical and subtropical regions with large areas of diversification in South America and Madagascar. Alkaloids have been found in most species analysed by modern methods; these are principally esters of the tropane type together with biosynthetically related bases such as hygrine, hygroline and cuscohygrine. Nicotine is of limited occurrence, cocaine and cinnamoylcocaine appear to be restricted to the cultivated species *E. coca* and *E. novogranatense*. The small trees or shrubs produce hard woods which constitute a rich source of diterpenoid compounds. Quinones and saponins probably contribute to the colour and durability of the wood. Phenolic constituents in the form of aromatic acids such as caffeic and chlorogenic acids, and flavonoids may have chemosystematic importance.

5. The Euphorbiaceae is a large family of about 300 genera and 6000 or more species. Most members are trees or shrubs, a few herbs. Some genera (e.g. *Euphorbia*) are xerophytic. The flowers are unisexual and regular with usually five perianth leaves; stamens may be numerous and are free or united. The superior ovary of three carpels forms a trilocular capsule. Genera include *Euphorbia* (about 2000 spp.), *Phyllanthus* (about 550 spp.), *Mallotus* (2 spp.), *Ricinus* (1 sp.), *Croton* (750 spp.), *Hevea* (12 spp.), *Jatropha* (175 spp.), *Manihot* (170 spp.), *Sapium* (120 spp.), *Poranthera* (10 spp.), *Securinega* (25 spp.), *Aleurites* (2 spp.) and *Hippomane* (5 spp.). In addition to castor seeds and castor oil (q.v.), products include the dye and taenicide kamala (from *Mallotus philippinensis*); rubber, from species of *Hevea*, *Manihot* and *Sapium*; manihot or cassava starch, from *Manihot esculentus* (*utilis*); Chinese tallow, a fat, from *Sapium sebiferum*; and a drying oil, from *Aleurites moluccana*. *Phyllanthus* is a widespread tropical genus and has been much employed in traditional medicines. Minor drugs are croton oil, from *Croton tiglium*, and cascarilla bark, from *C. cascarilla* and *C. eleuteria*. In some cases the latex is poisonous or irritant (e.g. that of *Hippomane*), and the resinous product 'euphorbium' was formerly much used as an antifouling agent for ships' hulls. Many species contain irritant or piscicidal substances. Some members such as cassava may contain cyanogenetic glycosides. This plant, *Manihot esculentus*, occurs in two varieties, sweet and bitter, only the latter yielding prussic acid. In addition to the constituents already mentioned, some members contain anthraquinones, triterpenoids, fatty acid epoxides, unsaturated fatty acids and antitumour agents. Alkaloids, when present, are usually of the aporphine, pyridine, indole, quinoline or tropane types. For a review of *Securinega suffruticosa* and its contained alkaloid securinine see D. Raj and M. Luczkiewicz, *Fitoterapia*, 2008, **79**, 419–427 (54 refs). Latices from *Euphorbia* species have widely varying biochemical properties with respect to their protein and carbohydrate properties, the type and amounts of enzymes present, and their haemagglutinating activities. For early reviews of the chemistry, taxonomy, and economic botany of the family, see *The Euphorbiales*, S. L. Jury, T. Reynolds, and D. F. Cutler (eds) (1987), London, UK: Academic Press and for a review (293 refs) of the phytoconstituents of *Euphorbia* spp. see A. K. Singla and K. Pathak, *Fitoterapia*, 1990, **61**, 483.

RUTALES

Rutaceae, Simaroubaceae, Burseraceae, Meliaceae, Malpighiaceae, Polygalaceae

This order is closely allied to the Geraniales. The chief difference is that in the Rutales the plants are mainly shrubs or trees. The flowers have a disc between the androecium and the gynaecium. Oil glands are of general occurrence. The order contains 12 families and is divided into three suborders. Of the families mentioned above, the Rutaceae, Simaroubaceae, Burseraceae and Meliaceae all belong to the same suborder, the Rutineae.

1. Rutaceae. The family consists of about 150 genera and 900 species; mainly shrubs and trees; distributed in both temperate and tropical countries, but particularly abundant in South Africa and Australia. Oil glands are present in the leaves and other parts. The flowers are usually in cymes with 4–5 sepals, 4–5 petals, 8 or 10 stamens and a superior ovary. The fruits are of various types, but in the orange subfamily, the Aurantioideae, it is a hesperidium. Fruits include orange and lemon (q.v.), lime (*Citrus limetta* and *C. medica* var. *acida*), citron, bergamot, shaddock and grapefruit. There are 12 different species of *Citrus*. Other genera include *Zanthoxylum* (20–30 spp.), *Fagara* (250 spp.), *Choisya* (6 spp.), *Ruta* (7 spp.), *Dictamnus* (6 spp.), *Diosma* (15 spp.), *Galipea* (13 spp.), *Cusparia* (*Angostura*) (30 spp.), *Ptelea* (3 spp.), *Toddalia* (1 sp.), *Skimmia* (7–8 spp.), *Limonia* (1 sp.), *Aegle* (3 spp.), *Moniera* (2 spp.), *Haplophyllum* (70 spp.), *Teclea* (30 spp.), *Esenbeckia* (38 spp.) and *Murraya* (12 spp.). Products not mentioned above are buchu leaves (*Barosma* spp.); jaborandi leaves and their alkaloid, pilocarpine (*Pilocarpus* spp.); Japan pepper (*Zanthoxylum piperitum*); elephant-apple (*Limonia acidissima*); Brazilian angostura (*Esenbeckia febrifuga*); and angostura or cusparia (*Galipea officinalis*). Species of *Haplophyllum*, *Evodia*, *Clausena*, *Phellodendron*, and *Zanthoxylum* have all been used in traditional medicine. Bael fruits (*Aegle marmelos*) are an important Ayurvedic medicine; they contain coumarins, flavonoids (rutin and marmesin) and a glucosylated propelargonidin containing up to five units of pelargonidin with immunomodulatory activity (A. M. Abeysekera *et al.*, *Fitoterapia*, 1996, **67**, 367). Southern Prickly Ash bark of the *BHP* 1996 is derived from *Zanthoxylum clava-herculis*; among other constituents it contains alkaloids e.g. chelerythrine and nitidine, a lignan-asarinin and an *n*-isobutyl polyeneamide. It is used as an antirheumatic. Northern Prickly Ash Bark (*BHP* 1983), *Z. americanum*, grows in the north-easterly parts of the USA. It contains similar alkaloidal constituents to the Southern species. Of 14 alkaloids of *Haplophyllum* screened for cytotoxic activity the furoquinoline, haplamine, was the most active (O. Jansen *et al.*, *J. Ethnopharm.*, 2006, **105**, 241). The bis-indole alkaloid yeuhchukene from *Murraya paniculata* has been studied for its anti-implantation, contraceptive activity; for information on the uses, activity and phytochemistry of this species, together with a report on the isolation of cinnamates and coumarins from the leaves, see Atta-ur-Rahman *et al.*, *Phytochemistry*, 1997, **44**, 683. Constituents of the Rutaceae include a wide variety of alkaloids, volatile oils, rhamno-glucosides, coumarins and terpenoids. Alkaloids include alkaloidal amines, imidazole, indole, isoquinoline, pyridine, pyrrolidine, quinazoline and quinoline types. Many of the fruits are rich in citric and other acids and in vitamin C.

2. Simaroubaceae. A family of 20 genera and about 120 species; tropical and subtropical shrubs and trees. Members differ from the Rutaceae in not containing oil glands. Bitter principles are a characteristic of the family. Genera include *Quassia* (*Simarouba*) (40 spp.), *Picrasma* (*Aeschrion*) (6 spp.), *Brucea* (10 spp.), *Soulamea* (10 spp.), *Ailanthus* (10 spp.), and *Perriera* (1 sp.). Quassia woods (q.v.) are used as bitters. *Ailanthus glandulosa*, Tree of Heaven, is widely cultivated and its leaves have been used to adulterate belladonna and mint. For a discussion of the quassinoids of the family see 'Quassia'.

3. Burseraceae. A family of about 16 genera and 500 species; tropical shrubs and trees. Many representatives in north-east Africa, Arabia and tropical America. The leaves, like the Rutaceae, are gland-dotted. Oleoresin canals are found in the phloem and sometimes in the pith. Genera include *Commiphora* (185 spp.), *Boswellia* (24 spp.), *Bursera* (80 spp.), and *Canarium* (75 spp.). The best-known product of the family is myrrh (q.v.). Other products are frankincense (*Boswellia* spp.), American elemi (*Bursera gummifer*), Manila elemi and Java almond from *Canarium luzonicum*.

4. Meliaceae. A family of 50 genera and about 1400 species; trees or shrubs. Some yield timber (e.g. mahogany from *Swietenia mahagoni*); others, seed oils. Genera include *Cedrela*, *Swietenia*, *Khaya*, *Carapa*, *Melia* and *Azadirachta*. *Azadirachta indica* (Neem) is an important Indian medicinal plant (q.v.); bark, leaves and seeds are used. For recent research, see Y. Fukuyama *et al.*, *Chem. Pharm. Bull.*, 2006, **54**, 1222. Significant constituents of the family are triterpenoids and limonoids.

5. Malpighiaceae. A family of 60 genera and 800 species; shrubs or small trees. Genera include *Malpighia* (35 spp.) and *Banisteriopsis*. Some members have stinging hairs. *Banisteriopsis* contains indole alkaloids, and plants may be hallucinogenic (q.v.).

6. Polygalaceae. A family of 12 genera and about 800 species, of which some 600 species belong to *Polygala*. It is represented in Britain by the milkwort, *Polygala vulgaris*. Other genera are *Monnina*, *Securidaca* and *Carpolobia*. Senega root (q.v.) is obtained from the North American *Polygala senega*. Characteristic constituents are triterpenoid saponins and, in *Polygala*, the sugar alcohol polygalitol. Methyl salicylate is common to a number of genera.

SAPINDALES

Anacardiaceae, Aceraceae, Sapindaceae, Hippocastanaceae

The Sapindales consist of 10 families.

1. Anacardiaceae. A family of 60 genera and some 600 species; mainly tropical trees and shrubs. Genera include *Mangifera* (40 spp.), *Anacardium* (15 spp.), *Rhus* (250 spp.), *Pistacia* (10 spp.), *Toxicodendron* (15 spp.), *Lannea* (70 spp.), *Cotinus* (3 spp.) and *Schinus* (30 spp.). Products include the mango, *Mangifera indica*; cashew nut, *Anacardium occidentale*; sumac leaves, used in dyeing and tanning, *Rhus coriaria*; the Japanese wax tree, *Thus succedanea*; mastic resin, *Pistacia lentiscus*; and pistachio nuts, *Pistacia vera*. The leaves of *Pistachia lentiscus* and *P. terebinthus* are a popular traditional medicine in Mediterranean regions; they contain vitamin E (α-tocopherol) for which a quantitative method for its determination has recently been published (B. Kivçak and S. Akay, *Fitoterapia*, 2005, **76**, 62). The family contains dyeing and tanning materials, and phenolic compounds some of which cause dermatitis (e.g. the vesicant constituents of the poison ivy, *Rhus toxicodendron*). Other species of *Rhus* yield Japanese lacquer and the fat known as Japan wax. Mastic resin contains triterpenoid acids and alcohols.

2. Aceraceae. A family of trees and shrubs. In the genus *Acer* (100 spp.) is *Acer saccharum*, which yields maple sugar.

3. Sapindaceae. A family of about 150 genera and 2000 species; tropical and subtropical. Genera include *Paullinia* (180 spp.), *Sapindus* (13 spp.), *Cardiospermum* (12 spp.), *Eriocoelum*, *Blighia* and *Radlkofera*. The seeds of *Paullinia cupana* are made into a paste and dried to form guarana; this contains caffeine and is used as a beverage. *Sapindus saponaria* has been used in Brazil and India as a soap and for the treatment of several diseases; it contains saponins with hederagenin (q.v.) as an aglycone. Constituents of the family include saponins, cyanogenetic glycosides, cyclitols (e.g. shikimic acid); the seed fats contain a high proportion of oleic acid. Alkaloids have been reported in a few species, including caffeine and theobromine in *Paullinia*.

4. Hippocastanaceae. A small family of only two genera and 15 species; tropical trees and shrubs of southern Africa. *Aesculus* (13 spp.) contains the horse chestnut, *A. hippocastanum*. Its seed fat, like the Sapindaceae, contains a high proportion, about 65–70%, of oleic acid. Several of the species examined contain phenolic acids, coumarins, cyclitols and saponins; alkaloids appear to be absent.

5 CELASTRALES

Aquifoliaceae, Celastraceae, Buxaceae

An order of 13 families; trees and shrubs with simple leaves.

1. Aquifoliaceae. The holly family consists of two genera and about 400 species, all but one of which belong to the genus *Ilex*. Members are trees and shrubs found in the temperate and tropical regions. Maté or Paraguay tea is obtained from *Ilex paraguariensis* and other species. A similar caffeine-containing product is cassina, the leaves of *Ilex cassine*. Constituents reported in the family include caffeine, theobromine, cyclitols (shikimic acid and inositol), triterpenes and triterpenoid saponins.

2. Celastraceae. A family of 55 genera and 850 species; tropical and temperate trees and shrubs. Genera include *Euonymus* (176 spp.), *Celastrus* (39 spp.), *Cassine* (40 spp.), *Maytenus* (225 spp.), *Prionstemma*, *Catha*, *Tripterygium* and *Peripterygia*. *Catha edulis* yields the leaves known as khat or Abyssinian tea; these contain the alkaloid cathine (norpseudoephedrine). The root bark of *Euonymus atropurpureus* contains cardioactive glycosides and is included in the *BHP* 1996. The large genus *Maytenus* has been widely used in traditional medicine and investigated for pharmacological and phytochemical properties. The alkaloid maytansine, isolated from *M. serrata* received considerable attention as a possible anticancer drug. Recently the morphology and histology of *M. ilicifolia* has been described (M. R. Duarte and M. C. Debur, *Fitoterapia*, 2005, **76**, 41). Constituents of the family include alkaloidal amines, alkaloids of the pyridine and purine types, sugar alcohols (dulcitol), saponins, cardenolides, terpenoids and substances having antitumour activity.

3. Buxaceae. A family of five genera and 100 species of tropical and temperate, usually evergreen, shrubs. The genera are *Buxus* (70 spp.), *Notobuxus* (7 spp.), *Sarcocolla* (16–20 spp.), *Pachysandra* and *Simmondsia*. Much research has been done on the steroidal alkaloids of the family, including the genus *Buxus*, some species of which find use in traditional medicine; see Atta-ur-Rahman *et al.*, *J. Nat. Prod.*, 1997, **60**, 976 for a study of *B. longifolia*. Other constituents include phenolic acids and waxes. The seeds of *Simmondsia chinensis* yield the liquid wax, jojoba wax, which consists of straight chain esters of 20:1, 22:1, 24:1 fatty acids (q.v.) and alcohols.

RHAMNALES

Rhamnaceae, Vitaceae

The order contains three families.

1. Rhamnaceae. A family of 59 genera and about 900 species; cosmopolitan, usually trees or shrubs. Genera include *Rhamnus* (110 spp.), *Zizyphus* (100 spp.), *Scutia* (9 spp.), *Discaria* (10 spp.), *Columbrina* (17 spp.), *Maesopsis* and *Hovenia*. British species are the alder buckthorn, *Rhamnus alnus*, and the buckthorn, *Rhamnus cathartica*. These, like *R. purshiana*, which produces cascara bark, contain quinones. The edible fruits of *Ziziphus jujuba* are known as French jujubes and are used in traditional Chinese medicine as a mild sedative; cytotoxic lupane-type triterpenes have been isolated from the fruits (S. M. Lee *et al.*, *Planta Medica*, 2003, **69**, 1051).

Z. vulgaris is similarly used in traditional medicine; ursane-type triterpenoids occur in the roots (H. M. Mukhtar *et al.*, *Pharm. Biol.*, 2005, **43**, 392). The constituents of the family include purgative quinones (anthraquinones, anthranols and their glycosides). Alkaloidal peptides occur in some genera; also terpenoids and triterpenoid saponins.

2. Vitaceae. The family contains about 65 spp. of *Vitis* (vines). *V. vitifera* produces grapes, wine, raisins and currants. There has been considerable recent interest in the beneficial effect of red wine arising from its antioxidant properties with respect to low-density lipoprotein and protection against atherosclerosis and coronary heart disease; see E. N. Frankel and A. S. Meyer, *Pharm. Biol.*, 1998, **36** (suppl.), 14. The compounds involved include flavonoids, anthocyanins, flavonols and phenolic acids. For a review of *Vitis vinifera* with 108 references, see E. Bombardelli and P. Morazzoni, *Fitoterpia*, 1995, **66**, 291.

MALVALES

Elaeocarpaceae, Tiliaceae, Malvaceae, Bombacaceae, Sterculiaceae

An order of seven families. Herbs, shrubs or trees; tropical and temperate. Many species contain mucilage; alkaloids are rare.

1. Elaeocarpaceae. A family of 12 genera and 350 species of tropical and subtropical trees and shrubs. Chief genera *Elaeocarpus* (200 spp.) and *Sloanea* (120 spp.). Indolizidine alkaloids occur in *Elaeocarpus*. Antibabesial ellagic acid rhamnosides, active against infections of dogs with parasitic *Babesia gibsoni*, have been isolated from *Elaeocarpus parvifolius* (A. Elkhateeb *et al.*, *Phytochemistry*, 2005, **66**, 2577).

2. Tiliaceae. A family of 50 genera and some 450 species; usually trees or shrubs. Genera include *Corchorus* (100 spp.) and *Tilia* (50 spp.). Jute fibre is obtained from *Corchorus capsularis* and *C. olitorius*. Lime Tree Flower *BHP* (1996), *BP/EP* is the dried inflorescences of *Tilia platyphyllos* or *T. cordata* (q.v.). The American lime yields phloem fibres, used by gardeners under the name of 'bass'. Cardiac glycosides are reported from *Corchorus*; alkaloids are absent.

3. Malvaceae. The family contains 75 genera and about 1000 species of herbs, shrubs and trees; tropical and temperate. Genera include *Malva* (40 spp.), *Gossypium* (20–47 spp., authorities differ), *Hibiscus* (300 spp.), *Althaea* (12 spp.), *Pavonia* (200 spp.) and *Thespesia* (15 spp.). The cottons, species of *Gossypium*, are important both for their seed hairs and seed oil (q.v.). Marshmallow root, from *Althaea officinalis*, is used as a demulcent (q.v.). The common hollyhock is *Althaea rosea*. Few species have been studied chemically, but saponins, tannins, leucoanthocyanins and phenolic acids occur; typical alkaloids appear to be absent.

4. Bombacaceae. A small family of about 20 genera and 180 species of tropical trees. Genera include *Bombax* (8 spp.), *Ceiba* and *Adansonia*. In tropical Africa the fruit pulp and bark of the baobab tree (*A. digitata*) are used medicinally and the edible seed oil is used in cooking and as a skin emollient. A range of constituents have been isolated; recently, procyanidins have been recorded in a methanolic extract of the pericarp (A. A. Shahat, *Pharm. Biol.*, 2006, **44**, 445). Kapok, which consists of the lignified, silky hairs which line the fruits of various species of *Bombax* and *Ceiba*, has been used for life-belts and as a stuffing material.

5. Sterculiaceae. A family of 60 genera and 700 species; mainly tropical. Genera include *Sterculia* (300 spp.), *Theobroma* (30 spp.), *Cola* (125 spp.) and *Brachychiton*. Cocoa, oil of theobroma and

chocolate are prepared from *Theobroma cacao*; kola or cola nuts come from *Cola vera* and *C. acuminata*; and sterculia or karaya gum come from *Sterculia urens*. As in the Malvaceae, mucilage is common; purine bases occur in *Theobroma* and *Cola*.

THYMELAEALES

Thymelaeaceae, Elaeagnaceae
An order of five families.

1. Thymelaeaceae. A family of 90 genera and 500 species; mostly temperate and tropical shrubs. Genera include *Gnidia* (100 spp.), *Daphne* (70 spp.) and *Pimelea* (80 spp.). Some species of *Daphne* are poisonous and contain vesicant resins. The bark of *Daphne mezereum* was formerly official; the floral fragrance is composed of about 95% s-(+)-linalool. Mucilage and coumarins common in the family; alkaloids absent.
2. Elaeagnaceae. A family of three genera and about 50 species, including *Hippophae* (3 spp.), *Elaeagnus* (45 spp.) and *Shepherdia* (3 spp.). Among the constituents are indole alkaloids and cyclitols.

VIOLALES

Flacourtiaceae, Violaceae, Turneraceae, Passifloraceae, Cistaceae, Bixaceae, Tamaricaceae, Caricaceae
An order of 20 families. It includes herbs, shrubs and trees; tropical and temperate. Cyanogenetic glycosides occur in some of the families (e.g. Flacourtiaceae, Turneraceae and Passifloraceae), but are absent from others (e.g. Violaceae).

1. Flacourtiaceae. A family of 93 genera and over 1000 species. Genera include *Erythrospermum* (6 spp.), *Hydnocarpus* (40 spp.), *Flacourtia* (15 spp.) and *Homalium* (200 spp.). The seed oils have been particularly studied, as species of *Hydnocarpus* contain cyclic, unsaturated acids which are bactericidal towards the micrococcus of leprosy. Other constituents of the family include cyanogenetic glycosides, tannins and phenolic acids. Alkaloids reported only in one genus, *Ryania*.
2. Violaceae. A family of 22 genera and about 900 species; cosmopolitan, herbs and shrubs. Genera include *Viola* (500 spp.), *Hybanthus* (150 spp.) and *Hymenanthera* (7 spp.). The pansy (*Viola tricolor*), sweet violet (*V. odorata*) and dog violet (*V. canina*) have been used medicinally. They contain volatile oil and anthocyanin, flavonoid (rutin) and carotenoid pigments. Cyclotoxic cyclotides (a family of small proteins) have been recorded in the aerial parts of a commercial sample of *V. tricolor* (E. Svängard *et al.*, *J. Nat. Prod.*, 2004, **67**, 114). *Hybanthus ipecacuanha* has occurred as an adulterant of genuine ipecacuanha.
3. Turneraceae. A family of seven genera and 120 species of trees, shrubs and herbs. *Turnera* has 61 species and *T. diffusa* is the source of damiana leaves.
4. Passifloraceae. A family of 12 genera and 600 species; tropical and warm temperate; shrubs and trees, often climbers. The main genera are *Passiflora* (500 spp.), *Adenia* (92 spp.) and *Tetrapathaea*, the latter a single species from New Zealand. Some of the fruits are edible (e.g. passion fruit, from *Passiflora edulis*). The dried aerial parts of *P. incarnata* are a popular herbal sedative; they contain flavonoids and traces of cyanogenetic glycosides, volatile oil and harmane-type alkaloids. Pharmacological tests have supported the traditional usage (R. Soulimani *et al.*, *J. Ethnopharmacology*, 1997, **57**, 11).
5. Cistaceae. A family of eight genera and 200 species. Members are herbs and shrubs, particularly found on chalk or sand. The genera include *Helianthemum* (100 spp.), *Cistus* (20 spp.) and *Halimium*. Species of *Cistus* yield the oleo-gum resin ladanum, used in perfumery and for embalming.
6. Bixaceae. This consists of the single genus *Bixa* with four species. *Bixa orellana* is cultivated for the colouring matter of its seeds. This, under the name of 'annatto', is used as an edible colourant, see Chapter 33.
7. Tamaricaceae. A family of four genera and 120 species; herbs and shrubs. *Tamarix* (54 spp.) includes *T. mannifera*, a plant which when punctured by scale insects yields the manna of the Bedouins.
8. Caricaceae. A family of four genera and 55 species; small trees mainly found in tropical America and Africa. *Carica* contains 45 species, and *Carica papaya* (papaw) is cultivated for the milky juice which is the source of the proteolytic enzyme papain.

CUCURBITALES

Cucurbitaceae
An order containing the single family Cucurbitaceae.

A family of about 110 genera and 640 species; abundant in the tropics; mostly herbs climbing by tendrils, with abundant sap and very rapid growth. Flowers are generally unisexual, regular and pentamerous, except in the gynaecium, which is reduced to three. The fruit is the fleshy type seen in the cucumber. Most members have bicollateral vascular bundles. Genera include *Cucurbita* (5 spp.), *Cucumis* (25 spp.), *Ecballium* (1 sp.), *Citrullus* (3 spp.), *Luffa* (6 spp.), *Bryonia* (4 spp.) and *Momordica* (45 spp.), *Cucurbita pepo* is vegetable marrow; *C. maxima*, great pumpkin; *Cucumis melo*, the melon; *C. sativus*, the cucumber; *Ecballium elaterium*, the squirting cucumber, yields the purgative elaterium; *Citrullus colocynthis* yields colocynth; *C. lanatus*, the water melon. The vascular network of the pericarp of *Luffa* is used as a bath sponge (loofah). The fruits and seeds of *L. acutangula* contain saponins and are used in Ayurvedic medicine. Bryony root, from *Bryonia dioica*, was formerly used as a purgative and for the treatment of gout; it contains saponins and sterols. *Bryonia alba* contains antitumour substances. The enzyme elaterase hydrolyses the bitter glucosides of the family to cucurbitacins and glucose. The cucurbitacins are triterpenoid bitter principles named A to Q, and the compound formerly known as α-elaterin is cucurbitacin-E. For their formation in tissue cultures of *Ecballium elatarium* see G. A. Attard and A. Scicluna-Spiteri, *Fitoterapia*, 2001, **72**, 146; G. Toker *et al.*, *Fitoterapia*, 2003, **74**, 618.

MYRTIFLORAE

Lythraceae, Myrtaceae, Punicaceae, Rhizophoraceae, Combretaceae, Onagraceae
An order of 17 families. Many members rich in tannins.

1. Lythraceae. A family of 25 genera and 550 species; herbs, shrubs and trees. Genera include *Rotala* (50 spp.), *Lythrum* (35 spp.), *Decodon* (1 sp.), *Lagerstroemia* (35 spp.), *Heimia* (3 spp.) and *Lawsonia* (1 sp.). The naphthoquinone lawsone occurs in henna, the leaves of *Lawsonia inermis*. Some species contain alkaloids.
2. Myrtaceae. A family of about 100 genera and 3000 species of evergreen shrubs and trees; well represented in Australia, the East Indies and tropical America. The family is divided into two subfamilies, the Myrtoideae (fruit a berry or drupe) and the Leptospermoideae (fruit a loculicidal capsule). Genera of the Myrtoideae include *Myrtus* (100 spp.), *Psidium* (140 spp.), *Pimenta* (18 spp.), *Eugenia* (1000 spp.), *Pseudocaryophyllus* and *Syzygium* (*Jambosa*). To the Leptospermoideae belong *Eucalyptus* (over 500 spp.), *Leptospermum*

(50 spp.) and *Melaleuca* (about 100 spp.). The large genus *Eucalyptus* has presented taxonomic problems and following a recent revision for *Flora of Australia* the nine, previously established, subgenera are each afforded generic status. Many of the genera provide important volatile oils and spices—for example, cloves and its oil (q.v.), eucalyptus oil, cajuput oil and pimento. *Psidium guajava* gives the edible fruit guava. Constituents of the family other than volatile oils are leucoanthocyanins, cyclitols, tannins (e.g. in eucalyptus kinos), phenolic acids and esters. Cyanogenetic glycosides and alkaloids are rare.

3. Punicaceae. The family contains the single genus *Punica* with two species. The fruit rind of *Punica granatum*, the pomegranate, contains tannin; in its stem and root bark tannin is accompanied by the liquid alkaloids pelletierine and isopelleterine. Pelletierine tannate was formerly official. Tannin-rich fractions have been investigated for their antioxidant, antimalarial and antimicrobial activities (M. K. Reddy *et al.*, *Planta Medica*, 2007, **73**, 461).

4. Rhizophoraceae. A family of 16 genera and 120 species; often trees of mangrove habit. *Rhizophora* (7 spp.) yields the tanning material mangrove cutch.

5. Combretaceae. A family of 20 genera and 600 species; tropical and subtropical trees and shrubs; usually rich in tannin. Genera include *Terminalia* (250 spp.), *Combretum* (250 spp.), *Quisqualis* (17 spp.) and *Anogeissus* (11 spp.). Myrobalans, the fruits of *Terminalia chebula*, are rich in tannin and are used both in tanning and in medicine. For an extensive microscopical examination of *T. australis*, used in traditional medicine in a number of S. American countries, see M. T. Castro *et al.*, *Pharm. Biol.*, 2005, **43**, 439; *Combretum butyrosum* yields a butter-like substance; and *Anogeissus latifolia* yields the gum known as ghatti gum.

6. Onagraceae. A family of 21 genera and 640 species; temperate and tropical; mostly perennial herbs, but a few shrubs and trees. Genera include *Fuchsia* (100 spp.), *Oenothera* (80 spp.), *Clarkia* (36 spp.) and *Epilobium* (215 spp.). Many are cultivated for their flowers. Seeds of *Oenothera* spp. have become important as sources of evening primrose oil (q.v.). Various species of *Epilobium* e.g. *E. angustifolium* and *E. hirsutum* are used traditionally for the treatment of benign prostate hyperplasia; the active components appear to be two macrocyclic ellagitannins oenothein A & B (B. Ducrey *et al.*, *Planta Medica*, 1997, **63**, 111). Tannins and a few cyanogenetic plants are recorded; alkaloids are rare or absent.

UMBELLIFLORAE

Alangiaceae, Cornaceae, Garryaceae, Araliaceae, Umbelliferae

An order of seven families. All, except the Umbelliferae and Araliaceae, are small. Acetylenic compounds occur throughout the order.

1. Alangiaceae. A family of 2 genera and 20 species, of which 17 belong to *Alangium*; tropical trees and shrubs. Alkaloids and triterpenoid saponins occur. *A. lamarkii* is an Indian medicinal plant.

2. Cornaceae. A family of 12 genera and 100 species; trees and shrubs, rarely herbs. Genera include *Cornus* (4 spp.) and *Acuba* (3 spp.).

3. Garryaceae. Contains only *Garrya*, with 18 species. Shrubs containing alkaloids.

4. Araliaceae. A family of 55 genera and 700 species; mainly tropical trees and shrubs, some climbing (e.g. ivy). Genera include *Panax* (8 spp.), *Tetrapanax* (1 sp.), *Aralia* (35 spp.), *Hedera* (15 spp.), *Cussonia* (25 spp.), *Pseudopanax* (6 spp.), *Fatsia* (1 sp.) and *Sciadodendron* (1 sp.). The best-known drug, which has been used for many centuries, is ginseng, from *Panax schinseng* (*P. ginseng*). *Tetrapanax*

papyriferum is the ricepaper tree, and *Hedera helix* the common ivy (q.v.). Resin passages occur in the family. Constituents include saponins, a few alkaloids, acetylenic compounds and diterpenoids and triterpenoids.

5. Umbelliferae. The family contains about 275 genera and 2850 species. Most members are herbs with furrowed stems and hollow internodes. Some are annuals (e.g. coriander), some biennials (e.g. hemlock) and some perennials (e.g. species of *Ferula*). The three subfamilies and main genera are as follows: (1) Hydrocotyloideae includes *Hydrocotyle* (100 species); (2) Saniculoideae includes *Eryngium* (230 spp.), *Astrantia* (10 spp.) and *Sanicula* (37 spp.); (3) Apioideae includes *Chaerophyllum* (40 spp.), *Coriandrum* (2 spp.), *Smyrnium* (8 spp.), *Conium* (4 spp.), *Bupleurum* (150 spp.), *Apium* (1 sp.), *Petroselinum* (5 spp.), *Carum* (30 spp.), *Pimpinella* (150 spp.), *Seseli* (80 spp.), *Foeniculum* (5 spp.), *Oenanthe* (40 spp.), *Ligusticum* (60 spp.), *Angelica* (80 spp.), *Ferula* (133 spp.), *Peucedanum* (120 spp.), *Pastinaca* (15 spp.), *Laserpitium* (35 spp.), *Thapsia* (6 spp.), *Daucus* (60 spp.), *Ammi* (10 spp.), *Heracleum* (70 spp.), *Prangos* (30 spp.) and *Anethum* (1 sp.). The leaves are usually large and have a sheathing base and much-divided lamina. The flowers are small and arranged in simple or compound umbels. Each has a five-lobed calyx, five petals, five stamens, and an inferior two-celled ovary. The fruit is a cremocarp, which is frequently crowned with a stigma-bearing disc known as the stylopodium. When ripe, the two mericarps separate from one another but frequently remain attached to the simple or forked carpophore which lies between them. The line separating the two mericarps is known as the commissure. Each mericarp contains a single seed which consists of a large endosperm, which has a small embryo embedded in it near the apex. Five primary ridges containing fibrovascular bundles run from base to apex in the pericarp, and secondary ridges sometimes alternate with these. Between the ridges are schizogenous oleoresin canals known as vittae. Members of the family differ in the number and arrangement of the vittae in each mericarp, but six is common, four on the dorsal surface and two on the commissural. Similar ducts occur in the stem and roots and in species of *Ferula* yield the oleo-gum resins and asafoetida, ammoniacum and galbanum.

The main umbelliferous fruits and their volatile oils used in pharmacy are fennel, *Foeniculum vulgare*; caraway, *Carum carvi*; dill, *Anethum graveolens*; coriander, *Coriandrum sativum*; aniseed, *Pimpinella anisum*; and cumin, *Cumminum cyminum*. *Bupleurum falcatum* roots contain oleanene saponins and are an important antihepatotoxic drug in oriental medicine. Visnaga, from *Ammi visnaga*, yields khellin, a dimethoxyfuranochromone. Among poisonous plants of the family may be mentioned *Conium maculatum*, the spotted hemlock, which contains the alkaloid coniine; and *Oenanthe crocata*, the hemlock waterdropwort, which contains oenanthotoxin. Other well-known plants of the family are celery, *Apium graveolens*; parsley, *Petroselinum crispum*; parsnip, *Pastinaca sativa*; and carrot, *Daucus carota*. Constituents of the family, other than volatile oils and resins, include coumarins (e.g. umbelliferone), furocoumarins, chromono-coumarins, terpenes and sesquiterpenes, triterpenoid saponins and acetylenic compounds. Alkaloids occur (e.g. coniine) but are rare.

SUBCLASS SYMPETALAE

The Sympetalae derive their name from the fact that their petals are fused. The subclass consists of 11 orders and 63 families, the chief of which have already been tabulated.

ERICALES

Ericaceae

An order of five families, including the Pyrolaceae, Epacridaceae and Ericaceae. Only the last family, the largest, will be described.

Ericaceae. A family of about 80 genera and 2000 species; particularly common on moors and peaty soils. Members are shrubs or small trees. The genera include *Rhododendron* (500–600 spp.), *Ledum* (10 spp.), *Erica* (over 500 spp.), *Calluna* (1 sp.), *Vaccinium* (300–400 spp.), *Gaylussacia* (49 spp.), *Gaultheria* (about 210 spp.), *Pieris* (10 spp.), *Lyonia* (30 spp.), *Arbutus* (20 spp.) and *Arctostaphylos* (71 spp.). In addition to the well-known garden plants, the family includes the wintergreen, *Gaultheria procumbens*, which yields natural oil of wintergreen (now generally replaced by synthetic methyl salicylate); and bearberry leaves from *Arctostaphylos uva-ursi*, which contain the phenolic glycoside arbutin and are again official. The medicinal properties of *Vaccinium myrtillus* (bilberry, blueberry, whortleberry) have been utilized since the Middle Ages and have been reviewed (P. Morazzoni and E. Bombardelli, *Fitoterapia*, 1996, **67**, 3); the fruits are included in the *BP/EP*. The family produces phenolic acids, phenolic glycosides (e.g. arbutin), aucubin glycosides, diterpenoids (grayanotoxin), triterpenoids (ursolic acid), cyclitols and leucoanthocyanins. A few species are cyanogenetic; saponins are absent.

PRIMULALES

Myrsinaceae, Primulaceae

An order of three families.

The Primulaceae consists of 20 genera and about 1000 species of herbaceous perennials with rhizomes or tubers. Especially common in the north temperate regions. Many members are cultivated as garden plants. Genera include *Primula* (500 spp.), *Cyclamen* (15 spp.), *Anagallis* (31 spp.) and *Dionysia* (41 spp.). The dried flowers of *Primula veris* (the cowslip) are used in herbal medicine for insomnia and as a sedative in combination with other herbs. The flowers are particularly rich in flavonoids. Saponins are present in some species; also phenolic esters and ethers. Alkaloids appear to be absent. Anthocyanin pigments are common, but not betacyanins or betaxanthins.

PLUMBAGINALES

Plumbaginaceae

The Plumbaginaceae is the only family of the order, and contains 19 genera and about 775 species. Members are herbs or shrubs often found on sea coasts or salt steppes. Genera include *Plumbago* (12 spp.) and *Ceratostigma*. Roots of *Plumbago* spp. are used in traditional Indian medicine; immunosuppressive and antitumour activities have been demonstrated. Constituents found in the family include phenolic acids, tannins, anthocyanin pigments and naphthoquinones (e.g. plumbagin).

EBENALES

Sapotaceae, Ebenaceae, Styracaceae

An order of seven families consisting mainly of trees and shrubs.

1. Sapotaceae. A family of some 35–75 ill-defined genera and about 800 species; most are tropical trees, often yielding good timber. Genera include *Mimusops* (57 spp.), *Madhuca* (*Bassia*) (85 spp.), *Achras* (70 spp.), *Pierreodendron* (2 spp.), *Palaquium* (about 115 spp.) and *Butyrospermum* (1 sp.). Latex sacs occur in the leaves, and in the cortex, phloem and pith of the stems. Gutta-percha is the coagulated latex from species of *Palaquium* and *Payena*. The oily seeds of *Butyrospermum parkii* are expressed to yield shea butter which can be used as an ointment and cream base for topical applications. Constituents of the family include latex, seed fats, cyanogenetic glycosides, saponins, tannins, leucoanthocyanins, pyrrolizidine alkaloids and the cyclitol D-quercitol.

2. Ebenaceae. A family of three genera and about 500 species; tropical trees and shrubs. The chief genera are *Diospyros* (about 500 spp.) and *Euclea* (20 spp.). Varieties of ebony are obtained from *Diospyros ebenum* and *Euclea pseudebenus*. In South-East Asia the fresh unripe fruits of *D. mollis* have long been used as an anthelmintic (hookworms and tapeworms). Other species yield edible fruits, 'date-plums'. For phytochemical research on the root- and stem-barks of *Diospyros* spp. involving the isolation of triterpenoids, diquinones and napthoquinones see M. R. Khan and D. Timi, *Fitoterapia*, 1999, **70**, 194; 209. Further details are given in Chapter 21 (naphthoquinones). Naphthoquinones are a characteristic of the family.

3. Styracaceae. A family of 12 genera and 180 species of trees and shrubs. Genera include *Styrax* (130 spp.) and *Halensia*. Benzoins (q.v.) are obtained from species of *Styrax*. Constituents of the family include balsamic resins, phenolic acids, tannins and the benzofuran egonol.

OLEALES

Oleaceae

The Oleaceae is the only family of the order. It is widely distributed, and contains 29 genera and about 600 species. Genera include *Olea* (20 spp.), *Forsythia* (7 spp.), *Fraxinus* (70 spp.), *Syringa* (30 spp.), *Osmanthus* (15 spp.), *Jasminum* (300 spp.) and *Ligustrum* (40–50 spp.). Many species are grown in Britain (e.g. *Syringa vulgaris*, the lilac). The manna of present-day commerce is obtained by making incisions in the stem of the manna ash, *Fraxinus ornus*. *F. oxyphylla* and *F. excelsior* afford Ash Leaf *BP/EP*. Of great economic importance is the olive, *Olea europoea*. In addition to olive oil (q.v.), the family produces sugar alcohols (e.g. the mannitol of manna), saponins, tannins, coumarins and iridoid glycosides. Alkaloids are rare.

GENTIANALES

Loganiaceae, Gentianaceae, Menyanthaceae, Apocynaceae, Asclepiadaceae, Rubiaceae

An order of seven families which is of medical and chemical interest. All the families contain alkaloids, but important glycoside-containing genera also occur.

1. Loganiaceae. A family of 18 genera and 500 species; trees, shrubs and herbs, some lianes. Genera include *Strychnos* (200 spp.), *Logania* (25 spp.), *Gelsemium* (2 spp.), *Geniostoma* (60 spp.), *Anthocleista* (14 spp.) and *Gardneria* (5 spp.). Nux vomica seeds (q.v.), the seeds of *Strychnos nux-vomica*, are the principal source of strychnine and brucine; calabash-curare (see 'Curare') owes its activity largely to *Strychnos* species. The family is rich in alkaloids of the indole and oxindole groups. Other constitutents are the aucubin glycoside loganin, and iridoids.

2. Gentianaceae. A family of 80 genera and about 1000 species; herbs and a few shrubs widely distributed. The leaves are opposite and decussate, the corolla lobes are contorted in the bud and the axis shows bicollateral bundles and interxylary phloem. Genera include *Gentiana* (400 spp.), *Exacum* (40 spp.), *Sebaca* (100 spp.), *Erythraea* (*Centaurium*) (30 spp.), *Chironia* (30 spp.), *Swertia* (100 spp.), *Halenia* (about 100 spp.) and *Enicostema* (3 or 4 spp.). Gentian root

5

(see 'Gentian'), from *Gentiana lutea*, has long been used in medicine. The herb of *Swertia chirata* (Chiretta) is described in the *BHP* (1983); it is used to stimulate the appetite in anorexia. *S. japonica* is used in Japan as a stomachic; hairy root cultures produce xanthone derivatives, the secoiridoids amarogentin and amaroswerin, and phenylglucosides. Some members, on account of their bitter principles, are used in liqueurs. The family contains alkaloids; iridoid glycosides; flavones, xanthones and their glycosides; phenolic acids; tannins; and the trisaccharide gentianose.

3. Menyanthaceae. This small family of five genera and 33 species is sometimes included in the Gentianaceae. It consists of aquatic or marsh herbs such as the British plant *Menyanthes trifoliata*, the buckbean (Bogbean Leaf *BHP* 1996, *BP/EP*). Like the Gentianaceae, the family contains bitter principles but the leaves instead of being opposite and decussate are alternate.

4. Apocynaceae. A family of about 250 genera and 2000 species which is closely allied to the Asclepiadaceae. Many members are woody climbers found in the tropics and subtropics. The only British species are the periwinkles, *Vinca major* and *V. minor*. Types of fruit are a pair of follicles, a berry, capsules or two indehiscent mericarps. The plants contain latex in non-articulated, branched or unbranched laticifers. The vascular bundles are bicollateral. Important genera, arranged under two subfamilies, are as follows: A. Plumieroideae: *Arduina–Carissa* (35 spp.), *Allamanda* (15 spp.), *Landolphia* (55 spp.), *Carpodinus* (50 spp.), *Hancornia* (1 sp.), *Pleiocarpa* (3 spp.), *Plumeria* (7 spp.), *Alstonia* (50 spp.), *Aspidosperma* (80 spp.), *Rhazya* (2 spp.), *Amsonia* (25 spp.), *Lochnera–Catharanthus* (5 spp.), *Vinca* (5 spp.), *Tabernaemontana* (100 spp.), *Voacanga* (25 spp.), *Rauwolfia* (100 spp.), *Ochrosia* (30 spp.) and *Cerbera* (6 spp.); B. Apocynoideae: *Mandevilla* (114 spp.), *Funtumia* (3 spp.), *Apocyanum* (7 spp.), *Nerium* (3 spp.), *Strophanthus* (60 spp.), *Wrightia* (23 spp.), *Parsonia* (100 spp.), *Lyonsia* (24 spp.) and *Malouetia* (25 spp.). Drugs include the Madagascaran periwinkle, *Catharanthus roseus* (also known as *Lochnera rosea* and *Vinca rosea*); strophanthus seeds; rauwolfia roots; kurchi or holarrhena bark; alstonia barks; and aspidosperma barks. Many species of *Landolphia, Carpondinus* and *Hancornia* yield rubber latex. [For a review (148 refs) of *Rhazya stricta* and *R. orientalis*, used in Unani medicine, see Atta-Ur-Rahman *et al.*, *Fitoterapia*, 1989, **60**, 291. For uses, chemistry and pharmacology of *Malouetia* spp. (41 refs) see N. G. Bisset, *J. Ethnopharm.*, 1992, **36**, 43.]
Constituents of the Plumieroideae include a vast range of indoline alkaloids; over 500 in *Alstonia, Aspidospermum, Catharanthus, Hunteria, Pleiocarpa, Tabernaemontana, Rauwolfia* and *Voacanga*. Steroidal alkaloids occur in *Holarrhena* and harman-type alkaloids in *Amsonia* and *Aspidosperma*. Cardioactive glycosides occur in *Acokanthera, Carissa* and *Melodinus* and in *Apocyanum, Nerium* and *Strophanthus*. Other constituents of the family are cyanogenetic glycosides, leucoanthocyanins, saponins, tannins, coumarins, phenolic acids, cyclitols and triterpenoids. Widely grown ornamental plants of the family include species of *Amsonia, Nerium* (oleander), *Vinca, Plumeria* (frangipani), *Thevetia* (yellow oleander) and *Mandevilla* (Chilean jasmine).

5. Asclepiadaceae. A family of 130 genera and 2000 species; tropical and subtropical shrubs, often twining, or perennial herbs. Genera include *Asclepias* (120 spp.), *Tylophora* (150 spp.), *Xysmalobium* (1 sp.), *Cryptostegia* (2 spp.), *Hoodia* (10 spp.), *Cynanchum, Marsdenia, Pergularia* and *Hemidesmus*. The latex cells usually contain a latex rich in triterpenes. Other constituents include: alkaloids of the indole, phenanthroindolizidine and pyridine groups; cardenolides; cyanogenetic glycosides; saponins, tannins, and cyclitols. Although the family yields no important drugs, Pleurisy Root,

Asclepius tuberosa, was official in the *BHP* 1983) many members are used in folk medicine in their countries of origin and others as arrow poisons. Among the better-known are Indian sarsaparilla, from *Hemidesmus indicus*, and condurango bark, from *Marsdenia condurango*. *Cryptostegia grandiflora*, the rubber vine or pink allamanda, contains poisonous cardenolides with some therapeutic potential; the plant, introduced to Australia as an ornamental, has become an aggressive weed. *Hoodia gordonii*, a succulent plant of the Kalahari desert, has been traditionally used by the San Bushmen as an appetite suppressant. In the West it has achieved popularity for the treatment of obesity, but it is now in danger of over-collection.

6. Rubiaceae. A family of about 500 genera and 6000 species, most of which are tropical trees and shrubs. A few members are herbs growing in temperate climates (e.g. species of *Galium*, such as the bedstraws, goosegrass or cleavers of Britain). The first subfamily is the Cinchonoideae, the carpels of which bear numerous ovules and which includes *Oldenlandia* (300 spp.), *Condaminea* (3 spp.), *Cinchona* (40 spp.), *Uncaria* (60 spp.), *Nauclea* (35 spp.), *Gardenia* (250 spp.) and *Mitragyna* (12 spp.). The second subfamily, Rubioideae, has only one ovule in each loculus; it includes the genera *Coffea* (40 spp.), *Ixora* (400 spp.), *Pavetta* (400 spp.), *Psychotria* (700 spp.), *Cephaëlis-Uragoga* (180 spp.), *Mitchella* (2 spp.), *Asperula* (200 spp.), *Galium* (400 spp.) and *Rubia* (60 spp.). Products include cinchona barks and their alkaloids such as quinine (q.v.), ipecacuanha root (see 'Ipecacuanha'), catechu, from *Uncaria gambier*, and coffee (q.v.), from *Coffea arabica* and other species. *Psychotria viridis* is a component of the hallucinogenic preparation ayahuasca (q.v); other species such as *P. brachypoda* and *P. colorata* are constituents of traditional painkillers (M. B. Leal and E. Elisabetsky, *Int. J. Pharmacognosy*, 1996, **34**, 267). It is of interest that, with *Psychotria*, analgesic activity is found in alkaloids with diverse structures as exemplified by the study of F. L. Both *et al.* on the alkaloid umbellatine from *P. umbellata* (*Pharm. Biol.*, 2002, **40**, 366). Of the many other alkaloid-containing species may be mentioned mitragyna leaves, from species of *Mitragyna*, and yohimbe bark, from *Pansinystalia yohimbe*. In the family, alkaloids of the indole, oxindole, quinoline and purine types are common; anthraquinones occur in *Morinda, Rubia* and *Galium*, and many have long been used as dyes (e.g. madder, from *Rubia tinctorum*). Anthocyanins occur in *Cinchona*; aucubin glycosides (e.g. asperulin), cyclitols (e.g. quinic acid), coumarins, depsides in *Coffea*; phlobatannins, catechins (e.g. in *Uncaria*); diterpenoids and triterpenoids and iridoid glycosides in *Genipa*. *Morinda reticulata* is interesting, as it accumulates selenium and is very toxic; *M. citrifolia*, *M. elliptica* and *M. lucida* are all employed in traditional medicine, some anthraquinones (e.g. alizarin-1-methyl-ether) have been shown to possess antifungal properties. For iridoids and anthraquinones of *M. citrifolia* fruits, see K. Kamiya *et al.*, *Chem. Pharm. Bull.*, 2005, **53**, 1597; the phytochemistry, pharmacology and safety of the fruits have been reviewed (O. Potterat and M. Hamburger, *Planta Medica*, 2007, **73**, 191).

TUBIFLORAE

Polemoniaceae, Convolvulaceae, Boraginaceae, Verbenaceae, Labiatae, Solanaceae, Scrophulariaceae, Bignoniaceae, Acanthaceae, Pedaliaceae, Gesneriaceae, Myoporaceae

An order of six suborders and 26 families containing many important drugs. The families considered below fall into the following suborders:

1. Convolvulineae: Polemoniaceae and Convolvulaceae.
2. Boraginineae: Boraginaceae.
3. Verbenineae: Verbenaceae and Labiatae.
4. Solanineae: Solanaceae, Scrophulariaceae, Bignoniaceae, Acanthaceae, Pedaliaceae and Gesneriaceae.
5. Myopineae: Myoporaceae.

Members of these families are usually herbs with alternate or opposite simple leaves. The flowers are generally bisexual and often zygomorphic. They usually have two or four epipetalous stamens and a bicarpellary superior ovary.

1. Polemoniaceae. A family of 15 genera and 300 species; herbs which are often cultivated as border plants. Genera include *Phlox* (67 spp.) and *Polemonium* (50 spp.). The chemistry of the family is imperfectly known, but constituents include saponins and tannins.

2. Convolvulaceae. A family of about 55 genera and 1650 species. Most are annual or perennial herbs, often with twining stems; a few shrubs and trees. Genera include *Convolvulus* (250 spp.), *Ipomoea* (500 spp.), *Pharbitis–Ipomoea*, *Argyreia* (91 spp.) and *Cuscuta* (170 spp.). The genus *Cuscuta* consists of parasites which are sometimes placed in a separate family, the Cuscutaceae. Species of dodder are parasitic on clover and on flax. *C. reflexa* found in the Indian subcontinent is used in a number of folk remedies; an alcoholic extract of the plant has hypotensive and bradycardiac effects.
Anatomical characters include the presence of latex cells, bicollateral bundles and frequently abnormal vascular development such as is found in drugs such as ipomoea and jalap (q.v.). Brazilian arrowroot is the starch obtained from the tubers of the sweet potato, *Ipomoea batatas*. Many species contain hallucinogens (q.v.) such as ololiuqui, from *Rivea corymbosa*, and morning glory seeds, from species of *Ipomoea*. The family contains indole, isoquinoline, pyrrolidine and tropane alkaloids, purgative resins, phenolic acids and triterpenoid saponins. Pyrrolizidine alkaloids have been reported in the family (seeds of *I. hederifolia*).

3. Boraginaceae. A family of about 100 genera and 2000 species; mostly herbs, often perennial. Inflorescence a coiled cincinnus. The flowers change colour during development. Genera include *Heliotropium* (250 spp.), *Cynoglossum* (50–60 spp.), *Symphytum* (25 spp.), *Borago* (3 spp.), *Anchusa* (50 spp.), *Alkanna* (25–30 spp.), *Pulmonaria* (10 spp.) and *Lithospermum* (60 spp.). Products include species of *Lithospermum*, which have hormone activity; alkanna or anchusa root, from *Alkanna tinctoria*, which contains red colouring matters. Both the *Lithospermum* species and *Alkanna* contain naphthoquinone derivatives. Formerly official were *Cynoglossum officinale* (hound's tongue), *Borago officinale* (borage) and *Pulmonaria officinalis* (lung-wort). The seed oil of borage is particularly rich in γ-linolenic acid (q.v.) and the plant is now being cultivated in England for its oil. Naphthoquinones, the ureide allantoin, pyrrolizidine alkaloids, cyclitols, phenolic acids and tannins, occur in the family. Allantoin is particularly abundant in the root of comfrey, *Symphytum officinale*. The common occurrence of pyrrolizidine alkaloids (*Alkana*, *Borago*, *Cynoglossum*, *Heliotropium*, *Symphytum*) has caused concern regarding the herbal use of a number of species.

4. Verbenaceae. A family of about 100 genera and 3000 species; herbs, shrubs and trees, many lianes. Genera include *Tectona* (3 spp.), *Lippia* (220 spp.), *Verbena* (250 spp.), *Callicarpa* (140 spp.), *Vitex* (250 spp.), *Nyctanthes*, *Duranta* and *Stilbe*. Teak is obtained from *Tectona grandis*; verbena oil from *Lippia citriodora*; and vervain, formerly official, from *Verbena officinalis*. *Vitex agnus-castus*, now included in the *BP/EP* 2007, has been used medicinally in Europe at least since classical Greek and Roman times and today is still available as a herbal preparation for the treatment of female conditions relating to the premenstrual syndrome and the menopause. (For a report of research see *Pharm. J.*, 2001, **265**, 106.) Among the constituents found in the family are volatile oils, saponins, tannins, quinones, iridoids, piscicidal substances; alkaloids appear to be rare.

5. Labiatae (Lamiaceae). A family of about 200 genera and 3300 species; aromatic, annual or perennial herbs or undershrubs. The family is well represented in the Mediterranean area and in Britain. The flowers are bisexual, zygomorphic, usually have the floral formula K(5), C(5), A4, G(2), and are arranged in verticillasters. The corolla is bilabiate and the stamens didynamous. With the exception of *Rosmarinus*, the genera have a gynobasic style and the four nutlets have only a small surface of contact with one another. Rosemary also differs from most genera in having only two stamens. The herbaceous members of the family have square stems. The leaves and other aerial parts have clothing hairs (see Fig. 42.4) and glandular hairs (Fig. 43.5), which secrete the volatile oil. The genera include *Ajuga* (40 spp.), *Teucrium* (300 spp.), *Rosmarinus* (3 spp.), *Scutellaria* (300 spp.), *Lavandula* (28 spp.), *Marrubium* (40 spp.), *Nepeta* (250 spp.), *Lamium* (40–50 spp.), *Ballota* (35 spp.), *Stachys* (300 spp.), *Salvia* (700 spp.), *Monarda* (12 spp.), *Satureja* (30 spp.), *Origanum* (15–20 spp.), *Thymus* (300–400 spp.), *Mentha* (18 spp. and 13 hybrid spp.), *Pogostemon* (40 spp.), *Ocimum* (150 spp.), *Leonurus* (14 spp.) and *Leonotis* (41 spp.). Many members of the family are used as culinary or medicinal herbs, as sources of volatile oils and in some cases for the preparation of constituents of the volatile oils such as menthol and thymol; chemical races are common. In addition to those drugs described elsewhere, note pennyroyal (*Mentha pulegium*), patchouli (*Pogostemon patchouli*), germander (*Teucrium chamaedrys*), wood sage (*T. scorodonia*), wood betony (*Stachys officinalis*), sweet basil (*Ocimum basilicum*), holy basil (*O. sanctum*), savory (*Satureja* spp.), and hyssop (*Hyssopus officinalis*). Also, thyme (*Thymus vulgaris*) and *Monarda punctata* are both important sources of thymol. Patchouli oil obtained from *Pogostemon cablin* (*P. patchouli*) is used medicinally in China, and also cultivated in India. Of the 41 constituents of the volatile oil, α-guaiene (*ca.* 21%) and α-bulnescene (*ca.* 16%) have been reported as the principal components, with α-bulnescene being active against PAF-induced platelet aggregation (Y.-C. Tsai *et al.*, *Fitoterapia*, 2007, **78**, 7).

α-Bulnescene

In addition to the volatile oils, constituents of the family include diterpenoids and triterpenoids, saponins, a few pyridine and pyrrolidine alkaloids, insect-moulting hormones, polyphenols and tannins, iridoids and their glycosides, quinones, furanoids, cyclitols, coumarin, and the sugars raffinose and stachyose.

6. Solanaceae. A family of about 90 genera and over 2000 species; tropical and temperate; herbs, shrubs or small trees. Genera include *Nicandra* (1 sp.), *Lycium* (80–90 spp.), *Atropa* (4 spp.), *Hyoscyamus* (20 spp.), *Physalis* (100 spp.), *Capsicum* (about 50 spp.), *Solanum* including *Lycopersicon* (1700 spp.), *Mandragora* (6 spp.), *Datura* (10 spp.), *Solandra* (10 spp.), *Cestrum* (150 spp.), *Nicotiana* (66 spp.), *Petunia* (40 spp.), *Salpiglossis* (18 spp.), *Schizanthus* (15 spp.), *Scopolia* (6 spp.), *Withania* (10 spp.), *Duboisia* (2 spp.), *Acnistus* (50 spp.) and *Fabiana* (25 spp.). Only five species are indigenous to Britain but many others are cultivated. The indigenous ones are *Datura stramonium*, thornapple; *Solanum dulcamara*,

5

bittersweet or woody nightshade; *Solanum nigrum*, black nightshade; *Atropa belladonna*, deadly nightshade; *Hyoscyamus niger*, henbane. Among species commonly cultivated in England are *Solanum tuberosum*, potato; *Solanum lycopersicum*, tomato; *Nicotiana tabacum*, tobacco; *Physalis alkekengi*, Chinese lantern; *Capsicum* spp., red and green peppers; *Solanum pseudocapsicum*, winter cherry; *Lycium halimifolium*, Duke of Argyll's Tea-plant; *L. barbarum*, wolfberry, and related spp. are traditional drugs of Chinese medicine for the treatment of age-related conditions (N. L. Etkin, Symposium Report, *Pharm. Biol.*, 2002, **40**, 80).

The flowers are bisexual and seldom markedly zygomorphic, although the carpels are placed obliquely. They have the floral formula K(5), C(5), A5, G(2). The ovary is typically bilocular, but frequently becomes falsely three- to five-locular (e.g. *Datura*). On the flowering branches adnation of the leaves with their axillary branches often occurs and the true origin of the parts is only made out by cutting sections. All members of the family have intraxylary phloem which is often accompanied by sclerenchymatous fibres. Products of the Solanaceae include: stramonium leaves; henbane leaves; belladonna herb and root; capsicums; potato starch from *Solanum tuberosum*; mandrake, from *Mandragora officinarum*; duboisia, from species of *Duboisia* which are used for the manufacture of tropane alkaloids; scopolia leaves and roots, sources of tropane alkaloids; tobacco from *Nicotiana tabacum*, the waste products of which are used for the extraction of the insecticide nicotine. The family contains a wide range of alkaloids which are of great taxonomic interest. Types of alkaloid recorded are tropane, alkaloidal amine, indole, isoquinoline, purine, pyrazole, pyridine, pyrrolidine, quinazolidine, steroid alkaloids and glycoalkaloids. Other constituents include steroidal saponins, withanolides, coumarins, cyclitols, pungent principles (e.g. in *Capsicum*), flavones, carotenoids and anthraquinones in *Fabiana*.

7. Buddlejaceae. A family of 6–10 genera are 150 spp.; principal genera are *Buddleja* (100 spp.) and *Nuxia* (40 spp.). Although *Buddleja* spp. have been used in traditional medicine in many parts of the world it was only relatively recently (e.g. P. J. Houghton, *J. Nat. Prod.*, 1985, **48**, 1005) that detailed phytochemical investigations were initiated. The genus produces flavonoids, iridoids and acylated iridoid glycosides, sesquiterpenoids, phenylethanoids, lignans and saponins (saikosaponins). Until the isolation of saikosaponins by Yamamoto *et al.* (*Chem. Pharm. Bull.*, 1991, **39**, 2764) these compounds were known only in *Bupleurum* spp. (Umbelliferae). Apparently, the eating habits of some insects indicate a similarity between *Buddleja* and the Scrophulariaceae.

8. Scrophulariaceae. A family of 220 genera and about 3000 species; annual or perennial herbs or undershrubs, a few trees; some semiparasites. Members differ from the Solanaceae in that they have carpels placed in an anterior–posterior plane, in the aestivation of the corolla and in not possessing bicollateral bundles. The flowers are usually zygomorphic and the stamens reduced to four. Anatomical characters include glandular hairs in which the head is divided by vertical walls only, and the stomata, which are surrounded by three or more epidermal cells. Calcium oxalate is relatively rare; when present, it occurs in small solitary crystals. Genera are *Verbascum* (306 spp.), *Calceolaria* (300–400 spp.), *Linaria* (150 spp.), *Antirrhinum* (42 spp.), *Scrophularia* (about 300 spp.), *Penstemon* (250 spp.), *Mimulus* (100 spp.), *Gratiola* (20 spp.), *Veronica* (300 spp.), *Digitalis* (20–30 spp.), *Isoplexis* (4 spp.), *Melampyrum* (35 spp.), *Euphrasia* (200 spp.), *Bartsia* (30 spp.), *Pedicularis* (500 spp.), *Rhinanthus* (50 spp.), *Odontitis* (30 spp.), *Chaenorrhinum* (20 spp.), *Bacopa* (100 spp.) and *Gratiola* (20 spp.). Important drugs are the leaves of *Digitalis*

purpurea and *D. lanata* and their cardiac glycosides. Picrorhiza rhizome or 'Indian gentian' from *Picrorhiza kurroa* contains bitter iridoid glycosides; it is used in India to treat liver ailments. *Verbascum thapsus* (mullein) (q.v.) commonly cited as an adulterant of digitalis, is used as a herbal medicine in Europe and India, particularly for bronchial conditions. The four species of *Isoplexis*, formerly placed in the genus *Digitalis*, are found only in the Canary Islands and Madeira. Cardenolides which are mono- and diglucosides only (cf. *Digitalis*), occur in both genera; the clonal propagation of *I. canariensis* has been described (F. Schaller and W. Kreis, *Planta Medica*, 1996, **62**, 450). Other constituents of the family include: steroidal and triterpenoid saponins; cyanogenetic glycosides in *Linaria* spp.; aucubin glycosides; naphthoquinones and anthraquinones; aurones; iridoids. Alkaloids are not very common, but monoterpenoid, quinazoline and quinolizidine types occur in some species.

9. Bignoniaceae. A family of about 120 genera and 650 species; mainly tropical trees, shrubs or lianes; particularly abundant in Brazil. Genera include *Jacaranda* (50 spp.), *Catalpa* (11 spp.), *Mussatia* (3 spp.), *Kigelia* (1 sp.) and *Tecomella* (1 sp.). *Kigelia pinnata* bark is used in traditional Nigerian medicine; it contains naphthoquinoids and iridoids and has been investigated for antibacterial activity by P. Houghton at King's College, London (*Pharm. J.*, 1993, **250**, 848). *K. africana*, the sausage tree, occurs across sub-Saharan Africa. Most parts of the tree are used indigenously and commercial fruit extract is used in skin-care products. Hippos distribute the seeds. In South America the leaves of *Mussatia hyacinthina* and other species are chewed alone or mixed with coca leaves for their sweetening, euphoric or medicinal effects. The above genera have received considerable phytochemical attention and constituents of the family include iridoids and iridoid glycosides, saponins, phenylpropanoids, tannins and quinones; alkaloids are rare.

10. Acanthaceae. A family of 250 genera and 2500 species. Shrubs and herbs, including some climbing plants and xerophytes. Abundant in the tropics but also found in the Mediterranean, Australia and the USA. Genera include *Acanthus* (50 spp.), *Andrographis* (20 spp.), *Blepharis* (100 spp.), *Adhatoda* (20 spp.) and *Barleria* (230 spp.). The leaves of *Adhatoda vasica* are used in India as a uterotonic and for the treatment of cough and allergies; they contain the alkaloid vascine (peganine); the antitussive activity has been demonstrated pharmacologically (J. N. Dhuley, *J. Ethnopharmacology*, 1999, **67**, 361), so too the hepatoprotective property in rats (D. Bhattacharyya *et al.*, *Fitoterapia*, 2005, **76**, 223). *Andrographis paniculata* (q.v.) is also an important Indian drug plant. In addition to alkaloids, the family contains tannins, diterpenoids, cyanogenetic compounds and saponins.

11. Pedaliaceae. A small family of 12 genera and 50 species; tropical herbs, or rarely shrubs; mostly shore or desert plants. The genera include *Harpagophytum* (8 spp.), *Pedalium* (1 sp.) and *Sesamum* (30 spp.). *Sesamum indicum* yields the fixed oil sesame or gingili oil. *Harpagophytum procumbens* (Devil's Claw) is found especially in the Kalahari desert and Namibian steppes. Its secondary tuberized roots are much used in traditional medicine and it is now included in western medicine (q.v.). Other constituents of the family include phenolics and flavonoids.

12. Gesneriaceae. A family of 120 genera and 2000 species; mainly tropical and subtropical herbs. The genus *Streptocarpus* has 132 species. Tannins, naphthoquinones, chalcones and anthraquinones but no alkaloids have been reported.

13. Myoporaceae. A family of three genera and some 240 species. The genus *Eremkophila* (209 spp.) is entirely Australian and has been used in aboriginal medicine. *Myoporum* (*c.* 30 spp.) occurs in the

S.W. Pacific area and the monotypic *Bontia* is found only in the West Indies. The family contains a striking range of terpenoids and also tannins, cyanogenetic glycosides and furans. (For a review (150 refs) see E. L. Ghisalberti, *Phytochemistry*, 1994, **35**, 7).

PLANTAGINALES

Plantaginaceae

An order containing the single family Plantaginaceae, which consists of three genera and about 270 species; annual or perennial herbs. All but four species belong to the genus *Plantago* (plantains). The seeds of several species are used in medicine; see 'Psyllium'.

DIPSACALES

Caprifoliaceae, Valerianaceae, Dipsacaceae

An order of four families; includes herbs, shrubs and small trees.

1. Caprifoliaceae. A family of 12 genera and about 450 species; mainly north temperate, herbs and small trees. Important genera are *Viburnum* (200 spp.), *Lonicera* (200 spp.) and *Sambucus* (40 spp.). British members include the common elder, *Sambucus nigra*; honeysuckles, species of *Lonicera*; the guelder-rose, *Viburnum opulus*. Elder flowers, usually in the form of an ointment, are used as a domestic remedy and are included in the *BP/EP*. The root bark of black haw, *Viburnum prunifolium*, is official in the *BHP* (1996). Constituents reported in the family are valerianic acid (compare Valerianaceae), aucubin glycosides, saponins, coumarins and cyanogenetic glycosides.
2. Valerianaceae. A family of 13 genera and about 360 species. Herbs, rarely shrubs. Genera include *Valeriana* (over 200 spp.), *Valerianella* (80 spp.), *Centranthus* (12 spp.) and *Patrina* (20 spp.). The first three of these genera are represented in Britain. The flowers of *Valeriana* and *Valerianella* have three stamens, those of *Centranthus* only one. *Centranthus ruber* is the common red valerian. The valerian roots of commerce are derived from the European *Valeriana officinalis* (q.v.) and the Indian valerian, *V. wallichii*. The family contains esters yielding isovalerianic acid (compare Caprifoliaceae), alkaloids and iridoids; valepotriates are characteristic of the tribe Valerianeae but are not found in the tribe Patrinieae.
3. Dipsacaceae. A family of eight genera and about 150 species. Genera include *Scabiosa* (100 spp.), *Knautia* (50 spp.) and *Dipsacus* (15 spp.). The ripe flower-heads of *Dipsacus fullorum* (fuller's teasel) are still used to a limited extent for raising nap on certain cloths. Constituents reported for the family include a *C*-glycoside, a few alkaloids, and tannins.

CAMPANULALES

Campanulaceae, Compositae

An order of eight families. In the families considered below, the anthers are either in contact with one another or fused so as to form a tube into which the pollen is shed. The flowers are hermaphrodite or unisexual by suppression. Mainly herbs with latex vessels or oil passages.

1. Campanulaceae. A family of about 70 genera and 2000 species. Tropical or subtropical herbs; a few trees or shrubs. The subfamily Campanuloideae contains *Campanula* (about 300 spp.) and has regular flowers, generally with free anthers. The subfamily Lobelioideae (which has sometimes been considered as a separate family, the Lobeliaceae) contains *Lobelia* (200–300 spp.). In this subfamily the flowers are zygomorphic and the anthers syngenesious. Family characters include the presence of latex vessels and inulin. Of medicinal importance is lobelia herb or Indian tobacco, *Lobelia inflata*, which contains alkaloids (q.v.). Indian lobelia, from *L. nicotianaefolia*, also contains lobeline. In addition to the constituents already mentioned, members of the family contain phenolic compounds, tannins and triterpenoid glycosides. The piperidine alkaloids found in the Lobelioideae have not been found in the other subfamilies, but they are not considered sufficiently significant to justify a separate family.

2. Compositae. The Compositae is the largest family of flowering plants and contains about 900 genera and some 13 000 species. Compared with some other large families such as the Leguminosae, the number of important economic products derived from it is relatively small. Chemical research in recent years has increased medical interest in the family and we now have a better knowledge of many almost-discarded folk remedies as well as hitherto uninvestigated plants. The latter include some having antitumour or antibacterial activity and others forming commercial sources of rubber latex. The two subfamilies and their main genera are as follows.

   (1) Tubuliflorae: In this subfamily latex vessels are absent, but schizogenous oil ducts are common. The corollas of the disc-florets are nonligulate. Genera include *Senecio* (1300 spp.), *Xanthium* (30 spp.), *Ambrosia* (30–40 spp.), *Zinnia* (20 spp.), *Helianthus* (110 spp.), *Dahlia* (27 spp.), *Helenium* (40 spp.), *Tagetes* (50 spp.), *Solidago* (100 spp.), *Bellis* (15 spp.), *Aster* (500 spp.), *Erigeron* (200 spp.), *Achillea* (200 spp.), *Anthemis* (200 spp.), *Chrysanthemum* (c. 200 spp.), *Matricaria* (40 spp.), *Tanacetum* (50–60 spp.), *Artemisia* (400 spp.), *Blumea* (50 spp.), *Inula* (200 spp.), *Doronicum* (35 spp.), *Calendula* (20–30 spp.), *Eupatorium* (1200 spp.), *Arnica* (32 spp.), *Vernonia* (600 spp.), *Echinops* (100 spp.), *Carlina* (20 spp.), *Arctium* (5 spp.), *Carduus* (100 spp.), *Centaurea* (600 spp.), *Carthamus* (13 spp.) and *Gerbera* (70 spp.). Omitting the huge number of cultivated garden plants, note chamomile or Roman chamomile flowers, from *Anthemis nobilis*; German chamomile, *Matricaria chamomilla*; insect flowers, *Chrysanthemum cinerariifolium*; wormseed or santonica, *Artemisia cina*; arnica flowers and rhizome, *Arnica montana*; calendula flowers, *Calendula officinalis*; yarrow herb, *Achillea millefolium*; grindelia herb, *Grindelia camporum*; blessed thistle leaves, *Cnicus benedictus*; coltsfoot leaves, *Tussilago farfara*; wormwood herb, *Artemisia absinthium*; pellitory or pyrethrum root, *Anacyclus pyrethrum*; elecampane root, *Inula helenium*; Ngai camphor, from *Blumea balsamifera*. The florets of the safflower, *Carthamus tinctorius*, are used as dye and as a substitute for saffron. Refined Sunflower Oil *EP/BP* is expressed from the seeds of *Helianthus annuus* and subsequently refined.

   (2) Liguliflorae: In this subfamily latex vessels are present but volatile oil is rare. All the flowers have ligulate corollas. Genera include *Cichorium* (9 spp.), *Crepis* (200 spp.), *Hieracium* (over 1000 spp.), *Taraxacum* (60 spp.), *Lactuca* (100 spp.), *Scorzonera* (150 spp.) and *Sonchus* (50 spp.). Vegetables obtained from this group include lettuce, scorzonera root, chicory and endive. Of members used medicinally may be noted dandelion root, *Taraxacum officinale*; lactucarium or lettuce-opium, *Lactuca virosa*; mouse-ear hawkweed, *Hieracium pilosella*—which has antibiotic activity and has been used for the treatment of Malta fever. Chicory root and dandelion root were used, particularly in war-time Europe, as adulterants of or substitutes for coffee.

As might be expected from its size, the Compositae contains a wide variety of chemical constituents and the literature is enormous. Already mentioned are the latex of the Liguliflorae and inulin which is

5

often present in very large amounts (e.g. in dahlia tubers). Some of the volatile oils found in the Tubuliflorae contain acetylenic compounds. Sesquiterpenes known as azulenes give the blue colour to freshly distilled oil of chamomile and yarrow. Many sesquiterpene lactones occur and are of varying types, including eudesmanolides (e.g. santonin), germacranolides, guaianolides and pseudoguaianolides; some of these have cytotoxic activity. The toxic *Senecio* alkaloids derived from pyrrolizidine have been much researched. Some cause liver damage and are therefore dangerous to livestock. Alkaloids of the pyridine, quinoline and diterpenoid types also occur in the family. Other constituents include the insecticidal esters of pyrethrum (q.v.) triterpenoid saponins of grindelia, cyclitols, coumarins and flavonols. *Stevia rebaudiana*, a herb indigenous to North Eastern Paraguay, is the source of stevioside, an ent-kaurene glycoside used as a sweetener for soft drinks, etc.

ANGIOSPERMS: MONOCOTYLEDONS

As the name indicates, monocotyledons have an embryo with one cotyledon. Many members are herbs, usually with parallel-veined leaves. The stele has scattered, closed vascular bundles; the flowers are usually trimerous.

As with the dicotyledons a much abbreviated form of Engler's classification indicating the main orders and families of pharmaceutical and phytochemical interest is given below.

Orders	Families
Liliiflorae	Liliaceae, Agavaceae, Amaryllidaceae, Hypoxidaceae, Dioscoreaceae, Iridaceae
Bromeliales	Bromeliaceae
Graminales	Gramineae
Principes	Palmae
Spathiflorae	Araceae, Lemnaceae
Cyperales	Cyperaceae
Scitamineae	Musaceae, Zingiberaceae, Cannaceae, Marantaceae
Microspermae	Orchidaceae

LILIIFLORAE

Liliaceae, Agavaceae, Hypoxidaceae, Amaryllidaceae, Dioscoreaceae, Iridaceae

The order is divided into five suborders and 17 families. Some botanists favour further subdivision—for example, the separation from the Liliaceae of *Smilax* and *Ruscus* into separate families, the Smilaceae and Ruscaceae respectively.

Many members of the group are perennial herbs having a bulb, corm or rhizome. The flowers are hermaphrodite, regular or zygomorphic, and typically have the floral formula P 3 + 3, A 3 + 3 or 3 + 0, G(3). The perianth is usually petaloid; the ovary superior (e.g. Liliaceae) or inferior (e.g. Iridaceae). Fruit a capsule or berry.

1. Liliaceae. A widely distributed family of about 250 genera and 3700 species; mostly perennial herbs with a rhizome or bulb. The flowers usually have six stamens and a superior (rarely semi-inferior) ovary, with numerous anatropous ovules attached to axile placentas. The fruit is a loculicidal or septicidal capsule, or a berry.
   Without troubling the reader with the names of subfamilies or tribes, the numbers inserted below will indicate the principal genera within each: 1. *Veratrum* (25 spp.), *Gloriosa* (5 spp.) and

Colchicum (65 spp.); 2. *Herreria* (8 spp.); 3. *Asphodelus* (12 spp.), *Bowiea* (2 spp.), *Funkia–Hosta* (10 spp.), *Kniphofia* (75 spp.) and *Aloe* (about 330 spp.); 4. *Gagea* (70 spp.), *Allium* (450 spp.); 5. *Lilium* (80 spp.), Fritillaria (85 spp.), *Tulipa* (100 spp.); 6. *Scilla* (80 spp.), *Urginea* (100 spp.), *Ornithogalum* (150 spp.), *Hyacinthus* (30 spp.), *Muscari* (60 spp.); 7. *Asparagus* (300 spp.), *Polygonatum* (50 spp.), *Convallaria* (1 spp.), *Trillium* (30 spp.), *Paris* (20 spp.); 8. *Ophiopogon* (20 spp.); 9. *Aletris* (25 spp.); 10. *Smilax* (about 350 spp.). For *Yucca*, *Dracaena* and *Agave* see below under 'Agavaceae'.

Some members of the family are cultivated for their flowers, others for food. Drugs include squill, sarsaparilla, veratrum, colchicum seed and corm, aloes and cevadilla seed. Garlic (*Allium sativum*), an age-old remedy frequently used for the treatment of colds, bronchitis, etc., has recently received much attention as a preventative of heart disease, as an antibiotic and as an anticancer drug.

Many members of the family contain alkaloids, which are of the steroidal, isoquinoline or purine types. Other steroidal substances include sterols, cardenolides, bufadienolides and steroidal saponins. The amino acid azetidine-2-carboxylic acid occurs in many genera and is also found in the Agavaceae. Other constituents include quinones (benzoquinones, naphthoquinones, anthraquinones and anthrones); flavonoids (anthocyanins and flavonols); the γ-pyrone chelidonic acid; cyanogenetic substances; and fructosan-type carbohydrates. Some volatile oils of the family have antimicrobial properties.

2. Agavaceae. A family of 20 genera and 670 species. The genera include *Yucca* (40 spp.), *Agave* (300 spp.), *Cordyline* (15 spp.), *Dracaena* (150 spp.), *Sansevieria* (60 spp.), *Phormium* (2 spp.), *Nolina* (30 spp.) and *Furcraea* (20 spp.). Dragon's blood is a dark red secretion from the leaves and trunk of *Dracaena draco* and *D. cinnabari*; the former is a native of the Canary Islands and Willis (*A Dictionary of the Flowering Plants and Ferns*, 1985) cites a tree blown down in 1868, 70 ft high and 45 ft in girth, that was supposed to be 6000 years old. Steroidal saponins have been reported as constituents of the resin (Y. Mimaki *et al.*, *Phytochemistry*, 1999, **50**, 805). *D. cinnabari* was the source of commercial Socotra dragon's blood, the flavonoids of which have been studied (M. Masaoud *et al.*, *Phytochemistry*, 1995, **38**, 745; 751). The resin is traditionally used as an astringent in the treatment of diarrhoea; it also has haemostatic and antiseptic properties. Chinese dragon's blood derived from *D. cochinchinensis* is reported to contain anti-*Helicobacter pylori* and thrombin inhibitory properties (Y. Zhu *et al.*, *J. Nat. Prod.*, 2007, **70**, 1570). For other products also known as dragon's blood, see *Daemonorops* spp. (Palmae) and *Croton lechleri* (Euphorbiaceae).

Steroidal saponins occur in species of *Yucca*, *Agave* and *Furcraea*; *Sansevieria zeylanica* yields bow-string hemp and *Furcraea gigantea* Mauritius hemp. The leaves of *Agave sisalana* yield the fibre sisal which is produced in large quantities in Central America and Kenya; the fermented sap of this plant forms the Mexican drink pulque. Species of *Sansevieria* are common house-plants under the name of 'mother-in-law's tongue'. Alkaloids and cardenolides appear to be absent from the family but the constituents otherwise closely resemble those of the Liliaceae.

3. Amaryllidaceae. A family of 85 genera and about 1100 species; mostly tropical or subtropical, and often xerophytes. Many have bulbs or rhizomes. Perianth petaloid, A 3 + 3, G(3). Fruit a loculicidal capsule or berry. Genera include *Galanthus* (20 spp.), *Leucojum* (12 spp.), *Amaryllis* (1 sp.), *Nerine* (30 spp.), *Pancratium* (15 spp.), *Hymenocallis* (50 spp.), *Narcissus* (60 spp.), *Ungernia* (6 spp.), *Hippeastrum* (75 spp.) and *Sternbergia* (8 spp.). The family contains types of alkaloid unlike those of any other family in

the order. One of these alkaloids, lycorine, has a marked fungicidal action; another, galanthamine, obtained from *Leucojum aestivum* and other species, is a newly marketed drug for the treatment of Alzheimer's disease.

4. Hypoxidaceae. A family of seven genera and 120 species. Herbs from a tuberous rhizome or corm. Several *Hypoxis* spp. have found use in traditional medicine as anti-inflammatory and antitumour drugs. A lipophilic extract is marketed in Germany, and the dried corm in South Africa, for treatment of prostate hypertrophy. The genus contains phenolic glycosides of the norlignan type.

5. Dioscoreaceae. A family of five genera and about 750 species; tropical or warm temperate climbing herbs or shrubs. The plants have fleshy tubers (called yams) or rhizomes. The leaves are often arrow-shaped. Flowers dioecious. Fruit a capsule or berry. The genera are *Dioscorea* (over 600 spp.), *Tamus* (5 spp.), *Rajana* (25 spp.), *Stenomeris* (2 spp.). *Tamus communis*, the black bryony, is exceptional in that it grows in Europe. It is common in English hedgerows and its scarlet berries are poisonous; a number of phenanthrone derivatives have been reported from the rhizome as well as dioscin and gracillin. The yams of *Dioscorea batatas* contain abundant starch and are important foodstuffs in the tropics. Steroidal saponins are present in many species of *Dioscorea* and *Tamus* and their extraction has become an important industry (see Chapter 23).

6. Iridaceae. A family of more than 60 genera and 800 species. Found in both tropical and temperate regions. Many perennial herbs with corm (e.g. *Crocus*) or rhizome (e.g. *Iris*). Flowers hermaphrodite, regular or zygomorphic; P3 + 3 petaloid, A3, G(3), inferior (or rarely superior). The fruit is a loculicidal capsule with numerous seeds. The genera include *Crocus* (75 spp.), *Romulea* (90 spp.), *Sisyrinchium* (100 spp.), *Tritonia* (55 spp.), *Freesia* (20 spp.) and *Iris* (about 300 spp.). Products of this family are saffron, from *Crocus sativus*, and orris root, from species of *Iris*. Constituents include quinones (naphthoquinones and anthraquinones), aromatic ketones (e.g. in *Iris*), carotenoid pigments (e.g. in saffron), terpenoids (mono-, sesqui-, di-and tetraterpenoids), and flavonoids (anthocyanins, flavones, flavonols and isoflavones).

BROMELIALES

Bromeliaceae

The Bromeliaceae is the only family of the order and contains about 44 genera and 1400 species; mainly tropical and subtropical, xerophytes and epiphytes. Fruit a berry or capsule. These interesting plants vary very much in size and habitat; many are grown as house-plants or in greenhouses. Genera include *Bromelia* (40 spp.) and *Ananas* (5 spp.). *Ananas comosus* (syn. *A. sativus*) is the pineapple, the juice of which contains bromelain, a protein-splitting enzyme which can be used as an adjunct in the treatment of trauma and oedema arising from surgery and for soft tissue inflammation. It is cited as an aid to digestion and studies (*Gut*, 1998, **43**, 196) have suggested it as a possible cure for travellers' diarrhoea. The chemistry of the family requires more study, but many species contain gums and mucilages and there are reports of tannins, phenolic acids and flavonoids.

GRAMINALES

Gramineae

An order of one family.

The Gramineae contains about 620 genera and 10 000 species. Mostly herbs with fibrous roots; rarely shrubs or trees. Annuals, biennials and perennials almost universally distributed and many of great economic importance. Leaves alternate, with sheath; blade usually long and narrow; veins normally parallel. Inflorescence of numerous spikelets, with scales. Flowers bisexual, protected by palea; stamens usually three; ovary unilocular with one ovule. Fruit one-seeded, usually a caryopsis (rarely a nut or berry). Some important genera are *Bambusa* (70 spp.), *Arundinaria* (150 spp.), *Oryza* (25 spp.), *Arundo* (12 spp.), *Triticum* (about 20 spp.), *Agropyron* (100–150 spp.), *Hordeum* (20 spp.), *Secale* (4 spp.), *Avena* (70 spp.), *Sorghum* (60 spp.), *Zea* (1 sp.), *Saccharum* (5 spp.) and *Andropogon* (113 spp.), *Cymbopogon* (60 spp.), *Phalaris* (20 spp.) and *Vetiveria* (10 spp.). Products include bamboos of many different sizes, from species of *Bambusa* and *Arundinaria*, rice from *Oryza sativa*, wheat from *Triticum*, barley from *Hordeum*, rye from *Secale*, millet or guinea corn from *Sorghum vulgare*, maize or Indian corn from *Zea mays* and sugar cane from *Saccharum officinarum*. The tribe Paniceae, which includes *Andropogon*, *Cymbopogon* and *Vetiveria*, is rich in volatile oils. These grass oils are relatively cheap and are much used in perfumery, especially for scenting soap. They include citronella oils, lemon-grass and palmarosa (geranium) oils from species of *Cymbopogon*; oil of vetivert from *Vetiveria zizanioides*. The roots of the latter plant, khus-khus, are used both in perfumery and as a drug and are also woven into fragrant-smelling mats and fans.

The Gramineae contains a very wide range of constituents but a large proportion of the chemical work has been devoted to the above-mentioned foodstuffs, starches, sugar and volatile oils. Other constituents include 11 different classes of alkaloid (for details see R. D. Gibbs, *Chemotaxonomy of Flowering Plants*, Montreal, Canada: McGill University Press), saponins, cyanogenetic substances, phenolic acids, flavonoids and terpenoids.

PRINCIPES

Palmae

The order contains the single family Palmae.

The Palmae has 217 genera and about 2500 species. Widely distributed in the tropics and subtropics. Mostly trees with an unbranched stem bearing a crown of large, often branched leaves. The flowers are usually unisexual and regular, consisting of two trimerous whorls of small perianth leaves, six stamens and three superior carpels. The carpels may be free or united and develop into a berry, drupe or nut. The seeds contain a very small embryo but abundant endosperm. Important genera are *Phoenix* (17 spp.), *Sabal* (25 spp.), *Copernicia* (30 spp.), *Metroxylon* (15 spp.), *Calamus* (375 spp.), *Areca* (54 spp.), *Elaeis* (2 spp.), *Cocos* (1 sp.), *Phytelephas* (15 spp.), *Serenoa* (1 sp.) and *Daemonorops* (100 spp.). Of economic interest are the date palm, *Phoenix dactylifera*; sago from the stems of *Metroxylon rumpii* and *M. laeve*; rattan canes from species of *Calamus*; areca or betel nuts from *Areca catechu*; palm oil and palm kernel oil from *Elaeis guineensis*; coconut from *Cocos nucifera*; carnauba wax from *Copernicia cerifera*. The resin from species of *Daemonorops* gives the East Asian dragon's blood and this appears (1997) to be the only available commercial source; the constituents investigated are of flavonoid origin, some derived from 5-methoxyflavan-7-ol and 5-methoxy-6-methylflavan-7-ol. Isolated compounds have been named dracoflavans (A. Arnone *et al.*, *J. Nat. Prod.*, 1997, **60**, 971). For the botany, chemistry and therapeutic uses of this, and other types of dragon's blood (species of *Croton*, *Dracaena* and *Pterocarpus*), see D. Gupta *et al.*, *J. Ethnopharm.*, 2008, **115**, 361. The fruits of *Serenoa repens* (saw-palmetto) native to the S.E. coastal states of North America are a popular remedy for male impotence and are used in the treatment of the symptoms of benign prostate hyperplasia (q.v.). Seeds of *Phytelephas* spp. (*P. aequatorialis* in Ecuador) are the basis of the vegetable ivory industry (for a report see A. S. Barfod *et al.*, *Econ. Bot.*, 1990, **44**, 293).

5

In addition to the fixed oil, carbohydrates and leaf wax mentioned above, the family contains saponins, tannins, catechins, flavonoids, terpenoids and ketones. Alkaloids occur in *Areca*, but few have been found in other genera. Steroidal substances occur (e.g. estrone in the pollen of *Phoenix*).

SPATHIFLORAE

Araceae
The order consists of two families, the Araceae and the Lemnaceae. The latter, which contains only six genera and 30 species of aquatic herbs, is of little importance.

The Araceae has 115 genera and about 2000 species; mainly herbs or climbing shrubs and over 90% tropical; many members contain poisonous latex, the poison being destroyed by heat. The genera include *Acorus* (2 spp.), *Arum* (15 spp.), *Monstera* (50 spp.), *Dracuncula*, *Amorphophallus* and *Cryptocoryne*. Calamus or sweet flag rhizome is derived from the perennial herb *Acorus calamus*, which is widely distributed in damp situations in Europe and North America. Arum, also known as lords and ladies, cuckoo-pint and wake robin, is *Arum maculatum*, a common hedgerow plant in England. It and other species of *Arum* are poisonous; these plants contain amines and cyanogenetic compounds. Species of *Monstera* are often grown as house-plants. The rhizome of *Cryptocoryne spiralis* is known as 'Indian ipecacuanha'. *Amorphophallus campanulatus* is the elephant-foot yam. Many members of the family are cyanogenetic. Alkaloids, either pyridine or indole types, are reported in a few genera. Other constituents include saponins, tannins, phenolic acids, amines and terpenoids.

CYPERALES

Cyperaceae
The order contains the single family.

The Cyperaceae has about 90 genera and 4000 species; widely distributed herbs. Genera include *Cyperus* (550 spp.), *Scirpus* (300 spp.) and *Carex* (150–200 spp.). Formerly official in a number of pharmacopoeias were the rhizomes of *Carex arenaria* and *Cyperus rotundus*. Papyrus, used in ancient times as paper, is derived from *Cyperus papyrus*. Like some members of the Gramineae, certain species of *Scirpus* and *Ampelodesma* serve as host plants for species of *Claviceps* and produce ergot-like sclerotia. Other family constituents include volatile oils, tannins, phenolic acids, flavonoids and sesquiterpenoids.

SCITAMINEAE

Musaceae, Zingiberaceae, Cannaceae, Marantaceae
An order of five families.

1. Musaceae. A family of two genera and 42 species, namely *Musa* (35 spp.) and *Enseta* (7 spp.). The plants are giant herbs with 'false' aerial stems and sheathed leaves arising from a rhizome. Fruit a berry. Of economic importance are the fruits of *Musa paradisiaca* (plantain) and *M. sapientum* (banana), which are rich in starch; bananas constitute a food source of potassium. Manila hemp or abaca is derived from *Musa textilis*. Constituents of the family include starch and fructosans, phenolic acids, anthocyanins, terpenoids and sterols; only isolated examples of alkaloids (alkaloidal amine and an indole alkaloid) are reported.

2. Zingiberaceae. A family of about 49 genera and 1300 species. Perennial aromatic herbs with fleshy rhizomes and tuberous roots; flowers in racemes, heads or cymes. Perianth 6-merous, the outer calyx-like, the inner corolla-like. Two of the stamens modified as a petaloid labellum. Fruit a loculicidal capsule. Seed with perisperm. Genera include *Curcuma* (5 spp.), *Alpinia* (250 spp.), *Zingiber* (80–90 spp.), *Amomum* (150 spp.), *Elettaria* (7 spp.), *Aframomum* (50 spp.) and *Hedychium* (50 spp.). *Costus* (150 spp.) is included by Engler in the Zingiberaceae, but is sometimes separated as a distinct family. Its main difference from the other genera listed is that its aerial parts are not aromatic. Products of the family include turmeric, the rhizomes of *Curcuma longa*; ginger, the rhizome of *Zingiber officinale*; cardamom fruits from *Elettaria cardamomum*; and grains of paradise, the seeds of *Aframomum melegueta*. Volatile oils and pungent principles such as are found in ginger (q.v.) are a feature of the family. Other constituents include the colouring matters known as curcuminoids (see 'Turmeric'), tannins, phenolic acids, leucoanthocyanins, flavonoids, ketones and terpenoids. Only a few isolated examples of alkaloids have been reported.

3. Cannaceae. This family contains only the single genus *Canna* (55 spp.). The rhizome of *Canna edulis* yields the starch, Queensland arrowroot.

4. Marantaceae. A family of 30 genera and 400 species of tropical herbaceous perennials. The genus *Maranta* (23 spp.) contains *Maranta arundinacea*, the rhizome of which yields West Indian arrowroot.

MICROSPERMAE

Orchidaceae
The order contains a single family.

The Orchidaceae is one of the largest families of flowering plants, with some 735 genera, over 17 000 species and many hybrids. Cosmopolitan perennial herbs, some terrestrial but many tropical epiphytes (e.g. *Vanilla*). The ovary is inferior and the fruit a capsule; seeds very small and light. Genera include *Orchis* (35 spp.), *Cypripedium* (50 spp.), *Phalaenopsis* (35 spp.), *Dendrobium* (1400 spp.), *Liparis* (250 spp.), *Malaxis* (300 spp.), *Vanda* (60 spp.), *Cryptostylis* (20 spp.) and *Vanilla* (90 spp.). The glycosides of vanilla, which produce vanillin and other aromatic substances by slow enzymic change, have long been known. More recently, attention has been directed to the numerous alkaloids present in the family. Some of these are of an unusual indolizidine type, others are derivatives of indole, pyrrolidine and pyrrolizidine. Other constituents include phenolic acids, tannin, flavonoids, coumarins and terpenoids.

ANIMAL PRODUCTS

As with the Plant Kingdom, animals are classified into Phyla, Classes, Orders, Families, Genera and Species. Although the number of pharmacognostical products derived from animal sources is limited there has been, in recent years, an immense interest in the chemistry of many marine creatures as potential sources of drugs and biologically active materials. In this respect much research has been published on the simpler marine organisms, see G. Blunden in Trease and Evans 2002 *Pharmacognosy*, 15th ed., p. 18.

Listed below are selected animal phyla which embrace species of interest (the many animal products used in traditional medicines of Africa, India and the Orient are not included).

PROTOZOA

Unicellular microorganisms including parasites causing malaria (*Plasmodium*), sleeping sickness (*Trypanosoma*) and dysentery (*Entamoeba*). Some dinoflagellates (*Prorocentrum*, *Dinophysis*) produce polyether toxins responsible for some shell-fish poisoning.

PORIFERA

(Sponges)

Metabolites include bromophenols (antibacterial properties), cyclic peroxides and peroxyketals (antimicrobial, ichthyotoxic, cytotoxic activities), modified sesquiterpenes (antimalarial, antifungal, antibacterial, anticancer activities). Siliceous sponge spicules are often found in samples of kieselguhr and agar (q.v.).

COELENTERATA

(Jellyfishes, sea anemones, corals)

The soft coral *Plexaura homomalla* is a rich source of prostaglandin A_2 and *Sarcophyton glaucum* contains diterpenoids (sarcophytols A and B) which inhibit tumour promotion. As with the sponges there is much current biochemical interest in this phylum.

PLATYHELMINTHES

(Flatworms)

This phylum includes the Trematodes (the parasitic flukes such as the liver fluke and *Schistosoma*) and the Cestoda (tapeworms).

NEMATODA

(Roundworms)

Some are parasitic in man and animals.

MOLLUSCA

Class Gastropoda includes the snails, slugs and limpets. Some snails are vectors of parasites such as *Schistosoma*.

Class Lamellibranchia includes scallops, mussels, oysters and clams.

Class Cephalopoda includes the squids, cuttlefishes and octopuses. Cuttlefish bone (from *Sepia officinalis*) has been employed in dentifrices and as an antacid.

ANNELIDA

(Segmented worms)

Earthworms, lugworms and leeches (q.v.) belong to this phylum. The potent neurotoxic agent nereistoxin is obtained from the Japanese species *Lumbriconereis heteropoda*.

ARTHROPODA

A very large phylum of jointed animals including the crustaceans, insects and arachnids.

Class Crustacea includes the shrimps, crabs, lobsters, centipedes and millipedes. Of little medicinal significance, nevertheless brine shrimps are being increasingly used in place of higher animals for the preliminary testing of phytochemicals for toxicity.

Class Insecta. Of the many orders of this taxon the following have medicinal interest:

1. Order Anoplura (Lice): Commonly infest birds and mammals. Important from human standpoint is *Pediculus humanus* encountered as the body louse (*corporis*) and the head louse (*capitis*); it is a proven carrier of typhus fever and an indirect transmitter of relapsing fever.

2. Order Hemiptera (Bugs): The cochineal beetle (q.v.) is an important colourant and shellac is a resinous substance prepared from a secretion that encrusts the bodies of a scale insect *Laccifer lacca*.

3. Order Coleoptera (Beetles): Beetles of the genera *Cantharis* and *Mylabris*, known as blistering beetles contain cantharidin derivatives and possess vesicant properties. Preparations of *C. vesicatoria* were at one time used in Western medicine in the form of plasters, collodions etc. as rubefacients and vesicants. Their use continues in the traditional medicine of Eastern Asia (R. W. Pemberton, *J. Ethnopharmacology*, 1999, **65**, 181). The Chinese blister beetle, *M. phalerata*, is used in Chinese traditional medicine for the treatment of cancer; various novel cantharidin-related compounds have recently been described (T. Nakatani *et al.*, *Chem. Pharm. Bull.*, 2004, **52**, 8079; 2007, **55**, 92).

Cantharidin

A number of small beetles are important infestants of stored drugs (see Chapter 15).

4. Order Lepidoptera (Butterflies and moths): Some moths infest stored drugs (see Chapter 15). Silk has been traditionally used in pharmacy in the form of oiled silk.

5. Order Hymenoptera (Ants, bees, wasps, etc.): Hive products derived from *Apis mellifica* include honey, beeswax, royal jelly and propolis (q.v.).

6. Order Diptera (Flies, gnats and midges): The successful use of maggots in the treatment of wounds infected with antibiotic-resistant *Staphylococcus aureus* has received recent attention. Sterile larvae of the common greenbottle *Lucilia sericata* are used. For a report see *Pharm. J.*, 1999, **262**, 422.

Class Arachnida. Arthropods with two divisions to the body (cephalothorax and abdomen) including spiders, scorpions and mites.

Order Acarina (Mites): the common housemite (q.v.) is a cause of allergy in humans; other species infest stored drugs (see Chapter 15).

CHORDATA

The most important subphylum of the Chordata is the Vertebrata (Craniata) composed of all those animals with backbones; a number of classification schemes will be found in the literature and two major groupings often referred to as superclasses are the Pisces (aquatic vertebrates) and the Tetrapoda (terrestrial vertebrates) each divided into four classes. The following four classes have medicinal significance:

1. **Class Osteichthyes** (Bony fish). The following families and species are important:

Gadidae: Cod	} Liver oils, sources of
Pleurnectidae: Halibut	vitamins A and D
Engraulidae: Anchovies	
Carangidae: Jacks and pompanos	
Clupeidae: Herrings	
Osmeridae: Smelts	} Body oils, rich in
Scombridae: Mackerels and tunas	omega-3 acids
Ammodytidae: Sand eels	
Salmonidae: Trout, salmon, whitefish and graylings	

2. **Class Amphibia** (Frogs and toads). Dried and powdered toadskins contain cardioactive principles and were used for the treatment of dropsy before the widespread adoption of digitalis.
3. **Class Reptilia** (Crocodiles, snakes and lizards). Snake venoms are important products.
4. **Class Mammalia** (Warm-blooded animals which suckle their young). Variously divided into subclasses, infraclasses and orders.

Subclass **Eutheria** embraces the placental mammals, e.g. bats, rodents, carnivores, whales, ungulates and primates. Formerly important was the whale-product spermaceti but its collection is now illegal. Other pharmaceuticals include lard, suet, wool fat, wool, gelatin, musk, catgut, heart-replacement valves from the pig, insulin, hormones, blood and liver products, vaccines and sera.

6

Pharmacological activities of natural products

As indicated in Chapter 2, a valid scheme for the study of medicinal plants and their products, and one which emphasizes pharmaceutical use, can be based on pharmacological action. The scheme can be extended to include numerous plants which, although eliciting a pharmacological response, are not, for varied reasons, used as drugs. In the latter category would be placed hundreds of alkaloid- and glycoside-containing plants.

Some major pharmacological groupings involve drugs which act on the nervous systems, heart and blood vessels, lungs, gastrointestinal tract, kidneys, liver, reproductive organs, skin and mucous membranes. Other categories include hormones, vitamins and chemotherapeutic drugs used for the treatment of infections and malignant diseases. Some plants (e.g. *Papaver*, ipecacuanha and liquorice) contain a range of compounds with differing pharmacological properties. Oliver-Bever's classical review (*J. Ethnopharmacol.*, 1983, **7**, 1) on West African plants which act on the nervous system well illustrates the problems of constructing a purely pharmacological classification for herbal materials. A system based on clinical usage may be more straightforward for the throughly studied allopathic drugs used in Western medicine but difficulties can arise for plants used in traditional medicine because of the often numerous conditions for which any one drug may be employed. However, this is a very active area of research and the situation for a particular drug becomes clearer as the chemical nature of the active constituents together with their pharmacological properties are elucidated.

DRUGS ACTING ON THE NERVOUS SYSTEM

The nervous system coordinates and regulates the various voluntary and involuntary activities of the body and is conveniently considered under two headings—the central nervous system (CNS) and the autonomic nervous system. The two are interlinked and some drugs which affect the CNS may also produce reactions associated with the autonomic system. In the case of others which act via the autonomic system it is sometimes more convenient to classify them under other headings appropriate to the organs involved; thus, those producing vasoconstriction or vasodilation may appear under the consideration of the circulatory and respiratory systems.

THE CENTRAL NERVOUS SYSTEM

The central nervous system comprises the brain (cerebrum, cerebellum, medulla oblongata) and the spinal cord. It coordinates the voluntary activities of the body and exhibits numerous interactions within the system together with linkages to the autonomic system. Drugs involved with the CNS can be broadly classified according to whether they have a general stimulatory or depressant action with further subdivision regarding specific actions such as anticonvulsant and psychopharmacological activities. Some of the most useful natural drugs of the group are the narcotic (opioid) analgesics; a number of herbal drugs are popular sedatives and others such as the hallucinogenic drugs have important sociological implications. See Table 6.1 for a summary of drugs acting on the central nervous system.

THE AUTONOMIC NERVOUS SYSTEM

The autonomic nervous system supplies the smooth muscle tissues and glands of the body. Its function is complex, involving ganglia situated outside the spinal cord; it is composed of two divisions, the sympathetic (thoracolumbar or adrenergic) division, which arises from the thoracic and lumbar regions; and the parasympathetic

6

Table 6.1   Drugs acting on the central nervous system.

Drugs affecting mental activity

Lysergic acid diethylamide	Hallucinogenic. Prepared by partial synthesis from ergot alkaloids or by artificial culture
Mescaline	Hallucinogenic. Obtained from peyote cactus
Cannabis	Hallucinogenic. Active constituents contained in the resin of *Cannabis sativa*
Purine bases (e.g. caffeine, theophylline, theobromine)	Stimulate mental activity; constituents of beverages—coffee, tea, cocoa, kola, maté
Cocaine	One of the earliest drugs used as a mental stimulant. Produces addiction. Contained in the leaves of *Erythroxylum coca*
Ginkgo biloba	Improves short term memory
Ginseng	Improves mental concentration particularly in the elderly
Galanthamine	Promising Amaryllidaceous alkaloid for treatment of Alzheimer's disease
Hops	Sedative, often combined with other herbs
Hypericum	Popular herbal remedy for relief of mild–moderate depression
Passiflora	Treatment of insomnia often in combination
Sage	Revived interest in its use for counteracting memory loss
St John's wort	Antidepressant, may adversely react with some mainstream drugs
Reserpine	Depresses mental activity. Used in psychiatric treatment. Obtained from *Rauwolfia* spp.
Yohimbine	Similar action to reserpine but its antiadrenaline reactions and effect on heart muscle render it of no clinical use. Found in various species of the Apocynaceae
Valerian	Sedative and hypnotic; aids sleeplessness and improves sleep quality

Analeptic drugs (stimulants of the CNS in addition to the mental stimulants indicated above)

Picrotoxin	Analeptic previously used in the treatment of barbiturate poisoning. Obtained from berries of *Anamirta cocculus*
Lobeline	Obtained from *Lobelia inflata*
Strychnine	Weak analeptic; toxic doses produce spinal convulsions. Obtained from the seeds of *Strychnos* spp.
Camphor	Weak analeptic. Obtained from *Cinnamomum camphora* and by synthesis

Central depressants of motor function

Tropane alkaloids (e.g. hyoscine, atropine, etc.)	Formerly the only drugs effective in the alleviation of the symptoms of Parkinson's disease. Used in treatment of travel sickness and delirium tremens
Gelsemium root	Rarely employed clinically owing to high toxicity. Galenical preparations occasionally used as antispasmodics

Analgesic drugs

Morphine	Effective for relief of severe pain. Depressant action on the cough and respiratory centres. The principal alkaloid of opium
Codeine	Although less active than morphine it is a much safer drug for the relief of mild pain and for use as a cough suppressant

(craniosacral or cholinergic) division, originating in the brain and in the sacral region. In general, an increase in activity of the sympathetic system gears the body for immediate action (fight and flight), whereas stimulation of the parasympathetic or vagal system produces effects more associated with those occurring during sleep and with energy conservation. Two important neurotransmitter substances of the autonomic nervous system are acetylcholine and noradrenaline and its derivatives; hence, other substances which either mimic or antagonize the action of either of these will produce a marked physiological response. Drugs acting on the autonomic nervous system are summarized in Table 6.2.

THE HEART, CIRCULATION AND BLOOD

In developed countries, coronary and associated circulatory diseases now constitute the principal cause of human mortality. Not surprisingly, therefore, this is an area of intensive research, not entirely devoted to treatment, but also to the prevention of these diseases. With increased public awareness of the importance of the latter, healthier living focused on diet, supplementary food factors, exercise, etc. has taken on a more important role, not least in the mind of the commercial world where

health food stores now supply many dietary supplements and medicinal plant products which overlap the traditional pharmaceutical range.

Many factors affect the complex regulation of the heart and the large group of drugs which is known to possess cardiovascular activity is not confined to action on the heart muscle itself. Thus those drugs possessing antiarrhythmic, antihypertensive, antihyperlipidaemic, vasoconstrictor, vasodilator, blood anticoagulant, and platelet aggregation activities must also be considered in this group. As with other important areas, there is an active search in the plant kingdom for compounds which may also serve as lead compounds for the semi-synthesis of new drugs. For some therapeutic groups, the lack of simple reliable screening techniques is a problem.

In a review (over 390 refs) E. L. Ghisalberti *et al.* (see Further Reading) have listed some 447 species from 109 families having cardiovascular activity, together with a compilation of over 700 secondary plant metabolites having such activity.

Cardioactive glycosides

A considerable number of plants scattered throughout the plant kingdom contain C_{23} or C_{24} steroidal glycosides which exert a slowing and strengthening effect on the failing heart. In Western medicine it is the glycosides of various *Digitalis* species that are extensively employed.

Table 6.2 Drugs acting on the autonomic nervous system.

Acetylcholine-like drugs	
Pilocarpine	From leaves of *Pilocarpus microphyllus*
Arecoline	From seeds of *Areca catechu*
Muscarine	From *Amanita* spp. and other fungi
Physostigmine	A cholinesterase inhibitor from seeds of *Physostigma venenosum*
Antagonists of acetylcholine	
Tropane ester alkaloids (e.g. hyoscine, atropine)	From a number of Solanaceae (e.g. *Duboisia, Atropa, Datura* etc.) They have widespread uses involving their gastrointestinal, bronchial, genito-urinary and ophthalmic effects in addition to the CNS activity (q.v.)
Neuromuscular blocking agents (e.g. tubocurarine) Ganglion blocking agents (e.g. tubocurarine in large doses) (not clinically important)	From leaves and stems of *Chondodrendron tomentosum*
Adrenaline-like drugs	
Ephedrine	From stems of *Ephedra* spp.; mainly synthetic
Antagonists of adrenaline	
Ergot alkaloids (e.g. ergotamine)	From sclerotia of *Claviceps* spp.
Noradrenaline depletion	
Reserpine	Has antihypertensive effect resulting from dilation of heart and circulatory vessels
Ophthalmic preparations The eye, being under the control of the autonomic nervous system, is affected by some of the drugs mentioned above; these include atropine, hyoscine, physostigmine and pilocarpine	

The pharmacological effectiveness of the cardioactive glycosides is dependent on both the aglycones and the sugar attachments; the inherent activity resides in the aglycones, but the sugars render the compounds more soluble and increase the power of fixation of the glycosides to the heart muscle.

The overall action of the digitalis glycosides is complicated by the number of different effects produced, and their exact mode of action on myocardial muscle in relation to current views on cardiac muscle physiology is still an area of investigation. Digitalis probably acts in competition with K^+ ions for specific receptor enzyme (ATPase) sites in the cell membranes of cardiac muscle and is particularly successful during the depolarization phase of the muscle when there is an influx of Na^+ ions. The clinical effect in cases of congestive heart failure is to increase the force of myocardial contraction (the positive inotropic effect) resulting in a complete emptying of the ventricles. As a result of depression of conduction in the bundle of His, the atrioventricular conduction time is increased, resulting in an extended P–R interval on the electrocardiogram. Arising from their vagus effects, the digitalis glycosides are also used to control supraventricular (atrial) cardiac arrhythmias. The diuretic action of digitalis, important in the treatment of dropsy, arises from the improved circulatory effect. However, following the introduction of safer diuretics in the 1950s, diuretic therapy for heart failure has become much more important and in some cases can replace digitalis treatment.

Among the many other plant genera containing cardioactive glycosides related to those of *Digitalis*, and used similarly, are *Strophanthus*, *Convallaria*, *Nerium*, *Thevetia* and *Erysimum*. For a full account of these drugs see Chapter 23.

Antiarrhythmic drugs

As mentioned above, the cardiac glycosides can be used to control supraventricular (atrial) cardiac arrhythmias. There are a number of other drugs such as the alkaloid quinidine (obtained from various cinchona barks, q.v.) which act on both supraventricular and ventricular arrhythmias. Quinidine is official in most pharmacopoeias as its salts and finds prophylactic use in recurrent paroxysmal dysrhythmias such as atrial fibrillation or flutter. Its therapeutic use for the attempted conversion of atrial fibrillation to sinus rhythm has now been largely replaced by electrical cardioversion.

Other drugs in this category include hawthorn and motherwort.

Antihypertensive drugs

The control of hypertension is an important element in the management of cardiovascular disorders. Primary hypertension, as distinct from other special forms which usually require hospitalization, represents about 90% of all cases ranging from mild conditions with the occasional rise in blood pressure to those with severe unrelieved high pressure. Of the hypotensive plant drugs rauwolfia and its principal alkaloid reserpine together with *Veratrum* extracts were recognized in allopathic medicine in the early 1950s. A number of plants regularly employed by Western herbal practitioners include mistletoe, *Crataegus*, Yarrow, *Tilia* and *Fagopyrum*. In fact, a large number of other herbal drugs, used to treat various conditions, have also been shown to possess antihypertensive activity. In Ayurvedic medicine *Piper betle*, *Jasminum sabac*, *Cardiospermum halicacabum* and *Tribulus terrestris*, used in the treatment of hypertension, have been shown to exhibit a high angiotensin converting enzyme inhibition suggesting a possible mechanism of action for these drugs (B. Somanadhan *et al.*, *J. Ethnopharmacology*, 1999, **65**, 103).

Platelet-activating factor (PAF) antagonists

In the circulatory system thrombi may be caused on the arterial side as a result of the adhesion of blood platelets to one another and to the walls of the vessels. This platelet aggregation is triggered by the platelet activating factor which is released from activated basophils. PAF from the rabbit was characterized in the 1970s as a 1-*O*-alkyl-2-acetyl-*sn*-glyceryl-3-phosphorylcholine. A number of prostaglandins and thromboxanes are also involved in the aggregation mechanism and thromboxane A_2 which is synthesized from arachidonic acid (q.v), is particularly potent. In undamaged vessels thromboxane A_2 is possibly balanced by a prostaglandin e.g. prostacyclin of the arterial intima which has deaggregation properties.

For the secondary prevention of cerebrovascular or cardiovascular disease, aspirin, which irreversibly acetylates the platelet enzyme cyclo-oxygenase has been employed at dosages of 300 mg daily with useful results. A large number of plants have been screened for anti-PAF activity. One of the first natural products so identified was the neolignan kadsurenone obtained from *Piper futokadsura*, a plant long used in Chinese traditional medicine for allergy treatments. Other plants of traditional medicine reported to have anti-PAF activity include species of *Forsythia*, *Arctium*, *Centipeda*, *Tussilago*, *Pyrola*, *Populus* and *Peucedanum*. The active constituents include lignans, sesquiterpenes, coumarins, pyrocatechol and salicyl alcohol.

Extracts of the maidenhair tree, *Ginkgo biloba* have proved especially interesting and are commercially available in Europe for the treatment of various circulatory disorders.

Certain fish oils (e.g. cod-liver, halibut-liver) once employed solely for their vitamin contents together with 'oily fish' body oils have recently received a resurgence in popularity as dietary supplements. One favourable response is that they decrease the ability of platelets to aggregate by virtue of their high eicosapentaenoic acid content; this acid tends to favour the biosynthesis of thromboxane A_3, a weaker stimulator of platelet aggregation than thromboxane A_2.

Drugs acting on blood vessels (Table 6.3)

These drugs are essentially either vasoconstrictor or vasodilator substances but their action may originate in a variety of ways (direct, central, peripheral or reflex). Some of the drugs (e.g. ergot, bronchodilators, diuretics), which are particularly useful in relation to specific systems, are classified elsewhere.

Oral anticoagulants

These compounds inhibit the clotting mechanism of the blood and are of value in arterial thrombosis; they have no effect on platelet aggregation. One group of active drugs constitutes the 4-hydroxy-coumarins which act by antagonizing the effects of vitamin K (see Chapter 31). Warfarin sodium is one of the most widely used drugs. Plants used in herbal medicine which contain coumarin derivatives and possess anti-vitamin K activity include *Melilotus officinalis*, *Galium aparine* and *Lavandula officinalis*.

Other anticoagulants are heparin, which is given by injection, and hirudin, produced by the leech; hirudin, a polypeptide of 65 amino acids, can also be obtained from genetically modified *Saccharomyces*.

Hypolipidaemic drugs

In recent years much prominence has been given to the association of high levels of blood cholesterol and plasma triglycerides with atherosclerosis and ischaemic heart disease. Treatment of hyperlipidaemia is preferably dietary accompanied by other natural regimens. Drug therapy is reserved for the more intractable conditions. Natural products having a beneficial action include nicotinic acid (Chapter 31) and those fish oils containing high quantities of ω-3-marine triglycerides. The latter involve eicosapentaenoic acid and docasahexaenoic acid which, when counting from the methyl end, possess the first double bond at C-3 (see Chapter 19).

The suggested beneficial properties of garlic (*Allium sativum*) for the treatment of various cardiovascular conditions remain a subject of extensive investigation. With reference to hyperlipidaemic patients, the majority of published data supports the hypothesis that garlic lowers serum total cholesterol and improves the lipid profile. There is a tendency towards reduction of low-density lipoprotein and an increase in high-density lipoprotein giving a more favourable HDL:LDL ratio. Similar hypocholesterolaemic properties have been demonstrated for globe artichoke. A reduction in the serum levels of total cholesterol, low-density lipoprotein cholesterol together with a lowered atherogenic index was observed with mild hypercholesterolic patients after a three-month course of psyllium seeds (K. Sagawa *et al.*, *Biol. Pharm. Bull.*, 1998, **21**, 184).

ACTION ON THE GASTROINTESTINAL TRACT

The gastrointestinal tract can be divided into three regions—the upper (mouth, stomach and upper portion of the duodenum), the

---

Table 6.3 Drugs acting on blood vessels.

Peripheral vasoconstrictor drugs	
Ergotamine (tartrate) from *Claviceps purpurea*	Produces a direct constrictor effect in vascular smooth muscle; the reversal of the dilation of cranial vessels leads to its use at the onset of classical migraine attack
Ergotoxine	Similar to ergotamine
Ephedrine (synthetic and from *Ephedra* spp.)	Prolonged action on blood pressure—see also 'Autonomic Nervous System'
Nicotine	Vasoconstrictor effects arise from its action on sympathetic ganglia, and by it promoting release of vasopressin and adrenaline
Central vasoconstrictor drugs	
Most of the drugs (e.g. picrotoxin) which stimulate the central nervous system also stimulate the vasomotor centre in the medulla, producing a rise in blood pressure. Although at one time used as respiratory stimulants, these drugs have been largely replaced by mechanical devices for artificial ventilation of the lungs	
Vasodilator drugs	
Papaverine (an opium alkaloid)	Acts directly on the blood vessels by causing relaxation of smooth muscle. An intravenous injection used for the treatment of pulmonary arterial embolism
Xanthine derivatives (caffeine, theobromine, theophylline)	As papaverine; they also have a central vasoconstrictor action counteracting the peripheral effect. Also diuretic
Ergotamine	Adrenaline antagonist—see 'Autonomic Nervous System'
Reserpine	Vasodilatation is produced by a peripheral and central action (q.v.)
Veratrum alkaloids (from *Veratrum* spp.)	Bradycardia and peripheral vasodilatation by sensitization of cardiac, aortic and carotid sinus baroreceptors

middle (lower half of the duodenum to the ileocolic sphincter) and the lower (caecum, colon and rectum). It is the upper and the lower portions that are most susceptible to disorder and are consequently associated with the greatest number of drugs for their treatment (see Table 6.4).

Table 6.4 Drugs acting on the gastrointestinal tract.

Bitters At one time these were extensively used in liquid medicaments to stimulate appetite. The bitter constituents stimulate the gustatory nerves in the mouth and give rise to an increase in the psychic secretion of gastric juice. Extracts of the following drugs have been so employed: gentian, quassia, calumba, cinchona (or quinine), nux vomica (or strychnine). Considerable recent research has involved the investigation of a number of these bitter compounds for other possible uses, e.g. the bitters of the Simaroubaceae as antitumour and antimalarial agents

Anticholinergic drugs In this capacity hyoscine and hyoscyamine help disturbances caused by gastric mobility and muscle spasm particularly with some ulcer patients

Emetics Ipecacuanha preparations, on oral administration, have a delayed emetic action produced by irritation of the mucous membranes (see 'Expectorants'). Picrotoxin stimulates the vomiting centre through its general effect on the central nervous system

Antiemetics Ginger has received scientific approval for the prevention of the symptoms of travel sickness. Cannabis affords sickness relief to patients undergoing chemotherapy

Carminatives These are aromatic substances which assist the eructation reflex; their mode of action is obscure. Dill oil is used for the relief of flatulence, especially in babies. Other plants or oils used as carminatives include caraway, fennel, peppermint, thyme, nutmeg, calamus, pimento, ginger, clove, cinnamon, chamomile, matricaria. Chalk is used as an antacid and charcoal as an adsorbent

Ulcer therapy Derivatives of glycyrrhetinic acid (a triterpenoid of liquorice root) prove effective in the treatment of peptic ulcer. Deglycyrrhizinized liquorice has also been employed. Other antiulcer agents include alginic acid, marshmallow and comfrey

Demulcents These soothe and protect the alimentary tract and overlap with some materials used in ulcertherapy. Iceland moss, orris and elm bark may be included here

Laxatives and purgatives Purgatives may be classed according to their mode of action

Agar, psyllium and ispaghula	Hydrophilic colloids which function as bulk-producing laxatives
Bran	An indigestible vegetable fibre which absorbs water and provides bulk
Senna (leaves and fruit)	Contains anthraquinone derivatives which are hydrolysed in the bowel to stimulate Auerbach's plexus in the wall
Cascara, rhubarb, aloes	As senna
Castor oil	Contains glycerides which on hydrolysis yield riconoleic acid, irritant to the small bowel
Podophyllum resin, jalap resin, colocynth	Drastic purgatives, now little used for this purpose. They were often prescribed with belladonna to reduce griping

Rectal and colonic drugs Arachis oil, esculin, hamamelis, pilewort and balsam of Peru are examples of this group; they include those used in suppositories

Antidiarrhoeal drugs Morphine and codeine act by increasing the smooth muscle tone of the bowel and by reducing its mobility. Commonly prescribed with kaolin

---

THE NASAL AND RESPIRATORY SYSTEMS

A large number of drugs of plant origin are to be found in this group. As infections of the respiratory tract are amongst the most common of illnesses, it is not surprising that there are numerous proprietary preparations for their treatment (Table 6.5).

THE LIVER

The liver, the principal organ of metabolism and excretion, is subject to a number of diseases which may be classed as liver cirrhosis (cell destruction and increase in fibrous tissue), acute or chronic hepatitis (inflammatory disease) and hepatitis (non-inflammatory condition). The most common drug of plant origin used in Western medicine for its antihepatotoxic properties is *Silybum marianum*. In Indian and Oriental medicine many plants are so used. For a discussion of this field of current interest see Chapter 29.

THE URINARY AND REPRODUCTIVE SYSTEMS

A number of plant materials are to be found in this group; the examples given in Table 6.6 are confined to Western usage.

THE SKIN AND MUCOUS MEMBRANES

In addition to acting as covering for the body, the skin performs a number of other physiological functions. Drugs affecting the skin may be of an emollient nature or they may act as absorbents, astringents, irritants or antiseptics (see Table 6.7). A number of substances are easily absorbed through the skin; this fact is utilized in transdermal medication but must also be borne in mind with respect to various poisons.

Table 6.5 Drugs acting on the nasal and respiratory systems.

Aromatic inhalations	Benzoin, cineole, eucalyptus oil, menthol and peppermint, pumilo pine oil, balsam of Tolu, thymol, turpentine, menthol, eucalyptus
Bronchodilators and nasal decongestants	Ephedra, ephedrine, xanthines (theophylline)
Expectorants	Ipecacuanha (in subemetic doses), senega root, liquorice root, squill bulb, tolu balsam, pulmilio pine oil, lobelia, grindelia, angelica root and leaf, storax, cocillana, coltsfoot, sweet violet, bloodroot, balm of Gilead
Antiexpectorants	Codeine, atropine
Cough depressants	Morphine, codeine, noscapine, wild cherry
Demulcents	Marshmallow, verbascum, plantago, Iceland moss, honey

6

Table 6.6 Drugs acting on the urinary and reproductive systems.

Diuretics	Xanthine derivatives as present in many beverages (tea, coffee, etc.) promote dilation of the renal medullary blood vessels. Digitalis glycosides improve the failing heart thereby increasing renal perfusion and glomerular filtration; hence, Withering's original introduction of digitalis for the treatment of dropsy. There is also a small but finite effect on tubular reabsorption of sodium ions
Diuretics and urinary antiseptics	Buchu, boldo, horsetail, Java tea, bearberry, juniper, copaiba. These include drugs used for the treatment of cystitis and urethritis
Drugs acting on the uterus	Preparations of ergot were traditionally used in childbirth and then largely replaced by the isolated alkaloid ergometrine. Administered as its salts it has a direct stimulant action on the uterine muscle and reduces the incidence of postpartum haemorrhage. Ergotamine acts similarly but is not suitable for obstetric use because of its marked peripheral vasoconstrictor action
	Black haw is a uterine tonic and sedative used for the prevention of miscarriage and for dysmenorrhoea after childbirth
	Hydrastis is employed for menorrhagia and other menstrual disorders
	Agnus castus has been traditionally employed for the treatment of menopausal disorders, premenstrual symptoms, dysmenorrhoea, etc.
Oral contraceptives	Female, see 'Steroids'. Male, gossypol (q.v.)
	Numerous plants have been, and are being, tested for antifertility activity
Male impotence	Papaverine (under careful medical supervision), yohimbine (erectile dysfunction)
Benign prostate hyperplasia (BPH)	A number of phytomedicinals are employed (often as admixtures) to treat the symptoms of BPH. Two metabolites associated with the condition are dihydrotestosterone and oestrogen which require two enzymes (5α-reductase and aromatase) for their synthesis in the body. It has been shown, for some of the drugs used, that they are inhibitors of these two enzymes. The following examples are well-established: *Cucurbita pepo* seeds (pumpkin), *Epilobium angustifolium* and other species, *Prunus africana* (*Pygeum africanum*) bark, *Serenoa repens* fruits (saw palmetto, sabal), *Urtica dioica* and *U. urens* root extracts

Table 6.7 Drugs used on the skin and mucous membranes.

Emollients and demulcents	These include a number of vehicles used in the preparation of ointments, creams, lotions, etc., and include fixed oils (e.g. olive, arachis, coconut, theobroma), fats (wool-fat, lard), waxes of animal origin (beeswax, spermaceti), gums (acacia, tragacanth) and mucilages (psyllium, elmbark)
Absorbents	Starch, alginates, charcoal
Astringents	Tannins (e.g. Tannic acid), krameria, catechu, galls, *Aspidosperma*, hamamelis, pomegranate rind, kinos
Counter-irritants	Camphor, turpentine, capsicum, aconite, methyl salicylate, mustard seed
Antiseptics	Tars, eucalyptus oil, thyme oil, eugenol, thymol, cajuput
Anti-inflammatory agents	Corticosteroids used locally, matricaria, arnica
Psoriasis and eczema treatment	Comfrey, allantoin, cadeoil, evening primrose oil, chrysarobin, *Lithospermum*, savin, myrrh, grindelia
Wound coverings	Type of wound covering (occlusive, non-occlusive, haemostatic) is important in the healing process. See alginates, cotton, etc.

STEROIDS AND ANTI-INFLAMMATORY DRUGS

Two types of corticosteroidal hormone are the glucocorticoids, which regulate carbohydrate and protein metabolism and which also possess a strong anti-inflammatory action, and the mineralocorticoids, which influence the electrolyte and water balance of the body. The clinical indications for systemic treatment with these drugs are complex, but include use in replacement therapy, Addison's disease, reduction of lymphatic tissues (leukaemias), suppression of lymphopoiesis (lymphomas) and as anti-inflammatory agents (a variety of conditions including rheumatoid arthritis, cerebral oedema and raised intracranial pressure).

These hormones are produced naturally in the adrenal cortex but a wide variety of semi-synthetic drugs of this type is commonly in use. These are synthesized using plant steroids as intermediates; diosgenin and hecogenin being the principal sources. To a lesser extent the steroidal alkaloids of the Solanaceae are employed. There is a large world demand for these compounds, particularly for the synthesis of oral contraceptives, and their distribution in nature and chemistry is considered in more detail in Chapter 23.

ACTION ON SUGAR METABOLISM

Many plants have been used in traditional systems of medicine for the oral treatment of diabetes and it is particularly important that Western practitioners be aware of any patients already taking such medication. Among the plants so used are karela fruit (*Momordica charantia*), cumin fruit, ginseng, *Teucrium oliverianum*, neem (*Azadirachta indica*), onion, *Aloe* spp., Job's tears (*Coix lachryma-jobi*) and *Galega officinalis*. For a discussion of the current position on plant-derived oral hypoglycaemic substances see Chapter 29.

NON-STEROIDAL ANTI-INFLAMMATORY DRUGS

Aspirin, first synthesized in 1853 by Carl Gerhardt, is still one of the most widely-used mild analgesic and non-steroidal anti-inflammatory drugs (NSAID). It had its medicinal origin in the salicylates and glycosides of willow bark, long used for the treatment of rheumatic diseases, gout and painful conditions of all types.

In view of the universal requirement for NSAIDs very many plants have been utilized for the purpose in traditional medicine and in recent years considerable research effort has been expended on their investigation.

Enzymes have been used to detect anti-inflammatory activity of plants—galangin, a flavonoid of *Alpinia officinarum* (Zingiberaceae; galangal rhizome) was found to be a cyclo-oxygenase inhibitor. Lipoxygenase inhibitors are present in *Spilanthes oleracea* (a S. American plant of the Compositae used for the treatment of rheumatic disorders) and also in *Echinacea purpurea* root, also Compositae, which contains a range of compounds including isobutylamides.

In a review of plants exhibiting anti-inflammatory activity Handa *et al.* (1992) cite that species of 96 genera belonging to 56 families are ascribed such activity.

In addition to the wide range of plants involved there is a similar diversity in the chemical nature of the active constituents. Flavonoids constitute one group widely associated with anti-inflammatory activity and are exemplified in the *BHP* (1996) by the monographs on Balm of Gilead Bud, Cimicifuga Rhizome, Equisetum, Jamaica Dogwood, Marigold, Matricaria Flowers, Meadowsweet, Poke Root, Red Clover Flower and Willow Bark. In the case of an infusion of matricaria flowers (*Chamomilla recutita*, German chamomile), used for its anti-inflammatory action in the treatment of acute gastritis, it has been shown by the mouse-ear test that it is the flavonoids and not the volatile oils that are responsible for activity; however, for *Calendula officinalis* the terpenoids were found to be active constituents (see Anon., *Pharm. J.*, 1992, **249**, 474). With liquorice root (*Glycyrrhiza glabra*) both the triterpenoid saponin glycyrrhizin and the flavonoids have, among their other pharmacological actions, anti-inflammatory activity.

Colchicine, an alkaloid of *Colchicum autumnale*, is the classical drug for the treatment of acute attack of gout. It may act by reducing the inflammatory response caused by deposits of urate crystals in the joint and by reduction of phagocytosis of the crystals. Its use has been somewhat replaced by allopurinol (inhibition of xanthine oxidase) and by phenylbutazone. Guaiacum resin (q.v) is cited for the treatment of chronic rheumatic conditions and gout; it contains a mixture of lignans. The dried root of *Harpagophytum procumbens* (Devil's claw) (Pedaliaceae), has recently received popular attention for the treatment of painful rheumatic conditions; iridoid glycosides, e.g. harpagoside, are the characteristic constituents. The juice of *Ananas comosus*, the pineapple (Bromeliaceae) contains a mixture of at least five proteolytic enzymes collectively called bromelin or bromelain. In Western medicine the enzyme has been introduced for its ability to dissolve fibrin in conditions of inflammatory oedema.

The action of ginkgolides (C_{20} terpenes from *Ginkgo biloba*) as potent antagonists of platelet activating factor has already been mentioned.

TREATMENT OF INFECTIONS

For natural products in this category, see Table 6.8.

TREATMENT OF MALIGNANT DISEASES

The last 50 years has witnessed a vast search of the plant kingdom for phytochemicals with anticancer activity, and medicaments derived from *Catharanthus*, *Taxus* and *Podophyllum* are among the most effective in current usage. Originally, most research centred on plants of Western origin but since 1986 focus has shifted towards the investigation of

Table 6.8 Drugs used for the treatment of infections.

Antibiotics Many higher plants possess constituents having antibacterial properties; none has been utilized clinically, mainly because of high toxicity. Moulds and streptomyces are the principal sources; see Chapter 30 for a consideration of antibacterial and antiviral drugs

Antimalarials Until the advent of the synthetic antimalarials, quinine, isolated from the bark of various *Cinchona* spp., constituted the most effective agent for the treatment of malaria; it is still used in Third World countries and is of some resurgent importance for combating malarial organisms resistant to other drugs. Artemisinin (Qinghaosa), an unusual sesquiterpene lactone, is the active constituent of an ancient Chinese drug derived from *Artemisia annua*. It is effective against chloroquine resistant strains of *Plasmodium vivax* and *P. falciparum* as well as against cerebral malaria; see Chapter 28

Amoebicides

Emetine	An alkaloid of ipecacuanha root, used as its hydrochloride or bismuthiodide in the treatment of amoebic dysentery. Complete eradication of the chronic infection is difficult and combined therapy with other drugs is often necessary

Anthelminthics

Extract of male fern	For tapeworm infections
Santonin	Possesses a powerful action in paralysing round-worms; although once extensively used its high toxicity has led to replacement by piperazine
Oil of Chenopodium	Like santonin; it has also been extensively used in hookworm disease but it gives variable results
Thymol	At one time much used in hookworm treatment

tropical and subtropical species. The introduction of new techniques designed to eliminate 'nuisance' compounds (see Chapter 9) has accelerated the process of screening many hundreds of specimens. Clinical trials continue on a number of promising compounds. For a fuller discussion, see Chapter 27.

TREATMENT OF ALLERGIES

A large number of materials give rise to allergic conditions in sensitive individuals. Extracts containing specific allergies are available as diagnostic kits or for desensitization. Examples of plant allergens are grass, flower and tree pollens, dried plants and moulds (see Chapter 39).

THE IMMUNE SYSTEM

Drugs affecting the immune system are termed immunomodulatory or adaptogenic. Some repress the system and are of value in, for example, preventing rejection of transplanted organs and others are stimulatory and can be used to help combat viral infections such as AIDS or assist in the treatment of cancer. Until relatively recently such herbal drugs were largely ignored by Western orthodox medicine, although they have always featured in traditional Chinese and Indian medicine in seeking to achieve homoestasis with regard to

6

bodily functions. Now, however, ginseng leads the market in herbal sales in Europe and the US and *Echinacea* spp., used by native N. American Indians, ranks around fifth in the US herb market sales and is widely used in Europe, with 800 preparations being quoted as available in Germany. For immunomodulators of Chinese origin see L.-H. Zhang *et al.*, *Phytotherapy Research*, 1995, **9**, 315, and for Indian drugs see A. A. Mungantiwar *et al.*, *J. Ethnopharmacology*, 1999, **65**, 125.

VITAMINS

These accessory food substances are considered in Chapter 31.

Further reading

Ghisalberti EL, Pennacchio M, Alexander E 1998 A review of drugs having cardiovascular activity (*nearly 400 refs*). Pharmaceutical Biology 36(4): 237–279

Handa SS, Chawla AS, Sharma AK 1992 Plants with anti-inflammatory activity (*a review with 278 references and 34 structural formulae*). Fitoterapia 63, 3

Wagner H (ed) 1999 Immunomodulatory agents from plants. Birkhauser Verlag, Basle

Williamson EM, Okpako DT, Evans FJ (eds) 1996 Pharmacological methods in phytotherapy research, Vol 1. Selection and pharmacological evaluation of plant material. John Wiley, Chichester

Wright CI, Van-Buren L, Kroner CI *et al* 2007 Herbal medicines as diuretics: a review of the scientific evidence. Journal of Ethnopharmacology 114(1): 1–31 (*around 120 references*)

7

Synergy and other interactions in phytomedicines

E. M. Williamson

The term 'synergy' (or synergism, from the Greek *syn-ergo*, meaning working together) refers to the phenomenon where two or more agents act together to produce an effect greater than would have been predicted from a consideration of individual contributions. Synergy is generally assumed to play a part in the effects of phytomedicines, and the use of combinations of herbs is fundamental to the philosophy of Western medical herbalism, traditional Chinese medicine (TCM) and Ayurveda. This attitude to their formulation and use differentiates herbal products from conventional medicines, even those originally obtained from plants. Modern phytomedicines are usually found as whole or semipurified extracts and should, ideally, be standardized for their active constituents, where known, to ensure clinical reproducibility. The likelihood of synergistic interactions is also recognized in reports from the European Pharmacopoeia Commission, where the most common type of extract, exemplified by *Hypericum perforatum*, is described as having 'constituents with known therapeutic or pharmacological activity which are not solely responsible for the overall clinical efficacy of the extract'. To complicate matters further, herbalists use preparations and mixtures that are not necessarily intended to target a particular organ, cell tissue or biochemical system. This kind of application has been described as the 'herbal shotgun' approach, as opposed to the 'silver bullet' method of conventional medicine, to distinguish the multitargeted approach of herbals from the single-target approach of synthetic drugs.

WHAT IS SYNERGY?

The term 'synergy' is now used very widely, and mainly inaccurately, to describe any kind of positive interaction between drugs. In pharmacology the term has a specific definition, but is often misapplied in practice. Whether an effect can truly be described as synergy, or is merely addition, is rarely established and evidence to prove it conclusively in herbal medicines is sparse. The opposite, antagonism, meaning 'working against', is a reduction in the overall expected effect. Put simply, both antagonism and synergism can be defined in relation to an additivity expectation, which can be calculated from the potency of individual mixture components. Synergism is an effect larger than additive, whereas antagonism is smaller than additive. There are two ways of calculating additivity expectations: dose addition and also independent action.

Interactions can also involve a potentiation of effects. The terms 'synergism', 'additivity' and 'antagonism' are applied to combinations where all components induce the effect of interest, whereas the term 'potentiation' should be applied where one or several 'inactive' compounds enhance or exacerbate the effect of other actives.

Synergy and other interactions can take place between the constituents of a single extract as well as in a mixture of herbs. Medical herbalists have always insisted that better results are obtained with whole plant extracts and combinations of these rather than with isolated compounds. TCM, in particular, uses complicated recipes and it has sometimes been thought that the inclusion of some herbs was unnecessary, but the rationale for such combinations is gaining increasing acceptance. A TCM herbal treatment for eczema was the subject of a clinical trial of 37 young patients (M. P. Sheehan and J. D. Atherton, *Br. J. Dermatol.*, 1992, **126**: 179–184), and investigations were carried out to identify the 'active constituent(s)' of the mixture. However, a programme of pharmacological tests failed to find a single active herb or compound: it was the herbal mixture that was so effective (J. D. Phillipson, reported in *European Phytotelegram*, 1994, **6**: 33–40).

MEASURING SYNERGY

Although the idea of synergy is easy to understand, the measurement of it is more problematic. It is fairly straightforward to identify synergy when one of the agents is inactive and a combination of this with an active agent produces an effect greater than that observed for the active alone (although this is more correctly termed potentiation), but difficulties in measurement arise when more than one (and there might easily be several) are active. Various methods for calculation have been devised over the years, but the following are now thought to be the most useful:

PREDICTION OF EFFECTS

Synergy is deemed present if the total effect of a combination is greater than would be predicted on the basis of expected additive effects of the mixture. Such additivity expectations can be derived from dose addition or independent action. Often, anticipated additivity is calculated by simply adding up the effects of individual mixture components, but this method can produce paradoxical and erroneous results and is therefore deemed unreliable (A. Kortenkamp and R. Altenburger, 1998; see legend for Fig. 7.1). The opposite applies for antagonism, which is observed less than would have been predicted.

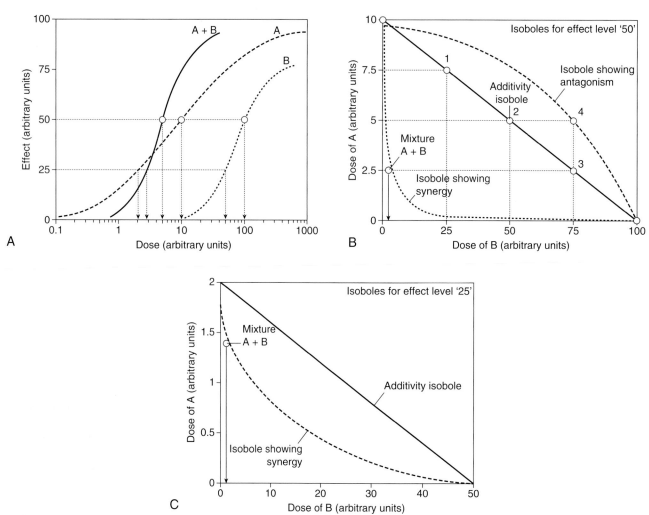

Fig. 7.1
An analysis of combination effects using the isobole method. A, Hypothetical dose–response curves for compounds A and B, and an equimolar mixture of A+B. An effect of 50 is produced by 10 (arbitrary) dose units of A or 100 dose units of B. The combination A+B yields this effect at 5 dose units (2.5 dose units A, 2.5 dose units B). Note that the curves for the individual compounds are dissimilar. B, Diagram showing isoboles for effect level '50' derived from Fig. 7.1A. The solid line (additivity isobole) joining 10 dose units on the A axis and 100 dose units on the B axis describes combinations of A and B that are expected to yield an effect level of '50', if the interaction between A and B is additive. For example, this should be the case with 7.5 dose units A plus 25 dose units B (point 1 on the additivity line), 5 dose units A plus 50 dose units B (point 2) or 2.5 dose units A plus 75 dose units B (point 3). However, the dose–response curves in Fig. 7.1A show that a combination of 2.5 dose units A and 2.5 dose units B is sufficient to produce this effect. Therefore a point below the additivity line is seen, yielding a concave-up isobole. It can be concluded that A and B interact with each other in a way that exacerbates their toxicity (synergism). Conversely, A and B antagonized each other if, e.g., 5 dose units of A plus 75 dose units of B were necessary to produce an effect level of 50 (open square 4). In this case, a point above the additivity line would appear, producing a concave-down isobole. C, Diagram showing isoboles for effect level '25' derived from Fig. 7.1A. (From A. Kortenkamp and R. Altenburger 1998 Synergisms with mixtures of xenoestrogens: a re-evaluation using the methods of isoboles. Science of the Total Environment 221(1): 59–73, with permission.)

THE ISOBOLE METHOD

The isobole method is an application of dose addition. It is unequivocal proof of synergy because it is independent of any knowledge of mechanisms and applies under most conditions. It makes no assumptions about the behaviour of each agent and is applicable to multiple components of up to three constituents, so can be applied to the analysis of effects in herbal mixtures. The isobole method uses graphs constructed to show curves (isoboles) describing combinations of two compounds, A and B, which produce the same specified action – which can be any measurable effect (Fig. 7.1A,B). The axes of the graph (Fig. 7.1B) represent doses of the two compounds on a linear scale. A line joining the iso-effective doses A and B of the single agents predicts the combinations of A and B that will yield the same effect, provided the interaction between A and B is only additive. This is the 'additivity line', in which case, there is no interaction between the two agents and they could be considered to be behaving like dilutions of each other.

For additivity (zero interaction), the relationship can be expressed algebraically by the equation of Berenbaum (*Pharmacol. Rev.*, 1989 **41**, 93–141; see Further reading):

$$d_A/D_A + d_B/D_B = 1$$

However, if synergy occurs, then smaller amounts are needed to produce the effect (i.e. the effect of the combination exceeds expectation) and the equation becomes $d_A/D_A + d_B/D_B < 1$, and the isobole is said to be 'concave-up'. The opposite applies for antagonism, and the equation becomes $d_A/D_A + d_B/D_B > 1$, producing a 'concave-down' isobole. It is actually possible to have synergy at a particular dose combination with antagonism at a different combination, and this would be reflected in the isobole. The position of isoboles varies depending on the effect level chosen for analysis (see Fig. 7.1B,C).

The isobole method can also be applied to mixtures in which only one of the two agents is active; in effect 'potentiation'. In this case, the iso-effective dose of the agent lacking activity can be regarded as being infinitely large, so the additivity isobole runs parallel to the respective dose axis. Synergism will again yield a concave-up isobole and antagonism a concave-down isobole, as shown in Fig. 7.2.

DEMONSTRATING SYNERGY AND POLYVALENT ACTION IN PHYTOMEDICINES

Proving the existence of true synergistic interactions, even within a single herbal extract, is remarkably difficult, and explains why this crucial aspect of herbal medicines is not well documented. To do so requires the extract to be fractionated, tested, recombined and retested in various permutations to see how each is interacting with the others. To complicate matters further, herbalists normally use mixtures of extracts, many of which are traditional combinations that are not necessarily intended to target a single biochemical system or enzyme (S. Y. Mills and K. Bone, *Principles and Practice of Phytotherapy*, Churchill Livingstone, 2000), making evaluation of additive or synergistic effects even more difficult. Simple examples of this practice would be the inclusion of laxative herbs in products used for haemorrhoids, or choleretic herbs in digestive preparations. This is not synergy but a way of approaching treatment from several angles concurrently, and could be described as 'polyvalent action'. This term is used to cover the various effects of multiple active constituents acting in combination, in harmony and possibly in synergy. It therefore overcomes some of the problems of defining the overall effect as synergistic even when it includes antagonism, if that applies to a reduction of undesir-

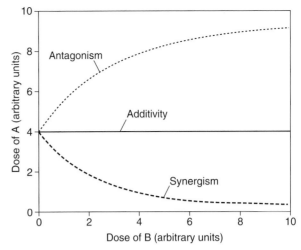

Fig. 7.2
The three types of combination effect for a mixture of an effective agent A and an ineffective compound B. When there is no interaction between A and B, the isobole is a straight line parallel to the dose axis of B (additivity). If there is a synergistic interaction, an isobole deviating towards the B axis is seen: in the presence of B smaller doses of A are sufficient to produce a predetermined effect. When there is antagonism, the isobole deviates away from the B axis. In this case, the presence of B requires higher doses of A to yield the same effect as in the absence of B. (From: A. Kortenkamp and R. Altenburger 1998 Synergisms with mixtures of xenoestrogens: a re-evaluation using the methods of isoboles. Science of the Total Environment 221(1): 59–73, with permission.)

able effects. As a preliminary step in looking for synergistic interactions, it is possible to test the effect of individual extracts singly and in combination, which will give an indication of synergy or antagonism although no real evidence as to which compounds are interacting.

In conventional medicine it is now common practice to use several drugs to treat a single complaint, such as in hypertension, psychoses and especially cancer, and this approach applies even more to plant extracts, because combinations are already present within the plant. There might be other sound reasons for not isolating individual components in some herbs such as ginkgo, St John's wort and ginseng, because these are traditionally used as standardized extracts for which there is positive clinical data. In some cases, the active ingredients may not even be fully known, and if synergy is involved, then bioassay-led fractionation (the usual method for identifying actives) would not even be possible (see P. Houghton, *Phytother. Res.*, 2000, **14**(6): 419–423). The identities of the main actives of many important herbs are still under discussion, and it would be unwise to exclude, by overpurification, any constituents that might contribute to efficacy. Even if the phytochemistry of a plant is well documented, the actual contribution of individual components to the overall effect might not have been ascertained. Examples include hawthorn (*Crataegus oxycantha*) as a cardiac tonic, hops (*Humulus lupulus*) as a sedative, black cohosh (*Cimifuga racemosa*) and chasteberry (*Vitex agnus-castus*) as hormone-balancing agents in women, saw palmetto (*Serenoa repens*) as an antiandrogen for prostatic hyperplasia, and devil's claw (*Harpagophytum procumbens*) as an anti-inflammatory agent. In other cases, the actives are unstable, and attempts to remove them from the 'protection' of the herb or whole extract could render them inactive. Here the obvious examples are garlic (*Allium sativum*) and valerian (*Valeriana* spp.). Garlic is often formulated as a product containing the precursor alliin, and the enzyme alliinase, which in solution (i.e. in the stomach) liberates the active allicin and other unstable, but still active, decomposition products. This is not synergy but, effectively, a drug-delivery system.

Interactions *in vivo* might also occur between combinations that enhance or hinder therapeutic activity by affecting absorption, metabolism or excretion. Some of these can be seen *in vitro*, such as the complexing of plant polyphenols and tannins with many drugs, which could theoretically reduce their effectiveness. This does not seem to be a real problem, otherwise tea drinkers would find many of their prescribed medicines inactive. Other interactions will only be seen clinically, such as the effects of cytochrome P450 enzyme induction, which are only seen after a period of treatment.

ENHANCEMENT OR REDUCTION OF ABSORPTION OR BIOAVAILABILITY

TCM and Ayurvedic formulae often have herbs such as liquorice or pepper included specifically to reduce or increase bioavailability of other ingredients, and this can be considered a form of synergy. Liquorice (*Glycyrrhiza* spp.) features as a synergist in a great many multiherbal preparations in TCM and the reason for its inclusion has not always been apparent. *Glycyrrhiza* extracts are used for their antiulcer, anti-inflammatory and antihepatotoxic properties and the saponin glycyrrhizin (formerly considered to be the 'active' constituent) exhibits activity in all of these areas. However, so also do the flavones, isoflavones and chalcones, and glycyrrhizin is certainly responsible for the more serious side effects related to its corticosteroid-like activity (such as Cushing's syndrome) associated with ingestion of large amounts of liquorice. A study on the bioavailability of glycyrrhizin, when given on its own or as part of a liquorice-root extract, showed that absorption of glycyrrhizin is lower when taken in the form of an extract (G. Cantelli-Forti *et al.*, *Environ. Health Perspect.*, 1994, **102** Suppl. 9: 65–68). Although the sample size was small, when a similar experiment was carried out in rats the results were in agreement. The authors suggest that differences are due to an unspecified interaction taking place during intestinal absorption.

Ayurveda also uses fixed combinations of herbs, and an important ingredient of many recipes, some of which date back to 6000 BC, is 'Trikatu' (Sanskrit, meaning 'three acrids'). *Trikatu* is a mixture of black pepper, *Piper nigrum;* long pepper, *Piper longum;* and ginger, *Zingiber officinale* and a theory for its use has been proposed that involves enhancement of bioavailability, not only by *Trikatu*, but especially by the alkaloid piperine, which is found in many *Piper* species (R. K. Johri and U. Zutshi, *J. Ethnopharmacol.*, 1992, **37**: 85–91). The effects on bioavailability probably result from the fact that piperine is a potent inhibitor of drug metabolism. Piperine also inhibits glucuronidation of epigallocatechin gallate in the small intestine, as well as slowing

gastrointestinal transit, which would increase its availability and residence time in the intestine, allowing for greater absorption (J. D. Lambert *et al.*, *J. Nutr.*, 2004, **134**(8): 1948–1952). Another example is the co-administration of piperine and curcumin to humans and rats, which enhanced the bioavailability of curcumin by 2000% and 154%, respectively, due to inhibition of the glucuronidation of curcumin (G. Shoba *et al.*, *Planta Med.*, 1998, **64**(4): 353–356.)

EXAMPLES OF SYNERGY, POLYVALENT ACTION OR ANTAGONISM IN HERBAL MEDICINES

SYNERGISTIC EFFECTS DEMONSTRATED IN SINGLE PLANT EXTRACTS

Synergy between ginkgolides present in *Ginkgo biloba* in a platelet aggregation test

Most ginkgo preparations are standardized for their terpene lactone (ginkgolide) and flavonoid content, and although these groups of compounds have discrete modes of action, it is likely that they work together. Recently, synergy has been demonstrated between ginkgolides A and B using a platelet aggregation assay. This is shown in the graph (Fig. 7.3) of the results obtained from investigating synergy between ginkgolides A and B as antithrombotic agents (Table 7.1). This is clinically significant because it means that if the most effective ratio of

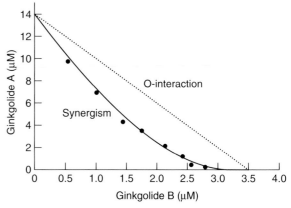

Fig 7.3
Synergy between ginkgolides A and B: the isobole drawn from values in Table 7.1. (From H. Wagner 2006 Multitarget therapy – the future of treatment for more than just functional dyspepsia. Phytomedicine 13: 122–129 with permission.)

Table 7.1 Synergy demonstrated by mixtures of ginkgolides A and B. IC$_{50}$ values of various ginkgolide A + B mixtures, obtained by an in-vitro platelet-aggregation test.

Mixture ratio GA:GB	IC$_{50}$ µg/ml	Concentration ginkgolide A		Concentration ginkgolide B	
		µg/ml	µM	µg/ml	µM
3:1	2.40	1.80	4.41	0.60	1.42
2:1	2.20	1.47	3.60	0.73	1.72
1:1	1.80	0.90	2.21	0.90	2.12
1:2	1.55	0.52	1.27	1.03	2.43
1:3	1.40	0.36	0.88	1.09	2.57
1:10	1.30	0.12	0.29	1.18	2.79

The IC$_{50}$ is the concentration causing a 50% inhibition of the platelet aggregation induced by platelet-activating factor (PAF) (n = 2–9).

ginkgolides is selected, a lower total dose of extract is needed. Ginkgo is used mainly for vascular insufficiency, especially in the brain, where it can result in impairment of cognition, and numerous studies have confirmed its efficacy. The effect can be partly related to the different constituents. The ginkgolides are diterpenes and are known to be platelet-activating factor (PAF) antagonists. Numerous studies have shown that the ginkgolides antagonize many of the effects of PAF, including inflammation, bronchoconstriction, bronchial hyperresponsiveness, platelet aggregation and allergic responses. The ginkgolides might thus contribute to the efficacy of ginkgo in cerebral insufficiency but may also produce some benefit in inflammatory disorders, including asthma. Ginkgo flavones are also anti-inflammatory, the combination being considered additive and possibly synergistic in effect, as well as increasing blood circulation to the brain, and a total ginkgo extract acts as an antioxidant activity in brain preparations. Clinical studies have shown ginkgo to be effective in improving cognitive function as well

as the early stages of dementia; the preparation used is a total extract not just the flavonoids. This suggests polyvalent as well as synergistic activity.

Potentiation of the effect of berberine by 5'-methoxyhydnocarpin in *Berberis* extract in prevention of bacterial resistance

Although this has been cited as a clear example of synergy between components of a single plant extract, it is more correctly termed potentiation. The phenomenon is demonstrated by a compound isolated from *Berberis fremontii* on the antimicrobial effects of berberine, another constituent, as shown in Fig. 7.4. Multidrug-resistance pumps (MDRs) protect bacteria from antimicrobials, and berberine is readily extruded by such MDRs. Several *Berberis* species were found also to synthesize an inhibitor of the norA (a membrane-associated efflux protein) MDR pump of a human pathogen *Staphylococcus aureus*. The inhibitor is

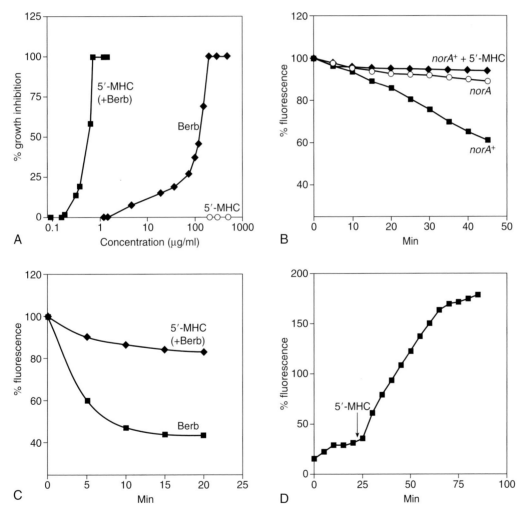

Fig. 7.4

Synergistic action of berberine and 5'-methoxyhydnocarpin (5'-MHC). A, Growth inhibition of *Staphylococcus aureus*. Berberine (Berb) was present at a concentration of 30 μg/ml when combined with 5'-MHC. Measurements were performed in triplicate, and the average values are shown. B, Inhibition of norA transport activity by 5'-MHC. *S. aureus* cells were loaded with ethidium bromide (EtdBr) and washed; the efflux was measured in the presence of 100 mM formate, a respiratory substrate. 5'-MHC was added at a final concentration of 10 μg/ml. C, Cells were loaded with berberine and efflux was measured in the presence of formate. D, Uptake of berberine added at time 0 by cells in the presence of formate. A small increase of fluorescence produced by 5'-MHC alone was subtracted from the plot. (From: F. R. Stermitz, P. Lorenz, J. N. Tawara, L. A. Zenewicz, K. Lewis 2000 Synergy in a medicinal plant: antimicrobial action of berberine potentiated by 5'-methoxyhydnocarpin, a multidrug pump inhibitor. Proceedings of the National Academy of Sciences of the USA 97(4): 1433–1437 (with permission). Copyright (2000) National Academy of Sciences, USA.)

5'-methoxyhydnocarpin (5'-MHC), originally found as a minor component of chaulmoogra oil. 5'-MHC had no antimicrobial activity alone but strongly potentiated the action of berberine and other norA substrates against *S. aureus*. MDR-dependent efflux of berberine and ethidium bromide (EtdBr; used for comparison because of its known mechanism of action and similarity in some properties to berberine) from *S. aureus* cells was completely inhibited by 5'-MHC. The level of accumulation of berberine in the cells was greatly increased in the presence of 5'-MHC, indicating that this compound effectively disabled the bacterial resistance mechanism. 5'-MHC has also been found to be present in *B. aquifolia* and *B. repens* suggesting that whole herbal extracts of these plants may have a superior antimicrobial effect to berberine alone where MDRs are involved (F. R. Stermitz *et al.*, *PNAS*, 2000, **97**(4): 1433–1437).

Enhancement of activity of Δ⁹–tetrahydrocannabinol in cannabis extract by other constituents

An example of the action of a known active compound being enhanced by the presence of other (inactive) compounds is shown by an experiment in which the antispastic effects of cannabis extract and isolated Δ^9-tetrahydrocannabinol (Δ^9-THC) were compared in an immunogenic model of multiple sclerosis. It can be seen from Fig. 7.5A that a cannabis extract (SCE) has a more rapid effect on relieving muscle spasticity than isolated Δ^9-THC at matched concentrations. Fig. 7.5B shows that the extract from which the Δ^9-THC has been removed (Δ^9-THC-free SCE) has no effect on spasticity, confirming that THC alone is responsible for the effect. The extract had been passed through a high-performance liquid chromatography preparative column, so to ensure that this had no effect on the effect of the extract, it was recombined to give extract TSCE, which had similar properties to SCE in the biological model (J. D. Wilkinson *et al.*, *J. Pharm. Pharmacol.*, 2003, **55**(12): 1687–1694).

ANTAGONISTIC OR OPPOSING EFFECTS DEMONSTRATED IN SINGLE PLANT EXTRACTS

Opposing effects on blood glucose levels of flavonoids in *Pterospartum tridentatum*

The isoflavonoid isoquercitrin and the flavonol sissotrin, both isolated from *Pterospartum tridentatum*, have been shown to have opposing actions on oral glucose tolerance in rats. The overall effect of the aqueous extract of *P. tridentatum* on blood glucose levels of normal rats given an oral glucose challenge was complex, in that it produced an antihyperglycaemic effect during the first 30 minutes, but subsequently blood glucose levels rose above those of control group (Fig. 7.6). This suggested the presence of compounds with different actions on glucose tolerance. An oral glucose tolerance test performed using isolated isoquercitrin and sissotrin, found these compounds to have opposing effects. Isoquercitrin showed a time-dependent antihyperglycaemic activity, by delaying the post-oral glucose load glycaemic peak, in a similar manner to the sodium-dependent glucose transporter inhibitor phloridzin (a flavonoid glucoside found in apples). By contrast, sissotrin produced an opposite effect by impairing glucose tolerance. These results show that the effect

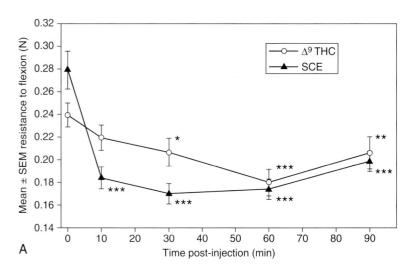

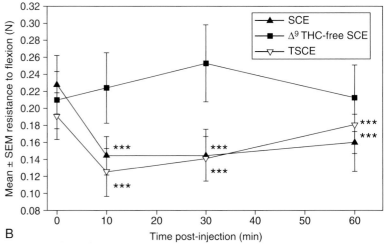

Fig 7.5
Effect of various cannabis extracts compared with isolated Δ⁹-tetrahydrocannabinol (Δ⁹-THC) on spasticity in an in-vivo model of multiple sclerosis.
Following the induction of chronic relapsing experimental allergic encephalomyelitis, spasticity of the hind limbs developed. This was measured by the resistance to full flexion of the hind limbs against a strain gauge before and following intravenous administration of: A, 1 mg/kg Δ⁹-THC and, 1 week later, in the same group of animals (n = 8 mice) with 5 mg/kg SCE (a cannabis extract) containing 20% Δ⁹-THC in vehicle; or B, 5 mg/kg SCE, Δ⁹-THC-free SCE and TSCE in the same group of animals (n = 6 mice), separated by at least 48 h. The data points represent mean ± SEM of resistance force (Newtons, N) of 12 individual spastic hind limbs in each experiment. *P < 0.05, **P < 0.01, ***P < 0.001 are significantly different means compared with baseline control of individual experiments. (From J. D. Wilkinson, B. J. Whalley, D. Baker, G. Pryce, S. Gibbons, A. Constanti, E. M. Williamson 2003 Medicinal cannabis: is Δ9THC responsible for all its effects? Journal of Pharmacy and Pharmacology 55(12): 1687–1694, with permission.)

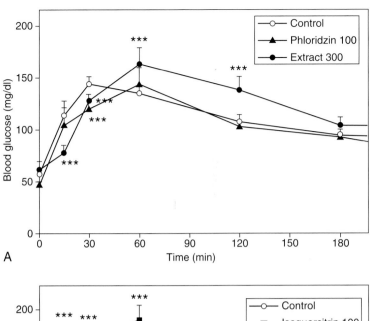

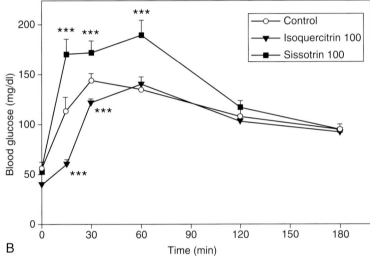

Fig 7.6
Opposing effects on blood glucose levels of flavonoids present in *Pterospartum tridentatum*.
Effect of (A) aqueous extract of *P. tridentatum* (300 mg/kg; n = 5) and phloridzin (100 mg/kg; n = 6); (B) isoquercitrin (100 mg/kg; n = 5) and sissotrin (100 mg/kg; n = 6) on oral glucose tolerance in normal Wistar rats compared with a control group (n = 6). * $P < 0.05$, ** $P < 0.01$, *** $P = 0.001$. (From: A. Paulo, S. Martins, P. Branco, T. Dias, C. Borges, A. Rodrigues *et al* 2008 The opposing effects of the flavonoids isoquercitrin and sissotrin, isolated from *Pterospartum tridentatum*, on oral glucose tolerance in rats. Phytotherapy Research, **22**(4), 539–543. © John Wiley & Sons Ltd. Reproduced with permission.)

of the extract on blood glucose may be either antihyperglycaemic or hyperglycaemic, and that it depends on the relative concentrations of isoquercitrin and sissotrin in the extract (A. Paulo *et al.*, *Phytother. Res.*, 2008, **22**(4), 539–543). This type of antagonism shows the importance of chemically characterizing an extract, because the relative flavonoid composition might vary among plant samples of the same species.

MULTIPLE PHARMACOLOGICAL EFFECTS DEMONSTRATED IN A SINGLE PLANT

Synergy and antagonism between compounds and fractions in Psyllium (ispaghula) husk

Psyllium husk, also known as ispaghula, is equally acceptable in traditional and modern medicine; it is also considered to be effective for use in both constipation and diarrhoea, which are two opposite disease states of the gut. The general perception is that its laxative effect is achieved mainly through its fibre content, which may be true, but what it makes more effective in chronic constipation than other fibre-containing remedies is not clear. However, evidence is now accumulating to suggest that it also contains constituents with gut-stimulatory properties, mediated partly through cholinergic activation, which is likely to supplement the laxative effect (A. H. Gilani *et al.*, *Phytother. Res.*, 1998, **12**(S1): S63–S65). Interestingly,

it also contains gut-inhibitory constituents, which not only are likely to offset the side effects associated with cholinergic components, but also provide a scientific explanation for the traditional use of ispaghula in diarrhoea (A. H. Gilani *et al.*, *Naunyn-Schmied. Arch. Pharmacol.*, 1998, **358**(S1): 40–73). In addition to gut-stimulatory and gut-inhibitory constituents, ispaghula also contains antiamoebic constituents, explaining its traditional use in amoebic dysentery (V. Zaman *et al.*, *Phytother. Res.*, 2002, **16**: 78–79), and thus demonstrating multiple effects, some supporting and some opposing a particular activity, in one medicinal plant.

SYNERGISTIC EFFECTS SHOWN BETWEEN TWO DIFFERENT PLANT EXTRACTS

Effect of soya and tea extracts on prostate tumour growth and angiogenesis in mice

A combination of a soya phytochemical concentrate (SPC) with tea extracts synergistically inhibited tumour growth and reduced serum concentrations of testosterone and dihydrotestosterone in a mouse model of androgen-sensitive human prostate cancer (Fig. 7.7). The inhibition of tumour progression was also associated with reduced tumour-cell proliferation and angiogenesis. SPC and black tea alone significantly reduced final tumour weights and, although green tea did

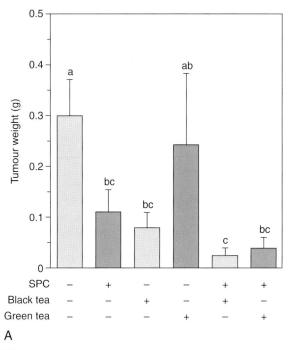

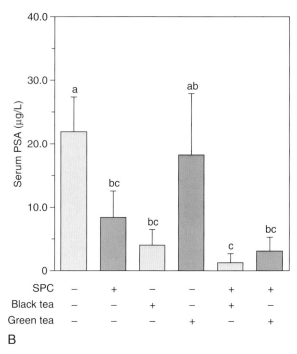

A

B

Fig. 7.7
Combined effects of soy phytochemicals and tea on final tumour weight and serum prostate-specific antigen (PSA) levels.
Effects of soy phytochemicals and tea combinations on final tumour weight (A) and serum prostate-specific antigen levels (B) in severe combined immune deficient (SCID) mice bearing LNCaP human prostate cancer cells. Compared with the control (Fig. 7.7A), all treatments other than green tea alone significantly reduced the final tumour weight. The combined effects of the soya phytochemical concentrate (SPC)/black tea combination (93%) and the SPC/green tea combination (88%) on final tumour weight reduction were greater than the expected additive effects (91% and 70%, respectively), suggesting that the combination of SPC with either black tea or green tea synergistically inhibited final tumour weight. In parallel, serum levels of PSA, a marker that is secreted by LNCaP cells and reflects tumour size, in mice in the experimental groups other than the green tea group were reduced (Fig. 7.7B), compared with the control. Comparisons of expected and observed values suggest that SPC combined with black tea or green tea synergistically reduced serum PSA concentration. Values are means ± SEM, n = 14–16. Means without a common letter differ, $P < 0.05$. (From: J.-R. Zhou, L. Yu, Y. Zhong, G. L. Blackburn 2003 Soy phytochemicals and tea bioactive components synergistically inhibit androgen-sensitive human prostate tumors in mice. Journal of Nutrition 133(2): 516–521, with permission.)

not reduce final tumour weight, it tended to elevate serum dihydrotestosterone concentrations. This study is significant because it supports the idea that the chemopreventive properties of the Asian diet might result from interactions between several components. In Asia, where the intake of soy products and tea consumption are very high, aggressive prostate cancer is significantly less prevalent than in other parts of the world.

NEW TECHNOLOGIES FOR LOOKING AT SYNERGY AND OTHER INTERACTIONS

One outcome of the recent development of informatics tools is the advancement of systems biology, which has the potential to revolutionize natural product research and scientific-based herbal medicine. The integration of data into systems biology can enable the understanding of living systems from a holistic perspective and facilitate the study of multitarget approaches. Evidence obtained from the new '-transcriptomic' technologies (genomics, proteomics and metabolomics) can hopefully support the identification of synergy and polyvalent pharmacological activities, as complex gene expression analysis by microarray can detect differences in cellular responses to drug combinations versus single agents (M. H. Cheok *et al.*, *Nat. Genet.*, 2003, **34**: 85–90). It could further demonstrate whether drug combinations can lead to the activation of entirely different genes to those activated by individual agents. Thus, the mode of action of a combination can

be, based on the gene expression, entirely different from the mode of action of the single agents contained in it. Although it is questionable whether the discriminating genes for treatment are the same as those responsible for the main action of the single agent, the method is still suitable for the discrimination of different treatments (see Further reading for reviews on the use of metabolomics and systems biology in research in phytomedicines).

CONCLUSION

There can be no doubt that most herbs rely for their effects on a variety of constituents, and the idea of synergy within and between them is also gaining acceptance. Whether they are acting in a truly synergistic way or by additive effects is not well documented, but it is important for both developing methods of standardization as well as furthering our knowledge of mechanisms of drug action. Clinical evaluation is also more difficult without knowing the extent to which synergy occurs within the herbal preparation, and it should be further investigated for all these reasons. In the meantime, evidence is accumulating to show that synergism does occur in extracts and mixtures, and that there is benefit in using whole extracts. However, it is still vital to ensure that extracts are standardized for the active principles known at the time and that any known synergistic interactions are taken into account. If done properly, this should lead to improved products with increased efficacy at lower doses and correspondingly reduced toxicity. Synergistic principles apply to all forms of drug treatment, not only those that are plant based, and although this is a well-known concept in phytotherapy, it is relatively new to other forms of conventional medicine.

Acknowledgement

The author wishes to thank Prof. Andreas Kortenkamp, University of London School of Pharmacy, for his expert advice on the different methods for the measurement of synergy.

Further reading
Synergy

Berenbaum MC 1989 What is synergy? Pharmacological Reviews 41: 93–141

Duke JA, Bogenschutz-Godwin MJ 1999 The synergy principle in plants, pathogens, insects, herbivores and humans. In: Kaufmann PB *et al* (eds) Natural products and plants. CRC Press, New York, pp. 183–205

Gilani AH, Atta-ur-Rahman 2005 Trends in ethnopharmacology. Journal of Ethnopharmacology 100: 43–49

Kortenkamp A, Altenburger R 1998 Synergisms with mixtures of xenoestrogens – a re-evaluation using the method of isoboles. Science of the Total Environment 221: 59–73

Wagner H 2001 Trends and challenges in phytomedicine: research in the new millennium. In: Yaniv Z, Bachrach U (eds) Handbook of medicinal plants. Haworth Medical Press, Binghamtown, NY, pp. 3–28

Williamson EM 2001 Synergy and other interactions in phytomedicines. Phytomedicine 8(5): 401–409

Metabolomics and systems biology

Ulrich-Merzenich G, Zeitler H, Jobs D, Panek D, Vetter H, Wagner H 2007 Application of the '-Omic-' technologies in phytomedicine. Phytomedicine 14: 70–82

Verpoorte R, Choi YH, Kim HK 2005 Ethnopharmacology and systems biology: a perfect holistic match. Journal of Ethnopharmacology 100: 53–56

Wang M, Lamers R-JAN, Korthout HAAJ, Nesselrooij JH, Witkamp RF, van der Heijden R *et al* 2005 Metabolomics in the context of systems biology: bridging traditional Chinese medicine and molecular pharmacology. Phytotherapy Research 19(3): 173–182

7

8

Traditional plant medicines as a source of new drugs

P. J. Houghton

DEFINITION

The scientific study of traditional plant medicines can be considered as a major part of ethnopharmacology, a term that was only introduced in 1967 but which describes an approach to the discovery of single biologically active molecules that has been used ever since the first compounds were isolated from plant material. Ethnopharmacology can be defined as the scientific study of materials used by ethnic and cultural groups as 'medicines'; in most instances, this is synonymous with the study of traditional medicines. These are usually the flowering plants, and so in most cases ethnopharmacology can be considered as a branch of ethnobotany: the study of the uses of plants by ethnic groups. However, it should be noted that some cultures, e.g. traditional Chinese medicine (TCM), also make use of animal and mineral matter, and so ethnopharmacology would also encompass the study of these.

Some discussion has taken place concerning the boundaries of what is meant by 'ethnic'. Some would include all ethnically based systems outside Western scientific medicine but the balance of opinion probably rests on a more restrictive definition, which includes only those bodies of knowledge that are restricted to a group that has lived in a locality for a long period of time but that does not have a sophisticated theoretical framework, formal education and a documented written history. This more rigid definition excludes the medical systems that have developed over thousands of years in cultures based in China and the Indian subcontinent, and emphasizes small ethnic groups where there is a threat of the rapid loss of knowledge due to globalization, loss of habitat migration and other factors that might lead to loss of cultural distinctiveness.

Some ethnographers would distinguish between folklore and ethnopharmacology, claiming that the former is common knowledge in the population as a whole, largely concerning remedies for minor conditions, based on relatively innocuous material. Ethnopharmacology is more concerned with the knowledge of a few specialists who are regarded by the society as able to correctly diagnose and treat disease states, generally using more potent products. In many situations, these specialists are also linked with the religious practices of the society.

It should also be noted that the discovery of new drugs might derive from a wider use of plants than for strictly medical purposes alone. Thus materials used as poisons, in pest control, in agriculture, as cosmetics, in fermentation processes and for religious purposes might also yield active substances that can be exploited as leads for drug development. It can thus be seen that ethnopharmacology is a very interdisciplinary subject and any thorough investigation will probably need the input of a variety of specialists, such as anthropologists, botanists, chemists and pharmacologists.

HISTORICAL DIMENSION

The isolation of some of the opium alkaloids in the early nineteenth century was a key event in the development of modern pharmacy. It showed that isolated compounds had much the same activity as the existing ethnopharmacological material and so paved the way for current orthodox Western medicine, which uses pure compounds for treatment. Since then, a vast amount of money has been spent on the synthesis of novel compounds but also on the isolation of molecules from natural sources and their development into medicines. The contribution of traditional plant medicines to this process has been significant and some notable examples are shown in Table 8.1.

It should also be remembered that the active molecules isolated from traditional medicinal plants might not only provide valuable drugs but

Table 8.1   Some common drugs originating from traditional medicinal plants.

Pharmaceutical	Structure	Plant source	Traditional use
Artemisinin (antimalarial)		Sweet wormwood *Artemisia annua*	In China for treating fever
Atropine (cholinergic blocker – used for dilating pupils and as gastrointestinal sedative)		Deadly nightshade *Atropa belladonna* and other Solanaceous drugs	Hallucinogenic brews in Europe, pupil enlargement in eye
Caffeine (CNS stimulant, diuretic)		Coffee *Coffea arabica*, Tea *Thea sinensis*	Stimulant drink or paste in Ethiopia (coffee), drink in China
Digoxin (anticardiac arrhythmia)		Foxgloves *Digitalis* spp.	*D. purpurea* leaves used in England and Wales for oedema due to congestive heart failure
Ephedrine (bronchial relaxant)		*Ephedra sinica* and other spp.	In China for respiratory complaints.
Ergometrine (contraction of uterus – used in childbirth)		Ergot *Claviceps purpurea*	In central Europe to aid childbirth

(Continued)

Table 8.1 Some common drugs originating from traditional medicinal plants. (Cont'd)

Pharmaceutical	Structure	Plant source	Traditional use
Galantamine (cholinesterase inhibitor, used to treat symptoms of Alzheimer's disease)		Snowdrop *Galanthus* spp.	In Balkans for muscle weakness
Pilocarpine (used to dilate pupils)		Jaborandi leaves *Pilocarpus jaborandi*	In Brazil to induce sweating
Reserpine (hypotensive, tranquillizer)		*Rauvolfia serpentina*	Extensively in Ayurvedic medicine (India) for mental illness
Scopolamine (Hyoscine) (CNS and gastrointestinal sedative)		Mandrake *Mandragora officinalis* and as for atropine	Preoperative sedative and analgesic, hallucinogenic preparations in many parts of the world

are also valuable as 'lead molecules', which might be modified chemically or serve as a template for the design of synthetic molecules incorporating the pharmacophore responsible for the activity. Examples of drugs having this origin are shown in Table 8.2.

Although the term 'drug discovery' is generally used to refer to the isolation of molecules with activity, it should also be remembered that there is increasing interest and recognition that a 'drug treatment' might consist of a mixture of compounds. This has always been the case for plant extracts (and most other natural substances), which contain several 'active ingredients'. It should be noted that such extracts, usually based on a reputed traditional use somewhere in the world, are being introduced and increasingly used as a complementary therapeutic approach in the West. A selection of common ones, together with their ethnopharmacological roots, is shown in Table 8.3.

Scientific interest in ethnopharmacology has increased over the last few years and this is reflected in the formation of the International Society for Ethnopharmacology in 1990 and the European Society for Ethnopharmacology at about the same time. Both of these groups hold regular meetings. Several scientific journals also publish papers on this topic, notably the *Journal of Ethnopharmacology*, founded in 1979. The 100th volume of this journal, published in 2005,

contains many useful 'state of the art' reviews on various aspects of ethnopharmacology.

This scientific interest is reflected by wider Western society, with its fascination with a much wider range of aspects of other cultures (e.g. dress, music, food, philosophy, as well as medicines) and this has been catalysed by large population migrations to the West and the relative ease of exposure to exotic cultures, which has been facilitated by large-scale international travel.

Although primarily concerned with human aspects, there has been a recent upsurge of interest in veterinary ethnopharmacology, i.e. methods and materials used to treat animals, particularly those important to the local economy as providers of food, transport and fibres. Other expansions from a strict definition of ethnopharmacology as being the study of medical practices include aspects of plants and other materials used in the diet, those used for ritualistic purposes, for poisons of various types, as cosmetics and as adjuncts to social gatherings. The increasingly blurred distinction between food and medicine, which has become a notable feature in 'Western' society, is a situation that has always been the case in other medical systems, such as Ayurveda and TCM, and it is now widely recognized that particular plants comprise part of the regular diet as much as for health maintenance as for

Table 8.2 Some important drugs developed from molecules found in traditional medicinal plants.

Drug	Structure	Template molecule, structure	Plant source and traditional use	Clinical use of drug
Atracurium (and other muscle relaxants)		Tubocurarine	*Chondodendron tomentosum* Paralysing dart poison from Guyana, north Brazil	Muscle relaxant during anaesthesia
Bromocryptine (also cabergoline, methysergide)		Ergotamine	*Claviceps purpurea* Used in central Europe to aid childbirth	Treatment of Parkinson's disease

Table 8.2 Some important drugs developed from molecules found in traditional medicinal plants. (Cont'd)

Drug	Structure	Template molecule, structure	Plant source and traditional use	Clinical use of drug
Dextromethorphan		Morphine	Papaver somniferum Analgesic, soporific from Mediterranean region	Cough suppressant Analgesic
Pethidine				
Etoposide		Podophyllotoxin	Podophyllum peltatum Used as purgative and wart treatment by native North Americans	Anticancer
Metformin		Galegine	Galega officinalis Used to treat diabetes in Europe	Antidiabetic in type 2 diabetes

Neostigmine

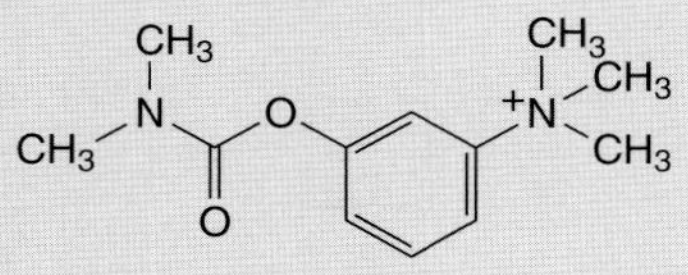

Rivastigmine

Sodium cromoglycate

2Na+

Verapamil

Physostigmine

Physostigma venenosum

Treatment of myasthenia gravis

Treatment of early symptoms of Alzheimer's disease

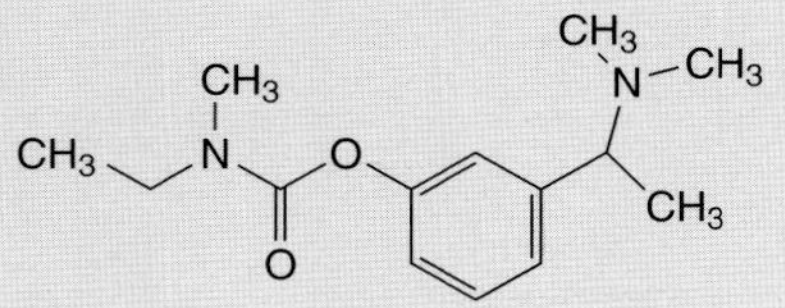

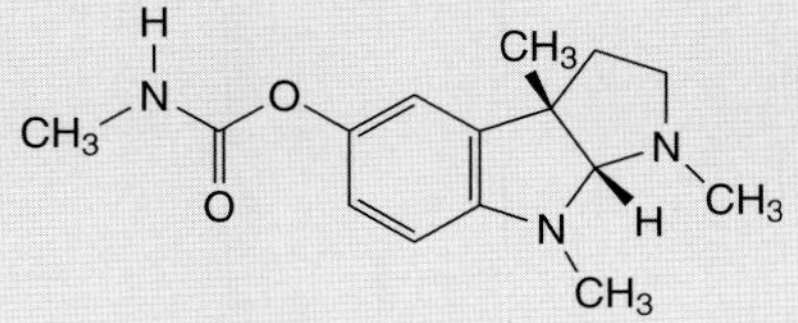

Ordeal poison from West Africa

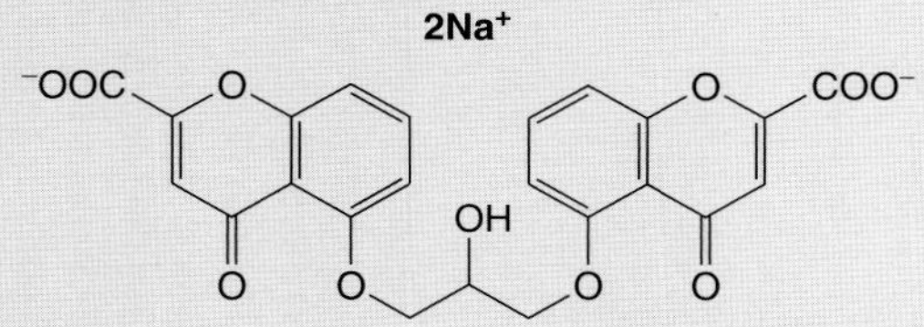

Khellin

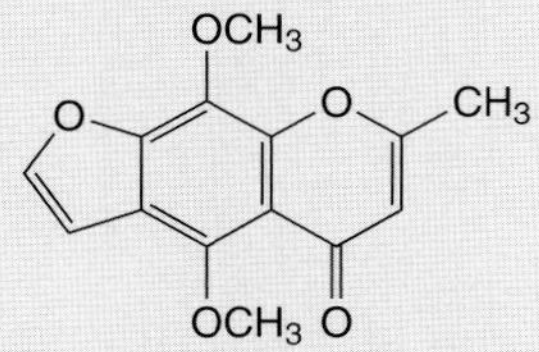

Ammi visnaga
Treatment of bronchial complaints in Egypt

Antiasthmatic

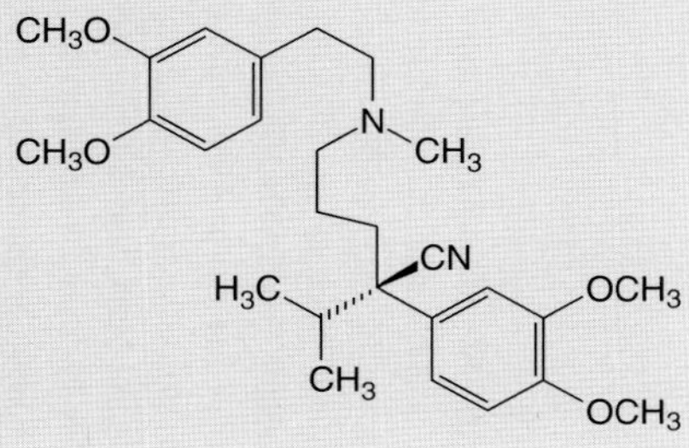

Papaverine

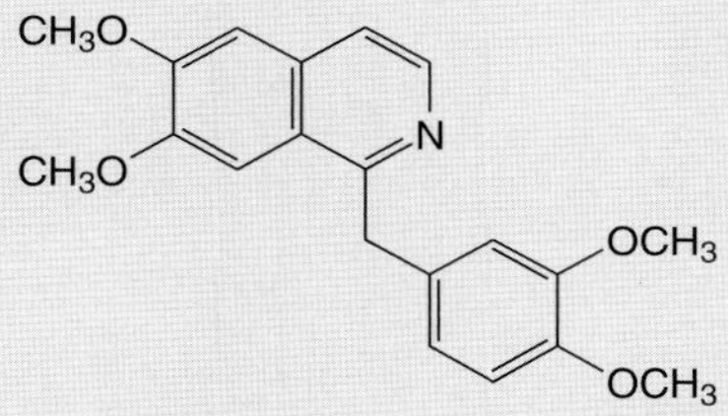

Papaver somniferum
Analgesic, soporific from Mediterranean region

Angina and anticardiac arrhythmia

8

Table 8.3 Ethnopharmacological origins (other then Europe) of some common herbal 'medicines'.

Herbal 'medicine' and botanical source	Current use	Geographical source	Traditional use (if different)
African prune bark *Pygeum africanum*	To reduce benign prostatic hyperplasia	Central African highlands	
Ashwagandha *Withania somniferum* roots	To enhance memory, general tonic	India	'Rasayana' general tonic
Black cohosh *Cimicifuga racemosa* roots	Depression associated with menstrual cycle and menopause	North America	Arthritis, neuralgia, menstruation disorders
Cat's claw *Uncaria tomentosa*. *U. guianensis* roots, stem bark, leaves	Rheumatism	Amazon area of South America	Antirheumatic and to treat infections and tumours
Dan shen, Chinese sage *Salvia miltiorrhiza* roots	Cardiovascular and cerebrovascular disease including ischaemic stroke	China	Cardiovascular diseases and cognitive decline
Devil's claw *Harpagophytum procumbens* fruit	Rheumatism	South-west Africa (Kalahari desert)	Purgative and for treating ulcers and boils
Dong quai *Angelica sinensis* root	Menopausal symptoms	China	Irregular menstruation, blood deficiency
Echinacea *Echinacea angustifolia*, *E. purpurea*, *E. pallida* roots and aerial parts	Common cold and other respiratory infections	North America	Anti-infective and to treat snakebite
Eleutherococcus, Siberian ginseng *Eleutherococcus senticosus* roots	Relief of fatigue, general health	Siberia	To help cope with stress
Ginkgo *Ginkgo biloba* leaves	To reduce CNS effects of ageing	China	For bronchitis
Ginseng *Panax ginseng* root	Relief of fatigue, general health	China, Korea	
Golden seal *Hydrastis canadensis* roots	Catarrh, appetite and digestion stimulant	North America	Gastrointestinal and skin disorders
Gotu Kola, hydrocotyle *Centella asiatica* herb	Wound healing and skin conditions	India	Rheumatism and skin conditions
Guarana *Paullinia cupana* seed kernels	Tonic	Northern Amazon forest	Stimulant drink
Hoodia *Hoodia gordonii* stems	Obesity	Southern Africa	Used to prevent hunger
Karela *Momordica charantia*	Antidiabetic	India and Southeast Asia	
Kava *Piper methysticum* roots	Anxiolytic and tranquillizer	Tonga, Fiji	Social drink to aid relaxation, treatment for skin conditions
Lapacho, Pau d'Arco *Tabebuia avelladanae* (and other *Tabebuia* spp.) inner bark	Stimulation of immune system to prevent infections	Tropical South America	General tonic
Maca *Lepidium meyenii* tuber hypocotyl	Erectile dysfunction, menopausal symptoms	High Andes of South America	Aphrodisiac
Saw palmetto *Serenoa repens* fruits	To reduce benign prostatic hyperplasia	South-east USA	

their macronutritional properties. Attention has also been focused on the ways in which the role of a substance can change through time or as it is transferred from one culture to another. Thus, coffee was thought of as primarily medicinal when it was first introduced into northwest Europe in the seventeenth century, but quite rapidly became a beverage. It is also of interest that cultural restraints might minimize abuse of a substance in its indigenous context but that, when these restraints are removed as the plant begins to be used in another part of the world or society, it becomes a problem to that society. An example of this situation is seen with the abuse of kava-kava in Australia by aboriginal peoples, who do not have the framework of ritualistic use of these roots in the Pacific islands of Fiji and Tonga, where it originates.

Several recent surveys have shown that using ethnopharmacology as a basis of selecting species for screening results in a significant increase in the 'hit rate' for the discovery of novel active compounds compared with random collection of samples. It should be noted that several 'classical' drugs stated to have derived from ethnopharmacological investigations, e.g. several shown in Table 8.1, arise from plants known as poisons rather than those with a more 'gentle' action, which comprise the bulk of many herbal medicine species. The latter group often relies on a mixture of compounds with a mixture of activities, where synergism and polyvalence might be occurring, and where the isolation of one 'active constituent' is much less likely.

With a very large number of living organisms still awaiting scientific investigation (about 90% of the estimated 250,000 species of flowering plants, probably the most studied part of the biosphere), ethnopharmacology appears to offer a reasonable selective strategy to be considered in deciding which organisms to study. An interesting overview of some ethnopharmacologically based molecules and the problems involved in their gaining regulatory status was published recently (T. W. Corson and C. M. Crews, *Cell*, 2007, **130**: 769–774).

THE PROCESS OF MODERN DRUG DISCOVERY USING ETHNOPHARMACOLOGY

The discovery process is composed of several stages. The first stage must be the reported use of a naturally occurring material for some purpose that can be related to a medical use. Consideration of the cultural practices associated with the material is important in deciding possible bases of the reputed activity. If there is an indication of a genuine effect, then the material needs to be identified and characterized according to scientific nomenclature. It can then be collected for experimental studies, usually comprising tests for relevant biological activity linked with isolation and determination of the structure of any chemicals present that might be responsible. The 'active' compounds are usually discovered by several cycles of fractionation of the extract linked with testing for the activity of each fraction, until pure compounds are isolated from the active fractions, a process known as bioassay-guided fractionation. These compounds, once their activity is proven and their molecular structure ascertained, serve as the leads for the development of clinically useful products. These various stages are discussed in detail below.

INFORMATION SOURCES

The most reliable type of information arises from in-depth studies carried out by field workers, living in the particular community of a particular ethnic group, on the use of the local plants and other materials. This usually comprises frequent communication with the local population, preferably in their own language. In should be noted, however, that an extensive knowledge of traditional medicines might reside with only a few people and a focus on this group would yield greater results. However, many such people are often reluctant to give away knowledge, which is regarded as 'protected' in some way, and this is exacerbated by concern that such knowledge could be exploited by drug companies, with little or no return to the original possessors of this knowledge.

Although the in-depth approach is most valuable, the fact is that most of the drugs that have been developed have arisen from less rigorous observations as a by-product of conquest or colonization. Thus, the more enlightened members of the Spanish *conquistadores* of Central and South America noted the practices of the various native American groups; and members of the British and French colonial administrations, together with non-governmental groups such as Christian missionaries, catalogued the uses of plants in Africa.

Most of these observations cannot now be checked in any way at first-hand, because the authors are long dead, but their records, books and other documents have been left as sources of information. This also applies to cultures that have left some type of written record, so that information on materials used in medicine in ancient Egypt, Babylonia, India and China is available. A recent paper (E. J. Buenz *et al., Trends in Pharmacological Sciences*, 2004 **25**: 494–498) describes some recent advances in electronic scanning of ancient texts that make information retrieval much easier, although the difficulties of linguistics and identifying the plants mentioned are not minimized as obstacles in such research.

Before such knowledge can be investigated scientifically, the information provided will often need clarification and translation into scientific terms. Of particular importance is the correct identification of the species used, which can be very difficult due to a lack of, or poor quality, illustrations as well as language difficulties. However, data on the part used, time of collection, methods of preparation, formulation and application are also necessary as they all affect the nature and amount of any biologically active compounds. Any restrictions on use due to time of year may be important, as they can indicate low levels (leading to inefficacy) or high levels (with concomitant risk of toxicity) of active compounds. Similarly, any types of individual excluded from treatment might indicate groups at risk due to age, gender or occupation.

Definition of the disease state in Western medical terms might also not be easy if the information is derived from a culture in which concepts of disease cause and symptoms are very different. In many records, the condition treated is described by a symptom that might be due to a number of disease states, e.g. a headache might be due to stress, tiredness, migraine attack or a brain tumour. Conversely, a particular disease state might be characterized by a number of symptoms, all of which have to be addressed when searching for possible leads to treating that illness. Thus, as an example, when searching an inventory of plants with a view to selecting those used for diabetes, those used for treating excess urination, weakness and ulcers should be considered, especially if diabetes is not recognized as a distinct illness diagnosed by sweet-tasting urine. Unfortunately, these factors are often ignored in current research, when a statement that 'plant species X is used to treat illness Y by people living in Z' is considered to provide adequate ethnopharmacological information. Such vague statements do not take into account all the possible sources of variation of biological activity that must be considered before any investigation proceeds.

SCIENTIFIC INVESTIGATION

Extraction

The extract used for testing should approximate as closely as possible that obtained by the traditional process used. Much research that has been published on the chemistry and activity of medicinal species is not very relevant to the traditional uses because it has concentrated on extracts made with non-polar solvents, such as ether or chloroform, whereas polar solvents are most commonly used. In many cases these will be simple extractions with hot water but a variety of other solvents can be used, as well as various additives or treatment of the material before use (see Table 8.4). In most instances, however, it is likely that fairly polar compounds will be extracted, although the solubility of less polar substances might be elevated considerably due to solubilizing compounds, e.g. saponins, also being present. Thus, an aqueous extract of the antimalarial plant, *Artemisia annua,* contains appreciable levels of the major antimalarial sesquiterpene artemisinin, which on its own has very low solubility in water.

Tests for activity

In most instances of modern drug discovery carried out by industrial and academic research groups, a particular bioassay, or series of in-vitro bioassays, designed on the basis of the biochemistry or molecular biology of the disease, is used to test extracts. In these situations, ethnopharmacology has little relevance to the tests used except that it provides a number of screening samples selected on the basis of their traditional use for the disease in question. However, this approach is valuable in selecting plants for further investigation from a list of those with a local reputation of treating serious diseases and this has been applied in screening programmes to detect antimalarial, antituberculosis and antidiabetic activity. These are not necessarily aimed at providing new lead compounds for 'conventional' drugs but have the goal of providing a scientific basis for the more effective use of extracts and mixtures. The Global Initiative for Traditional Systems (GIFTS)

Table 8.4 Effect of pretreatment and extraction processes on plant constituents.

Treatment	Effect	Equivalent scientific process	Example from traditional medicines
Before extraction			
Roasting	Destruction of unwanted components	Heating at regulated temperature	Removal of toxic proteins from seeds of *Cassia occidentalis* (West Africa)
Soaking in water	Hydrolysis of glycosides	Boiling	Removal of cyanogenic glycosides from cassava
Storage	Enzymatic activity leading to formation of desired compounds or removal of unwanted compounds	Incubation with purified enzymes under standardized conditions	Formation of vanilla flavour Removal of toxic anthrones from cascara
Extraction process			
Water + ashes	Alkaline medium favours extraction of phenols and acids, slows release of alkaloids	Use of ammonia or dilute alkali	Traditional 'quid' used for coca 'chewing'. Used in 'paan', shredded Betel nut (*Areca catechu* seeds) wrapped in leaf of *Piper betel*
Water + acidic fruit juice	Favours extraction of alkaloids	Use of dilute acids	
Local alcoholic beverages	Extraction of less polar compounds	Dilute alcohol extraction	Many traditional tinctures
Animal fats or plant oils	Lipophilic compounds	Petrol or chloroform extraction	*Hypericum perforatum* oil extract for treating burns

of Health is one example. It arose from academia and cooperates with the Tropical Disease Research programme of the World Health Organization (WHO) in finding new antimalarials in a collaborative network of research, government and community organizations named RITAM, the Research Initiative on Traditional Antimalarial Methods.

In spite of the common use of in-vitro bioassays, ethnopharmacological research can adopt a different approach when a particular biological effect of the traditional medicine or poison has been noted but the causes are not known. This is often the case when historical data are consulted and ailments are described in terms of their symptoms rather than underlying causes (see above). The biological effect might be essentially toxicological, e.g. use of poisoned arrows, and so it is important to seek to ascertain the basis of the toxic effect.

The best type of test to verify a reputed activity (and any toxicity) is a well-designed clinical trial, but this does not lend itself to bioassay-guided fractionation! It has been argued that long-term use of a material in traditional medicine is a good indicator of therapeutic efficacy but many are cautious about making such claims, preferring the suggestion that a long history of use is more an indicator of lack of obvious toxicity. In-vivo animal models of disease states are the next-best approach but expense and ethical considerations preclude this type of experiment in many countries, particularly for a fractionation process.

Most test systems for biological activity therefore utilize in-vitro systems using animal tissue, cultured cells, cloned receptors or enzyme systems. Many tests have been developed in recent years, and these offer the opportunity to carry out large numbers of tests using small amounts of material in a short time and are, therefore, well-suited to bioassay-guided fractionation. To be of most value, the range of tests chosen should be closely related to the possible underlying causes of the disease, e.g. tests for the efficacy of a preparation for an inflammatory disease such as arthritis should encompass key mechanisms associated with the formation of the various mediators involved, such as the lipoxygenases and cyclooxygenases involved in eicosanoid synthe-

sis, histamine antagonists, secondary messenger systems such as the cytokine NFκB, as well as more general oxidation processes involving free radical damage. The advantages and disadvantages of in-vitro testing have been summarized in a paper presented at a recent meeting of the International Society for Ethnopharmacology (Houghton *et al.*, *J. Ethnopharmacol.*, 2007 **110**: 391–400).

It should be noted that biological testing for the traditional use might reveal a different, but nevertheless interesting, activity. Such was the case in the discovery of the anticancer compounds from *Catharanthus roseus*, a plant originally investigated because of its reputation in Jamaica as a treatment for diabetes. Deaths of animals treated with the extract were traced to dramatic reductions in leucocyte count, and it was from this that the application to treatment of leukaemic cancers was made.

Chemical examination

Chemical examination should be linked with tests for biological activity and it is probably only a happy accident of history that the many alkaloidal drugs were developed from traditional medicines, without the need for bioassay-guided fractionation, because the alkaloids were present in fairly high amounts and they were relatively easy to obtain in a purified state. For many other traditional medicines, where activity is not due to alkaloids, it has been much more difficult to separate the actives from all the other compounds. Chemotaxonomic considerations can often provide a reasoned guess to the nature of the active components and thus a short cut to their isolation. Thus, insecticidal or anti-inflammatory activity noted in a member of the Asteraceae could be ascribed to the sesquiterpene lactones that are present in many members of this family.

The presence of common classes of naturally occurring compounds can be screened by the use of appropriate chromogenic reagents after separation using thin-layer chromatography or by more sophisticated techniques, such as gas chromatography or liquid chromatography linked with mass spectrometry. These techniques are also valuable in dereplication, the process by which known active compounds present in the extract are detected, and so time is not wasted in a long bioassay-guided process that culminates in the 'discovery' of a well-known compound.

SOME MODERN EXAMPLES OF DRUG DISCOVERY BASED ON THE ETHNOPHARMACOLOGICAL APPROACH

SINGLE COMPOUNDS

Although the list of existing drugs introduced as a result of ethnopharmacological leads is impressive, some newer interesting examples of compounds arising from this approach have appeared in recent years, including galantamine and artemisinin (see Table 8.1). Others, which have attracted considerable research interest, are described below.

Prostratin

An ethnobotanical survey of Samoa carried out by the American Paul Cox in the late 1980s revealed the traditional use of a hot-water infusion of the stem wood of *Homalanthus nutans* for the viral disease yellow fever. Work carried out in conjunction with the National Cancer Institute in USA resulted in the isolation of a phorbol named prostratin, which was found to be effective against the killing of human host cells by HIV. Prostratin appeared to stimulate protein kinase C, which was a novel mode of action for an anti-HIV drug. Although extensive trials were commenced, prostratin has since been dropped from the anti-HIV drug development programme due to some toxic effects.

Flavopiridol

The bark of the Indian tree *Dysoxylum malabaricum* (Meliaceae) was traditionally used to treat arthritis and investigations into the related *D. binectariferum* provided rohitukine, a chromone alkaloid that exhibited anti-inflammatory activity in laboratory animals. Studies into the mechanism of action found that it was different from many other natural anti-inflammatory compounds in that it inhibited tyrosine kinase. A series of analogous compounds was developed to optimize the effect and the flavonoid derivative flavopiridol was shown to have superior activity. As numerous oncogenes encode for the production of protein with such kinase activity, inhibition might decrease tumour growth and this was found to be the case with flavopiridol, which is now in advanced stages of clinical testing as an anticancer agent.

Huperzine A

A tea from *Huperzia serrata,* a club moss, was a traditional drink for elderly people in several areas of China. Over the last twenty years, huperzine A, an alkaloid with cholinesterase inhibitory properties, has been isolated and shown to have significant beneficial effects on memory in patients. As memory appears to be impaired in patients with low levels of acetylcholine (ACh) in the brain, inhibition of the enzyme that degrades ACh will have the net effect of raising ACh levels and thereby improving memory. Huperzine A is in clinical use in China for treatment of elderly patients showing loss of memory and clinical trials in other countries are being planned.

PURIFIED AND STANDARDIZED EXTRACTS

There has been a renaissance of interest in using mixtures of compounds rather than single chemical entities in orthodox therapy (see Schmidt *et al.*, *Nature Chemical Biology*, 2007 **3**: 360–366); this has always been the approach in herbal systems of medicine. The acceptance of such products is still in its infancy as regards Western regulatory procedures but is at an advanced stage in some of the emerging economies such as India and China. Even in Western countries such as USA and UK, funds are being released by government agencies, non-profit-making funding organizations and industry for clinical trials of characterized and standardized extracts, practically all of them having an ethnopharmacological basis and many are from Asia. Some of the interesting products being investigated are listed in Table 8.5 but it should be noted that, in some cases, the compounds thought to be most active are also being investigated for use as single chemical drugs or as lead compounds for development of the same.

THE VALUE OF THE ETHNOPHARMACOLOGICAL APPROACH

EFFICACY AND SAFETY

The argument most often used to support the ethnopharmacological approach to drug discovery is the fact that a plant material has been used for generations in a particular culture. Lack of technological sophistication is not synonymous with a lack of appreciation of efficacy or safety and so it is likely that there would be no serious adverse effects associated with the regular use of the material. In many cases it has been shown that potential harm is minimized through a selected method of preparation of the material, by its administration being restricted to trained personnel (most commonly the 'medicine men (or women)' of the community), or by its being used in special ways, particularly by the addition of other materials that might decrease the toxicity by countering unwanted pharmacological effects or by altering the bioavailability or metabolism of the material. The addition of alkaline ash to coca leaves in the traditional method of 'chewing' them is a good example of this. The high pH favours the less water-soluble form of cocaine, so affecting its release into the saliva and uptake into the bloodstream, and possibly reducing the addictive potential.

ECONOMIC AND SOCIOPOLITICAL CONSIDERATIONS

Although not closely related to the process of 'drug discovery' by the industrially developed countries, the scientific validation of a local remedy from a developing country can encourage its use and introduction into therapy in its original habitat, or its growth and adoption as therapy in areas with similar growing conditions. Cultivation and production of extracts from such plants might be a substitute for more expensive Western drugs and medicines, especially in countries where healthcare resources are stretched.

A notable example of this is Plantas do Nordeste, a collaboration between the Royal Botanic Gardens Kew, UK, and a consortium of scientists and agriculturists in the impoverished region of north-eastern Brazil. The project has evaluated some of the local medicinal plants and promoted the cultivation of them across the region as an aspect of healthcare, together with the training of personnel in their use.

The possible validation of their traditional remedies by the scientific ethnopharmacological approach is also valuable in helping small ethnic groups retain or recover their sense of identity and value, especially when threatened by globalization and cultural imperialism by more politically or commercially powerful groups.

Table 8.5 Standardized herbal extracts under clinical investigation.

Botanical source (commercial name of extract)	Ethnopharmacological link	Clinical effect under investigation	Major active ingredients
Artemisia dracunculus Russian tarragon	Used as antidiabetic plant in Russia	Insulin resistance as a cause of diabetes	2,4-Dihydroxy-4-methoxydihydrochalcone
Cannabis sativa Indian hemp (Sativex®)	Used as an anaesthetic and analgesic in central Asia for many centuries	As analgesic and antispasmodic in multiple sclerosis	Tetrahydrocannabinol Cannabidiol
Capsicum annuum Chilli pepper	Used by Incas and Aztecs in America for coughs and bronchitis	As analgesic in arthritis and neuralgia	Capsaicin
Coix lachryma-jobi lijen, Job's tears (Kanglaite)	Used in TCM for various purposes	As adjuvant in anticancer chemotherapy	Not specified, may be fatty-acid derivatives
Ginkgo biloba Ginkgo	Used in TCM for asthma and bronchitis	As cognitive enhancer in old age and Alzheimer's disease	Ginkgolides, e.g. Biflavonoids, e.g.

Table 8.5 Standardized herbal extracts under clinical investigation. (Cont'd)

Botanical source (commercial name of extract)	Ethnopharmacological link	Clinical effect under investigation	Major active ingredients
Curcuma longa Haldi, Turmeric	Used in India as an anti-inflammatory in skin and gastrointestinal tract	Psoriasis, wound healing, anticancer, Alzheimer's disease	Curcumin
Tripterygium wilfordii Lei gong teng, Thunder God Vine	Used in TCM for inflammatory diseases	Rheumatoid arthritis	Triptolide Celastrol

TCM, traditional Chinese medicine.

PROBLEMS WITH THE ETHNOPHARMACOLOGICAL APPROACH

RELIABILITY OF INFORMATION

Some of the difficulties of obtaining accurate and reliable information have been discussed above. It should also be noted that the use of a plant might not be due to rational observation or experimental evidence, but instead be based on a subjective consideration. Probably the most notorious example of an irrational approach is the 'doctrine of signatures' whereby some sensory aspect of the plant was thought to indicate its medicinal usefulness, e.g. a plant with yellow juice might be considered for treating jaundice, one with heart-shaped leaves for cardiac complaints, etc. Although, in some cases, relevant activity has been found for plants identified in this way, these are usually the exceptions rather than the rule.

BIOLOGICAL VARIATION

On a scientific level, the chief concerns are the difficulty of knowing the chemical composition of a plant or its extract due to its complexity and also due to the variation caused by genetic or environmental factors. This complicates elucidation of the active compounds and also makes the activity of different batches less reliable. Indigenous knowledge often has subtle ways of distinguishing 'best' plant species or varieties and only thorough investigation will uncover the criteria used.

LOSS OF SPECIES

It is estimated that 25% of the flowering plant species of the world might become extinct within the first 25 years of the twenty-first century. Climate change, increasing population making demands on land and resources, as well as commercial exploitation of the environment all play a part in this and result in a loss of habitats. It is not unusual to record the presence of an interesting species in one locality only to return a few months later to find that the whole area has been cleared for some commercial activity. Although many ethnic groups in all parts of the world are affected, and most have a rich fund of knowledge about the medicinal uses of local organisms, it is probably those small groups in the centres of biodiversity, especially tropical rainforests, who are most vulnerable to irretrievable loss of species. Although the imminent extinction or increasing rarity of species are often promoted as a loss of potential new drugs for the developed world, it should be remembered that the local inhabitants could lose many of their basic affordable or available medicines.

In light of this, many medicinally important species have been subjected to some form of cultivation and, in several places, gardens of medicinal plants, formerly collected from the wild, are now being cultivated to provide local healers with species that they formerly collected from the wild.

LOSS OF KNOWLEDGE

The current opportunity to exploit ethnopharmacology might not last long. Whereas much concern has been quite rightly expressed over the

8

disappearance of the world's biodiversity and habitats, less attention has been paid to the threat to the immense wealth of knowledge about the medicinal uses of the local flora that exists amongst threatened ethnic groups. The irretrievable loss of large amounts of this knowledge is possible, due not only to the extinction of plant species due to climate change, urban expansion and destruction of habitat, but also to the breakdown in traditional societal structures of the transmission of such knowledge. The threat is especially acute in cultures in which information is oral rather than written, and is exacerbated by urban drift, particularly of young people, neglect of local materials, adoption of Western globalized products and health structures, and by war, famine and other causes of migration and consequent disruption of traditional society.

THE NEED FOR DEREPLICATION

Extracts from plants can show an interesting activity and, conventionally, this is followed by laborious, prolonged, bioassay-guided fractionation to isolate the compounds responsible. However, such considerable effort might result in the isolation of known compounds, or the activity might be found to be due to substances, such as polyphenols, which have a general inhibitory activity on many enzymes. This problem might be overcome by the use of dereplication procedures, whereby suspected known active compound types are removed by fractionation and purification procedures. Alternatively, active extracts and fractions can be examined by techniques, such as chromatography linked to mass spectrometry, which can afford substantial amounts of information about each component and data from the peaks obtained can be screened against a data library of known compounds.

INTELLECTUAL PROPERTY RIGHTS (IPR) ISSUES

The commercial aspects of the ethnopharmacological approach have aroused much controversy in recent years with regard to the intellectual property rights of the groups having the knowledge. Several international agreements, particularly the Rio Declaration and Convention of Biological Diversity (CBD) of 1992, have concentrated on sharing with the source countries the benefits and profits that might arise from the development of new drugs based on ethnopharmacological leads. The effect that such measures might have on their patent rights and returns from investment have been considered closely by pharmaceutical companies and some have decided not to take the risks involved. Some other companies, however, have been willing to sign agreements aimed at sharing profits directly or making substantial payments to countries in exchange for access to their flora for testing purposes.

CONCLUSION

The study of plants used in traditional medicine has received new impetus with the introduction of a wide variety of small-scale bioassay methods and improved methods for fractionation, isolation and characterization of compounds. In some cases, individual compounds responsible for the reputed activity have been isolated and used as lead molecules. However, it is also apparent that, in many cases, the observed effects seen in patients or animals are due to a mixture of constituents, perhaps each contributing a different biological effect to the overall activity. Thus it is likely that not only will traditional medicines continue to provide new molecules for drug discovery, but that they might also form the basis for the wider acceptance of crude extracts, in a standardized form, as another type of medicine in orthodox practice.

Further reading

Balick MJ, Cox PA 1997 Plants, people and culture: the science of ethnobotany. Freeman, London

Chadwick DJ, Marsh J (eds) 1994 Ethnobotany and the search for new drugs. Ciba Foundation Symposium 185, Wiley, Chichester, UK

Heinrich M, Barnes J, Gibbons S, Williamson EM 2004 Traditional systems of herbal medicine. In: Fundamentals of pharmacognosy and phytotherapy. Churchill Livingstone, Edinburgh, pp. 169–183

Journal of Ethnopharmacology 2005 Perspectives of ethnopharmacology. 100: issues 1–2

Lewis WH 2003 Ethnobotany in new drug discovery – a review. Economic Botany 57: 126–134

Phillipson JD, Anderson LA 1989 Ethnopharmacology and Western medicine. Journal of Ethnopharmacology 25: 61

Pieroni A, Price LL 2006 Eating and healing: traditional food as medicine. Haworth Medical Press, Binghamtown, NY

Prendergast HDV, Etkin NL, Harris Houghton PJ 1998 Plants for food and medicine. Royal Botanic Gardens, Kew, UK

Proceedings of the First International Congress of Ethnopharmacology, Strasbourg, 1990. Journal of Ethnopharmacology 1992 32: 1–235

Proceedings of the Second International Congress of Ethnopharmacology, Uppsala, 1992. Journal of Ethnopharmacology 1993 38: 89–225

9

Discovering new lead compounds in pharmaceutical research and development

*M. J. O'Neill and J. A. Lewis**

*Disclaimer: the information in this chapter represents the authors' personal views. In no way does it represent the views of GlaxoSmithKline.

Traditional remedies invariably involve crude plant extracts containing multiple chemical constituents, which vary in potency from highly active (e.g. *Digitalis* leaf) to very weak (e.g. cinnamon bark). By contrast, orthodox medicine relies heavily on single (or a very small number of) chemically well-characterized active ingredients exhibiting selective activities at, in many cases, well-characterized biological targets. These medicines are generally very potent and many exhibit fairly narrow windows between an effective and a toxic dose. Orthodox medicines are formulated into doses that are carefully standardized for bioavailability.

Compounds derived from higher plants continue to feature among the most widely used orthodox medicines we have today (*Martindale*, see Further reading). These include analgesic agents (e.g. morphine, codeine and the non-steroidal anti-inflammatory drugs based originally on the structure of salicin), antimalarial treatments (e.g. quinine), antitumour drugs (e.g. vincristine and taxol) and asthma therapies (e.g. cromoglycate). Other plant-derived compounds are currently being evaluated in pharmaceutical development, an example of which is artemisinin, an extract of the sweet wormwood plant (*Artemisia annua*), which is being assessed in combination with chlorproguanil and dapsone as a new antimalarial treatment.

In some cases, natural materials continue to be the only viable commercial source of the active compound. For example, GlaxoSmithKline harvests up to 10 000 metric tons dry weight of poppy capsule per year to provide a source of opiate alkaloids.

'High-throughput screening' (HTS) is a major strategy for the discovery of new lead chemicals in the pharmaceutical industry. HTS uses miniaturized assay formats, usually microtitre plates in which, for example, 384 or 1536 different samples can be assayed, in volumes of less than 50 and 5 μl, respectively in one run. Using sophisticated automation equipment, typically, hundreds of thousands of samples are screened against each biological target of interest every day: the final numbers for each usually being dictated by the overall cost of the assay, which can vary from < 1 p per well to > 20 p per well. Screening collection sizes range from 400 000 to over 4 million.

HTS is often portrayed, by people who know little about it, as an activity requiring very little intellectual input. The reality is that HTS is a complex process that demands an understanding of the role of specific biological targets in disease progression; the development of bioassays capable of discovering modulators of the target; the design, miniaturization and automation of bioassays (which are automation friendly); an understanding of the macro- and micro-structure of the biological target so that the sample selection strategy is optimized; the engineering of custom-built robots capable of storage, retrieval and bioassay of millions of samples per annum and the development of software systems that can enable scientists involved to make sense of the mass of data that emerges.

BIOLOGICAL ASSAYS AND HIGH-THROUGHPUT SCREENING

Ideal biological assays for screening are those that enable identification of compounds acting on specific biological targets, involve a minimum number of reagent addition steps, perform reliably and predictably, are easily amenable to miniaturization and automation, and involve low-cost ingredients and detection technology. Biochemical targets of interest in pharmaceutical lead discovery range from enzymes to receptors (nuclear and transmembrane) to ion channels and, in the case of infectious disease, to whole microorganism cells.

An example of a biological assay that has the characteristics needed in a good screen is the squalene synthase enzyme assay, which was

9

developed to look for inhibitors of squalene synthesis, a potential target for the identification of novel cholesterol lowering agents (Tait, 1992). Using either [1-^{14}C] isopentenyl diphosphate as a precursor for squalene or [2-^{14}C] farnesyl diphosphate as a direct substrate of squalene synthase, the production of radiolabelled squalene is determined after adsorption of assay mixtures onto silica gel thin-layer chromatography sheets and selective elution of the diphosphate precursors into a solution of sodium dodecyl sulfate at alkaline pH. The use of [2-^{14}C] farnesyl diphosphate, and of an endogenous oxygen consumption system (ascorbate/ascorbate oxidase) to prevent further metabolism of squalene, allows the method to be applied as a dedicated assay for squalene synthase activity. The assay can be readily operated in microtitre plate format, which allows 96 or 384 samples to be screened per plate. It can be deployed either in a quantitative, low-throughput mode or in a qualitative, high-throughput mode, which has proved to be resistant to interference by compounds other than selective inhibitors.

The endogenous neuropeptide bradykinin (BK) is implicated in the mediation of various types of pain in the mammalian CNS. Antagonism of bradykinin to its receptors is a potential target for the development of new analgesic agents. An assay has been devised to detect compounds that antagonize binding of radio-labelled bradykinin to BKII receptors expressed in Chinese hamster ovary (CHO) cells (Sampson *et al.*, 2000). Compounds under test are added to the wells of microtitre plates to which CHO cells have adhered. After incubation with radiolabelled bradykinin, the excess labelled ligand is removed by washing. The plates are then counted in a scintillation counter so as to assess binding of labelled bradykinin to the receptors expressed on the surfaces of the cells. This particular screen suffers interference from compounds that possess cytotoxicity through a variety of mechanisms. It is therefore essential to run follow-up control assays against other cell types to distinguish false positives.

In the infectious disease arena, it is still common to run high-throughput, whole-cell antifungal or antibacterial assays to detect samples that inhibit growth of the designated strain, e.g. *Candida albicans*, *Staphylococcus aureus*. Optical density or colour changes using a redox indicator are the most frequently used assay technologies. Assays in this therapeutic area may be mechanism based. For example, a *C. albicans* cell-free translation system using polyurethane as a synthetic template, has been established to search for compounds that inhibit fungal protein synthesis (Kinsman *et al.*, 1998).

Screening plant extracts for antitumour activity involves assays against a wide variety of cancer cell lines and mechanism-based *in vitro* targets, which have been documented extensively (Pezzuto, 1997). Among the most frequently used mechanism-based assays are those assessing activity against the biological targets of existing antitumour drugs, such as topoisomerases I and II, collagenase, tubulin binding and stabilization, endocrine hormone synthesis and androgen and oestrogen receptor binding. Mechanism-based assays often require sophisticated or expensive reagents: an assay for activity of DNA ligase I involves incubating plant extracts with recombinant human DNA ligase I cDNA and its radiolabelled substrate, and measuring uptake 5′-^{32}P labelled phosphomonoesters into alkaline-phosphatase-resistant diesters (Tan *et al.*, 1996).

SAMPLE AVAILABILITY FOR HIGH-THROUGHPUT SCREENING

During the 1980s and early 1990s, natural product samples were the mainstay of HTS programmes within the pharmaceutical industry, due at least in part to the lack of availability of large numbers of synthetically derived chemicals. Over recent years, this situation has changed dramatically. The highly competitive arena of drug discovery provides pharmaceutical companies with a clear incentive to be first to discover and patent new lead molecules. Thus, a range of technologies has evolved to facilitate ever-increasing numbers of samples to be rapidly generated and evaluated.

Most large pharmaceutical houses have built up a compound bank containing hundreds of thousands of chemical compounds, which reflect the chemistries of earlier medicines developed by the company. Chemical diversity in these collections can be supplemented by acquisition of new compound types from the growing ranks of specialist compound vendors. Computational modelling techniques are utilized to generate sets of specific interest for given biological targets. Methods are available for electronically filtering out 'undesirable' compounds and techniques such as pharmacophore analysis, two- or three-dimensional structure searching or chemical clustering can be used to derive sets of the required size. Ready access to these compound collections is facilitated by the use of robotic storage and retrieval facilities, which can present the samples in formats appropriate for HTS bioassays.

Combinatorial chemistry techniques are widely applied in the drug-discovery process, especially for generating large numbers of compounds for lead discovery and in the optimization of lead compounds. Using robotic systems, tens of thousands of compounds can be synthesized from a small number of reagents in a few days. To date, however, it appears that the most successful of these compound libraries, in terms of yielding interesting bioactive molecules, have utilized focused chemistry based on structural knowledge of the biological target and the pharmacophoric features required to affect it.

To supplement the chemical diversity of the compound banks and the chemically focused combinatorial libraries, a number of pharmaceutical companies continue to screen natural extracts. Historically, large collections of microbial organisms (notably fungi and filamentous bacteria) were built up from a diversity of environmental niches and emphasis was placed on the development of a range of fermentation conditions capable of eliciting the microbes to produce a variety of secondary metabolites. The extracts generated for HTS from this source can be reproduced on demand, should further studies on bioactivity of interest be required. In particular, industry found microbial fermentations to be a prolific source of antibiotics. More recently, from the same source, valuable immunosuppressant drugs and lipid-lowering agents have been added to the medicine chest.

Plant samples also feature in the HTS programmes of a small number of pharmaceutical discovery organizations. The feasibility of using plants in a drug-discovery programme depends on ensuring that effective procurement strategies are in place to source both the primary material and additional supplies should these be required.

SELECTING SAMPLES FOR SCREENING

Advances in screening technology have increased the throughput capacity of an average HTS from tens of thousands of samples to hundreds of thousands of samples over the last decade. Even so, the availability of so many samples for HTS means that choices might need to be made about the most appropriate sub-set of samples for each particular target. The sample selection strategy may then be 'diversity-based', i.e. samples are chosen to represent as wide a spectrum of chemical diversity as possible, or 'focused', i.e. the samples represent specific chemical types only.

Both strategies are likely to play a role in a pharmaceutical company's methodology. Diversity screening may yield an unexpected interaction between a compound and a biological target, although the question of what constitutes 'representative' chemical diversity in the vast area of potential chemical space remains unanswered. Focused screening requires a large amount of prior information about a target, and this might not always be available. A combination of both approaches may be adopted. Computational methodologies for hit identification are continuously being developed. For example, compound databases enabling three-dimensional chemical structure searching are often used. If there are known ligands for a target, these can be used to construct a pharmacophore, which can then be utilized to search further chemical databases and select molecules with desired features. Chemical clustering can be used to derive sets of the required size. In the case of combinatorial chemistry-derived libraries, targeted sets can be generated with desired chemical properties, by using appropriately selected chemical building blocks. Natural products offer a potentially infinite source of chemical diversity unmatched by synthetic or combinatorially derived compound collections (Strohl, 2000), thus making them a desirable tool for diversity based screening. If a focused strategy is adopted, however, it is necessary to develop different techniques for natural product sample selection in order that the most appropriate samples are accessed for relevant targets.

The United Nations Convention on Biological Diversity (CBD) of 1992 has, to date, 191 parties, including 168 signatories (see its website http://www.cbd.int and the references therein). The key objectives of the Convention are to ensure the conservation of biological diversity, the sustainable use of natural resources and to implement fair and equitable sharing of benefits. Within the framework of the Convention are the concepts of the sovereignty of states over genetic resources and their obligation to facilitate access. The contracting parties are expected to establish measures for benefit sharing in the event of commercial utilization. This involves collaboration between the collector, the source country and the commercial partner. It is now normal practice to draw up a legal agreement to cover these issues and many companies have issued policy statements relating to this area.

As an example, a statement on GlaxoSmithKline's website (http://www.gsk.com) describes how a pharmaceutical company addresses such issues. The policy recognizes the importance of matters considered at Rio and subsequent meetings of the Congress of the Parties and goes on to state that GlaxoSmithKline will collaborate only with organizations that can demonstrate both the expertise and the authority to supply natural materials. Only relatively small quantities of plant material are collected, from sustainable sources. GlaxoSmithKline supports the CBD's role in providing a framework for the conservation of biological diversity and the sustainable use of its components and the CBD objective 'to provide fair and equitable sharing of the benefits arising from the use of genetic resources'. GlaxoSmithKline further supports the approach laid down in the CBD and in the Bonn Guidelines of leaving it to national governments to determine the conditions under which access to genetic resources should be given and for the parties concerned mutually to agree on the benefits to be shared. Agreements will cover such matters as the permitted use of the resources and the nature and timing of any benefits that are to be shared. This approach allows national governments the flexibility to determine what rules will best serve their national interests and allows the stakeholders involved to reach agreement appropriate to each particular case.

STRATEGIES FOR THE SELECTION OF PLANT MATERIAL FOR HIGH-THROUGHPUT SCREENING

Before a decision is made on what natural materials will be evaluated in a given screen, it is essential to gather some information on whether a target is indeed appropriate for input of natural product extracts.

For example, if the biological target is very highly tractable, if there are significant time constraints and cost of goods issues, and if data suggest it is likely to be relatively straightforward to obtain synthetically derived, small-molecule lead compounds then it might be inappropriate to screen natural products against that target. However, if a target is of a class where it is difficult to find small molecule hits, e.g. involving protein–protein interactions, or if there is a strong precedent or rationale for natural-product-derived actives, then natural product input should be considered. The latter may be exemplified by, for example, the antimicrobial area, where the track record of drug discovery from microbial sources is beyond dispute. The same rationale would apply to the superb track record of plant species in yielding analgesic medicines.

If the target appears to be suitable for natural product input, the sample selection for the screen needs to be considered. Various strategies can be adopted, depending on the extent of the available natural materials collections and on the capacity and 'robustness' of the target itself.

Some companies have access to large and diverse natural materials collections. Such collections are likely to include samples acquired to add diversity to the potential collection (and inherent in the desire for taxonomic diversity is the assumption that this will be reflected in chemical diversity of extracts subsequently generated). Most collections will also include samples particularly selected for various reasons, e.g. a microbial producer of a given compound or a plant used ethnomedically for a given condition. These large collections probably still only reflect a fraction of the world's potential biodiversity. It has been estimated that only around 70 000 fungal species are known, out of an estimated 1 500 000 (see the UN CBD website http://www.cbd.int and the references therein). Further, it has been estimated that only about 1% of microbial biodiversity actually comprises 'culturable' organisms (Amman et al., 1995). Thus, a huge number of strains may not be amenable to conventional isolation and cultivation methodologies, and many groups are now working on applying cloning techniques to harness the potential chemical diversity of these organisms.

A diversity-based approach requires acquisition of pre-selected taxonomic groups. The strategy may utilize the assumption that taxonomic diversity will inherently be reflected in the chemical diversity of the extracts subsequently prepared and screened. Various techniques can be employed to analyse the taxonomic spread of a plant collection and then make efforts to fill gaps so that the collection more completely reflects available diversity.

A more focused approach depends on having prior knowledge about selected samples, which might suggest that they contain particular chemical classes of interest or that they possess desirable biological properties. This strategy can be considered under two headings 'chemical targeting' and 'biological targeting'.

Chemical targeting

This utilizes natural materials as sources of specific compounds of interest to a particular disease area, or as sources of chemical classes deemed to have suitable pharmacophores. In this way, chemical types that are under-represented in an existing sample collection can be identified. Plant-derived chemicals can provide an effective means of filling any 'gaps', thereby enhancing the overall diversity of available chemistry. It may not always be necessary to expend resource taking this process to full isolation and structure elucidation. In some cases, a set of plants can be selected on the basis that they are reported to produce a general chemical class of interest and appropriate crude or semi-purified extracts can be prepared in order to enrich the extract with the desired chemical types.

9

Biological targeting. This adopts what may be thought of as a disease-driven process. Plant samples can be selected for biological evaluation using some type of information associated with them that suggests their relevance for evaluation in a given therapeutic target. Perhaps the most striking observations available are ethnobotanical reports of traditional medicinal uses of plants. A number of orthodox medicines available commercially today were discovered by following leads provided from indigenous knowledge (Cox, 1994).

PROCESS FOR IDENTIFICATION OF PLANTS FOR TARGETED SETS

Various approaches are adopted in assimilating the information needed to select plants of particular relevance for a given disease target. Some research groups rely on developing a network of ethnobotanists, who work closely with indigenous colleagues and traditional doctors in various countries. The outcome of this approach is a low number of plant samples identified for evaluation in the laboratory and a great deal of information on their use. Some pharmaceutical companies prefer only to use information that is already in the public domain. Various journals and books hold a significant amount of information relating to the ethnobotanic uses of various plants; for example, there are many publications describing the properties of plants used in Chinese Traditional Medicine (e.g. Chang and But, 1986). Perhaps the most time-effective way of searching for information relating to reported biological or chemical properties of plants is to use electronic data stored in a range of databases. One key example of this is the NAPRALERT (Natural Products Alert) database (Loub et al., 1985). This system was initiated and is maintained at the University of Illinois at Chicago. It contains a wealth of information in the form of a huge number of references relating to reports of biological activity in the scientific literature, ethnobotanical reports and phytochemical data.

For chemical information, databases such as the Chapman and Hall *Dictionary of Natural Products* (2000) can be useful tools. This database contains information on well over 100 000 natural products, often including the species from which the compound originates. Searches can be carried out on the basis of chemical structure, sub-structure, structural similarity, presence of particular functional groups, etc. in order to build a set of organisms reported to produce these compounds. Alternatively, the database can be searched on the basis of species or genus, so as to build a list of compounds reported to derive from particular organism groups. This can be particularly useful in the process of de-replication and compound identification (see later). In addition, searches can be carried out on a range of other fields, such as molecular weight, which are also useful in compound identification following identification of a molecular ion by mass spectrometry analysis, reported uses of the natural product, literature references, log P, etc. The database comprises not just plant metabolites but compounds from all natural sources, and although the data are not complete, it can represent a valuable starting point by which to build chemically focused sets of samples for screening.

In the case of preparing samples that might be expected to contain specific chemical entities, phytochemical procedures reported in the literature can be used to generate semi-purified extracts, or extracts enriched in the compound or chemical class of interest. In the case of plants with an ethnomedical use, it might be possible to prepare extracts using methodology as recommended for use in traditional medicine.

These 'targeted' approaches are likely to involve smaller numbers of plant samples than a high throughput, random screening programme. However, the actual numbers of plants selected and screened can be tailored by the scientist, by making the selection criteria more or less stringent. For example, a selection process may result in a small number of plants reported to produce specific compounds of interest, but if the assay is capable of screening much larger numbers of samples, the set can be extended to include all those plants reported to produce metabolites of the much broader chemical class. Similarly, a set can be extended taxonomically to an optimum size by including plants of related species or genera, on the basis that they might also produce related chemistry. Making the selection criteria slightly more 'fuzzy' in this manner also allows a greater role for the element of luck—always important in the drug discovery process!

SAMPLE PREPARATION

Preparation methods are tailored towards the type of natural material being processed and the strategy for analysis being undertaken. For plant samples, the standard approach is to acquire and store dried plant material. In rare cases, for example if an ethnomedical report dictates use of fresh material, then this may be undertaken, but would not be the norm. Although a very small amount of plant material—less than half a gram—may provide sufficient extract to allow testing in many hundreds of bioassays, it is only sensible to collect a larger amount of material. For natural product samples to remain competitive sources of lead compounds, it is necessary to be able to very rapidly follow-up any active extracts. For this reason, collection of a few hundred grams of dry material is more typical. Plant material is finely ground using techniques ranging from pestle and mortar to industrial grinding apparatus, as appropriate.

Microbial strain collections are maintained either as freeze-dried cultures or are preserved by low-temperature storage. Required strains are generally revived by inoculation onto agar and/or growth media, and then are cultivated on a medium—or, more often, a range of media—that have been developed with the aim of promoting secondary metabolite production. Factors like incubation times and temperature, media composition and agitation rates can all have a significant effect on growth and metabolite synthesis. The next step is to generate an extract for analysis in a range of bioactivity screens. Often, there will be no prior knowledge of which chemical types may be present in the samples, and which will be active in any given bioassay. Techniques will therefore be aimed at solubilizing as wide a range of compounds as possible, typically using an alcoholic solvent, such as methanol or ethanol, or an aqueous alcoholic solvent. Extraction may take the form of a cold infusion or it may involve hot-solvent extraction using a Soxhlet apparatus (Silva et al., 1998). If the natural source material is under investigation because it has been reported to contain a desired compound or chemical class, then a bespoke extraction procedure will be adopted, probably using a literature report. If the target molecule is less specific, for example if the aim is to access any alkaloid molecules that might be present, then alkaloid-enriched extracts can be generated by following a method such as acid–base partitioning.

An alternative approach might favour the development of fractionation methods, so that several fractions originating from a single sample are generated prior to biological testing. Although more labour intensive, this can have the benefit of eliminating many of the problems that can be seen when testing crude extracts in some bioassays, e.g. frequent actives caused by commonly occurring interfering compounds such as tannins, saponins, flavonoids, etc. Such actives can take a significant time to de-replicate amd eliminate and, in some circumstances, it may be desirable to reduce this resource by spending time before biological testing to do some semi-purification of extracts. Techniques used can include solvent partitioning or chromatographic fractionation.

DE-REPLICATION AND ISOLATION OF ACTIVE COMPONENTS

Biological analysis is likely to yield a number of active extracts, as defined by showing a certain level of activity in a given screen. A process then needs to begin that will either lead to a full identification of a fully characterized, active compound or to a partial identification of activity to the level of a family of known compounds.

Before commencing full bioassay-guided fractionation of the active samples it is necessary to review the tolerance of a given assay to crude or semi-purified extracts of natural materials. The aim of evaluating such samples in a biological assay is to identify compounds that interact with a particular biological target, e.g. an enzyme or receptor. However, in practice, most assays utilize a measurable system, such as colour, light or radioactivity, enabling a high throughput of samples. This leads to the possibility of detection of non-specific interactions, which are particularly problematic when investigating multi-component, uncharacterized extracts as opposed to single chemical entities. Examples of natural products that generate such effects are detergent-like compounds, which disrupt cell membranes, polyphenolics, which form complexes with a wide array of proteins, antioxidants and ultraviolet (UV) quenchers. It is vital to be able to detect, and eliminate, such actives as rapidly as possible (VanMiddlesworth and Cannell, 1998). This process can be speeded up by testing a standard set of known interfering compounds and extracts in an assay prior to the full screen. This provides data to indicate the tolerance of the assay to such samples, and can at times lead to a decision not to proceed with testing of crude extracts against that target. The physicochemical properties of a compound can give useful clues as to its identity. The most commonly used properties include high-performance liquid chromatography (HPLC) retention time and UV spectra data that are readily acquired through standard analytical techniques. By comparing these data with those of known compounds, it may be possible to characterize the components of a mixture without the need for full isolation—or at least, it may be possible to narrow the possibilities. If a library of such data from a relatively large number of natural products is used, this can be very effective in identifying those compounds that are present in more than one organism. If full isolation of the active component is warranted, various methods may be adopted. There is no single, best isolation technique, nor is there any single, correct method for any given compound. Most separation methods involve some form of chromatography—typically preparative HPLC. An isolation method would normally involve solvent partitioning, followed by a crude chromatography step such as a silica column or counter-current chromatography with a relatively small number of fractions based on polarity, followed by final purification through a high-resolution separation step such as HPLC. At each stage of the purification, the active compound is tracked by bioassay of the fractions. The only sure way to identify the structure of a bioactive metabolite is to demonstrate activity using the isolated compound and then to determine its structure by nuclear magnetic resonance (NMR) and mass spectrometry (MS). Until a compound is isolated, it is also impossible to determine its concentration and, hence, its potency in a given assay. It is also prudent to check that the concentration of the metabolite in the extract and the activity in the unpurified extract tally, so that a minor but active component does not go unaccounted for. Secondary testing will then be undertaken on the active compound to determine the mechanism and the selectivity of action and eventually, to evaluate *in vivo* activity. The chemical structure of the compound will also be evaluated to give some indication of the classical 'drug-like' qualities of the molecule. These are to some extent subjective but include consideration of whether the compound is of sufficiently low molecular weight to allow ready chemical modification, and not prevent drug uptake; of whether the compound is likely to be stable with respect to oral uptake, whether it has sites that may be suitable for modification, whether it is likely to have a suitable log P, and so on. In fact, some classes of natural product are not suitable as drug candidates by these criteria, as they are too big and complex or possess unsuitable redox properties. If the molecule is deemed to be of interest, related metabolites from the sample, or related species, may be accessed for structure activity determination. Even if the structure of the metabolite is not novel, this does not preclude it becoming a lead molecule, particularly if the mode of action is novel.

AN EXAMPLE OF THE SUCCESS OF HIGH-THROUGHPUT SCREENING OF PLANTS FOR NEW LEAD COMPOUNDS

The discovery of a series of novel and highly potent euphane triterpenes illustrates the potential of plant extracts to generate useful chemical leads in a high-throughput screening programme.

During a 'random' screening programme to search for novel inhibitors of human thrombin, which were capable of blocking the formation of blood clots and hence could be of value in treating and preventing deep vein thrombosis, some 150 000 samples, including synthetic compounds and bacterial, fungal and plant extracts, were evaluated. Methanolic extracts of *Lantana camara* (Verbenaceae) leaves, obtained from a UK garden, were found to display potent activity.

Large-scale extraction and bioassay-guided chromatographic fractionation led to the identification of a series of novel compounds, which were characterized by NMR and MS as 5,5-*trans*-fused cyclic lactone-containing euphane triterpenes (O'Neill *et al.*, 1998). The compounds showed IC_{50} values of the order of 50 nm against thrombin.

After the initial activity was detected, literature searches on *Lantana camara* revealed this plant species to be reported to be toxic to grazing animals, which, on ingestion of the leaves, develop hepatotoxicity and photosensitization (Sharma and Sharma, 1989). These toxic effects have been attributed to the lantadenes, a series of pentacyclic triterpenes. A further study of haematological changes in sheep following *Lantana* poisoning demonstrated a significant increase in blood coagulation time and prothrombin time, with an associated decrease in blood sedimentation rate, total plasma protein and fibrinogen (Uppal and Paul, 1982). This observation might be associated with the thrombin inhibitory translactone-containing euphane triterpenes described above.

The biological activity of these compounds has been reported in detail (Weir *et al.*, 1998). Their mechanism of action as inhibitors of blood clotting is via acylation of the active site Ser 195 residue of thrombin. This acylating activity has been found to be generic against other serine protease enzymes and this finding forms the basis for exploitation in drug discovery.

Further reading

Amman RL, Ludwig W, Schleifer KH 1995 Phylogenetic identification and in situ detection of individual microbial cells without cultivation. Microbiological Reviews 59: 143–169

Chang H-M, But P-H 1986 Pharmacology and applications of Chinese materia medica. World Scientific Publishing Co, Singapore

Cox P 1994 The ethnobotanical approach to drug discovery: strengths and limitations. In: Ethnobotany and the search for new drugs. Wiley, Chichester (Ciba Foundation Symposium 185), pp 25–41

Dictionary of natural products, 5th edn, 2000 Chapman and Hall/CRC Press

Kinsman OS, Chalk PA, Jackson HC *et al* 1998 Isolation and characterisation of an antifungal antibiotic (GR 135402) with protein synthesis inhibition. Journal of Antibiotics 51 (I): 41–49

Loub WD, Farnsworth NR, Soejarto DD, Quinn ML 1985 NAPRALERT: Computer handling of natural product research data. Journal of Chemical Information and Computing Sciences 25: 99–103

9

Martindale, the complete drug reference. Internet version: http//www.csi. micromedex.com

O'Neill MJ, Lewis JA, Noble HM *et al* 1998 Isolation of translactone containing triterpenes with thrombin inhibitory activity from the leaves of *Lantana camara.* Journal of Natural Products 61(11): 1328–1331

Pezzuto JM 1997 Plant derived anticancer agents. Biochemical Pharmacology 53(2): 121–133 *and references therein*

Sampson JH, Phillipson JD, Bowery N *et al* 2000 Ethnomedically selected plants as sources of potential analgesic compounds: indications of in vitro biological activity in receptor binding assays. Phytotherapy Research 14: 24–29

Sharma OMP, Sharma PD 1989 Natural products of the Lantana plant—the present and prospects. Journal of Scientific Industrial Research 48: 471–478

Silva GL, Lee I-S, Kinghorn AD 1998 Special problems with the extraction of plants. In: Cannell RJP (ed) Natural products isolation. Humana Press, Totowa, NJ, pp 343–363

Strohl WR 2000 The role of natural products in a modern drug discovery program. Drug Discovery Today 5(2): 39–41

Tait RM 1992 Development of a radiometric spot-wash assay for squalene synthase. Analytical Biochemistry 203(2): 310–316

Tan GT, Lee S, Lee I-S *et al* 1996 Natural product inhibitors of human DNA ligase I. Biochemical Journal 314: 993–1000

Uppal RP, Paul BS 1982 Haematological changes in experimental Lantana poisoning in sheep. Indian Veterinary Journal 18–24

VanMiddlesworth FW, Cannell RJP 1998 Dereplication and partial identification of natural products. In: Cannell RJP (ed) Natural products isolation. Humana Press, Totowa, NJ, pp 343–363

Weir MP, Bethell SS, Cleasby A 1998 Novel natural product 5,5-*trans*-lactone inhibitors of human a-thrombin: mechanism of action and structural studies. Biochemistry 37: 6645–6657

PART

3 Principles related to the commercial production, quality and standardization of natural products

10

Commerce in crude drugs

R. Baker

Like almost all other basic commodities, the trade in crude drugs is of great antiquity. The necessity for goods to be collected, graded, transported and distributed effectively has rarely been considered by the pharmacist as part of his or her remit, and thus it has been left to the trader or merchant to perform this less scientific, but by the same token important, group of tasks. The essentials of the trade are still very much as they were 10, 100 or 1000 years ago, although the speed and efficiency with which they can be performed has improved exponentially with time. It is well within quite young living memory that one had to book a telephone call to one's supplier in Brazil, China or India some hours or perhaps a day in advance: now communications by fax or more frequently now by e-mail take moments to perform, and replies come with similar alacrity. The advent of 'VOIP' (Voice Over Internet Protocol) and the various messaging services, which are essentially free of charge, has improved at least the availability of means of communication.

HISTORICAL DEVELOPMENTS

The absolute origins of the trade in crude drugs are lost in the mists of time. One supposes the first contract for the collection and supply of a drug with a third party, whether in exchange for specie or not, came about when physicians or pharmacists found themselves too busy to do this relatively menial task themselves. The trust that physicians had in the collectors must have been remarkable, as unadulterated drug was essential, if only to avoid poisoning the patient! It is probable that the first commercial dealers in botanical drugs were apprentices or freed slaves, who preferred to take on that role rather than becoming pharmacists themselves: we shall never know for certain. References from antiquity to the drug trade are rare, although some mural inscriptions from Ancient Egypt, dating back to 3000 BC, evidence knowledge of the effect of medicinal plants and, in the British Museum, clay tablets from the library of King Ashurbanipal (668–626 BC) of Assyria suggest that, around 2500 BC, the Sumerians had a form of Herbal. By 660 BC, around 250 drugs were recognized by the Assyrians themselves, some of which were actively cultivated. Hippocrates (467 BC) was well acquainted with a variety of drugs (although it is improbable that any of the works attributed to him are actually 'of his hand'). Theophrastus, like Alexander the Great, was a pupil of Aristotle, and later became chief of the Aristotelian school. He listed some 500 plants known to him, and distinguished cinnamon from cassia (an art that, apparently, is being lost in this day and age, at least by some manufacturers of foodstuffs!). It is instructive to note that the use of the Mercury's or Hermes' winged staff with entwined snakes or caduceus, nowadays a widely understood symbol for medicine, was originally a symbol for commerce.[1] The whole economy of the ancient city state of Kyrene (Cyrene, near Shahhat in present-day Libya) was predicated on the supply of silphium, a now (probably) extinct species of giant fennel.[2] The importance of this plant was so great that it was habitually depicted on the coins of this city, both in the form of the plant itself and also as its heart-shaped seeds. It is said by some that the last specimen of a stalk of this plant was presented to the Emperor Nero, who promptly ate it. Mohammed was said to be a spice trader, and at that time spice traders were invariably concerned with crude drugs, particularly as many products were used for both culinary and medicinal purposes, as they are today. The adventures of all of the major explorers, such as Marco Polo,

---

[1] The true symbol for medicine in this context is the rod of Asclepius, one snake and no wings

[2] It is believed by some to be *Ferula indiana*

Columbus, Henry the Navigator and the like were undertaken partly with a view to the sourcing of botanical crude drugs. The establishment of the great National Trading Companies, for instance The Honourable East India Company, The Netherlands United East India Company and the Danish Asiatic Company, were undertaken with a similar view.

Prior to modern times, there was no real distinction between the drug and spice trades, and thus during London's development as an entrepôt, the Guild of Pepperers of London (later the Grocers' Company) was charged with the overseeing of both trades. The importance of the trade is evidenced on the Grocers' Company coat of arms, which features nine cloves (Flores Eugenia Caryophilia). The foundation of the East India Company in 1600 placed a near monopoly in the import of 'East India produce' into England, and it was from this that the modern general produce trade emerged. Initially in *ad hoc* form, and later by way of the famous 'coffee houses', trade in drugs, even until the Second World War, was conducted in the main by auction. The problem was that the shippers at origin had no direct representation in the consuming countries, and thus had to engage the services of a broker. The usual format was for the goods, whether sent 'on consignment' (i.e. sent speculatively to London in the reasonable hope of a sale) or 'ex stock' (being the property of an importing merchant), to be put up for show in the warehouse prior to auction, or for samples to be drawn and placed on view in the brokers' offices. The various broking firms then attempted to sell the merchandise entrusted to them by public auction (the order in which the various brokers did so being decided by lot). Towards the end of the popularity of auctions in London, it was common for no, or almost no, goods actually to be sold at the auction; instead the auctioneer would invite a customer to see him after the auction and would subsequently negotiate a mutually acceptable price between the shipper and the potential customer.

During the Second World War, when lines of communication with the various origins were disrupted, a certain amount of regulation was imposed by the government. This saw an end both to the auctions and, due to licensing controls, to the supply of goods to London on consignment. The trade then took a new form: samples were displayed in brokers' offices for all to see. The traders, brokers and buyers met in the Corn Exchange and deals were done by word of mouth (and sometimes in covert whispers) in the best traditions of the trade. By the 1960s, with improving communications and increased volumes, this method became impractical and the trade finally took to conducting most of its business by telecommunications.

Obviously, early on, when the trade between the dealers and brokers was small and almost self-regulating, little regulatory interference was required. However, the increasing numbers of firms involved in the trade required a system of settling disputes in an inexpensive and swift manner. Thus, in 1876 the General Produce Brokers' Association (GPBA) of London was formed. This body performed a number of functions: it presented a united voice to those outside the trade, it regulated the trade by means of a system of arbitration and appeal and it provided a forum in which to voice concerns of interest to members in general. The GPBA thrived initially, but suffered as time went on and various trade groups formed their own Associations, leaving the GPBA with only the smaller parts of London Commodity Trading as its remit. More recently, broking as part of the London trade became less relevant and the name was accordingly changed in 1981 to the 'General Produce Association of London'. Finally, in 1985, the name was again changed, this time to the 'International General Produce Association', to reflect the current true nature of the trade. Forms of contract are issued by the Association for the use of members and others (it is probably true to say that the IGPA contracts, terms and conditions are those most generally used world-wide), and there is a thriving, and relatively swift and inexpensive, system of arbitration and appeal.

CURRENT ASPECTS

London's pre-eminence as the drug-trading centre has diminished substantially over the years. Although still undeniably the largest market for the trade in essential oils and aromatic chemicals (a trade misnomer frequently used to denote flavour and perfumery chemicals and isolates such as menthol, camphor, piperonal, vanillin and the like, be they natural or synthetic), its role concerning crude herbs and botanicals (such as rhubarb, ipecacuanha and boldo, for instance) has decreased to Hamburg's benefit, and the trading of spices has moved substantially to Rotterdam. Nonetheless, when disputes need to be settled, most eyes still invariably turn to London to obtain a 'fair deal'.

The North American trade is, as it always has been, substantially different. Unlike most of Western Europe, Canada and the United States of America, as well as being large consumers of crude drugs, are also large producers. Many products regularly traded in the European drug markets emanate almost exclusively from North America. A number of American firms hold stocks of drugs (many of native origin, but not exclusively so) speculatively, being confident that there will be demand for the product held on their books in the near term. Granted, there is a trend towards the European market usages of trade, but nonetheless, consumers in North America should be thankful that, because of this pattern of business, it is still usually possible to obtain materials for immediate delivery from a trader's stock, rather than waiting for shipment from origin. There has been a certain amount of consolidation in the trade in the USA and, consequently, the North American market is edging, however reluctantly, towards the European model.

Consuming patterns in Europe have also changed. There has been substantial consolidation of companies concerned with crude and processed botanical drugs, particularly but not exclusively within Germany, to the extent that nowadays one large conglomerate, while not controlling the business, has great influence. A number of recent closures and rationalization have caused concern, particularly on the part of consuming companies. What effect all of this will eventually have on the world markets for crude drugs has yet to be seen, but the current mood of the market could well be described as 'melancholic'.

Trade nowadays has changed substantially. In relatively recent times, many drugs were imported speculatively with a view to selling them either 'afloat' (i.e. once confirmed the goods were aboard ship) or from 'the spot' (i.e. with the goods in store in a European warehouse, available for immediate delivery). With the changing requirements of buyers, be it either for the quality of the goods required or with changing trends in the particular drugs used, this has become less common, and nowadays it is more likely that a customer will request of a trader an offer for a specific quantity of crude drug for shipment from origin and delivery after safe arrival of shipment, be that in one delivery or in parts, either against a sample or (more rarely) a mutually agreed level of quality. Whereas the customer is, of course, at liberty to approach the origin direct for supplies, the advantages of purchasing from a trader are those of transference of risk. If the quality or condition of goods is such that on arrival the goods are either of lower quality than that contracted or damaged in some way, or if delivery is delayed beyond the agreed period, recourse is to the local trader, from whom one is far more likely to obtain settlement than the origin, where satisfaction of a claim might be far more difficult or, in some cases, impossible to perform, due for instance to local currency regulations. Also, if the trader concerned supplies the same material to various buyers it can frequently be possible to rearrange the allocations on his book to provide the buyer with an 'emergency' delivery should production demands require this. In return for this service, the trader asks a small premium over the price paid to origin and requires absolute adherence to the contract terms, such as delivery dates and terms of payment, for it is on this basis that the price has been calculated and thus, by inference, the margin. Margins in the crude drug trade are currently probably as small as they have ever been. For the customer to delay or cancel an order placed, or to delay payment once goods are delivered, is unacceptable, as would be the trader defaulting, delivering goods late or of poor quality. A fallacy still holds in the consumer industries that 'rapacious' traders make vast sums from their livelihood. This might once have been the case, centuries ago, but almost invariably nowadays margins are confined to low, single-figure percentage levels, representing a small fraction of those that the customer usually makes. This point cannot be overemphasized: contracts (which, after all are based on the concept of 'equity' or fairness) work both ways and, in London at least, the old adage *Verba mea pacta* still holds with the traders; it must also do so with the customer. Is it reasonable that a trader who has purchased a specific product for a customer, for which that trader has no other potential outlet, should without recourse be required not to deliver goods because of an error on the part of the customer, or a whim of the customer's customer?

The question of quality from the trader's point of view is improving. Strong competition at origin has seen a general increase in quality across the board. Many goods are still traded on the old descriptions such as the 'Common Round' or 'Flat' grades of Chinese rhubarb or 'Mossel Bay' or 'Port Elizabeth' aloes from South Africa. One can always be sure that 'Mossel Bay' aloes will pass the requirements of the *British Pharmacopoeia*, whereas 'Port Elizabeth' will rarely, if ever, do so. Nonetheless, more and more trading is being undertaken on the basis of pre-shipment samples, and shippers at origin feel happier to do so now that the world-wide networks of courier services are in place, as a sample of the specific lot in question can be on the desk of the trader two or three days after it was dispatched from origin, rather than the two or three weeks it used to take, or the two or three months before the advent of airmail. Some products are still traded on the basis of out-turn analysis, there being defined a nominal content of isolate on which the price of the contract is calculated, a minimum level below which the parcel is rejectable, and an agreed pro-rata formula for adjusting the invoice value once the quality has been independently established.

From a commercial point of view, the world has changed dramatically over the past few years. The change in Eastern Europe from state capitalism (less accurately, communism) to free-market economies has also changed supply patterns from these countries. Fifteen years ago, traders had one or two source companies to contact in a country, whereas now there is a plethora of suppliers. Reliability has changed as well: formerly, contracts were sacrosanct but nowadays attitudes are a little more relaxed. Further, to increase income, commercially valuable crude drugs are being produced in countries that previously had not done so; India is an excellent case in point. This country had for many years been a large nett importer of ipecacuanha root (*Cephaelis acuminata*), for both internal consumption and re-export of finished alkaloids. Granted, there has been a small local cultivation of this material, but the quality, until recently, had been relatively poor. Over the past few years, however, India has been able to offer ipecacuanha of high quality and at very competitive levels. These developments all tend to reduce the price of the drugs in question. But at what point does this become deleterious to the market? The answer must be directly related to economics. Subsequent to the changes in Eastern Europe, the prices of some drugs have fallen consistently. Thus, in a place where aspirations for personal income are rising fast (not unreasonably, considering past history and current circumstances), the income from their produce is consistently falling. Perhaps due to increased competition, or conversely from factors at the point of consumption, the price falls.

Frequently, the initial effect of lower prices is, in the short term, to raise the quality of the product delivered, with a view to securing the next order. However, if low prices are sustained then eventually the quality of the crop slowly falls as the producer is unable to fertilize or tend the crop to the optimum levels. Adulteration, either with admixed drug or, more subtly, with water (i.e. increasing the moisture content) sometimes takes place. Finally, the farmer or collector is presented with the decision of either continuing the cultivation of the product in the absence of profit or changing crop in favour of one that gives a return. In the worst case, supplies of a drug could well cease for lack of profit to the producer, which, when taken in the context of the price at which the finished product is retailed to the public, is almost insignificant.

It might be that the reader is taken aback by what appears to be a hard-nosed trader making a plea for a fair deal to the producer; this, however, is not the case. The writer would far rather have a steady, sustained business over an extended period than a phenomenal short trading 'boom' and thereafter be out of business.

Be it desirable or otherwise, there has been a move over recent years for the goods to be extracted at origin and the isolate, rather than the bulk drug, being shipped. At first glance this has many advantages for all concerned; the less technically demanding work is performed at origin, where labour and facilities are less expensive and where local regulations as regards, say, effluent are less stringent. This adds value to the goods and increased foreign exchange earnings for the country of origin. It is of advantage to the trader, as there are fewer freight, warehousing and handling costs involved and, finally, it gives the customer an (at least semi-) prepared product with which to work, thus eliminating the expensive and laborious initial extraction processes. However, this concept is a double-edged sword. One may be tempted to be a little more cursory as regards quality control of the inward product, particularly after a long run of good experience. If a parcel of material is found to be of inferior quality for whatever reason, the resulting loss tends to be the greater as concentration of the product frequently leads to the acquisition of fewer, larger parcels and (most important) deprives the consuming country, over time, of the knowledge and equipment with which to perform the complete process. In relatively peaceful times this last consideration might be irrelevant; but if lines of communication with the traditional suppliers are disrupted by war, terrorism or natural disaster, then even though it would be possible to obtain the raw material from elsewhere, this would be of little use if the know-how and/or equipment required for the complete extraction process is lost. Commercially, this is of little moment, but for the greater good it is vital not to lose the expertise that has been built up over many centuries in the consuming countries for a small cost saving. A middle road to this position has evolved in recent years. Goods are procured by the user of the finished product and shipped to an extractor in a third country that usually has low wages and lenient pollution and employment regulations, to be extracted on a 'toll' basis. The drawbacks are two-fold: the 'carbon footprint' of the goods is increased substantially and, again, the expertise of extraction is still maintained out of the country. There is of course a cost saving, but in the long term is this adequate compensation?

Another problem has arisen recently, which also gives cause for concern. It was brought to the author's attention by a friend who is a practitioner in speech and language therapy, that atropine delivered by way of a patch (used for control of the secretion of saliva) was proving difficult to source. A few phone calls led to the conclusion that the reason why this medicine was unavailable was that it was perceived that there was insufficient profit in the manufacture of the said patches, and thus production had ceased. Half a century or more ago this would not have been regarded as serious, for the pharmacist would simply

10

have obtained a supply of the raw material in question, performed his own extraction and concocted it into the required carrier. Now, with the majority of pharmacists at best unwilling (and at worst unable) to perform this act, the patient will have to go without.

CHANGING DEMANDS

The pattern of demand is changing, as it has always done. Recent inroads into the market by 'nutraceuticals' (bio-active products presented as 'dietary supplements' or similar) have changed the demand for various botanicals. Products of which one would have heard rarely some 10 or 20 years ago are now objects of daily discussion. The lack of licensing of these products is a point of major concern. The majority of the botanicals involved are well documented and every company that the writer has come across to date has been responsible and reputable. However, the relatively high margins that these products attract when offered to the consumer with this cachet, and the comparative lack of technical expertise needed to manufacture the product for presentation to the public, could probably in time attract (or perhaps has already attracted) undesirable elements into the trade, with potentially disastrous consequences. Origins are offering prepared extracts that need little more than mixing with an excipient and tableting or filling into freely available capsules. If nutraceuticals, originally and naturally the domain of the chemist's shop, the supermarket or the health-food store, appear at more unlikely venues (such as open-air markets and car boot sales—as this trader has seen, on occasion) then the potential problems multiply. It is almost inconceivable that well-known branded products within their stated shelf life would emerge at these sites, but given a substantial price advantage to the public, is it not reasonable to speculate, be it by accident or design, that any problem starting with a retail outlet of this type attached to goods of questionable origin would reflect badly on the industry as a whole? Licensing, both of the manufacturer and the retailer, would minimize this risk, even if that licensing were far less stringent than that required for dispensing. EU regulations are currently being shaped to tackle this problem, but their implementation has and will attract substantial opposition. Furthermore, there has been a number of recent examples of products included in various traditions of oriental medicine having found their way into Europe, where the said ingredients are simply prohibited as noxious if not positively poisonous. One practitioner was seen on the news defending the use of the product and pronouncing the prohibition to be 'prejudiced' against that person's ethnic traditions. The author will leave readers to make up their own mind on that score.

Fair Trade is set to become important in this trade. Although one can, of course, see the advantages of the concept, there are a couple of problems. A recent policy change has caused the Fair Trade authorities to begin to charge suppliers at origin for registration and audit. This ensures that only the better-financed suppliers will be able to afford registration, which to my mind rather negates the point of the Fair Trade in the first place. Thus, on the one hand, we in the West are pouring vast sums of money into the less well-developed parts of the world to enable people to reach beyond poverty, but with the other hand we are stopping those who most need our help by placing financial hurdles in the way.

THE FUTURE

In my few years in the trade I have seen the total demise of the telegram as a trading tool; telex is going the same way. If the rate of change continues as it is, by the time this appears in print the fax will be considered a quaint, slow form of communication; e-mail may well be superseded within a short time. The tools of the trade change, but the methods and principles do not. Trade is based on mutual trust. If the supply of a raw material needs to be guaranteed then there is only one possible method of obtaining that guaranteed supply, and that is from one's preferred trader. If the trader from whom you obtain your raw materials says that the goods will be delivered at a certain time then, within the terms of the contract, that trader will move heaven and earth to do so, just as the trader's predecessors did 10, 50 or 100 years ago. Many is the time that I have listened to the complaint that, 'Origin has let me down, I need 5 tons of XYZ root next week'. If support is not forthcoming in ordinary times, then where is the impetus on the trader's part to provide support to those who require it in difficult times? Perhaps accounting and purchasing departments in manufacturing organizations should carefully consider this question when looking at the 2% or so saving they make (or more often appear to make) when purchasing direct from origin. As an insurance policy, the trader is very inexpensive.

11

Production of crude drugs

The crude drug that reaches the pharmaceutical manufacturing line will have passed through various stages, all of which influence the nature and amount of active constituents present. These aspects will be considered under the headings 'Source Materials', 'Environmental Conditions', 'Cultivated and Wild Plants', 'Collection', 'Drying', 'Storage' and 'European Regulations'.

SOURCE MATERIALS

It is imperative that correct identification of the source material is made. Adulteration may be accidental, particularly if collection is made from wild plants, or it may be deliberate. Failure in this area can result in poisoning (e.g. hemlock fruits mistaken for other umbelliferous fruits) or inactive products (e.g. substitution of St John's wort with other vegetable material when demand exceeds supply). For pharmacopoeial drugs, precise macroscopic and microscopic characters are available.

For the isolation of specific constituents, the source can vary, e.g. particular steroids may be obtained from various diverse plants (q.v. Chapter 25) or hyoscine from a number of solanaceous species. Recently a potential problem concerning the production of the oral antiviral against avian flu—Tamiflu® (oseltamivir)—arose from a shortage of Chinese staranise (q.v.), the source of the starting material (shikimic acid, see Fig. 18.8) for the synthesis. However, the toxic Japanese star anise, regarded as an adulterant of the Chinese drug, also contains shikimic acid and could provide an alternative source (D. V. C. Awang and M. Blumenthal, *HerbalGram*, 2006, **70**, 58).

In the article 'Plant part substitution—a way to conserve endangered medicinal plants' S. Zschocke *et al.* (*J. Ethnopharm.*, 2000, **71**, 281) explore the possibility of using the leaves of plants that are traditionally used for their barks, bulbs and roots, thus conserving the plant.

ENVIRONMENTAL CONDITIONS

Plant growth and development, and often the nature and quantity of secondary metabolites, are affected by temperature, rainfall, aspect, length of day (including the quality of light) and altitude. Such effects have been studied by growing particular plants in different climatic areas and observing variations. The findings of such research are illustrated by work on cannabis by El-Kheir *et al.* in 1986 in which seeds of cannabis, grown in England and rich in CBD and devoid of THC, when cultivated in Sudan started to produce THC in the first generation and in the second generation contained up to 3.3% THC with a further decrease (down to 0% in some plants) of CBD (see 'Cannabis' for explanation of chemistry). However, it is impossible to control all the variables in such experiments, and special laboratories (phytotrons) have been constructed in which all the factors are independently controllable. Even so, a meaningful expression of the results can often present some difficulty. For example, a particular factor may lead to the development of a small plant which, when analysed on a percentage dry weight basis, indicates a high proportion of metabolite, even though the overall yield per plant could be quite low. Conversely, certain nutrients may result in the production of large plants with a somewhat low analytical figure for constituents on a percentage dry weight basis, but yield per plant may exceed that of the control.

Temperature

Temperature is a major factor controlling the development and metabolism of plants. Although each species has become adapted to its own natural environment, plants are frequently able to exist in a considerable range of temperature. Many tropical and subtropical plants will grow in temperate regions during summer months, but lack frost resistance to withstand the winter. In general, the highest temperatures are experienced near the Equator, but as the temperature falls about 1°C for every 200 m of elevation, it is possible in, say, Jamaica to have a tropical climate on the coast and a temperate one in the mountains. The annual variations in temperature are just as important as the temperature of the hottest month. At Singapore the annual range of temperature is as little as 1.5°C, whereas Moscow, with its hot summers and cold winters, has a range of 29.3°C. In general, the formation of volatile oils appears to be enhanced at higher temperatures, although very hot days may lead to an excess physical loss of oil. The mean optimum temperature for nicotine production in *Nicotiana rustica* is 20°C (lower at 11–12°C and at 30°C). Several authors have indicated that fixed oils produced at low temperatures contain fatty acids with a higher content of double bonds than those formed at higher temperatures.

Rainfall

The important effects of rainfall on vegetation must be considered in relation to the annual rainfall, its distribution throughout the year, its effect on humidity and its effect coupled with the water-holding properties of the soil. Variable results have been reported for the production of volatile oils under different conditions of rainfall and may in some instances be coupled with the development of glandular hairs. Continuous rain can lead to a loss of water-soluble substances from leaves and roots by leaching; this is known to apply to some plants producing alkaloids, glycosides and even volatile oils. This could account for low yields of some active constituents in wet seasons from plants whose general condition appears to be good.

With *Cassia angustifolia* (Tinnevelly senna) it has been shown that short-term drought increases the concentration of sennosides A+B but in the longer term causes loss of leaf biomass (H. Ratnayaka *et al.*, *Planta Medica*, 1998, **64**, 438).

Day-length and radiation characteristics

Plants vary much in both the amount and intensity of the light which they require. In the wild state the plant will be found where its shade requirements are met, and under cultivation similar shade must be provided. In certain cases research has shown that light is a factor which helps to determine the amount of glycosides or alkaloids produced. With belladonna, stramonium and *Cinchona ledgeriana* full sunshine gives a higher content of alkaloids than does shade. At Gif-sur-Yvette experiments indicated that with *Datura stramonium* var. *tatula* long exposure to intense light brought about a sharp increase in hyoscine content at the time of flowering. An important *in vivo* reaction in the formation of the antitumour alkaloids of *Catharanthus roseus* is exemplified by the dimerization of the indole alkaloids catharanthine and vindoline leading to vinblastine; Hirata *et al.* (*Planta Med.*, 1993, **59**, 46) demonstrated that irradiation of intact plants with near ultraviolet light in the range 290–380 nm (peak 370 nm) stimulates the synthesis of dimeric alkaloids, probably by inducing catharanthine oxidation as a trigger reaction. This observation has support from *in vitro* studies.

It has been shown that under long-day conditions peppermint leaves contain menthone, menthol and traces of menthofuran; plants grown under short-day conditions contain menthofuran as a major component of the volatile oil. Furthermore a long photoperiod for young leaves activates the reduction pathway with conversion of menthone to methol. In studies on the day–night changes in the relative concentrations of volatiles from flowers of *Nicotiana sylvestris* and other species a marked increase (about tenfold) in aromatic compounds including benzyl alcohol was detected at night, whereas no increase in the volatiles (e.g. linalool, caryophyllene) originating from the

mevalonic acid pathway (q.v.) was noted (J. H. Loughrin *et al.*, *Phytochem.*, 1990, **29**, 2473).

The daily variation in the proportion of secondary metabolites is probably light-controlled and is discussed more fully under 'Collection Times'. Many plants initiate flowers only in certain day-lengths, and where flowering is essential this factor must be carefully considered before planting in a new region. Presence or absence of light, together with wavelength range, have a marked effect on the secondary metabolite production of some plants in tissue culture.

The type of radiation which plants receive is also important. With *Ocimum basilicum*, C. B. Johnson *et al.* (*Phytochemistry*, 1999, **51**, 507), have found, in relation to herbs raised under glass and receiving no UV-B radiation, that supplementary UV-B radiation increases levels of both the phenyl-propanoids and terpenoids of the leaves. Flavonoids and anthocyanins are also known to be influenced by UV-B radiation. Depletion of the ozone layer and the consequent effect of increased radiation at the earth's surface has been a topic of much recent speculation. Concerning medicinal plants, R. Karouson *et al.* (*Phytochemistry*, 1998, **49**, 2273) raised two chemotypes of *Mentha spicata* which were subjected to increased UV-B radiation equivalent to a 15% ozone depletion over Patras, Greece. In one chemotype essential oil production was stimulated by the treatment while a similar non-significant trend was noted with the other.

Altitude

The coconut palm needs a maritime climate and the sugar cane is a lowland plant. Conversely, tea, cocoa, coffee, medicinal rhubarb, tragacanth and cinchona require elevation. In the case of *Cinchona succirubra* the plants grow well at low levels but produce practically no alkaloids. The bitter constituents of *Gentiana lutea* increase with altitude, whereas the alkaloids of *Aconitum napellus* and *Lobelia inflata* and the oil content of thyme and peppermint decrease. Other oil-producing plants may reach a maximum at certain altitudes. Pyrethrum gives the best yields of flower-heads and pyrethrins at high altitudes on, or near, the Equator. It is therefore produced in East Africa and north-west South America. However, vegetative growth is more lush under irrigated conditions at lower altitude, so the propagation farms (for the vegetative multiplication of plants) are, in Ecuador, situated at lower levels than the final commercial farms.

G. A. Statti *et al.* (*Fitoterapia*, 2004, **75**, 212–216) studied bergamot (*Citrus bergamia*) grown at different altitudes and solar exposures in Calabria, Italy; they found both chemical (linalool, linalyl acetate composition) and biological (antioxidant and antifungal activities) diversities.

The flowering heads of *Arnica montana*, grown in Austria in experimental plots at altitudes between 590 and 2250 m showed no altitude effect on the total contents of sesquiterpene lactones and flavonoids but the latter with vicinal-free hydroxy groups in ring B increased with altitude relative to the other flavonoids. Caffeic acid derivatives were 85% higher at the summit compared with the valley (R. Spitaler *et al.*, *Phytochemistry*, 2006, **67**, 407). For a study of the effect of altitude on the podophyllotoxin content of the aerial parts and underground organs of *Podophyllum hexandrum* populations from the Kumaun region of the Indian Central Himalayas, see M. Nadeem *et al.*, *Planta Med.*, 2007, **73**, 388.

CULTIVATED AND WILD PLANTS

Certain drugs are now obtained almost exclusively from cultivated plants. These include cardamoms, Indian hemp, ginger, and peppermint and spearmint for oil production. Others include Ceylon cinnamon, linseed, fennel, cinchona and opium. In other cases both wild and cultivated plants are used. Some plants have been cultivated from time immemorial (e.g. flax, opium poppy and coca). Others are now grown because supplies of the wild plants are insufficient to meet the demand or because, owing to sparse distribution or inaccessibility, collection is difficult. Cultivation is essential in the case of drugs such as Indian hemp and opium, which are subject to government control, and recently for those wild plants in danger of over-exploitation and which have now been given CITES (q.v.) listing. In many cases cultivation is advisable because of the improved quality of the drug which it is possible to produce. The improvement may be due to the following.

1. The power to confine collections to species, varieties or hybrids which have the desired phytochemical characters (e.g. aconite, cinnamon, fennel, Duboisia, cinchona, Labiate drugs and valerian).
2. The better development of the plants owing to improved conditions of the soil, pruning, and the control of insect pests, fungi, etc.
3. The better facilities for treatment after collection. For example, drying at a correct temperature in the cases of digitalis, colchicum, belladonna and valerian, and the peeling of cinnamon and ginger.

For success in cultivation it is necessary to study the conditions under which the plant flourishes in the wild state and reproduce these conditions or improve on them. Small changes in ecology can affect plant products; thus, satisfactory rubber trees grow wild in the Amazon basin but cleared areas converted to rubber plantations have been a failure.

Soils

Different plant species vary enormously in their soil and nutritive requirements, and this aspect has received considerable attention with medicinal plants. Three important basic characteristics of soils are their physical, chemical and microbiological properties.

Variations in particle size result in different soils ranging from clay, via sand, to gravel. Particle size is one factor influencing water-holding capacity, and some plants (e.g. *Althaea officinalis*) which produce mucilage as a water-retaining material contain less mucilage when grown on soil with a high moisture content. Although particular species have their own soil pH tolerances (*Datura stramonium* 6.0–8.2, *Majorana hortensis* 5.6–6.4), no marked influence of pH value within the tolerance range has been demonstrated for essential oils (*Mentha piperita*) and alkaloids (*D. stramonium*). All plants require calcium for their normal nutrition but plants known as caliphobous plants (e.g. *Pinus pinaster* and *Digitalis purpurea*) cannot be grown on chalky soils, probably owing to the alkalinity. In other cases different varieties of the same species may grow on different soils. For example, in Derbyshire, UK, *Valeriana officinalis* var. *sambucifolia* is common on the coal measures, but avoids the limestone, where it is replaced by *Valeriana officinalis* var. *mikanii*.

The effect of nitrogen-containing nutrients on alkaloid production has received considerable study (solanaceous drugs including *Nicotiana*, opium); generally nitrogen fertilizers increase the size of the plants and the amounts of alkaloids produced but, as indicated elsewhere, the method of expressing the results of such experiments is important. The effects of nitrogen on glycoside and essential oil contents appear variable; presumably in these cases the final result arises from the general effect of nitrogen on the plant's metabolism. Nitrogen fertilization has been shown to increase the silymarin content of the fruits of *Silybum marianum* grown on reclaimed ground. The effect of potassium on alkaloid production shows no consistent trend, but an interesting example is the increase in putrescine production in barley grown on a potassium-deficient medium, where it is possible that the organic base has been formed to act as a substitute for potassium ions.

It has long been maintained that trace amounts of manganese are necessary for the successful production of *Digitalis purpurea* and more recently it was shown that a regimen of manganese and molybdenum feeding over the two years of development of *D. grandiflora* gives significant increases in glycoside yield.

Propagation from seeds

To ensure success the seeds must be collected when perfectly ripe. If not planted immediately, they should normally be stored in a cool and dry place and must not be kiln-dried. Some seeds such as cinnamon, coca and nutmegs rapidly lose their power of germination if allowed to dry or if stored for quite short periods. Long storage of all seeds usually much decreases the percentage which germinate.

Although seeds are naturally sown at the season when they ripen, it is frequently more convenient, especially in the case of the less hardy exotic species, to defer sowing until the spring. In some cases, however, immediate sowing of the fresh seed is advisable. For example, it has been shown that if the seeds of *Colchicum autumnale* are air-dried even for a few days, only about 5% germinate in 1 year and some may not germinate for 5 years; whereas if sown as soon as the capsules dehisce, 30% will germinate in the first year. In some instances, as with *Datura ferox* and foxglove, seeds may remain viable in the ground for many years before germinating. With *Erythroxylum coca* and *E. novogranatense* the seeds stored at 4°C for 24 days gave, respectively, 29% and 0% germination (E. L. Johnson, *Planta Med.*, 1989, **55**, 691). Seeds may, if slow germinating, be soaked in water or a 0.2% solution of gibberellic acid for 48 h before sowing; more drastic methods, such as soaking in sulphuric acid in the case of henbane seeds, or partial removal of the testa by means of a file or grindstone, have also been recommended. With *Ipomoea purga* (jalap) scarification of the seeds has been the secret of success in obtaining 95% germination in eight days (A. Linajes *et al.*, *Economic Botany*, 1994, **48**, 84).

Time of seed-sowing may affect the active constituents, as illustrated by *Chamomilla recutita*—for 17 cultivars investigated most gave a significantly higher yield of oil if they were spring-sown rather than autumn-sown and the oil composition also varied (O. Gasic *et al.*, *J. Ess. Oil Res.*, 1991, **3**, 295, through *Chem. Abs.*, **116**, 37955).

Propagation by vegetative means

The following examples of vegetative propagation may be mentioned.

1. By the development of *bulbs* (e.g. squill); *corms* (e.g. colchicum); *tubers* (e.g. jalap and aconite); or *rhizomes* (e.g. ginger).
2. By *division*, a term usually applied to the separation of a plant which has a number of aerial stems or buds, into separate parts each having roots and a growing point. This method may be used for althaea, rhubarb, gentian and male fern.
3. By *runners* or *offsets* (e.g. chamomile and the mints).
4. By *suckers* or *stolons* (e.g. liquorice and valerian).
5. By *cuttings* or portions of the plant severed from the plant and capable of developing roots. Success by this method has been extended to a large number of plants by the use of rooting hormones (see Chapter 12) and by the employment of mist propagation.
6. By *layers*. A layer is a branch or shoot which is induced to develop roots before it is completely severed from the parent plant. This is done by partly interrupting the food supply by means of a cut or ligature and embedding the part. Alternatively the slit portion of the branch is enclosed in moist peat, surrounded by moss, and the whole enclosed in polythene. This method has been used successfully for the propagation of cascara.

7. By *grafting* and *budding*. Grafting is an operation in which two cut surfaces, usually of different but closely related plants, are placed so as to unite and grow together. The rooted plant is called the *stock* and the portion cut off the *scion* or *graft*. In Guatemala young *Cinchona ledgeriana* scions are grafted on *Cinchona succirubra* root-stocks, eventually giving a tree which produces bark rich in the alkaloid quinidine. Grafting of female scions of *Myristica fragrans* on male stocks may be used to increase the proportion of fruit-bearing trees in the plantation. The method has been used considerably in phytochemical research to study sites of synthesis of metabolites etc. *Budding* consists of the introduction of a piece of bark bearing a bud into a suitable cavity or T-shaped slit made in the bark of the stock. Budding is largely used for *Citrus* species, selected strains of sweet orange, for example, being budded on sour stocks.

8. By *fermentation*. This process applies particularly to the production of moulds and bacteria, and is extensively used in the manufacture of antibiotics, lysergic acid derivatives and some vitamins.

9. By *inoculation*. Specific to ergot whereby the spores of the fungus are artificially cultured and injected into the rye heads by special machines,

10. By *cell culture* followed by differentiation; see Chapter 13.

Hydroponics

Plants can be cultivated without soil by the use of an artificial aqueous nutrient medium. The system is suitable for raising plants under laboratory conditions for biogenetic and other studies. It is used commercially for such crops as tomatoes and strawberries but is uneconomic for the large-scale production of common medicinal plants.

S. J. Murch *et al.* (*Planta Med.*, 2002, **68**, 1108) have obtained data showing that a greenhouse hydroponic system can be effectively used for the production of St John's wort containing the active constituents hypericin, pseudohypericin and hyperforin.

COLLECTION

Drugs may be collected from wild or cultivated plants, and the task may be undertaken by casual, unskilled native labour (e.g. ipecacuanha) or by skilled workers in a highly scientific manner (e.g. digitalis, belladonna and cinchona). In the USA the explosive demand for some herbs has led to concern over wholesale uncontrolled collection, so-called wildcrafting, resulting in the over-harvesting of such plants as *Panax quinquefolium*, *Polygala senega*, *Echinacea* spp. and *Cimicifuga racemosa* (black cohosh). Elsewhere *Prunus africana* (pygeum bark) found from Nigeria to Madagascar, *Rauwolfia serpentina* from India, and *Turnera diffusa* (damiana) from Mexico are other examples of over-exploitation.

A strategy for the sustained harvesting of *Camptotheca acuminata* (Nyssaceae), the source of the anticancer drug camptothecin, has been described by R. M. Vincent *et al.*, (*J. Nat. Prod.*, 1997, **60**, 618). The alkaloid is accumulated in young leaves and by their repeated removal axillary bud outgrowth is stimulated giving an increased harvestable amount of camptothecin in a non-destructive manner. Further studies by S. Li *et al.* (*Planta Med.*, 2002, **68**, 1010) showed that camptothecin accumulates primarily in the glandular trichomes of the leaves and stems with overall variation among *Camptotheca* species and varieties, and significantly, according to tissue ages and seasons. Details of the two best strains for cultivation are given.

With *Hypericum perforatum* it has been shown that from the first bud phase to the open flower stage the contents of dianthrones, quercetin derivatives and hyperforin increase; in the unripe fruits dianthrones and quercetin glycosides decrease whereas the hyperforin content increases (D. Tekelová *et al.*, *Planta Med.*, 2000, **66**, 778).

The season at which each drug is collected is usually a matter of considerable importance, as the amount, and sometimes the nature, of the active constituents is not constant throughout the year. This applies, for example, to the collection of podophyllum, ephedra, rhubarb, wild cherry and aconite. Rhubarb is reported to contain no anthraquinone derivatives in winter but anthranols which, on the arrival of warmer weather, are converted by oxidation into anthraquinones; also the contents of *C*-glycosides, *O*-glycosides and free anthraquinones in the developing shoots and leaves of *Rhamnus purshiana* fluctuate markedly throughout the year.

The age of the plant is also of considerable importance and governs not only the total quantity of active constituents produced but also the relative proportions of the components of the active mixture. A few examples are given in Table 11.1 but some ontogenetic variation of constituents must exist for all plants.

There is increasing evidence that the composition of a number of secondary plant metabolites varies appreciably throughout the day and night. In some cases—for example, with digitalis and the tropane alkaloid-containing plants which have been extensively studied—the evidence has been somewhat conflicting in this respect. However, this may be largely due to the methods of analysis employed; thus, throughout the day the overall amount of alkaloid or glycoside may not change to any extent but there may be an interconversion of the various alkaloids or glycosides present. Daily variations of the alkaloids of the poppy, hemlock, lupin, broom, the solanaceous plants and ergot have been reported, also with the steroidal alkaloids of 'industrial shoots' of *Solanum laciniatum*, the cardiac glycosides of *Digitalis purpurea* and *D. lanata*, the simple phenolic glycosides of *Salix* and the volatile oil content of *Pinus* and *Salvia*.

Generally speaking, leaves are collected as the flowers are beginning to open, flowers just before they are fully expanded, and underground organs as the aerial parts die down. Leaves, flowers and fruits should not be collected when covered with dew or rain. Any which are discoloured or attacked by insects or slugs should be rejected. Even with hand-picking, it is difficult, certainly expensive, to get leaves, flowers or fruits entirely free from other parts of the plant. In cases such as senna leaf and digitalis the official monographs allow a certain percentage of stalks to be present or a limited amount of 'foreign matter' (for definition, see *BP/EP* and Chapter 16). Similarly, with roots and rhizomes a certain amount of aerial stem is often collected and is permitted in the case of senega root. The harvesting of umbelliferous fruits resembles that of wheat. Reaping machines are used, and the plants, after drying in shocks, are threshed to separate the fruits. Special machines are used to harvest ergot and lavender flowers (illustrations will be found in earlier editions). Barks are usually collected after a period of damp weather, as they then separate most readily from the wood. For the collection of gums, gum resins, etc., dry weather is obviously indicated and care should be taken to exclude vegetable debris as far as possible.

Underground organs must be freed from soil. Shaking the drug before, during and after drying, or brushing it, may be sufficient to separate a sandy soil, but in the case of a clay or other heavy soil washing is necessary. For example, valerian collected from the wild is washed in the streams on the banks of which it usually grows. Before drying, any wormy or diseased rhizomes or roots should be rejected. Those of small size are often replanted. In certain cases the rootlets are cut off; rhubarb, ginger and marshmallow are usually peeled. All large organs, such as calumba root and inula rhizome, should be sliced to facilitate drying. Before gentian root is dried, it is

Table 11.1 Examples of the ontogenetic variation of some metabolites.

Example	Ontogenetic variation
Volatile oils	
Mentha piperita	Relatively high proportion of pulegone in young plants: replaced by menthone and menthol as leaves mature
M. spicata	Progression from predominance of carvone in young plants to dihydrocarvone in older ones
Cloves	Contain about 14–21% of oil; mother 'blown' cloves contain very little oil
Coriandum sativum	Marked changes in oil composition at the beginning of flowering and fruiting
Achillea millefolium	During flowering, monoterpenes (principally 1,8-cineole) predominate in oils from leaves and flowers. Oil obtained during the vegetative period contains principally sesquiterpenes (92%) with germacrane D the major component
Laurus nobilis	Highest yield: end of August (Portugal), July (China), Spring (Israel), coinciding with highest level of 1,8-cineole
Valeriana officinalis	Highest content in September (valerenic acid and derivatives, and the valepotriates reached maximum in February–March)
Cinnamomum camphora	Camphor accumulates in heartwood as tree ages; ready for collection at 40 years
Diterpenes	
Taxus baccata	Needles contain up to 0.1% 10-deacetylbaccatin which is replaced by large amounts of 2,4-dimethoxyphenol in winter
Cannabinoids	
Cannabis sativa	Young seedlings contain principally cannabichromene; Δ^9-tetrahydrocannabinol is major cannabinoid of adult plants
Cardioactive glycosides	
Digitalis purpurea	Glycoside content varies with age; purpurea-glycoside A is formed last but eventually reaches a constant maxiumum of 50% of the total glycoside
D. lanata	Although highest levels of total glycosides are observed in first-year leaves, those glycosides most important medicinally (e.g. lanatoside C) attain their highest levels in second-year plants
Cyanogenetic glycosides	
Linum usitatissimum seeds	Monoglucosides (linamarin and lotaustralin) and diglucosides (linustatin and neolinustatin) in developing embryos; diglucosides only accumulate in mature seeds
Steroidal sapogenins	
Agave sp.	Steroidal sapogenins isolated from young, mature, old and flowering plants had successively fewer hydroxyl groups
Yucca sp.	Similar to Agave
Dioscorea tokoro	Changes in sapogenin content in first season's growth
Alkaloids	
Papaver somniferum	Morphine content of capsule highest 2½–3 weeks after flowering; the secondary alkaloids (codeine, thebaine, narcotine and papaverine) reach their maximum somewhat earlier
Datura stramonium	The hyoscine/hyoscyamine ratio falls from about 80% in young seedlings to about 30% in mature fruiting plants
Duboisia myoporoides	The hyoscine/hyoscyamine ratio depends both on the developmental stage of the plant and on the position of the leaves on the stem
Ipomoea violacea seeds	Lysergic acid amide/chanoclavine ratio increases as the seed matures
Steroidal alkaloids	
Solanum dulcamara fruits	Solasodine content fluctuates during maturation of fruit; tomatidenol and soladulcidine eventually predominate
Citrus glycosides and limonoids	Limonin and naringin levels in grapefruit fall as fruit matures
Furanocoumarins	
Ammi visnaga	Unripe fruits richest in both khellin and visnagin
Tannins	
Liquidambar formosana	Seasonable variation of hydrolysable leaf tannis, most rapid changes in the Spring
Vanillin	
Vanilla planifolia	Highest rate of vanillin biosynthesis occurs 8 months after flower pollination

made into heaps and allowed to ferment. Seeds such as nux vomica and cocoa, which are extracted from mucilaginous fruits, are washed free from pulp before drying.

DRYING

If enzymic action is to be encouraged, slow drying at a moderate temperature is necessary. Examples of this will be found under 'Orris Rhizome', 'Vanilla Pods', 'Cocoa Seeds' and 'Gentian Root'. If enzymic action is not desired, drying should take place as soon as possible after collection. Drugs containing volatile oils are liable to lose their aroma if not dried or if the oil is not distilled from them immediately, and all moist drugs are liable to develop mould. For these reasons, drying apparatus and stills should be situated as near to the growing plants as possible. This has the further advantage that freightage is much reduced, as many fresh drugs contain a considerable amount (60–90%) of water.

The duration of the drying process varies from a few hours to many weeks, and in the case of open-air drying depends very largely on the weather. In suitable climates open-air drying is used for such drugs as clove, colocynth, cardamom and cinnamon. Even in warm and dry climates arrangements have to be made for getting the drug under the cover of sheds or tarpaulins at night or during wet weather. For drying in sheds the drugs may be suspended in bundles from the roof, threaded on strings, as in the case of Chinese rhubarb, or, more commonly, placed on trays made of sacking or tinned wire-netting. Papers spread on a wooden framework are also used, particularly for fruits from which it is desired to collect the seeds.

Drying by artificial heat is more rapid than open-air drying and is often necessary in tropical countries (e.g. West Africa, where the humidity is very high, and Honduras for drying cardamom fruits). In Europe continuous belt driers are used for large crops such as digitalis. Alternatively heat may be applied by means of open fires (e.g. nutmegs), stoves or hot-water pipes. In all drying sheds there must be a space of at least 15 cm between superimposed trays, and air must circulate freely.

H. N. ElSohly *et al.* (*Planta Medica*, 1997, **63**, 83) have studied the effect of drying conditions on the taxane content of *Taxus* needles. When the length of drying extended up to 10 and 15 days as in a shadehouse or in the laboratory the recovery of taxanes was adversely affected. Drying in a tobacco barn, greenhouse or oven, and freeze-drying was generally satisfactory for taxol and cephalomannine recoveries but the recoveries for 10-deacetyltaxol and 10-deacetylbaccatin III were only 75–80% of those expected.

Rapid drying helps flowers and leaves to retain their colour and aromatic drugs their aroma, but the temperature used in each case must be governed by the constituents and the physical nature of the drug. As a general rule, leaves, herbs and flowers may be dried between 20 and 40°C, and barks and roots between 30 and 65°C. In the cases of colchicum corm and digitalis leaf it will be noted that the *BPC* and *BP* specify the temperatures at which drying is to be done. For rural tropical areas, solar dryers have some distinct advantages over conventional artificial heat dryers and have been introduced into some countries.

Exactly how far drying is to be carried is a matter for practical experience. If leaves and other delicate structures are overdried, they become very brittle and tend to break in transit. Drugs such as aloes and opium may require further drying after importation.

STORAGE

The large-scale storage of drugs is a considerable undertaking. Except in a few cases, such as cascara bark, long storage, although often unavoidable, is not to be recommended. Drugs such as Indian hemp and sarsaparilla deteriorate even when carefully stored. It has been reported that the content of taxol in *Taxus baccata* leaves and extracts stored at room temperature for one year decreased by 30–40% and

70–80% respectively; storage in a freezer and out of direct sunlight produced no adverse deterioration (B. Das *et al.*, *Planta Medica*, 1998, **64**, 96).

Similarly the alkamides of the popular immunostimulant herb *Echinacea purpurea* decrease rapidly on storage; N. B. Perry *et al.* (*Planta Medica*, 2000, **66**, 54) have shown that although drying has little effect on the quantity of alkamides, storage for 64 weeks at 24° produces an 80% loss, and a significant loss even at −18°. Drugs stored in the usual containers—sacks, bales, wooden cases, cardboard boxes and paper bags—reabsorb about 10–12% or more of moisture. They are then termed 'air-dry'. Plastic sacks will effectively seal the contents. The permissible moisture contents of starch, acacia gum and others will be found in the *BP* and *European Pharmacopoeia*. The combined effects of moisture and temperature on humidity and the subsequent water-condensation when the temperature falls, must be considered in drug storage. Drugs such as digitalis and Indian hemp should never be allowed to become air-dry or they lose a considerable part of their activity. They may be kept in sealed containers with a dehydrating agent. For large quantities the bottom of a case may be filled with quicklime and separated from the drug by a perforated grid or sacking. If the lime becomes moist, it should be renewed. Volatile oils should be stored in sealed, well-filled containers in a cool, dark place. Similar remarks apply to fixed oils, particularly cod-liver oil. In the latter case the air in the containers is sometimes replaced by an inert gas. Air-dry drugs are always susceptible to the attack of insects and other pests, so they should be examined frequently during storage and any showing mould or worminess should be rejected.

In order to reduce undesirable microbial contamination and to prevent the development of other living organisms, some plant materials may require sterilization before storage.

EUROPEAN REGULATIONS

To ensure that satisfactory standards for the growing and primary processing of medicinal and aromatic (culinary) herbs are achieved throughout the European Union 'Guidelines for Good Agricultural Practice of Medicinal and Aromatic Plants' was issued as a final European version in August 1998. It covers seeds and propagation, cultivation, harvesting, primary processing, packaging, storage and transport, personnel and facilities, documentation, education and quality assurance. Details can be found in *ICMAP News*, No 6, April 1999 (ICMAP = International Council for Medicinal and Aromatic Plants). Legal requirements covering the manufacture of herbal medicines in Europe have now (2007) been implemented (see Chapter 16: Quality control).

12

Plant growth regulators

The growth and development of plants is regulated by a number of chemical substances which together exert a complex interaction to meet the needs of the plant. Five groups of plant hormones are well established; they are the auxins, gibberellins, cytokinins, abscisic acid and its derivatives, and ethylene. These substances are of wide distribution and may, in fact, occur in all higher plants. They are specific in their action, are active in very low concentrations, and regulate cell enlargement, cell division, cell differentiation, organogenesis, senescence and dormancy. Their action is probably sequential. Other hormones concerned with flower formation and reproduction, but as yet uncharacterized, have also been envisaged. The essential role of these substances is illustrated by cell and tissue cultures; without the addition of suitable hormones no development or cell division occurs.

The effects of these very active substances on the production of secondary metabolites, particularly with a view to producing plants containing an enhanced proportion of active constituent, are of interest to pharmacognosists. In such studies the manner in which the results are recorded is all-important, particularly as the treatment may also influence the size of the test plant compared with the controls. For commercial purposes yield per hectare is an obvious criterion, whereas for biosynthetic studies yield per plant or per cent fresh weight may be of more significance. For final drug evaluation per cent dry weight is the most likely requirement.

In spite of the early enthusiasm for research on drug enhancement by the use of hormones applied to medicinal field crops, very little in the way of useful practical application emerged; the results were, however, of interest and selected examples of this older work continue to be retained in this chapter.

AUXINS

These growth-promoting substances were first studied in 1931 by Dutch workers who isolated two growth-regulating acids (auxin-a and auxin-b, obtained from human urine and cereal products, respectively). They subsequently noted that these had similar properties to indole-3-acetic acid (IAA), the compound now considered to be the major auxin of plants, and found particularly in actively growing tissues. Several similar acids, potential precursors of indoleacetic acid, have also been reported as natural products; they include indoleacetaldehyde, indoleacetonitrile and indolepyruvic acid. These compounds and IAA are all derived, in the plants, from tryptophan.

Typical effects of auxins are cell elongation giving an increase in stem length, inhibition of root growth, adventitious root production and fruit-setting in the absence of pollination. A number of widely used synthetic auxins include indole-3-butyric acid, naphthalene-1-acetic acid (NAA) and 2,4-dichlorophenoxyacetic acid (2,4-D).

Indole-3-acetic acid

2,4-Dichlorophenoxyacetic acid

In the plant, oxidative degradation of IAA to give a number of products is controlled by IAA oxidase. Some substances such as the ortho-diphenols (e.g. caffeic and chlorogenic acids and quercetin) inhibit the action of the enzyme and, hence, stimulate growth themselves. Conversely, monophenols such as *p*-coumaric acid promote the action of IAA oxidase and so inhibit growth. IAA may also be conjugated in the plant with aspartic acid, glutamic acid, glycine, sugars and cyclitols; such bound forms may represent a detoxication mechanism or are inactive storage forms of the hormone.

The main practical uses of auxins are: (1) in low concentrations to accelerate the rooting of woody and herbaceous cuttings; and (2) in higher concentrations to act as selective herbicides or weed-killers. Placed for 24 h in a 1:500 000 solution of NAA, cuttings will subsequently develop roots. This includes cuttings from trees such as holly, which were formerly very difficult to propagate in this way and had to be raised from seed or by grafting. Similarly, indole-3-butyric acid was successful with *Cinchona* cuttings, saving some 2 or 3 years compared with growth from seed. Similar results have been obtained with cuttings of *Carica, Coffea, Pinus* and other species. In biogenetic studies, use has been made of auxins to induce root formation on isolated leaves such as those of *Nicotiana* and *Datura* species. Auxins used in suitable concentration (usually stronger than when used for rooting cuttings) selectively destroy some species of plant and leave others more or less unaffected. They have, therefore, a very important role as selective weed-killers in horticulture and agriculture. Thus 2,4-D is particularly toxic to dicotyledonous plants while, in suitable concentration, having little effect on monocotyledons. It can, therefore, be used to destroy such dicotyledonous weeds as dandelion and plantain from grass lawns. (N.B. Certain carbamate and urea derivatives have an opposite effect and can be used to destroy grass without serious injury to dicotyledonous crops.)

There have been several reports on the effects of auxins on the formation of secondary metabolites on medicinal plants.

Seedlings and young plants of *Mentha piperita*, when treated with derivatives of NAA, gave in the mature plants an increased yield (30–50%) of oil which itself contained 4.5–9.0% more menthol than the controls. The study of the effects of auxins on alkaloid formation has concentrated principally on the tropane alkaloids of *Datura* species. Morphological changes in the plants were observed (2,4-D, for example, produced abnormal and bizarre forms of *D. stramonium*; an increase in trichome production, particularly in branched non-glandular forms; smooth fruits as distinct from those with spines; and a proliferation of vascular tissue). Generally, workers found no marked effect on alkaloid production or on the type of alkaloids produced, although a Russian paper records that with thornapple and scopolia tissue cultures a stimulating effect on alkaloid production was obtained with NAA and an inhibiting effect with 2,4-D; similar results were reported for *Rauwolfia serpentina* tissue cultures with these two hormones. An increased alkaloid production has been reported for submerged cultures of certain ergot strains when treated with various auxins (IAA; NAA; 2,4-D; indole propionic acid; indole butyric acid), whereas unpredictable irregular quantitative and qualitative effects on ergoline alkaloid production were observed with the same hormones in *Ipomoea, Rivea* and *Argyreia* (Convolvulaceae) suspension cultures. Experiments carried out in Hungary involving the injection of IAA into poppy capsules 1 and 2 days after flowering produced a relatively elongated capsule form and, in general, a reduced alkaloid content. In studies on anthraquinone production by cell suspension cultures of *Morinda citrifolia*, Zenk and co-workers have shown that cells grown in the presence of NAA have a substantial anthraquinone production but those with 2,4-D as sole auxin do not. IAA appears to have no beneficial effect on the production of sennosides in *Cassia angustifolia*.

GIBBERELLINS

This group of plant growth regulators was discovered by Japanese workers in connection with the 'bakanae' (foolish seedlings) disease of rice. In this, the affected plants become excessively tall and are unable to support themselves; through a combination of the resulting weakness and parasite damage they eventually die. The causative organism of the disease is *Gibberella fugikuroi*, and in 1926 Kurosawa found that extracts of the fungus could initiate the disease symptoms when applied to healthy rice plants. Some 10 years later, Yabuta and Hayashi isolated a crystalline sample of the active material which they called 'gibberellin'. Preoccupation with the auxins by western plant physiologists, the existence of language barriers and the advent of World War II meant that a further 10 years elapsed before the significance of these findings was appreciated outside Japan. In the 1950s groups in Britain, the USA and Japan further investigated these compounds, which were shown to have amazing effects when applied to plants. It soon became apparent that a range of gibberellins was involved, and they are now distinguished as GA_1, GA_2, GA_3, etc. GA_3, commonly referred to as gibberellic acid and produced commercially by fungal cultivation, is probably the best-known of the series; its structure was finally determined in 1959. The first good indications that gibberellins actually existed in higher plants came with West and Phinney's observation in 1956 that the liquid endosperm of the wild cucumber (*Echinocytis macrocarpa*) was particularly rich in substances possessing gibberellin-like activity and Radley's report of a substance from pea-shoots behaving like gibberellic acid on paper chromatograms. Finally, in 1958 MacMillan and Suter isolated crystalline GA_1 from *Phaseolus multiflorus*. By 1980, 58 gibberellins were known of which about half were derived from the *Gibberella* fungus and half from higher plants. GA_{117} was characterized from fern gametophytes in 1998 (G. Wynne *et al.*, *Phytochemistry*, 1998, **49**, 1837). Of these many GAs most are either dead-end metabolites or are intermediates in the formation of active compounds; only a limited number have hormonal activity *per se*. It is now considered possible that these substances are present in most, if not all, plants.

Gibberellins are synthesized in leaves and they accumulate in relatively large quantities in the immature seeds and fruits of some plants. The most dramatic effect of gibberellins can be seen by their application to short-node plants—for example, those plants producing rosettes of leaves (*Digitalis, Hyoscyamus*)—when bolting and flowering is induced; also, dwarf varieties of many plants, when treated with the hormone, grow to the same height as taller varieties. Other important actions of the gibberellins are the initiation of the synthesis of various hydrolytic and proteolytic enzymes upon which seed germination and seedling establishment depend.

The growth effect of gibberellins arises by cell elongation in the subapical meristem region where young internodes are developing. The effects of gibberellins and auxins appear complementary, the full stimulation of elongation by either hormone necessitating an adequate presence of the other.

As with auxins, gibberellins appear also to occur in plants in deactivated forms; thus, β-D-glucopyranosyl esters of GA_1, GA_4, GA_8, GA_{37} and GA_{38} are known. As such they may serve a depot function. The glucosyl ester of GA_3 has been prepared in several laboratories.

The biogenetic pathways of the gibberellins appear to be similar in both higher plants and *Gibberella*. They arise at the C_{20} geranylgeranyl pyrophosphate level of the isoprenoid mevalonic acid pathway (q.v.) with cyclizations giving the C_{20} tetracyclic diterpernoid entkaurenoic acid, which by a multistep ring contraction furnishes the gibbane ring system as exemplified by the key intermediate GA_{12}-aldehyde. Several

Gibberellic acid (GA₃)

GA₁₂ aldehyde.
Key diversification point for synthesis of GAs

pathways diverge from GA_{12}-aldehyde to give the known 90 or so gibberellins. All GAs have either the ent-gibberellane (C_{20} GAs) or the ent-20-norgibberellane (C_{19} GAs) (loss of C-20) carbon skeleton. Both types are modified by the position and number of OH groups, oxidation state of C-18 and C-20, lactone formation, presence and position of double bonds on ring A, epoxide formation, the presence of a carboxyl group and hydration of the C16–C17 double bond.

The gibberellins have been used to treat many plants which contain useful secondary metabolites. A summary of some of the findings, for different groups, is given below.

Volatile oils and terpenoids

Early work involving GA treatment of volatile oil-containing plants was concerned with resultant changes in morphological characters in genera such as *Citrus, Eucalyptus* and *Foeniculum*. GA spraying of the flowers of *Humulus lupulus* advanced the maturity of the hops by 10 days and gave a more evenly developed crop. Although the cones of treated flowers were more subject to wind burn than normal, their yield was increased by about 40%. The α-resin content of the hops, on which their commercial value depends, however, was 1.8% compared with 10.2% for the controls; the volatile oil composition also differed. Several studies have been made of the effects of GA treatment on *Mentha piperita*. The detailed results vary, but the general result is a lowering of the oil content (possibly by reduction of the number of glandular hairs) with little change in the oil composition. In contrast to the above, Kaul and Kapoor have reported favourably on the GA treatment of *Chenopodium ambrosioides* and *Anethum* spp. with respect to volatile oil content. The former afforded a 33% increase in volatile oil with no appreciable change in ascaridole content. With *Anethum graveolens* specific doses of GA increased the oil content by up to 50% and with *A. sowa* (Indian dill) by up to 30%. At the lower doses of GA treatment there was no significant change in the carvone content of the oil, but at higher concentrations there appeared to be a slight increase over the (then) official limit (53%, *BP* 1958). With *Foeniculum vulgare* and *Coriandrum sativum* Gjerstad found that foliar sprays of 100 parts/10⁶ GA, applied bi-weekly, gave a difference in cauline length of 200–300% but no differences were detected in yield of fruits and quantity and quality of volatile oil.

Alkaloids

The seeds of the tropane alkaloid-producing species of *Atropa, Hyoscyamus* and *Datura* often exhibit protracted dormancy or erratic germination; GA treatment of the seeds can be used to assist in obtaining uniform germination and total emergence. Considerable work has been published on the effects of the hormone on the morphology and alkaloid content of treated plants. *Hyoscyamus niger* is a perennial and

the hormone effects included stem elongation giving a two- to threefold increase in height; a spindly and vine-like growth; slightly chlorotic and narrow leaves; a more rapid onset of flowering; increases in the stem dry weights but decreases in the dry weights of leaves, tops and roots. The overall yield of alkaloids in the treated plants was reduced by about a half and the concentration of alkaloids in various morphological parts ranged from 43 to 84% of that of the controls, with the stems showing the greatest reduction. Subsequent experiments showed that with belladonna, increased alkaloid yields could be obtained by adjusting the dose of GA treatment to favour overall growth in the older plant.

Similar results have been reported with *Datura* spp., plants showing the predictable morphological effects and giving a reduced alkaloid yield. The effects were not transmitted to the second-generation plants. With *Nicotiana tabacum* and *Duboisia* hybrids, treatment again gave a generally reduced alkaloid content accompanied by characteristic morphological effects.

Other alkaloid-containing plants which have been subjected to GA treatment include *Catharanthus roseus* (generally a lowering of alkaloid content and some change in the relative proportion of vinblastine to other alkaloids); *Rauwolfia serpentina* (lowering of alkaloid concentration in the roots, the effect increasing with dose); and *Thea sinensis* (slight difference in caffeine content of leaves). It would appear, therefore, that with the alkaloid-containing plants so far tested, the substantial internodal growth produced by GA is offset by a lower overall accumulation of alkaloid.

Glycosides

In 1959 Sayed and Beal reported the effects of the daily GA treatment of first-year rosette *Digitalis purpurea* plants. Flowering occurred in the first year with treated plants and the leaves became longer and more linear, with an increase in dry weight. An increase in cardioactive glycosides was obtained but no increase in the digitoxose content was observed. Similar experiments by Burton and Sciuchetti in 1961 involving weekly treatments of *D. lanata* produced similar results, with 'bolting' after the twelfth week. The total glycoside per shoot of the treated plants was considerably increased in the first 8 weeks, and at harvest time showed about 30% increase with the lower dose of hormone (10 μg week⁻¹), and a 50% decrease with the higher (50 μg week⁻¹). The authors concluded that the effect of the treatment of glycoside production correlated more closely with the growth response than with the effect on carbohydrate formation. With both leaf and root cultures Lui and Staba (1981) found GA to have a positive effect on the production of digoxin.

Application of GA to *Cassia angustifolia* (Bhatia *et al.*, *Planta Med.*, 1978, **34**, 437) appeared to reduce the sennoside content of the leaves at all concentrations used, but slightly increased the dry weight of the shoot.

Fixed oils

Gjerstad obtained castor plants (*Ricinus communis*) five times the height of controls as a result of GA treatment. No significant differences were observed regarding the quantity and quality of the fixed oil of the seed.

CELL DIVISION HORMONES: CYTOKININS

Auxins and gibberellins are concerned largely with cell enlargement; and although they influence cell-multiplication processes, there are other substances which have a more specific effect on cell division (cytokinesis). The activity of the latter is not only confined to cell division in a tissue *per se*; they also regulate the pattern and frequency of organ production as well as position and shape. They have an inhibitory effect on senescence. The presence of such compounds has been suspected for many years, the German botanist Haberlandt in 1913 having noted that phloem tissues contained water-soluble substances capable of promoting cell division in parenchymatous cells of wounded potato tubers. It was not until many years later (1954) that Miller, working at Wisconsin on tissue cultures, discovered that aged or autoclaved DNA from herring sperm stimulated cell division. This active degradation product was called kinetin and in 1955 was identified as 6-furfurylaminopurine (6-furfuryladenine). Kinetin itself has not been isolated from plants, but in 1964, after the indication of cytokinins in liquid endosperm of the coconut and in extracts of maize embryos at the milky stage, an active substance named zeatin was isolated from the latter source. Like most other cytokinins, it is a 6-substituted adenine derivative, 6·(4-hydroxy-3-methylbut-2-eny1)-aminopurine. It has since been shown to be associated in maize with zeatin riboside (1 β-D-ribofuranose) and with a phosphate ester of this compound. The hormone complex has been detected in the cambial region of various woody plants. Isopentenyladenine and dihydrozeatin are examples of cytokinin isolated from other sources; many more have been detected but not identified. The sidechain of cytokinins is of isoprenoid origin.

Kinetin

Cytokinins have been much employed in tissue culture work, in which they are used to promote the formation of adventitious buds and shoots from undifferentiated cells. In cell cultures, they have been shown to promote the biosynthesis of berberine (*Thalictrum minus*), condensed tannins (*Onobrychis viccifolia*) and rhodoxanthin (*Ricinus*).

A limited study only has been made of the effects of cytokinins on secondary metabolism in intact plants. Concerning plants producing tropane alkaloids, Ambrose and Sciuchetti have compared the action of kinetin and GA on *Datura meteloides*. Plants received weekly doses of 25 μg kinetin; in relation to the controls the following differences were noted:

Kinetin treatment	Gibberellic acid treatment
Shorter and bushier plants	Taller and spindly plants
Decreased growth	Increased growth
No change in alkaloid content in plant organs	Decreased alkaloid production
Delayed response	Rapid response

Luanratana and Griffin (*J. Nat. Prod.*, 1980, **43**, 546, 552; 1982, **45**, 270) observed the beneficial effects of a commercial seaweed extract containing cytokinin activity on *Duboisia* hybrids grown both hydroponically and in a commercial plantation. In the latter there was an 18% increase in leaf yield and a 16% increase in hyoscine content compared with the controls. A further pointer to the usefulness of the treatment was that in field plants it led to a delay in the usual seasonal fall in alkaloid content (February–April in Australia), thus permitting an economically useful, extended collection period. Shah *et al.*

(1990) reported favourable increases in growth and alkaloid yield with *Hyoscyamus muticus* treated with kinetin (50 p.p.m.).

Verzár-Petri injected benzyladenine and kinetin separately into developing poppy capsules; the effects were similar to those observed with auxins. Leaves of the coffee plant after kinetin treatment developed a transient increase of up to 10% in their caffeine content. The effect was transitory and passed after 6–12 days. With *Cassia angustifolia* plants low concentrations of hormone were found to increase slightly the sennoside content and to favour an increase in the dry weight of shoots.

Zeatin

GROWTH INHIBITORS

Natural growth inhibitors are present in plants and affect bud opening, seed germination and development of dormancy. One such substance, abscisic acid [3-methyl-5-(1-hydroxy-4-oxo-2,6,6-trimethyl-2-cyclohexane-1-y1)-*cis*,*trans*-2,4-pentadienoic acid] was isolated and characterized in 1965; it has also been isolated from the fungus *Cenospora rosicola*.

The structural similarity of abscisic acid (ABA) to the carotenoids prompted research on the relationship of these two groups of compounds and it has now been demonstrated that some xanthophylls, particularly violaxanthin, produce a germination inhibitor on exposure to light. Evidence has now accumulated in support of an indirect 'apo-carotenoid' pathway for ABA biosynthesis, the most likely precleavage precursors being 9′-*cis*-neoxanthin and 9-*cis*-violaxanthin which fracture across the 11,12 (11′,12′) double bond to produce xanthoxin which in plant tissues is readily transformed into ABA (see A. D. Parry and R. Horgan, *Phytochem.*, 1991, **30**, 815). However, it is also possible that ABA arises from farnesol at the C_{15} sesquiterpenoid level of the MVA pathway (q.v.). The theoretical postulation involves a number of steps in which, as with the apo-carotenoid pathway, *cis*-Δ^2-xanthoxin could also be involved. In accord with isoprenoid biosynthesis, mevalonic acid (MVA) has been demonstrated to be stereochemically incorporated into ABA in higher plants, and likewise labelled acetate in *Cenospora rosicola*. Other substances related to abscisic acid have

Abscisic acid (ABA)

cis-Δ^2-Xanthoxin

been isolated from plants and include vomifoliol (several sources), which lacks the 2,4-pentadiene side-chain; it has the same activity as abscisic acid in stomatal closure tests. Little or no work appears to have been reported on the effects of abscisic acid on the production of pharmacognostically interesting substances.

A number of synthetic growth inhibitors have been studied; the first to be described was maleic hydrazide in 1949. *N*-Dimethyl-aminosuccinamic acid can be considered as a hydrazine derivative and acts as a shoot-elongation inhibitor by suppressing the oxidation of tryptamine to IAA. Sciuchetti and colleagues showed that this compound sprayed on to *Datura stramonium* and *D. innoxia* plants reduced the eventual height of the plants and lowered, overall, their total alkaloid content; however, significant increases were noted in the concentrations of stem alkaloid (56% increase in the second week and 90% in the fourth week compared with the controls). The inhibitor, tributyl 2,4-dichlorobenzylphosphonium chloride (phosphon) produced similar results with *D. ferox*. Trigonelline, an alkaloid of fenugreek seeds, promotes cell arrest in G_2 (a specific period preceding mitotic division of the nucleus) in various legumes.

ETHYLENE

It has been known for many years that ethylene induces growth responses in plants, and in 1932 it was demonstrated that the ethylene evolved by stored apples inhibited the growth of potato shoots enclosed with them; it has a role in fruit ripening. Current thought maintains that this simple compound should be included among the natural plant hormones. Ethylene is synthesized in the plant from *S*-adenosylmethionine via the intermediate 1-aminocyclopropane-1-carboxylic acid (ACC). The gene for ACC synthase has been cloned from tomato squash (H. Klee and M. Estelle in *Annu. Rev. Plant Physiol.*, 1991, **42**, 529). One biochemical action of ethylene is the stimulation of the *de novo* synthesis and secretion of cell-wall dissolving enzymes such as cellulase during leaf abscission and fruit ripening. A compound that gives rise to a typical ethylene response in plants is (2-chloroethyl)phosphonic acid (ethephon) applied in aqueous solution in concentrations of the order of 100–5000 p.p.m. In the cell sap, at pH values above 4.0 it is broken down to ethylene and phosphate. It is marketed as Ethrel.

At low concentration ethylene has been shown to increase the sennoside concentration in *Cassia angustifolia*, and applied to tobacco leaves it stimulates production of the stress compounds phytuberin and phytuberol (these are compounds produced in response to tobacco mosaic virus); with *Digitalis lanata* tissue cultures, cardenolide accumulation is decreased. Ethephon is now increasingly used as standard practice for enhancing the flow of rubber latex. Sprayed on to the scraped bark (tapping groove) of the rubber tree it increases latex yields by from 36 to 130%.

Other growth regulators

In addition to the well-known plant growth substances discussed above, a very large number of other compounds have been isolated from natural sources which in some way influence plant growth. Some are widely distributed and others are of restricted occurrence. Generally they have a less specific action than the regulators already mentioned above. They have no common chemical structure and only a few recurrent functional groups (e.g. phenolic hydroxy groups and α-methylene-γ-butyrolactone moieties). This implies that these substances may be acting at many different sites along the growth regulatory process. Substances involved include aliphatic and aromatic carboxylic acids, phenolic and neutral compounds, salicylate, polyamines, *S*- and *N*-heterocyclic compounds, including alkaloids and terpenes. *Acorus calamus* produces a number of sesquiterpenes having the skeletal structures of cadinane, acorane and eudesmane which inhibit the germination of lettuce seeds (K. Nawamaki and M. Kuroyanagi, *Phytochemistry*, 1996, **43**, 1175). A new class of plant growth regulators known as brassinosteroids is found in the seeds, pollens, galls, leaves, flower-buds and shoots of a considerable range of plants. Some 40 of these compounds are known; they stimulate cell enlargement and cell division and influence gene expression and nucleic acid metabolism at the molecular level, see V. A. Khripach *et al.* (1999), *Brassinosteroids, a New Class of Plant Hormone*, San Diego: Academic Press.

13

Plant cell and tissue culture; biochemical conversions; clonal propagation

One of the rapidly expanding areas of pharmacognosy has involved the application of the artificial culture of plant cells, tissues and organs to the study of medicinal plants. Principal topics include the development of commercial production of expensive biomedicaments, the discovery of new metabolites, the selection of superior strains of medicinal plants, the elucidation of biosynthetic pathways of secondary metabolites with isolation of corresponding enzymes, and the improvement of medicinal plant species by genetic engineering.

INDUSTRIAL SIGNIFICANCE

A number of factors militate against dependence by the pharmaceutical industry on the use of botanical sources of drugs, and these have been, to some extent, responsible for the reluctance of industry to invest in the exploitation of the plant kingdom. These factors include the following.

1. *Availability of raw material.* Some plants, although highly desirable as sources of biochemicals, just cannot be produced in an economically sufficient quantity to satisfy demand. An example is *Strophanthus sarmentosus* seeds, which, early in the search for corticosteroid precursors (1950s), were known to contain a very suitable compound, sarmentogenin, conveniently substituted in the steroid C ring (see Chapter 23). But the plants, tropical lianes existing as different chemical races (Chapter 14), are not particularly abundant and are difficult to cultivate. More recent examples include the very limited supply of the Pacific yew (*Taxus brevifolia*) the principal source of taxol, a diterpene with considerable potential as a starting material for the semisynthesis of promising anticancer drugs and also *Coleus forskohlii*, an Indian species now listed as vulnerable to extinction in the wild as a result of indiscriminate collection for the isolation of forskolin, a diterpenoid used in the treatment of glaucoma and heart disease.
2. *Fluctuation of supplies and quality.* The production of crude drugs is subject to the vagaries of the climate, to crop disease, to varying methods of collection and drying which influence quality, and to the inherent variation of active constituents arising from plants of the same species having different genetic characteristics.
3. *Political considerations.* New compounds of promising medicinal value are increasingly reported in previously uninvestigated tropical or subtropical species situated in countries of uncertain political persuasion. Industry is not prepared to undertake the prolonged and expensive development of such material.
4. *Patent rights.* Generally, it is not possible to patent a naturally occurring plant metabolite as such, only a novel method for its extraction and isolation. Hence, there is little incentive for a pharmaceutical company to spend many years and vast sums of money on launching a new natural product over which it has no patent rights.

Following from the above, it is not surprising that industry worldwide takes a close interest in the commercial possibilities of cultivating particular species of plant cells, under conditions analogous to the production of antibiotics, that will yield biomedicinals. By this means, production could at all times be geared to demand, and a product of standard quality assured. Furthermore, a highly sophisticated and specific method of production can be patented.

Shikonin, a dye and antibacterial, is commercially produced by the cultivation of *Lithospermum* plant cells and the production of the ginsenosides and antitumour alkaloids of *Catharanthus roseus* are currently being developed; Japanese patents exist concerning the manufacture of many secondary metabolites including the purple pigment from *Melissa officinalis*, the production of catharanthine and ajmalicine by cell cultures derived from *C. roseus* anthers, the manufacture of an analogue of taxol (q.v.) by callus cultures of *Taxus* spp., and tropane alkaloids from *Duboisia* tissue cultures. A vast amount of work has been reported during the last decade and the majority of common medicinal plants, and many less common ones, have been subjected to cell culture investigation. Nevertheless, in the majority of cases, yields of metabolites have been commercially disappointing. Staba, a pioneer in the investigation of medicinal plant cell culture, stated (*J. Nat. Prod.*, 1985, **48**, 203) 'there are arguably as many gravestones as milestones along the way in developing plant tissue culture systems for the production of secondary metabolites'. Ultimately, of course, as Fowler pointed out over 25 years ago (*Chem. Ind.*, 1981, 229), 'no matter how elegant the science, the fundamental criterion has to be price comparability coupled with profitability', a fact clearly obviated by subsequent events.

CULTIVATION OF PLANT CELLS

Although the feasibility of artificially cultivating plant cells had long been recognized, and White had propagated isolated tomato roots for periods of over 30 years, it was only some few decades ago that modern developments in the cultivation of cells of higher plants as a callus, or as a suspension liquid culture, really began. In this connection the publication of P. R. White's *Cultivation of Plant and Animal Cells* in 1954 and H. E. Street's developmental work at Leicester University deserve mention.

Cultures of single cells growing under controlled conditions in a liquid medium, or callus cultures consisting of undifferentiated masses of cells developing on a semi-solid medium, can be initiated from parenchymatous tissues of shoots, roots and other plant structures (see Fig. 13.1). The maintenance of such cultures depends on an adequate supply of nutrients, including growth factors, and a controlled sterile environment. The cells, although undifferentiated, contain all the genetic information present in the normal plant. By suitable manipulation of the hormone content of the medium, it is possible to initiate the development of roots, shoots, and complete plants from the callus cell culture and to encourage the division of cells in a suspension culture.

Several forms of suspension culture are commonly utilized, as follows.

1. *Batch suspension cultures.* In this technique the cells multiply in a liquid medium which is being continuously agitated to break up any cell aggregates. Except for the circulation of air, the system is 'closed' with respect to additions or subtractions from the culture. Typically, the original inoculation of cells into the medium is followed by a lag period and then, after increasing in mass, the cells undergo a period of exponential growth and division. Finally, a stationary growth phase is reached, at which point some component of the medium, essential for growth, has probably been exhausted. Growth will recommence when cells are transferred to a fresh medium or when more medium is added to the original culture.

2. *Semicontinuous cultures.* In this instance the system, an 'open' one, is designed for the periodic removal of culture and the addition of fresh medium, by which means the growth of the culture is continuously maintained.

3. *Continuous cultures.* Two forms of this 'open' system are the chemostat and turbostat systems, in which the volume of culture remains constant and fresh medium and culture are, respectively, continuously added and withdrawn. The essential feature of these two systems is that cell proliferation takes place under constant conditions. In the chemostat arrangement, a steady state is achieved by adding medium in which a single nutrient has been adjusted so as to be *growth-limiting*; this contrasts with the batch culture method, in which the transient conditions in which the cells find themselves lead to continuous changes in their growth rate and metabolism.

The problems associated with plant-cell culture are not completely identical with those encountered in the fermentation of microorganisms and fungi. With the former there is much slower cell proliferation and it takes about 3–6 weeks to progress from the shake-flask level (300 ml) to production capacity (20 000 litres). Also in plant cell cultures, large aggregates of cells may form, which then exist under different environmental conditions from the suspended cells. Dispersal of aggregates by the use of the usual fermenter paddles was originally considered too vigorous for fragile plant cells, resulting in their rupture. To overcome this, various designs of low-shear fermenters including the air-lift or drum types were designed. However, such refinements are not always necessary and the shikonin production mentioned above is, in fact, carried out in conventional stirred-tank vessels. As R. Verpoorte *et al.* have pointed out (*J. Nat. Prod.*, 1993, **56**, 186), for the industrial application of plant cell cultures, the recognition that shear-tolerant plant cell cultures exist is important because the fermentation industry at present uses stirred tanks almost exclusively. Investment in new ingenious bioreactors, as reported for experimental cell cultures in recent years, would place a major constraint on the commercialization of plant cell biotechnology.

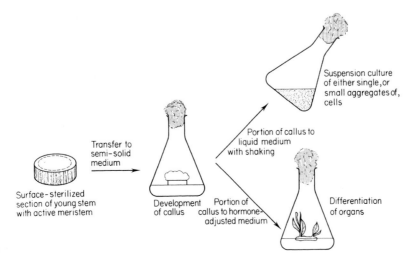

Fig. 13.1
Origin of plant cell cultures.

To maximize on the cell mass produced, the cell suspension culture eventually becomes very dense and this presents problems of even aeration.

Most pilot studies have utilized fermenters of 5–15 litres capacity and the reported scaling up to 20 000 and more recently 75 000 litres in West Germany and Japan presents chemical engineering problems of considerable complexity.

PRODUCTION OF SECONDARY METABOLITES

The genetic information required for the manufacture of secondary metabolites is also present in the undifferentiated cells of the species concerned, and when activated should lead to the production of these materials. Much interest has been aroused by this aspect of cell culture with the aim of growing particular plant cells on a commercial scale for the production of valuable metabolites.

A pioneer in the cell culture of medicinal plants was E. J. Staba of Minnesota University, and his group was the first to demonstrate that many medicinal plants did produce in cell culture their characteristic secondary metabolites, albeit often in low yield. Notable advances were made by Zenk and colleagues who in 1975 demonstrated a 10% (dry weight) production of anthraquinone derivatives in a *Morinda citrifolia* culture—at that date the highest yield of secondary metabolite achieved by cell culture. By 1991 (M. H. Zenk, *Phytochemistry*, 1991, **30**, 3861) almost 1000 species of callus were deposited in the collection at Braunschweig. Commercially orientated research has concentrated on those species that produce high-value speciality phytochemicals. Obvious examples are *Catharanthus roseus* (dimeric antitumour alkaloids), ginseng (ginsenosides) and *Taxus* species (taxol).

Apart from the general problem of low yield of product other factors which need to be addressed with cell cultures as a source of phytopharmaceuticals are: instability of cell lines, compartmentalization and isolation of the products, and the nature of the metabolites produced. Some points concerning these problems are given below.

Low production of desired metabolites

Knowledge of the enzymology of secondary metabolite formation, although rapidly expanding, is still incomplete. Secondary metabolic processes compete with primary metabolism for precursors and potential bottlenecks for the former may involve those enzymes linking the primary and secondary pathways, for example, tryptophan decarboxylase converting tryptophan to tryptamine in the formation of indole alkaloids and cyclase enzymes involved in the synthesis of cyclohexanoid monoterpenes from geranylpyrophosphate. With cell cultures, as distinct from whole plants, particular genes may be repressed and need to be activated by suitable elicitors, a technique which is currently an important area of research and is discussed below.

The **compositions of the media** in which culture cells are grown have been extensively investigated with a view to increasing both the biomass and secondary metabolites. Often, as reported with *Dioscorea deltoidea* for instance, rapidly dividing cells produce little or no metabolites of interest and a change from a growth medium (high biomass) to a production medium is required to effect the necessary biosynthesis. In this connection Zenk's 'alkaloid production medium' for ajmalicine in *C. roseus* may be noted, together with the effects of long-term starvation of phosphate on levels of purine nucleotides and related compounds (F. Shimano and H. Ashihara, *Phytochemistry*, 2006, **67**, 132).

Variations in the relative hormonal contents of the growth medium can also affect metabolism. It has been reported that reduced concentrations of 2,4-D increased alkaloid formation in *C. roseus* cultures and that abscisic acid and antigibberellin compounds have similar effects. With *Thalictrum minus*, ethylene has been shown to activate the production of berberine in cell cultures from the key intermediate (*S*)-reticuline and the ethylene-producing reagent 2-chloroethylphosphoric acid stimulates anthraquinone production in callus cultures of *Rheum palmatum*. Conversely, cardenolide accumulation in *Digitalis lanata* tissue cultures is decreased by ethylene. Cytokinins have been found to enhance secondary metabolite accumulation in a number of tissue culture studies—indole alkaloids (*C. roseus*), condensed tannin (*Onobrychis* sp.), coumarins (*Nicotiana* sp.), rhodozanthin (*Ricinus* sp.), berberine (*Thalictrum minus*). Rhodes *et al.* found a five-fold increase in alkaloid content of a culture of *Cinchona ledgeriana* occurs when cells are transferred from a 2,4-D, benzyladenine medium to one containing IAA and zeatin riboside. For information on plant hormones, see Chapter 12.

Although alkaloids from a wide range of medicinal plants have been produced satisfactorily by cell culture in the laboratory, a singular lack of success has been experienced in obtaining quinine and quinidine from *Cinchona* cultures and morphine and codeine from those of *Papaver somniferum* although, in both cases, other alkaloids are formed. To some extent the problems with the former are being overcome by the use of transformed roots (see below) but the growth rate is very slow. With morphine biosynthesis it appears that lack of developed laticiferous tissue in the unorganized cell culture may be responsible because cytodifferentiation leading to latificer-type cells leads to morphinan alkaloid production. One problem with *Catharanthus* cell cultures has been their inability to dimerize the requisite indole monomers to form the medicinally important anticancer alkaloids vinblastine and vincristine. In a similar way the accumulation of monoterpenes in cell cultures of some volatile oil-producing plants is severely limited, probably because of the absence of such storage structures as glands, ducts and trichomes. Thus, in *Rosa damascena* callus and suspension cultures, negligible amounts of monoterpenes are accumulated, although enzymes with high activity for the conversion of mevalonate and IPP into geraniol and nerol (see Chapter 18) are extractable from the apparently inactive callus. In this case, non-compartmentalization of the metabolites probably leads to their further metabolism. This is supported by the finding that, when added to cultures of *Lavandula angustifolia*, the monoterpenoid aldehydes geranial, neral and citronellal are reduced to their corresponding alcohols, geraniol, nerol and citronellol which, once formed, disappear from the cultures over about 15 h.

In studies on the phenolic antioxidant compounds produced by *in vitro* cultures of rosemary, A. Kuhlmann and C. Rohl (*Pharm. Biol.*, 2006, **44**, 401) find the content of carnosic acid, carnosol and rosmaric acid to be dependent on the differentiation grade of the cell culture type. Higher concentrations of rosmaric acid were measured in suspension cultures than in shoot and callus cultures, whereas the former on average produced three-fold less carnosic acid than the two latter cultures. Carnesol could not be detected in suspension cultures.

With *Ginkgo biloba* although a satisfactory biomass of undifferentiated cells could be produced on a manufacturing scale, the poor level of ginkgolides produced renders it of scant importance.

It has been observed that the **origin (stem, root, etc.) of the callus** can play an important part in determining the biochemistry of the subsequent culture.

Improved metabolite production may sometimes be achieved by the **addition of precursors** to the culture medium. Thus, addition of coniferin (a phenylpropane) to cell suspension cultures of *Podophyllum* *hexandrum* improved podophyllotoxin production 12.8-fold and an increase in quinoline alkaloids was obtained with *Cinchona ledgeriana* cultures fed with L-tryptophan. With transformed root cultures of *Catharanthus roseus*, the addition of the precursor loganin to the culture medium has been shown to increase the production of both ajmalicine and serpentine at the early stationary phase of growth, although it produced no increases during the early and late exponential growth phases. Catharanthine production was unaffected but was increased, together with the other alkaloids, by multiple feedings of loganin (see E. N. Gaviraj and C. Veeresham, *Pharm. Biol.*, 2006, **44**, 371 and references cited therein).

Light intensity and selective wavelengths of light have been shown to have a stimulating effect on the production of some secondary metabolites in various tissue cultures. Thus, in one report (1990) blue light enhanced, whereas red light decreased, diosgenin production in *Dioscorea deltoidea* callus cultures. A recent example of the stimulant effect of UV-B radiation on secondary metabolism in callus cultures is the research of F. Antognoni *et al.* (*Fitoterapia*, 2007, **78**, 345) on *Passiflora quadrangularis*. Daily doses of UV-B radiation (12.6, 25.3, 37.9 KJ m^{-2}) produced increases in the flavonoid production of orientin, isoorientin, vitexin and isovitexin. Isoorientin accumulation in the callus after 7 days reached levels comparable to those found in the fresh leaves of greenhouse-raised plants. However, such beneficial treatments are difficult to accommodate with conventional stirred-tank fermentors.

The selection of **high-yielding cell lines** has been a major factor in countering low productivity. Such selection, perhaps involving a few plants from several thousand, has been greatly facilitated by the use of modern immunoassays (q.v.). In the case of *Catharanthus roseus* cultures, for example, recent research has concentrated on the production of the dimeric alkaloids vinblastine and vincristine (q.v.), the important anticancer drugs. The alkaloids are produced at the end of a complex biogenetic pathway in which the monomers are first produced. The latter, as corynanthe-, strychnos- and aspidosperma-type alkaloids can all be produced (0.1–1.5%) in culture using Zenk's alkaloid production medium. Different cell cultures derived from any one species of plant may vary enormously in their synthetic capacities, so that, in the above case, distinct high ajmalicine-producing and high serpentine-producing strains are possible.

Examples of other plants for which somaclonal variation has been exploited include *Nicotiana rustica* (nicotine) (of no commercial interest), *Coptis japonica* (berberine), *Anchusa officinalis* (rosmarinic acid), *Lithospermum erythrorhizon* (shikonin) and *Hyoscyamus muticus* (hyoscine). For *Thalictrum minus* (berberine) a strain giving a 350-fold increase in alkaloid production has been reported.

Instability of cell lines. It is well known that changes in the genetic characteristics of cells occur within a culture so that callus selected for specific biochemical properties may need reselection after a period of time. In a few cases, for example anthraquinone formation, selection may be achieved on a colour basis but, more usually, assays such as radio-immunoassay are necessary. Gross changes in chromosome number may occur in cultured cells; thus, Tabata and colleagues noted in 1974 that with a particular suspension culture of *Datura innoxia* cells there was a 32% level of diploid cells, with the remainder mostly at the tetraploid level, ranging in constitution from $4n-5$ to $4n+3$ (see Chapter 14 for extra chromosomal types). Another strain contained no diploid cells but cells with 46 or 44 chromosomes occurring in the proportions of 79% and 21%, respectively. Nevertheless, for alkaloid production, Kibler and Neumann in 1979 found that haploid ($1n$) and diploid ($2n$) cell suspension cultures of

D. innoxia showed no difference in tropane alkaloid production (c.f. leaves of $1n$ and $2n$ plants; Table 14.1), but for protoplast-derived cell-culture clones of *Hyoscyamus muticus*, Oksman-Caldentey *et al.* have found that cultures from $1n$ plants are richer in hyoscine than those from $2n$ plants.

Isolation of product. For continuous cultivation and production of active metabolites it is preferable, for isolation purposes, that the metabolites be excreted into the medium rather than be retained within the cells. The biomass can then be separated from the nutrient liquid from which the active constituents are extracted. Two-phase culture systems have been described. With these an immiscible non-toxic liquid phase, e.g. a silicone product, is added to the fermentation tank to extract the metabolites and in this way the development of the culture is not disturbed. The removal of entrapped metabolites from immobilized cells (q.v.) without killing the cells is another innovation.

Nature of metabolites produced. Sometimes compounds not detected in the original plant appear in the cultures; thus, a new coumarin, rutacultin, has been isolated from suspension cell cultures of *Ruta graveolens*, two new chalcones have been characterized from static (callus) cultures of *Glycyrrhiza echinata*, sesquiterpene lactones from *Andrographis paniculata* cultures, new minor alkaloids and anthraquinones from *Cinchona ledgeriana* and *C. pubescens*, and tropane alkaloids, not previously obtained from the species, from belladonna root-cell suspension cultures. Recently the novel compound (2-glyceryl)-*O*-coniferaldehyde has been obtained from cultures of *Artemisia annua* and *Tanacetum parthenium* (L. K. Sy and G. D. Brown, *Phytochemistry*, 1999, **50**, 781) and the quinone-methide triterpenes, tingenone and 22-hydroxytingenone, from callus cultures of *Catha edulis* (E. Abdel Sattar *et al.*, *Saudi Pharm. J.*, 1998, **6**, 242). Other plants yield cultures which produce a different spectrum of secondary metabolites from those found in the intact plant. These aspects of cell culture, although generally unhelpful for the promotion of this technique for industrial purposes, have important implications for other areas of phytochemistry. However, in the case of cell cultures of *Papaver somniferum* and *P. bracteatum* which do not produce morphinan alkaloids, sanguinarine, a benzophenanthridine alkaloid of commercial importance, is obtained in yields sufficiently high to allow industrial exploitation.

INDUCED SECONDARY METABOLISM IN CELL CULTURES

Although the undifferentiated cells of a plant suspension culture are generally totipotent, i.e. they possess the complete genetic make-up of the whole plant, many genes, including those involved in secondary metabolism, are repressed with the consequence that the yields of desired compounds in such cultures are disappointingly low. However, it is becoming increasingly apparent that a large number of secondary metabolites belong to a class of substances termed phytoalexins. These are stress-related compounds produced in the normal plant as a result of damaging stimuli from physical, chemical or microbiological factors. When cell cultures are subjected to such elicitors, some genes are derepressed, resulting, among other things, in the formation of the secondary metabolites which are found in the entire plant. The technique is being increasingly employed in cell-culture studies and examples giving a range of both abiotic acid and biotic inducers are given in Table 13.1.

Table 13.1 Induced production of metabolites in cell cultures by various elicitors.

Elicitor	Plant-cell suspension culture	Effect
Arachidonic acid	*Taxus* spp.	Production of taxol
Chitosan	*Polygonum tinctorium*	Production of indirubin
Colchicine	*Valeriana wallichii*	Sixty-fold increase in valepotriates with six new compounds (not due to higher ploidy level)
Copper sulphate	*Lithospermum erythrorhizon*	Greatly increased shikonin production
	Various Solanaceae	Induced formation of sesquiterpene phytoalexins of lubimin type
Calcium	*Alkanna tinctora*	Stimulation of sanguinarine and chelerythrine biosynthesis
Acetylsalicylic acid	*Catharanthus roseus*	Increased production of tumour cell suspensions (505%), total phenolics (1587%), furanocoumarins (612%), anthocyanins (1476%)
Methyl jasmonate	*Sanguinaria canadensis*	Dihydrobenzophenanthridine oxidase activated in last step of sanguinarine biogenesis
	Cinchona robusta	Production of novel anthraquinones (robustaquinones) with a rare oxygenation pattern in ring A
	Nicotiana tabacum	Production of anatalline
Thiosemicarbazide	*Panax ginseng*	Promotes biosynthesis of saponins and inhibits phytosterol production
Sterilized fungal mycelia (*Pythium, Phytophthora, Verticillium*), etc. or extracts	*Pimpinella anisum* *Petroselinium crispum* *Ammi majus*	Stimulation of coumarin synthesis
	Catharanthus roseus	Production of catharanthine and other major indole alkaloids stimulated
	Cephalotaxus harringtonia	Dramatic increase in alkaloid content
	Cinchona ledgeriana	Increase in anthraquinone production
	Gossypium arboreum	One hundredfold increase in gossypol after 120 h incubation
Yeast, yeast extracts and carbohydrate preparations	*Eschscholtzia californica*	Large and rapid increase of benzophenanthridine alkaloid production
	Thalictrum rugosum	Up to fourfold enhancement of berberine
	Ruta graveolens	Increased production of acridone expoxides but not rutacridone
	Orthosiphon aristatus	Stimulation of rosmarinic acid production

BIOCHEMICAL CONVERSIONS BY PLANT CELL CULTURES

In much the same way that modification of a particular substrate can be effected by microbial fermentation so, too, can plant suspension cultures be employed for the same purpose.

Of possible commercial significance is the ability of some cell cultures of *Digitalis lanata* to effect glucosylations, hydroxylations, and acetylations. Reinhard and colleagues demonstrated that their cell culture, strain 291, cultivated in air-lift bioreactors, was particularly efficient in the conversion of β-methyldigitoxin into β-methyldigoxin (a 12β-hydroxylation). Commercial exploitation of this process would enable utilization of the large stocks of digitoxin which accumulate as a byproduct in the manufacture of digoxin from *D. lanata*. More recently, Stricker (*Planta Med.*, 1986, 418) reported on a highly efficient 12β-hydroxylation of digitoxin itself using *D. lanata* cell suspensions with a two-stage process involving first, the proliferation of cells in a growth medium and then a transfer to a suitable production medium. With cell cultures of both *D. lanata* and *Thevetia neriifolia* a number of new cardenolides have been biosynthesized from added precursors. Cell suspension cultures of *Strophanthus gratus* will effect various biochemical conversions of digitoxigenin, as will cultured ginseng cells.

Monoterpene bioconversions have been demonstrated with *Mentha* cell lines capable of transforming pulegone to isomethone, and (−)-menthone to (+)-neomenthol. Cultured cells of *Eucalyptus perriniana* have been shown to biotransform thymol, carvacrol and eugenol into glycosides (glucosides and gentiobiosides), which accumulated within the cells (K. Shimoda *et al.*, *Phytochemistry*, 2006, **67**, 2256).

The rue plant (*Ruta graveolens*) and its normal tissue cultures contain a number of constituents, including furanocoumarins derived from 7-hydroxycoumarin (Fig. 13.2, series A). In 1974, Steck and Constabel showed that two chemical mimics of the 7-hydroxycoumarin precursor, the 4-methyl and 8-methyl derivatives, when fed to the *Ruta* cell culture, gave rise to a number of the corresponding unnatural analogues (Fig. 13.2, series B and C).

Possibilities for the production of anticancer drugs are illustrated by the biotransformation of synthetic dibenzylbutanolides to lignans suitable for conversion to etopside (Chapter 27) by a semi-continuous process involving cultures of *Podophyllum peltatum* (J. P. Kutney

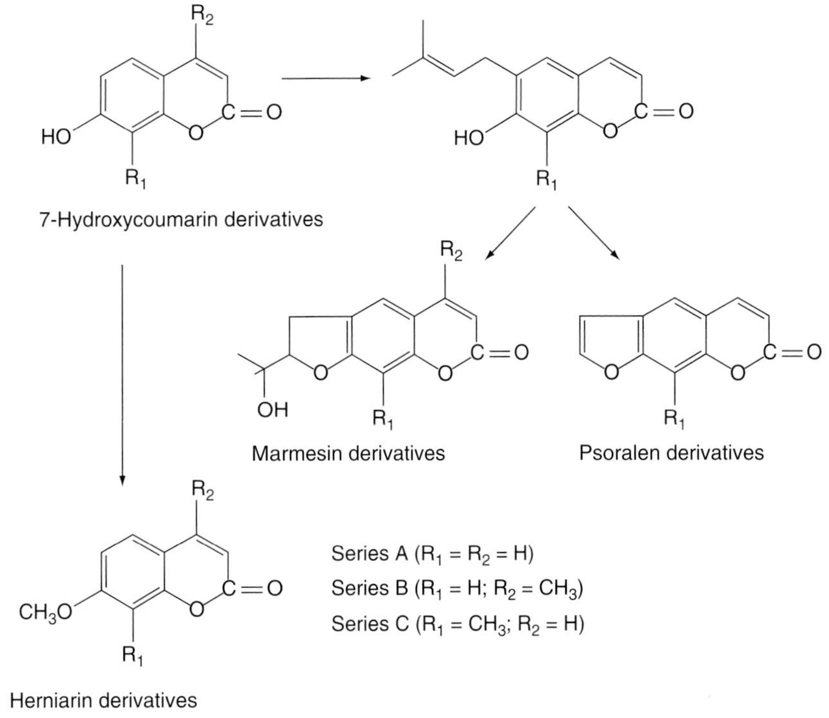

Fig. 13.2
Biochemical conversions involving *Ruta graveolens* cell cultures.

et al. Heterocycles, 1993, **36**, 13). Interesting and potentially useful hydroxylation and oxidation reactions have also been demonstrated for the biotransformation of podophyllum lignans in cell suspension cultures of *Forsythia intermedia* (A. J. Broomhead and P. M. Dewick, *Phytochemistry*, 1991, **30**, 1511).

The principal alkaloid produced by the cultivation of *Rauwolfia serpentina* cells is the glucoalkaloid raucaffricine. However, feeding with high levels of ajmaline leads to the production of a new group of alkaloids, the raumaclines.

Some biotransformations are stereo-specific and have potential for the isolation of optically active compounds from the racemate; thus, *Nicotiana tabacum* cell cultures can selectively hydrolyse the *R*-configurational forms of monoterpenes such as bornyl acetate and isobornyl acetate.

Many other biochemical transformations by cell cultures have been demonstrated, and include epoxidations, ester formation and saponification, glycosylation, hydroxylation, isomerization, methylation, and demethylation and oxidation.

For this technique to be commercially viable, the product must be sufficiently important, the substrate must be available in reliable amounts, and the reaction should not be one that is more easily performed by microorganisms or by chemical means.

IMMOBILIZED PLANT CELLS

Immobilized plant cells can be used in the same way as immobilized enzymes to effect chemically difficult reactions. Reinhard and coworkers have reported on the immobilization of *Digitalis lanata* cells by suspending them in a sodium alginate solution, precipitating the alginate plus entrapped cells with calcium chloride solution, pelleting, and allowing the product to harden. The granules catalysed the conversion of digitoxin to purpurea glycoside A (formula, see Table 23.7) and hydroxylated β-methyldigitoxin to give β-methyldigoxin. Although

the hydroxylating activity of the entrapped cells was about half that of suspended cells, the pellets had the advantage that the biocatalyst was re-usable for periods extending to over 60 days. Other workers report the biotransformation of codeinone to codeine by immobilized cells of *Papaver somniferum* and the release of papaverine, codeine and morphine to the medium (3240–4050 mg 1^{-1}); decarboxylation of L-tyrosine and L-DOPA has also been recorded. Japanese workers have studied seaweed immobilized cell cultures for the production of flavour constituents. Glyoxal cross-linked polyacrylamide-hydrazide has been used as the immobilizing agent for *Mentha* cells which effect the monoterpene reductions mentioned above and the technique has been further developed by arresting unwanted cell division of the entrapped cells by gamma irradiation. Other immobilization supports which have been used include polyurethane foam, acrylamide and xanthan-acrylamide.

A technique which has been found useful for the study of alkaloid formation in *Coffea arabica* is to use a membrane of polypropylene sheeting of specified pore size, porosity and thickness on which to immobilize the cells in a 3-mm thick layer; the nutrient medium circulates below the membrane. *Catharanthus roseus* cells have also been considerably studied and progress has been made in developing methods for the release of alkaloids sequestrated in the cell vacuoles without killing the culture.

It has been suggested that the immobilization of mycelia-forming microorganisms (e.g. *Claviceps paspali*) by alginic acid might be effective in the biotechnological production of complex metabolites such as the ergot alkaloids.

ORGAN CULTURE

In the same way that it is possible to culture undifferentiated plant cells, so aseptic suspension cultures of leaves and roots can be maintained. The organs can be obtained in the culture either by differenti-

13

ation from callus tissue cultures by suitable hormonal manipulation, or by the use of sterilized roots or growing points from whole plants or seedlings. Often, these cultured organs will synthesize secondary metabolites which may be either non-existent or in poor yield in the normal cell culture. Thus, cardenolide production in *Digitalis lanata* and *D. purpurea* cultures increases as tissue differentiation proceeds. Enhanced production of alkaloids occurs when roots develop from the callus cultures of the tropane alkaloid-producing Solanaceae. In contrast to the latter, in which leaf differentiation alone produces little alkaloid, leaf organ cultures of *Catharanthus roseus* and *Rauwolfia serpentina* synthesize a variety of alkaloids. Dimeric alkaloids have been detected in organ cultures of *C. roseus*, suggesting the possibility of an efficient production system for these valuable alkaloids. The dimers occurred only in those cultures which also contained vindoline and catharanthine. Whereas cell suspension cultures of *Papaver bracteatum* were found to synthesize orientalidine and sanguinarine, the root and shoot cultures produced thebaine. For ginsenoside production, ginseng root cultures have been grown in 20 000-litre bioreactors.

As with cell culture, elicitation can give increased yields of secondary metabolites. Thus both normal and hairy (q.v. below) root cultures of *Hyoscyamus muticus* when treated with jasmonic acid and its methyl ester at concentrations of 0.001 to 10 μM produced large increases in the levels of methyl putrescine and conjugated polyamines. However the increase of tropane alkaloid production was not remarkable (S.-Bionde *et al.*, *Plant Cell Rep.*, 2000, **19**, 691).

Transformed root culture—'hairy root' culture

Certain soil bacteria of the genus *Agrobacterium* cause a transformation of plant cells by introducing into their genome t-DNA from a bacterial plasmid. Such transformed roots, produced by inoculat-

ing the host plant, when grown in a hormone-free medium give rise to copious roots referred to as 'transformed roots' or 'hairy roots' (see Chapter 14). On removal of the *Agrobacterium* the roots continue to develop profusely and for some plants which normally produce secondary metabolites the hairy roots accumulate these metabolites in quantities comparable to those found in the normal intact plant.

Agrobacterium rhizogenes and *A. tumefaciens* are the bacterial species most commonly used to effect transformation.

Compared with the few examples given in the 13th edition of this book there is now a considerable bibliography on transformed root cultures of medicinal plants. Some examples are given in Table 13.2.

As with ordinary cell cultures and root cultures it is possible to utilize transformed roots to carry out biological conversions not normally associated with the intact plant. The rapid growth rate of hairy roots offers the possibility of rapid conversions. Ginseng hairy root cultures have been shown to convert digitoxigenin (the aglycone of a number of *Digitalis* cardiac glycosides, q.v.) into new compounds by esterification at C-3 with stearate, palmitate and myristate, and by the formation of gentiobiosides and sophorosides. Parr *et al.* (*Phytochemistry*, 1991, **30**, 2607) in studies on the biosynthesis of tropane alkaloids fed the *S*-analogue of tropinone (8-thiabicyclo[3.2.1] octan-3-one) to transformed root cultures of *Datura stramonium* and obtained the *S*-analogue of tropine, together with the 3-*O*-acetyl ester.

Cell cultures derived from *A. rhizogenes*-transformed *Papaver somniferum* tissue have been studied for alkaloid production (R. D. Williams and B. E. Ellis, *Phytochemistry*, 1993, **32**, 719). As with normal cultures, no morphinan alkaloids were produced but large amounts of sanguinarine were.

Table 13.2   Metabolites of some transformed (hairy) roots.

Alkaloid-containing plants	
Atropa belladonna	Increase in growth rate compared with untreated roots
Catharanthus roseus	Optimization of selected lines may give source of catharanthine and vindoline
Cinchona ledgeriana	Quinoline alkaloid production comparable with that of intact plants
Datura stramonium	Alkaloid content comparable with normal roots of intact plants; increased by use of various elicitors, e.g. methyl jasmonate
Hyoscyamus albus	New piperidone alkaloid obtained together with tropane alkaloids
H. muticus	Culture treated with chitosan accumulated hyoscyamine 2.5 to 3-fold compared with untreated hairy roots
Narcissus confusus	Improved production of galanthamine in shake cultures by use of methyl jasmonate as elicitor
Solanum laciniatum	Solasodine yield increased about four-fold
Flavonoids	
Glycyrrhiza glabra	Known and new flavonoids produced; also a new prenylated biaurone
Iridoids	
Valeriana officinalis	Yield of valepotriates four times that found in normal 9-month-old roots
Lignans	
Linum flavum	5-Methoxypodophyllotoxin production 2–5 times that of untransformed roots; 5–12 times higher than cell suspension culture; comparable with natural roots
Polyacetylenes	
Lobelia inflata	Polyacetylenes produced, some having a gentiobiose moiety. These compounds have anticancer activity
Quinones	
Sesamum indicum	Yield of antimicrobial naphthoquinone increased by more than 50 times that found in intact plant
Steroids	
Panax ginseng	Japanese patent for production of ginsenosides; diol and triol type ginsenosides produced. Production more effective than with ordinary root cultures
Trigonella foenum-graecum	By optimization of the cultural conditions, up to three times the production of diosgenin compared with non-elicited roots

CLONAL PROPAGATION

As noted earlier (Fig. 13.1), by adjustment of the plant growth regulators in the cell culture medium it is possible to promote differentiation of organs from callus tissues and to carry these forward to produce entire plants. As all cells of the callus are derived from a single meristem, all regenerated plants should be genetically identical. This fact has obvious commercial implications for the production, in a short period of time, of uniform crops derived from a small number of desirable plants (or even a single individual).

In 1980, Levy reported from Ecuador on the first large-scale commercial application of *in vitro* culture for the mass propagation of clones of pyrethrum plants. The scale of such projects is evident from the original objective, which was to produce, from 57 superior clones isolated over a 10-year research period up to 1976, 12 million plants per year to reach a plantation target of the number required for 1000 ha of land over 4 years. Further details of the process are given in the 15th edition of this book. Similar techniques are now practised for other crops of pharmaceutical interest, benefits being the ability to introduce selected high-yielding strains on a commercial scale in a short time, the creation of improved growth characteristics and a greater ease of plantation planning.

Clonal propagation is a potentially valuable method for producing high-yielding crops of species which tend to be variable when grown from seed. Fennel (*Foeniculum vulgare*), for instance, is genetically heterozygous and produces wide variations in oil yield and composition. In 1987, Miura *et al.* (*Planta Med.*, 1987, **53**, 92) recorded a 2-year trial involving the production of uniform clonal plants derived from somatic embryoids of suitable parent plants. In the normal sexually propagated plants the anethol content of fruits varied from 0 to 12.9% (mean 2.82%), whereas in the clonal plants it showed a narrower distribution of 0.7–3.0% (mean 1.92%).

Genetic homogeneity

In practice, genetic changes can occur in cells during their artificial culture, and careful regulation of the medium is necessary. However, it has been shown, at least for *Datura innoxia*, that on differentiation it is the normal 2*n* plants, as distinct from the abnormal chromosomal types, that are favoured. Clonally propagated species for which the homogeneity of the secondary metabolites has been shown include *Aconitum carmichaelii*, *Angelica acutiloba*, *Bupleurum falcatum*, *Gentiana scabra*, *Rehmannia glutinosa* and *Stevia rehaubiana*.

Further reading

Verpoorte R, Heijden R van der, Schripsema J 1993 Plant cell biotechnology for the production of alkaloids: present status and prospects (*review with 130 refs*). Journal of Natural Products 56: 186

Zafar R, Aeri V, Datta A 1992 Application of plant tissue and cell culture for production of secondary metabolites (*review with 80 refs*). Fitoterapia 63: 33

14

Phytochemical variation within a species

As was indicated in Chapter 3, the species represents the unit of plant classification; it may constitute a homogeneous taxon of plants with little variation from one specimen to another or it may include various varieties or races which each have some distinctive feature(s). Thus with *Datura stramonium* four varieties are described: var. *stramonium*—white flowers, thorny capsules; var. *inermis*—white flowers, bald capsules; var. *tatula*—lilac flowers, thorny capsules and var. *godronii*—lilac flowers, bald capsules. Often such varieties represent single gene mutations (in the above case two independent genes are involved) and are morphologically recognizable. In other instances the mutation gives rise to a variant having a different secondary metabolite profile—not necessarily discernible in the morphological form; these are termed chemical races or chemodemes. The mutation may involve the presence or absence of a single component or, if acting at an early stage of the biosynthetic route, may involve a whole series of compounds.

Knowledge of the existence of such chemical races is not new and A. Tschirch (1856–1939) in his *Handbuch der Pharmakognosie* deals with the various 'physiological forms' of *Vanilla planifolia*, *Cinchona* spp., fennel, *Piper nigrum* and the balsam-containing trees. Also, 60 years ago A. R. Penfold and co-workers were describing chemical races of various Australian oil-producing species of *Leptospermum*, *Boronia* and *Eucalyptus*.

In addition to the above which involve submicroscopic point mutations associated with an alteration in the DNA chromosomal material, there are other genetic variations which may affect chemical constituents of the species. These include (a), the existence of polyploids in which chromosome sets become doubled, tripled, quadrupled etc., (b), the addition of one or a few chromosomes above the normal complement (extrachromosomal types), (c), gross structural changes to a chromosome, (d), artificially produced transgenic plants.

Two consequences of the above are, on the positive side, it provides the possibility for the selection and establishment of superior strains with respect to the chemical constituents as described in this chapter. The negative aspect concerns the arrival on the drug market of material which is low in active constituents. This, together with other factors, necessitates the need for strict quality control (Chapter 16) which is being vigorously addressed by various legislative bodies (Chapter 2). Transgenic crops present their own problems.

CHEMICAL RACES, CHEMOTYPES, CHEMODEMES

The plant kingdom has been subjected to an extensive, but not exhaustive, chemical investigation. Thousands of samples have been screened for substances of medicinal value or for suitable precursors of therapeutically active compounds. Many other plants have been studied chemically from the viewpoints of manural treatments, plant resistance and biosynthesis of active constituents. From such observations has emerged evidence for the existence of 'chemical races', 'chemotypes' or 'chemodemes'. These are defined as chemically distinct populations within a species and have similar phenotypes but different genotypes and as such are identical in external appearance but differ in their chemical constituents.

Before the existence of a chemical race can be established, certain fundamental observations are necessary. A chemical analysis of a number of random samples of a particular species may show a variation between the samples but would be insufficient to demonstrate any genetical differences, since factors such as age, climate and soil can all exert profound effects on the result of the ultimate analysis. Samples of seed, or clones from different plants, must be raised together under uniform conditions, and to exclude hybrids, which do not breed true, cultivation for a number of generations is desirable. It may then be possible to demonstrate that differences occur in either the nature or quantity of a particular constituent and that these differences are of a hereditary nature.

Such observations necessitate numerous assays and precise horticultural work, to which must be added the difficulties of dealing with plants which may take years to mature. Furthermore, many of the more important vegetable drugs cannot be successfully cultivated in temperate climates, so that it is not surprising that the number of medicinal plants fully investigated under ideal conditions is still limited. However, with the world-wide increase in genetic studies on medicinal plants, progress is being made towards the isolation of those enzymes associated with the existence of specific chemical races; recently, for example, the cloning of an enzyme involved in ginkolide biosynthesis (K. SangMin, *Phytochemistry*, 2006, **67**, 1435).

The clinical significance of chemical races is illustrated by Valerian; the plant normally contains both volatile oil and iridoid compounds, the latter with reported cytotoxic activity. As the sedative properties of the drug are ascribable to the valerenic acid and valerone constituents the cultivation of chemical races lacking the iridoids was introduced.

Fixed oils. Agriculturally, the cultivation of seed oil plants is second only in importance to that of cereals. Most of the fixed oil produced is used by the food industry but there are also important industrial and other, including pharmaceutical, uses. It is not surprising therefore that sustained breeding programmes for the improvement of yields and quality of oil have been in progress over many years. Normal rapeseed oil contains, as an acylglycerol, 20–40% of erucic acid, an acid having an extra long carbon chain (C_{22}) and one double bond. Its presence in quantity renders the oil unsuitable for edible purposes but varieties are now extensively grown which contain no erucic acid. The value of the crop has been further enhanced by coupling low erucic acid content with one giving low glucosinolates in the protein meal thus improving the animal feed properties. However, erucic acid is industrially important for the manufacture of lubricants, artificial fibres and plasticizers, so that varieties of rape developed for their high erucic acid content are also important agricultural crops.

The production of oil from sunflower seed has been improved by varieties that yield linoleic acid-enriched oil and which are more convenient for harvesting by having a large single flower head and no side-shoots. Groundnuts, the source of Arachis Oil *BP*, exist as various strains with different relative proportions of fatty acids.

Safflower constitutes an important oil-seed crop and its genetic variability has facilitated the breeding of varieties with widely differing oil constitutions. High oleic varieties are used for oil for human consumption and high linoleic varieties are important for oils used as industrial coatings and lubricants.

The above examples involve plants with a short life-span so that breeding by classical methods is a relatively rapid procedure. However, this is not so with plants such as the coconut palm, olive and cocoa so that in these cases modern techniques involving gene transfer would have an obvious advantage for the introduction of new or modified oil characteristics.

Cyanogenetic glycosides. A well-known chemical race in the cyanogenetic series is the almond. There are many varieties of *Prunus communis* showing different morphological forms, with and without amygdalin, but some varieties have similar characters and differ only in the presence or absence of the glycoside. Also in this group the clovers, especially *Trifolium repens*, have been extensively studied and *Linaria* has been shown by Dillemann to produce a chemical race by introgressive hybridization. *L. striata* contains cyanogenetic glycosides, and, crossed with the non-active *L. vulgaris*, gives rise to hybrids which, on repeated back-crossing with *L. vulgaris*, give some plants difficult to distinguish from *L. vulgaris* but which contain the cyanogenetic principles of *L. striata*.

Alkaloids. The *Duboisia* species form an important commercial source of the tropane alkaloids and have been extensively studied by Australian workers. With both *D. myoporoides* and *D. leichhardtii*, trees from natural stands in various locations were examined and their progeny were raised side by side in experimental plantations. The trees produce hyoscine, hyoscyamine, norhyoscyamine, tigloidine and valeroidine, and the proportion of any one alkaloid to total alkaloid may vary greatly. It was shown not only that seasonal and environmental factors are involved in this variation, but also that within a species there exists a wide range of alkaloid genotypes. Other varieties containing nicotine and nornicotine were also reported. Interspecific hybrids between the two species were studied and four hybrid clones were selected for possible exploitation as high alkaloid yielding strains. Thus, in this genus we have the possibility of two distinct types of chemical race—different alkaloid types within a species and different alkaloid types among hybrid phenotypes.

An example of the improvement of the morphine content of opium poppies by genealogical selection is furnished by the work of Lecat. The original seed gave capsules having an average morphine content of 0.385%. From this heterogeneous population were selected six individuals whose capsules analysed about 0.7% morphine. The seeds of these plants formed the heads of the lines cultivated in successive years, during which the best plants were collected and all those containing less than 0.7% morphine were rejected. The harvest of 1955 gave capsules with an average morphine content of 0.765%, thus doubling the original morphine content of the population. Such a method of breeding does not produce a race of plants surpassing individual morphine contents from the original heterogeneous population; it merely produces a homogeneous race of the alkaloid-rich plants.

Phillipson and colleagues reported at least three different chemical races of *Papaver fugax* and *P. armeniacum* in which either (1) 1-benzyltetrahydroquinoline, proaporphine, aporphine, (2) morphinane or (3) rhoeadine types are the major alkaloids; there are at least two different chemical strains of *P. tauricola* containing either the first or third types of the above. Three different isoquinoline alkaloid chemotypes of *Thalictrum minus* have been reported from Bulgaria. *Papaver bracteatum* is a species exhibiting races with respect to thebaine.

From *Claviceps purpurea* a number of races have been isolated containing different groups of ergot alkaloids and these have obvious implications for the commercial production of alkaloids.

One fodder crop in which the presence of alkaloids is undesirable is lupin seed. Ordinary wild forms are bitter and contain alkaloids of the lupinane series but over the years a number of sweet forms have been developed for commercial purposes in Europe. The strains depend for their low alkaloid content on the presence of a particular recessive gene. However, as a number of such genes exist, cross-fertilization between two different sweet strains will again give bitter progeny. To avoid this happening, considerable care is necessary in regions where different strains are grown side by side. Other plants for which there is evidence of alkaloid varieties include *Ephedra distachya* and the *Lycopodium* species.

Chemical races appear to be lacking in the pharmaceutically important indole alkaloid-containing genera *Strychnos*, *Rauwolfia* and *Catharanthus*.

Anthraquinones. The purgative anthraquinone drugs owe their activity to complex mixtures of the 1,8-dihydroxy derivatives of anthranols, their glycosides and free anthraquinones. The relative proportions of the constituents of the mixture, which greatly influence the pharmacological activity, depend not only on time of collection, age of plant, drying conditions and geographical source, but also on genetical factors. In a programme involving *Rheum palmatum*, van Os produced races varying in their rhein/chrysophanol ratio and other hereditary strains for high- and low-yielding total anthraquinones. The analysis of individual *Cassia angustifolia* plants has indicated that selection of individuals for high sennoside B-yielding strains is a possibility.

Cardiac glycosides. With *Digitalis purpurea* the property of high glycoside content is hereditary. The proportion of glycosides derived from digitoxin and gitoxin is also very different in plants of different origin and remains so during subsequent cultivation under standardized conditions. The strains were distinguished chemically as digipurpurin, strospeside and digitoxin types. It now remains to prove that these characters are independent of the phenotype (i.e. that they are not inseparably associated with other characters of the parent plant). One race, 'Cambridge', which is relatively rich in digitoxin, is easy to distinguish; the other digitoxin race found in the Vosges differs little from the other selections. Variation in the proportion and quantity of glycosides in *D. lanata* has also been noted in mixed populations and, by the selfing of selected individuals, strains rich in a particular glycoside have been produced, the inherited character being strongly developed. Valuable physiological forms could thus be produced and Ligeti has recommended that these strains be designated by such names as '*D. lanata* Ehrh, chemo-varieties A and C', depending on the respective predominance of lanatosides A and C. It appears that with such inbred lines continuous selection is still required to prevent reversion to the normal character level of the species.

The great value of the radioimmunoassay (q.v.) for the rapid selection of high-yielding strains of *Digitalis lanata* has been demonstrated by Weiler and Westekemper. After two selection steps involving the analysis of over 10 000 individual plants, the average digoxin content of the plants could be raised two to threefold and several strains with average digoxin concentrations in the leaf of 0.6% were isolated. Individual plants were found with 0.9–1.0% digoxin content. As is usual with this type of selection, no plants better than the few best of the original selection were obtained.

Following intensive chemical investigation of the genus *Strophanthus*, Reichstein and his colleagues differentiated four chemical varieties of the polymorphous *S. sarmentosus* from different geographical sources. They are sarverogenin-, sarmentogenin- and sarmutogenin-producing types with glycosides of these, and a fourth form which has a low glycosidal content (Fig. 14.1). Although the locality of growth may produce quantitative differences in the constituents of the various races, the overall type is genetically controlled. Similar variation may exist among those plants that yield steroidal saponins, several thousand of which, from different localities have been screened for their sapogenin content.

Withanolides. The plant *Withania somnifera* (Solanaceae), in addition to producing alkaloids, contains steroidal lactones. Investigations over the years, carried out on various sources of plant material, and concerning the non-alkaloidal constituents, had given differing results, which were explained by the work of Abraham *et al.* (1968) on Israeli plants. Three chemotypes were discovered among 24 populations of *W. somnifera* collected in various parts of the country. Chemotype I contained predominantly withaferin A (0.2% of the dry weight), which is the principle responsible for the plant's bacteriostatic and antitumor properties. Chemotype II contains a compound of similar structure, and chemotype III a mixture of related compounds comprising a group

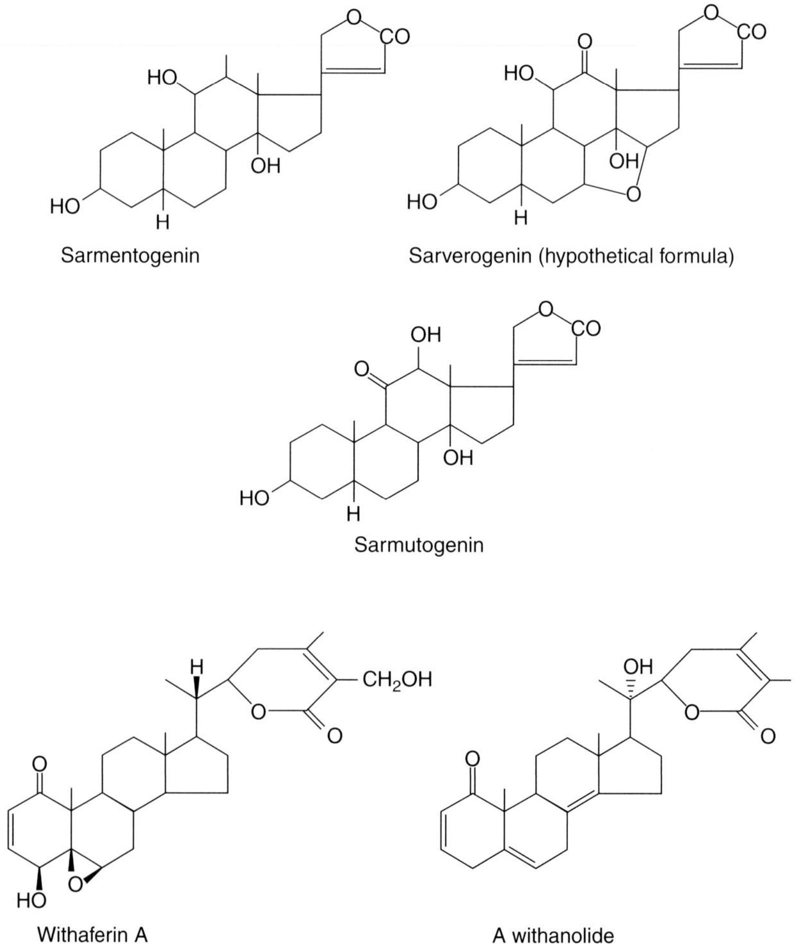

Fig. 14.1
Steroidal constituents of chemical races of *Strophanthus* and *Withania*.

Sarmentogenin

Sarverogenin (hypothetical formula)

Sarmutogenin

Withaferin A

A withanolide

Table 14.1 Chemical races of *Solanum dulcamara*.

Aglycone	Sugars	Glycoside
Soladulicidine (25D)	Galatose (1 mol) Glucose (2 mol) Xylose (1 mol)	Soladulcidine-tetraoside
Solasodine (25D)	Galactose (1 mol) Glucose (1 mol) Rhamnose (1 mol)	Solasonine
Δ5-Tomatidenol (25L)	Galactose (1 mol) Glucose (1 mol) Rhamnose (1 mol)	α-Solamarine

of steroidal lactones—the withanolides (Fig. 14.1). The only morphological difference observed between the chemotypes was a difference in flowering time (12 days early) for chemotype III. Since then, other chemotypes of *W. somnifera* have been reported from India and South Africa.

Steroidal alkaloids. *Solanum* spp. (Solanaceae) contain steroidal glycosidic alkaloids some of which have been investigated as potential intermediates in corticosteroid synthesis. In *S. dulcamara* (the woody nightshade) Sander has distinguished a west European tomatidenol group and an east European soladulcidine-solasodine group (Table 14.1). Although polyploid forms do occur in the genus, these chemical varieties all had $2n = 24$ chromosomes and were genetically stable. Subsequent work demonstrated that the different chemotypes can occur in the same locality. With the commercial species, about 3500 individual 6-month-old *Solanum laciniatum* and *S. aviculare* were analysed by radioimmunoassay (q.v.) and found to contain average leaf concentrations of 1.6–1.7% solasodine; from these a few individuals were selected for future breeding work.

Essential oils. The biochemical group of plants offering evidence of the largest number of chemical races is that containing volatile oils.

Here, again, many of the differences within a species which have been reported may be due to factors other than genetic ones. Australia offers unique opportunities for the investigation of this problem as the flora is rich in oil-bearing plants. As an example, the common form of *Eucalyptus dives* contains piperitone as the chief constituent of the oil, but other races are known which produce principally phellandrene or cineole, while still others produce oils intermediate in composition.

There are three races of *Melaleuca bracteata* producing volatile oils containing chiefly methyl eugenol, methyl iso-eugenol and elemicin, respectively. They can be transformed one into the other by simple chemical steps, which suggests that one of the compounds (e.g. methyl eugenol) occurs in all the races. With the appropriate enzyme, methyl iso-eugenol could be formed by a simple double-bond shift and elemicin by the addition of a hydroxyl group and subsequent methylation. Because of this a one-gene-one-enzyme hypothesis suggests itself and it would be possible to test this by breeding experiments.

In the American turpentine industry, breeding investigations have shown that oleoresin yields in pines are inherited. Two chemotypes differing in their Δ^3-carene content of the oil have been recognized for *Pinus sylvestris*.

Methyl eugenol   Methyl iso-eugenol   Elemicin

14

Plants of the Labiatae have long been cultivated for their volatile oils and many varieties of a single species may exist; these are not, however, necessarily true chemical races because morphological differences may also be involved. Chemical races in the genera *Ocimum*, *Melissa*, *Micromeria* and *Thymus* have been studied. As one example, Rovesti's observations on the Ethiopian plant *Ocimum menthaefolium* are shown in Table 14.2. These forms occurred at different altitudes and exhibited a correlation between humidity of atmosphere and the constituents but cultivation of all four types at Asmara showed the chemical races to be stable and not transitory phenotypes varying with the environment. Similar wide variations of constituents of *Melissa officinalis* have been noted. Sixteen genotypes cultivated in the same field in former Yugoslavia for 2 years contained 0.046–0.246% oil. The constituents were the same for all oils but there was wide variation in relative amounts between the genotypes, namely citronellal 2.711–12.141%, linalool 1.501–6.380%, caryophyllene 1.210–19.073%, geranyl acetate + citronellol 9.710–26.913; (through *Chem. Abs.*, 1991, **114**, 58920). In Spain a 5-year selection and improvement programme for *M. officinalis* raised the essential oil content from 0.2–0.3% to more than 0.5% (T. Adzet *et al.*, *Planta Med.*, 1992, **58**, 558).

Chemotypes of *Acorus calamus*, sweet flag (Acoraceae), having differences in essential oil composition, have been DNA profiled.

Cinnamomum camphora (Lauraceae) exists as various chemical races which vary in their volatile oil composition, and a similar situation prevails for *C. zeylanicum* (*C. verum*). In the same family *Ocotea pretissa* gives oils of the sassafras type which may or may not contain camphor.

Chemical races appear to occur very widely in some Compositae. For *Tanacetum vulgare* (Tansy) ten different chemotypes have been reported for Finland with others for Piedmont (Italy) and Central Europe. Some principal components of these forms are thujone, isothujone, camphor, chrysanthenyl acetate and sabinene. *Achillea millefolium* (Yarrow) occurs as various chemical races and *Artemisia dracunculus* (Tarragon) has yielded, from plants originating mainly in France, an oil containing estragol, whereas from plants of Germany and Russia, sabinene, elemicin and *trans*-isoelemicin are the principal components. Wormwood *BP/EP* (*A. absinthium*) has a number of chemotypes with respect to its volatile oil content which may contain over 40% of any one of *p*-thujone, *trans*-sabinyl acetate *cis*-epoxyocimene or chrysanthenyl acetate. A clone of *Artemisia annua* giving a high yield of the important antimalarial artemisinin has been recorded (D. C. Jain *et al.*, *Phytochemistry*, 1996, **43**, 1993).

Further examples of chemical races among volatile oil-containing drugs of the Labiatae can be found in Chapter 22.

Miscellaneous. Other groups of active compounds which exist as chemical races are the phloroglucinol derivatives of *Dryopteris*, cannabinoids in cannabis, the bitter principles (e.g. amaragentin, sugars and volatile oil) of *Gentiana lutea* and the glycosides of *Salix*. The existence of two discrete chemotypes of *Equisetum arvense* with respect to flavonoid content is noted in the *British Herbal Compendium* Vol. 1. *Artemisia annua* plants raised in Holland from seeds obtained from a number of countries gave plants exhibiting distinct geographic chemotypes (T. E. Wallaart *et al.*, *Planta Medica*, 2000, **66**, 57).

These examples serve to show that the occurrence of chemical races in plants, whether they be of natural origin or produced by plant breeding, can offer considerable scope for the improvement of the therapeutic value of the drug either by adjustment of the individual constituents or by increase in the overall yield.

CHANGES IN CHROMOSOME NUMBER

Polyploidy. In some organisms the chromosomes can be grouped, not in pairs but in threes, fours or higher numbers; these are polyploid individuals—triploid, tetraploid, octaploid, etc. Such polyploids can be derived by the multiplication of the chromosomes of a single species (*autoploids*) or as a result of the multiplication of the chromosomes following hybridization between two species (*alloploids*). The latter case furnishes a mechanism whereby a hybrid of two species, itself infertile, may give rise to a constant fertile type by polyploid formation. In the new polyploid form, pairing of the chromosomes at meiosis is possible which was probably not so in the original hybrid. Types such as this arise naturally: *Primula kewensis* formed as above from the infertile hybrid *P. verticillata* × *P. floribunda* was first recorded in 1912; since then many new species have been synthesized as well as some Linnean species (e.g. the production of the hemp nettle, *Galeopsis tetrahit* Linn. from *G. pubescens* × *G. speciosa*). Of pharmacognostical interest is the stabilization of the (fertile) F₁ hybrid of *Datura ferox* × *D. stramonium* by polyploid formation as indicated later in this chapter. In some species the somatic chromosome number

Table 14.2 Oil composition of *Ocimum menthaefolium*.

Race	Oil content	Composition of oil (%)
Var. *camphorata*	0.285	Camphor 23, cineole 13, pinene 10, estragol 40, sesquiterpene 10
Var. *estragolata*	0.248	Estragol 73, linalool 9, anethole 5, sesquiterpene 5, limonene 1.8
Var. *anisata*	0.236	Anethole 39, estragol 31, limonene 10, linalool 9, sesquiterpene 1.1
Var. *citrata*	0.212	Citral 56, estragol 20, terpene alcohol 10, terpene (as limonene) 9, sesquiterpene 5
Var. *intermedia* (between camphorata and estragolata)	0.267	Camphor 7, cineole 3, estragol 58

Colchicine   Isocolchicine   Colchicine

varies irregularly within wide limits (e.g. the blue grass *Poa pratensis* from 20 to over 100). Such plants, termed *aneuploids*, do not breed true and often exhibit apogametic (asexual) reproduction.

Among the natural polyploids of medicinal interest may be mentioned the mints and valerian; many of the former are alloploids. Valerian occurs across Europe in a variety of forms (2*n*, 4*n* and 8*n*); it is possible that the wide variability in pharmacological action of different samples of Valerianae Radix is associated with these different forms and a more rigid definition of the botanical source might be desirable. As indicated in Table 14.3, the oil compostion of *Acorus calamus*, the sweet flag, varies with the ploidy. For pharmaceutical purposes the 2*n* variety, containing no detectable toxic β-asarone is preferable.

Polyploidy can be artificially induced in many plants by suitable treatment with the alkaloid colchicine. The cytological effect of colchicine on dividing cells was reported by Dustin, Havas and Lits in 1937 and in the same year used practically by Blakeslee in his *Datura* studies. In the presence of colchicine, chromosomes in a cell undergoing mitosis will continue to divide without the formation of a mitotic spindle figure. Sister cells therefore are not formed, and in the growing root tips of onion (2*n* = 16), a 72-h treatment with colchicine solution has given rise to cells containing as many as 256 chromosomes. This 'C-mitotic' activity of colchicine may arise from its interaction with the disulphide bonds of the spindle protein and by inhibition of the conversion of globular proteins to fibrous proteins. On cessation of treatment, the spindle figure again forms in the normal way.

C-mitotic activity is greatly influenced by modifications of the colchicine molecule. Thus, colchicine is 100 times more active than its isomer isocolchicine and colchiceine is virtually inactive.

Modification of substituents in other rings may not have such a marked effect on activity—colcemid, which possesses a methylamino substituent in place of the acetylamido group of colchicine, is reported to have effects the same as colchicine but with toxicity to animal cells.

Plant materials can be treated with colchicine in a number of ways. Seeds are frequently soaked in an aqueous solution of colchicine (0.2–2.0% solution for 1–4 days) before planting, and seedlings can be inverted onto filter paper soaked in the solution so that the growing points are not damaged. Alternatively, the soil around the roots of young seedlings can be moistened with the alkaloid solution. Young buds and shoots can be treated by immersion, and lanolin pastes and agar gels are useful for general application to tissues.

Newly formed polyploids usually require a number of generations to stabilize themselves and treatments of the above type often fail to give a uniform plant regarding chromosome number; such mixochimeric conditions may involve different chromosome numbers in the three germ layers of the plant.

Typical effects of polyploidy compared with the diploid state are larger flowers, pollen grains and stomata. The influence of polyploidy on the constituents of a number of drug plants is indicated in Table 14.3; some figures quoted are taken from extensive studies and are given as an approximate indication of the differences obtained. As can be seen, the effects of polyploidy are not generally predictable and each species

Table 14.3   Influence of chromosome number on constituents of medicinal plants.

Plant	Constituents	Form 2n	Form 4n	Form Others
Atropa belladonna	Total tropane alkaloids		Increase of about 68% over 2n	
Datura innoxia	Hyoscine, dry weight (%)	0.21		0.14, 0.11 (1n)
	Atropine, dry weight (%)	0.03		0.01, 0.01 (1n)
Datura stramonium	Total tropane alkaloids		Increases of about 60–150% over 2n	
Hyoscyamus niger	Total tropane alkaloids		Increase of 22.5% over 2n	Mainly 8n increase of about 34% over 2n
Cinchona succirubra	Quinine, dry weight (%)	0.53	1.12	0.27 (1n)
Opium poppy	Morphine yield per unit area			Increases of up to 100%: 3n plants especially high
Lobelia inflata	Alkaloid content: dry weight (%) per plant	0.25	0.32–0.46 52–152% that of 2n	
Acorus calamus	Volatile oil content (%)	2.1 (light oil, no detectable β-asarone)	6.8 (yellow-brown viscous oil. 2–8% β-asarone)	3.1 (3n) (yellow oil, 0.3% β-asarone)
Achillea millefolium complex	Azulene in volatile oil	Very variable	Most promising source	No azulene (8n)
Carum carvi	Volatile oil content (%)	6.0	10.0	
Mentha spicata	Volatile oil content (%)	0.48	0.05	
Fenugreek seeds	Diosgenin	0.68	0.60	
Digitalis purpurea	Total glycosides (%)		Lower or same as in 2n	
Digitalis lanata	Total glycosides (%)		Lower or same as in 2n. Relatively high content of lanatosides A and B	3.0 (3n)
Urginea indica	Proscillaridin A and scillaren (%)	0.004–0.26	0.02–0.45	0.04–0.07 (3n)
Capsicum sp.	Ascorbic acid (%)	0.04–0.09	0.04–0.15	
Cannabis sativa	Ratios of marihuana-like activity (toxicity to fish)	1.4	2.6	

must be examined individually. Care must be taken that the method used to express the results does not give a deceptive effect. Thus, with lobelia, tetraploid plants are smaller than diploid ones, so that, in spite of an increased percentage of alkaloid in $4n$ plants expressed on a dry weight basis, the total alkaloid content per plant may not exceed that of the $2n$ plants. A similar situation exists with tetraploid *Artemisia annua* with respect to artemisinin content (T. Wallaart *et al.*, *Planta Medica*, 1999, **65**, 728). With tetraploid caraway plants, notwithstanding a 13% smaller crop of fruits from one plant, the total volatile oil content of this plant was increased by 100%; the $4n$ caraway was also found to be perennial ($2n$ = biennial) and to possess an increased frost resistance.

Berkov reported (*Pharm. Biol.*, 2001, **39**, 329) that for autotetraploids of *Datura innoxia*, *D. stramonium* and *Hyoscyamus niger*, the $4n$ seeds contained, respectively, 1.8, 1.65 and 1.96 times the alkaloid content of the $2n$ seeds. Also (S. Berkov and S. Philipov, *Pharm. Biol.*, 2002, **40**, 617), for *D. stramonium* roots, concentrations of the principal alkaloids together with the 13 minor ones were higher in the $4n$, compared with the $2n$, roots.

In some species polyploidy does not affect the relative proportions of the individual constituents—for example, solanaceous herbs produce increased quantities of tropane alkaloids in the $4n$ state and reduced amounts as haploids but the proportion of hyoscine to hyoscyamine remains unaltered; the proportion of carvone in oil of caraway derived from $4n$ plants is also unchanged. However, $4n$ *Digitalis lanata* is reported to contain a relatively high proportion of lanatosides A and B compared with the $2n$ form. Haploid *D. lanata* plants raised from androgenic cell cultures are reportedly smaller than the $2n$ form, have some morphologically abnormal flowers and show very variable cardenolide contents (B. Diettrich *et al.*, *Planta Medica*, 2000, **66**, 237). The sesquiterpene lactones of *Ambrosia dumosa*, family Compositae, exhibit marked differences between the diploid and polyploid forms.

V. Lebot and J. Levesque (*Phytochemistry*, 1996, **43**, 397) record that some 100 tons of kava root (*Piper methysticum*) (q. v.) are imported annually into Europe. The plants are all sterile decaploids ($2n$ = $10x$ = 130) and are raised by smallholders throughout the Pacific Islands. Unfortunately the yields of kavalactones from different sources vary enormously and there is a real need for clonal selection for genetic improvement. The above authors have examined by HPLC the chemical composition of 121 cultivars originating from 51 Pacific Islands.

Extrachromosomal types. Sometimes plants occur with one or more chromosomes extra to the somatic number and these are known as extrachromosomal types. They were first noticed by Blakeslee's group in 1915, although their genetic constitution was not immediately apparent, when they sporadically appeared in pure line cultures of *Datura stramonium*. Such plants were later shown to possess 25 chromosomes in the somatic cell and with *Datura* (n = 12), twelve $2n + 1$ types are possible, each one containing a different extra chromosome. The chromosomes were designated by numbering their halves (or ends), so that the largest chromosome is 1.2 and the smallest 23.24. All 12 types eventually appeared in Blakeslee's cultures and were originally named according to some obvious characteristic of the plant (e.g. Globe, Rolled, Ilex, etc.) although the end-numbering system can also be used to identify them; thus, Globe = $2n + 21.22$. Other $2n + 1$ types are also produced and are termed secondaries, tertiaries and compensating. Secondary types have the extra chromosome made up of two identical halves of a chromosome (e.g. $2n + 1.1$) and in tertiary types it is composed of two halves of different chromosomes. Compensating types lack one of the normal chromosomes, which is compensated for by two others each carrying a different half of the missing one (e.g. $2n - 1.2 + 1.9 + 2.5$). At meiosis $2n + 1$ types produce a mixture of n and $n + 1$ gametes and so do not breed true; they proved particularly useful to geneticists for gene location.

Table 14.4 Alkaloids of some primary and secondary types of *Datura stramonium**.

Type		Alkaloid content, compared with controls, at vegetative state (calculated on a dry weight basis)
$2n + 1.2$	'Rolled'	136% increase
$2n + 9.10$	'Echinus'	143% increase
$2n + 3.4$	'Glossy'	
$2n + 5.5$	'Strawberry'	
$2n + 11.11$	'Wedge'	155–227% increases
$2n + 17.17$	'Dwarf'	
$2n + 19.19$	'Divergent'	
$2n + 10.10$	'Thistle'	
$2n + 13.14$	'Microcarpic'	35–40% decreases
$2n + 21.22$	'Globe'	

*From Mechler and Haun (*Planta Med.*, 1981, **42**, 102)

In 1963, Stary reported the analysis of the primary types Poinsettia ($2n + 17.18$) and Globe ($2n + 21.22$) and showed them to possess more hyoscine than hyoscyamine in the leaves of mature plants, whereas in diploid strains the reverse is true. Mechler and Haun have reported on the total alkaloid content of other $2n + 1$ types, including some secondary types. Their abstracted results are given in Table 14.4.

ARTIFICIAL PRODUCTION OF MUTATIONS

The mutagenic properties of X-rays and radium emissions were exploited as early as 1921 by Blakeslee at the commencement of his classical studies on the genetics of the genus *Datura*. Since then, all types of ionizing radiation (α-particles, β-rays, γ-rays, thermal and fast neutrons) have been extensively studied in this respect and a number of new varieties of crop plants have been produced (barley, peas, soya beans, mustard and rape). In barley approximately one-fifth of all viable mutations produced by ionizing radiations are of the 'erectoides' (dense spike, stiff straw) type; in other crops increased yields, early maturity and mildew resistance have been achieved.

Subsequent to a small number of investigations on chemical mutagens dating from 1910, the avalanche of research on this subject started during and after World War II, following observations by Auerbach and Robson on the production of mutations in *Drosophila* (fruit fly) by mustard gas. Further stimulus was given to this work by the discovery that many chemical mutagens also possess carcinogenic or anticarcinogenic properties. These substances vary enormously in their molecular complexity and chemical properties, and it is only more recently that their mode of action has been elucidated.

Collectively, ionizing radiations and chemicals will produce a mutation spectrum which covers all of the groups listed earlier. The former, however, produce in the chromosomes aberrations of a more random nature than do chemicals, which often act principally at certain loci—particularly at those areas of the chromosome which stain differently at mitosis (heterochromatin). Also, the distribution of effects between nuclei is more random with X-rays than with chemicals.

Mutagenic agents act at various stages of nuclear organization. Thus, at that stage of the interphase (non-dividing) nucleus when DNA synthesis is taking place, aberrations involving chromatid exchanges and isochromatid breaks occur. These effects do not become immediately (0–8 h) manifest in the cell but appear as delayed effects 8–48 h after treatment. Ionizing radiations and most chemicals produce aberrations of this type. Clearly, breaks which occur in the interphase nucleus chromosomes before DNA synthesis occurs (chromosomes unsplit) would be of the chromosome type and these are induced by X-ray treatment and by a few chemicals (e.g. ethoxycaffeine and streptonigrin). Other mutations may be induced during the DNA post-synthetic stage of the interphase nucleus and during mitosis itself—as in the production of polyploids by colchicine and in the inducement of binucleate or polynucleate conditions due to inhibition of cell plate formation by cyclic organic compounds (e.g. halogenated derivatives of benzene and toluene, hydrazinotropone compounds, aminopyrine). Most mutagens produce more than one type of fragmentation or exchange effect (e.g. ethoxycaffeine and streptonigrin, besides producing chromosome exchanges, also induce sub-chromatid exchanges). A few of the many known mutagens are given in Table 14.5.

Factors which may influence the effect of mutagenic treatment include oxygen tension within the tissues, temperature and pH. Chemical mutagens can be applied in a similar way to colchicine (q.v.). Seeds, whole plants, isolated organs, growing points, etc., are suitable for direct irradiation. In order to obtain single mutations in a plant, irradiation of pollen, which is subsequently used to fertilize a normal flower, is often advantageous. It is unlikely that a pollen grain will retain its viability if it undergoes more than one mutational change.

Among plants of medicinal interest, the production of polyploid forms has already been discussed. Blakeslee's radiation work on *Datura stramonium* resulted in the production of many single gene mutation types (e.g. Zigzag, Quercina, Bunchy, Equisetum—names derived from some characteristic aspect of the plant). These mutants are not isolated individuals but are produced regularly by radiation treatment. Some forms such as 'pale' (chlorophyll-deficient) are more frequent than others. In many cases Blakeslee was able to map the position of the genes responsible for these effects. Other mutants obtained in these studies were of the extra-chromosomal type (q.v.).

Several workers have studied, without a full genetic analysis, alkaloid production in various species of *Datura* raised from irradiated seeds; types have been produced which show differences in the relative proportions of the alkaloids synthesized but no new alkaloids have been detected by this treatment.

By the irradiation of poppy seeds with [60]Co a number of mutations have been produced, including ones producing plants with an increased morphine content; these increases were maintained in the X_2 generation with an average morphine content of 0.52% compared with 0.32% for the controls.

As mentioned earlier, races of sweet lupins (almost free of bitterness) can be obtained by selection. More recently, bitter lupin seeds of an X-ray-induced early-maturing mutant of *Lupinus digitatus* were treated with ethylmethanesulphonate solution, and, of the 440 progeny, 11 were mutants which could be classed as sweet. Four of these were of normal vigour and near-normal fertility.

Breeding experiments have been performed with irradiated *Mentha piperita* in the USA in an endeavour to produce a dominant mutation (bud sport) for *Verticillium* (wilt) resistance, a disease to which mints are particularly prone; a successful strain, *Todd's Mitcham Peppermint*, is now cultivated. A radiation-induced mutant of Scotch peppermint (*Mentha × gracilis*) has been shown to produce an oil typical of the ordinary peppermint (C-3 oxygenated monoterpenes) instead of the C-6 oxygenated monoterpenes characteristic of spearmint (see Fig. 22.4 for formulae). The results have given further insight into the biogenesis of these compounds (R. Croteau *et al.*, *Plant Physiol.*, 1991, **96**, 744).

In India mutant strains of *Capsicum annuum* with increased yields (20–60%) of capsaicin have been isolated from M_3 and M_4 generations originating from seed treated with sodium azide and ethylmethanesulphonate.

In the future, haploid plants will undoubtedly find increasing use for the study of induced mutations; in many cases whole plants can now be regenerated from haploid tissue cultures of pollen. Such material has the advantage that induced recessive mutations, which in the diploid organism require subsequent breeding experiments for their study, are immediately apparent in the phenotype.

HYBRIDIZATION

In plant breeding hybridization forms a possible means of combining in a single variety the desirable characters of two or more lines, varieties or species, and occasionally of producing new and

Table 14.5 Cytological action of some chemical mutagens.

Group	Examples	Cytological effect
DNA precursors and related compounds	Adenine	Inhibition of early stages of DNA synthesis, purine formation
	Deoxyadenosine	Inhibition of deoxyribonucleotide synthesis
	Ethoxycaffeine	Complex formation with inhibition of the DNA-polymerase reaction, degradation and denaturation of DNA
DNA base analogues	Thymidine analogue 5-bromodeoxyuridine	Production of abnormal DNA
Antibiotics	Streptomycin	As ethoxycaffeine
	Actinomycin	As ethoxycaffeine
Alkylating agents	Nitrogen mustard	Production of abnormal DNA
	Diepoxypropyl ether	
Nitroso compounds and chelating agents	Many compounds (e.g. cupferron, 8-hydroxy-quinoline)	Possibly combine with some trace heavy metals (Fe, Cu) which may be bound with the DNA molecule
Miscellaneous	Inorganic cyanides	Inhibition of cytochrome oxidase with resultant peroxide formation
	Maleic hydrazide	Reaction with sulphydryl groups
	Hydroxylamine	Combination with cytosine component of DNA

desirable characters not found in either parent. Hybridization, particularly between homozygous strains which have been inbred for a number of generations, introduces a degree of heterozygosity with resultant hybrid vigour (heterosis) often manifest in the dimensions and other characteristics of the plant. Several methods of breeding crops by the use of sexual hybridization are available and for these the reader is referred to standard works on the subject. Although this chapter is devoted principally to chemical variants of a particular species it is convenient to include here, in addition to intervarietal hybridization, interspecific hybridization in which hybrid vigour is also apparent.

The hybrid nature of a number of drugs (e.g. cinchona, q.v.) is well known. The commercial mints are hybrids and must therefore be propagated vegetatively, as the plants will not breed true and the progeny vary in their oil composition. Hegnauer considers that with the spearmint-type oil (high carvone content) genes of *Mentha longifolia* or of *M. rotundifolia* seem to be necessary. The cultivated peppermint (*M. piperita*) is probably a hybrid derived from *M. aquatica* and *M. spicata* and it is the former that contributes the menthofuran characteristics. Hybrids between various species of *Mentha* have been used to study the inheritance of a number of essential oil components, including menthol, carvone and pulegone.

Hybrids of species producing tropane alkaloids have received considerable study. In the genus *Datura* the effect of hybridization on chemical constituents is illustrated by the cross *D. ferox × D. stramonium*. The aerial organs of the latter normally contain hyoscyamine and hyoscine (2:1 ratio) at the flowering period; and those of the former, hyoscine with some meteloidine. The F_1 of the cross consists of plants larger than either of the parents, and containing hyoscine as the principal alkaloid with only small amounts of other bases. In the F_2, segregation occurs as regards both morphological characters and alkaloid constituents. With *D. leichhardtii* and *D. innoxia* the former plant produces hyoscyamine and hyoscine (2:1) and the latter species usually mainly hyoscine but sometimes, according to conditions of growth, appreciable quantities of hyoscyamine. In this instance the F_1 hybrid contains a hyoscyamine:hyoscine ratio intermediate between that of the two parents. Various hybrids of tree daturas have also given favourable alkaloid yields and have been subjected to field trials in Ecuador. These plants are self-sterile but can be propagated by cloning (Chapter 13).

In experiments performed in Australia on hybrids of *Duboisia leichhardtii* and *D. myoporoides* no uniform dominance of either hyoscine or hyoscamine in the F_1 was obtained, although the ratio generally favoured hyoscyamine even in geographical areas conducive to the production of hyoscine. Investigations of this type on *Duboisia* are complicated by the occurrence of chemical races and by the marked susceptibility of alkaloid content to environment. However, single desirable hybrids can be vegetatively propagated and have now become established as commercial crops (q.v.). Experiments in Japan on artificial crosses of *Duboisia* produced some F_1 hybrids which contained more than twice the amount of alkaloids (hyoscine and hyoscyamine) than that contained by the parents. Greatest increases were found when *D. myoporoides* was the female parent. Naturally occurring intergeneric hybrids involving *Duboisia* spp. and other Anthocercideae have been analysed (El-Imam *et al.*, *Int. J. Pharmacog.*, 1991, **29**, 263) and the alkaloid metabolism in callus and regenerating shoot cultures of the commercial hybrid *D. leichhardtii × D. myoporoides* studied (Gritsanapan and Griffin, *Phytochemistry*, 1992, **31**, 3069).

Nicotiana tabacum (Solanaceae), as now cultivated, must have been derived from at least two different parent species, and 'synthetic' tobaccos can be prepared by using suspected species as parents. Although it has not been possible to produce in this way species exactly comparable to *N. tabacum*, such synthetic plants are most useful for the study of alkaloid inheritance characteristics. This is important in the commercial production of tobacco, in which both the quantity and the nature of the alkaloid produced are important. Demethylation of nicotine may take place in the leaves of some species, and by hybrid studies this reaction has been shown to be due, in the groups of plants studied, to either one pair of dominant factors or two pairs of dominant and independent factors.

The inheritance of the opium alkaloids (morphine, codeine, thebaine, narcotine and papaverine) has been studied in the cross *Papaver somniferum × P. setigerum*. A heterotic increase in codeine and thebaine was found in different F_1 plants, and in the F_2 plants, with the exception of codeine, some increase in alkaloid content was noted. An absence of narcotine was generally dominant over its presence (Khanna *et al.*, *Planta Med.*, 1986, p. 157). A continuation of this work to the F_8 generation (Shukla *et al.*, *Int. J. Pharmacognosy*, 1995, **33**, 228) resulted in a population that was completely diploid but which showed considerable diversity with regard to the opium contents of morphine, narcotine and papaverine. The pattern of alkaloids was closer to that of *P. somniferum* than to that of *P. setigerum* with morphine contents ranging from 8.0 to 30.0%. The authors envisaged that a suitable breeding programme could result in opium with a higher level of morphine than that normally encountered. F_1 hybrids of *P. bracteatum* and *P. orientale* contained a lower thebaine content and higher oripavine content than in either parent, a result which provided genetic evidence for the biosynthetic linkage between these alkaloids (Fig. 26.15).

In a continuation of the Israeli work on withanolides Eastwood *et al.* reported that a cross of a South African chemotype of *Withania somnifera* with the Israeli chemotype II produced three new withanolides not detected in either parent. The outstanding feature was the presence of a new oxidizing system in the hybrid which apparently oxidizes ring A to a diketone in the presence of either the saturated or the unsaturated lactone (Fig. 14.2). A further notable feature was the isolation of a compound having a saturated C2–C3 link, a feature which had only been noticed in a minor constituent of chemotype I. In *Datura*, too, hybrids may contain different withanolides from those of either parent and involve different oxidation states of ring C.

Solasodine occurs in *Solanum incanum* up to the extent of 1.8% whereas *S. melongena* contains only traces of steroidal alkaloids. Work in Jammu, India, has shown the F_1 hybrid of these species to be much more prolific in fruit-bearing than either of its parents, with a content of 0.5% solasodine. The diversity of glycoalkaloids found in *Solanum*

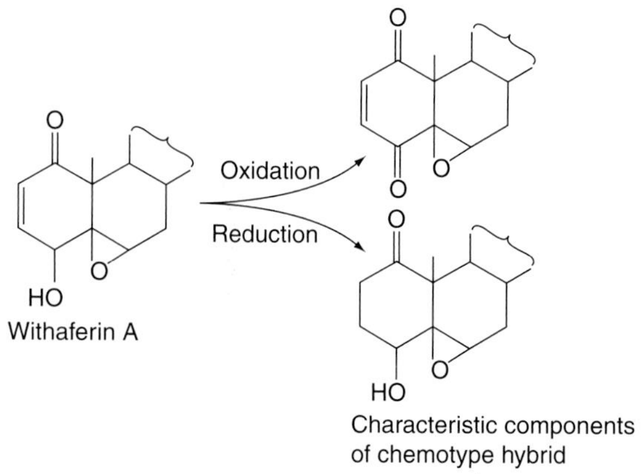

Fig. 14.2

Withanolide oxidations and reductions characteristic of a *Withania somnifera* chemotype hybrid (for complete structure of withaferin A see 'Withanolides').

Table 14.6 Lanatoside formation in *Digitalis* hybrids.

♀	Parents	♂	Glycosides of the F_1
D. purpurea	×	D. lanata	Lanatoside A (principal glycoside). Also lanatosides B and E. Small amount of glucogitaloxin. No lanatoside C or purpurea glycoside A
D. purpurea	×	D. lutea	Similar to the above
D. lutea	×	D. lanata	Same composition as the parent plants which resemble one another. Lanatoside A the principal glycoside but lanatoside C, which occurs in large amounts in *D. lanata*, could not be detected

species is, in part, the result of the independent inheritance of the aglycone and glycosidic moieties and explains the occurrence of a new alkaloid, sisuine, found in the hybrid of *S. acaule* and *S. ajanhuiri*. This group of hybrid clones is cultivated by the Aymara people of Western Bolivia.

In 1961, Calcandi and coworkers demonstrated (Table 14.6) that in the hybridization of *Digitalis* species, lanatoside formation is dominant to purpurea glycoside formation; in 1984 these observations were largely confirmed for some crosses and extended with more detailed analysis by Wichtl and Mangkudidjojo (*Pharm. Zeit.*, 1984, **129**, 686). For the glycoside content of other *Digitalis* F_1 hybrids including those of *D. ferruginea* and *D. cariensis*, see Fingerhut *et al.*, *Planta Med.*, 1991, **57** (Suppl. No. 2), A70; A71.

Preliminary studies by Cornish *et al.* in 1983 indicated that foenugreek seed, a potential source of diosgenin (Chapter 23), is capable of genetic improvement regarding the monohydroxysapogenin yield by hybridization of various races of *Trigonella foenum-graecum*.

Pyrethrum hybrids have been used in Kenya for pyrethrin production (see Chapter 40); these hybrids are produced either by crossing two clones assumed to be self-sterile or by planting a number of desirable clones together and bulking the seed. The aim is to obtain progeny which, owing to hybrid vigour, will increase pyrethrin yield per acre. Unfortunately, it appears that increased production of pyrethrins is not always associated with hybrid vigour. Research at the Pyrethrum Marketing Board, Kenya, indicated that clonal selection, based on vigour and individual pyrethrin content of hybrids raised from seed, followed by vegetative propagation, would give better results.

TRANSGENIC MEDICINAL PLANTS

Until recently the transfer of genetic material from one plant to another was dependent on hybridization as has been discussed above and its application is limited to those relatively few species which are intercompatible and give fertile F_1 hybrids.

Developments in molecular biology and chemical genetics have provided new vistas for genetics and it is now possible to explain, in terms of the DNA molecule, chromosome duplication and the structure of the gene itself—two mysteries involving the nature of life which intrigued and baffled scientists for many years. From such fundamental studies the science of genetic engineering explosively emerged in 1973, when it became possible, by the formation of recombinant DNA, to transfer certain DNA sequences from the chromosomes of one organism to those of another. Since DNA assemblages represent the genes or hereditary characters of an organism, this led the way for the artificial transfer of a particular character from one organism to another.

Nature itself does effect genetic transfers between very dissimilar organisms as evidenced by the well-known crown gall and hairy root diseases of plants. Both are caused by bacterial infection of the plant and involve, respectively, the soil organisms *Agrobacterium tumefaciens* and *A. rhizogenes*. Crown gall disease is essentially a plant cancer and hairy root disease is also a proliferation manifestation in which there is an excessive development of the root system. A further characteristic associated with both diseases is the production, by the host, of a group of substances called opines, the actual compounds synthesized being specific for the particular parasite involved. Many opines are dicarboxylic acids, the majority being formed by condensation of an amino acid (lysine, arginine, ornithine, histidine) with either pyruvate or α-ketoglutarate; others involve simple sugars such as mannose and sucrose, see Fig. 14.3. (For a review on opines (129 refs) see Y. Dessaux *et al.*, *Phytochemistry*, 1993, **34**, 31.) Another important feature concerning these diseases, first noted in the late 1960s, was that *Agrobacterium* strains would degrade only those opines for whose occurrence in the host they were responsible. Thus opines, of no value to the plant cell, constitute an exclusive food substrate for the particular bacterial strain. When, however, the bacterium is eliminated from the host plant (e.g. by treatment with an antibiotic) the characteristic morphological features and the production of opines continue to be maintained. This is because genetic material (T-DNA) of the bacterium carrying the genes which express the disease has been transported to, and integrated into, the plant DNA. These genes are carried on large plasmids which have been named Ti (Tumour-inducing) and Ri (Root-inducing) plasmids. Such transgenic plant material is of particular medicinal and phytochemical interest when grown as transformed cell cultures or hairy root cultures in studies involving the production of secondary metabolites and has already been discussed in some detail in Chapter 13.

A further development has been to utilise *Agrobacterium* in a vector system for transferring genes from one species of higher plant to another. Such transfers usually involve just a single enzyme system; multiple enzyme systems involved in secondary metabolism and originating from different chromosomes obviously present great problems. Of pharmacognostical significance is the work of Hashimoto's group at Kyoto University on *Atropa belladonna*: the conversion of

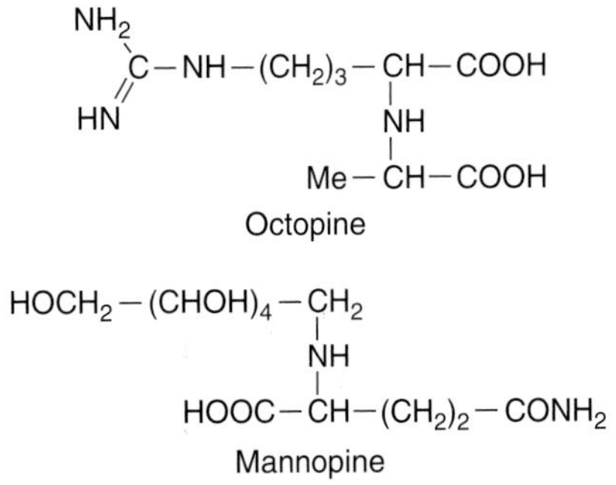

Fig. 14.3
Examples of opines.

hyoscyamine to hyoscine (Chapter 26) in the plant involves the enzyme hyoscyamine-6-hydroxylase and in the normal belladonna plant the gene is not strongly expressed and plants are hyoscyamine dominant. Conversely, although *Hyoscyamus niger* contains less alkaloid (% dry weight) than belladonna it contains a higher proportion of hyoscine. The hydroxylase gene of *H. niger* was placed under the control of the cauliflower mosaic virus 35S promoter and introduced to *A. belladonna* roots by a binary vector system using *Agrobacterium rhizogenes* (*Phytochemistry*, 1993, **32**, 713). The belladonna hairy roots produced showed increased amounts, and increased enzyme activities, of the hydroxylase and contained up to fivefold higher concentrations of hyoscine than the wild-type hairy roots. A second paper (*Proc. Natl. Acad. Sci. USA*, 1992, **89**, 11799) reported that whole plants regenerated from the transformed roots showed, in the first transformant and its selfed progeny, an alkaloid composition of the leaves and stems that was almost exclusively hyoscine. Such a plant, if developed commercially, would be a valuable temperate-region source of hyoscine.

In the same area K. Jouhikainen *et al.* (*Planta*, 1999, **208**, 545) have demonstrated enhancement of scopolamine production in *Hyoscyamus muticus* hairy root cultures by introducing the above 35S-*h6h* transgene that codes for the enzyme hyoscyamine-6β-hydroxylase (EC 1.14.11.11). *H. muticus* is a species producing up to 6% dryweight of tropane alkaloids, normally hyoscyamine; the introduction of the above transgene moved alkaloid production towards scopolamine (but not entirely) and indicated the potential for greater conversion by the use of more efficient promoter systems.

With belladonna, the first successful application of transferring an agronomically useful trait to a medicinal plant has been reported (K. Saito *et al.*, *Plant Cell Rep.*, 1992, **11**, 219). It involved the production of transgenic fertile *A. belladonna* plants integrated with a herbicide-resistant *bar* gene by means of *Agrobacterium*–Ri vector. The regenerated plants were produced via hairy roots and the *bar* trait was transferred to progeny, which showed resistance to bialaphos and phosphinothricin.

An example of the possible potential for increasing alkaloid yield in *Cinchona* is illustrated by the successful integration of two genes from *Catharanthus roseus* into the hairy roots of *Cinchona officinalis* (A.-Geerlings *et al.*, *Plant Cell Reports*, 1999, **19**, 191). These two genes, responsible for the respective production of the enzymes tryptophan decarboxylase and strictosodine synthase, are crucial to the synthesis of both the cinchona and catharanthus alkaloids (Chapter 26). As a result of the transfer both the quinine and quinidine levels were raised above the normal for *C. officinalis* hairy roots; in this instance however, after one year, the roots had lost their capacity to produce alkaloids.

Transgenic plants of *Panax ginseng* which develop abundant roots have been produced and could therefore be of commercial significance (D.-C. Yang and Y.-E. Choi, *Plant Cell Reports*, 2000, **19**, 491).

Further reading

Lindsey K (ed) 2000 Transgenic plant research. Harwood Academic, Amsterdam

15

Deterioration of stored drugs

The factors which must be considered in relation to drug deterioration are moisture content, temperature, light and the presence of oxygen; when these conditions are suitable, living organisms (bacteria, moulds, mites and insects) will rapidly multiply, using the drug as a source of nutrient. Drugs affected in this way are excluded by national pharmacopoeias.

PRIMARY FACTORS

As indicated in Chapter 11, air-dry drugs contain about 10–12% of moisture, and in some instances (e.g. digitalis) this may be sufficient to activate enzymes present in the leaves and bring about decomposition of the glycosides. Other drugs, such as powdered squill, which contain mucilage quickly absorb moisture and become a sticky mass. The containerized shipment of drugs which is now common practice can lead to spoilage due to excessive condensation of moisture on the inner metal walls. It is a particular problem with cargoes in transit from humid moist climates to temperate regions. An increase in temperature, in combination with moisture, may accelerate enzyme activity; a large temperature rise will obviously lead to a loss of volatile constituents (e.g. essential oils from dried plant material) and in the case of absorbent cotton-wool cause a reorientation of the small amount of fatty material present leading to non-absorbency or lower absorbency. Direct sunlight can cause decomposition of certain constituents (e.g. vitamins in cod-liver oil) as well as producing a bleaching of leaves and flowers. Oxygen assists in the resinification of volatile oils and in the rancidification of fixed oils.

MOULD AND BACTERIAL ATTACK

The moulds found in deteriorating drugs are usually the same as those associated with poorly stored food products. Species of *Rhizopus, Mucor, Penicillium* and *Eurotium* are common. Their presence is indicated by a mass of hyphae which bind the particles of drug and by a characteristic smell. Deterioration of drugs is only one aspect of the importance of moulds in pharmacognosy—see Chapter 30. Bacterial attack of crude drugs is less obvious unless chromogenic species are involved or effects produced such as dustiness in cotton-wool by attack on the fibres. Although not a cause of deterioration, certain pathogenic bacteria such as salmonellae and *Escherichia coli* are tested for in some crude drugs taken internally (digitalis, sterculia, tragacanth, gelatin). Also, as plant materials which have been dried under normal conditions contain viable bacteria and mould spores in variable amounts, the pharmacopoeias set limits for the total viable aerobic count per gram of drug (see Quality Control, Chapter 16).

COLEOPTERA OR BEETLES

Beetles are insects and constitute the largest order of the animal kingdom, comprising some 250000 species, of which about 600 have been found associated with stored food products or drugs. Not all of these utilize the stored product itself but may be found in the wood of packing-cases or living predaciously. Beetles have a body which is divided into head, thorax and abdomen. To the lower side of the thorax are attached three pairs of legs, while the upper surface usually bears two membranous hind-wings which are folded beneath horny elytra (forewings). They show complete metamorphosis of egg, larval, pupal and adult stages, and those which constitute pests in stored products cause damage both as adults and as larvae. Among the characters which distinguish the larvae of most species which attack foodstuffs and vegetable drugs are the well-developed biting mouth-parts and a head which is darker in colour than the rest of the body. Table 15.1 lists beetles commonly found in stored drugs; for illustrations see Fig. 15.1.

Table 15.1 Beetles commonly found in stored drugs.

	Description
Family Nitidulidae (sap-feeding beetles)	
Carpophilus spp., e.g. *C. hemipterus* (dried fruit beetles)	Obovate or oblong 2–4.5 mm long; 11-segmented antennae with a compact club. Elytra somewhat shortened exposing two–three apical abdominal segments. In this country about three species are found in granaries, food-stores and warehouses
Family Silvanidae	
Oryzaephilus mercator (merchant grain beetle)	Dark brown, narrow, distinctly flattened beetles, about 3 mm long. Clubbed antennae. Attack nuts and dried fruits
O. surinamensis (saw-toothed grain beetle)	
Family Curculionidae (weevils)	
Calandra granaria (granary weevil)	Dark brown to black insects, about 3–4 mm long. Hind-wings absent, characteristic snout and antennae. Bore into seeds and fruits and lay an egg in the cavity by means of the ovipositor. Larvae develop and pupate within the seeds
Calandra oryzae (rice weevil)	Similar, hindwings present. 2.3–4.5 mm long
Family Anobiidae ('furniture beetles')	
Stegobium paniceum (*Sitodrepa panicea*) *Anobium paniceum* (drugroom beetle)	Pale reddish-brown in colour, greyish hairs, 2–3 mm long. Antennae 11-segmented, with three terminal segments forming a loose club. Common in many stored vegetable drugs, formerly frequent in ships' biscuits
Anobium punctatum (common furniture beetle)	Similar to *Stegobium paniceum*, 3–5 mm long. Viewed laterally, the prothorax exhibits a distinct hump. Does not attack drugs but may occur in wood of packing-cases, floors, etc.
Lasioderma serricorne (tobacco, cigar or cigarette beetle)	Reddish colour, 2–2.5 mm long. Found in many stored products, including ginger and liquorice
Family Ptinidae ('spider beetles')	
Ptinus fur (white-marked spider beetle) *P. tectus* (Australian spider beetle) *P. hirtellus* (brown spider beetle) *Trigonogenius globulus* *Niptus hololeucus* (goldenspider beetle, cloth bug) *Gibbium psylloides*	All rather similar, somewhat resembling spiders, with long legs and antennae, stout bodies and hairy covering, 2–4 mm long. Some species (e.g. *Niptus hololeucus*) are densely covered with hairs; others (e.g. *Gibbium* spp.) are glabrous with a shining cuticle. Of wide occurrence in stored products—food, spices, cocoa, cereals, almonds, capsicum, ginger, nutmegs, etc.
Family Tenebrionidae	
Tribolium confusum (confused flour beetle) *T. castaneum* (rust red flour beetle)	Reddish-brown beetles, 2–4 mm long. Found in many foodstuffs including flour and nuts. Infested flour has lingering pungent odour. Reported as becoming more common in crude drugs e.g. rhubarb

LEPIDOPTERA

The Lepidoptera include the moths and butterflies, and although the number of species is large, only a relatively small number of moths cause injury to drugs. As in the case of the clothes moth, the damage is caused by the larva and not by the mature insect; but since moths are very mobile and lay eggs, infestation tends to spread rapidly. Moths reported in stored drugs are listed in Table 15.2.

Ephestia kuehniella, the Mediterranean flour moth; *E. cautella*, the fig moth; *E. elutella*, the cocoa moth, and *Plodia interpunctella*, the Indian meal moth, all belong to the same family, the Phycitidae.

Table 15.2 Moths of stored drugs.

Moth	Products attacked
Ephestia kuehniella	Almond, capsicum, cocoa, cotton seed, ground-nut
E. cautella	Tonco bean, cocoa
E. elutella	Cocoa, tobacco, rose petals, pomegranate root bark
Plodia interpunctella	Cinnamon bark and yeast cake
Tinea pellionella	Aconite root, almonds, capsicums, mustard seed, ginger, linseed, orris, saffron and tobacco

Various members of the family Tineidae, which cause damage to clothes, carpets, etc., are also found in drugs.

Ephestia kuehniella is about 25 mm long. It has dark brownish-grey scaly forewings and dirty-white hindwings. The larvae are whitish except for the brownish anterior and the dark hairs on each segment; when fully grown, they remain in the food material, where they overwinter and form pupae. In contrast, the grubs of *E. elutella* migrate away from the food and in so doing often leave the food containers completely 'webbed' with their silky threads; they enter cracks in walls, etc., where they spin cocoons and remain until they pupate in the spring to finally emerge as adults in May.

ARACHNIDA

The arachnids or 'mites' differ from the true insects in that the mature forms have eight legs but possess no antennae. The members of the Tyroglyphidae (e.g. *Tyroglyphus dimidiatus*, the cheese-mite) are much smaller than the insects, and individuals can only be seen with a lens. If the suspected 'dust' is scraped into a pile, it will be seen to move and will gradually become flat if mites are present in considerable numbers.

Tyroglyphus farinae (*Acarus siro*) (Fig. 15.2A), the flour or meal mite, is 0.4–0.7 mm long. The body is oval in outline, with a truncated posterior, and is clearly divided into two regions—the anterior propodosoma and the posterior hysterosoma. It is common in cereal products, oil-seed cakes and many other commodities.

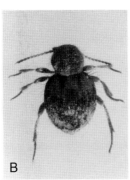
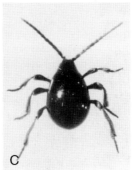
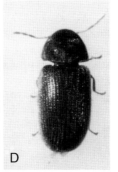

Fig. 15.1
Insect pests found in crude drugs. A, *Calandra granaria*; B, *Ptinus* spp; C, *Gibbium* spp.: (all × 10). D, *Stegobium paniceum* (× 12). (Photos: Dr M. E. Brown)

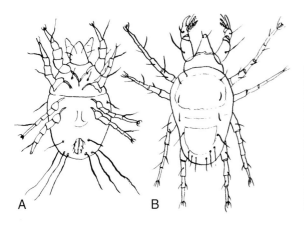
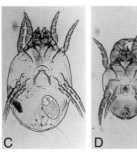

Fig. 15.2
Arachnids. A, *Tyroglyphus farinae*, female, ventral view, × 40. B, *Cheyletus eruditus*, female, dorsal view, × 40. C, *Dermatophagoides culinae*, female, ventral view. D, *D. culinae*, male, ventral view.

The Tyroglyphidae may themselves be attacked by other mites such as *Cheyletus eruditus* (Fig. 15.2B).

A number of different mites commonly attack cantharides, causing considerable damage. Ergot, quince and linseed are other drugs which seem very liable to attack.

Mites commonly exist in ordinary house dust as found under carpets, in mattresses, etc.; and these include *Dermatophagoides pteronyssinus*, *D. culinae*, *Glycyphagus domesticus* (the house mite) and *Tyroglyphus farinae* (the flour mite). It has been shown, comparatively recently, that these mites are the allergens responsible for house dust sensitivity, an allergy from which many people suffer. It is now possible to diagnose this condition by prick tests which utilize an extract prepared from *Dermatophagoides culinae*. This mite (Fig. 15.2C) does not show the marked division of the body into two parts exhibited by *Tyroglyphus* spp.

CONTROL OF INFESTATION

The detection, prevention and eradication of mite and insect infestation is an important hygienic and economic consideration for all who have occasion to store and use crude drugs. Effective preventive measures involve *good hygiene* in the warehouse (removal of spillages, old debris and packaging materials; elimination of sources of infections such as floor cracks and crevices), *effective stock control* (regular inspection, rotation of stock, early recognition of infestation), *optimum storage conditions* (maintenance of cool, dry environment) and *good packaging* (woven sacks and bags, multi-ply paper sacks stitched at the seams, paper, polythene film, flimsy cardboard are all penetrable by insects and mites)

If material becomes infested it may be wiser to sacrifice a small consignment rather than to risk contamination of other materials. After a contaminated drug has been removed, pallets, shelves, walls and floors should be thoroughly cleaned and sprayed with a contact insecticide such as chlorpyriphos-methyl or pirimiphos-methyl. Weekly air-spraying with pyrethrins or synthetic pyrethroids, and the use of slow-release dichlorvos strips, control air-borne insects. Various dust formulations may be used in cracks.

Fumigation is the only practical means of killing insects and mites in bulk consignments. Methyl bromide and ethylene oxide have been commonly used and the treatment needs to be applied under gas-proof sheets or in other suitable gas-tight enclosures or chambers. However in Europe the use of ethylene oxide has now been prohibited.

Owing to the possible hazards involved, the work should be performed by professional operators in compliance with the Health and Safety at Work Acts. Before drugs are subsequently used the fumigants must be completely removed as, if they are consumed, they may constitute a health hazard.

Low-temperature storage appears to offer great possibilities. It not only reduces insect attack, but also will, if a sufficiently low-temperature be employed, gradually destroy insects, larvae and eggs. The eggs of *Ephestia elutella* and *E. kuehniella* are rapidly destroyed at −15°C and more slowly at rather higher temperatures.

The eggs of the flour mite can withstand exposure to −10°C for up to 12 days or 0°C for several months; development is possible within the range 2.5–30°C, depending on humidity.

Studies on the effects of ionizing radiations (e.g. from a ⁶⁰Co source) on cereal pests such as *Tyroglyphus* mites and various beetles show that small doses inhibit reproductive ability and larger ones destroy both mites and their eggs.

The quantitative determination of insect infestation in powdered vegetable drugs is of some significance. Melville (*J. Pharm. Pharmacol.*, 1949, **1**, 649; 1951, **3**, 926) developed a method based on the acetolysis of the weighed sample for the quantitative isolation of the insect fragments present. These fragments are suspended in a suitable medium with a weighed quantity of lycopodium spores. Using the fact that the number of strial punctures per elytron is characteristic for a particular beetle, one can, by counting the strial punctures evident on the fragments of elytra present under the microscope, arrive at a figure for the number of beetles present. The use of lycopodium spores (94 000 spores mg^{-1}) eliminates the necessity for counting all the strial punctures present in a particular volume (or weight) of the suspension; the use of lycopodium powder in this respect is described under 'Quantitative Microscopy' (Chapter 43).

SPOILAGE BY RODENTS

Rodent faeces usually contain the animal's hairs, so that drugs which on microscopical examination show the presence of these hairs should be rejected.

Further reading

Dales MJ 1996 A review of plant materials used for controlling insect pests of stored products. Bulletin 65, Natural Resources Institute, Chatham, UK

Pedigo LP 2002 Entomology and pest management, 4th edn. Prentice Hall, Upper Saddle River, NJ

Rees D 2004 Insects of stored products. CSIRO, Collingwood, Victoria and Manson, London

Sabramanyam B (ed) 1995 Integrated management of insects in stored products. Marcel Dekker, New York

16

Quality control

The quality control of crude plant drugs is of paramount importance. In the past, the monographs of national pharmacopoeias adequately covered this aspect for drugs used in the allopathic system of medicine and the *British Herbal Pharmacopoeias* (1983, 1990, 1996) contained descriptions, tests and quantitative standards for those species commonly employed by medical herbalists. However, there was no control on the plant materials used in the many herbal products manufactured for general retail sale. Under current EU regulations, herbal products can only be manufactured under licence in conformity with the 'Rules and Guidance for Pharmaceutical Manufacturers and Distributors 2007', as set out by the Medicines and Healthcare products Regulatory Agency (MHRA) and published by the Pharmaceutical Press, London. Also, the *BP/EP* 2007 includes a monograph 'Herbal Drugs', which gives requirements relating to definition, production, identification, various tests, pesticide residues, heavy metal content, microbiological quality and, where necessary, limits for aflatoxins and radioactive contamination. Quality control personnel are required to have particular expertise in herbal medicinal products in relation to the above.

One possible problem in devising standards for crude drugs concerns the requirement for an assay of the active constituents when the latter may not have been precisely ascertained. Furthermore, one of the tenets of herbal medicine is that the maximum effectiveness of the drug derives from the whole drug or its crude extract rather than from isolated components. In cases where an assay is lacking it is therefore important that the crude drug is properly authenticated, its general quality verified and all formulations of it prepared in accordance with good manufacturing practice. Attention should also be paid to the shelf-life of the crude drug and its preparations.

Although official standards are necessary to control the quality of drugs their use does raise certain problems. Of necessity, to accommodate the considerable variation that occurs between different batches of a natural product it is necessary to set reasonable standards which allow the use of commercial material available in any season. This has resulted in a tendency for producers or manufacturers to reduce all of their material to the lowest requirement; for example, in a good year the majority of the alkaloid-rich leaves of belladonna herb may be removed and used for the economical manufacture of galenicals and the residue of the herb, containing much stem, used to give the powdered drug. Similarly, high-quality volatile oils may be mixed with lower grades and still remain within official limits.

STANDARDS APPLICABLE TO CRUDE DRUGS

There are a number of standards, numerical in nature, which can be applied to the evaluation of crude drugs either in the whole or the powdered condition.

Sampling

Before a consignment of a drug can be evaluated, a sample must be drawn for analysis; considerable care must be exercised to ensure that this sample is truly representative. With large quantities of bulky drugs a different method of sampling is required from that involving broken or powdered drugs. The *BP* gives no specific instructions for this but the methods of sampling used in the USA are fully described in older editions of the *USP*. EU guidelines specify that sampling should be carried out by those with particular expertise.

Preliminary examination

In the case of whole drugs the macroscopical and sensory characters are usually sufficient to enable the drug to be identified. The general appearance of the sample will often indicate whether it is likely to comply with such standards as percentage of seed in colocynth, of ash in valerian or of matter insoluble in alcohol in asafoetida. However, drugs may comply with the descriptions given in the pharmacopoeias and yet be unsatisfactory, as it is often difficult specifically to describe deterioration of drugs owing to faulty harvesting, shipment or storage or deterioration due to age. In such cases the trained worker will be able to infer much of the history of the sample from its appearance. The following examples will serve to indicate the type of evidence to look for.

If leaves and similar structures are baled before being properly dried, much discoloured material may be found in the middle of the bale. Overdrying, on the other hand, makes leaves very brittle and causes them to break in transit. If starch-containing drugs break with a horny fracture, it may usually be inferred that the temperature of drying has been too high and that the starch has been gelatinized. A pale colour in the case of chamomiles indicates that the drug has been collected in dry weather and carefully dried, while the colour of the fractured surface of gentian is a good indication as to whether it has been correctly fermented. Some drugs are particularly liable to deterioration if, during shipment or storage, they become damp (e.g. cascara). Under moist condition moulds readily establish themselves on drugs having a high mucilage content (e.g. psyllium, linseed, squill and cydonia). Evidence of insect attack must also be looked for.

The price of certain drugs depends largely on such factors as size and colour, which are not necessarily related to therapeutic value. This applies to such important drugs as senna leaflets, senna pods, chamomile flowers, ginger, nutmegs and rhubarb.

Foreign matter

The difficulty of obtaining vegetable drugs in an entirely pure condition is fully recognized, and pharmacopoeias contain statements as to the percentage of other parts of the plant or of other organic matter which may be permitted. Table 16.1 gives examples of various official types of limit applicable to specific drugs. Drugs containing appreciable quantities of potent foreign matter, animal excreta, insects or

mould should, however, be rejected even though the percentage of such substances be insufficient to cause the rejection of the drug on the percentage of foreign matter.

In the case of whole drugs a weighed quantity (100–500 g, according to the type of drug), of a carefully taken sample is spread in a thin layer on paper. It is examined at ×6 magnification and the foreign matter is picked out and weighed and the percentage recorded. Details will be found in the appropriate *BP* Appendix. For foreign organic matter in powdered drugs, see 'Quantitative Microscopy'.

Moisture content

Not only is the purchase of drugs (e.g. aloes, gelatin, gums) which contain excess water, uneconomical, but also in conjunction with a suitable temperature moisture will lead to the activation of enzymes and, given suitable conditions, to the proliferation of living organisms. As most vegetable drugs contain all the essential food requirements for moulds, insects and mites, deterioration can be very rapid once infestation has taken place.

A large number of methods are now available for moisture determination, many being employed in industries unrelated to pharmacy.

Loss on drying.   This is employed in the *BP/EP* and *USP*. Although the loss in weight, in the samples so tested, principally is due to water, small amounts of other volatile materials will also contribute to the weight loss. For materials (digitalis, hamamelis leaf, yarrow, hawthorn berries, starch, aloes, fibres) which contain little volatile material, direct drying (100–105°C) to constant weight can be employed. The moisture balance combines both the drying process and weight recording; it is suitable where large numbers of samples are handled and where a continuous record of loss in weight with time is required. For materials such as balsams which contain a considerable proportion of volatile material, the drying may be accomplished by spreading thin layers of the weighed drug over glass plates and placing in a desiccator over phosphorus pentoxide. Vacuum drying over an absorbent may be utilized, possibly at a specified temperature.

Table 16.1   Examples of BP limits for foreign matter.

Drugs	Foreign matter limits
Leaves and herbs	
Bearberry leaf	≯8% Foreign matter of which ≯5% stems and ≯3% other foreign matter. Leaves of different colour to official description ≯10%
Birch leaf	≯3% Fragments of female catkins, ≯3% other foreign matter
Lemon balm	≯10% Stems having a diameter 1 mm, ≯2% other foreign matter
Wild thyme	≯3% Foreign matter (involves recognition of *Thymus vulgaris* and *T. zygis*)
Wormwood	≯5% Stems with diameter greater than 4 mm, ≯2% other foreign matter
Fruits and seeds	
Hawthorn berries	≯2% Foreign matter, ≯5% deteriorated false fruits
Juniper berries	≯5% Unripe or discoloured cone berries, ≯2% other foreign matter
Psyllium seeds	≯1% Foreign matter including greenish unripe fruits. No seeds of other *Plantago* spp.
Inflorescences	
Calendula flowers	≯5% Bracts, ≯2% other foreign matter
Elder flowers	≯8% Fragments of coarse pedicels and other foreign matter, ≯15% discoloured brown flowers
Lime flowers	≯2% Foreign matter, absence of other *Tilia* spp.
Rhizomes and roots	
Couch grass rhizome	≯15% Greyish-black pieces of rhizome in cut drug
Marshmallow root	≯2% Brown deteriorated root, ≯2% cork in peeled root
Valerian root	≯5% Stem bases, ≯2% other foreign matter
Barks	
Quillaia bark	≯2% Foreign matter
Cascara bark	≯1% Foreign matter

Separation and measurement of moisture. The 'loss on drying' methods can be made more specific for the determination of water by separating and evaluating the water obtained from a sample. This can be achieved by passing a dry inert gas through the heated sample and using an absorption train (specific for water) to collect the water carried forward; such methods can be extremely accurate, as shown in their use for the determination of hydrogen in organic compounds by traditional combustion analysis.

Methods based on distillation have been widely used for moisture determination. The sample to be analysed is placed in a flask together with a suitable water-saturated immiscible solvent (toluene, xylene, carbon tetrachloride) and pieces of porous pot and is distilled. The water in the sample has a considerable partial pressure and co-distils with the solvent, condensing in the distillate as an immiscible layer. A simple apparatus (Fig. 16.1A) originally devised by Dean and Stark permits the direct measurement of the water obtained and the less dense solvent (toluene, xylene) is continuously returned to the distillation flask. The method is employed in the *USP* and in the *BP/EP* for some volatile oil-containing drugs (Roman chamomile flowers, lovage root, eucalyptus, peppermint and sage leaves) and aniseed and star-anise fruits. To accommodate the loss of water due to solubility in the solvent the *BP* specifies a preliminary distillation of the solvent with added water (about 2 ml); the exact volume of water separating as a layer is read off and then the drug (sufficient to give a further 2–3 ml water) added to the flask and distillation resumed. Water separated from the drug is calculated from the combined final volume. Heavier-than-water solvents require the receiver shown in Fig. 16.1B. The method is readily applicable to crude drugs and food materials but has the disadvantage that relatively large quantities of the sample (5–10 g) may be required.

Gas-chromatographic methods have become increasingly important for moisture determination because of their specificity and efficiency. The water in the weighed, powdered sample can be extracted with dry methanol and an aliquot submitted to chromatography on a column on either 10% carbowax on Fluoropak 80 or Porapak, a commercial polymer suitable for gas–liquid chromatography (GLC). The water separated by this means is readily determined from the resulting chromatogram. Teflon-6 coated with 10% polyethylene glycol 1500, with *n*-propanol as an internal standard has also been employed for the determination of moisture in crude drugs.

Chemical methods. The most extensively employed chemical method for water determination is probably the Karl Fischer procedure, which finds use not only in the pharmaceutical, but also in the food, chemical and petrochemical industries. It is used in the *BP* and is particularly applicable for expensive drugs and chemicals containing small quantities of moisture [very small quantities of water (10 μg to 10 mg) are determined quantitatively by coulometric titration, see below]. Dry extracts of alkaloid-containing drugs, alginic acid, alginates and fixed oils (e.g. arachis, castor, olive and sesame oils for *BP* parenteral use) may usefully be evaluated. For crude drugs such as digitalis and ipecacuanha the powdered material can first be exhausted of water with a suitable anhydrous solvent (dioxan) and an aliquot taken for titration.

The Karl Fischer reagent consists of a solution of iodine, sulphur dioxide and pyridine in dry methanol. This is titrated against a sample containing water, which causes a loss of the dark brown colour. At the end-point when no water is available, the colour of the reagent persists. The basic reaction is a reduction of iodine by sulphur dioxide in the presence of water. The reaction goes to completion by the removal of sulphur trioxide as pyridine sulphur trioxide, which in turns reacts with the methanol to form the pyridine salt of methyl sulphate, see formulae below.

$$H_2O + I_2 + SO_2 \rightleftharpoons 2HI + SO_3$$

In the absence of methanol, the pyridine sulphur trioxide reacts with another molecule of water. The reagent requires standardization immediately before use and this can be done by employment of a standard solution of water in methanol or by use of a hydrated salt—for example, sodium tartrate ($Na_2C_4H_4O_6 \cdot 2H_2O$). To eliminate interference from atmospheric moisture, the titration is carried out under an atmosphere

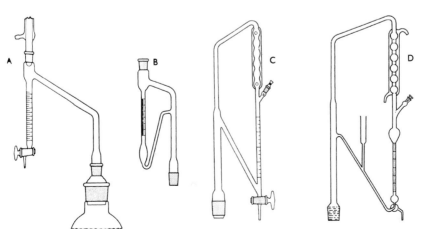

Fig. 16.1
A, Apparatus for the determination of moisture in crude drugs by distillation and for volatile oils heavier than water; B, receiver of apparatus for the determination of water in crude drugs (heavy entrainment) and for volatile oils in drugs; C, receiver for determination of volatile oil in drugs as used by the *BP* 1980; D, receiver for determination of volatile oil in drugs as used by both the *EP* and the *BP*.

of dry nitrogen, the end-point being recorded amperometrically. Equipment is now available for a completely automated determination, thus eliminating the manual aspects of sample handling and weighing, introduction to the Karl Fischer cell, titration and data completion. Although the *BP* Karl Fischer reagent contains pyridine, as above, the latter has been replaced by other bases (e.g. imidazoles) in some commercial reagents. Alternatives to methanol, such as diethylene glycol monoethyl ether, have been introduced to improve reagent stability.

The principal drawbacks of the Karl Fischer method are the instability of the reagent and the possibility of substances in the sample, other than water, which may react with the reagent.

The coulometric method for the quantitative determination of water relies on the same basic reactions as indicated above for the Karl Fischer procedure. However, the iodine is produced electrochemically at the anode by oxidation of iodide and reacts immediately with the sulphur dioxide and water from the sample. When all the water is used up, iodine is produced in excess and this is the electrochemical end-point. If necessary, moisture in a solid sample can be evaporated and passed into the reaction vessel in a stream of dry inert gas. The method is employed for the measurement of the very small amounts of water permissible in fixed oils used for the preparation of parenteral dosage forms; examples include a maximum of 0.1% for soya, olive and evening primrose oils.

Other chemical methods for water determination include treating the sample with various carbides, nitrides and hydrides and measuring the gas evolved; gas chromatography has been employed for the analysis of the liberated gas.

Spectroscopic methods. Water will absorb energy at various wavelengths throughout the electromagnetic spectrum and this fact can be made a basis for its quantitative determination (see later in this chapter for a general discussion on spectroscopy). Measurements can be made in both the infrared and ultraviolet regions; interfering substances must be absent. The method is particularly suitable for very small quantities of water (e.g. trace quantities in gases). Nuclear magnetic resonance (NMR) spectroscopy has been employed for the determination of moisture in starch, cotton and other plant products.

Electrometric methods. Conductivity and dielectric methods have both been utilized for moisture determination but have not, as yet, found extensive application to pharmaceutical products.

Extractive values

The determination of water-soluble or ethanol-soluble extractive is used as a means of evaluating drugs the constituents of which are not readily estimated by other means. But as suitable assays become available (e.g. with the anthraquinone-containing drugs), some of the previously used extractive tests are no longer required as pharmacopoeial standards. In certain cases extraction of the drug is by maceration, in others by a continuous extraction process. For the latter the Soxhlet extractor is particularly useful and has been in use for many years, not only for the determination of extractives (e.g. fixed oil in seeds) but also for small-scale isolations (Fig. 16.2). A development of the Soxhlet technique is also shown in Fig. 16.2; in this apparatus extraction is by boiling solvent followed by percolation; finally, evaporation yields the extract and the recovered solvent ready for the next sample. Some examples of the types of extractive used are given in Table 16.2.

Ash values

When vegetable drugs are incinerated, they leave an inorganic ash which in the case of many drugs (e.g. rhubarb) varies within fairly wide limits and is therefore of little value for purposes of evaluation. In other cases (e.g. peeled and unpeeled liquorice) the *total ash* figure is of importance and indicates to some extent the amount of care taken in the preparation of the drug. In the determination of total ash values the carbon must be removed at as low a temperature (450°C) as possible without producing flames. If carbon is still present after heating at a moderate temperature, the water-soluble ash may be separated and the residue again ignited as described in the *BP*, or the ash may be broken

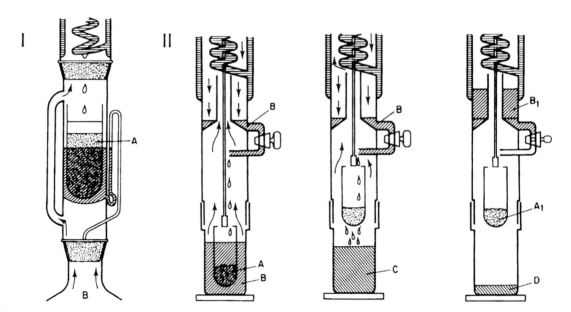

Fig. 16.2
I, Soxhlet continuous extraction apparatus. A, powdered drug for extraction in thimble and plugged with suitable fibre e.g. defatted tow or cotton wool; solvent refluxes into thimble and syphons into flask B, containing boiling solvent, when receiver is full. II, Three-stage continuous extraction and solvent recovery: left, extraction by boiling with solvent; centre, percolation stage; right, removal of solvent. A, sample for extraction; A₁, exhausted drug; B, solvent; B₁, recovered solvent; C, solvent containing soluble plant constituents; D, final extract. (Soxtec System, Tecator Ltd.)

Table 16.2 Extractives employed for drug evaluation.

Drug	Method of evaluation
Gentian, liquorice, many drugs of *BHP*	Percentage of water-soluble extractive
Quillaia	Percentage of ethanol (45%) extractive
Valerian, cocillana, asafoetida	Percentage of ethanol (60%) extractive
Ginseng, hop strobiole	Percentage of ethanol (70%) extractive
Ginger, ipomoea and jalap	Percentage of ethanol (90%) extractive
Benzoin, catechu and Tolu balsam, myrrh	Limits of ethanol-insoluble matter
Colocynth	Limit of light petroleum extractive
Crushed linseed	Percentage of ether-soluble extractive

up, with the addition of alcohol, and again ignited. The total ash usually consists mainly of carbonates, phosphates, silicates and silica.

To produce a more consistent ash, the *Pharmacopoeia* utilizes a *sulphated ash*, which involves treatment of the drug with sulphuric acid before ignition, whereby all oxides and carbonates are converted to sulphates. Two methods are given. The first, employed unless otherwise directed, involves moistening a weighed quantity of the drug with (concentrated) sulphuric acid followed by gentle ignition and then repeating the moistening of the charred drug with subsequent firing at 800°C. The ignition is repeated until a constant weight of ash is achieved. The second method utilizes sulphuric acid R for moistening the drug, followed by gentle heating until the drug is charred; after cooling, a second 1 ml of sulphuric acid R is added and the ignition is continued at 600°C ± 50°C until complete incineration is achieved. If the residue exceeds the prescribed limit the process is repeated until a constant weight (within 0.5 mg) is obtained or until the residue complies with the prescribed limit.

If the total ash be treated with dilute hydrochloric acid, the percentage of *acid-insoluble ash* may be determined. This usually consists mainly of silica, and a high acid-insoluble ash in drugs such as senna, cloves, liquorice, valerian and tragacanth indicates contamination with earthy material. Senna leaf, which may be used directly as the powdered drug, is required to have a low acid-insoluble ash (2.5%); hyoscyamus, however, which unavoidably attracts grit on to its sticky trichomes, is allowed a higher value (12%). Horsetail *BP/EP*, the dried sterile stems of *Equisetum arvense*, has a natural content of silica and the acid-insoluble ash value should lie within the limits 10–15%. In the case of ginger a minimum percentage of *water-soluble ash* is demanded, this being designed to detect the presence of exhausted ginger.

Crude fibre

The preparation of a crude fibre is a means of concentrating the more resistant cellular material of drugs for microscopical examination. It is particularly useful for rhizomes such as ginger which contain relatively large amounts of oleoresin and starch. The technique involves defatting the powder and boiling in turn with standard acid and alkali with suitable washing of the insoluble residue obtained at the different stages (see Chapter 43). The crude fibre so obtained can also be employed quantitatively to assay the fibre content of foods and animal feedstuffs and also to detect excess of certain materials in powdered drugs, e.g. clove stalk in clove. For further details see the 14th edition of this book.

Determination of volatile oil

Minimum standards for the percentage of volatile oil present in a number of drugs are prescribed by many pharmacopoeias. A distillation method is usually employed, and the apparatus first described by Meek and Salvin in 1937 is still widely used in laboratories; the receiver for this apparatus is very similar to that for water estimation by heavy entrainment (Fig. 16.1B). The weighed drug is placed in a distillation flask with water or a mixture of water and glycerin and connected to the receiver (cleaned with chromic acid), which is filled with water and connected to a condenser. On distillation, the oil and water condense and the volatile oil which collects in the graduated receiver as a layer on top of the water is measured. For oils with relative densities around or greater than 1.00, separation from the water is assisted by placing a known volume of xylene in the receiver and reading off the combined oil and xylene. Alternatively, for oils with relative densities greater than water (e.g. clove oil, 1.05), a receiver similar to the type shown in Fig. 16.1A can be used and no xylene is necessary. The *BP* 1980 employed the apparatus illustrated in Fig. 16.1C; it differs from the above in that the distillate passes through the condenser and so is cooler than with the reflux type. The *BP* (2007) employs an apparatus similar to that shown in Fig. 16.1D. The time taken to complete the distillation of the oil varies with the nature of the drug and its state of comminution but about 4 h is usually sufficient. Solution of the volatile oil in a fixed oil (e.g. in powdered fruits of the Umbelliferae) may retard distillation. Note that the pharmacopoeial standards for volatile oil contents of powdered drugs are lower than those for the corresponding whole drugs.

Tannin content

A number of drugs (Agrimony, Alchemilla, Hamamelis, Loosestrife, Oak bark, Rhatany, Tormentil) are assayed for their tannin contents (*BP* 2007). The method refers to those polyphenols adsorbed by hide powder and giving a colour reaction with sodium phosphomolybdotungstate reagent. See individual drugs.

Bitterness value

This standard is relevant to Bogbean leaf, Centaury, Gentian and Wormwood of the *BP*. These drugs are used for their bitter effect and specific directions for the determination of the standard are given under each monograph. The bitterness value is determined organoleptically by comparison with a quinine hydrochloride solution which acts as the standard.

Swelling index

This is defined in the *BP* as the volume in millilitres occupied by 1 g of a drug, including any adhering mucilage, after it has swollen in an aqueous liquid for 4 h. The drug is treated with 1.0 ml ethanol (96%) and 25 ml water in a graduated cylinder, shaken every 10 min for 1 h and allowed to stand as specified. In some instances, as with linseed and psyllium seed where the mucilage is in a layer near the surface of the drug, the standard can be determined on the whole drug; in other cases such as marshmallow root where the mucilage is distributed throughout the tissues, the powdered drug is used. Examples are: Agar ≮10, Cetraria ≮4.5, Fenugreek ≮6, Fucus ≮6.0, Ispaghula husk ≮40 (determined on 0.1 g powder), Ispaghula seed ≮9, Linseed ≮4 (whole drug) and ≮4.5 (powdered drug), Marshmallow root ≮10, Psyllium ≮10.0.

Some variations in the method of determination have given rise to other terminology. Thus Skyrme and Wallis in their original work on seeds of *Plantago* spp. in 1936 used the term *swelling factor* (24-h standing period) and the *BP* (1993) cites *swelling power* in respect of

Ispaghula husk (variation in shaking procedure and standing time). Yet again, for Iceland moss the *BP 2007* cites *swelling value, ≮4.5.*

R_F values

Pharmacopoeias are increasingly employing thin-layer chromatography as a means for assessing quality and purity. For a discussion of chromatographic analysis, see Chapter 17. It suffices to mention here that the R_F value (rate of flow, i.e., distance moved by solute divided by distance moved by solvent front) of a compound, determined under specific conditions, is characteristic and can be used as an aid to identity. R_F values vary from 0.0 to 1.00; the hR_F ($R_F \times 100$) values are in the range 0–100. Quantitative extracts of crude drugs are prepared and compared chromatographically with standard reference solutions of the known constituents. Intensities of the visualized chromatographic spots can be visually compared and the method can be used to eliminate inferior or adulterated drugs. In this way semiquantitative tests for the principles of drugs (peppermint, saffron, German chamomile, digitalis) not rapidly evaluated by other means have been developed.

In an analogous manner, gas chromatographic retention times and peak areas can be employed for the examination of volatile oils and other mixtures.

Microbial contamination

The *BP* requires a number of drugs (e.g. acacia, agar, pregelatinized starch, sterculia, tragacanth, powdered digitalis etc.) to be free of *Escherichia coli* in the quantity of material stated; others (e.g. alginic acid, cochineal, guar, tragacanth) are also tested for the absence of *Salmonella*. Upper limits for total viable aerobic count, commonly 10^3, 10^4 microorganisms g^{-1}, are being increasingly applied to crude drugs including the gums, Agar, Tragacanth, Acacia, Guar and Guar Galactomannan. Xanthan gum (q.v.) produced by fermentation has limits of 10^3 for bacteria and 10^2 for fungi, g^{-1}. Generally, manufacturers will ensure that, for crude drugs to be taken internally, the limits for bacterial and mould contamination as applied to foodstuffs are adhered to.

In an investigation by Lutomski and Kedzia (*Planta Med.*, 1980, **40**, 212) of mould contamination of crude drugs, 246 samples were examined and 24% were contaminated at the level of 10 000 organisms g^{-1}. From 50 crude drugs, 75 *Aspergillus* and 28 *Penicillium* strains were isolated; other common genera were *Mucor, Rhizopus* and *Thamnidium*. There was no evidence to show that moulds were producing strongly toxic substances in the crude drug and herbal preparations, in contrast to the embryotoxic, teratogenic, mutagenic and carcinogenic substances produced by some species of the above in peanuts, corn, wheat and rice (see Chapter 39). However, in a series of papers Roy and colleagues (*Int. J. Crude Drug Res.*, 1990, **28**, 157; *Int. J. Pharmacognosy*, 1991, **29**, 197 and references cited therein) have shown that roots (e.g. *Acorus calamus, Picrorrhiza kurroa*) and seeds (Neem and *Datura*) stored under traditional storage conditions in India develop unacceptable levels of mycotoxins, principally aflatoxin B₁; the effects of temperature, relative humidity and light on the elaboration of aflatoxin B₁ have also been studied. By the use of mass spectrometry, mycotoxins in food products such as cereals, oil seeds and milk are regularly determined at levels of one part per billion and below.

For a review on the microbial contamination of medicinal plants, see W. Kneifel *et al.*, *Planta Medica*, 2002, **68**, 5.

Toxic residues

These may arise in crude drugs as a result of pesticide application during cultivation of the drug and at a later stage from fumigation of the stored product. The problems and the nature of the toxic residues are essentially those encountered in the food industry and in a number of countries regulations exist to cover limits of these residues in foods, cosmetics, drugs and spices. Appendix XI L of the *BP* 2007 gives the requirements relating to pesticide residues for herbal drugs; specific directions for the sampling of bulk materials are given and the various insecticides and their assays listed. In certain instances it may be necessary to test for aflatoxins and radioactive impurities. It has been reported that many spices, chamomile and valerian obtained commercially contain pesticide residues, but mainly within acceptable levels.

Thin-layer chromatography (TLC) and gas chromatographic methods are available for the determination of organochlorine and urea derivatives, enzymatic methods for organophosphorus compounds, colorimetric methods for urea derivatives, and spectroscopic techniques for paraquat, triazines and heavy metals.

Toxic residues may be substantially reduced or eliminated by the use of infusions of the dried plant material and by the extraction of the useful plant constituents. Storage at 30°C has been shown to reduce rapidly the ethylene oxide residues in senna pods to tolerable levels. Much research has been devoted to the harmful effects of ethylene oxide which is a very effective insecticide and acaricide; for an in-depth report see Golberg (1986), *Hazard Assessment of Ethylene Oxide*, Boca Raton, FL., USA: CRC Press.

Heavy metal accumulation

Herbal drugs, like foods, should comply with the WHO guidelines, and the Pharmacopoeial monograph 'Herbal Drugs', with respect to heavy metal content. Small quantities of trace elements are invariably present in plant materials and, indeed, some, such as zinc, copper and molybdenum, appear to be necessary microcomponents of a normal diet. However, under certain circumstances the levels of some metals, particularly those of lead, cadmium, copper and mercury, can increase to unacceptable concentrations. This may arise either by the deliberate inclusion of, for example, mercury compounds in a particular herbal formulation or by the natural accumulation of heavy metals in herbs growing under particular environmental conditions. Mercury was once accepted as a common ingredient of Western medicines (see the *BPC* of 1949) and, more recently, has appeared in Asian medicines exported world-wide to immigrant communities. In the second instance, increased levels of heavy metals can arise from the nature of the soil and via atmospheric pollution. It is of interest to note that one method of prospecting for metals has involved the analysis of the above-ground flora of the area involved; in this respect, some plants are more prone to metal accumulation than others.

The published work on this aspect of herbal drugs is somewhat limited. For recent studies readers are referred to research by V. Rai *et al.* (*Pharm. Biol.*, 2001, **39**, 384) on the accumulation of lead, cadmium, copper and zinc in nine important drugs of Indian medicine. Samples were obtained from various localities in India and consisted of both authenticated material as well as market samples. In most cases, the concentrations of lead and cadmium exceeded the permissible WHO limits; concentrations varied in the same plant obtained from different localities and the authors attributed this to the industrial activity of the region and possible vehicular pollution.

Limitations for particular metals are placed on some products that have been chemically manipulated, for example, nickel in hydrogenated soya and arachis oils. There are pharmacopoeial limits for iron, chromium and zinc in gelatin, cadmium in linseed oil and iron in pilocarpine salts. Determination is by atomic adsorption spectroscopy after acid digestion of the sample with concentrated nitric, hydrochloric and sulphuric acids. Adsorption is measured at the following wavelengths: Cd 228.8 nm, Cu 324.8 nm, Fe 248.3 nm, Ni 232 nm, Pb 283.5 nm and Zn 213.9 nm; separate techniques are given for As 193.7 nm and Hg 253.7 nm.

Test for aristolochic acids

This test is included in the *Pharmacopoeia* primarily to detect the presence of these acids in unlicensed herbal medicines. They are present in various species of *Aristolochia* and *Asarum*, which may be used either as substitutes or adulterants in certain traditional Chinese medicines. Because of the nephrotoxic and carcinogenic properties of aristolochic acid, the use of *Aristolochia* has been prohibited in the UK since 1991, see 'Serpentary'; with a further statutory prohibitive order in 2001. Other regulatory orders are in force world-wide. In spite of this, such products periodically appear on the market, a recent example being the availability of Xie Gan Wan pills in South Wales (see MHRA warning, *Pharm. J.*, 2007, **279**, 224).

For the pharmacopoeial test, the sample is shaken with 0.1 M sodium hydroxide for at least 2 hours and the filtered solution purified using a solid-phase extraction column. It is then subjected to liquid chromatography and the eluate monitored at 225 nm. No peaks due to aristolochic acid I and arictolochic acid II should appear, as evidenced by comparison with the chromatogram of a reference solution of these two acids.

STANDARDS APPLICABLE TO VOLATILE AND FIXED OILS

Certain standards are particularly appropriate to volatile oils and fixed oils.

Refractive index

The refractive index of a substance is the ratio between the velocity of light in air and the velocity in the substance under test. For light of a given wavelength (it is usual to employ the D line of sodium, which has a doublet of lines at 589.0 nm and 589.6 nm), the refractive index of a material is given by the sine of the angle of incidence divided by the sine of the angle of refraction. The refractive index varies with the temperature, and pharmacopoeial determinations are made at 20°C.

A convenient instrument is the Abbé refractometer, in which the angle measured is the 'critical angle' for total reflection between glass of high refractive index and the substance to be examined. By this means, and by selecting a particular wavelength of light at which to make the measurements, it is possible to calibrate the instrument directly in terms of refractive index. It is the emergent beam that is viewed in the instrument, and the critical angle is indicated by the edge of the dark part of the field of view. In this instrument the need for a monochromatic light source is eliminated by the inclusion of a dispersion 'compensator' placed at the base of the telescope tube of the refractometer. This consists of two direct-vision prisms made accurately direct for the D sodium line; the prisms can be made to rotate in opposite directions. The system of variable dispersion which these prisms form can be made to counterbalance the resultant dispersion of the refractometer prism and the material being examined. The temperature of the sample is adjusted by a water jacket.

Automatic refractometers such as the Leica Auto Abbé refractometer are now available. Advantages over the traditional 'visual' transmitted light instruments are: (1) they measure refractive index with precision to the fifth decimal place, compared with four decimal places for the visual refractometer (however, current pharmacopoeias require only three decimal places in standards for volatile oils); (2) a reflected light principle is employed meaning that light is not transmitted through the sample and hence problems with dark or coloured samples are avoided; (3) the shadow-line location is determined by the instrument software, eliminating variations in readings caused by individual subjective interpretations of the placement of the shadowline border on a crosswire; (4) no mechanical components are involved, thus reducing wear with time. However, if the increased sensitivity of such instruments is to be fully utilized then additional care and consideration must be given to the measurement of temperature and to the correction for effect of temperature on refractive index.

Measurements of refractive index are particularly valuable for purity assessments of volatile and fixed oils, and many values can be found in the *EP*, *BP*, *BPC* and other pharmacopoeias. Oils of cassia, cinnamon and cinnamon leaf have refractive indices of about 1.61, 1.573–1.600 and about 1.53, respectively, making possible the differentiation of the oils. The refractive index of lemon oil is 1.474–1.476 and that for terpeneless lemon oil 1.475–1.485.

Optical rotation

The optical rotation of a liquid is the angle through which the plane of polarization of light is rotated when the polarized light is passed through a sample of the liquid; this rotation may be either clockwise or anticlockwise. Along with the fundamental effects of the molecules of liquid under investigation, the observed rotation is dependent on the thickness of the layer examined, its temperature and the nature of the light employed. The *BP* uses the D-line of sodium (λ = 589.3 nm), a layer 1 dm thick and a temperature of 20°C. With 'half-shadow' or 'triple-shadow' polarimeters in which the two or three fields are viewed simultaneously and matched to the same intensity, rotations can be measured with an accuracy of at least ± 0.01 degree.

Most volatile oils contain optically active components and the direction of the rotation, and its magnitude, is a useful criterion of purity. Examples to illustrate the range of values found are caraway oil, +74° to +80°; lemon oil, +57° to +70°; terpeneless lemon oil, −5° to +2°; cinnamon oil, 0° to −2°; citronella oil, Java, −5° to +2°; citronella oil, Ceylon, −9° to −18°; nutmeg oil, +8° to +18°; peppermint oil, −10° to −30°; spearmint oil, −45° to −60°.

Many solid materials of natural origin are optically active and the rotation of their solutions (water, ethanol and chloroform are common solvents) can be measured in a similar way to the above. The specific rotation of the solid is given by

$$\frac{\text{Angular rotation per dm of solution}}{\text{Grams of optically active substance per ml of solution}}$$

$$= \frac{100\alpha}{lc} = \frac{100\alpha}{ldp}$$

where α is the observed rotation in degrees, l is the length of the observed layer in dm, c is the number of grams of substance contained in 100 ml solution, d is the density and p is the number of grams of substance contained in 100 g of solution. The record of the specific rotation of a compound should include the solvent used and the concentration, in addition to the type of light employed (sodium D line of 589.3 nm or mercury green line of 546.1 nm)—for example, $[\alpha]_D^{20°}$ (2.0% in ethanol) = −15°.

For examples of the use of specific rotation as a physical constant, students can consult the *BP* or other pharmacopoeial monographs on alkaloidal salts.

The visual polarimeter requires the use of solutions which are not highly coloured or to any extent opaque, and sometimes, with plant extracts, such solutions are difficult to obtain. Because angular rotation falls off linearly, whereas absorption does so exponentially with decrease in path length, the use of short sample tubes has an obvious advantage if it is possible to measure accurately the correspondingly small rotations. Automatic polarimeters employ a sample tube about 1/10th the length of that required by a visual polarimeter. Measurement of small rotations is made possible by utilization of the Faraday electro-optic effect; this involves the rotation of the plane of a polarized beam of light in a magnetic field, the degree of rotation being proportional to the field strength. The instrument is zeroed by means of two solenoids through which passes the polarized beam. The insertion of an optically active solution between the solenoids affords a recordable signal, either (−) or (+), which is generated by a photomultiplier at the end of the light path.

Chiral purity

Optical rotation as described above arises within molecules having at least one asymmetric carbon atom. Such molecules have two possible configurations (enantiomers), which are non-superimposable mirror images of one another and exhibit opposite light-rotational properties [(−) and (+)]. Plants synthesize just one enantiomer, which, under certain conditions, may partially change to the opposite isomer. Equal quantities of both are known as racemic mixtures and have zero rotation; thus, for the alkaloid hyoscyamine, $[\alpha]_D$ in 50% ethanol = −22° and its racemate atropine is optically inactive. Synthetically produced compounds are normally racemates. The relatively recent introduction of chiral chromatography has provided a method for the quantitative separation of enantiomers and has found use as a standard for volatile oils, which are susceptible to adulteration with the synthetic product. The *Pharmacopoeia* uses chiral gas chromatography employing fused silica columns 30 m in length with a stationary phase of modified β-cyclodextrine. Chiral purity tests are specified for the volatile oils of caraway, neroli and lavender, and also for carvone.

Quantitative chemical tests

A number of quantitative chemical tests—acid value, iodine value, saponification value, ester value, unsaponifiable matter, peroxide value, anisidine value, acetyl value, volatile acidity—are mainly applicable to fixed oils and are mentioned in Chapter 19. Some of these tests are also useful in the evaluation of resins (acid value, sulphated ash), balsams (acid value, ester value, saponification value), volatile oils (acid value, acetyl value, peroxide value, ester value) and gums (methoxyl determination, volatile acidity).

ASSAYS

A crude drug may be assayed for a particular group of constituents—for example, the total alkaloids in belladonna or the total glycosides of digitalis. Alternatively, it may be necessary to evaluate specific components—for example, the reserpine content, as distinct from the total alkaloid content, of *Rauwolfia* spp. Biological assays, which can be time-consuming, were at one time employed for the assay of those potent drugs (e.g. digitalis) for which no other satisfactory assay was available. In pharmacopoeias these have now been largely replaced by chemical and physical assays for routine standardization. However, the biological assay remains important for screening plant materials and their fractionated extracts in the search for new drugs. In this respect there is a role for simple biological assays (e.g. brine shrimp toxicity) which can be carried out by the phytochemist without the specialist procedures used by pharmacologists. Some types of assay commonly employed are given in Table 16.3. Often a preliminary purification or fractionation of the active constituents of the drug is required and for this chromatography is finding increasing use. Examples of chromatographic systems employed are listed in Table 16.4 and are more fully explained in Chapter 17. Spectrometric methods, particularly in conjunction with chromatography, are finding increasing use and are dealt with more fully below.

Spectroscopic analysis

The electromagnetic vibrations utilized in spectroscopic analysis can be roughly divided, according to wavelength, into the ultraviolet (100–400 nm), the visible (400–800 nm), the near-infrared (800–3000 nm) and the infrared (3–40 μm) regions. The ultraviolet region can be subdivided into three further categories—UVC (100–290 nm), UVB (290–320 nm) and UVA (320–400 nm). These are often quoted in connection with sunlight—all UVC is absorbed by the ozone layer of the atmosphere, UVB is present in small amount but is primarily responsible for major skin damage and UVA, although the major component, is far less damaging. In spectroscopic analysis we are concerned with the capacity of certain molecules to absorb vibrations

Table 16.3 Types of assay employed for crude drugs.

Types of assay	Examples
Separation and weighing of active constituents	Colchicine in colchicum corm and seed. Resins of podophyllum and of the Convolvulaceae. Crude filicin in male fern. Total balsamic esters of Peru balsam
Chemical	'Total alkaloids' of many drugs (e.g. acid–base titrations). Non-aqueous titrations of alkaloid salts. Strychnine in nux vomica. Morphine in opium. Cinnamic aldehyde in oil of cinnamon. Free alcohols in peppermint oil. Carvone in oil of caraway. Assay of fumitory
Physical	Cineole in eucalyptus oil (f.p. of o-cresol complex)
Spectrometric, including colorimetric and fluorescence	Most groups of active constituents
Biological	Cardioactive drugs, antibiotics, vitamins, taenicides, anthraquinone derivatives, mydriatic drugs, saponins, antitumour drugs, antiamoebic drugs, ginkgolides (anti-PAF activity)
Radioimmunoassay (RIA)	Hesperidin, limonin and naringin (*Citrus*), cardenolides (*Digitalis lanata*), loganin (plant cell cultures), sennosides (*Cassia angustifolia*), tropane alkaloids (medicinal Solanaceae), morphine and related alkaloids (poppy capsules), lysergic acid derivatives (ergot), quinine (cultured plant tissues), ajmaline (*Rauwolfia* spp.), vincristine and related alkaloids (*Catharanthus roseus*), solasodine (*Solanum* spp.)
Enzyme-immunoassay (ELISA)	Quassin, neoquassin, 18-hydroxyquassin (*Quassia* and *Picrasma* spp.), podophyllotoxin, tropane alkaloids (Solanaceae), artemisinin in *Artemisia annua*, pyrrolizidine alkaloids, ergot alkaloids, galanthamine in *Leucojum aestivum*, saikosaponina in *Bupleurum*, ginsenosides

Table 16.4 Chromatographic systems employed in the analysis of drugs.

Type	Employment
Liquid chromatography; *BP* uses stainless steel columns of varying size; typical packing is chromatographic octadecylsilyl silica gel	Arnica flower, Cola, Devil's claw, Garlic, Goldenseal root, Opium, Papaveretum, triglycerides of fixed oils (e.g. Refined sesame oil)
Gas chromatography	Volatile oils; *BP* gives chromatographic profiles for some drugs e.g. to aid distinction between Aniseed oil from star-anise and that from *Pimpinella anisum*. Separation of fatty acids derived from fixed oils. Fatty acid content of fruits, e.g. Saw Palmetto Fruit
Thin-layer chromatography	Extensively used in *BP* and *BHP* as an identification test and test for purity. Separated constituents can be removed from chromatogram and determined spectrometrically

at specific wavelengths. Thus, the butenolide side-chain of cardiac glycosides is responsible for a strong absorption at 215–220 nm, the conjugated double bonds of lycopene (a pigment of tomatoes and other fruits) give rise to the absorption of light at a wavelength of 470 nm, thus giving a red colour, and the carbonyl group of ketones, carboxylic acids and esters is responsible for a strong absorption in the infrared at about 5.7–6.1 µm. In the ultraviolet and visible regions the characteristic absorption spectrum of a molecule is produced by changes in the electronic energy levels associated with various chromophoric groups within the molecule. These changes involve the absorption of relatively high amounts of energy (in precise quanta), and they are also accompanied by changes in vibrational and rotational energy changes within the molecule. The result is a banded absorption spectrum showing no sharply defined peaks. By comparison, the absorption spectrum of a molecule in the infrared region is much more complex, because here the energies involved are too small to bring about electronic transitions but large enough to produce numerous vibrational and associated rotational energy changes. Each of these changes is associated with a characteristic wavelength and the spectrum shows a much finer structure than in the visible or ultraviolet regions. The infrared spectrum of a molecule can be divided into the 'fingerprint' region (7–11 µm), which is characteristic of the molecule under examination but in which it is difficult to assign peaks to specific vibrations, and the remainder of the spectrum, in which many functional groups can be recognized. The *BP* employs the comparison of infrared spectra of phytochemicals (pilocarpine, physostigmine, etc.) with *European Pharmacopoeia Chemical Reference Substances* (EPCRS) as a test of identity.

The *BP* uses ultraviolet absorption characteristics as standards for benzylpenicillin, lanatoside C and a number of alkaloids—for example, morphine, reserpine, cocaine, colchicine and tubocuraine chloride.

If light of a particular wavelength is passed through a solution of a substance, the transmission $T = I/I_0$, where I_0 is a measure of the light reaching the detector (a photoelectric cell) when solvent alone is used in the light-path and I is the light reaching the detector when a solution of the substance under investigation is examined. T is measured in experiments but the most useful value is $\log_{10}(I_0/I)$, the decimal optical density or simply the optical density (E). The optical density, but not the transmission, is proportional to the number of absorbing units in the light-path. For solutions this is Beer's law. The absorption spectrum of a pure substance under defined conditions of solvent and temperature is a set of values of E observed at different wavelengths in a solution of unit concentration (1 mol l^{-1}) when the thickness of the layer traversed by the light is 1 cm. Alternatively, any other solution of known strength may be used. For example, for a 1% w/v solution with a layer thickness of 1 cm the optical density is indicated by $E_{1cm}^{1\%}$. Such absorption spectra are valuable for the identification, determination of

the structure and purity and analysis of compounds. Some substances will absorb ultraviolet light of a certain wavelength and during the period of excitation re-emit light of a longer wavelength and often in the visible region. This is fluorescence, and the fluorescence spectrum is characteristic for those substances which exhibit the phenomenon. The applications of fluorescence analysis are discussed below.

For the *quantitative evaluation* of a substance, a standard curve is first prepared by measuring the optical densities of a series of standard solutions of the pure compound by use of light of a suitable wavelength, usually that at which the compound gives an absorption maximum. The solutions must be sufficiently dilute to obey Beer's law. The optical density of the solution to be evaluated is then determined and its composition ascertained from the standard curve. Individual components of a mixture can be determined by ultraviolet absorption, provided that the different compounds exhibit different absorption maxima. Thus, for strychnine and brucine the reported $E_{1cm}^{1\%}$ values at the wavelengths (λ) indicated are:

	$E_{1cm}^{1\%}$	
λ	Strychnine	Brucine
262 nm	322	312
300 nm	5.16	216

By measurement of the extinctions of the mixed alkaloid solution at the above wavelengths, a two-point spectrophotometric assay is available for the determination of both alkaloids. This method, official in the *BP* (1980) for the assay of nux vomica seeds and preparations, replaced the older, chemical method. A similar type of assay is employed by the *EP* for quinine-type alkaloids and cinchonine-type alkaloids in cinchona bark; measurements are made at 316 and 348 nm. Occasionally it is useful to examine the ultraviolet spectrum of a more complex mixture; thus, the *USP* includes an ultraviolet absorbance test for the absence of foreign oils in oils of lemon and orange and the *BP* an extinction limit test between 268 and 270 nm for castor oil.

In most cases it is essential that no interfering substances are present during the measurements; these can be particularly troublesome in the ultraviolet region, particularly with materials extracted from thin-layer and paper chromatograms. For this reason, if pure solutions are not available for analysis, some form of colorimetric analysis is often preferable, particularly if the reaction used to produce the colour is highly specific for the compound under consideration.

Colorimetric analyses can be carried out with a suitable spectrophotometer—most instruments which operate in the ultraviolet range also have facilities for work in the visible region—but much simpler colorimeters in which suitable filters are used to select the correct wavelengths of light required are quite satisfactory for most purposes.

In these instruments a simple light-source is used and, between the lamp and the solution to be analysed, a filter is placed which transmits that range of wavelengths absorbed by the compound under test (i.e. a colour complementary to that of the solution under test). The transmitted light is recorded by a photoelectric cell and the composition of the solution determined by reference to a standard curve. The *BP/EP* tests the colouring power of Roselle (*Hibiscus sabdariffa*) by measurement of the absorbance of a water-soluble extract at 520 nm; similarly for an acid extract of Red Poppy Petals at 525 nm.

Characteristic absorption maxima from the more complex infrared spectra can also be utilized in quantitative analysis in the same way as ultraviolet and visible absorptions. Mixtures of substances can also be evaluated; thus, by measurements at 9.80, 9.15 and 9.00 μm it is possible to evaluate separately the 25β- and 25α-epimeric steroidal sapogenins present in plant extracts. A few of the many examples of the application of spectrometric analysis to constituents of drugs are given in Table 16.5.

Table 16.5 Some examples of the application of spectrometric analysis to the constituents of drugs.

Region of spectrum	Constituents	Wavelength for measurement of optical density
Ultraviolet	Alkaloids:	
	Lobeline	249 nm
	Reserpine	268 nm
	Vinblastine	267 nm
	Vincristine	297 nm
	Tubocurarine chloride	280 nm
	Morphine	286 nm
	Colchicine	350 nm
	Cardioactive glycosides with butenolide side-chain	217 nm
	Saponins—glycyrrhizinic acid	250 nm
	Iridoids—harpagoside in Devil's claw	278 nm
	Quassinoids	254 nm
	Cassia oil—aldehyde content	286 nm
	Bergamot oil—bergapten content	313 nm
	Flavaspidic acid from male fern	290 nm
	Capsaicin	248 and 296 nm
	Vanillin	301 nm
	Allicin—garlic	254 nm
	Vitamin A (cod-liver oil)	328 nm
Visible	Alkaloids:	
	Ergot (total alkaloids)	550 nm by the use of *p*-dimethylaminobenzaldehyde reagent; 532 nm by the reaction with vanillin in concentrated hydrochloric acid
	Morphine	442 nm by the nitroso reaction
	Reserpine	390 nm by the treatment of alkaloid with sodium nitrite in dilute acid
	Tropic acid esters of hydroxytropanes	555 nm by treatment of alkaloid with fuming nitric acid followed by evaporation to dryness and addition of methanolic potassium hydroxide solution to an acetone solution of the nitrated residue (Vitali–Morin reaction)
	Anthraquinones	500 nm after treatment with alkali (see 'Senna leaf *BP*' for the determination of sennoside; also aloes (512 nm), cascara and rhubarb (515 nm)); 530 nm for the cochineal colour value
	Capsaicin in capsicum	730 nm after reaction with phosphomolybdic acid and sodium hydroxide solution; 505 nm after treatment with diazobenzene-sulphonic acid in 10% sodium carbonate solution
	Cardioactive glycosides:	
	based on digitoxose-moiety	590 nm by Keller–Kiliani reaction
	based on lactone ring	620 nm by reaction with *m*-dinitrobenzene
	Ouabain	495 nm by reaction with alkaline sodium picrate
	Cyanogenetic glycosides: (cyanide determination)	630 nm by the pyridine-parazolone colour reaction
	Tannins:	
	Rhatany, hamamelis leaf	715 nm using phosphotungstic acid and sodium carbonate solution (see *BP*)
	Procyanidins (as cyanidin chloride) in hawthorn berries	545 nm
	Volatile oils:	
	Menthol from peppermint oil	500–579 nm (green filter) by use of *p*-dimethylaminobenzaldehyde reagent
	Proazulenes (as chamazulene) in yarrow	608 nm measured on the blue oil obtained by distillation

(Continued)

Table 16.5 Some examples of the application of spectrometric analysis to the constituents of drugs. (Cont'd)

Region of spectrum	Constituents	Wavelength for measurement of optical density

Infrared	Flavonoids:
	  Birch leaf, calendula flowers (hyperoside), elder flowers (isoquercitrin)
	Alkaloids:
	  Quinine and strychnine mixtures
	Steroidal sapogenins
	Volatile oils:
	  o-Methoxycinnamaldehyde in cassia oil
	
	Water
		425 nm with aluminium chloride and glacial acetic acid
		
		6.2 and 6.06 μm
		11.11 μm and 10.85 μm; see text
		
		Measurements at 7.18 μm and 7.62 μm to distinguish bark oil from leaf and twig oils
		1.9 μm; fairly specific for water without interference from other –OH groups

Fluorescence analysis

Many substances—for example, quinine in solution in dilute sulphuric acid—when suitably illuminated, emit light of a different wavelength or colour from that which falls on them. This emitted light (fluorescence) ceases when the exciting light is removed.

Analytical tests based on fluorescence *in daylight* are not much used, as they are usually unreliable, owing to the weakness of the fluorescent effect. An exception to this is the well-known umbelliferone test, which can be applied to ammoniacum, galbanum and asafoetida. A strongly fluorescent solution of umbelliferone can be prepared by boiling galbanum with acid and filtering into an excess of alcoholic ammonia. Other fluorescent solutions are those of quinine (in dilute acid), aesculin (by infusing horse chestnut bark), chlorophyll (from nettle or parsley leaves), β-naphthol (dissolved in alkali) and aqueous solutions of the dyes eosin and fluorescein.

A very important generalization made by Stokes in 1852 stated that 'in fluorescence the fluorescent light is always of greater wavelength than the exciting light'. Light rich in short wavelengths is very active in producing fluorescence and for this reason strong ultraviolet light (such as can be obtained from a tungsten arc or mercury vapour lamp) produces fluorescence in many substances which do not visibly fluoresce in daylight. Fluorescence lamps are usually fitted with a suitable filter which eliminates visible radiation from the lamp and transmits ultraviolet radiation of the desired wavelength. Convenient long- and short-wave ultraviolet hand lamps are available for chromatographic observations; **it is most important that the eyes are properly protected in the presence of ultraviolet radiation**.

For examination, *solids* may be placed directly under the lamp, whereas *liquids* may be examined in non-fluorescent dishes or test-tubes or after spotting on to filter paper. Many alkaloids in the solid state show distinct colours—for example, aconitine (light blue), berberine (yellow) and emetine (orange). Pieces of cinchona bark when placed under the lamp show a number of luminous yellow patches and a few light blue ones. If the inner surface of the bark is touched with dilute sulphuric acid the spot immediately turns blue. Ipecacuanha root has a brightly luminous appearance wherever the wood is exposed, while the wood of hydrastis rhizome shines golden yellow. Areca nuts when cut show a light blue endosperm. Slices of calumba appear intensely yellow, with the cambium and phloem distinguished by their dark-green colour. Precipitated and prepared chalks may readily be distinguished from one another.

Most *oils, fats* and *waxes* show some fluorescence when examined in filtered ultraviolet light. In general, fixed oils and fats fluoresce least, waxes more strongly, and mineral oils (paraffins) most of all.

Powders may be examined macroscopically as above or microscopically by means of a fluorescence microscope. In connection with powdered drugs may be mentioned the detection of ergot in flour, of cocoa shells in powdered cocoa, and of rumex in powdered gentian. Different varieties of rhubarb may be distinguished from one another. The *BP* 1973 included a fluorescence test on the entire or powdered drug for the detection of rhapontic rhubarb but this is now replaced by a TLC test.

The location of separated compounds on paper and thin-layer chromatograms by the use of ultraviolet light has been extensively employed. With plant extracts it is often worthwhile to examine the chromatogram in ultraviolet light even if the constituents that one is investigating are not themselves fluorescent. In this way the presence of fluorescent impurities may be revealed which, if otherwise undetected, could interfere with a subsequent absorption analysis. Sometimes fluorescence-quenching can be employed to locate non-fluorescent substances on thin-layer chromatograms. For this, an ultraviolet fluorescent background is produced by the incorporation of a small amount of inorganic fluorescent material into the thin layer. The separated substances cause a local quenching of the background fluorescence and they therefore appear as dark spots on a coloured background.

Quantitative fluorescence analysis. This technique utilizes the fluorescence produced by a compound in ultraviolet light for quantitative evaluation. The instrument employed is a fluorimeter and consists of a suitable ultraviolet source and a photoelectric cell to measure the intensity of the emitted fluorescent light. Within certain limits of concentration the intensity of the fluorescence for a given material is related to its concentration. It is usual to select a narrow range of wavelengths for measurement by inserting a filter between the fluorescing solution and the photoelectric cell. The concentration of a substance in solution is obtained by reference to a standard curve prepared by subjecting standard solutions to the fluorimetric procedure. With plant extracts it is important to ascertain that (1) the substance being determined is the only one in the solution producing a fluorescence at the measured wavelength and (2) there are no substances in the solution which absorb light at the wavelength of the fluorescence. Refined instruments are now available in which the fluorescence spectrum is automatically analysed and in which the wavelength of the incident radiation can also be varied.

Quinine can be conveniently assayed by the measurement of the blue fluorescence (366 nm) produced by irradiation of the alkaloid in a dilute sulphuric acid solution at about 450 nm. The method can be used for the assay of quinine in the presence of other alkaloids (e.g. strychnine). Alexandrian senna has been assayed by measurement of the fluorescence produced in the Bornträger reaction under specified conditions. The hydrastine content of hydrastis root may be determined by oxidizing an extract of the drug with nitric acid and measuring the fluorescence of the hydrastinine produced; by this method berberine and canadine, other alkaloids of hydrastis, are excluded from the assay. Emetine and papaverine may be determined fluorimetrically after oxidation with acid permanganate and noscapine after oxidation with persulphate. Fluorimetric methods have also been published for the estimation of the ergot and rauwolfia alkaloids, umbelliferone, aflatoxin and a number of drugs in body fluids.

NMR spectroscopy

Although this technique is usually associated with structure-determinations of organic compounds the use of ^{1}H-NMR spectroscopy has been described for the assay of atropine and hyoscine in extracts of belladonna, hyoscyamus and stramonium. It has also been used for the quantitative determination of strychnine and brucine in *Strychnos nux-vomica*, affording a number of advantages over other methods (M. Frédérich *et al.*, *Planta medica*, 2003, **69**, 1169). Another application has been the classification and correlation of extracts of St John's wort, involving multivariate data analysis and pharmacological activity (G. Ross *et al.*, *Planta medica*, 2004, **70**, 771).

^{13}C-NMR spectroscopy has been used to distinguish the exudates of various resin-producing families and, together with ^{1}H-nmr spectroscopy, to characterize those of *Pinus* (Pinaceae) and of other Coniferae families (Cupressaceae, Araucariaceae and Podocarpaceae) (J. B. Lambert *et al.*, *J. Nat. Prod.*, 2005, **68**, 625; 2007, **70**, 1283).

Immunoassays

Such assays are highly sensitive and usually very specific and have been developed as a powerful analytical tool for the quantitative determination of many compounds in biological fluids.

Radioimmunoassays (RIA). The assay depends on the highly specific reaction of antibodies to certain antigens. There are various modifications of the technique and it is the saturation method that has been developed for phytoanalysis. Usually the relatively small molecules (below MW 1000) constituting the secondary plant metabolites are not involved in such immunoresponses, but when bound covalently to protein carriers, as haptens, they do become immunogenic. (Haptens are molecules which combine with antibodies but do not stimulate their production unless linked to a carrier molecule.) If such a hapten is prepared in the labelled condition (e.g. ^{3}H- or ^{125}I-labelled) with a known specific activity, mixed with an unknown amount of unlabelled hapten and added to a limited amount of antibody in the form of a serum, then there will be competition between the labelled and unlabelled antigen for the restricted number of binding sites available. This results in some bound and some unbound hapten; these can be separated and a determination of the radioactivity in either fraction, with reference to a standard curve, enables the amount of unlabelled antigen to be calculated. The antiserum is raised in suitable animals (e.g. rabbits).

Following the rapid development of RIA procedures in clinical analyses, and largely owing to the work of Weiler, Zenk and colleagues in Germany since 1976, the method has been satisfactorily applied to a range of plant medicinals as illustrated in Table 16.3.

RIA has the advantage that only small amounts of plant material are required; it is usually specific for a single, or small range of metabolites; relatively crude, unprocessed plant extracts can usually be used; and the process can be mechanized. Thus, it is an efficient tool for the screening of large numbers of plants, some 200–800 specimens being assayed in 1 day. For the application of the method to the selection of high-yielding strains of *Digitalis* and *Solanum*, see Chapter 14. With herbarium material, assays can be performed on quantities of sample ranging from 0.5 mg to a few milligrams and in the examination of individual plants, structures as small as anther filaments (e.g. in digitalis) can be accommodated.

Possible disadvantages of the method are the considerable specialized expertise required to set up the assays and the possibility of cross-reactions with components of the plant extract other than those under investigation. Problems arising from the latter need to be ascertained before the assay. The RIA for hyoscine, for example, is highly specific but norhyoscine will react even more strongly; the cross-reaction with 6-hydroxyhyoscyamine is considerably less, and with hyoscyamine, very much less. Similarly, in the assay for solasodine, tomatidine, if present, will cross-react.

Enzyme-linked immunosorbent assays (ELISA). In this method, competition for an immobilized antibody takes place with a modified form of the compound under analysis that has an enzyme bound to it. Release of the compound–enzyme complex from the binding site and determination of the enzyme activity enables the original solution to be quantified.

Examples of applications to medicinal plants are given in Table 16.3. As with RIAs, the method is very sensitive; thus, for the pyrrolizidine alkaloid retronecine it can be measured in the parts per billion range and one sclerotium of ergot is detectable in 20 kg of wheat.

Tandem mass spectroscopy (MS–MS)

In phytochemistry to date, mass spectroscopy is usually associated with the structure elucidation of compounds rather than with their assay. However, by the simultaneous use of two mass spectrometers in series it is possible to determine quantitatively the amount of a particular targeted compound in complex mixtures, plant extracts or even in dried plant material. Plattner and Powell in their report on maytansinoid identification (*J. Nat. Prod.*, 1986, **49**, 475) refer to it as an important analytical tool for 'needle-in-a-haystack' analytical problems. Sensitivity to picograms of targeted compounds can be achieved with high specificity and nearly instantaneous response; for sensitivity it compares with RIA but is much more rapidly performed. The method has been used for the analysis of cocaine in plant materials, pyrrolizidine in *Senecio* and other genera, taxanes from single needles of *Taxus cuspidata*, aflatoxin B_1 in peanut butter, xanthones, steroids and antibiotics. Hoke *et al.* (*J. Nat. Prod.*, 1994, **57**, 277) consider it the best overall method for the determination of taxol, cephalomannine and baccatin in *T. brevifolia* bark and needle extracts. The chemotaxonomy of the Cactaceae has been investigated by this method.

Quantitative microscopy

Powdered drugs or adulterants which contain a constant number, area or length of characteristic particles/mg (e.g. starch grains, epidermis, trichome ribs respectively) can be determined quantitatively by microscopy using lycopodium spores as an indicator diluent. The method, formerly official in the *BP*, is described in Chapter 43.

PART

4 | Phytochemistry

17

General methods associated with the phytochemical investigation of herbal products

Before about 1800 only slow progress was made in phytochemistry. A few compounds such as cane-sugar, starch, camphor and benzoic acid had long been known, as their preparation was extremely simple; also complex mixtures such as fats, fixed oils, volatile oils, tars and resins had been prepared and used, although virtually nothing was known of their composition. The early scientific workers in the phytochemical field failed to appreciate the extreme complexity of the materials they were trying to investigate and almost entirely lacked the techniques necessary for real progress. Many hundreds of plants were burnt to yield ashes and these early investigators were disappointed to find no significant differences between the ashes of poisonous and those of non-poisonous plants. Expression, aqueous extraction and evaporation had long been used for the preparation of sugar from sugar-cane and the French apothecary Nicholas Leméry (1645–1715) extended the use of extraction processes and made use of alcohol as a solvent. Robert Boyle (1627–91) disposed of the ancient theory of Aristotle that matter was composed of four elements, and although he never isolated an alkaloid, he was obviously moving in the right direction when he treated opium with potassium carbonate and alcohol. In 1747 sucrose was isolated from many plants, including sugarbeet, by the German apothecary A. S. Marggraf (1709–80). K. W. Scheele (1742–86) was highly successful in the phytochemical field and isolated citric, gallic, malic, oxalic, tartaric and prussic acids.

In the nineteenth century progress became more rapid. In 1803 narcotine, the first alkaloid, was isolated; morphine, strychnine, emetine and many others followed rapidly. Between 1813 and 1823 Chevreul elucidated the chemical nature of fats and fixed oils. Until well into the middle of the twentieth century the main emphasis in natural-product chemistry remained the isolation and structure determination of a wide variety of compounds. At this point it became apparent that the principal structural types commonly found in plants had been largely elucidated. Indeed, by this time the attention of natural-product chemists was turning to the elucidation of the actual biosynthetic pathways found in the plant. Such studies were made possible by the introduction of new techniques of separation and analysis. This emphasis has continued until today, when most of the major pathways, including stereochemical aspects, have been studied in some depth. Interest has now moved on to plant biochemistry involving enzymatic and DNA studies related to the biosynthesis of natural products. There has also developed a renewed interest in the patterns of occurrence of compounds in plants (comparative phytochemistry).

Not all the chemical compounds elaborated by plants are of equal interest to the pharmacognosist. Until relatively recently the so-called 'active' principles were frequently alkaloids or specific glycosides usually with pronounced pharmacological properties; these therefore received special attention, and in large measure constituted the principal plant drugs of the allopathic system of medicine. It is now realized that many other constituents of plants, particularly those associated with herbal medicine, have medicinal properties which manifest themselves in more subtle and less dramatic ways than the obviously poisonous plants. This has considerably widened the scope of plant metabolites considered worthy of more detailed investigation. Other groups such as carbohydrates, fats and proteins are of dietetic importance, and many such as starches and gums are used in pharmacy but lack any marked pharmacological action. Substances, such as calcium oxalate, silica, lignin and colouring matters, may be of assistance in the identification of drugs and the detection of adulteration.

As a result of the recent interest in the plant kingdom as a potential source of new drugs, strategies for the fractionation of plant extracts based on biological activity rather than on a particular class of compound, have been developed. The chemical examination follows after the isolation of the active fraction.

17

The phytochemical investigation of a plant may thus involve the following: authentication and extraction of the plant material; separation and isolation of the constituents of interest; characterization of the isolated compounds; investigation of the biosynthetic pathways to particular compounds; and quantitative evaluations. Parallel to this may be the pharmacological assessment of the separated components, which may, in some investigations, precede the characterization.

EXTRACTION OF PLANT MATERIAL

All plant material used should be properly authenticated, as much time and money can be wasted on the examination of material of doubtful origin. The choice of extraction procedure depends on the nature of the plant material and the components to be isolated. Dried materials are usually powdered before extraction, whereas fresh plants (leaves, etc.) can be homogenized or macerated with a solvent such as alcohol. The latter is also particularly useful for stabilizing fresh leaves by dropping them into the boiling solvent. Alcohol is a general solvent for many plant constituents (most fixed oils excepted) and as such may give problems in the subsequent elimination of pigments, resins, etc. Water-immiscible solvents are widely used—light petroleum (essential and fixed oils, steroids), ether and chloroform (alkaloids, quinones). The extraction of organic bases (e.g. alkaloids) usually necessitates basification of the plant material if a water-immiscible solvent is to be used; for aromatic acids and phenols acidification may be required. Extraction itself may be performed by repeated maceration with agitation, percolation or by continuous extraction (e.g. in a Soxhlet extractor, Fig. 16.2). Special methods for volatile oils, such as the *enfleurage* process, are considered in Chapter 22. Ultrasound may enhance the extraction process for some plant materials and the *BP* uses this in the preparation of a 50% ethanolic solution of opium for the assay of alkaloids and in the assay procedure of Agnus Castus. Its use has been studied for the extraction of atropine from *Hyoscyamus muticus* using various solvent systems (A. Djilana and B. Legseir *Fitoterapia*, 2005, **76**, 148).

Spouted bed extraction

In certain instances, as in the production of annatto powder from the seeds of *Bixa orellana*, the physical removal of the pigment layer of the seed-coat can yield a less impaired product than that produced by solvent extraction. Such methods can involve the use of a ball mill or a spouted bed unit. A development of the latter, the conical spouted bed extractor, has been investigated for annatto production. Basically it consists of a cylinder tapered at both ends and containing the seeds at the lower end through which a jet of hot air is forced. Seeds and pigment-loaded fine particles are propelled into the space above from whence the seeds fall back to be recirculated and the annatto powder moves to a cyclone from which it is collected. For full details see M. L. Passos *et al.*, *Drying Technology*, 1998, **16**, 1855.

Supercritical fluid extraction

The use of supercritical fluids for the extraction of a range of materials including plant products of medicinal, flavouring and cosmetic interest has, during the last decade, become of increasing economic and research interest.

In 1822, Cagniard de la Tour reported that above a certain temperature, and pressure, single substances do not condense or evaporate but exist as a fluid. Under these conditions the gas and liquid phases both possess the same density and no division exists between the two phases. This is the critical state. For water, the critical conditions for temperature (t_c) and pressure (p_c) are 374°C and 220 atmospheres respectively

and for carbon dioxide $t_c = 31$°C and $p_c = 74$ atm. In practice conditions somewhat above the critical temperature and pressure for a particular substance are usually used and these *supercritical fluids* exhibit properties intermediate between those of the liquid and gaseous phases. In phytochemistry these properties can be exploited to maximize the extraction of plant constituents. For industrial purposes supercritical fluid carbon dioxide has an environmental advantage over many common organic solvents and leaves no solvent residues in the product. It also allows a low temperature process and has proved of value for the extraction of labile expensive fragrances and medicinal phytochemicals. To render it more polar a small amount of modifier, e.g. methanol, may be added to the carbon dioxide. The high pressures, and for some substances the high temperatures, involved in supercritical fluid extraction are the principal disadvantages of the technique.

Pioneer work on medicinal plants was carried out by Stahl and coworkers (*Planta Med.*, 1980, **40**, 12, and references cited therein). They studied the use of liquefied and supercritical carbon dioxide and liquefied nitrous oxide for the extraction of various plant constituents, including various types of alkaloids, the pyrethrins and the components of chamomile. With pyrethrum flower extract, the content of pyrethrins is substantially higher (up to 50%) than in commercially available petroleum ether extracts. By a two-step precipitation the active ingredients can be raised to up to 60% without decomposition of the thermolabile pyrethrins.

Further examples involving the extraction of phytochemicals with supercritical carbon dioxide follow:

1. Acylphloroglucinols: Oxygenated hyperforin derivatives of *Hypericum*
2. Alkaloids: Decaffeination of green coffee (industrial application)
   Isolation of vindoline from *Catharanthus roseus*
3. Diterpene: Extraction of taxol from *Taxus brevifolia* (extraction more selective than conventional ethanol extraction), also from *T. cuspidata*
4. Fixed oils: Extraction of oil from evening primrose (subtle shift in triglyceride composition; oxidation of γ-linolenic acid during extraction reduced)
5. Pigments: Extraction of annatto seeds
6. Sapogenins: *Smilax china* (increased yield of diosgenin)
7. Sesquiterpene lactones: In conjunction with gas chromatography for the isolation of parthenolide from feverfew. Addition of methanol or methyl cyanide as CO_2 modifiers gave higher yields but produced co-extractives
   The use of 10% methanol in CO_2 for the extraction of trilactones from ginkgo could be of commercial significance
8. Volatile oils and resins: Hops (commercial application); frankincense and myrrh (efficient extraction); juniper berries (significant difference in composition compared with distilled oil, the latter being significantly more enriched with monoterpenoid hydrocarbons)
   Piper nigrum muntok (superior aroma of oil; yield 2.8 per cent volatile oil compared with 0.6 per cent by steam

distillation); rose petals (product richer in relevant fragrance compounds compared with steam distillation); rosemary (aroma more closely resembles plant fragrance than distilled oil); also studied: angelica root, celery, coriander, *Illicium verum*, *Maytenus illicifolia*, pimento

For a review covering the extraction of flavour and fragrance compounds, see M. Gotto *et al.*, *Aroma research* 2007, **8**, 110

For additional information on the method, consult the 'Further reading'.

Solid phase microextraction

The method is suitable for some volatile oil-containing drugs. T. J. Betts (*Planta Medica*, 2000, **66**, 193), using methyl polysiloxane solid phase microextraction fibres, has extracted the volatile oil from the headspace above fresh cut eucalyptus leaves (37° for 10 min.). The fibres were then desorbed at 200° for capillary gas chromatography of the oil. Not surprisingly, the oil composition differs from that of steam-distilled oils. The method, coupled with gas chromatography and mass spectrometry, has been recently employed for the analysis of the flowers and essential oils from *Lavandula angustifolia* cultivated in N.E. Italy (C. Da Porto and D. Decorti, *Planta Medica*, 2008, **74**, 182).

SEPARATION AND ISOLATION OF CONSTITUENTS

As the instrumentation for the structure elucidation of organic compounds becomes ever more effective, and allows the use of increasingly small amounts of material, the most difficult operation in phytochemical research becomes that of the isolation and purification of plant constituents. Although the chemical properties of functional groups and moieties contained in compounds such as acids, aldehydes, phenols and alkaloids can be exploited for their separation from other materials, such methods might not fractionate components of the same class; it is in this latter area that new techniques are constantly being developed.

Sublimation

Sublimation may sometimes be possible on the whole drug, as in the isolation of caffeine from tea or for the purification of materials present in a crude extract. Modern equipment employs low pressures with a strict control of temperature.

Distillation

Fractional distillation has been traditionally used for the separation of the components of volatile mixtures; in phytochemistry it has been widely used for the isolation of the components of volatile oils. On a laboratory scale it is not easy by this method to separate minor components of a mixture in a pure state and gas chromatography is now routinely used (q.v.).

Steam distillation is much used to isolate volatile oils and hydrocyanic acid from plant material. The TAS oven (see 'Thin-layer chromatography') involves steam distillation on a semi-micro scale for the direct transfer of volatile materials from a powdered drug to a thin-layer plate.

Fractional liberation

Some groups of compounds lend themselves to fractional liberation from a mixture. As an example, a mixture of alkaloid salts in aqueous solution, when treated with aliquots of alkali, will give first the weakest base in the free state followed by base liberation in ascending order of basicity. If the mixture is shaken with an organic solvent after each addition, then a fractionated series of bases will be obtained. A similar scheme can be used for organic acids soluble in water-immiscible solvents; in this case, starting with a mixture of the acid salts, it is possible to fractionally liberate the acids by addition of mineral acids.

Fractional crystallization

A method much used in traditional isolations and still valuable for the resolution of often otherwise intractable mixtures. The method exploits the differences in solubility of the components of a mixture in a particular solvent. Frequently, derivatives of the particular components are employed (picrates of alkaloids, osazones of sugars).

Adsorption chromatography

Of the various methods of separating and isolating plant constituents, the 'chromatographic procedure' originated by Tswett is one of the most useful techniques of general application. The use of charcoal for the decolorization and clarification of solutions is well known; coloured impurities are *adsorbed* by the charcoal and a colourless solution results on filtration. All finely divided solids have the power to adsorb other substances on their surfaces to a greater or lesser extent; similarly, all substances are capable of being adsorbed, some much more readily than others. This phenomenon of selective adsorption is the fundamental principle of adsorption chromatography, the general process of which may be described with reference to one of Tswett's original experiments.

A light petroleum extract of green leaves is allowed to percolate slowly through a column of powdered calcium carbonate contained in a vertical glass tube. The pigmented contents of the solution are adsorbed on the substance of the column and undergo separation as percolation proceeds. The more strongly adsorbed pigments, xanthophyll and the chlorophylls, accumulate in distinct, characteristically coloured bands near the top of the column, while the less strongly adsorbed pigments, the carotenes, accumulate lower down.

Frequently, complete separation of all the constituents into distinct bands does not result during the first 'adsorption stage', but the bands remain crowded together near the top of the column. Such a column may be *developed* by allowing more of the pure solvent to percolate through the column when the adsorbed materials slowly pass downwards and the separate bands become wider apart. In many cases the process may be rendered more efficient by the use of a different solvent, one from which the substances are less strongly adsorbed. If, for example, light petroleum containing a little alcohol is percolated through the chromatogram obtained in the experiment described above, the bands become wider apart and pass down the column more rapidly than when pure light petroleum is used. As percolation continues, the lower bands reach the bottom of the column and disappear; the pigment is then obtained in the solution leaving the bottom of the column. This process of desorption is termed *elution* and the solution obtained is the *eluate*.

It was from such classic experiments of Tswett on the separation of coloured compounds that the term 'chromatography' arose and it has remained to describe this method of fractionation although its application to colourless substances is now universal.

Substances are more readily adsorbed from non-polar solvents such as light petroleum and benzene, while polar solvents—alcohol, water and pyridine, for example—are useful eluting media; many substances are adsorbed at one pH and eluted at another.

Various substances may be used as adsorbing materials; alumina is the most common and other materials include kaolin, magnesium oxide, calcium carbonate, charcoal and sugars.

When colourless substances are chromatographed, the zones of adsorbed material are not visible to the eye, although they may, in some cases, be rendered apparent as fluorescent zones when the column is examined under ultraviolet light. Failing this, it becomes necessary to divide the chromatogram into discrete portions and elute or extract each portion separately. Sometimes it is more convenient to collect the eluate from the whole column in fractions for individual examination.

The apparatus required is simple and consists essentially of a vertical glass tube into which the adsorbent has been packed; a small plug of glass wool or a sintered glass disc, at the base of the tube, supports the column. With volatile developing solvents it is usually preferable to use a positive pressure at the head of the column. Numerous modifications of the apparatus are used for large-scale operations, for use with heated solvents and for chromatography in the absence of air or oxygen.

Adsorption chromatography has proved particularly valuable in the isolation and purification of vitamins, hormones, many alkaloids, cardiac glycosides, anthraquinones, etc. It is commonly employed as a 'clean-up' technique for the removal of unwanted materials from plant extracts prior to assay.

Thin-layer chromatography with adsorbents such as alumina is an adaptation of the method and is discussed separately in this chapter.

Partition chromatography

Partition chromatography was introduced by Martin and Synge in 1941 for the separation of acetylated amino acids and was first applied to the separation of alkaloids by Evans and Partridge in 1948. The method has now been largely superseded by the more sophisticated HPLC (see below) but it retains the advantage of being inexpensive to set up and operate. The separation of the components of a mixture is, as in counter-current extraction, dependent on differences in the partition coefficients of the components between an aqueous and an immiscible organic liquid.

The aqueous phase is usually the stationary phase and is intimately mixed with a suitable 'carrier' such as silica gel, purified kieselguhr or powdered glass and packed in a column as in adsorption chromatography. The mixture to be fractionated is introduced on the column, in a small volume of organic solvent, and the chromatogram is developed with more solvent or successively with different solvents of increasing eluting power. When water is the stationary phase, the solutes undergoing separation travel down the column at different speeds depending on their partition coefficient between the two liquid phases; the use of a buffer solution as aqueous phase widens the scope of the technique, as ionization constants and partition coefficients are exploited in effecting separation.

The separated zones may be located by methods similar to those employed in adsorption chromatography. With water as the aqueous phase, the positions of separated zones of acids or alkalis may be shown by employing a suitable indicator dissolved in the water. This method is clearly not applicable to buffer-, acid- or alkali-loaded columns, and in these cases complete elution (elution development) of the separated zone is often necessary. The eluate is collected in aliquot portions and estimated chemically or physically for dissolved solute. A graph of the analytical figure (titration, optical rotation, optical density, refractive index, etc.) for each fraction of eluate may then be plotted to show the degree of separation of the solutes.

The fractionations obtained in partition chromatography are influenced to a considerable degree by the displacement effect of one solute on another and advantage is taken of this in displacement development, in which the chromatogram is developed with a solution of an acid or a base that is stronger than any in the mixture to be separated. The effect is for the stronger acids or bases to displace the weaker ones, resulting in a rapid clear-cut separation of the constituents. For the elution development of these separated zones it is essential that there is no distortion of the zones, since the front of one band follows immediately on the tail of the preceding less acidic or less basic component.

There have been several theoretical treatments of partition chromatography, all involving certain approximations, since a theory taking into account all known variables would be extremely complicated. For general purposes, one of the most satisfactory treatments of columns loaded with water is that of Martin and Synge, in which the theoretical plate concept of fractional distillation is applied to partition chromatography. In this theory, diffusion from one plate to another is taken as negligible and the partition of solute between two phases is independent of concentration and the presence of other solutes.

Partition chromatography on paper

In 1944 Consden, Gordon and Martin introduced a method of partition chromatography using strips of filter paper as 'carriers' for the analysis of amino acid mixtures. The technique was extended to all classes of natural products, and although to a large measure replaced by thin-layer chromatography (TLC), it remains the method of choice for the fractionation of some groups of substances.

The solution of components to be separated is applied as a spot near one end of a prepared filter-paper strip. The paper is then supported in an airtight chamber which has an atmosphere saturated with solvent and water, and a supply of the water-saturated solvent. The most satisfactory solvents are those which are partially miscible with water, such as phenol, n-butanol and amyl alcohol. Either the paper may be dipped in the solvent mixture so that the solvent front travels up the paper (ascending technique) or the trough of solvent may be supported at the top of the chamber, in which case the solvent travels down the paper (descending technique). The BP 2007 gives details of both methods. As the solvent moves, the components also move along the paper at varying rates, depending mainly on the differences in their partition coefficients between the aqueous (hydration shell of cellulose fibres) and organic phases. After the filter-paper strips have been dried, the positions of the separated components can be revealed by the use of suitable developing agents: ninhydrin solution for amino acids; iodine solution (or vapour) or a modified Dragendorff's reagent for alkaloids; ferric chloride solution for phenols; alkali for anthraquinone derivatives; antimony trichloride in chloroform for steroids and some components of volatile oils; aniline hydrogen phthalate reagent for sugars. The relative positions of the components and the size of the spots depend upon the solvent, and this should be selected to give good separation of the components with well-defined, compact spots. Improved separation of mixtures can often be obtained by adjusting the acidity of the solvent with ammonia, acetic acid or hydrochloric acid or by impregnating the paper with a buffer solution or formamide solution.

For the separation of some substances it is necessary to use a two-dimensional chromatogram: first one solvent is run in one direction, then, after drying of the paper, a second solvent is run in a direction at right angles to the first—this is particularly applicable to mixtures of amino acids.

The ratio between the distance travelled on the paper by a component of the test solution and the distance travelled by the solvent is termed the R_F value and, under standard conditions, this is a constant for the particular compound. However, in practice, variations of R_F often occur and it is desirable to run reference compounds alongside unknown mixtures.

The quantity of substance present determines the size of the spot with any one solvent and can be made the basis of quantitative evaluation. Also, the separated components of the original mixture can be separately eluted from the chromatogram, by treating the cut-out spots with a suitable solvent, and then determined quantitatively by some suitable method—for example, fluorescence analysis, colorimetry or ultraviolet adsorption. Drugs so evaluated include aloes, digitalis, ergot, hemlock, lobelia, nux vomica, opium, rauwolfia, rhubarb, broom, solanaceous herbs and volatile oils.

High-performance liquid chromatography (HPLC)/ high-speed LC

HPLC is a liquid column chromatography system which employs relatively narrow columns (about 5 mm diameter for analytical work) operating at ambient temperature or up to about 200°C at pressures up to 200 atm (20 000 kPa).

The columns are costly and it is usual to employ a small precolumn containing a cartridge of packing material to remove adventitious materials which might otherwise damage the main column. Normal flow rates of eluate are 2–5 ml min⁻¹ but can be up to 10 ml min⁻¹, depending on the diameter of the column and the applied pressure. The apparatus is suitable for all types of liquid chromatography columns (adsorption, partition by the use of bonded liquid phases, reversed phase, gel filtration, ion exchange and affinity). The arrangement of such an apparatus, suitable for use with two solvents and giving graded elution, is illustrated in Fig. 17.1. Detection of the often very small quantities of solute in the eluate is possible by continuous monitoring of ultraviolet absorption, mass spectrum, refractive index, fluorescence and electrical conductance; nuclear magnetic resonance can now be added to this list. To improve detection, solutes may be either derivatized before chromatography (this technique can also be used to improve separations) or treated with reagents after separation (post-column derivatization). A transport system for monitoring is commercially available; in this a moving wire passes through the flowing eluate (coating block) and the dissolved solute, deposited on the wire, is pyrolysed and its quantity automatically recorded. It will be noted that, for any particular fractionation, some detector systems would be selective for certain groups of compounds and others would be universal.

HPLC can give much improved and more rapid separations than can be obtained with the older liquid chromatography methods and it is therefore finding increasing use in numerous areas. As with GLC apparatus, it is available from many manufacturers and can be completely automated.

Many stationary phases are available, the most widely used being silica based. In these, which consist of porous particles 5–10 μm in diameter, the silanol groups (Si-OH) afford a polar surface which

can be exploited in separations using an organic mobile phase as in ordinary adsorption chromatography.

Reversed-phase packing material (Spherisorb ODS) is produced by the bonding of octadecylsilyl groups ($C_{18}H_{37}Si-$) to silica gel. In the commercial material there appears to be a considerable proportion of residual silanol–OH groups, so that adsorption and partition effects may operate during separation. The hydrocarbon chains probably allow non-polar interaction to take place. The structure of the packing material might be represented as:

To reduce tailing effects which might be caused by the remaining free hydroxyl groups the latter can be masked by treatment with a short-chain silane, usually trimethylchlorosilane. Silica-based columns are restricted to use in the range pH 3–8 and to overcome this polymer phases operating at pH 1–13 are available; these, however, have the disadvantage of exhibiting a high column back-pressure.

Of relatively recent introduction are chiral stationary phases which are utilized to separate the enantiomers of racemic mixtures. These have great potential for the study of natural products, many of which are optically active, and for isolating the pharmacologically active enantiomer from the racemic mixture of a synthetic drug. Pharmacognostical examples include, among many others, the assay of partially racemized hyoscine extracted from plants, the separation of aromatics and the resolution of mixtures of (+)- and (−)-epicatechin and other proanthocyanidin enantiomers of *Cassia fistula* and *C. javanica*. The mode of action of chiral stationary phases is not fully understood; typical materials are cyclodextrins, cellulose- and amino acid-derivatives suitably bonded. Two products are sorbents made of spherical silica gel particles to which β-cyclodextrin (ChiraDex®) or γ-cyclodextrin (Chira-Dex® GAMMA) are covalently bonded via a carbamate bond and long spacer.

For a review on the rapid detection and subsequent isolation of bioactive constituents of crude plant extracts with schemes for LC/UV, LC/MS, LC/MS/MS and LC/NMR see K. Hostettman *et al.*, *Planta Medica*, 1997, **63**, 2.

Supercritical fluid chromatography

This technique, developed over recent years for both the qualitative and quantitative analysis of medicinal products, utilizes supercritical

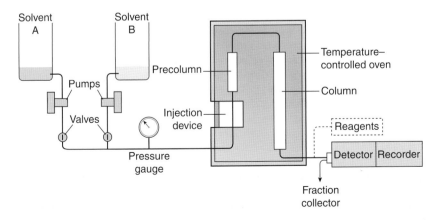

Fig. 17.1
Schematic representation of apparatus for high-performanance liquid chromatography utilizing two solvents.

fluids, particularly carbon dioxide, as the mobile phase in liquid chromatography. The low viscosity of the supercritical liquid provides a faster flow rate than standard HPLC and higher diffusivity of the materials to be separated. The plate height in the column, the length of the column and the time required for a particular separation are all reduced compared with the established technique. Sharper elution peaks give increased separation efficiency. Waste-disposal of used solvents is eliminated. Changes to the instrumental set-up have been devised to accommodate the properties of a supercritical liquid.

Counter-current extraction

This is a liquid–liquid extraction process and the principles involved are similar to those of partition chromatography. Developed by Craig in 1944, the extraction machine used (for that time) small amounts of extract and overcame the tedious multiple extraction processes then employed. Now, however, for research purposes, only the smallest of samples for fractionation and analysis are required, making the use of the cumbersome counter-current apparatus largely unnecessary.

Briefly, a lower, stationary phase is contained in a series of tubes and an upper, moving immiscible liquid is transferred from tube to tube along the series, the immiscible liquids being shaken and allowed to separate between each transference. The mixture to be fractionated is placed in the first tube containing the immiscible liquids and the apparatus is agitated and the layers are allowed to separate. The components of the mixture will be distributed between the two layers according to their partition coefficients. The upper phase is moved along to the second tube containing lower phase and more moving phase is brought into contact with the lower phase of tube 1. Shaking and transference again takes place and continues along a sufficient number of tubes to give a fractionation of the mixture.

The applications of counter-current extraction covered many fields of plant chemistry, including alkaloids, amino acids, antibiotics, antitumour compounds, phenols including anthraquinone derivatives, cardiac glycosides, essential oils, fatty acids, plant auxins, prostaglandins, steroids and vitamins.

Other more recent developments involving the counter-current principle are high-speed counter-current chromatography (planet coil centrifugal CCC), droplet counter-current chromatography (DCCC) and centrifugal droplet CCC. Details of these can be found in the 15th edition of this book. For a review (245 refs) giving the background and up-to-date methodology employed in the counter-current separation of natural products see G. F. Pauli *et al.*, *J. Nat. Prod.*, 2008, **71**, 1489–1508.

Thin-layer chromatography

In 1958 Stahl demonstrated the wide applicability of TLC, a technique which had been known in principle for many years but was never developed. It has now achieved remarkable success in the separation of mixtures of all classes of natural products and is established as an analytical tool in modern pharmacopoeias.

In outline the method consists of preparing, on a suitable glass plate, a thin layer of material, the sorbent, which may be either an adsorbent as used in column adsorption chromatography or an inert support which holds an aqueous phase as in column partition chromatography. The mixtures to be resolved are dissolved in a suitable solvent and placed as a series of spots on the film towards one end of the plate; this end is then dipped in a suitable solvent mixture and the whole enclosed in an airtight container. The solvent front travels up the film and after a suitable time the plate is removed, the solvent front is marked, the solvent is allowed to evaporate and the positions of the separated compounds are determined by suitable means.

TLC has certain advantages over paper chromatography. Fractionations can be effected more rapidly with smaller quantities of the mixture; the separated spots are usually more compact and more clearly demarcated from one another; and the nature of the film is often such that drastic reagents, such as concentrated sulphuric acid, which would destroy a paper chromatogram, can be used for the location of separated substances.

With adsorption TLC various substances exhibit different adsorptive capacities and any one material may vary in its activity according to the pretreatment. The adsorbent must be chosen in relation to the properties of the solvent and the mixture to be fractionated. In general, for a given substance, if a highly active adsorbent is used, then a solvent with a correspondingly high power of elution for this substance is required. Alumina (acid, basic and neutral) of different activity grades is very commonly employed. In order to produce a film with reasonable handling properties, the adsorbent may be mixed with about 12% of its weight of calcium sulphate ($CaSO_4.1/2H_2O$) to act as a binder. Ready-mixed powders are obtainable commercially; they require mixing with a given quantity of water and the slurry needs to be spread by a mechanical device or with a glass rod on to glass plates. The film sets within a few minutes and is then activated by heating at a suitable temperature (105°C for 30 min is common). Commercial ready-spread plates are available. The thickness of the film is characteristically of the order of 250 μm, but for preparative work layers of up to several millimetres thickness are employed. The thick films must be carefully dried to avoid cracks.

Solutions of substances to be examined are applied to the film with the aid of capillary tubes or, for quantitative work, with microsyringes and micrometer pipettes which permit volumes to be read off to ±0.05 μl. A useful innovation for applying steam-volatile components of a powdered drug directly to a thin-layer plate is the Stahl TAS oven. The drug sample is placed in a cartridge together with a suitable propellant (e.g. hydrated silica gel) and inserted in the TAS oven maintained at a predetermined temperature. The tapered exit of the cartridge is situated a short distance from the base-line of a TLC plate and 'steam-distilled' components from the drug are deposited ready for immediate development (for illustration see 12th edition). Stahl (*Planta Med.*, 1976, **29**, 1) has described a development of this apparatus whereby 18 samples can be simultaneously deposited on a plate under uniform conditions. A more recent application has involved the study of tannin-containing drugs.

The solvents used for running the chromatogram must be pure, and common ones are methanol, ethanol and other alcohols, chloroform, ether, ethyl acetate, *n*-hexane, cyclohexane, petroleum spirit and mixtures of these. For routine assays automatic multiple development with polarity graduation of the developing solvent can be used. It must be remembered that chloroform ordinarily contains up to 1% of ethanol, which gives it quite different elution properties from those of pure chloroform. Benzene, formerly frequently used as a component of the mobile phase, has now for health reasons been routinely replaced with other non-polar solvents. Similarly, inhalation of chloroform-containing mixtures should be avoided.

TLC, which involves the partition of a substance between two immiscible phases, is again analogous to the column procedure and to paper chromatography. In the latter, the hydration shell of the cellulose fibres forms the stationary phase and thin-layer chromatograms utilizing powdered cellulose give comparable results. Kieselguhr and silica gel are also commonly employed, and their properties as thin layers can be modified by the inclusion of acids, bases and buffer solutions. The thin layers may also include a substance fluorescent in ultraviolet light and this facilitates the detection of solutes which cause a quenching of the background fluorescence. Much used is Kieselgel GF_{254} 'Merck' which gives a background green fluorescence when irradiated with ultraviolet light of wavelength 254 nm. Small quantities of ammonia solution, diethylamine, acetic acid, dimethylformamide and pyridine are often present as constituents of the developing solvents for silica plates. Other layers used include polyamide, which is particularly suitable for phenolic compounds, 'Sephadex' (Pharmacia,

Uppsala), a cross-linked dextran used as a molecular sieve (gel filtration), and ion exchangers. 'Reversed-phase' plates are now available commercially and are stated to be useful in that they will indicate the type of separation which a mixture would undergo by reversed-phase HPLC (q.v.).

As with paper chromatography, the method can be extended to two-dimensional chromatography, to electrophoretic separations, to quantitative evaluations and to work involving radioactive substances.

Compounds resolved on the TLC plate are visualized using either general or specific methods; thus, ultraviolet light will indicate fluorescent compounds (these should be examined in both long- (*c.* 365 nm) and short- (*c.* 263 nm) wavelength ultraviolet light. Fluorescence-quenching compounds (a very large number) are detected by the use of impregnated sorbents (see above). Iodine and Dragendorff's reagents are used in the form of sprays for the general detection of alkaloids although they (iodine in particular) are not absolutely specific for alkaloids. For indole alkaloids, the reagent *p*-dimethylaminobenzaldehyde is useful for ergot and a phosphomolybdic acid reagent for others. Antimony trichloride in chloroform is used as a spray reagent for steroidal compounds and other terpenoids, similarly anisaldehyde in sulphuric acid; both these require the sprayed chromatograms to be heated at 100°C for varying times (5–20 min) in order to develop the colours. Ammonia vapour can be used for free anthraquinone compounds and Fast Blue Salt B 'Merck' for cannabinoids and phloroglucides. Sugars separated by TLC using phosphate buffered amino layers (e.g. precoated plates of silica gel–Merck NH_2) can be located by *in-situ* thermal reaction (150°C for 3–4 min.) and fluorescence monitoring.

The *European* and *British Pharmacopoeias* employ thin-layer chromatographic tests for most vegetable drugs; illustrations of the chromatograms of the fatty acids derived from fifteen different fixed oils are given.

Preparative TLC. As mentioned above, thicker layers of sorbent are employed for preparative work and the separated bands of compounds are scraped from the plate and subjected to solvent extraction. With modern spectrometric methods for structure-determination available, this technique generates quantities of material sufficient for a complete analysis.

To speed up separations and to make them on-line for continuous recording, various modifications of preparative TLC have been developed. These include *centrifugally accelerated layer chromatography* and *overpressure layer chromatography*. The latter involves the complete covering of the sorbent layer with an elastic membrane under external pressure thus eliminating the vapour phase from the chromatographic plate. The mobile phase is forced up the sorbent layer through a special inlet. This method, introduced by Tyihák *et al.* in 1979–80, was subsequently adapted to *on-line overpressure layer chromatography* for the preparative separation of a number of natural products (the isolation of frangula-emodin; noscapine and papaverine fractionation; furocoumarin isomers of *Heracleum sphondylium* (Umbelliferae); the preparation of the secoiridoid glycosides of *Gentiana purpurea*). See J. Pothier *et al.* (*Fitoterapia*, 1997, **68**, 42) for the semi-preparative isolation of the alkaloids of *Strychnos nux-vomica*, opium, *Datura stramonium* and *Lupinus*.

Gas–liquid chromatography

The use of a liquid stationary phase and a mobile gaseous phase in chromatography was first suggested by Martin and Synge in 1941 and developed by James and Martin in 1952 for the separation of the lower fatty acids. Gas–liquid chromatography is now extensively used in all branches of analytical chemistry. Many commercial instruments are available, the more sophisticated being completely automated. For a schematic diagram see Fig. 17.2.

The *empty columns* are made of glass or metal and are either straight, often up to about 1.3 m in length, or coiled and up to 16 m in length. James and Martin used a tube of 4 mm internal diameter. The liquid *stationary phase* is held on an *inert material*, commonly partially fused diatomite. A uniform particle size, with a minimum of dust, is essential, for the inert support and the particles should be as small as possible to give a large surface area but sufficiently large to allow even packing of the column. The choice of stationary phase is governed by the temperature at which the column is to operate and the nature of the material to be fractionated; it should be non-volatile at the operating temperature and should not react with either the stationary and mobile phases or the solutes. Some materials commonly used, with their recommended temperature of operation, include: (1) non-polar compounds—silicone oils 200–250°C, apiezon oils and greases 275–300°C, silicone gum rubber 400°C, high-boiling-point paraffins such as mineral oil 100°C, squalene 75°C; (2) moderately polar compounds—high boiling point alcohols and their esters 100–225°C; (3) strongly polar compounds—polypropylene glycols and their esters 225°C. Up to 25% by weight of stationary phase is commonly employed on columns; one method of dispersing the stationary phase over the inert support is to dissolve it in a low boiling point solvent such as ether, mix thoroughly with the support and spread out the powder to allow the solvent to evaporate. The powder is then packed into the empty column a little at a time and as evenly as possible and then enclosed in a uniformly heated oven.

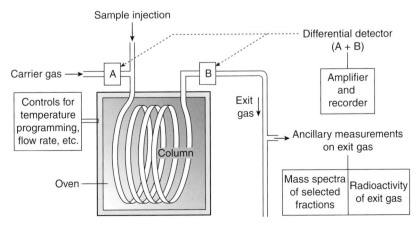

Fig. 17.2
Schematic diagram of gas–liquid chromatograph with ancillary attachments.

A combined support and stationary phase which can replace the above is furnished by cross-linked polymers of specified pore size. These are produced as beads from styrene-like compounds and are marketed under the trade name 'Porapak'. Advantages of such columns are that they remove undesirable adsorption sites present in diatomite, bleeding of the column (gradual leakage of stationary phase from the column) is reduced, and the rapid elution of water and other highly polar molecules is achieved with little or no tailing.

The *operating temperature* of the column is critical. Mixtures of low-boiling-point substances can be fractionated at low temperatures; some ethers, for example, can be dealt with at room temperature. Other materials require much higher temperatures—volatile oils 150–300°C, steroids 250°C and pesticides 400°C. Modern instruments can be temperature-programmed so that the column temperature increases as chromatography proceeds. This has the advantage that good separations of mixtures containing compounds with widely different properties can be obtained in one operation and long waits for the emergence of the more strongly retained fractions, with correspondingly less resolution, are lessened.

The *mobile phase* is a gas which is inert in so far as the other components of the chromatogram are concerned. The choice of gas is dependent on the detector system (see below), and gases commonly used are hydrogen, nitrogen, helium and argon. The *flow rate* of the gas is important; too high a flow rate will give incomplete separations and too slow a rate will give high retention times and diffuse peaks. Typical flow rates for short columns are 10–50 ml min^{-1}.

By means of a suitable injection device, the sample to be analysed is introduced on to the top of the column; 1.0–5.0 μl is a typical volume but with some detectors it can be considerably less. The measurement of such small volumes is difficult, especially if quantitative results are required, and often the sample is dissolved in a low-boiling-point solvent such as ether; the ether passes rapidly through the column and emerges with the gas front. The mixture to be analysed should volatilize immediately it comes into contact with the stationary phase. Some compounds, not themselves volatile, may be converted into volatile derivatives before chromatography. Thus, sugars, flavonoids including anthocyanins, morphine, codeine and the cardioactive glycosides and aglycones can be chromatographed as their trimethylsiloxy derivatives, which are formed as below:

$$2ROH + (CH_3)_3SiNHSi(CH_3)_3 \rightarrow 2ROSi(CH_3)_3 + NH_3$$

Non-volatile plant acids can first be converted to their methyl esters by treatment with diazomethane.

Along with the analytical columns of the above type, larger preparative columns can be used for the isolation of the separated components in quantities sufficiently large for subsequent examination. Sample sizes of 0.1–20 ml and column lengths of up to 60 m and internal diameters of 1–2 cm illustrate the dimensions involved.

The *detector system* analyses the effluent gas from the column. It may be of the integral type, in which some property—for example, titration value—of the eluate is recorded or it may be of the differential type, in which some property of the effluent gas is compared with that of a reference gas, often the mobile phase. The latter type is the most commonly used and examples are the katharometer, gas density balance, flame ionization, β-argon ray and electron-capture detectors. For details of these detectors the student is referred to one of the several standard books on gas chromatography. All these differential detectors give an electrical signal which is recorded graphically by a suitable recorder. Because not all detectors give the same relative response to given compounds under the same conditions, some columns are fitted with a double detector system.

The volume of gas that emerges from the column before the arrival of the gas front into which the sample was introduced at the head of the column is termed the 'hold-up' volume and it is dependent on the capacity of the column. It is obtained by multiplying the time which the gas front takes to pass through the column by the flow rate; the arrival of the front is often indicated on the recorder by a negative peak caused by the small amount of air injected with the sample. The observed retention volume $V_{R,obs}$ of a component is calculated from its retention time, and the $V_{R,obs}$ less the 'hold-up' volume is the adjusted retention volume ($V_{R,ad}$). By taking into account the pressure drop along the length of the column the net retention volume ($V_{R,net}$) is obtained. This volume is characteristic for a given compound under the defined conditions of the amount of stationary phase and temperature. Of more universal value is the specific retention volume ($V_{R,sp}$), which is the $V_{R,net}$ reduced to 0°C g^{-1} of stationary phase:

$$V_{R,sp} = \frac{V_{R,net} \times 273}{\text{weight of stationary phase on column} \times \text{temperature (K) of column}}$$

Reference compounds are used to aid the identification of components of a mixture. For quantitative work with differential detectors, the areas enclosed by the peaks are proportional to the quantities of compounds which they represent. To obtain the percentage composition of components within a mixture, without the necessity of placing known amounts of sample on the column, internal standards can be used. These are pure substances, mixed in known proportion with a sample of material to be analysed, which give sharp peaks on the chromatogram not overlapping those of the mixture. Before use, internal standards must be calibrated for detector response against individual components of the mixture.

Sophisticated attachments are available for some equipment. It is thus possible to record the radioactivities and mass spectra of the separated components of a mixture as they emerge from the column. Such instruments have immense potential in biological research. Data storage and retrieval units are now available as standard accessories.

Some pharmacognostical examples of the applications of gas chromatography include the examination of many volatile oils (see, for example the *BP* assay of Clove Oil), camphor, plant acids, some alkaloids (opium, tobacco and *Conium* and tropane derivatives), the resins of the Convolvulaceae and of *Cannabis*, and steroidal compounds such as the sapogenins and cardioactive glycosides and aglycones. The *BP* test for foreign oils in fixed oils involves the gas-chromatographic separation of the methyl esters of the fatty acids produced by hydrolysis of the sample. The detection and estimation of cocaine and its metabolites in the body is an important forensic application. The estimation of pesticide residues on crops is of utmost importance, and here the sensitivity of detector systems, such as the electron capture detector, has made possible the determination of the chlorinated pesticides down to the parts-per-billion range.

Capillary-column gas chromatography

As the name implies, capillary bore columns are used rather than the standard columns described above. They afford marked improvements in resolving power and in speed of analysis.

The internal diameters of the columns range from about 0.15 mm to about 0.53 mm and the columns can be 1 to 60 m in length. They were originally made of stainless steel and then glass, but fused-silica columns are now considered the obvious choice as they are strong, easy to use, highly inert and give excellent performance. They can be conveniently used in the coiled condition, held, for example, in a 150 mm diameter cage. Such columns hold the stationary phase in a number of ways.

(1), Wall-coated open tubular (WCOT) columns have the inner wall of the tube coated with stationary phase up to about 1 μm in thickness. Greater thickness leads to column bleeding in which the stationary phase moves down the column and eventually leaks into the detector. Thicker layers, and hence increased sample capacity, can be achieved with silica columns having specially bonded phases. WCOT columns have the highest efficiency but a low sample capacity. (2), Support-coated open tubular (SCOT) columns have the inner wall lined with a thin layer of support material coated with immobile phase. This has the effect of increasing the available area of immobile phase, affording the column a greater load capacity. The efficiency, while lower than that of the WCOT columns is much higher than that for packed columns. (3) Micropacked columns involve a coated support packed into narrow-bore columns. In all ways they represent a compromise, being more efficient than the normal packed columns but having the same problem in that column length is restricted by the high back-pressure.

Another difference between capillary column chromatography and standard gas chromatography concerns the method of introducing the sample to the column. The volume of sample dissolved in solvent for analysis by the capillary method is too small for a microsyringe and so special injection heads are necessary which either split the sample (e.g. 25:1 with the smaller portion passing to the column) or are of the so-called splitless-injector type which are able to accommodate the relatively large volume of solvent and deliver the dissolved solute to the column.

As with other chromatographic techniques (see HPLC) the introduction of chiral stationary phases has given an added dimension to gas chromatography. Examples include the separation of the two enantiomers of linalool enabling the detection of reconstituted bergamot oil in the genuine oil (A. Cotroneo *et al.*, *Flavour Frag. J.*, 1992, 7, 15) and the detection of added reconstituted lemon oil in the genuine cold-pressed essential oil (G. Dugo *et al.*, *J. Essent. Oil Res.*, 1993, 5, 21). Some volatile oils of the *Pharmacopoeia* are tested for chiral purity (q.v).

Gel filtration chromatography, gel permeation chromatography (molecular sieves)

These techniques are used for the separation of substances in solution according to their molecular size. The former refers to the use of aqueous mobile phases and the latter to organic mobile phases.

Hydrophilic gels such as those prepared from starch, agar, agarose (a component of agar), polyacrylamide, polyvinylcarbitol and cross-linked dextrans have been used for the fractionation of proteins, peptides, amino acids and polysaccharides.

The particles of these gels possess pores formed by the molecular structure of the gel, and when packed into a column and percolated with a solution, they permit large molecules of solute, which do not enter the pores, to pass rapidly down the column with the solvent via the intergranular interstices. Conversely, small molecules which are able to enter the gel pores become evenly distributed (on equilibrium) across the column and pass more slowly down its length. Thin layers of the sorbent can be used as in TLC.

The dextran gels (Sephadex) are formed by cross-linking dextrans (polymers of glucose in which linkages are almost entirely of the 1,6-α type) with α-epichlorohydrin (Fig. 17.3).

Individual pore sizes are determined by the distance apart of the cross-links, and gels covering a molecular weight range of up to about 200 000 are produced. Each gel type possesses a range of pore sizes, so that below the size limit of complete exclusion of the large molecules, different-sized solute molecules will enter the gel to a greater or lesser extent and so will vary in their elution rates. Similar principles are involved in the use of controlled-pore glass as sorbent; this gives a rigid column with continuous uniform pores. Obviously, the method is most applicable to mixtures containing large molecules of various sizes and to the separation of large molecules from small ones (as in desalting operations on partially hydrolysed proteins). The technique is important in DNA analysis for the separation of those fragments that result from the treatment of DNA with specific restriction enzymes.

Under the heading 'Size-exclusion chromatography', the *Pharmacopoeia* also uses rigid supports as packing material for columns; these may consist of glass, silica or a solvent-compatible cross-linked organic polymer.

Size-exclusion chromatography is used for the determination of those smaller fatty acids (oligomers) that need to be limited in fish oils, such as Fish Oil, Rich in Omega-3-Acids *BP/EP*, (oligomers, maximum 1.5%).

Electrochromatography

For the electrophoretic separation of mixtures, a filter-paper strip is impregnated with a solution of an electrolyte (usually a buffer solution) and supported in the centre; its two ends are dipped into solutions in which electrodes are immersed. A spot of the material to be fractionated is placed on the paper, the whole apparatus sealed and a potential difference of about 2–10 volts per centimetre applied along the paper. Some separations are carried out at much higher voltages than the above. According to the nature of the charge on the ions of the solute mixture, the solutes will move towards either the anode or the cathode. Thus, the amino acids can be separated either into groups (acid group, neutral group, basic group) or into individual amino acids. The migration velocity for a given substance depends on the magnitude of the ionic charge and the size and shape of the particular molecule. If preferable, paper can be replaced by thin layers of the gels described under 'Gel filtration', above. Many alkaloidal mixtures have been separated by this method and also plant acids, the component sugars of cardiac glycosides and anthraquinone derivatives.

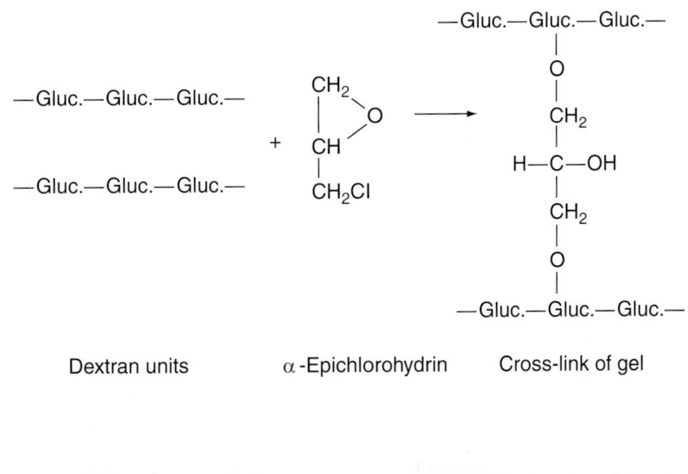

Dextran units   α-Epichlorohydrin   Cross-link of gel

Fig. 17.3
Formation of dextran gels.

17

A development which combines the advantages of both gel filtration and electrophoresis is that of polyacrylamide gradient gel electrophoresis. It is a two-dimensional electrophoresis system which separates according to mobility of solutes in one direction and according to size in the other.

Capillary electrophoresis is a technique of relatively recent introduction and can give separation efficiencies of the order of 4×10^5 theoretical plates. It provides a more rapid analysis than gel electrophoresis and with detector systems such as the laser-induced fluorescence detector combines a high resolution with a 500-fold increase in sensitivity over UV detection. The method has been used for the analysis of flavonoids.

Affinity chromatography

This method has been developed largely for the resolution of protein mixtures, and it depends on the specific, reversible binding of individual proteins with a particular ligand such as an enzyme substrate or inhibitor. The ligands are coupled with a suitable carrier (cellulose, beaded agarose, controlled-pore glass, polyacrylamide or cross-linked dextrans), possibly with the introduction of a spacer—a suitable chemical moiety such as a hydrocarbon chain—between the ligand and matrix. Excess ligand is removed by washing and the material is packed in a column. A protein mixture in a suitable buffer solution is passed down the column and a protein with sufficient affinity for the bound ligand is retarded and may later be eluted in a purified state by a change in ionic strength or pH of the column buffer. The method has the advantage of preparing in one step a particular component in a high state of purity.

Affinity chromatography has been applied to the purification of enzymes for potential clinical application, for the isolation of certain antibodies and for the specific fractionation of different types of cells (e.g. erythrocytes and lymphocytes).

CHARACTERIZATION OF ISOLATED COMPOUNDS

It is outside the scope of this book to consider in any detail the structure elucidation of natural products. It is sufficient to state that although still utilizing classical chemical methods of degradation, chemists are coming to rely more and more on the use of physical techniques to establish structures of new compounds and to identify known compounds in plant sources. Ultraviolet, infrared, mass and nuclear magnetic resonance spectroscopy together with X-ray crystallographic and optical rotatory dispersion methods have all played a significant role in these developments. Various modifications of mass spectrometry (MS) have become of increasing importance for the structural characterization and determination of the active constituents of plants; these include electron ionization MS, chemical ionization MS, field desorption MS, fast atom bombardment MS and electrospray ionization MS. For an example of the application of electrospray MS combined with sequential tandem mass spectrometry to the investigation of the steroidal saponin mixture of the Chinese and Indian drug *Tribulus terrestris*, see S. Fang *et al.*, *Planta Medica*, 1999, **65**, 68. Many problems of structure elucidation which 40 years ago were incapable of investigation, either through paucity of material or through lack of suitable chemical methods, can now readily be solved in a standard research laboratory. J. Schmidt *et al.* (*Phytochemistry*, 2007, **68**, 189), using liquid chromatography and similar combined MS techniques to the above, have demonstrated the importance of such methods for evaluating biosynthetic pathways and for studying the fate of distant natural product precursors in specific plants. They fed [ring-^{13}C-6] tyramine to *Papaver somniferum* seedlings and elucidated the structures of some twenty alkaloids into which the tyramine was incorporated; the alkaloids included those of the morphinan, benzoisoquinoline, protoberberine, benzo[*c*]phenanthridine, phthalide, isoquinoline and protopine classes. The routine analytical application of some of these techniques to plant drug analysis has been considered in Chapter 16.

BIOGENETIC INVESTIGATIONS

The living material used in biochemical research is extremely varied. Some work is possible which utilizes the whole organism with a minimum of disturbance—for example, bacteria, yeasts and moulds can be cultivated and investigated biochemically, and with animals, test substances can be added to the food and the blood and excreta analysed. With intact higher plants, however, the ultimate destruction of the plant for analysis is usually necessary. Minces, breis and homogenates are examples of preparations in which the tissues and the cell wall structures have been destroyed but in which the intracellular particles are still intact. The components of such a mixture can be isolated by centrifugation and the biological activity of each fraction can be tested. The penultimate stage in a biogenetic study is the isolation of the enzymes involved in the pathways under consideration and the *in vitro* demonstration of their properties. Finally, it is becoming increasingly possible to locate and clone the gene responsible for the synthesis of a particular enzyme. Now that the principal overall pathways associated with secondary metabolism have been largely established, it is the enzymic studies that currently receive considerable attention.

The techniques discussed below have been used for the study of secondary metabolism and their application dates from the middle of the last century; they relate principally to the search for the intermediates involved in particular pathways rather than to reaction mechanistics. It must be remembered however that many of the primary metabolic pathways, e.g. the Krebs (TCA) cycle, were established using classical biochemical methods.

TRACER TECHNIQUES

Tracer technology, now widely employed in all branches of science, had its origin in the early part of the last century, when it was realized that elements existed with identical chemical properties but with different atomic weights. Such isotopes may be stable (^{2}H, ^{13}C, ^{15}N, ^{18}O), or the nucleus may be unstable (^{1}H, ^{14}C) and decay with the emission of radiation. If it is possible to detect these isotopes by suitable means, then they can be incorporated into presumed precursors of plant constituents and used as markers in biogenetic experiments.

Radioactive tracers.   In biological investigations the use of radioactive carbon and hydrogen, and to a lesser extent and for more specific purposes sulphur, phosphorus and the alkali and alkaline-earth metals, enables the metabolism of compounds to be followed in the living organism. For studies on proteins, alkaloids and amino acids a labelled nitrogen atom may give more specific information than a labelled carbon, but the two available isotopes of nitrogen are both stable, necessitating the use of a mass spectrometer for their use as tracers.

Natural carbon possesses two stable isotopes with mass numbers 12 and 13, the latter having an abundance of 1.10 atoms per cent. Radioactive isotopes of carbon have mass numbers of 10, 11 and 14. ^{10}C has a half-life of 8.8 s and ^{11}C a half-life of 20 min., which limits their usefulness in biological research. However, ^{14}C has an estimated half-life of over 5000 years and in the atomic pile it may be produced by the bombardment of ^{14}N with slow neutrons, the target material usually being aluminium or beryllium nitride.

The immense possibilities in biological research for the use of organic compounds with specific carbon atoms labelled led to the synthesis of many compounds from the inorganic carbon compounds produced in the pile by routes not before commercially utilized. In these syntheses the purity of the product is of great importance, since a small proportion of a strongly radioactive impurity might seriously jeopardize the results of any subsequent experiments.

Many compounds which are most conveniently prepared from natural sources (e.g. certain amino acids by the hydrolysis of proteins) are produced by growing *Chlorella* in an atmosphere containing $^{14}CO_2$. All the carbon compounds of the organism thus become labelled, each compound possessing a uniform labelling of its carbon atoms.

Many tritium (^3H)-labelled compounds are commercially available. Tritium labelling is effected by catalytic exchange (platinum catalyst) in aqueous media, by irradiation of organic compounds with tritium gas and by hydrogenation of unsaturated compounds with tritium gas. Tritium is a pure β-emitter of low toxicity, half-life 12.43 years, with a radiation energy lower than that of ^{14}C.

Detection and assay of radioactively labelled compounds. When radioactive tracers are used in biogenetic studies, adequate methods for the detection and estimation of the label are essential. For the soft and easily absorbed radiation from ^3H-and ^{14}C-labelled compounds the instrument of choice is the liquid scintillation counter. It depends on the conversion of the kinetic energy of a particle into a fleeting pulse of light as the result of its penetrating a suitable luminescent substance. Rutherford successfully used this method in his early studies on radioactivity and he counted the flashes of light produced by bombardment with α-particles on a fluorescent screen prepared from zinc sulphide. The usefulness of the detector was tremendously heightened by the development of the photomultiplier tube, which replaced the human eye in recording the scintillation. Liquid scintillation media, consisting of a solvent in which the excitation occurs and a fluorescent solute which emits the light to actuate the photomultiplier, have also been devised for the purpose of enabling the sample to be incorporated in the same solute, and, hence, attain optimum geometry between sample and scintillator.

Modern instruments are fully automatic (e.g. for 100 samples at a time) and will also measure mixed radiations such as ^3H and ^{14}C (this is possible because, although both are β-emitters, they have different radiation energies. With all counters, the instrument is connected to a suitable ratemeter which records the counts over a given time. With ^{14}C, because of its long half-life, no decay corrections are necessary for normal biogenetic experiments. However the half-life is important in carbon dating of old materials. With ^3H-labelled material some correction for decay may be necessary if samples are stored for any length of time.

The traditional unit of radioactivity has been the *curie*, defined as that quantity of any radioactive nuclide in which the number of disintegrations per second is 3.7×10^{10}. Subunits are the millicurie (3.7×10^7 disintegrations per second) and the microcurie (3.7×10^4 d.p.s.). The SI unit now used for radioactive disintegration rate is the *becquerel* (Bq), which has a disintegration rate of $1 \ s^{-1}$, and its multiples include the gigabecquerel (GBq), at $10^9 \ s^{-1}$ (27.027 millicuries), and the megabecquerel (MBq), at $10^6 \ s^{-1}$ (27.027 microcuries).

For information on the theoretical basis of radioactive isotope utilization and the regulations governing the use of radioactive substances in universities and research establishments the reader is referred to the standard works and official publications on these subjects.

Autoradiography. A technique used for the location of radioactive isotopes in biological and other material is autoradiography. In this the specimen is placed in contact with a suitable emulsion (e.g. X-ray sensitive film) and after exposure the latter is developed in the usual manner. The resulting autoradiograph gives the distribution pattern of the radioactive substances in the specimen. The method can be applied to whole morphological parts (e.g. leaves) or to histological sections, for which the resulting negative is viewed under a microscope. In a similar manner, radioactive compounds on paper and thin-layer chromatograms can also be detected and the relative amounts of radioactivity in different spots determined by density measurements or by the use of calibrated films.

Precursor–product sequence. For the elucidation of biosynthetic pathways in plants by means of labelled compounds, the precursor–product sequence is commonly invoked. In this a presumed precursor of the constituent under investigation, in a labelled form, is fed to the plant and after a suitable time the constituent is isolated and purified and its radioactivity is determined. If specific atoms of the precursor are labelled, it may be possible to degrade the isolated metabolite and ascertain whether the distribution of radioactivity within the molecule is in accordance with the hypothesis under test. Radioactivity of the isolated compound alone is not usually sufficient evidence that the particular compound fed is a direct precursor, because substances may enter the general metabolic pathways of the plant and from there become randomly distributed through a whole range of products. If this happens, degradation of the isolated constituent and the determination of the activity of the fragments would probably show that the labelling was random throughout the molecule and not indicative of a specific incorporation of the precursor. Further evidence for the nature of the biochemical incorporation of precursors arises from double- and triple-labelling experiments; either different isotopes, or specific labelling by one isotope at two or more positions in the molecules, are employed. The method has been applied extensively to the biogenesis of many plant secondary metabolites. Leete, in his classical experiment, used two doubly labelled lysines to determine which hydrogen of the lysine molecule was involved in the formation of the piperidine ring of anabasine in *Nicotiana glauca*. His feeding experiments gave the incorporations shown in Fig. 17.4, indicating the terminal N to be involved.

It will be appreciated that with the above lysine precursors it is not necessary to have *individual* molecules labelled with both ^{14}C and

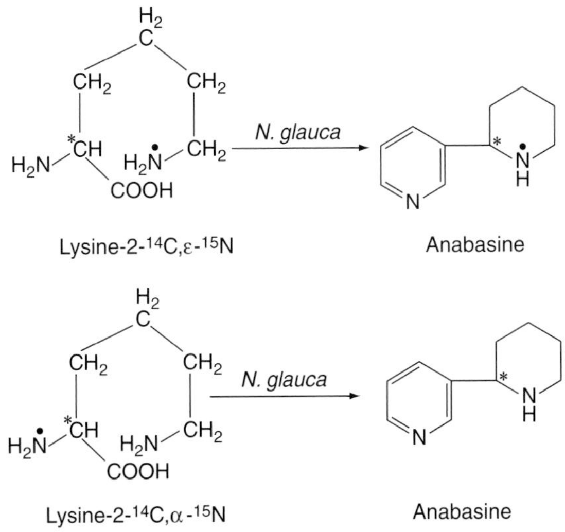

Fig. 17.4
Incorporation of doubly-labelled lysines into anabasine.

[15]N but that the same result is obtained by using standard mixtures of specifically labelled [^{14}C]lysine and [^{15}N]lysine. (Note: [15]N is a stable isomer.) Extensive use has been made of ^{3}H/^{14}C ratios in the study of stereospecific hydrogen elimination reactions.

Competitive feeding.   If incorporation is obtained, it is still necessary to consider whether this is in fact the normal route of synthesis in the plant and not a subsidiary pathway, invoked as a result of the atypical availability to the plant of the administered compound. Competitive feeding experiments can be of value in determining which of two possible intermediates is normally used by the plant. In its simplest form, without taking into account a number of other factors, competitive feeding could distinguish whether B or B′ was the normal intermediate in the formation of C from A as below:

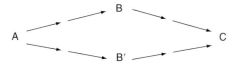

Inactive B and B′ are fed with labelled A to separate groups of plants and a control is performed by feeding labelled A only to another group. If the incorporation of activity into C is inhibited in the plants receiving B, but is unaffected in the group receiving B′, then we may conclude that the pathway from A to C probably proceeds via B. In such experiments involving intact plants, the biological variation between normal plants is often so great that it is difficult to perform a controlled investigation. In comparative studies on the rates of demethylation of codeine and unnatural codeine derivatives in *Papaver orientale*, Kirkby and colleagues in 1972 overcame this problem by using the same plant simultaneously as the control and as the test plant. They did this by administering to the plant a mixture of ^{3}H-labelled codeine and ^{14}C-labelled unnatural codeine derivative. The products of the conversion of both could be independently followed by their characteristic radiations, even when the metabolites produced were chemically identical. (For the use of competitive feeding in the elucidation of the biogenesis of tropane alkaloids, see Beresford and Woolley, *Phytochemistry*, 1975, **14**, 2209.)

Administration of precursors.   Negative results arising from feeding experiments must also be interpreted with caution; thus, the administered precursor may never have reached the necessary site of synthesis in the plant, or the plant may not, at the time of the experiments, have been synthesizing the constituent under investigation. Two examples of the latter situation which, until discovered, were the cause of misleading results in alkaloid studies were the cessation of hordenine production in barley seedlings 15–20 days after germination and the restricted synthesis of hyoscine, as distinct from hyoscyamine, in old plants of *Datura stramonium*.

Often, the actual weight of labelled material fed to the plant is extremely small and contamination of the solution by microorganisms, during infiltration, can lead to a loss, or even the complete disappearance, of the original compound. This situation is very likely to arise with infiltrations into non-sterile roots—it can, in some instances, be controlled by the use of broad-spectrum antibacterial agents.

A number of methods can be employed to introduce labelled substances into plants. Root feeding is particularly suited to plants which can be grown in hydroponic culture solution and which synthesize the compounds under investigation in the roots. Direct injection of precursor solutions is sometimes possible; this is particularly applicable to plants with hollow stems (Umbelliferae) and to capsules (opium poppy). For the introduction of [1-^{13}C]glucose solution into chamomile flowers K.-P. Adam and J. Zapp (*Phytochemistry*, 1998, **48**, 953) used a microsyringe, injected into the hollow receptacle of the inflorescence. With rigid tissues it is difficult to avoid a loss of solution from the site of injection by this method. Infiltrations can be made into rigid stems by using a wick consisting of a thread drawn through the stem and dipping into the labelled solution; alternatively, a flap can be cut in the stem and this dipped into the solution to be inflitrated.

Sequential analysis.   A second method of investigation with ^{14}C is to grow plants in an atmosphere of [14]CO$_2$ and, by analysis of the plants at given time intervals, to obtain the sequence in which various related compounds become labelled. From the results obtained, certain biosynthetic routes may become apparent and others rejected. Here, again, degradation of the isolated radioactive compounds is important, because some units of the molecule may become labelled more rapidly than others. This method has been very successfully used in the elucidation of the path of carbon in photosynthesis and also for determining the sequential formation of the opium, hemlock and tobacco alkaloids. Exposure periods to [14]CO$_2$ as short as 5 min. have been used to obtain evidence of the biosynthetic sequence piperitone → (−)-menthone → (−)-menthol in *Mentha piperita*. In a number of instances the pathways suggested by these experiments have been at variance with those obtained by feeding labelled intermediates; it would seem that the latter are therefore examples of non-obligatory intermediates.

Use of stable isotopes.   The stable isotopes ^{2}H, ^{13}C, ^{15}N, and ^{18}O, which have a low natural occurrence, can be used in the same way as radioactive elements for labelling compounds to be used as possible intermediates in biosynthetic pathways. The usual methods of detection are mass spectroscopy (^{15}N and ^{18}O) and nuclear magnetic resonance (NMR) spectroscopy (^{1}H and ^{13}C). It is the latter which is becoming of increasing significance for biosynthetic studies (the use of mass spectroscopy and NMR spectroscopy in biogenetic studies should not be confused with their extensive use in structural analysis of organic compounds).

ISOLATED ORGANS, TISSUES AND CELLS

The cultivation of isolated organs and tissues of plants eliminates interference from other parts of the plant which may produce secondary changes in the metabolites. It can be used for feeding experiments in conjunction with labelled compounds and is also useful for the determination of the site of synthesis of particular compounds.

Isolated shoots of plants, when placed in a suitable solution or in water, will usually remain turgid for some days and during this time presumably have a normal metabolism; soon, however, a pathological metabolism commences. The technique can be refined by aseptically connecting the cut end of the shoot to a reservoir of suitable sterile nutrient, when the shoots will remain normal for much longer periods. Such shoots often develop roots at the cut ends—a factor which could invalidate the results of an experiment. The technique has been recently (2007) used for the study of the biogenesis of hyperforin and adhyperforin in *Hypericum performatum* (q.v.). Isolated leaves can be similarly maintained. *Rooted leaves* have been used in studies on *Nicotiana* and *Datura*. By this method a large quantity of root is obtained with a relatively small amount of aerial parts. It has the advantage that the nutrient solution requires no sugar, as sufficient starch is synthesized in the leaf and consequently bacterial and fungal growth in the nutrient solution is minimized. *Petal discs* have been used in the investigation of the biosynthesis of oil of rose. *Isolated roots* have been extensively used. Surface-sterilized seeds are germinated under aseptic conditions, and the root is severed and transferred to a sterile nutrient solution. Under suitable conditions a rapid growth is obtained and subcultures may be produced as necessary. In this way strains of tomato roots have been maintained for many years. For biogenetic and growth studies, selected compounds can be added to the culture as necessary. It has been demonstrated by this method that tropane alkaloids are formed in the roots of a number of Solanaceae. Also, the incorporation of a number of precursors into the alkaloids has been followed.

The technique can be extended to the cultivation of *isolated tissues and cells* (see Chapter 13), the use of which affords considerable potential in the investigation of biogenetic pathways. They offer the prospect of absolutely uniform plant material, obtainable at all times and manageable under regulated and reproducible conditions—factors rarely possible in work with entire living plants. Furthermore, potential precursors of the metabolite under investigation can easily be added to the system and samples can be taken repeatedly for analysis. The aseptic nature of the culture means that bacterial and fungal modifications of the precursor are eliminated. The method has recently been used to study the bifurcation of the taxoid biosynthetic pathway in *Taxus caspidata* by the administration of early precursors to the cell culture (R. E. B. Ketchum *et al.*, *Phytochemistry*, 2007, **68**, 335).

GRAFTS

Grafting techniques have considerable use in biosynthetic studies, particularly for the determination of the sites of primary and secondary metabolism of some secondary plant products.

Alkaloid formation by grafted plants has been extensively studied in *Nicotiana* and the tropane alkaloid-producing Solanaceae. Thus, tomato scions grafted on to *Datura* stocks accumulate tropane alkaloids, whereas *Datura* scions on tomato stocks contain only a small amount of tropane alkaloids. This suggests the main site of alkaloid synthesis to be the *Datura* roots. However, interspecific grafts involving *D. ferox* and *D. stramonium* demonstrate that secondary modifications of alkaloids do occur in the aerial parts of these plants. This has been demonstrated conclusively by feeding alkaloid-free scions of *D. ferox* on *Cyphomandra betacea* stocks with hyoscyamine; on subsequent analysis, hyoscine was isolated from the leaves. More details of this conversion are given in the appropriate section.

In other genera it has been shown by grafts involving tomato that the alkaloid anabasine is produced in the leaves of *Nicotiana glauca*, nicotine in the roots of *N. tabacum* and the pungent principle of capsicum, capsaicin, in the developing fruits. Reciprocal grafts of high and low resin-yielding strains of *Cannabis* have shown this biochemical character to be determined by the aerial parts.

MUTANT STRAINS

Large numbers of mutant strains of microorganisms have been produced which lack a particular enzyme, which results in their metabolism being blocked at a particular stage. Such an organism may accumulate the intermediate compound immediately before the block and for its survival may require an artificial supply of another intermediate which arises after the block. Such organisms are obviously useful materials in biosynthetic studies and have proved of major importance in some investigations.

A mutant of *Lactobacillus acidophilus*, by its ability to utilize a constituent of 'brewer's solubles' but not acetate, led to the isolation of mevalonic acid, an important intermediate of the isoprenoid compound pathway.

Ultraviolet-induced mutants of ergot auxotrophic with respect to a number of amino acids have been produced; cultures of these have been used to inoculate rye and the resulting alkaloid contents of the sclerotia have been investigated. *Gibberella* mutants have been used to obtain novel isoprenoid compounds. With higher plants, in spite of repeated attempts with chemicals and irradiation, less success has been obtained in producing mutants useful for the study of biogenesis of therapeutically active compounds; the production of mature haploid plants from cell cultures of pollen (see Chapter 14) may offer a more satisfactory starting material for future work.

Further reading

Harborne JB 1998 Phytochemical methods—a guide to modern techniques. Chapman and Hall (now under Kluwer Academic Publishers imprint), Dordrecht, Nl

Houghton PJ, Raman A 1998 Laboratory handbook for the fractionation of natural products. Chapman and Hall (now under Kluwer Academic Publishers imprint), Dordrecht, Nl

Khaledi MG 1998 High performance capillary electrophoresis. J. Wiley, New York, NY

Meyer V 1999 Practical high-performance liquid chromatography, 3rd edn. J. Wiley, Chichester, UK

Mukhopadhyay M 2000 Natural extracts using supercritical carbon dioxide. CRC Press, Boca Raton, FL

Phillipson JD 2007 Phytochemistry and pharmacognosy. Phytochemistry 68: 2960–2972. *Review with 63 references*

Reich E, Schibli A 2007 High-performance TLC for the analysis of medicinal plants. Thieme, Stuttgart

Taylor LT 1996 Supercritical fluid extraction. J. Wiley and Sons, New York, NY

Wagner H, Bladt S, Rickl V 2003 Plant drug analysis. A thin-layer chromatography atlas. Springer, Berlin

18

Basic metabolic pathways and the origin of secondary metabolites

The biosynthesis of both primary and secondary metabolites is dependent on the highly organized structure of the plant and animal cell. Unlike animal cells, those of plants possess a rigid cell wall and are separated one from another by an intercellular structure, the middle lamella. Direct connection between adjacent cells is maintained by primary pit fields through which pass the plasmodesmata. Within the cell wall is the protoplast consisting of cytoplasm, nucleus and various organelles.

The light microscope shows the nucleus to contain various inclusions such as nucleoli, chromosomes (stainable during cell division) and the nuclear sap. The nucleus appears to be suspended within the cell by the cytoplasm, in which there may be large vacuoles with their own characteristic contents (crystals, aleurone grains, etc.). Other cytoplasmic inclusions are mitochondria, Golgi bodies, lysosomes and plastids (chloroplasts, chromoplasts, leucoplasts), but their structure is not resolvable, because of their small size. Electron microscopy shows a number of the subcellular organelles to have a highly organized fine structure suited to the many and varied biochemical processes which they perform.

Although, because of varied form and function, it is not possible to illustrate a 'typical' plant cell Fig. 18.1A shows diagrammatically the structures that might be expected in an unspecialized young root cell. Such a cell possesses a rigid wall, which immediately distinguishes it from an animal cell, but no chloroplasts and only small vacuoles are present. In a green plant cell (Fig. 18.1B) the same components are present but the large vacuole has oppressed the nucleus and cytoplasm towards the wall; green plastids often with starch granules are common.

The organelles allow the creation of different chemical environments within one cell, and furthermore, by their structure they increase the area available for surface reactions which are all-important in biological systems. A description of the various organelles is given in the 14th edition of this book and Fig. 18.1C illustrates some aspects of their interdependence in the normal functioning of the cell. The molecular structures of these bodies have been extensively studied and details will be found in standard botanical texts.

Some basic metabolic pathways appear to be similar in both plants and animals, whereas others are more restricted in their occurrence. It is to the secondary plant products (i.e. those not necessarily involved in the essential metabolism of the cell) that the majority of vegetable drugs owe their therapeutic activity and so it is in these that pharmacognosists are particularly interested. However, as illustrated in Fig. 18.2, the production of these secondary metabolites is dependent on the fundamental metabolic cycles of the living tissue and so a brief indication of the latter will also be given; for fuller accounts of these, the student should consult a standard work on plant biochemistry.

ENZYMES

Many reactions occurring in the cell are enzyme-dependent, and before anything was known of the chemical nature of these substances it was recognized that they were organic catalysts produced by animal and vegetable cells. Their wide distribution and the delicacy of their operation has long been appreciated; they engineer reactions at normal temperatures and at pH values around neutral in a manner not possible in the laboratory.

An enzyme usually acts on one substance or class of substances, since it is specific for a particular atomic group or linkage. Specificity, however, varies; lipases are, in general, not highly specific, whereas fumarase acts only upon L-malate and fumarate, while D-malate is a competitive inhibitor of fumarase. Enzymes are also stereo- and regiospecific in their actions and, as it becomes possible to prepare more rare examples, organic chemists are becoming increasingly aware of enzyme potential for carrying out single-step transformations with complete

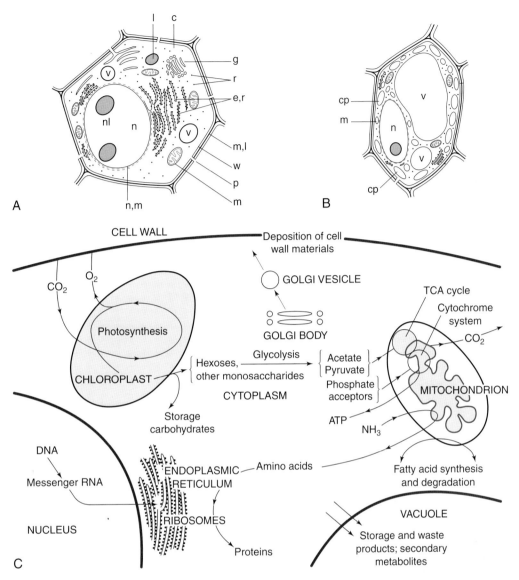

Fig. 18.1
The plant cell. A, diagrammatic representation of an undifferentiated cell: c, cytoplasm; e.r, endoplasmic reticulum; g, Golgi apparatus; l, lysosome; m, mitochondrion; m.l, middle lamella; n, nucleus; nl, nucleolus; n.m, nuclear membrane; p, pit in wall; r, ribosomes, w, primary cell wall; v, vacuole. B, green plant cell: cp, chloroplast; m, mitochondrion, n, nucleus; v, vacuole. C, Flow chart of some cell metabolites.

stereochemical exactitude, an aspect important in the synthesis of many drugs. An enzyme will convert many thousand times its own weight, and the gradual diminution in activity which takes place is probably due to secondary reactions which bring about destruction of the enzyme.

The enzymology of the secondary metabolic pathways in plants has still been little investigated but progress is being made and here again cell cultures have proved useful in that they are often a better source for the isolation of enzymes than is the differentiated plant. In some cases, e.g. cell cultures of volatile oil-containing plants, little or no oil accumulates in the culture owing to the absence of storage receptacles but the relevant enzymes for terpenoid synthesis are still manufactured and preparations of them can be made.

New horizons for the study of the enzymology of secondary metabolism have now opened up as a result of advances in gene technology. In suitable instances, by cloning, the cDNA responsible for an enzyme's synthesis can be expressed in another organism such as a bacterium and large amounts of enzyme prepared. By conventional methods only very small amounts of purified enzyme could be obtained from the original plant material. Of particular interest has been the isolation,

characterization and cloning of the enzyme strictosidine synthase. This governs the key reaction for the commencement of the biosynthesis of the very many monoterpenoid indole alkaloids, namely the condensation of tryptamine and secologanin to give $3\alpha(S)$-strictosidine (see Chapter 26); for a review (126 references) on this enzyme see T. M. Kutchan, *Phytochemistry*, 1993, **32**, 493.

By means of relatively new technology, enzymes can be immobilized on a suitable carrier either in whole plant cells or as the isolated enzyme. In this way these biocatalysts can be repeatedly used in analytical and clinical chemistry, or to effect specific chemical transformations.

Like other catalysts, enzymes influence the rate of a reaction without changing the point of equilibrium. For example, lipase catalyses either the synthesis of glycerides from glycerol and fatty acids or the hydrolysis of glycerides, the final point of equilibrium being the same in either case. Similarly, β-glucosidase (prunase) has been used for both the synthesis and the hydrolysis of β-glucosides. In plants such reversible reactions may proceed in one direction or the other under different conditions, often resulting in daily and seasonal variations in the accumulation of metabolites.

18

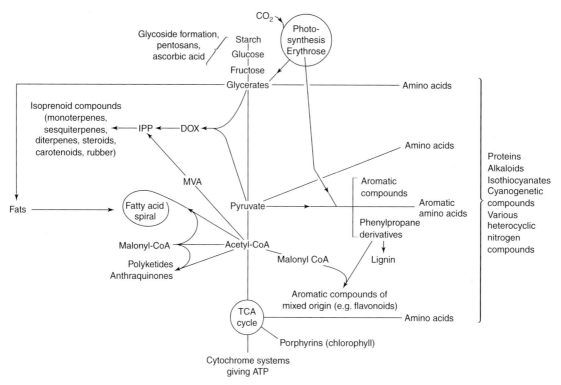

Fig. 18.2
Origins of some secondary metabolites in relation to the basic metabolic pathways of plants. DOX=deoxyxylulose; IPP=isopentenyl diphosphate; MVA=mevalonic acid.

Enzymes are colloidal in nature and consist of protein or contain protein as an essential part. They may be partly purified, and in some cases isolated, by the methods of protein chemistry (i.e. by fractional precipitation, dialysis and, more recently, gel and affinity chromatography, see Chapter 17). Most enzymes are soluble either in water or in dilute salt solutions and are precipitated by alcohol or acetone (acetone powders) and by high concentrations of salts. They are inactivated by heat, ultraviolet light and X-rays or by any treatment which brings about denaturation of proteins.

The activity of enzymes is markedly affected by the reaction of the medium and the presence of substances such as salts. It is well known, for example, that pepsin works only in an acid medium and trypsin in an alkaline one. In general, carbohydrases have pH optima of 3.8–7.5 and lipases optima of pH 5–8, while enzymes which act on bases all have optima more alkaline than pH 7.

The effect of heat on enzymes is of considerable importance in the drying of drugs. At low temperatures enzymic changes are not usually marked, although the proteolytic or protein-splitting enzymes in cod livers do bring about some hydrolysis at temperatures approaching zero. The optimum working temperatures of different enzymes vary, but they usually lie between 35 and 50°C. At temperatures of about 60°C destruction of the enzymes is usually fairly rapid, although considerable loss may take place below this temperature. When dry, enzymes show increased resistance to heat; thus, zymase, which in the presence of moisture is rapidly inactivated at 50°C, will, when dry, resist a temperature of 85°C.

Chemical nature

Following the isolation of urease in crystalline form by Sumner in 1926, many other enzymes have been prepared in a crystalline form and their protein nature has been established. Their molecular weights are high, but vary from about 9000 (hydrogenase) to about 1 000 000. In many cases the component amino acids are known and in some cases (e.g. ribonuclease) the amino acid sequence within the molecule has been determined. During the isolation of an enzyme, the purified protein (apoenzyme) may be inactive but regains its activity in the presence of an essential coenzyme or activator, which may be organic or inorganic.

Coenzymes

Some enzymes which require the presence of smaller organic molecules, called coenzymes, before they can function are of very common occurrence and participate in a large number of important biochemical reactions. One group of coenzymes consists of esters of phosphoric acid and various nucleosides. The adenosine and uridine phosphates contain one basic unit each (mononucleotides); they serve to transport energy in the form of high-energy phosphate bonds and this energy is made available for biochemical reactions in the presence of the appropriate enzyme by hydrolysis of the bond. Thus, the terminal phosphate bond of the adenosine triphosphate (ATP) on hydrolysis to adenosine diphosphate (ADP) affords 50 000 J mol^{-1}.

Uridine triphosphate (UTP) is involved in the synthesis of sucrose via diphosphate glucose which is also associated with the formation of uronic acids and cellulose.

Nicotinamide-adenine dinucleotide (NAD) and nicotinamide-adenine dinucleotide phosphate (NADP) contain two basic units each and are termed dinucleotides. They function in oxidation–reduction systems with appropriate enzymes; the oxidized forms are written NAD$^+$ and NADP$^+$ and the reduced forms NADH and NADPH respectively.

Another important coenzyme is coenzyme A (CoA), which contains the units adenosine-3,5-diphosphate, pantothenic acid-4-phosphate and thioethanolamine. It participates in the transfer of acetyl and acyl groups, acetyl-CoA (active acetate) having a central role in plant and animal metabolism.

Coenzyme A

Riboflavine (Fig. 31.2) is a component of the two coenzymes flavin mononucleotide (FMN) and flavin adenine dinucleotide (FAD). They participate in the biological oxidation–reduction system, and FAD facilitates the transfer of H$^+$ ions from NADH to the oxidized cytochrome system.

Other coenzymes are the decarboxylation coenzymes thiamine, biotin and pyridoxine (Fig. 31.2). Folic acid (Fig. 31.2) derivatives participate in enzymatic reactions which involve one-carbon fragment transfers.

A series of quinones e.g. plastoquinone and ubiquinone are widely distributed in plants, animals and microorganisms and function in biological electron transfer processes.

Classification of enzymes

As more enzymes are isolated, it becomes important to have a precise scheme of classification and nomenclature. Many long-established names such as pepsin, prunase, diastase and names for enzyme mixtures, such as emulsin and zymase, continue in use. A step towards uniform nomenclature was made when they were denoted by the name of the substrate and the termination '-ase'. Classes of enzymes were named similarly. Thus, the general term 'esterase' includes lipases, which hydrolyse fats; chlorophyllase hydrolyses chlorophyll; etc. The 1961 *Report of the Commission on Enzymes** made the recommendation that the chemical reactions catalysed be generally adopted for classification and nomenclature. This, of course, presupposes that the exact chemical reaction is known; see also the 1984 International Union of Biochemistry publication (London, UK: Academic Press) *Enzyme Nomenclature* and any later reports. Enzymes are classified into six main groups (Table 18.1).

Oxidoreductases. As any oxidation implies a simultaneous reduction, the names 'oxidase' and 'reductase' may be applied to a single type of enzyme. Eleven different groups of oxidoreductases are recognized. Many oxidases (that is, enzymes that utilize molecular oxygen as acceptor) convert phenolic substances to quinones. They act on guaiacum resin to produce a blue colour which is used as a test for their detection. Oxidases include laccase (1.10.3.2), present in lac, and ascorbate oxidase (1.10.3.3), which is widely distributed in plants. Oxalate oxidase (1.2.3.4), a flavoprotein present in mosses and the leaves of higher plants, oxidizes oxalic acid into carbon dioxide and hydrogen peroxide. Peroxidases (1.11) are distinguished by the fact that they use hydrogen peroxide and not oxygen as the hydrogen acceptor. Catalase (1.11) must be regarded as an exception, since it catalyses the decomposition of hydrogen peroxide. An oxidoreductase of the morphine biosynthetic pathway (Chapter 26) has recently been purified and characterized; it catalyses the stereoselective reduction of salutaridine to 7(*S*)-salutaridinol using NADPH as cosubstrate.

Hydrolases. These include many different types, of which the following are some of pharmaceutical importance.

1. Hydrolysing esters. These include lipases (3.1), which may be of vegetable or animal origin and which hydrolyse glycerides.

---

* This report has a numbered classification for each enzyme. For example, the enzyme present in garlic, alliine-lyase, is numbered 4.4.1.4. The first number denotes the fourth of the six main groups already mentioned and the other numbers further subdivisions. Thus:

    4 = lyases
    4.4 = carbon-sulphur lyases
    4.4.1 = In this example a further subdivision is not required.
4.4.1.4 = the fourth enzyme listed in the group, namely alliine-lyase (formerly known as alliinase) or allyl sulphinate-lyase.

Table 18.1 Classification of some enzymes.

Group	Trivial name	Systematic name
1. Oxidoreductases	Glucose dehydrogenase	β-D-Glucose: NAD(P)-oxidoreductase
	p-Diphenyl oxidase (lactase)	p-Diphenol: O_2 oxidoreductase
	Peroxidase	Donor: H_2O_2 oxidoreductase
	Catalase	H_2O_2: H_2O_2 orthoreductase
2. Transferase	α-Glucan phosphorylase	α-1,4-Glucan: orthophosphate glucosyl-transferase
3. Hydrolases	Lipase	Glycerol ester hydrolase
	Chlorophyllase	Chlorophyll chlorophyllidohydrolyase
	Tannase	Tannin acyl-hydrolase
	α-Amylase	α-1,4-Glucan 4-glucano-hydrolyase
	Inulase	Inulin 1-fructanohydrolase
4. Lyases	Aldolyase	Ketose-l-phosphate aldehydelyase
	Decarboxylase	L-Tryptophan-decarboxylase
5. Isomerases	Maleate isomerase	Maleate cis-trans-isomerase
6. Ligases (Synthetases)	Asparagine synthetase	L-Aspartate: ammonia ligase (ADP)

Mammalian lipases also hydrolyse other esters, such as phenyl salicylate, acetylcholine and atropine. Other esterases are chlorophyllase (3.1.1.14), which hydrolyses chlorophyll, and tannase (3.1.1.20), which hydrolyses ester links in tannins. Other esterases probably occur in many drugs which contain esters in their volatile oils (e.g. valerian).

2. Hydrolysing sugars and glycosides. To the important group of glycoside hydrolases (3.2.1) belong all those enzymes that hydrolyse sugars, carbohydrates and glycosides. Those hydrolysing sugars include β-fructofuranosidase (sucrase or invertase), lactase, maltase, gentiobiase and trehalase. Polysaccharide enzymes are represented by α-amylase (3.2.1.1), β-amylase, cellulase, lichenase, inulase. Among the glycoside-hydrolysing enzymes are β-glucosidase or β-D-glucoside glucohydralase (3.2.1.20), which has a wide specificity for β-D-glucopyranosides. More specific glucoside-hydrolysing enzymes are those acting on salicin, amygdalin, sinigrin and cardiac glycosides.

3. Hydrolysing the C–N linkage. Many enzymes act on peptide bonds. To this group belong the well-known animal enzymes pepsin, rennin, trypsin, thrombin and plasmin, and the vegetable enzymes papain (from *Carica papaya*) and ficin (from species of fig). All the above belong to the group 3.4.4. Other enzymes acting on linear amides (3.5.1) are asparaginase (present in liquorice and many other plants) and urease. Cyclic amides are acted on by penicillinase (3.5.2.6).

Lyases. Two important decarboxylases in the biosynthesis of monoterpenoid indole alkaloids and benzylisoquinoline alkaloids are L-tryptophan-decarboxylase (EC 4.1.1.27) amd L-tyrosine/L-dopa-decarboxylase (EC 4.1.1.25), respectively.

Isomerases. Two enzymes important in pathways leading to medicinally important metabolites are isopentenyl diphosphate (IPP) isomerase (EC 5.3.3.2) amd chalcone isomerase (EC 5.5.1.6). The former is involved in the isomerization of IPP and dimethylallyl diphosphate (Fig. 18.18), an essential step in the formation of terpenoids, and the latter is a key enzyme catalysing the isomerization of chalcones to their corresponding flavanones (Fig. 18.11).

PHOTOSYNTHESIS

Photosynthesis, by which the carbon dioxide of the atmosphere is converted into sugars by the green plant, is one of the fundamental cycles on which life on Earth, as we know it, depends. Until 1940, when investigations involving isotopes were undertaken, the detailed mechanism of this 'carbon reduction' was unknown, although the basic overall reaction,

$$CO_2 + H_2O \xrightarrow{\text{light}} (CH_2O) + O_2$$

had been accepted for many years.

Photosynthesis occurs in the chloroplasts: green, disc-shaped organelles of the cytoplasm which are bounded by a definite membrane and which are autoreproductive. Separated from the rest of the cell, the chloroplasts can carry out the complete process of photosynthesis. Bodies with similar properties are found in cells of the red algae but these contain, in addition to chlorophyll as the principal pigment, other tetrapyrrole derivatives—the phycobilins.

The light microscope reveals no definite internal structure of the chloroplasts, but electron microscopy shows these bodies to have a highly organized structure in which the chlorophyll molecules are arranged within orderly structures (grana), each granum being connected with others by a network of fibres or membranes. According to one theory, the flat chlorophyll molecules themselves are orientated between layers of protein and lipid molecules so that the whole chloroplast can be looked upon as a battery containing several cells (the grana), each cell possessing layers of plates (the chlorophyll molecules).

Two fundamental processes which take place in photosynthesis, both of which require light, are the production of adenosine triphosphate (ATP) from adenosine diphosphate (ADP) and phosphate and the light-energized decomposition of water (the Hill reaction; named after the English biochemist Robert Hill, 1899–1991):

$$H_2O \xrightarrow{h\nu} 2[H] + \tfrac{1}{2}O_2$$

ATP is a coenzyme and the high energy of the terminal phosphate bond is available to the organism for the supply of the energy necessary for endergonic reactions. The Hill reaction produces free oxygen and hydrogen ions which bring about the conversion of the electron carrier, NADP, to its reduced form NADPH (see 'Coenzymes').

In this complicated process, two systems, Photosystem I and Photosystem II (also known as pigment systems I and II) are commonly referred to; they involve two chlorophyll complexes which absorb light at different wavelengths (above and below $\lambda = 685$ nm). Photosystem II produces ATP and Photosystem I supplies all the reduced NADP and some ATP. In these light reactions the chlorophyll molecule captures solar energy and electrons become excited and move to higher energy levels; on returning to the normal low-energy state, the electrons give up their excess energy, which is passed through a series of carriers (including in the case of Photosystem II plastoquinone and several cytochromes) to generate ATP. Photosystem I involves an electron acceptor and the subsequent reduction of ferredoxin in the production of NADPH. Reference to the current literature indicates that the nature and organization of the photosystems remains a very active research area. Students will have observed that an alcoholic solution of chlorophyll possesses, in sunlight, a red fluorescence—no carriers are available to utilize the captured energy and it is re-emitted as light. Hill first demonstrated in 1937 that isolated chloroplasts, when exposed to light, were capable of producing oxygen, provided that a suitable hydrogen acceptor was present. Work with isotopes has since proved that the oxygen liberated during photosynthesis is derived from water and not from carbon dioxide.

Following the light reactions, a series of dark reactions then utilize NADPH in the reduction of carbon dioxide to carbohydrate.

Current research suggests that terrestrial plants can be classified as C_3, C_4, intermediate C_3–C_4 and CAM plants in relation to photosynthesis.

C_3 plants

The elucidation of the carbon reduction cycle (Fig. 18.3), largely by Calvin and his colleagues, was in large measure determined by methods dependent on exposing living plants (*Chlorella*) to ^{14}C-labelled carbon dioxide for precise periods of time, some very short and amounting to a fraction of a second. The radio-active compounds produced were then isolated and identified. In this way a sequence for the formation of compounds was obtained. 3-Phosphoglyceric acid, a C_3 compound, was the compound first formed in a labelled condition but it was only later in the investigation, after a number of 4-, 5-, 6- and 7-carbon systems had been isolated, that ribulose-1,5-diphosphate was shown to be the molecule with which carbon dioxide first reacts to give two molecules of phosphoglyceric acid. An unstable intermediate in this reaction is 2-carboxy-3-ketopentinol.

C_4 plants

Some plants which grow in semi-arid regions in a high light intensity possess an additional carbon-fixation system which, although less efficient in terms of energy utilization, is more effective in its use of carbon dioxide, so cutting down on photorespiration and loss of water. Such plants are known as C_4 plants, because they synthesize, in the presence of light, oxaloacetic and other C_4 acids. Carbon assimilation is based on a modified leaf anatomy and biochemistry. Its presence in plants appears haphazard and has been linked with the so-called Kranz syndrome of associated anatomical features. In the mesophyll cells pyruvate is converted via oxaloacetate to malate, utilizing carbon dioxide, and the malate, or in some cases aspartate, is transported to the vascular bundle cells, where it is oxidatively decarboxylated to pyruvate again, carbon dioxide and NADPH, which are used in the Calvin cycle. Pyruvate presumably returns to the mesophyll cells. Plants possessing this facility exhibit two types of photosynthetic cells which differ in their chloroplast type. Intermediate C_3–C_4 pathways are also known.

CAM plants

This term stands for 'crassulacean acid metabolism', so called because it was in the Crassulaceae family that the distinctive character of a build-up of malic acid during hours of darkness was first observed. Other large families, including the Liliaceae, Cactaceae and Euphorbiaceae, possess members exhibiting a similar biochemistry. As with C_4 plants, this is an adaptation of the photosynthetic cycle of plants which can exist under drought conditions. When water is not available, respiratory carbon dioxide is recycled, under conditions of darkness, with the formation of malic acid as an intermediate. Carbon dioxide and water loss to the atmosphere are eliminated, a condition which would be fatal for normal C_3 plants.

From fructose, produced in the Calvin cycle, other important constituents, such as glucose, sucrose and starch, are derived: erythrose is a precursor in the synthesis of some aromatic compounds. Glucose-6-phosphate is among the early products formed by photosynthesis and it is an important intermediate in the oxidative pentose phosphate cycle and for conversion to glucose-1-phosphate in polysaccharide synthesis.

CARBOHYDRATE UTILIZATION

Storage carbohydrate such as the starch of plants or the glycogen of animals is made available for energy production by a process which involves conversion to pyruvate and then acetate, actually acetyl-coenzyme A, the latter then passing into the tricarboxylic acid cycle (Fig. 18.4). As a result of this, the energy-rich carbohydrate is eventually oxidized to carbon dioxide and water. During the process, the hydrogen atoms liberated are carried by coenzymes into the cytochrome system, in which energy is released in stages, with the possible formation of ATP from ADP and inorganic phosphate. Eventually the hydrogen combines with oxygen to form water.

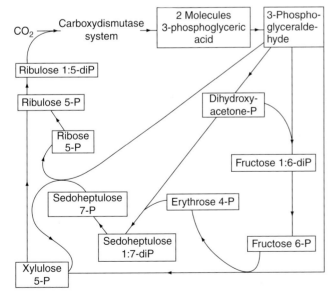

Fig. 18.3
The path of carbon in photosynthesis (after Calvin); the formulae of the sugars involved are given in Chapter 20.

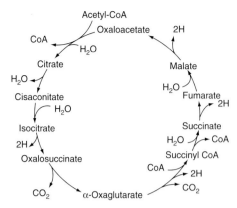

Fig. 18.4
The tricarboxylic acid cycle (TCA) or Krebs cycle.

A number of pathways for the initial metabolism of glucose are known for various living tissues. One involves compounds which are found in the photosynthetic cycle, and it appears as a reversal of this cycle but the mechanism is apparently quite different. Another pathway is the Embden–Meyerhoff scheme of glycolysis (Fig. 18.5).

The kinetics and enzyme systems involved in the above pathways have been studied extensively. It will be noted that one molecule of glucose can give rise to two molecules of pyruvate, each of which is converted to acetate, and one molecule of carbon dioxide. One turn of the TCA cycle represents the oxidation of one acetate to two molecules of carbon dioxide, giving rise to twelve molecules of ATP. The overall reaction for the metabolism of one molecule of glucose in terms of ADP and ATP is

$$C_6H_{12}O_6 + 6CO_2 + 38ADP + 38P \text{ (inorganic)}$$
$$\longrightarrow 6H_2O + 6CO_2 + 38ATP$$

The above schemes, given in barest outline, are fundamental not only for the building up and breaking down of reserve foodstuffs, but also in that the intermediates are available for the biosynthesis of all other groups of compounds found in plants. The levels at which some of the important groups arise are indicated in Fig. 18.2.

GLYCOSIDES

Glycosides are formed in nature by the interaction of the nucleotide glycosides—for example, uridine diphosphate glucose (UDP-glucose)—with the alcoholic or phenolic group of a second compound. Such glycosides, sometimes called *O*-glycosides, are the most numerous ones found in nature. Other glycosides do, however, occur in which the linkage is through sulphur (*S*-glycosides), nitrogen (*N*-glycosides) or carbon (*C*-glycosides).

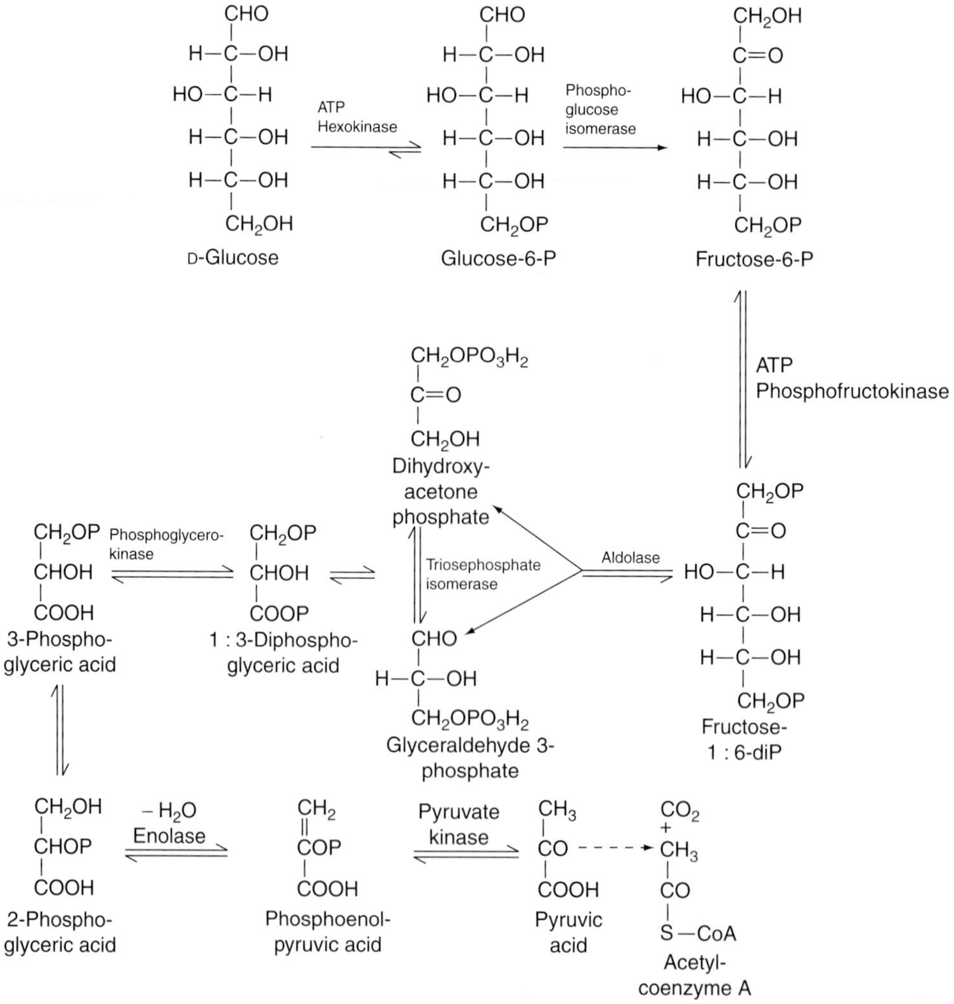

Fig. 18.5
Outline of the Embden–Meyerhoff scheme of glycolysis.

The formation and hydrolysis of an *O*-glycoside such as salicin may be represented:

$$R.\boxed{OH} + \boxed{H}O.X \rightleftharpoons R.OX + H_2O$$

Sugar   Aglycone   Glycoside

or

$$C_6H_{11}O_5OH + HO.C_6H_4.CH_2OH \rightleftharpoons C_6H_{11}O_5.O.C_6H_4.CH_2OH + H_2O$$

Glucose   Salicyl alcohol   Salicin
(saligenin)

It will be noted that such reactions are reversible and in plants glycosides are both synthesized and hydrolysed under the influence of more or less specific enzymes. While glycosides do not themselves reduce Fehling's solution, the simple sugars which they produce on hydrolysis will do so with precipitation of red cuprous oxide.

The sugars found in glycosides may be monosaccharides such as glucose, rhamnose and fucose or, more rarely, deoxysugars such as the cymarose found in cardiac glycosides. More than one molecule of such sugars may be attached to the aglycone either by separate linkages, which is rare, or, more commonly, as a di-, tri- or tetrasaccharide. Such complex glycosides are formed by the stepwise addition of sugars to the aglycone molecule.

Since sugars exist in isomeric α- and β-forms, both types are theoretically possible. Practically all natural glycosides, however, are of the β-type, although the α-linkage is found in nature in some carbohydrates such as sucrose, glycogen and starch. In *k*-strophanthoside, a glycoside formed from the aglycone strophanthidin and strophanthotriose (cymarose + glucose + glucose) the outer glucose molecule has the α-linkage and the inner glucose the β-linkage. Isomeric glycosides may be prepared synthetically; for example, from glucose and methyl alcohol one obtains both the α- and β-methyl glucosides by introducing methyl groups into the OH groups printed in heavy type in the formulae of glucose below.

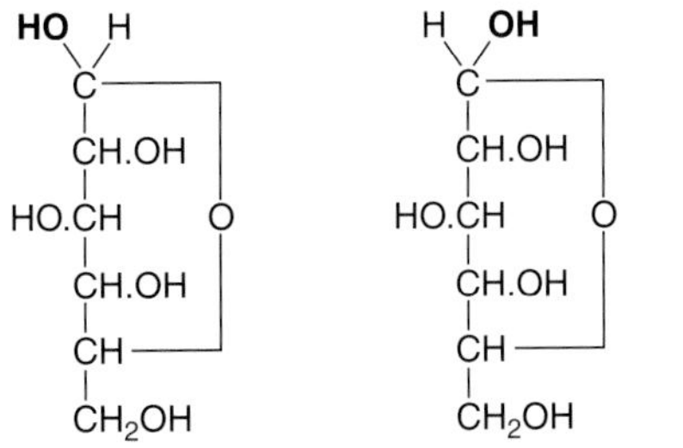

β-Glycoside forming structure   α-Glycoside forming structure

The term 'glycoside' is a very general one which embraces all the many and varied combinations of sugars and aglycones. More precise terms are available to describe particular classes. Some of these terms refer to the sugar part of the molecule, others to the aglycone, while others indicate some well-defined physical or pharmacological property. Thus, a *glucoside* is a glycoside having glucose as its sole sugar component; a *pentoside* yields a sugar such as arabinose; *rhamnosides* yield the methyl-pentose rhamnose; and *rhamnoglucosides* yield both rhamnose and glucose. Terms used for aglycones are generally self-explanatory (e.g. phenol, anthraquinone and sterol glycosides). The names 'saponin' (soap-like), 'cyanogenetic' (producing hydrocyanic acid) and 'cardiac' (having an action on the heart), although applied to these substances when little was known about them, are useful terms which do in fact bring together glycosides of similar chemical structure.

The older system of naming glycosides using the termination '-in' (e.g. senegin, salicin, aloin, strophanthin) is too well established to be easily changed. It is not ideal, however, since many non-glycosidal substances (e.g. inulin and pectin) have the same termination. Modern workers more frequently use the termination '-oside' (e.g. sennoside) and attempt to drop the older forms by writing sinigroside for sinigrin, salicoside for salicin and so on.

Although glycosides form a natural group in that they all contain a sugar unit, the aglycones are of such varied nature and complexity that glycosides vary very much in their physical and chemical properties and in their pharmacological action. In Part 5 they are classified according to that aglycone fragment with which they often occur in the plant.

FATS AND FATTY ACIDS

Fats, considered in more detail in Chapter 19, are triglycerides involving long-chain saturated or unsaturated acids and, as such, constitute an important food reserve for animals and plants (particularly in seeds). Related to the simple fats are the complex lipids, most of which are diesters of orthophosphoric acid; they have the status of fundamental cellular constituents.

The fatty acids, on liberation from the fat, are available for the production of acetyl-CoA by the removal of C_2 units. The elucidation of this spiral (Fig. 18.6) owes much to the work of Lynen and it was primarily investigated with animal tissues. In this β-oxidation sequence one turn of the spiral involves four reactions—two dehydrogenations, one hydration and a thiolysis liberating a two-carbon unit of acetyl-CoA. All these reactions can be shown by isolated enzyme studies to be reversible, and until about 1953 it was generally assumed that the biosynthetic route of fatty acids operated in the reverse direction, starting from acetyl-CoA. This, however, is not precisely so, as indicated below.

Biosynthesis of saturated fatty acids

From the above it was generally assumed that the biosynthetic route for fatty acids operated in the reverse direction to the β-oxidative sequence for the degradation of these acids and started with acetyl-CoA. However, the unfavourable equilibrium of the initial thiolase reaction in such a pathway:

$$2CH_3-\overset{O}{\underset{\|}{C}}-SCoA \rightleftharpoons CH_3-\overset{O}{\underset{\|}{C}}-CH_2-\overset{O}{\underset{\|}{C}}-SCoA + CoA$$

$$K_{eq} = 1.6 \times 10^{-5}$$

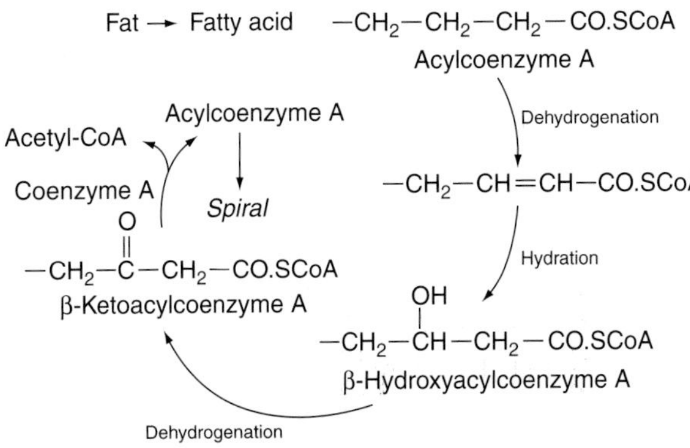

Fig. 18.6
Degradation of fatty acids. Reactions involved in one turn of the spiral.

and the poor yield of long-chain fatty acids obtained with purified enzymes of the β-oxidation pathway together with other observations suggested the possibility that this was not necessarily the principal biosynthetic pathway. It was then shown, with animal tissues, that malonyl coenzyme A was necessary for the initial condensation with acetate. In fact, in palmitic acid (C_{16},) only one of the eight C_2 units (i.e. the C15 + C16 carbons) is derived directly from acetyl-CoA; the other seven C_2 units are attached by malonyl-CoA, which is formed by carboxylation of acetyl-CoA.

One feature of this anabolic pathway is the involvement of the acyl carrier protein (ACP) to produce fatty acyl thioesters of ACP. This conversion serves (1) to activate the relatively unreactive fatty acid and (2) to provide a carrier for the fatty acid acyl group. Thus, these ACP thioesters appear to be obligatory intermediates in fatty acid synthesis, whereas it is the fatty acid thioesters of coenzyme A which operate in the catabolic oxidation pathway. The synthesis is explained by the reactions shown in Fig. 18.7. Reactions 4–7 are then repeated, lengthening the fatty acid chain by two carbons (derived from malonyl-S-ACP) at a time. Eight enzymes have been identified as being involved in the synthesis of palmitoyl-ACP and stearoyl-ACP from acetyl-CoA.

In purified enzyme systems, when propionyl-CoA replaced acetyl-CoA, the product was a C_{17} acid and, similarly, butyryl-CoA gave primarily a C_{18} (stearic) acid. Thus, the formation of these C_{16}, C_{17} and C_{18} acids may well depend on the availability of acetyl-, propionyl- and butyryl-CoA.

The system of biosynthesis of fatty acids in plants appears to operate in the same way as in animal tissues, but whereas in the latter the enzymes are located in the cytoplasm, in plants they are found in the mitochondria and chloroplasts. The mitochondria derived from the mesocarp of the avocado fruit have been used to demonstrate the incorporation of [^{14}C]acetate into esterified long-chain fatty acids.

Biosynthesis of unsaturated fatty acids

As a number of unsaturated fatty acids have a particular significance in pharmaceutical products, a treatment of their formation is deferred until Chapter 19.

AROMATIC BIOSYNTHESIS

The shikimic acid pathway

This appears to be an important route from carbohydrate for the biosynthesis of the C_6–C_3 units (phenylpropane derivatives), of which phenylalanine and tyrosine are both examples. A scheme of biogenesis for these aromatic amino acids, as elucidated in various organisms, is given in Fig. 18.8; for higher plants, the presence of the enzyme system responsible for the synthesis of shikimic acid has been confirmed.

An important branching point arises at chorismic acid; anthranilate synthase uses chorismic acid as a substrate to give anthranilic acid which is a precursor of tryptophan. The synthesis is controlled by the latter acting as a feedback inhibitor; chorismate mutase converts chorismic acid to prephenate, the precursor of phenylalanine and tyrosine, and a variety of control mechanisms appear to operate at the branching point. The opium alkaloids are synthesized via this pathway (Chapter 26) and two isoforms of chorismate mutase have been isolated and characterized from poppy seedlings (M. Benesova and R. Bode, *Phytochemistry*, 1992, **31**, 2983).

Although there are only small differences in the sequence of reactions for the shikimate pathway in bacteria, fungi and plants there are considerable differences in the molecular organization of the pathway. (For a review (123 refs), see J. Schmid and N. Amrhein, *Phytochemistry*, 1995, **39**, 737.)

The shikimic acid pathway is also important in the genesis of the aromatic building blocks of lignin and in the formation of some tannins, vanillin and phenylpropane units of the flavones and coumarins (see Chapter 21). For a review see 'Further reading'.

The acetate hypothesis

The central position of acetate in relation to the general metabolism of plants has already been indicated and it is possible to devise many possible routes by which acetate condensation could occur to give a variety of aromatic compounds. The general validity of the mechanism has been established by the use of labelled compounds but the detailed steps for many compounds remain to be established. Thus, the incorporation of [1-^{14}C]acetate into 6-methylsalicylic acid by *Penicillium griseofulvum* takes place as below:

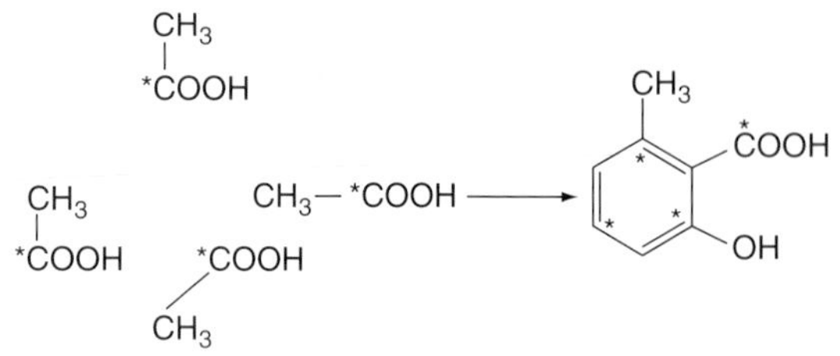

and the production of the mould anthraquinone metabolite endocrocin, from eight C_2 units, is represented in Fig. 18.9. Decarboxylation of endocrocin affords emodin. The original chain lengthening, which can be represented as a condensation of acetate units, is the same as in fatty acid production (q.v. above) but does not require the reduction of =CO to =CH$_2$. Thus, malonic acid plays a similar role in this aromatic synthesis to that in fatty acid formation and the chain is built up from the combination of malonyl units with a terminal acetyl (the starter) unit. Sometimes the starter unit is not acetate, as indicated with the

1. $CH_3CO\text{-}S\text{-}CoA + CO_2 + ATP \xrightarrow[\text{Biotin enzyme}]{Mn^{2+}} HOOCCH_2CO\text{-}S\text{-}CoA + ADP + Pi$

2.   acetyl-S-CoA + ACP-SH $\longrightarrow$ acetyl-S-ACP + CoASH

3.   malonyl-S-CoA + ACP-SH $\longrightarrow$ malonyl-S-ACP + CoASH

4.   malonyl-S-ACP + acetyl-S-ACP $\longrightarrow$ acetoacetyl-S-ACP + CO$_2$ + ACP-SH

5.   acetoacetyl-S-ACP + NADPH + H$^+$ $\longrightarrow$ D(–)-3-hydroxybutyryl-S-ACP + NADP$^+$

6.   D(–)-3-hydroxybutyryl-S-ACP $\longrightarrow$ crotonyl-S-ACP + HOH

7.   crotonyl-S-ACP + NADPH + H$^+$ $\longrightarrow$ butyryl-S-ACP + NADP$^+$

Fig. 18.7
Initial stages in the biosynthesis of fatty acids.

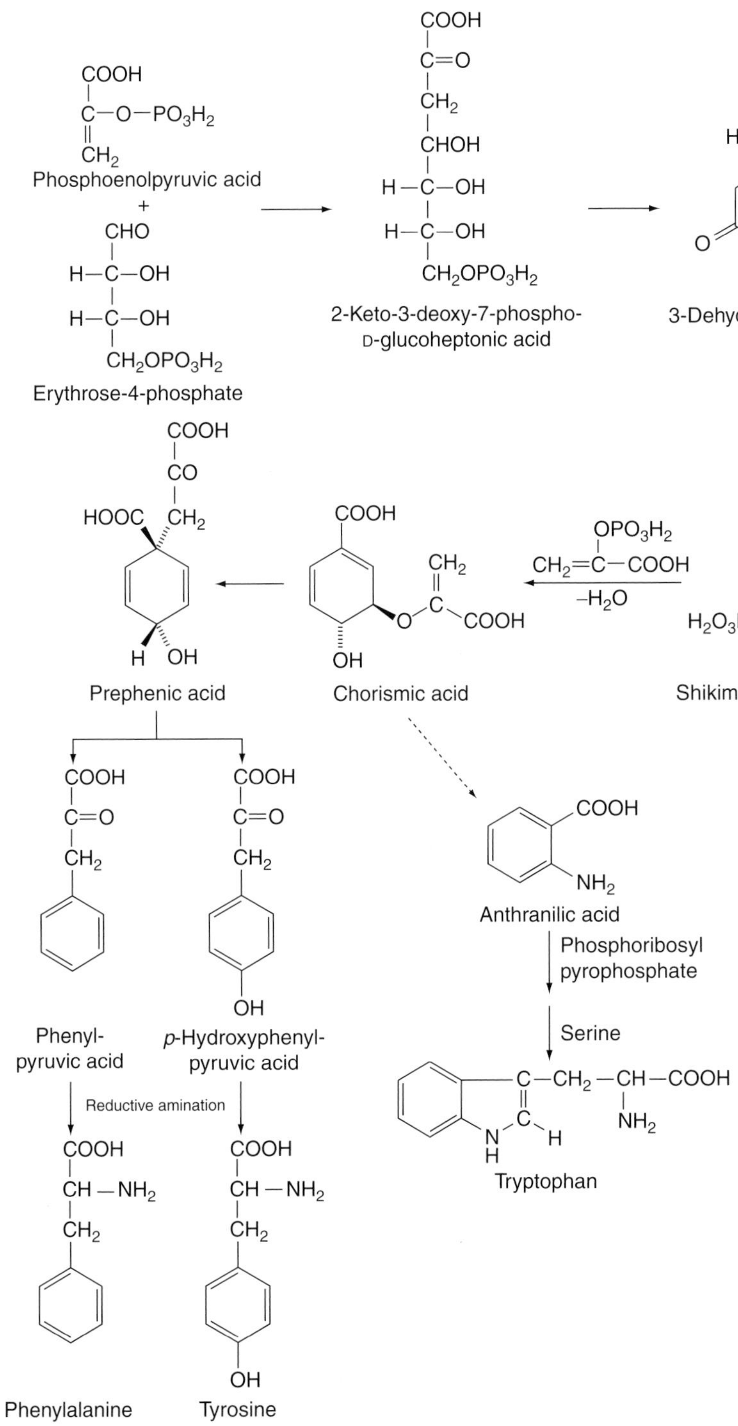

Fig. 18.8
Biosynthesis of aromatic compounds via the shikimic acid pathway.

formation of the tetracycline antibiotics from nine units; here malon-amide-SCoA is the starter unit and by invoking standard biochemical reactions tetracycline is formed (Fig. 18.10). Higher plants also utilize the polyacetate–malonate pathway for the biosynthesis of emodin-type anthraquinones, such compounds all having substituents on both outer rings.

From the anthraquinones listed in Chapter 21, it will be seen that the structures of some anthraquinones are not fully explained by the acetate–malonate pathway and these are discussed below. However,

there appear to be many exceptions to the rules in applying the general pathways to specific anthraquinones.

Compounds containing aromatic rings of different origin

The structures of anthraquinones such as alizarin, rubiadin, pseudopur-purin and morindadiol, pigments of the Rubiaceae and other families, cannot be readily explained on the acetate hypothesis.

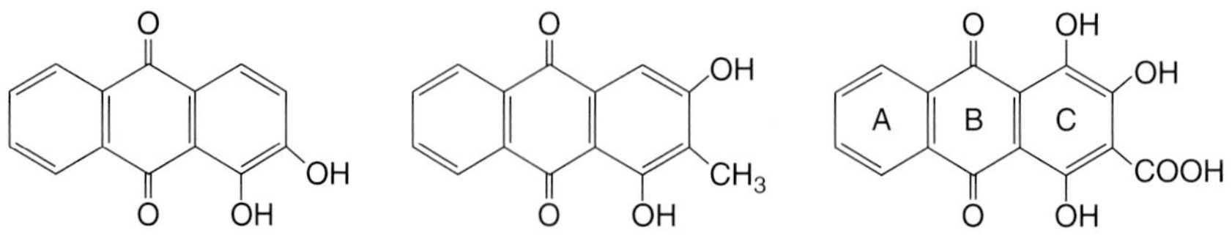

18

Alizarin   Rubiadin   Pseudopurpurin

Circumstantial evidence that these compounds might be formed from naphthoquinones with the participation of mevalonic acid (a key precursor in the formation of isopentenyl units, q.v.) was provided by their co-occurrence in teak and other plants with naphthoquinones having an isopentenyl residue (e.g. formula below).

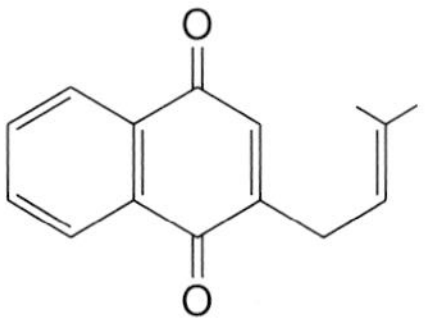

That mevalonate (itself derived from acetate) is involved in this formation has been shown by tracer experiments with *Rubia tinctorum*; ring C and carbon side-chain of pseudopurpurin and rubiadin are derived from mevalonate, and in the same plant shikimic acid has been shown to be incorporated into ring A of alizarin.

The aromatic rings of some compounds can be derived from both the shikimic acid and the acetic acid pathways. Thus, a phenylpropane formed by the former route may undergo chain lengthening by the addition of acetate units (via malonyl; see 'Fatty Acids', above) to give a polyketide and then, by ring closure, give a flavonoid derivative (Fig. 18.11).

Isoflavones are formed in the same manner, with a rearrangement of the aryl-B ring in relation to the three carbons (Fig. 18.11). The flavonoids, in addition to their importance in plants as pigments, have interesting medicinal properties and are discussed in more detail in Chapter 21.

Rotenoids (insecticides of *Derris* and *Lonchocarpus* spp.) show a structural relationship to the isoflavones; see Chapter 40.

Stilbenes (q.v.) are also compounds containing aromatic units of different biogenetic origin.

AMINO ACIDS

Amino acids occur in plants both in the free state and as the basic units of proteins and other metabolites. They are compounds containing one or more amino groups and one or more carboxylic acid groups.

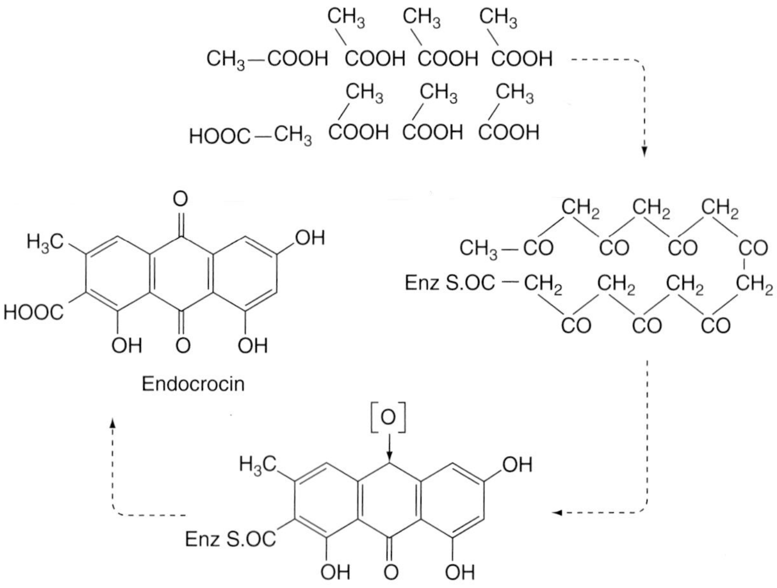

Fig. 18.9
Biogenesis of endocrocin.

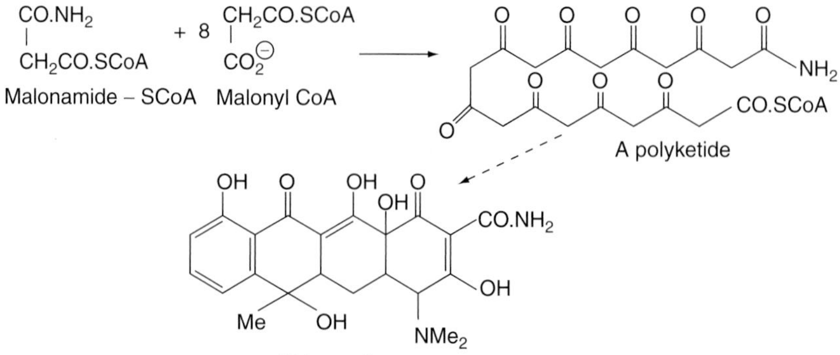

Fig. 18.10
Formation of tetracycline.

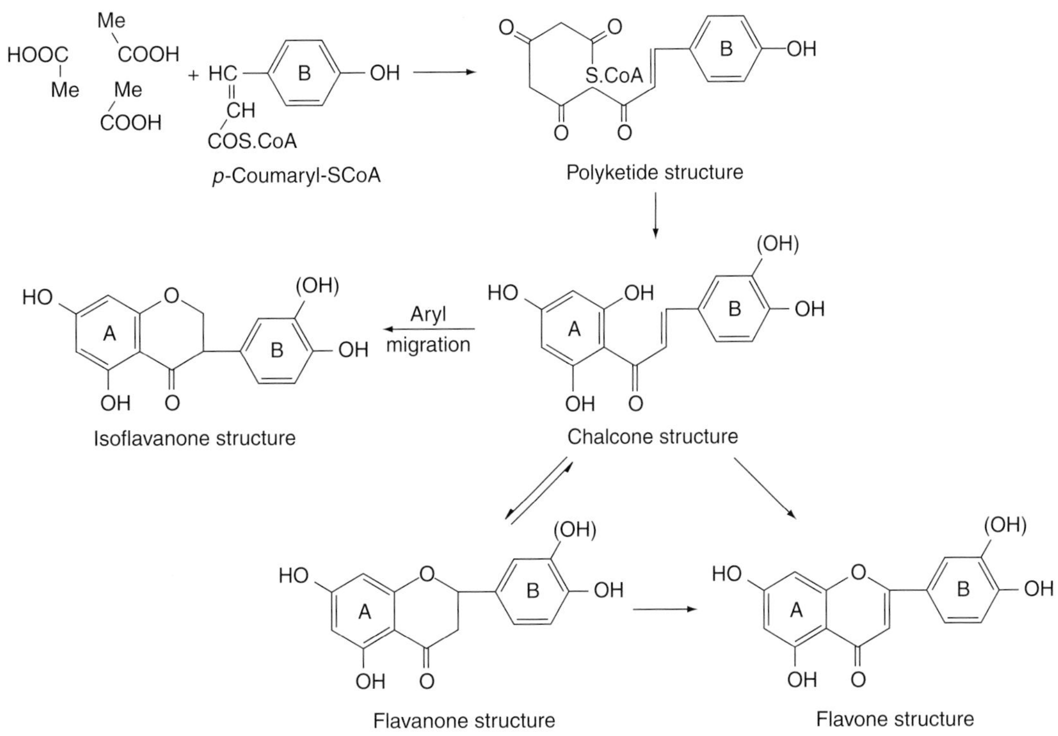

Fig. 18.11
Origin of flavanones, isoflavanones and flavones.

Most of those found in nature are α-amino acids with an asymmetric carbon atom and the general formula R–CH(NH$_2$)COOH. Some 20 different ones have been isolated from proteins, all having an L-configuration. Other amino acids occur in the free state and some having the D-configuration have been isolated from plants and microorganisms, where they may form antibiotic polypeptides.

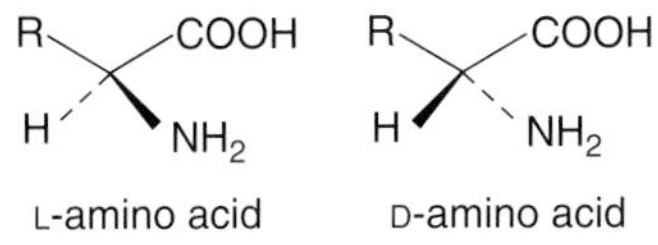

Many amino acids contain only carbon, hydrogen, oxygen and nitrogen, but other atoms may be present (e.g. sulphur in cystine, and iodine in thyroxin). As already mentioned, more than one amino group may be present (e.g. lysine, diaminocaproic acid) and more than one carboxylic acid group (e.g. aspartic or aminosuccinic acid). Some amino acids are aromatic such as phenylalanine, or heterocyclic such as proline (pyrrolidine nucleus), tryptophan (indole nucleus) and histidine (imidazole nucleus).

Amino acids are generally soluble in water but only slightly soluble in alcohol. A general test is to warm with ninhydrin, when, with the exception of proline, which gives a yellow, they give a pink, blue or violet colour. Amino acids do not respond to the biuret test (compare polypeptides and proteins). Certain amino acids are detected by more specific tests (e.g. histidine gives colour reactions with diazonium salts).

Amino acids found in proteins

These include α-alanine; arginine; asparagine (amide of aspartic acid), abundant in many plants, particularly etiolated seedlings; aspartic acid; aminosuccinic acid, involved in the biosynthesis of purines; cysteine, which contains sulphur; cystine or dicysteine (in hair and insulin); 3,5-di-iodotyrosine (in thyroid); glutamic acid (a component of the folic acid vitamins); glutamine (free in animals and plants, e.g. sugarbeet); glycine (aminoacetic acid); histidine; δ-hydroxylysine (in gelatin); hydroxyproline (in gelatin); leucine (α-aminocaproic acid); isoleucine;

lysine; methionine (contains a sulphur atom); 3-monoiodotyrosine (in thyroid); phenylalanine; proline; serine (in phosphoproteins such as casein); threonine (in casein); thyroxin (the iodine-containing thyroid-hormone); 3,5,3′-triiodothyronine (in thyroid); tryptophan; tyrosine and valine.

Amino acids found free and not occurring in proteins

Following the pioneer research of Fowden, several hundred of these amino acids have been characterized and only a few (e.g. γ-aminobutyric acid, α-aminoadipic acid, pipecolic acid and δ-acetylornithine) are of wide occurrence. Seeds or fleshy organs of plants are the principal sites for the accumulation of these compounds where they may serve as a nitrogen reserve. Other examples in this class are: β-alanine (β-aminopropionic acid); citrulline (an intermediate in the cycle of urea synthesis); creatine; ergothioneine (a sulphur-containing constituent of some animal tissues and of ergot); and taurine (a component of bile acids). A number have teratogenic properties (see Chapter 39). 3-N-Oxalyl-L-2, 3-diaminopropanoic acid is a neurotoxin present in the seeds of *Lathyrus sativus*, the grass pea; it is the causal agent of human neurolathyrism, an irreversible paralysis of the lower limbs, which occurs in some drought prone areas of Ethiopia, India and Bangladesh (see Yu-Haey Kuo *et al.*, *Phytochemistry*, 1994, **35**, 911 for references and biosynthetic studies). Other non-protein amino acids provide plant protection from insects.

Non-protein amino acids, considered oddities of plant biosynthesis 40 years ago, now constitute a group receiving increasing attention because of their possible physiological and ecological significance.

Biosynthesis of amino acids

As amino acids are also the precursors of some secondary metabolites, their biosyntheses will be considered below. They arise at various levels of the glycolytic and TCA systems.

Nitrogen appears to enter the metabolism of the organism by reductive amination of α-keto acids; pyruvic, oxalacetic and α-ketoglutaric acids give alanine, aspartic acid and glutamic acid, respectively (Fig. 18.12).

By transamination reactions with other appropriate acids, alanine, aspartic acid and glutamic acid serve as α-amino donors in the formation of other amino acids. The general transamination reaction may be written:

$$R\text{—}CH(NH_2)\text{—}COOH + R'\text{—}CO\text{—}COOH \rightleftharpoons$$
$$R\text{—}CO\text{—}COOH + R'\text{—}CH(NH_2)\text{—}COOH$$

Glutamic acid, in particular, appears to be a central product in amino-acid metabolism and glutamic acid dehydrogenase has been reported in a number of plant tissues. The enzyme functions in conjunction with NAD:

$$\alpha\text{-ketoglutaric acid} + NH_3 + NADPH \rightleftharpoons \text{glutamic acid} + NAD$$

That the nitrogen of ammonia first appears in the dicarboxylic amino acids and is later transferred to other nitrogen compounds was demonstrated in some of the earliest plant biochemistry experiments (around 1940), which utilized ^{15}N.

Proline, hydroxyproline, ornithine and arginine

These amino acids are of importance in the secondary metabolism of some plants in that they are precursors of a number of alkaloids. They are metabolically connected to glutamic acid (Fig. 18.13) and their formation in plant cells is complex in that the reactions are strictly compartmentalized. The enzymes involved have been characterized, and for the formation of ornithine it is the *N*-acetyl derivatives which are involved. Arginine appears to be synthesized from ornithine in all organisms via the reactions of the urea cycle. (For a review giving the role of the mitochondria, cytoplasm and plastids in these reactions, see P. D. Shargool *et al.*, *Phytochemistry*, 1988, **27**, 1571.)

Serine and glycine

Together with cysteine and cystine, these amino acids arise at the triose level of metabolism. Preparations from rat liver use the pathway indicated in Fig. 18.14 for the formation of serine.

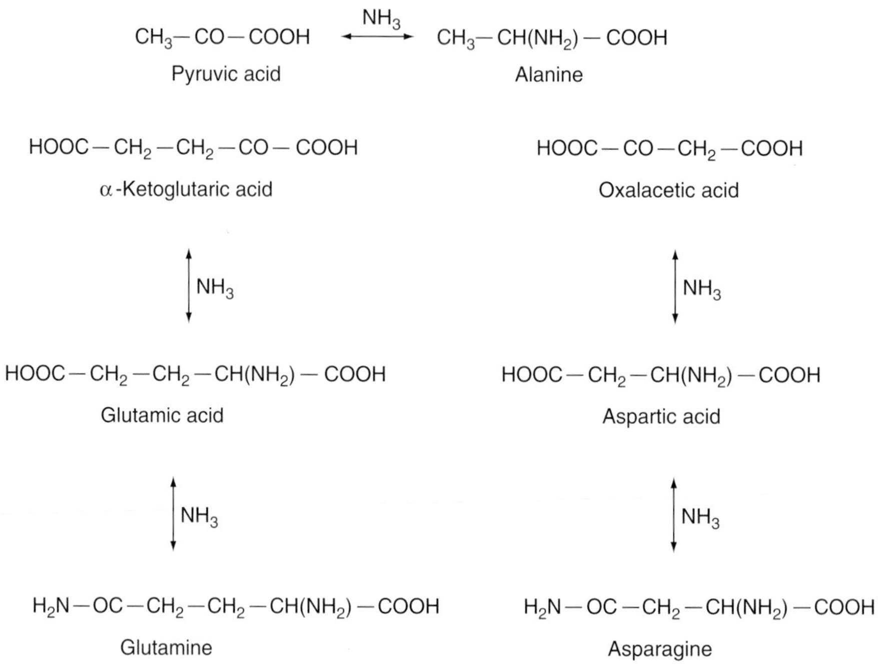

Fig. 18.12
Reductive- and trans-amination in the formation of amino acids.

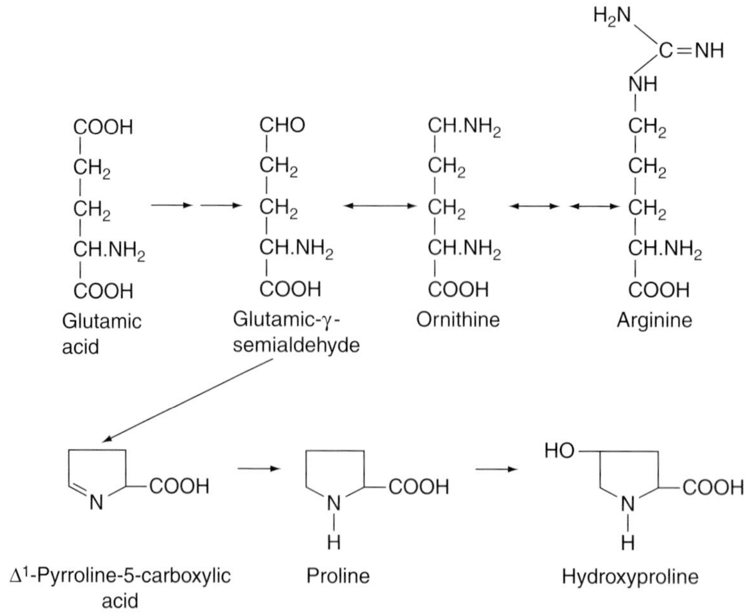

Fig. 18.13
Origin of proline, hydroxyproline, ornithine and arginine.

$$COOH-CHOH-CH_2OPO_3H_2 \longrightarrow COOH-CO-CH_2OPO_3H_2$$

3-Phosphoglyceric acid   3-Phosphohydroxypyruvic acid

$$COOH-CH.NH_2-CH_2OH \longleftarrow COOH-CH.NH_2-CH_2OPO_3H_2$$

Serine   3-Phosphoserine

Fig. 18.14
Formation of serine and glycine.

Serine and glycine are readily interconvertible:

$$CH_2OH-CH.NH_2-COOH \rightarrow HCHO + CH_2.NH_2-COOH$$

In animal tissues it has been shown that tetrahydrofolic acid (THFA) is responsible for the removal of the hydroxymethyl group of serine to form hydroxymethyltetrafolic acid. As this compound serves as a source of formate and methyl groups in many reactions, the β-carbon of serine may be their original source; this applies to the formation of methionine (Fig. 18.15), itself an important methyl donor in plant biochemistry.

Alanine, valine and leucine

Studies with microorganisms and yeasts have shown these amino acids to be derived from pyruvate. There is evidence that α-ketoisovaleric acid is aminated to form valine and that it can also condense with acetate to form an intermediate which on decarboxylation and amination affords leucine (Fig. 18.16).

Isoleucine

This amino acid

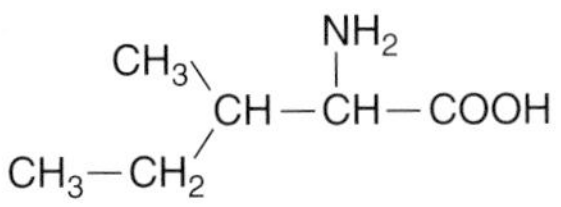

CH_3—CH—CH—COOH with NH_2 and CH_3—CH_2 branches

$$\begin{matrix} CH_3 \diagdown \\ \quad\quad CH-CH-COOH \\ CH_3-CH_2 \diagup \quad \overset{|}{NH_2} \end{matrix}$$

is formed by a similar series of reactions to valine but commencing with α-aceto-α-hydroxypropionic acid instead of α-acetolactic acid.

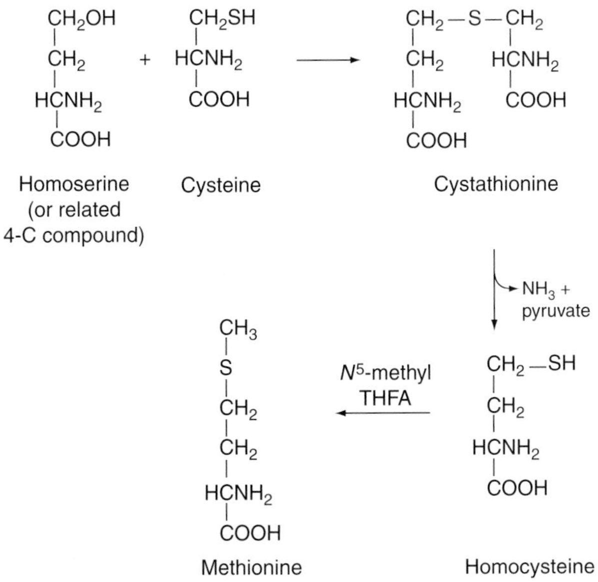

Fig. 18.15
Origin of methionine.

Lysine

Lysine, $H_2N–(CH_2)_4–CH(NH_2)–COOH$, is derived, in plants, from aspartate involving a pathway utilizing 2,3-dihydropicolinic acid and diaminopimelic acid. It is the precursor of some alkaloids of *Nicotiana*, *Lupinus* and *Punica*.

For a review of the biosynthesis and metabolism of aspartate-derived amino acids (lysine, threonine, methionine, *S*-adenosyl methionine) see R. A. Azevedo *et al.*, *Phytochemistry*, 1997, **46**, 395.

Aromatic amino acids

These have already been mentioned in the discussion of the biosynthesis of aromatic compounds.

PEPTIDES AND PROTEINS

The term 'peptide' includes a wide range of compounds varying from low to very high molecular weights and showing marked differences in physical, chemical and pharmacological properties. The lowest members are derived from only two molecules of amino acid, but higher members have many amino-acid units and form either peptides, simple proteins (albumins, globulins, prolamines, glutalins, etc.) or more complex proteins, conjugated proteins, in which other groupings form part of the molecule—for example, carbohydrate in mucoproteins, the very complex chlorophyll molecule in the protein of chloroplasts, phosphorus-containing proteins such as casein, nucleoproteins, in which proteins are combined with nucleic acid, and the lipoproteins of the cytoplasm, in which protein is combined with lipids. Among such substances with relatively low molecular weight are some antibiotics which have a cyclic polypeptide structure (e.g. gramicidin, bacitracin and polymyxin); peptide hormones such as oxytocin and vasopressin from the posterior pituitary gland; and glutathione, which is found in nearly all living cells.

All these more or less complex compounds have two or more molecules of amino acid united by a peptide linkage which results from the elimination of water, an OH coming from one amino acid and an H from the other.

Thus, a dipeptide is formed:

$$R-CH(NH_2)COOH + R'-CH(NH_2)COOH \longrightarrow$$

Amino acid   Amino acid

$$R-CH(NH_2)CO-NH-\underset{\underset{COOH}{|}}{CH}-R' + H_2O$$

Dipeptide

A dipeptide of the Sapindaceous plant *Blighia sapida* has hypoglycaemic properties and although more complex, penicillin also has a

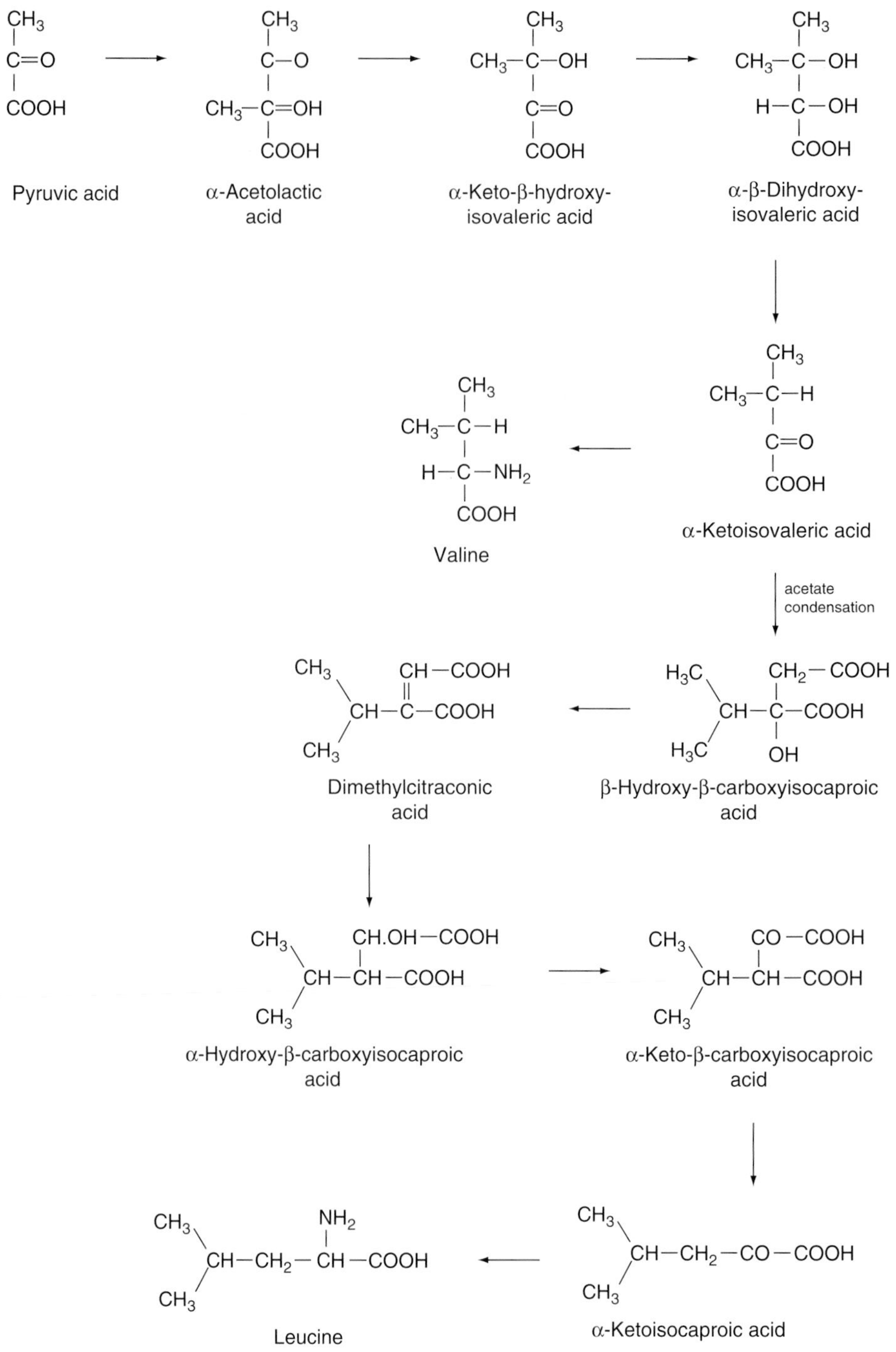

18

Fig. 18.16
Formation of valine and leucine.

dipeptide structure. Tripeptides have three amino-acid components and polypeptides from ten upwards. Peptides are usually defined as protein-like substances having molecular weights below 10 000. In typical proteins the molecular weight is higher, ranging from about 30 000 to 50 000 in the relatively simple prolamines and glutelins and reaching very high values, sometimes several million, in the complex proteins such as those in sheep's wool.

Protein synthesis takes place in association with the ribosomes, which are small bodies found in the cytoplasm and particularly in the endoplasmic reticulum area (see Fig. 18.1). The amino acids are brought to the ribosomes associated with a transfer-RNA molecule and by the action of the ribosomes, using a sequence dictated by a

particular messenger-RNA molecule, are linked to form the peptide chains of the particular protein. Although not directly relevant to most pharmacognostical studies, the story of the nucleic acids and their vital role in the control of cell metabolism is a fascinating one which it is suggested students study from a standard work on biochemistry.

ISOPRENOID COMPOUNDS

Studies on the pyrogenic decomposition of rubber led workers in the latter half of the nineteenth century to believe that isoprene could be regarded as a fundamental building block for this material. As a result of the extensive pioneering investigations into plant terpene structures, Ruzicka published in 1953 his 'biogenetic isoprene rule', which indicated that the apposition of isoprenoid units could be used to explain not only the formation of rubber and the monoterpenes, but also many other natural products, including some, such as sterols and triterpenes, with complex constitutions. The value of the rule lay in its broad unifying concept, which allowed the postulation of a rational sequence of events which might occur in the biogenesis of these otherwise unrelated compounds. Examples of various structures to which the rule can be applied are indicated in Fig. 18.17.

The task set biochemists was to investigate the validity of the rule, and the work on this subject constitutes a brilliant example of modern biochemistry; however, as will be seen below, this chapter of research is still unfinished. By 1951 it had been established that acetic acid was intimately involved in the synthesis of cholesterol, squalene, yeast sterols and rubber. The use of methyl- and carboxyl-labelled acetic acid with animal tissues indicated that the methyl and carboxyl carbons alternated in the skeleton of cholesterol or squalene and that the lateral carbon atoms all arose from the methyl group of acetic acid.

The discovery, in 1950, of acetyl-coenzyme A, the so-called 'active acetate', gave further support to the role of acetate in biosynthetic processes.

The mevalonic acid pathway. The next major advance in the elucidation of the isoprenoid biosynthetic route was the discovery in 1956 of mevalonic acid and the demonstration of its incorporation, by living tissues, into those compounds to which the isoprene rule applied. Mevalonic acid (3,5-dihydroxy-3-methylvaleric acid) is a C_6 acid and, as such, is not the 'active isoprene' unit which forms the basic building block of the isoprenoid compounds. During the next four years, by research involving the use of tracer techniques, inhibitor studies, cell-free extracts, partition chromatography and ionophoresis as well as synthetic organic chemistry, it was established that the C_5 compound for which biochemists had been seeking so long was isopentenyl pyrophosphate; it is derived from mevalonic acid pyrophosphate by decarboxylation and dehydration. Isoprenoid synthesis then proceeds by the condensation of isopentenyl pyrophosphate with the isomeric dimethylallyl pyrophosphate to yield geranyl pyrophosphate. Further C_5 units are added by the

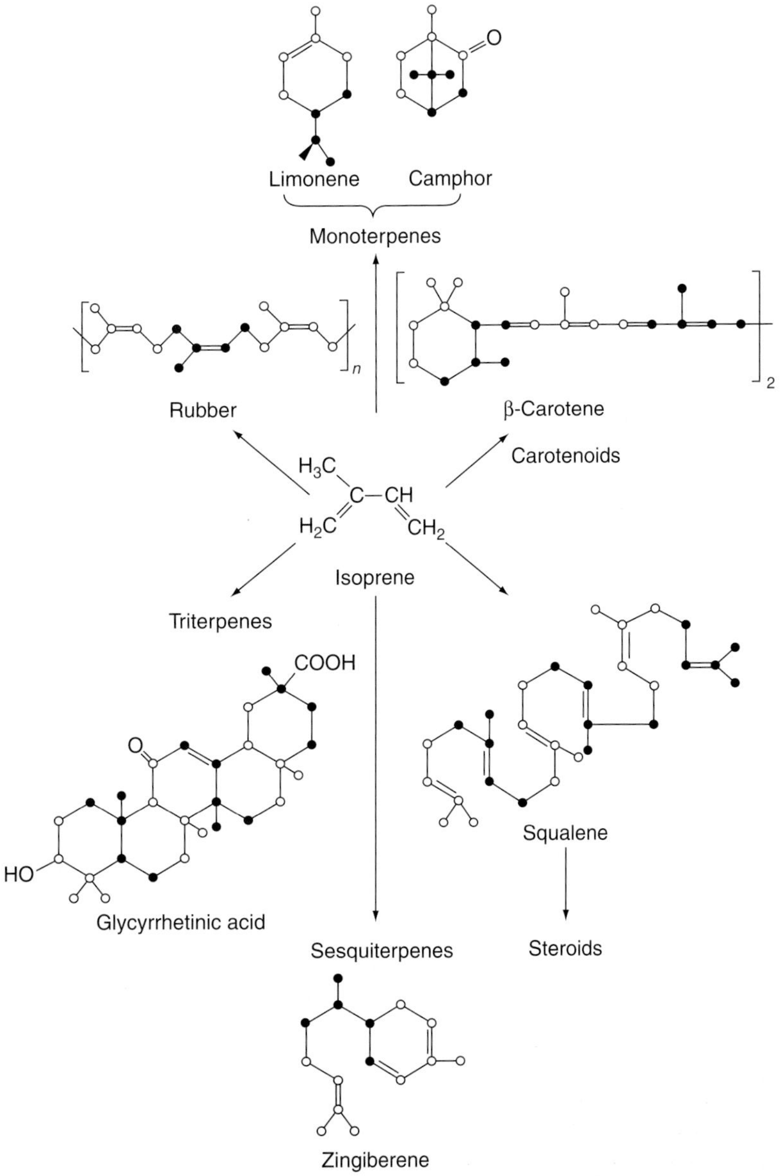

Fig. 18.17
Application of the isoprene rule illustrating incorporation of C_5 units.

addition of more isopentenyl pyrophosphate. These preliminary stages in the biosynthesis of isoprenoid compounds are shown in Fig. 18.18.

From geranyl and farnesyl pyrophosphates various structures can be built up (see Fig. 18.19).

Studies, particularly by Cornforth and Popják, involving the use of stereospecifically ^{3}H- and ^{14}C-labelled mevalonic acid, have demonstrated the stereochemical mechanism of the initial stages of isoprenoid formation. Only the (R)-form of mevalonic acid gives rise to the terpenoids, the (S)-form appearing to be metabolically inactive. In the formation of isopentenyl pyrophosphate, the elimination is *trans* and the elimination of the proton in the isomerization to the dimethylallyl pyrophosphate is also stereospecific (Fig. 18.20A).

In the subsequent additions of the C_5 isopentenyl pyrophosphate units to form the terpenoids the elimination of hydrogen is *trans*. Figure 18.20B shows the stereochemistry of the addition of one isopentenyl pyrophosphate unit. In the biogenesis of rubber, however, the hydrogen elimination produces a *cis* double bond (Fig. 18.20C).

It is considered that a simple change in orientation of the isopentenyl pyrophosphate on the enzyme surface could produce this change without altering the reaction mechanism. In neither rubber nor gutta are hybrid molecules containing both types of bond detectable. The first

direct evidence for the presence of isopentenyl diphosphate isomerase in rubber latex was reported in 1996 (T. Koyama *et al.*, *Phytochemistry*, 1996, **43**, 769).

In recent years the enzymology of the isoprenoid pathway has been extensively studied and for details the reader is referred to a standard text on plant biochemistry. One key regulatory enzyme is hydroxymethylglutaryl-CoA reductase (EC 1.1.1.34, mevalonate kinase); it has been extensively studied in animals and more recently in plants. As with many enzymes the situation is complicated by the existence of more than one species of enzyme and a plant may possess multiple forms each having a separate subcellular location associated with the biosynthesis of different classes of terpenoids. For a review of the functions and properties of the important isomerase enzyme isopentenyl diphosphate isomerase see 'Further reading'.

It should be noted that some metabolites of mixed biogenetic origin involve the mevalonic acid pathway; prenylation for example is common, with C_5, C_{10} and C_{15} units associated with flavonoids, coumarins, benzoquinones, cannabinoids, alkaloids, etc.

The validity of the mevalonate pathway in the formation of all the major groups noted in Fig. 18.19 has been shown, and until recently no other biosynthetic route to isoprenoids had been discovered.

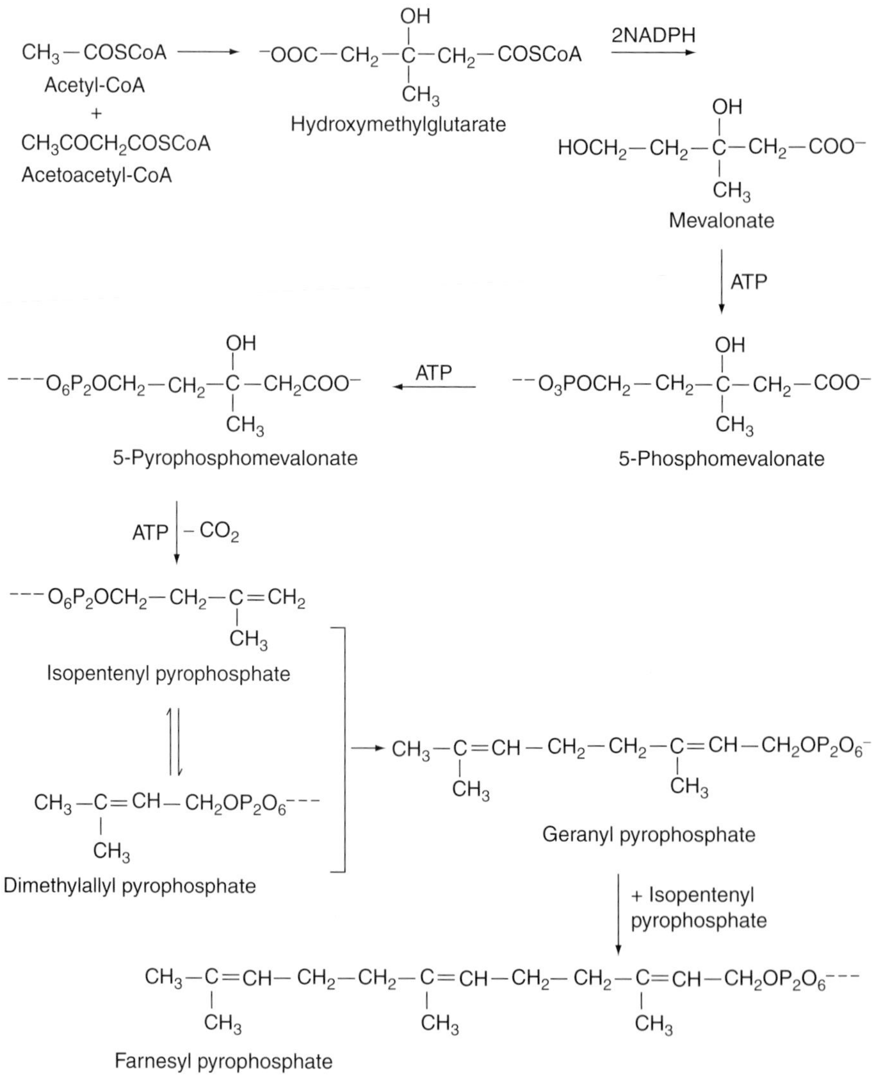

Fig. 18.18
Preliminary stages in the biosynthesis of isoprenoid compounds.

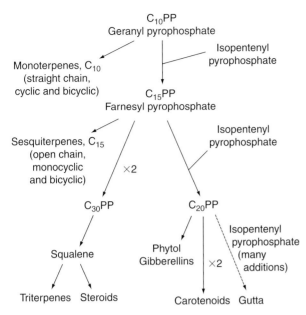

Fig. 18.19
Biosynthesis of isoprenoid compounds.

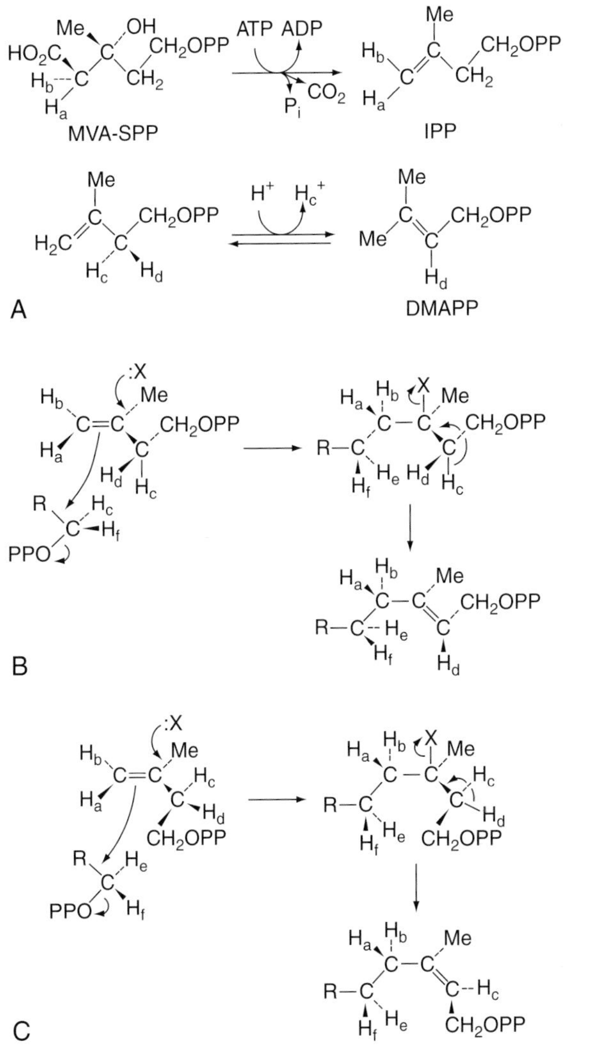

Fig. 18.20
Stereospecific reactions in terpenoid biogenesis. A, Formation from mevalonic acid (MVA) of isopentenyl pyrophosphate (IPP) by *trans* elimination; isomerization to dimethylallyl pyrophosphate (DMAPP). B, Association of the two 5-C units with *trans* elimination of hydrogen. C, As B but involving formation of *cis* double bonds as found in rubber.

The 1-deoxy-D-xylulose (triose/pyruvate) pathway. Following its discovery in 1956 mevalonic acid came to be considered the essential precursor for all isoprenoid syntheses. However, in 1993 M. Rohmer *et al.*, (*Biochem. J.*, 1993, **295**, 517) showed that a non-mevalonate pathway existed for the formation of hopane-type triterpenoids in bacteria. The novel putative precursor was identified as 1-deoxy-D-xylulose-5-phosphate, formed from glucose via condensation of pyruvate and glyceraldehyde-3-phosphate. Subsequent steps including a skeletal rearrangement afford isopentenyl pyrophosphate—the same methyl-branched isoprenoid building block as formed by the MVA route.

It was soon demonstrated that this novel route to IPP was also operative in the formation of monoterpenes (*Mentha piperita*, *Thymus vulgaris*), diterpenes (*Ginkgo biloba*, *Taxus chinensis*) and carotenoids (*Daucus carota*). This raised the question of to what extent the two pathways co-existed in the plant and it was hypothesized that the classical acetate/mevalonate pathway was a feature of cytoplasmic reactions whereas the triose/pyruvate sequence was a characteristic of the plastids. This did not exclude either the movement of plastid-synthesized IPP and DMAPP from the organelle to the cytoplasm or the translocation of a suitable C₅-acceptor to the plastid. Evidence accumulating indicates a cooperative involvement of both pathways. Indeed recent work on the biosynthesis of the isoprene units of chamomile sesquiterpenes (K.-P. Adam and J. Zapp, *Phytochemistry*, 1998, **48**, 953) has shown that for the three C_5 units of both bisaboloxide A and chamazulene, two were mainly formed by the non-mevalonate pathway and the third was of mixed origin.

The deoxyxylulose (DOX) pathway has helped explain the previously reported rather poor incorporations of MVA into certain isoprenoids. Thus V. Stanjek *et al.* (*Phytochemistry*, 1999, **50**, 1141) have obtained a good incorporation of labelled deoxy-D-xylulose into the prenylated segment of furanocoumarins of *Apium graveolens* leaves, suggesting this to be the preferred intermediate.

Fig. 18.21 illustrates how [1-¹³C]-glucose, when fed to plants, can be used to differentiate IPP and subsequent metabolites, formed either by the MVA pathway or the DOX route.

SECONDARY METABOLITES

As indicated earlier in Fig. 18.2, the basic metabolic pathways constitute the origins of secondary plant metabolism and give rise to a vast array of compounds; some of these are responsible for the characteristic odours, pungencies and colours of plants, others give a particular plant its culinary, medicinal or poisonous virtues and by far the greatest number are, on current knowledge, of obscure value to the plant (and to the human race). However, a number of modern authors suggest that secondary metabolites, rather than constituting waste products of metabolism, are biosynthesized to aid the plant's survival. Notwithstanding, it may be that in some instances the purpose for which these compounds were produced no longer exists but the biosynthetic pathway has survived. For an interesting discussion and references, see E. J. Buenz and S. J. Schepple, *J. Ethnopharmacol*, 2007, **114**, 279. The possible functions in the plant of one large group of secondary metabolites, alkaloids, are discussed in Chapter 26.

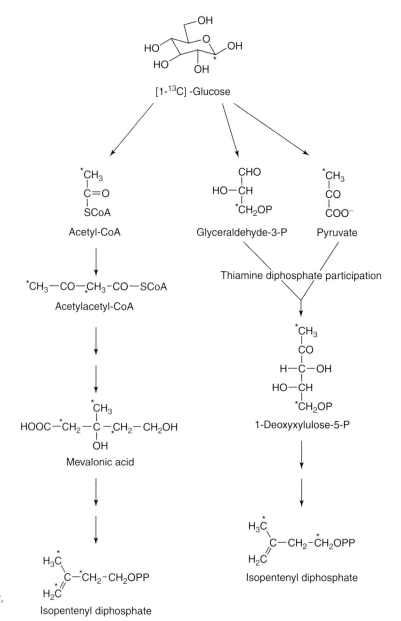

Fig. 18.21
The incorporation of [1-¹³C]-glucose into isopentenyl diphosphate: left, via the mevalonic acid pathway; right, via the deoxyxyulose pathway.

Recently, considerable attention has been directed to the possible ecological implications of secondary metabolites not only in relation to plant–plant interaction but also concerning the interrelationship of plants and animals. Various insects sequester specific alkaloids, iridoids, lactones and flavonoids which serve as defensive agents or are converted to male pheromones. The literature concerning chemical ecology is regularly reviewed and the volatile isoprenoids that control insect behaviour and development have been reported on (J. A. Pickett, *Nat. Prod. Rep.*, 1999, **16**, 39). The enzymology associated with secondary metabolism is now receiving considerable attention and, with respect to alkaloid formation, a number of enzymes associated with the biosynthesis of the tropane, isoquinoline and indole groups have been prepared. The biosynthetic origins of those metabolites of medicinal interest are considered in more detail in Part 5, which is arranged principally according to biogenetic groups.

Although a number of the biogenetic groups are characterized by particular skeletal structures, the actual chemical properties of particular compounds are determined by the acquisition of functional groups.

Thus, terpenes may occur as alcohols (menthol), ethers (cineole), ketones (carvone), etc., and as such have similar chemical properties to non-terpenoid compounds possessing the same group; aldehydes, as an example of a functional group, may be of aliphatic origin (citronellal), aromatic (cinnamic aldehyde), steroidal (some cardioactive glycosides); and resulting from the introduction of a heterocyclic system one biogenetic group may possess some of the chemical properties of another (e.g. steroidal alkaloids).

A particular group of compounds may also involve different biogenetic entities; thus, the complex indole alkaloids contain moieties derived from both the shikimate and isoprenoid pathways. In contrast, the same structure, as it occurs in different compounds, may arise from different pathways, as has been previously indicated with the formation of aromatic systems.

Stress compounds

These are compounds which accumulate in the plant to a higher than normal level as a result of some form of injury, or disturbance to the metabolism; they may be products of either primary or secondary metabolism. Common reactions involved in their formation are the polymerization, oxidation or hydrolysis of naturally occurring substances; many however, are entirely secondary in their formation. A number of environmental and biological factors promote the synthesis of stress compounds and these include mechanical wounding of the plant, exposure to frost, ultraviolet irradiation, dehydration, treatment with chemicals, and microbial infection (see phytoalexins below). The production of such compounds has also been observed in cell cultures subjected to antibiotic treatment and in cells immobilized or brought into contact with calcium alginate. Examples of the latter include the formation of acridone alkaloid epoxides by *Ruta graveolens*, and the increased production of echinatin and the novel formation of a prenylated compound by *Glycyrrhiza echinata* cultures.

Stress compounds are of pharmaceutical interest in that they may be involved in various crude drugs formed pathologically (e.g. some gums and oleoresins) and potential drugs (gossypol); they are implicated in the toxicity of some diseased foodstuffs and they play a role in the defensive mechanism of the plant. In the latter area, the phytoalexins have received considerable attention in recent years and can be regarded as antifungal compounds synthesized by a plant in greatly increased amounts after infection. The antifungal isoflavonoid pterocarpans produced by many species of the Leguminosae are well known, see 'Spiny restharrow'. Other phytoalexins produced in the same family are hydroxyflavanones, stilbenoids, benzofurans, chromones and furanoacetylenes. Sesquiterpene phytoalexins have been isolated from infected *Ulmus glabra* and *Gossypium*. In the vine (*Vitis vinifera*) the fungus *Botrytis cinerea* acts as an elicitor for the production of the stilbenes resveratrol (q.v.) and pterostilbene.

Chemically, stress compounds are, in general, of extreme variability and include phenols, resins, carbohydrates, hydroxycinnamic acid derivatives, coumarins, bicyclic sesquiterpenes, triterpenes and steroidal compounds. For the promotion of stress compounds in cell cultures see Chapter 13 and Table 13.1.

Further reading

Facchini PJ, Huner-Allnach KL, Tari LW 2000 Plant aromatic L-amino acid decarboxylases: evolution, biochemistry, regulation and metabolic engineering applications. Phytochemistry 54(2): 121–138

Grayson DH 2000 Monoterpenoids (*a review covering mid-1997 to mid-1999*). Natural Product Reports 17(4): 385

Knaggs AR 1999, 2000 The biosynthesis of shikimate metabolites. Natural Product Reports 16(4): 525–560; 17(3): 269–292

Kruger NT, Hill SA, Ratcliffe RG (eds) 1999 Regulation of primary metabolic pathways in plants. Kluwer, Dordrecht, Netherlands

Ramos-Valdivia AC, Van der Heijden R, Verpoorte R 1997 Isopentenyl diphosphate isomerase: a core enzyme in isoprenoid biosynthesis. Natural Product Reports 14(6): 591–604

Rohmer M 1999 The discovery of a mevalonate-independent pathway for isoprenoid biosynthesis in bacteria, algae and higher plants. Natural Product Reports 16(5): 565–574

Seigler DS 1998 Plant secondary metabolism. Kluwer, Dordrecht, Netherlands

Singh BK 1999 (ed) Plant amino acids—biochemistry and biotechnology. Marcel Dekker Inc, New York

Wink M (ed) 1999 Biochemistry of plant secondary metabolism. Sheffield Academic Press

18

PART

5 | Pharmacopoeial and related drugs of biological origin

Introduction

Drugs of the European and British Pharmacopoeias together with some related plant materials are considered in some detail in Chapters 19–26. They are arranged according to the biosynthetic origins of their principal constituents. An indication of how these drugs can also be grouped on a pharmacological/clinical usage basis is given in Chapter 6.

A large number of plant species, particularly those used in various traditional medicines, have been, and still are being, screened for specific pharmacological activities. Overviews involving some areas of this research, with its notable successes, are given in Chapters 26–29 and illustrate in conjuction with Chapters 8 and 9 the current approach to the search for 'new' drugs of potential value to the allopathic system of medicine.

Some products such as nutraceuticals, vitamins, antibiotics, hormones and flavourings are conveniently treated as heterogeneous biochemical groups (Chapters 31–33).

In Part 5, to help distinguish the monographs on drugs of the *BP* 2007 and *EP* from those of non-official drugs, the usual conventions relating to hierarchical headings have not been strictly observed; headings for the former are printed in bold capitals whereas the latter are in smaller typesize.

19

Hydrocarbons and derivatives

Hydrocarbons contain carbon and hydrogen only and, from these, by the addition of functional groups and by interaction, all other natural compounds can theoretically be derived. In a particular class of compounds such as volatile oils, the components of any one member may be biosynthetically related (e.g. menthol and menthone in oil of peppermint) although because of their different functional groups they may undergo different sets of chemical reactions and possess different pharmacological properties. Among the most common functional groups are carboxylic acids, alcohols, ketones, aldehydes and phenols; biochemical interactions produce esters, lactones etc.

In this book most examples of medicinal plants containing the above are considered under their respective biogenetic groupings and in this chapter the detailed description of drugs is restricted to those examples in which simple acids, alcohols and esters comprise the principal medicinal components.

HYDROCARBONS

Although not featuring strongly in the pharmaceutical armamentarium, hydrocarbons are important in nature as components of cuticular waxes. The majority of these are odd-numbered long-chain alkanes within the range C_{25-35} formed by decarboxylation of the next higher, even-numbered, free fatty acid. In recent years the long-chain polyenes of the Compositae have been systematically investigated in relation to their chemotaxonomic importance. Isoprene (C_5H_8), the unsaturated hydrocarbon moiety from which the terpenoids (isoprenoids) can be constructed (Fig. 18.17), has not to date been found free in nature. A number of cyclic terpenoid hydrocarbons including limonene, pinene, phellandrene and cadinene are components of essential oils. Rubber, gutta and the carotenes are polyunsaturated terpenoids.

MONOBASIC ACIDS

Organic acids possess one or more carboxyl groups and a monobasic acid may be represented as RCOOH. The very high frequency of the biochemical occurrence of the carboxyl group means that acids are found in all living organisms and as derivatives of all the major metabolic groups. They participate in essential metabolism and in this capacity range from the simple acids of the respiratory sequence to the complex deoxyribonucleic acids associated with the storage and transmission of hereditary characters. In the metabolic cycles they frequently function in association with coenzymes, and may accumulate as simple salts, esters and amides, or less frequently in the free state. Amino acids are discussed in Chapter 18.

C_1–C_6 Monocarboxylic acids

A number of these acids together with hydroxy- and keto-derivatives are intermediates in the early stages of the biosynthesis of fats, isoprenoid compounds and various amino acids (q.v.). In the free state they are not found abundantly in nature but occur scattered throughout the plant kingdom in the esterified form as a feature of some volatile oils, resins, fats, coumarin derivatives and alkaloids.

Some common acids are illustrated in Table 19.1.

Fatty acids

These acids are important as components of plant oils (acyl lipids) in which they occur as esters with the trihydric alcohol glycerol. They are also components of the resins of the Convolvulaceae and of waxes in which they are esterified with long-chain alcohols. Most are C_{10} to C_{20}

Table 19.1   Examples of C_1–C_6 monocarboxylic acids.

Name	Structure	Comments
Formic acid	HCOOH	Name derives from its first isolation from the ant, *Formica rufa*. A decomposition product of many vegetable materials. Occurs free in the hairs of the stinging nettle; combined in the gitaloxigenin series of cardioactive glycosides. *N*-formyl-L-methionine is involved in the initiation of protein synthesis on ribosomes
Acetic acid	MeCOOH	An essential primary metabolite, particularly as acetyl-CoA. Common in the esterified form
Propionic acid	MeCH₂COOH Me(CH₂)₂COOH	Produced in the fatty acid oxidative cycle when an acyl-CoA with an odd number of carbon atoms is involved. Esterified as a tropane alkaloid
n-Butyric acid iso-Butyric acid	Me–CH–Me ∣ COOH	Occurs in traces in many fats. Occurs free in carob beans (*Ceratonia siliqua*) and as its ethyl ester in croton oil. Component of resins of the Convolvulaceae and minor tropane alkaloids. Intermediate in the metabolism of valine
n-Valeric acid iso-Valeric acid	Me(CH₂)₃COOH Me–CH–Me ∣ CH₂ ∣ COOH	Not common; component of Convolvulaceous resins. Free and esterified in *Valeriana* spp. Combined in some tropane alkaloids (e.g. valeroidine) and in the pyranocoumarin, dihydrosamidin. Intermediate in the metabolism of leucine
2-Methylbutyric acid	Me ∣ CH₂ ∣ CHMe ∣ COOH	Component of some tropane and *Veratrum* alkaloids, Convolvulaceous glycosides and the pyranocoumarin visnadin
Caproic acid Crotonic acid (*trans*-butenoic acid)	Me(CH₂)₄COOH Me–C(H)=C(H)–COOH	Occurs in traces in many fats. Constituent of croton oil
Tiglic acid	Me–C(H)=C(Me)–COOH	Occurs in croton oil (glycoside) from *Croton tiglium*. The acid of many minor tropane alkaloids, e.g. tigloidine. Component of Convolvulaceous resins and *Symphytum* alkaloids. Biosynthetically derived from isoleucine
Angelic acid	H–C(Me)=C(Me)–COOH	Occurs in the rhizome of *Angelica*. Esterifying acid of the *Schizanthus* alkaloid schizanthine X and of some volatile oils, e.g. chamomile oils. Component of the Cevadilla seed alkaloid cevadine and *Symphytum* alkaloids
Senecioic acid	Me–C(Me)=C(H)–COOH	First isolated from a species of *Senecio* (Compositae). Occurs as the esterifying acid of some alkaloids of *Dioscorea* and *Schizanthus*. Component of the pyranocoumarin samidin

straight-chain monocarboxylic acids with an even number of carbon atoms. Over 200 have been isolated from natural sources but relatively few are ubiquitous in their occurrence. They may be saturated (e.g. palmitic and stearic acids) or unsaturated (e.g. oleic acid). The double bonds, with a few minor exceptions such as the seed oil of pomegranate, are *cis*.

Less commonly they are cyclic compounds such as hydnocarpic acid and the prostaglandins. The latter are a group of physiologically active essential fatty acids found in most body tissues and are involved in the platelet-aggregation and inflammatory processes. They promote smooth muscle contraction making them of clinical use as effective abortifacients and for inducing labour. All the active natural prostaglandins are derivatives of prostanoic acid (see Table 19.4).

A rich source of prostaglandin A_2 (PGA_2) is the soft coral *Plexaura homomalla*. Although recognized in the 1930s, and their structures determined in 1962, it was not until 1988 that prostaglandins were unequivocally established as components of some higher plants (cambial zones and buds of *Larix* and *Populus* spp.)

The characteristic acid of castor oil, ricinoleic acid (hydroxyoleic acid) has both a hydroxyl group and an unsaturated double bond. A range of acetylenic fatty acids occurs throughout the plant kingdom and some of them possess antifungal and antibacterial properties. The biogenetic relationship between these, the olefinic fatty acids and the saturated fatty acids is outlined later in this chapter.

Examples of fatty acids are listed in Tables 19.2–19.4. It will be noted that some have more than one unsaturated bond, the bonds being interspersed by methylene groups. These polyunsaturated acids have received much attention in recent years both regarding their role in dietary fats and as medicinals. All the common acids have trivial names but in order to indicate more precisely their structures without recourse to the full systematic chemical name each can be represented by a symbol. Thus α-linolenic, systematic name all-*cis*-$\Delta^{9,12,15}$-octadecatrienoic acid, has 18 carbons and three double bonds which can be represented by 18:3. The position of the double bonds is then indicated by the *n-x* convention where *n* = number of carbon atoms in the molecule and *x* is the number of inclusive carbon atoms from the methyl (ω) end to the first carbon of the first double bond, in this case 3, so that the symbol for α-linolenic acid is 18:3(*n-3*). The positions of the two remaining double bonds are deduced by the fact that they will follow on from each other being separated only by one methylene (-CH$_2$-) group. In this area students may find the literature situation somewhat confusing because in some texts the acids may be symbolized on the basis of conventional chemical systematic numbering—for fatty acids the carboxyl carbon being C1. For α-linolenic acid this is represented as 18:3(*9c.12c.15c*), *c* indicating a *cis*-bond. The advantage of the first system is that it indicates any bioequivalence of the double bonds in acids of different chain-length, bearing in mind that chain elongation *in vivo* proceeds at the carboxyl end of the molecule by the addition of 2C units. Thus it can be seen from Table 19.3 that γ-linolenic acid and arachidonic acid both fall into the biochemical ω-6 family of unsaturated fatty acids and their respective symbols 18:3(*n-6*) and 20:4(*n-6*) reflect this whereas symbols based on chemical nomenclature for these acids *viz* 18:3(*6c,9c,12c*) and 20:4(*5c,8c,11c,14c*) do not. A comparison of symbols for some common unsaturated acids is shown in Table 19.5.

Under certain conditions, which are specified in pharmacopoeias, iodine or its equivalent is taken up at these double bonds and the so-called *iodine value* is thus a measure of unsaturatedness. The iodine value is the number of parts of iodine absorbed by 100 parts by weight of the substance. Near-infrared spectroscopy can also be used to

determine this value as it is directly related to the HC=CH stretch bands at 2130 nm in the spectrum. Iodine values are useful constants for acids, fixed oils, fats and waxes, and help to indicate the composition of complex mixtures as well as pure substances.

Table 19.4 Cyclic unsaturated acids.

Common name	Structural formula
Hydnocarpic	
Chaulmoogric	
Gorlic	
Prostanoic	
PGA2	

Table 19.5 Comparison of symbols ascribed to unsaturated fatty acids.

Common name of acid	Symbol employing biochemical equivalence of double bonds	Symbol based on chemical nomenclature
Palmitoleic	16:1 (*n-7*)	16:1 (9c)
Oleic	18:1 (*n-9*)	18:1 (9c)
Petroselinic	18:1 (*n-12*)	18:1 (6c)
Ricinoleic	18:1 (*n-9*) (hydroxy at *n-7*)	D(+)-12h-18:1(9c) (h = hydroxy)
Erucic	22:1 (*n-9*)	22:1 (13c)
Linoleic	18:2 (*n-6*)	18:2 (9c,12c)
Eicosadienoic	20:2 (*n-6*)	20:2 (11c,14c)

Table 19.2 Straight-chain saturated acids.

Common name	Systematic name	Structural formula
Caprylic	*n*-Octanoic	$CH_3(CH_2)_6COOH$
Capric	*n*-Decanoic	$CH_3(CH_2)_8COOH$
Lauric	*n*-Dodecanoic	$CH_3(CH_2)_{10}COOH$
Myristic	*n*-Tetradecanoic	$CH_3(CH_2)_{12}COOH$
Palmitic	*n*-Hexadecanoic	$CH_3(CH_2)_{14}COOH$
Stearic	*n*-Octadecanoic	$CH_3(CH_2)_{16}COOH$
Arachidic	*n*-Eicosanoic	$CH_3(CH_2)_{18}COOH$

Table 19.3 Straight-chain unsaturated acids.

Common name	Number of unsaturated bonds	Structural formula
Palmitoleic	1	$CH_3(CH_2)_5CH=CH(CH_2)_7COOH$
Oleic	1	$CH_3(CH_2)_7CH=CH(CH_2)_7COOH$
Petroselinic	1	$CH_3(CH_2)_{10}CH=CH(CH_2)_4COOH$
Ricinoleic	1	$CH_3(CH_2)_5CH(OH)CH_2CH=CH-(CH_2)_7COOH$
Erucic	1	$CH_3(CH_2)_7 CH=CH(CH_2)_{11}COOH$
Linolenic	2	$CH_3(CH_2)_4CH=CHCH_2CH=CH-(CH_2)_7COOH$
α-Linoleic	3	$CH_3CH_2CH=CHCH_2CH=CHCH_2-CH=CH(CH_2)_7COOH$
γ-Linolenic	3	$CH_3(CH_2)_4CH=CHCH_2CH=CHCH_2CH=CH(CH_2)_4COOH$
Arachidonic	4	$CH_3(CH_2)_4CH=CHCH_2CH=CHCH_2-CH=CHCH_2CH=CH(CH_2)_3COOH$

Biosynthesis of saturated fatty acids.   See Chapter 18.

Biosynthesis of unsaturated fatty acids.   Before the elucidation of the overall chemistry of formation of polyunsaturated fatty acids such as linoleic in the early 1960s by Bloch, knowledge concerning the biosynthesis of these compounds lagged behind that of the saturated acids. Recent progress has been much more rapid and, in general, it now appears that in aerobic organisms, monoenoic acids with the double bond in the 9,10-position arise by direct dehydrogenation of saturated acids. In higher plants, for this reaction, coenzyme A may be replaced by the acyl carrier protein (ACP), and Bloch has demonstrated that stearoyl-S-ACP is an effective enzyme substrate of the desaturase system of isolated plant leaf chloroplasts. The reduced forms of nicotinamide adenine dinucleotide (NADH) or nicotinamide adenine dinucleotide phosphate (NADPH) and molecular oxygen are cofactors.

$$CH_3(CH_2)_{16}CO—S—ACP + O_2 + NADPH \longrightarrow$$
(stearoyl-S-ACP)

$$CH_3(CH_2)_7CH = CH(CH_2)_7—CO—S—ACP + H_2O + NADP$$
(oleoyl-S-ACP)

The position of the introduced double bond in respect to the carboxyl group is governed by the enzyme; hence, chain length of the substrate acid is most important. The hydrogen elimination is specifically *cis* but a few unusual fatty acids such as that in the seed oil of *Punica granatum* with the structure 18:3 (9*c*,11*t*,13*c*) have *trans* bonds. As

illustrated in Fig. 19.1, further double bonds may be similarly introduced to give linoleic and linolenic acid.

Unsaturated fatty acids can also be formed in plants by elongation of a medium-chain-length unsaturated acid. This appears to occur by the formation of an intermediate, β,γ-unsaturated acid rather than the α,β-unsaturated acid normally produced in saturated fatty acid biosynthesis; the β,γ-bond is not reduced and more C_2 units are added in the usual way (Fig. 19.2).

Sterculic acid, a component of seed oils of the Malvaceae and Sterculiaceae, is a cyclopropene and is also derived from oleic acid, with methionine supplying the extra carbon atom to give, first, the cyclopropane. Ricinoleic acid is a hydroxy fatty acid found in castor oil seeds and is again biosynthesized from oleic acid (Fig. 19.3).

Some of the natural acetylenes and acetylenic fatty acids have obvious structural similarities to the more common fatty acids. The hypothesis that triple bonds are formed from double bonds by a mechanism analogous to that for the formation of double bonds and involving structurally and stereochemically specific enzymes has now received experimental support. By this means (Fig. 19.4) the range of acetylenes found in Basidiomycetes and in the Compositae, Araliaceae and Umbelliferae can be derived from linoleic acid via its acetylenic 12,13-dehydroderivative, crepenynic acid, an acid first isolated from seeds oils of *Crepis* spp.

Aromatic acids

Two common aromatic acids are benzoic acid and cinnamic acid (unsaturated side-chain), which are widely distributed in nature and

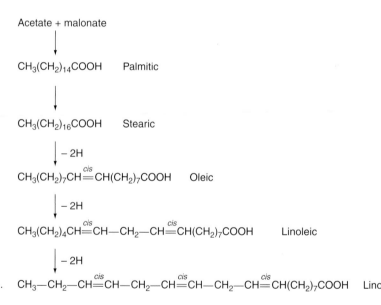

Fig. 19.1
Sequence of formation of olefinic fatty acids in plants.

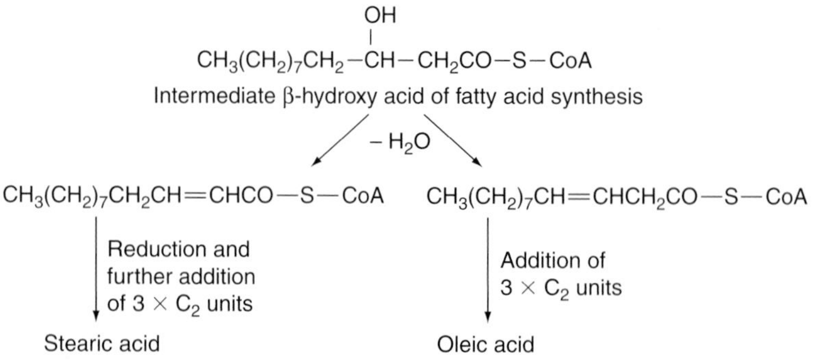

Fig. 19.2
Alternative pathways for synthesis of unsaturated fatty acids.

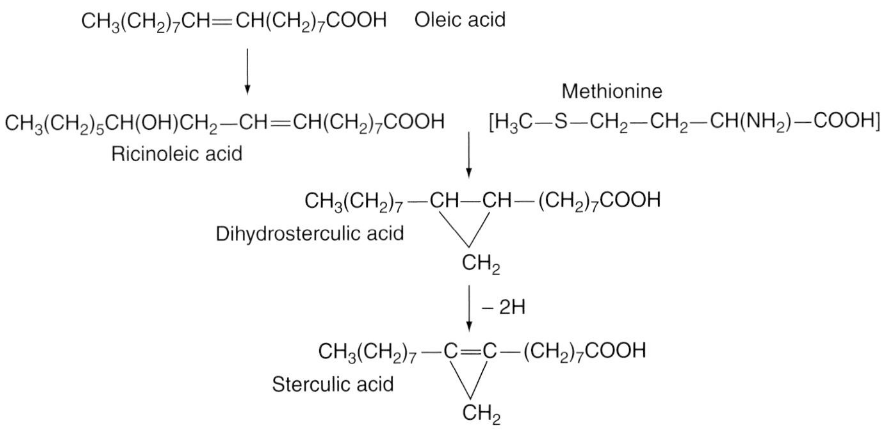

$$CH_3(CH_2)_7CH=CH(CH_2)_7COOH \quad \text{Oleic acid}$$

$$CH_3(CH_2)_5CH(OH)CH_2-CH=CH(CH_2)_7COOH \qquad \text{Methionine}$$
$$\text{Ricinoleic acid} \qquad\qquad\qquad [H_3C-S-CH_2-CH_2-CH(NH_2)-COOH]$$

$$CH_3(CH_2)_7-CH-CH-(CH_2)_7COOH$$
Dihydrosterculic acid

$$CH_2$$

$$\downarrow -2H$$

$$CH_3(CH_2)_7-C=C-(CH_2)_7COOH$$
Sterculic acid

$$CH_2$$

Fig. 19.3
Oleic acid as the precursor of ricinoleic and sterculic acids.

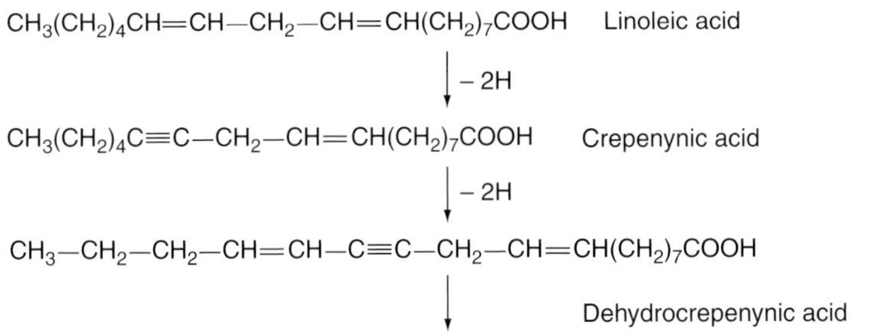

$$CH_3(CH_2)_4CH=CH-CH_2-CH=CH(CH_2)_7COOH \quad \text{Linoleic acid}$$

$$\downarrow -2H$$

$$CH_3(CH_2)_4C\equiv C-CH_2-CH=CH(CH_2)_7COOH \quad \text{Crepenynic acid}$$

$$\downarrow -2H$$

$$CH_3-CH_2-CH_2-CH=CH-C\equiv C-CH_2-CH=CH(CH_2)_7COOH$$

Dehydrocrepenynic acid

Range of acetylenes formed by further introduction of acetylenic bonds at the 'distal' part (furthermost from carboxyl group) of molecules and by chain shortening in 'proximal' part of molecule.

Fig. 19.4
Formation of acetylenic fatty acids.

often occur free and combined in considerable amounts in drugs such as balsams. Truxillic acid, a polymer of cinnamic acid, occurs in coca leaves. Other related acids of fairly common occurrence are those having phenolic or other groupings in addition to a carboxyl group; such are: salicyclic acid (*o*-hydroxybenzoic acid), protocatechuic acid (3,4-dihydroxybenzoic acid), veratric acid (3,4-dimethoxybenzoic acid), gallic acid (3,4,5-trihydroxybenzoic acid) and 3,4,5-trimethoxybenzoic acid. Similarly, derived from cinnamic acid, one finds *p*-coumaric acid (*p*-hydroxycinnamic acid), ferulic acid (hydroxymethoxycinnamic acid), caffeic acid (hydroxycinnamic acid) and 3,4,5-trimethoxycinnamic acid. Unbelliferone, which occurs in combination in asafoetida, is the lactone of dihydroxycinnamic acid.

Acids having an alcohol group are quinic acid (tetrahydroxyhexahydrobenzoic acid), which occurs in cinchona bark and in some gymnosperms; mandelic acid, C$_6$H$_5$CHOHCOOH, which occurs in combination in cyanogenetic glycosides such as those of bitter almonds and other species of *Prunus*; and shikimic acid, an important intermediate metabolite (see Fig. 18.8). Shikimic acid has itself acquired recent pharmaceutical importance as the starting material for the semisynthesis of the antiviral drug oseltamivir (Tamiflu®) for use against bird flu infections in humans. Its principal source has been star-anise fruits (q.v.), leading to a supply shortage of the plant material. Other natural sources rich in this acid and of potential future use are needles of the Pinaceae (S. Marshall, *Pharm. J.*, 2007, **279**, 719) and the fruits (gumballs) of the American sweet gum tree *Liquidamber styraciflua* (q.v.). The acid is also produced commercially by the fermentation of genetically modified *Escherichia coli*. Tropic acid and phenyllactic acid are two aromatic hydroxy acids that occur as esters in tropane alkaloids (q.v.). For examples of the above see Fig. 19.5.

Chlorogenic or caffeotannic acid is a condensation product of caffeic acid and quinic acid. It occurs in maté, coffee, elder flowers,

lime flowers, hops and nux vomica and is converted into a green compound, which serves for its detection, when an aqueous extract is treated with ammonia and exposed to air. See also 'Pseudotannins' (Chapter 21).

The biogenesis of the aromatic ring has been discussed in Chapter 18.

DIBASIC AND TRIBASIC ACIDS

Oxalic acid, (COOH)$_2$, forms the first of a series of dicarboxylic acids which includes malonic acid, CH$_2$(COOH)$_2$, and succinic acid, (CH$_2$)$_2$(COOH)$_2$. Closely related to malonic acid is the unsaturated acid fumaric acid, COOH–CH=CH–COOH. Malic acid contains an alcohol group and has the formula COOH–CH$_2$–CHOH–COOH. It is found in fruits such as apples and tamarinds. A high percentage of tartaric acid, COOH–(CHOH)$_2$–COOH, and its potassium salt occurs in tamarinds and other fruits.

The tribasic acids, citric, isocitric and aconitic are closely related to one another. The Krebs' citric acid cycle, which is discussed in Chapter 18, is very important. Citric acid is abundant in fruit juices, and aconitic acid, which occurs in *Aconitum* spp., is anhydrocitric acid. It forms part of the Krebs' cycle and the glyoxalate cycle in microorganisms.

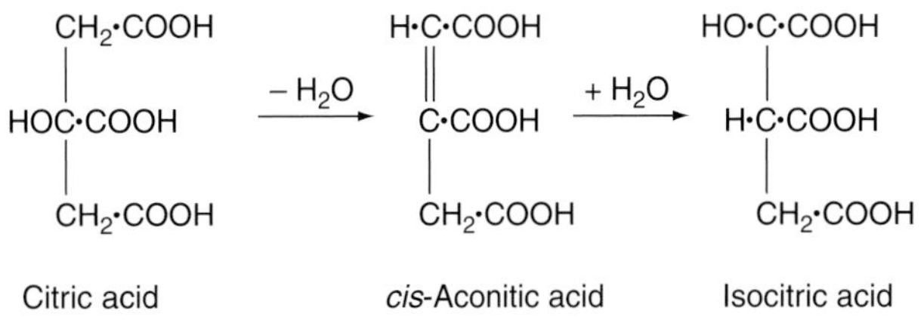

$$\begin{array}{ccc}
CH_2\cdot COOH & H\cdot C\cdot COOH & HO\cdot C\cdot COOH \\
| & \| & | \\
HOC\cdot COOH \xrightarrow{-H_2O} & C\cdot COOH \xrightarrow{+H_2O} & H\cdot C\cdot COOH \\
| & | & | \\
CH_2\cdot COOH & CH_2\cdot COOH & CH_2\cdot COOH \\
\text{Citric acid} & \textit{cis}\text{-Aconitic acid} & \text{Isocitric acid}
\end{array}$$

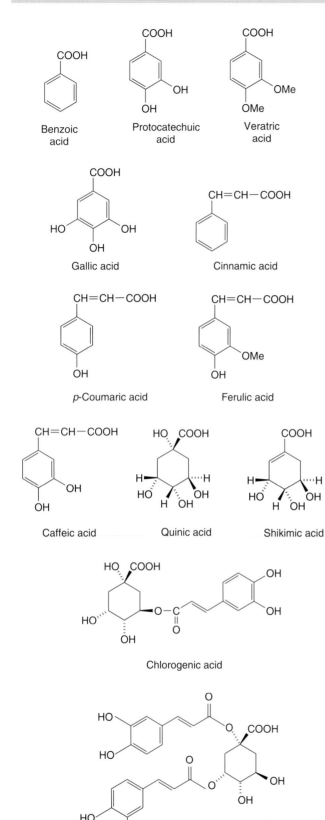

Fig. 19.5
Aromatic and other cyclic acids.

Of interest are opines, a group of substances formed by a host plant after infection with *Agrobacterium* spp.; a number of these compounds are di- and tri-carboxylic acids. For further details see Chapters 13 and 14.

ALCOHOLS

Alcohols possess one or more hydroxyl groups and exist naturally in either the free state or combined as esters. Like phenols they generally have common names ending in 'ol' (e.g. ethanol, glycerol and mannitol). They can be classed according to the number of hydroxyl groups present: monohydric alcohols-one hydroxyl, dihydric-two, trihydric-three and polyhydric-four or more. Furthermore each hydroxyl group may be classed as *primary*: –CH$_2$OH (e.g. ethanol), *secondary*: –CHOH– (e.g. isopropanol) or *tertiary*: ≡COH (e.g. *t*-butanol). The remainder of the molecule may be saturated or unsaturated, aliphatic or aromatic. Numerous examples will be encountered throughout the text.

Monohydric aliphatic alcohols
Lower members of the series are found principally combined as esters e.g. methyl salicylate in oil of wintergreen and methyl and ethyl esters responsible for some fruit aromas. Esterified long-chain alcohols are constituents of some pharmaceutically important animal waxes and include cetyl alcohol (C$_{16}$H$_{33}$OH), ceryl alcohol (C$_{26}$H$_{53}$OH) and myricyl alcohol (C$_{30}$H$_{61}$OH). Such alcohols also participate in the formation of esters which are constituents of leaf cuticular waxes; an example is Carnauba Wax *BP* which contains myricyl cerotate.

Monohydric terpene alcohols
These are alcohols associated with that large group of compounds which arise from mevalonic acid and have isoprene as a fundamental structural unit. Pharmacognostically they are particularly evident as constituents of volatile oils namely: (1) non-cyclic terpene alcohols occur in many volatile oils—for example, geraniol in otto of rose, its isomer nerol in oils of orange and bergamot and linalol both free and combined as linalyl acetate in oils of lavender and rosemary; (2) monocyclic terpene alcohols are represented by terpineol and its acetate in oil of neroli and menthol and its acetate in oil of peppermint; (3) dicyclic terpene alcohols are particularly abundant in the Coniferae (e.g. sabinol and its acetate in *Juniperus sabina*). In the dicotyledons oil of rosemary contains borneol and its esters.

Monohydric aromatic alcohols
Benzyl alcohol, C$_6$H$_5$CH$_2$OH, and cinnamyl alcohol, C$_6$H$_5$CH=CHCH$_2$OH, occur both free and as esters of benzoic and cinnamic acids in balsams such as Tolu and Peru. The latter balsam is sometimes adulterated with cheap synthetic benzyl benzoate.

Included in this class is coniferyl alcohol, which forms an important component of the lignin molecule. Lignins are extremely complex phenylpropane polymers; they form an important strengthening material of plant cell walls and vary in composition according to their source, see Chapter 21, section on 'Lignans and Lignin'.

Dihydric alcohols
Dihydric alcohols or *glycols* are compounds containing two hydroxyl groups; they are found naturally in many structural classes of compounds. The bicyclic amino alcohol 3,6-dihydroxytropane occurs

free and as esters in a number of species of the Solanaceae and Erythroxylaceae, the dihydric alcohol panaxadiol is a component of some ginseng steroids, and oenanthotoxin, the poisonous constituent of the hemlock water dropworts (*Oenanthe* spp.), is a polyene diol.

Trihydric alcohols

As with the glycols these compounds occur in a range of structural types. An important example is glycerol (propan-1,2,3-triol), an essential component of fixed oils and fats which are discussed in more detail below.

Polyhydric aliphatic alcohols

The following are alcohols with either four or six hydroxyl groups. The *meso* form of erythritol, $CH_2OHCHOHCHOHCH_2OH$, is found in seaweeds and certain lichens both free and combined with lecanoric acid. The hexahydric sugar alcohols (e.g. sorbitol, mannitol and dulcitol) are formed in nature by the reduction of either an aldehyde group of an aldose or the keto groups of a ketose. Sorbitol is abundant in many rosaceous fruits, mannitol in manna and dulcitol in species of *Euonymus*.

ESTERS

Esters arise from the union of an alcohol and an acid with loss of water:

$$R^1CH_2OH + R^2COOH \rightleftharpoons R^1CH_2OCOR^2 + HOH$$

The reaction is reversible and in plants esterase enzymes control the reaction.

Many different types of esters are known, and those formed by an acetylation of an alcoholic group are very common and are found in many biosynthetic groups of metabolites including volatile oils, e.g. linalyl acetate in lavender. Esters which involve aromatic acids such as benzoic and cinnamic acids with corresponding alcohols are sometimes found associated with free acids, other volatile metabolites and resins, in such products as balsams (see drugs described at the end of this chapter). A number of alkaloids (e.g. atropine and reserpine) are esters.

A particularly important group of esters from the pharmaceutical viewpoint is that comprising the lipids or fatty esters. These involve a long-chain fatty acid of the type described earlier and alcohols such as glycerol and the higher monohydric alcohols.

The term 'lipid' includes not only fixed oils, fats and waxes (simple lipids), but also phosphatides and lecithins (complex lipids), which may contain phosphorus and nitrogen in addition to carbon, hydrogen and oxygen. These substances are widely distributed in both the vegetable and animal kingdoms, and in plants they are particularly abundant in fruits and seeds. In animals the depot fats resemble those found in plants, while the complex lipids occur mainly in the more active tissues such as the brain and liver. The latter group plays an important role in the structure of cellular membranes, the hydrophobic nature of the fatty acids being all-important to their biological role.

The lecithins are esters of glycerophosphoric acid in which the two free hydroxyls of the glycerol are esterified with fatty acids while one of the two remaining groups of the phosphoric acid is esterified to an alcohol (choline, ethanolamine, serine, glycerol or inositol). Because plants have no mechanism for controlling their temperature, they must possess membrane lipids that remain mobile at relatively low temperatures. This property is conferred by the methylene-linked *cis* double

bonds of the polyunsaturated acids bound as esters with the polar lipids. Conversely, in simple lipids, all three hydroxyl groups are esterified with fatty acids and these compounds have been traditionally referred to as triglycerides, although with current nomenclature triacylglycerols is preferred. The prefix *sn* is now employed to denote the *stereospecific numbering* of the molecule.

A complex lipid
(a 1,2-diacyl-*sn*-glycero-3-phosphorylcholine)

A simple lipid or triacylglycerol
(tripalmitin)

Fats and fixed oils

As agricultural crops, seeds used for the extraction of fixed oils rate in importance second only to cereals. Over the last 60 years the production of oils for the food industry has increased enormously, whereas consumption by industrial and other users has remained relatively static but, in the pharmaceutical industry at least, not without interesting developments. Fixed oils are also obtained from fruit pericarps and in some instances such as the palm, *Elaeis guineensis* (Palmae), two oils differing in properties and chemical composition are obtained— the pleasantly flavoured palm kernel oil from the endosperm and palm oil from the orange-yellow fleshy pericarp. Oil seed crops are particularly advantageous commercially as following the expression of the oil a valuable high protein cattle feed remains. Also, such crops have benefited from plant breeding both regarding the yield and nature of the oil produced, and the morphology of the plant itself (see Chapter 14).

A naturally occurring mixture of lipids such as olive oil or oil of theobroma may be either liquid or solid and the terms 'oil' and 'fat' have, therefore, no very precise significance. Coconut oil and chaulmoogra oil, for example, leave the tropics as an oil and arrive in Western Europe as a solid. Even an oil such as olive oil will largely solidify in cold weather. In general, acylglycerols involving saturated fatty acids are solid and those of unsaturated acids are liquids. When both types are present, as in crude cod-liver oil, cooling results in the deposition of saturated acylglycerols such as stearin. In most medicinal cod-liver oils these solid materials are removed by freezing and filtration. Acylglycerols are represented by the general formula given below and can be hydrolysed by heating with caustic alkali to form soaps and glycerin.

If the fatty acids represented by R^1, R^2 and R^3 are the same, the triacylglycerol is known as a simple triacylglycerol—for example, tripalmitin on hydrolysis yields three molecules of palmatic acid. In nature, however, R^1, R^2 and R^3 are usually different and the ester is known as a mixed triacylglycerol. On hydrolysis they frequently yield both saturated and unsaturated acids (Fig. 19.6); there is a strong tendency for unsaturated acids, particularly the C_{18} olefinic acids, to be linked to the secondary hydroxyl.

Biogenesis. Acylglycerols are formed from the fatty acyl-CoA or, more probably, the fatty acyl carrier protein (ACP) and L-α-glycerophosphate, as indicated in Fig. 19.7.

Extraction. Most commercial oils are derived from either seeds or fruits and nowadays are mostly extracted by the producing country and exported as the crude oil. Sophisticated derivatizations of oils are mainly carried out by the importing countries.

The initial treatment before extraction depends on the botanical structure—for example, American cotton seeds require delinting and castor seeds and ground nuts require decorticating. Special machines are available for these purposes. Removal of the oil may take the form of cold or hot expression, centrifuging or solvent extraction, again depending on the commodity. With seeds the remaining cake usually forms a valuable cattle feed and for this reason complete removal of the oil is not always necessary. The crude oil requires refining, however, as for example with olive oil, the first expressed oils, *extra virgin* and *virgin* constitute the premium grades and require no further purification. Cold-drawn oils usually require nothing further than filtration; castor oil requires steaming to inactivate lipase; the addition of a determined amount of alkali may be required to remove free acid; and washing and decolorization may be performed. An antioxidant may be added and its nature and concentration stated on the label. Specific points concerning preparation are mentioned under the individual oils described at the end of the chapter. Where appropriate, the *refined* pharmaceutical oils are suitable for use in the manufacture of parenteral dosage forms.

Quantitative tests. A number of quantitative tests are commonly used to evaluate fixed oils and fats. *Acid value* refers to the number of mg of potassium hydroxide required to neutralize the free acids in 1 g of the oil; high acid values arise in rancidified oils. Particularly low values are officially specified for those oils to be used in parenteral dosage forms; for refined wheat-germ oil, for example, the value is ≯0.3, whereas for the refined oil for general use the value is ≯0.9 and for the unrefined oil ≯20.0. Similar figures apply to other fixed oils so used. *Saponification value*: the hydrolysis reaction of lipids

(above) can be used to determine the saponification value of the oil and is expressed as the number of mg of potassium hydroxide required to neutralize the free acids in, and to hydrolyse the esters in, 1 g of the substance. *Ester value* is the difference between the saponification and acid values. *Iodine value* (see 'Fatty acids') gives a measure of the unsaturation of the oil. Oils which partially resinify on exposure to air are known as semidrying or drying oils. Such oils (e.g. linseed oil) have high iodine values. In some cases, particularly for animal fats such as butter, the determination of *volatile acidity* is useful, since the lower fatty acids such as butyric acid are volatile in steam and this may be used for their separation and estimation. It is frequently useful to determine *unsaponifiable matter*, which consists of compounds such as sterols which remain after saponification of the acylglycerols and removal of the glycerol and soaps by means of solvents. The content of brassicasterol in the sterol fraction of fixed oils is limited by the *Pharmacopoeia* for some oils, e.g. maximum 0.3% for evening primrose oil and borage oil.

The *acetyl value* is the number of milligrams of potassium hydroxide required to neutralize the acetic acid freed by the hydrolysis of the acetylated fat or other substance. The oil is first acetylated with acetic anhydride, which combines with any free hydroxyl groups present, and the product is then isolated after thorough removal of acid resulting from the reagent; its saponification value is determined together with that of the original oil. The acetyl value is calculated from the difference between these two figures.

The *hydroxyl value* of a substance depends on the number of free hydroxyl groups present. It is expressed as the number of milligrams of potassium hydroxide required to neutralize the acid combined by acylation of the sample. Most fixed oils have low values, which arise from small quantities of sterols present; castor oil is an exception (minimum value 150), arising from the high proportion of ricinoleic acid present.

Under unsuitable storage conditions, such as exposure to light and air, fixed oils undergo secondary oxidation to give peroxides that then generate aldehydes and ketones. Such deterioration is detected by measurement of the *peroxide value* and *anisidine value*. The former is described by the *Pharmacopoeia* as 'the number that expresses in milliequivalents of oxygen the quantity of peroxide contained in 1000 g of the substance, as determined by the prescribed methods'. These methods involve the liberation of iodine from a potassium iodide solution by the peroxides present in the sample and titration with 0.01 M

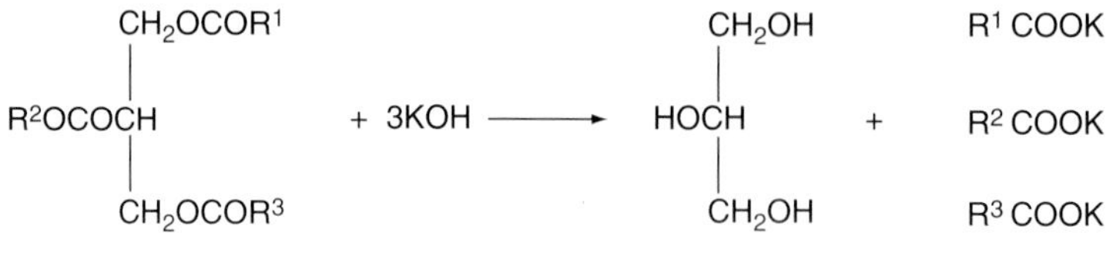

Fig. 19.6
Hydrolysis of a mixed triacylglycerol.

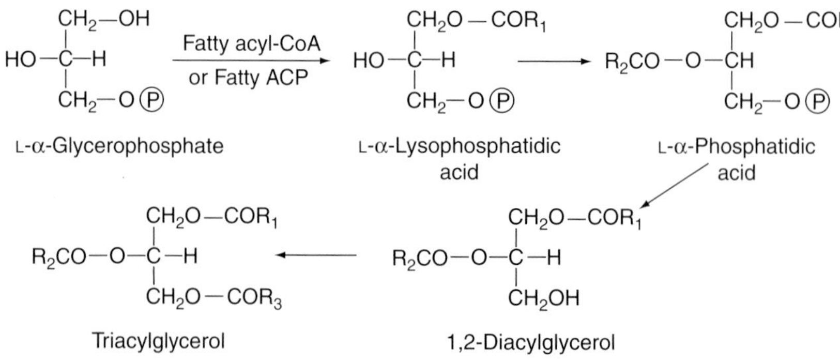

$$CH_2OCOR^1$$
$$R^2OCOCH \quad + \ 3KOH \longrightarrow$$
$$CH_2OCOR^3$$

$$CH_2OH \qquad R^1 COOK$$
$$HOCH \qquad + \quad R^2 COOK$$
$$CH_2OH \qquad R^3 COOK$$

Fig. 19.7
Formation of acylglycerols; R¹, R² and R³ may or may not be the same acyl groups.

L-α-Glycerophosphate → L-α-Lysophosphatidic acid → L-α-Phosphatidic acid

Triacylglycerol ← 1,2-Diacylglycerol

sodium thiosulphate solution. For refined oils such as olive, borage, evening primrose and wheat-germ the typical value is 10; if these oils are to be used for parental dosage forms the maximum is 5. The maximum permissible value is higher for the virgin oils, e.g. olive = 20. Peroxide values are also used for fish oils, e.g. maximum value for farmed salmon oil, 5.0.

Anisidine values are determined photometrically (350 nm) and depend on the coloured complex produced by the interaction of *p*-anisidine (the methyl ether of *p*-aminophenol) with aldehydes and ketones. They are used principally for the evaluation of fish oils, including type-A cod-liver oil and farmed salmon oil (maximum 10).

Certain physical constants of fixed oils and fats are significant: specific gravity, melting point, refractive index and sometimes optical rotation (e.g. castor oil). Table 19.6 shows how chemical standards are related to chemical composition. The gas chromatographic separation and quantification of the acids produced by the hydrolysis of specific fixed oils is an official method for their identification and quality control; type chromatograms are included in the *BP/EP*. Such detailed analyses often eliminate the necessity of routinely applying all the above quantitative standards. Some examples of this application are given for the oils in Table 16.4. Comments on the detection of adulterants in the more expensive oils can be found under individual headings.

Waxes

The term 'wax', although sometimes applied to the hydrocarbon mixture hard paraffin, is best confined to those natural mixtures containing appreciable quantities of esters derived from higher monohydric alcohols of the methyl alcohol series combined with fatty acids. In this series of alcohols the members change from liquids to solids, become less soluble in water and have higher melting points with increase in molecular weight. The first solid of the series is dodecyl alcohol, $C_{12}H_{25}OH$. Waxes include vegetable products such as carnauba wax and animal products such as spermaceti, beeswax and so-called 'wool-fat'.

Although waxes are abundant in nature (e.g. on epidermal surfaces), a limited number only are of commercial importance; some of the best-known and their chief alcohols are given at the end of the chapter.

An important practical difference between fats and waxes is that fats may be saponified by means of either aqueous or alcoholic alkali but waxes are only saponified by alcoholic alkali. This fact is used for the detection of fats when added as adulterants to waxes (e.g. for detecting the fat 'Japan wax' as an adulterant in beeswax). Saponification of the wax ester cetyl palmitate may be represented as:

$$C_{15}H_{31}.COOC_{16}H_{33} + alcoholic\ KOH \rightarrow C_{16}H_{33}OH$$

Cetyl palmitate   Cetylalcohol
$$+ C_{15}H_{13}.COOK$$
Potassium palmitate

While fats consist almost entirely of esters, waxes, in addition to esters of the cetyl palmitate type, often contain appreciable quantities of free acids, hydrocarbons, free alcohols and sterols. The hydrocarbons and sterols are unsaponifiable and both spermaceti and wool fat, which contain considerable quantities of these, have high saponification values. If analytical data for fats and waxes are compared, it will be noted that the acid values of waxes tend to be higher—for example, beeswax contains about 15% of free cerotic acid, $C_{26}H_{53}COOH$. In most waxes, iodine values are relatively low and unsaponifiable matter is high (Table 19.7).

Table 19.6 Numerical properties of fixed oils.

Fat or oil	Melting point, °C	Saponification value	Iodine value	Approximate fatty composition	
				Saturated (%)	Unsaturated (%)
Almond	−18	183–208	99–103	12	88 Ol. Ln.*
Castor	−18	175–183	84	0.3–2.5	88–94 Ricinoleic; 5–15 Ol. Ln.
Olive	†	185–196	79–88	7–20	75–93 Ol. Ln.
Arachis	−5 to +3	188–196	86–106	18	82 Ol. Ln.
Coconut	23–26	250–264	7–11	92	8 Ol.
Cottonseed	0 (Before winterizing)	190–198	109–116	27	73 Ln. Ol.
Palm	30	248	13.5	50	50 Ol. Ln.
Theobroma	31–34	193–195	33–42	59	41 Ol. Ln.
Lard	34–41	192–198	50–66	60	40 Ol.
Cod-liver	Clear at 0	180–190	155–180	Under 15	Over 85 with up to six unsaturated bonds

*Ol. = oleic; Ln. = linoleic; †deposits palmitin at 2°C.

Table 19.7 Chemical standards of waxes.

Wax	Acid value	Saponification value	Iodine value	Important constituents
Spermaceti	Below 1	120–136	Below 5	Cetyl palmitate and cetyl myristate
Beeswax	18–24	70–80 (ester value)	8–11	72% esters, mainly myricyl palmitate; free cerotic acid; steryl esters
Carnauba	4–7	79–95	10–14	
Wool-fat	Below 1	90–106	18–32	Steryl esters, esters of other aliphatic alcohols, fatty acids and hydrocarbons

19

DRUGS CONTAINING ACIDS, ALCOHOLS AND ESTERS

ROSELLE

The dried calyces and epicalyces of *Hibiscus sabdariffa* L., family Malvaceae, collected during the fruiting period, constitute the drug 'roselle'. As an ornamental, the plant is grown globally in subtropical areas and the leaves, stems and seeds also find use as colourants, flavourings and as a source of fibre (rosella hemp). Its common name, Jamaica sorrel, arose following its early introduction to that country. Commercial supplies of the drug come principally from S.E. Asia, Egypt and the Sudan.

Characters.   The easily broken, crimson to violet drug consists of the flower portions comprising a pitcher-shaped calyx with five recurved teeth and, below, and attached to it, an epicalyx of up to about twelve obovate leaflets. The powder, examined microscopically, exhibits coloured parenchymatous cells containing cluster crystals of calcium oxalate, mucilage-containing cells, vascular tissue, epidermal cells, anisocytic stomata, covering trichomes, a few glandular trichomes and pollen grains with spiney exines.

Constituents.   Roselle contains a considerable quantity of free acids including citric, tartaric and malic acids and the lactone of hydroxycitric acid. The *BP/EP* requires a minimum content of 13.5% of acids expressed as citric acid determined by potentiometric titration. Phenolic compounds include anthocyanins involving the glycosides of delphinidin and cyanidin for which the *Pharmacopoeia* specifies and absorbance of ≮0.350 for the whole drug and ≮0.250 for the cut drug when measured at 520 nm in a prescribed aqueous extract. A spectrophotometric assay for total anthocyanins has been reported (T. Sukwattanasinit *et al.*, *Planta Medica*, 2007, **73**, 1517). Various polysaccharides have been recorded; for a report on their stimulation of proliferation and differentiation of human keratinocytes see C. Brunold *et al.*, *Planta Med.*, 2004, **70**, 373.

Use.   A colourant and flavouring component for herbal preparations. Traditionally, all parts of the plant have been employed as an astringent and cooling agent; it has a diuretic action. Antioxidant and hypocholesterolemic activities have been investigated (V. Hirunpanich *et al.*, *J. Ethnopharmacol.*, 2006, **103**, 252).

Further reading
Vasudeva N, Sharma SK 2008 Biologically active compounds from the genus *Hibiscus*. Pharmaceutical Biology 46: 145–153. *A review with 68 references*

Tamarind pulp

The drug consists of the fruit of the tree *Tamarindus indica* (Leguminosae) deprived of the brittle, outer part of the pericarp and preserved with sugar. The fruits are about 5–15 cm long. They have a brittle epicarp, a pulpy mesocarp, through which run from the stalk about five to nine branched fibres, and a leathery endocarp. The latter forms from four to twelve chambers, in each of which is a single seed.

In the West Indies the fruits ripen in June, July and August. The epicarps are removed, the fruits are packed in layers in barrels, and boiling syrup is poured over them; alternatively, each layer of fruits is sprinkled with powdered sugar.

Tamarind pulp occurs as a reddish-brown, moist, sticky mass, in which the yellowish-brown fibres mentioned above are readily seen. Odour, pleasant and fruity; taste, sweet and acid.

The seeds, each enclosed in a leathery endocarp, are obscurely four-sided or ovate and about 15 mm long. They have a rich brown testa marked with a large patch or oreole. Within the testa, which is very thick and hard, lies the embryo. The large cotyledons are composed very largely of hemicellulose which stains blue with iodine.

The pulp contains free organic acids (about 10% of tartaric, citric and malic), their salts (about 8% of potassium hydrogen tartrate), a little nicotinic acid and about 30–40% of invert sugar. It is reported that the tartaric acid is synthesized in the actively metabolizing leaves of the plant and then translocated to the fruits as they develop. The addition of sugar to the manufactured pulp, to act as a preservative, somewhat lowers the natural proportion of acids.

Flavonoid *C*-glycosides (vitexin, isovitexin, orientin and isoorientin) occur in the leaves. The fixed oil of the seeds contains a mixture of glycerides of saturated and unsaturated (oleic, linoleic) acids.

Tamarind pulp is a mild laxative and was formerly used in Confection of Senna; it has traditional medicinal uses in the W. Indies and in China and the leaves have been suggested as a commercial source of tartaric acid.

Manna

The name 'manna' is applied to a number of different plant products. The biblical manna was probably the lichen *Lecanora esculenta*, which can be carried long distances by wind. The only manna of commercial importance is ash manna, derived from *Fraxinus ornus* (Oleaceae). The drug is collected in Sicily. When the trees are about 10 years old, transverse cuts are made in the trunk. A sugary exudation takes place and when sufficiently dried is picked off (flake manna) or is collected on leaves or tiles.

Manna occurs in yellowish-white pieces up to 15 cm long and 2 cm wide or in agglutinated masses of broken flakes, with a pleasant odour and sweet taste. It contains about 55% of the hexahydric alcohol mannitol, relatively small amounts of hexose sugars but larger amounts of the more complex sugars mannotriose and mannotetrose (stachyose). The triose on hydrolysis yields glucose (1 mol) and galactose (2 mol), while the tetrose yields glucose (1 mol), fructose (1 mol) and galactose (2 mol). Manna has a mild laxative action.

SUMATRA BENZOIN

Two commercial varieties of benzoin—Sumatra benzoin and Siam benzoin—are included in the *BP/EP*. Sumatra benzoin (*Gum Benjamin*) is a balsamic resin obtained from the incised stem of *Styrax benzoin* Dryand, and *Styrax paralleloneurus* Perkins (Styracaceae). It is produced almost exclusively from cultivated trees grown in Sumatra, although the tree is also native to Java and Borneo.

History.   The drug was noted by Ibn Batuta, who visited Sumatra in the fourteenth century, but was not regularly imported into Europe until the sixteenth century.

Collection and preparation.   Sumatra benzoin is a purely pathological product and there is some evidence to show that its formation is brought about not only by the incisions made, but also by fungi (see 'Stress Compounds', Chapter 18). In Sumatra the seeds are sown in rice fields, the rice shading the young trees during their first year. After the harvesting of the rice the trees are allowed to grow until they are about 7 years old.

Tapping.   The rather complicated process consists of making in each trunk three lines of incisions which are gradually lengthened.

The first triangular wounds are made in a vertical row about 40 cm apart, the bark between the wounds being then scraped smooth. The first secretion is very sticky and is rejected. After making further cuts, each about 4 cm above the preceding ones, a harder secretion is obtained. Further incisions are made at 3-monthly intervals and the secretion instead of being amorphous becomes crystalline. About 6 weeks after each fresh tapping the product is scraped off, the outer layer (finest quality) being kept separate from the next layer (intermediate quality). About 2 weeks later the strip is scraped again, giving a lower quality darker in colour and containing fragments of bark. Fresh incisions are then made and the above process is repeated. After a time the line of incisions is continued further up the trunk.

Grades.   The above three qualities are not sold as such but are blended in Palembang to give the benzoin grades of commerce. The best grade contains the most 'almonds' and the worst contains a few almonds but abundant resinous matrix. The blending is done by breaking up the drug, mixing different proportions of the three qualities and softening in the sun. It was formerly exported after stamping into tins but now the commercial drug arrives in plaited containers with a plastic wrapping.

Characters.   *Sumatra benzoin* occurs in brittle masses consisting of opaque, whitish or reddish tears embedded in a translucent, reddish-brown or greyish-brown, resinous matrix. Odour, agreeable and balsamic but not very marked; taste, slightly acrid. *Siamese benzoin* occurs in tears or in blocks. The tears are of variable size and flattened; they are yellowish-brown or reddish-brown externally, but milky-white and opaque internally. The block form consists of small tears embedded in a somewhat glassy, reddish-brown, resinous matrix. It has a vanilla-like odour and a balsamic taste.

When gradually heated, benzoin evolves white fumes of cinnamic and benzoic acids which readily condense on a cool surface as a crystalline sublimate. On warming a little powdered benzoin with solution of potassium permanganate, a faint odour of benzaldehyde is noted with Sumatra benzoin but not with the Siamese. When an alcoholic solution of ferric chloride is added to an alcoholic extract of Siamese benzoin, a green colour is produced. Sumatra benzoin does not give this test. The *BP/EP* includes a TLC test for the absence of Dammar gum, a copal resin, used in the manufacture of varnishes and apparently derived from species of *Hopea, Shorea* and *Vateria* family Dipterocarpaceae.

Constituents.   Sumatra benzoin contains free balsamic acids (cinnamic and benzoic) and esters derived from them. Also present are triterpenoid acids such as siaresinolic acid (19-hydroxyoleanolic acid) and sumaresinolic acid (6-hydroxyoleanolic acid). For the formula of oleanolic acid see under 'Triterpenoid Saponins'. The content of total balsamic acids (calculated as cinnamic acid) is at least 20%, and the amount of cinnamic acid is usually about double that of benzoic acid. Up to about 20% of free acids may be present. High-grade material from *S. paralleloneurum* contains benzoic acid 3%, vanillin 0.5% and cinnamic acid 20–30%.

Allied drug.   *Palembang benzoin,* an inferior variety produced in Sumatra, may be collected from isolated trees from which the resin has not been stripped for some time. It is easily distinguished, being very light in weight and breaking with an irregular porous fracture. It consists almost entirely of reddish-brown resin, with only a few very small tears embedded in it. Palembang benzoin is used as a source of natural benzoic acid.

Uses.   Benzoin, when taken internally, acts as an expectorant and antiseptic. It is mainly used as an ingredient of friar's balsam, or as a cosmetic lotion prepared from a simple tincture. It finds considerable use world-wide in the food, drinks, perfumery and toiletry industries; it is a component of incense.

SIAM BENZOIN

Siam benzoin *BP/EP* is obtained by incision of the trunk of *Styrax tonkinensis* (Pierre) Craib ex Hartwich; it contains 45.0–55.0% of total acids calculated as benzoic acid (dried drug). It is the traditional source of benzoin for a number of European pharmacopoeias.

The drug is produced in relatively small areas in the Thai province of Luang Prabang, northern Laos and northern Vietnam from trees growing in the wild at an altitude of between 600 and 2500 m. It seems that this height is necessary for resin production; not all trees are productive.

The method of collection appears similar to that for Sumatra benzoin, the resin being produced at the interface of the bark and wood layers only after injury. The collected tears are sorted into grades based on size and colour, the most esteemed being the largest and palest. Length of tears commonly varies from a few millimetres to 3 cm, flattened or sometimes, if large, concavo-convex as would be expected if the resin collected between the bark and the wood of the tree. They are yellowish-white to reddish on the outer surface, often in the commercial drug cemented together by the brownish resin, which increases due to oxidation as the material is stored. The fracture of the tears is waxy-white with an agreeable odour resembling vanilla.

Constituents.   The combined acid content of Siam benzoin consists principally of coniferyl benzoate and a very small amount of coniferyl cinnamate (coniferyl alcohol, see Fig. 21.2, is found in the cambial sap of both gymnosperms and angiosperms). Free benzoic acid amounts to some 10% of the drug. Other constituents are triterpenoid acids and esters, and vanillin.

Tests.   Compared with Sumatra benzoin, Siam benzoin is expensive and is liable to adulteration with the former, which can be detected by the *BP/EP* TLC test; this indicates an absence of cinnamic acid in the genuine drug. This absence also means that no odour of benzaldehyde is produced when the powdered drug is warmed with a solution of potassium permanganate *cf.* Sumatra benzoin. Also, Siam benzoin in ethanol, on treatment with ferric chloride solution, gives a green, not yellow, colour. The pharmacopoeial assay for total acids involves the back-titration with hydrochloric acid of a hydrolysed solution of the drug in alcoholic potassium hydroxide solution.

Uses.   Similar to those of Sumatra benzoin.

ASH LEAF

Ash leaf *BP/EP* consists of the dried leaves of *Fraxinus excelsior* L., the common ash, or *Fraxinus oxyphylla* M. Bieb., family Oleaceae, having a minimum content of 2.5% total hydroxycinnamic acid derivatives expressed as chlorogenic acid.

The common ash is found throughout temperate Europe, in Western Asia and extending northwards into Scandanavia; it is common in Britain. The leaves are up to 30 cm in length, opposite, pinnate and consisting of a rachis bearing 9–13 leaflets. It is the latter that constitute the official drug; they are about 7 cm long with short petiolules, lanceolate to ovate, apex apiculate to acuminate and a sharp, shallow forward-toothed margin. Colour dark green on the upper surface, lighter below.

Elements of the powdered drug include: upper epidermis with some striated cuticle and a lower surface with anomocytic stomata, occasional covering trichomes and, rarely, glandular trichomes.

Constituents of the leaf embrace the coumarin glycoside fraxin (formula shown in Table 21.2), various hydroxycinnamic acid derivatives, e.g. chlorogenic acid (see Fig. 19.5), tannins, the sugar alcohol mannite and bitter principles. The *BP* assay is based on the colour reaction of an acidified methanolic extract of the sample with solutions of sodium nitrite and sodium molybdate followed by alkali. Absorbance is measured at 525 nm.

Ash leaf has a mild laxative and diuretic action.

Allied species. *Fraxinus ornus* is a commercial source of manna (q.v.) and its leaflets can be substituted for the above. It may be distinguished by not affording the characteristic zones of acteoside, chlorogenic acid and rutin (see Fig. 21.15) when subjected to TLC examination. Hydroxycoumarins, secoiridoid glycosides, phenylethanoids and flavonoids have been reported in the plant. For a review, including biological activities, see I. Kostova, *Fitoterapia*, 2001, **72**, 471; similarly for the genus (39–63 spp., depending on the classification) and featuring over 150 compounds, biological activities and 150 references, see I. Kostova and T. Iossifova, *Fitoterapia*, 2007, **78**, 85–106.

ARTICHOKE LEAF

The leaves of the globe artichoke, *Cynara scolymus* L., family Asteraceae/Compositae, have been long-used in traditional medicine and are now included in the *BP/EP*, the *BHP* and the *Complete German Commission E Monographs*. The plant is native to the Mediterranean region and northern Africa and probably evolved from *C. cardunculus* at an early date (D. Bown, *Encyclopedia of Herbs*, 1995, Dorling Kindersley, London).

Leaves, up to *ca* 70 cm long and 30 cm wide, are collected and dried just before the flowering stage. The leaf lamina is deeply lobed, reaching to 1–2 cm of the midrib but becoming pinnatifid towards the petiole. The margin is coarsely toothed and trichomes cover both surfaces, being particularly dense and twisted on the lower surface. Hairs also cover the petioles, which, together with the main veins, are flat on the upper surfaces and raised and ridged on the lower.

The greyish-green to brown powder exhibits epidermi of straight- or sinuous-walled cells and many anomocytic stomata. Covering, multicellular, uniseriate trichomes occur scattered or in felted masses together with fewer glandular trichomes having brown contents in a monoseriate or biseriate head. Groups of lignified fibres and reticulately thickened vessels arise from veins of the petiole and midrib. The drug has a slight odour and a salty taste followed by bitterness.

Phenolic acids are important constituents and include chlorogenic acid, caffeic acid and cynarin (1, 5-di-*O*-caffeoylquinic acid) (see Fig. 19.5). The *BP* specifies a minimum requirement for chlorogenic acid of 0.8%, which is determined by liquid chromatography using chlorogenic acid reference solution for peak area comparison. Flavonoids include luteolin-7β-D-glucoside and the 7β-D-rutionoside. The former, together with chlorogenic acid, are used in the official TLC test for identity. Other constituents include volatile oil, sesquiperpene lactones, e.g. cynaropicrin, inulin, tannins and phytosterols.

Artichoke leaf is used for the treatment of indigestion and dyspepsia; for its use as a hepatic, see Chapter 29.

NETTLE LEAF

All parts of the nettle are used medicinally, the dried roots and herb in the *BHP* and the dried leaves in the *BP/EP*. The latter specifies two species—*Urtica dioica* L., the stinging nettle, and *U. urens* L., the small nettle. Both species are common throughout North temperate regions.

U. urens is an annual herb with the lower leaves shorter than their petioles, whereas *U. dioica* is a coarse hispid perennial with the lower leaves longer than their petioles.

The green powdered drug has a slight odour and bitter taste. Cells of both epidermises have sinuous anticlinal walls and the lower epidermis includes numerous anomocytic stomata. Cystoliths containing large calcium carbonate masses are present in the epidermal layers (see Fig. 42.1A). Clothing trichomes, stinging hairs and glandular trichomes are numerous. In the powder, the upper cells of the stinging trichomes are usually broken off.

The constituents of nettle have been extensively researched. They include a number of acids such as chlorogenic, caffeoylmalic, caffeic, malic and fumaric. Flavonoids include quercetin and its glycosides isoquercitrin and rutin (see Fig. 21.15). 5-Hydroxytryptamine (serotonin) is a component of the stinging hairs. Other metabolites include lignans, scopoletin (see Table 21.2) and choline acetyltransferase.

Scopoletin and chlorogenic acid are used as reference compounds in the *BP* TLC identification test. The assay is by liquid chromatography, requiring a minimum of 0.3% for the sum of the caffeoylmalic acid and chlorogenic acid content, expressed as chlorogenic acid. The high total ash limit for the drug (20.0%) is dictated by the considerable natural inorganic content, particularly silicic acid and calcium and potassium salts, which are present in the leaves.

Nettle has been used traditionally to treat many disorders. It is a diuretic and is employed in various rheumatic conditions and to assist micturition in cases of benign prostatic hyperplasia.

Further reading

Kavalali GM (ed), Hardman R (series ed) 2003 Urtica: therapeutic and nutritional aspects of stinging nettles. CRC Press UK, London

ECHINACEA SPP.

Echinacea species (coneflowers), are perennial herbs of the Compositae/Asteraceae native to the prairie regions of Ohio where they were used by the Plains tribes to treat a variety of conditions, particularly wounds. Three species are currently important. Roots of *Echinacea augustifolia* DC., the narrow-leaved coneflower, and *E. pallida* Nutt., the pale coneflower, are included in the *BP/EP*. The whole plant of *E. purpurea* (the purple coneflower) is much used for the commercial preparation of herbal medicaments, it being the largest of the three species and easy to cultivate. All continue to receive research attention in connection with their phytochemical, pharmacological and clinical attributes.

Particular groups of compounds can be found in all three species but variations occur concerning specific metabolites. Some aspects of earlier research must also be treated with caution because it is now known that some commercial batches of so-called *E. augustifolia* grown in Europe were in fact *E. pallida* (R. Bauer *et al.*, *Planta Medica*, 1988, **54**, 426; *Sci. Pharm.*, 1987, **55**, 159; P. R. Bradley, *Brit. Herb. Comp.*, 1992, **1**, 81).

The roots of the two official drugs are not easily differentiated by their morphological and microscopical characteristics; in the powders, numerous sclereids and phytomelanin deposits occur in both. However, TLC can be used for the identification and also for the detection of *E. purpurea* in adulterated *E. augustifolia*, and to detect other *Echinacea* spp. and *Parthenium integrifolium* in *E. pallida*. A recent DNA study [sequence characterized amplified region (SCAR) analysis] has demonstrated the distinction of *E. purpurea* from the other two species (B. Adinolfi *et al.*, *Fitoterapia*, 2007, **78**, 43).

Constituents. A caffeic acid derivative, echinacoside, is present in the roots of both *E. augustifolia* and *E. pallida*. Cynarin, a quinic acid derivative, occurs only in the former. Esters involving tartaric acid, such as caftaric acid and cichoric acid, occur in small amounts in both species. Other constituents include high-molecular-weight polysaccharides, alkylamides, acetylenes, volatiles including humulene (see Fig. 21.4) and traces of pyrrolizidine alkaloids (F. Pellati *et al.*, *Phytochemistry*, 2006, **67**, 1359 and references cited therein).

The *BP/EP* requires minimum contents of echinacoside for *E. augustifolia* root (0.5%) and *E. pallida* root (0.2%) determined by liquid chromatography with spectrometric detection at 330 nm.

Actions. Echinacea is considered to have immunostimulant properties based on its alkylamide, polysaccharide and cichoric acid components. Preparations of the drug have become popular for the prevention and treatment of the common cold and other respiratory complaints. A recent meta-analysis of fourteen studies (S. A. Saah *et al.*, *The Lancet Infectious Diseases*, 2007, **7**, 473) indicated that Echinacea reduced both the incidence (by 58.0%) and the duration (by 1.4 days) of the common cold. For a mini-review on the role of alkamides as an active principle, see K. Woelkart and R. Bauer, *Planta Medica*, 2007, **73**, 615; for a report on this controversial aspect, see B. Barrett, *HerbalGram*, 2006, **70**, 36. Other traditional uses involve its anti-inflammatory and antibacterial properties.

Further reading

Miller SC (ed), Hardman R (series ed) 2004 Medicinal and aromatic plants – industrial profiles. Vol. 39, Echinacea: the genus *Echinacea*. CRC Press, Taylor and Francis Group, London

PYGEUM BARK

Pygeum bark is obtained from the stems and branches of *Prunus africana* (Hook f.) Kalkm. syn. *Pygeum africanum* Hook f., family Rosaceae, a tree indigenous to the rain-forests of Africa. Cameroon is the principal exporter. The increased demand for the drug from Europe and the US has led, as with other trees not easily cultivated commercially, to the danger of over-collection.

The whole or cut bark is now included in the *BP/EP* and consists of dark- to reddish-brown pieces with an outer wrinkled cork with some lichens attached and an inner longitudinally striated surface. The powder exhibits typical bark characteristics: cork cells, sclereids in groups or singly, fibres principally in groups, pigmented cells, small starch grains and cluster crystals of calcium oxalate.

Constituents. Identified constituents include aliphatic alcohols occurring as ferulic acid esters, phytosterols, triterpenoid pentacyclic acids and a lipid fraction involving C_{12}–C_{24} fatty acids. Pharmacopoeial tests include a minimum extractive value of 0.5% (continuous Soxhlet-type extraction with methylene chloride as solvent) and a TLC separation to show characteristic bands including those of β-sitosterol and ursolic acid.

Uses. Traditionally for the symptomatic treatment of benign prostatic hyperplasia. The activity appears to be comparable to that of *Serenoa repens* fruit extracts.

PERU BALSAM

Balsam of Peru is obtained from the trunk of *Myroxylon balsamum* var. *pereirae* (Leguminosae), after it has been beaten and scorched.

The drug is produced in Central America (San Salvador, Honduras and Guatemala) and is now included in the *European Pharmacopoeia* and the *BP* (2000).

History. The drug derives its name from the fact that when first imported into Spain it came via Callao in Peru. It was known to Monardes and the method of preparation was described as early as 1576, although afterwards forgotten. In 1860 the collection was described and illustrated by Dorat.

Collection and preparation. In November or December strips of bark, measuring about 30 × 15 cm, are beaten with the back of an axe or other blunt instrument. The bark soon cracks and may be pulled off after 2 weeks. As in the case of Tolu balsam, the secretion is purely pathological in origin and very little balsam can be obtained from the bark unless it is charred with a torch about 1 week after the beating. The balsam produced in the bark is obtained by boiling the bark in water and is known as *tacuasonte* (prepared without fire) or *balsamo de cascara* (balsam of the bark).

The greater part of the balsam, however, is prepared, after the removal of the bark, by the second method. The balsam which exudes is soaked up with rags, which, after some days, are cleaned by gently boiling with water and squeezing in a rope press. The balsam sinks to the bottom and, the water having been decanted, the balsam (*balsamo de trapo*) is poured off and strained.

Less destructive methods of preparation have been investigated and include the removal of narrow strips of bark and the replacement of scorching with the use of a hot iron. With this treatment the tree recovers in 6 months, compared with 8 years after the drastic traditional method. The drug is chiefly exported from Acajutla (San Salvador) and Belize (British Honduras) in tin canisters holding about 27 kg.

Characters. Balsam of Peru is a viscid liquid of a somewhat oily nature, but free from stickiness and stringiness. When seen in bulk, it is dark brown or nearly black in colour, but in thin layers it is reddish-brown and transparent. The original containers have a whitish scum on the surface. The balsam has a pleasant, somewhat vanilla-like odour and an acrid, slightly bitter taste.

The drug is almost insoluble in water. It is soluble in one volume of alcohol (90%), but the solution becomes turbid on the addition of further solvent. The relative density, 1.14–1.17, is a good indication of purity, and if abnormal indicates adulteration with fixed oils, alcohol, kerosene, etc. The *BP/EP* includes tests for the absence of artificial balsams (solubility characteristics in petroleum spirit), fixed oils (solubility in chloral hydrate solution) and turpentine (odour test).

Constituents. The official drug is required to contain not less than 45.0% w/w and not more than 70% w/w of esters, assayed gravimetrically. The chief balsamic esters present are benzyl cinnamate (cinnamein) $C_6H_5CH=CHCOOCH_2C_6H_5$ (sap. value 234), benzyl benzoate (sap. value 264.3) and cinamyl cinnamate (styracin). The drug also contains about 28% of resin, which is said to consist of peruresinotannol combined with cinnamic and benzoic acids, alcohols (nerolidol, farnesol and benzyl alcohol) and small quantities of vanillin and free cinnamic acid.

Work on the isoflavonoids contained in the trunk-wood has indicated that considerable chemical differences characterize the various forms or species of the *M. balsamum* group.

Uses. Balsam of Peru is used as an antiseptic dressing for wounds and as a parasiticide. Now that it is no longer used in Tulle gras dressings, it is of less current interest in Western medicine. Taken internally it is used to treat catarrh and diarrhoea. Allergic responses are possible.

Prepared storax

Prepared storax is a balsam obtained from the wounded trunk of *Liquidambar orientalis* (Hamamelidaceae) and subsequently purified. This is known as Levant storax and is obtained from a small tree found in the south-west of Turkey.

Collection and preparation. In the early summer the bark is injured by bruising or by making incisions. After a time the outer bark may be pared off, or the whole bark may be left until the autumn, when it is removed. The pieces of bark are pressed in horse-hair bags, first in the cold and again after steeping in hot water. Sometimes the bark is boiled with water and again pressed. The exhausted bark is used in the East for fumigation. The crude or liquid storax is exported in casks from Izmir.

Storax is obtained by dissolving the crude balsam in alcohol, filtering and recovering the solvent at as low a temperature as possible so as not to lose any of the volatile constituents. The alcohol-insoluble matter consists of vegetable debris and a resin.

Characters. *Crude storax* is a greyish, viscous liquid with a pleasant odour and bitter taste. It usually contains about 20–30% of water. About 82–87% is alcohol soluble.

Purified storax forms a brown, viscous, semisolid mass which loses not more than 5% of its weight when dried on a water-bath for 1 h. It is completely soluble in alcohol and partially in either. It has a characteristic balsamic odour and taste.

Constituents. Storax is very rich in free and combined cinnamic acid. After purification it yields 30–47% of total balsamic acids.

By steam distillation storax yields an oily liquid containing phenylethylene (styrene), $C_6H_5CH=CH_2$, cinnamic esters, vanillin and free cinnamic acid. The resinous portion of the drug consists of resin alcohols present both free and combined with cinnamic acid. The presence of cinnamic acid in the drug is shown by the odour of benzaldehyde which is produced when the drug is mixed with sand and warmed with a solution of potassium permanganate.

Recent research carried out in Turkey has shown the presence of many compounds not previously reported; these include monoterpenes, phenylpropanes and aliphatic acids.

Allied drug. American storax obtained from *L. styraciflua*, a large tree found near the Atlantic coast from Central America to Connecticut, is also used in the USA. This balsam resembles the Levant storax in constituents. Thirty-six compounds have been identified in the leaf-oil of the plant and tannins and related phenolics obtained from cell cultures. American researchers have reported the fruits as a rich source of shikimic acid, starting material for the synthesis of the antiviral drug oseltamivir. The yield is greatly superior to that from star-anise fruits, the accepted source material.

Uses. Storax is chiefly used in the preparation of friars' balsam and benzoin inhalation.

TOLU BALSAM

Tolu Balsam is obtained by incision from the trunk of *Myroxylon balsamum* (L.) Harms. var. *balsamum* (Leguminosae), a large tree that differs but little from that yielding balsam of Peru. Wild trees occur in Colombia and Venezuela and in the former country large quantities of balsam were produced in the neighbourhood of the Magdalena and Cauca rivers. The trees are cultivated in the West Indies, particularly in Cuba.

History. Balsam of Tolu was described by Monardes in 1574 and its collection was observed by Weir in 1863.

Collection. The drug is collected by making V-shaped incisions in the bark, the secretion being received in a calabash placed in the angle of the V. Many such receivers are fixed on each tree, the yield per tree being 8–10 kg. Periodically, the balsam is transferred to larger containers. It is exported in tins from Cartagena, Sabanilla and Sta. Marta.

Characters. When freshly imported, tolu is a soft, yellow semisolid. On keeping it turns to a brown, brittle solid. It softens on warming, and if a little is then pressed between two glass slides, microscopical examination shows crystals of cinnamic acid, amorphous resin and vegetable debris. Odour is aromatic and fragrant; taste, aromatic; the drug forms a plastic mass when chewed.

It is almost entirely soluble in alcohol, the solution being acid to litmus, and giving a green colour with ferric chloride (the latter possibly owing to the presence of resinotannol). Like other drugs containing cinnamic acid, it yields an odour of benzaldehyde when a filtered decoction is oxidized with potassium permanganate solution.

Constituents. Tolu contains about 80% of resin derived from resin alcohols combined with cinnamic and benzoic acids. The drug is rich in free aromatic acids and contains about 12–15% of free cinnamic and about 8% of free benzoic acid (acid value from 100–160). Other constituents are esters such as benzyl benzoate and benzyl cinnamate and a little vanillin. Recent investigations have shown the presence of other esters, styrene, eugenol, vanillin, ferulic acid, 1,2-diphenylethane, mono- and sesquiterpene hydrocarbons and alcohols. The balsam also contains numerous triterpenoids. Total balsamic acids (*BP/EP*, 25–50%) are determined by titration following hydrolysis of the esters.

Uses. Balsam of Tolu has antiseptic and flavouring properties and is commonly added to cough mixtures in the form of a syrup of tincture.

PHARMACEUTICAL FIXED OILS AND FATS

ALMOND OIL

Almond oil is a fixed oil obtained by expression from the seeds of *Prunus dulcis* (Miller) E. A. Webb (Rosaceae) var. *dulcis* (sweet almond) or *P. dulcis* (Miller) D. A. Webb var. *amara* (D.C.) Buchheim (bitter almond) or a mixture of both varieties.

The oil is mainly produced from almonds grown in the countries bordering the Mediterranean (Italy, France, Spain and North Africa).

Characters of plants and seeds. Almond trees are about 5 m in height and the varieties, except for differences in the seeds, are almost indistinguishable. The young fruits have a soft, felt-like pericarp, the inner part of which gradually becomes sclerenchymatous as the fruit ripens to form a pitted endocarp or shell. The shells, consisting mainly of sclerenchymatous cells, are sometimes ground and used to adulterate powdered drugs.

The sweet almond is 2–3 cm in length, rounded at one end and pointed at the other. The bitter almond is 1.5–2 cm in length but of similar breadth to the sweet almond. Both varieties have a thin, cinnamon-brown testa which is easily removed after soaking in warm water, a process which is known as blanching. The oily kernel consists of two large, oily planoconvex cotyledons, and a small plumule and radicle, the latter lying at the pointed end of the seed. Some almonds have cotyledons of unequal sizes and are irregularly folded. Bitter almonds are sometimes found in samples of sweet almonds, particularly those of African origin; their presence may be detected by the sodium picrate test for cyanogenetic glycosides.

Constituents. Both varieties of almond contain 40–55% of fixed oil, about 20% of proteins, mucilage and emulsin. The bitter almonds contain in addition 2.5–4.0% of the colourless, crystalline, cyanogenetic glycoside amygdalin (see Chapter 25).

Refined almond oil is obtained by grinding the seeds and expressing them in canvas bags between slightly heated iron plates. They are sometimes blanched before grinding, but this does not appear to be of any particular advantage. The oil is clarified by subsidence and filtration. It is a pale yellow liquid with a slight odour and bland, nutty taste. The *BP/EP* specifies oleic acid 62–86%, linoleic acid 20–30%, palmitic acid 4–9% together with lesser amounts of other acids as produced by the hydrolysis of the oil using GLC analysis. There are tests for the absence of other oils and sterols; the sterol fraction of the genuine oil consists principally of β-sitosterol (73–87%).

Virgin almond oil BP/EP conforms to similar tests as above but is not refined.

Hydrogenated almond oil is also included in the *BP/EP*.

Essential or volatile oil of almonds is obtained from the cake left after expressing bitter almonds. This is macerated with water for some hours to allow hydrolysis of the amygdalin to take place. The benzaldehyde and hydrocyanic acid are then separated by steam distillation.

Bitter almond oil contains benzaldehyde and 2–4% of hydrocyanic acid. Purified volatile oil of bitter almonds has had all its hydrocyanic acid removed and therefore consists mainly of benzaldehyde.

Uses. Almond oil is used in the preparation of many toilet articles and as a vehicle for oily injections. When taken internally, it has a mild, laxative action. The volatile almond oils are used as flavouring agents.

ARACHIS OIL

Arachis oil is obtained by expression from the seeds of *Arachis hypogaea* L. (Leguminosae) (*earth-nut, ground-nut, peanut*) a small annual plant cultivated throughout tropical Africa and in India, Brazil, southern USA and Australia. Various genotypes exist which show differences in the relative amounts of fatty acids contained in the oil. Enormous quantities of the fruits and seeds are shipped to Marseilles and other European ports for expression. Ground-nuts are the world's fourth largest source of fixed oil.

Preparation. During ripening the fruits bury themselves in the sandy soil in which the plants grow. Each fruit contains from one to three reddish-brown seeds. The fruits are shelled by a machine. The kernels contain 40–50% of oil. Owing to the high oil content the seeds, when crushed, are somewhat difficult to express. After the initial 'cooking', part of the oil is removed in a low-pressure expeller and the cake is solvent extracted. The two oil fractions are then mixed before purification. The press cake forms an excellent cattle food. The ground pericarps have been used as an adulterant of powdered drugs.

Constituents. Arachis oil consists of the glycerides of oleic, linoleic, palmitic, arachidic, stearic, lignoceric and other acids. When saponified with alcoholic potassium hydroxide, crystals of impure potassium arachidate separate on standing. Arachis oil is one of the most likely adulterants of other fixed oils (e.g. olive oil). The *BP* examination of the oil is similar to that mentioned under 'Olive Oil' below; the temperature at which the cooling, hydrolysed oil becomes cloudy should not be below 36°C. As with olive oil more stringent standards are required for oil to be used parenterally.

Uses. Arachis oil has similar properties to olive oil. It is an ingredient of camphorated oil but is used mainly in the production of margarine, cooking fats, etc.

Hydrogenated arachis oil is produced by refining, bleaching, hydrogenating and deodorizing the above. As with other hydrogenated oils it is much thicker than the parent oil, constituting a soft, off-white mass. There are various types of the hydrogenated oil with so-called nominal drop points determined as prescribed in the *Pharmacopoeia*; these fall within the range 32–42°C and, within this range, the drop point should not differ by more than 3°C from the nominal value. Again, as with other hydrogenated oils there is a limit for nickel (≯1 ppm) determined by atomic absorption spectrometry. The peroxide value should not exceed 5.0%.

COCONUT OIL

The expressed oil of the dried solid part of the endosperm of the coconut, *Cocos nucifera* L. (Palmae) is a semisolid, melting at about 24°C and consisting of the triglycerides of mainly lauric and myristic acids, together with smaller quantities of caproic, caprylic, oleic, palmitic and stearic acids. This constitution gives it a very low iodine value (7.0–11.0) and a high saponification value.

The particularly high proportion of medium chain-length acids means that the oil is easily absorbed from the gastrointestinal tract, which makes it of value to patients with fat absorption problems.

Fractionated coconut oil. Fractionated and purified endosperm oil of the coconut *C. nucifera*, or Thin Vegetable Oil of the *BPC*, contains triglycerides containing only the short and medium chain-length fatty acids (e.g. octanoic, decanoic; see Table 19.2). It maintains its low viscosity until near the solidification point (about 0°C) and is a useful non-aqueous medium for the oral administration of some medicaments.

Medium-chain Triglycerides BP/EP, synonymous with the above, may also be obtained from the dried endosperm of *Elaeis guineensis* (Palmae). The fatty acid composition of the hydrolysed oil, determined by GC, has the following specifications: caproic acid ≯2%, caprylic acid 50–80%, capric acid 20–50%, lauric acid ≯3.0%, myristic acid ≯1.0%.

COTTONSEED OIL

Cottonseed oil is expressed from the seeds of various species of *Gossypium* (Malvaceae) in America and Europe. In the UK, Egyptian and Indian cottonseed, which do not require delinting on arrival, are largely used. See under 'Cotton'.

The preparation of cottonseed oil is one of hot expression and a pressure of about 10 000 kPa is used. The crude oil is thick and turbid and is refined in various ways, that known as 'winter bleached' being the best of the refined grades. Cottonseed oil is a semi-drying oil and has a fairly high iodine value. When used to adulterate other oils its presence may be detected by the test for semidrying oils described in the *BP* monograph for Arachis Oil.

The hydrogenated oil, only, is official.

LINSEED AND LINSEED OIL

Linseed (*flaxseed*) is the dried ripe seed of *Linum usitatissimum* L. (Linaceae), an annual herb about 0.7 m high with blue flowers and a globular capsule. The flax has long been cultivated for its pericyclic fibres and seeds. Supplies of the latter are derived from South America, India, the USA and Canada. Large quantities of oil are expressed in England, particularly at Hull, and on the Continent.

Macroscopical characters. The seeds are ovate, flattened and obliquely pointed at one end; about 4–6 mm long and 2–2.5 mm broad. The testa is brown, glossy and finely pitted. Odourless; taste, mucilaginous and oily. If cruciferous seeds are present, a pungent odour and taste may develop on crushing and moistening. A transverse section shows a narrow endosperm and two large, planoconvex cotyledons.

Microscopical characters. Microscopical examination of the testa shows a mucilage-containing outer epidermis; one or two layers of collenchyma or 'round cells'; a single layer of longitudinally directed elongated sclerenchyma; the hyaline layers or 'cross-cells' composed in the ripe seed of partially or completely obliterated parenchymatous cells with their long axis at right angles to those of the sclerenchymatous layer; and an innermost layer of pigment cells. The outer epidermis is composed of cells, rectangular or five-sided in surface view, which swell up in water and become mucilaginous. The outer cell walls, when swollen in water, show an outer solid stratified layer and an inner part yielding mucilage, itself faintly stratified. The radial layers or 'round cells' are cylindrical in shape and show distinct triangular intercellular air spaces. The sclerenchymatous layer is composed of elongated cells, up to 250 μm in length, with lignified pitted walls. The hyaline layers often remain attached to portions of the sclerenchymatous layer in the powdered drug (see Fig. 41.7I). The pigment layer is composed of cells with thickened pitted walls and containing amorphous reddish-brown contents (Fig. 41.7H). The cells of the endosperm and cotyledons are polygonal with somewhat thickened walls, and contain numerous aleurone grains and globules of fixed oil. Starch is present in unripe seeds only.

Constituents. Linseed contains about 30–40% of fixed oil, 6% of mucilage (*BP* swelling index for whole seeds ≮4.0), 25% of protein and small quantities of the cyanogenetic glucosides linamarin and lotaustralin. Other constituents are phenylpropanoid glycosides (L. Luyengi *et al.*, *J. Nat. Prod.*, 1993, **56**, 2012), flavonoids, the lignan (–)-pinoresinol diglucoside (a tetrahydrofurofuran-type lignan—see Table 21.7) and the cancer chemoprotective mammalian lignan precursor secoisolariciresinol diglucoside (S.-X. Qiu *et al.*, *Pharm. Biol.*, 1999, **37**, 1). Recently, 22 different lignans, mainly of the aryltetralin type, have been identified from Bulgarian species of *Linum*, section Syllinum (N. Vasilev *et al.*, *Planta Medica*, 2008, **74**, 273).

Cell cultures of *Linum album* are able to synthesize and accumulate the lignans podophyllotoxin and 5-methylpodophyllotoxin (T. Smollny *et al.*, *Phytochemistry*, 1998, **48**, 975).

Linseed oil. The extraction of linseed oil is one of hot expression of a linseed meal and the press is adjusted to leave sufficient oil in the cake to make it suitable as a cattle food.

Linseed oil of *BP* quality is a yellowish-brown drying oil with a characteristic odour and bland taste; much commercial oil has a marked odour and acrid taste. On exposure to air it gradually thickens and forms a hard varnish. It has a high iodine value (≮175) as it contains considerable quantities of the glycosides of unsaturated acids. Analyses show α-linolenic acid, $C_{17}H_{29}COOH$ (36–50%), linoleic acid $C_{17}H_{31}COOH$ (23–24%), oleic acid $C_{17}H_{33}COOH$ (10–18%), together with some saturated acids—myristic, stearic and palmitic (5–11%). For the formation of the unsaturated acids, see Figs. 19.1 and 19.2.

For use in paint, linseed oil was boiled with 'driers' such as litharge or manganese resinate which, by forming metallic salts, caused the oil to dry more rapidly. Such 'boiled oils' must not be used for medicinal purposes.

Uses. Crushed linseed is used in the form of a poultice and whole seeds are employed to make demulcent preparations. The oil is used in liniments, and research has suggested that hydrolysed linseed oil has potentially useful antibacterial properties as a topical preparation in that it is effective against *Staphylococcus aureus* strains resistant to antibiotics. Linseed cake is a valuable cattle food.

OLIVE OIL

Olive oil (*salad oil, sweet oil*) is a fixed oil which is expressed from the ripe fruits of *Olea europoea* L. (Oleaceae). The olive is an evergreen tree, which lives to a great age but seldom exceeds 12 m in height. It produces drupaceous fruits about 2–3 cm in length. The var. *latifolia* bears larger fruits than the var. *longifolia*, but the latter is said to yield the best oil. The oil is expressed in all the Mediterranean countries and in California. Italy, Spain, France, Greece and Tunisia produce 90% of the world's production.

Olive oil has been ranked sixth in the world's production of vegetable oils (F. D. Gunstone *et al.*, 1994, *The Lipid Handbook*, Chapman and Hall).

History. The olive appears to be a native of Palestine. It was known in Egypt in the seventeenth century BC, and was introduced into Spain at an early period.

Collection and preparation. The methods used for the preparation of the oil naturally vary somewhat according to local conditions. In the modern factories hydraulic presses are widely used but in the more remote districts the procedure is essentially that which has been followed for hundreds of years and is described in earlier editions of this book. The first oil to be expressed from the ground fruits is known as virgin oil; subsequently the marc may be solvent extracted to obtain the lower quality oil. The superior grades of oil are extra virgin, virgin and pure or refined. The *Pharmacopoeia* includes monographs for both the virgin oil and refined oil.

Characters. Olive oil is a pale yellow liquid, which sometimes has a greenish tint. The amount of colouring matter present, whether chlorophyll or carotene, appears to determine the natural fluorescence of the oil in ultraviolet light.

The oil has a slight odour and a bland taste. If the fruits used have been allowed to ferment, the acid value of the oil will be higher than is officially permitted. It should comply with the tests for absence of arachis oil, cotton-seed oil, sesame oil and tea-seed oil. The latter oil, which is obtained from China, is not from the ordinary tea plant but from a tree, *Camellia sasanqua*.

Constituents. Olive oils from different sources differ somewhat in composition. This may be due either to the use of the different varieties of olive or to climatic differences. Two types of oil may be distinguished: (a) that produced in Italy, Spain, Asia Minor and California, which contains more olein and less linolein than type; and (b), produced in the Dodecanese and Tunisia. Typical analyses of these types are:

	Type (a)	Type (b)	BP limits
	%	%	%
Oleic acid	78–86	65–70	56–85
Linoleic acid	0–7	10–15	3.5–20.0
Palmitic acid	} 9–12	15	{ 7.5–20.0
Stearic acid			0.5–5.0

The characteristic odour of olive oil, particularly the virgin oils, arises from the presence of volatile C_6 alcohols (hexanol, *E*-2-hexenol, *Z*-3-hexenol), C_6 aldehydes and acetylated esters. Oils arising from different chemotypes can be distinguished by headspace gas–liquid chromatography (M. Williams *et al.*, *Phytochemistry*, 1998, **47**, 1253). The dehydrogenases which produce the unsaturated alcohols have been studied in the pulp of developing olive pericarps (J. J. Salas and J. Sánchez, *Phytochemistry*, 1998, **48**, 35).

The *BP/EP* examination of the oil includes a TLC test for identity and, to detect foreign oils, the GC determination of the individual methyl esters of the acids produced by hydrolysis. Limits of the principal acids are given above: other percentage limits, which exclude foreign oils, include saturated fatty acids of chain length less than C_{16}(≯0.1), linolenic (≯1.2), arachidic (≯0.7), behenic (≯0.2). There are also limits for a number of sterols in this fraction of the oil including campestrol ≯4.0%, cholesterol ≯0.5%, Δ^7-stigmasterol ≯0.5% and $\Delta^{5, 24}$-stigmastadienol.

For the biosynthesis of the acids, see the introduction to this chapter.

The saturated glycerides tend to separate from the oil in cold weather; at 10°C the oil begins to become cloudy and at about 0°C forms a soft mass.

Uses.   Olive oil is used in the preparation of soaps, plasters, etc., and is widely employed as a salad oil. Oil for use in the manufacture of parenteral preparations is required to have a lower acid value and peroxide value than that normally required, and to be almost free of water (0.1%) as determined by the specified Karl Fischer method.

Recent research has suggested that olive oil may protect against colonic carcinogenesis by virtue of its action on prostaglandins: rats fed on a diet containing olive oil, as distinct from those receiving safflower oil, were protected (R. Bartoli *et al.*, *Gut*, 2000, **46**, 191).

Both fruits and oil are now widely promoted in health-food stores on account of their α-linolenic acid content.

PALM OIL AND PALM KERNEL OIL

Palm oil.   The oil is obtained by steaming and expression of the mesocarp of the fruits of *Elaeis guineënsis* Jacq. (Palmae). This palm occurs throughout tropical Africa but over half of the world production of oil originates from Malaysia. In terms of world production palm oil had by 2003 overtaken that of sunflower and rapeseed oils (Table 19.8). It will be noted that for the oils listed, palm oil is superior regarding land use and productivity.

Palm oil is yellowish-brown in colour, of a buttery consistency (m.p. 30°C) and of agreeable odour. Palmitic and oleic acids are the principal esterifying acids.

Table 19.8 World production of some fixed oils (2003).

Crop	Production (10^6 ton)	Oil yield ton/ha/year	Area of plantations (10^6 ha)
Soybean	31.4	0.46	88.4
Sunflower seed	9.0	0.66	22.6
Rapeseed	12.5	1.33	25.2
Palm oil	28.7	3.30	8.5

Source: Malaysian Oil Palm Association.

Palm kernel oil.   Palm kernel oil is obtained by heating the separated seeds for 4–6 hours to shrink the shell, which is then cracked and the kernels removed whole. The oil is then obtained by expression. It differs chemically from palm oil (above) in containing a high proportion (50%) of the triglycerides of lauric acid, a saturated, medium chain-length fatty acid (Table 19.2). The mixture of other acids resembles that found in coconut oil.

Fractionated Palm Kernel Oil *BP*   is palm oil which has undergone selective solvent fractionation and hydrogenation. It is a white, brittle solid, odourless or almost so, with m.p. 31°–36°C making it suitable for use as a suppository base.

RAPESEED OIL

Refined Rapeseed Oil *BP/EP* is obtained by mechanical expression or by extraction from the seeds of *Brassica napus* L. and *B. campestris* L.

The crop is now extensively cultivated in Europe and oils with various properties depending on glyceride composition are commercially available. As was indicated in Chapter 14 not all varieties yield an oil suitable for medicinal purposes so that the specified pharmacopoeial limits of the various esterifying acids are important standards as are relative density (*c.* 0.917) and refractive index (*c.* 1.473). Oleic, linoleic and linolenic acids are the principal esterifying acids, with eicosenoic acid and erucic acid limited to 5.0 and 2.0% of the acid fraction, respectively.

As with some other oils, the addition of a suitable antioxidant is permitted, the name and concentration of which must be stated on the label together with a statement as to whether the oil was obtained by mechanical expression or by extraction.

SAFFLOWER OIL

Safflower oil is obtained by expression or extraction from the seeds (achenes) of *Carthamus tinctorius* L. (Compositae) or hybrids of this species. Commonly known as safflower, false saffron, saffron thistle, the plant is native to Mediterranean countries and Asia and has been used for colouring and medicinal purposes from Ancient Egyptian and Chinese times. The pigment from the flowers (carthamin) is yellow in water and red in alcohol and was the traditional dye for the robes of Buddhist monks. It is now cultivated largely for the seed oil in its countries of origin, as well as in the US, Australia, Africa and S.E. Asia.

As produced commercially, safflower oil is of two types—type 1 coming from the original species and type 2 from hybrid forms producing an oil rich in oleic acid; the acid fraction of the type 1 oil has oleic acid limits of 8–12% and the type 2 oil 70–84%. Other acids are palmitic, stearic and linoleic acids generally proportionately higher for the type 1 oil.

The pharmacopoeial oil is refined and may have an added antioxidant; it should comply with the usual tests for fixed oils with brassicasterol limited to 0.3% of the sterol fraction.

Safflower oil, like linseed oil, is a drying oil and has found commercial use in paints and varnishes. It is used in the food industry and is recommended for its cholesterol-lowering properties.

SESAME OIL

Sesame oil (*Gingelly oil, Teel oil*) is obtained by refining the expressed or extracted oil from the seeds of *Sesamum indicum* L. (Pedaliaceae), a herb which is widely cultivated in India, China, Japan and many tropical countries. The oil is official in the *EP* and *BP*.

The seeds contain about 50% of fixed oil which closely resembles olive oil in its properties and which it has, in some measure, replaced. It is a pale yellow, bland oil which on cooling to about −4°C solidifies to a buttery mass; it has a saponification value the same as that for olive oil and a somewhat higher iodine value (104–120).

Principal components of the oil are the glycerides of oleic and linoleic acids with small proportions of palmitic, stearic and arachidic acids. It also contains about 1% of the lignan sesamin, and the related sesamolin. The characteristic phenolic component is the basis of the *BP* test for identity and also the test for the detection of sesame oil in other oils. The original test involved the production of a pink colour when the oil was shaken with half its volume of concentrated hydrochloric acid containing 1% of sucrose (Baudouin's test). However, some commercially refined oils may not give a positive Baudouin's test. With the current *BP* test for the absence of sesame oil in other oils, e.g. olive oil, the reagents are acetic anhydride, a solution of furfuraldehyde and sulphuric acid; a bluish-green colour is a positive result. The composition of triglycerides in sesame oil is determined by liquid chromatography, those triglycerides having as acid radicals oleic 1 part and linoleic 2 parts, and those having oleic 2 parts and linoleic 1 part being among the most predominant.

As stated above, sesame seeds and oil also contain lignans; these are antioxidants of the tetrahydrofurofuran-type (Table 21.7) and include sesamin, sesamolinol and sesamolin. Another lignan, sesaminol, is formed during industrial bleaching of the oil. The biological activities of these compounds include reduction in serum cholesterol levels and increased vitamin E activities. For the biogenesis of such lignans see M. J. Kato *et al.*, *Phytochemistry*, 1998, **47**, 583.

SOYA OIL

Soya oil is obtained from the seeds of *Glycine soja* Sieb. and Zucc. and *Glycine max* (L.) Merr (*G. hispida* (Moench) Maxim).

Refined soya oil. Processing involves deodorization and clarification by filtration at about 0°C. It should remain bright when kept at 0°C for 16 h. The principal esterifying fatty acids are linoleic (48–58%), oleic (17–30%), linolenic (5–11%) and stearic (3–5%). There is an official limit test of not more than 0.5% for the brassicasterol content of the sterol fraction of the oil.

Hydrogenated soya oil occurs as a white mass or powder; it consists principally of the triglycerides of palmitic and stearic acid.

SUNFLOWER OIL

Sunflower oil is obtained from the seeds of *Helianthus annuus* L. by mechanical expression or by extraction; it is then refined. Principal components of the fatty-acid mixture produced by hydrolysis of the oil are linoleic acid (48–74%), oleic acid (14–40%), palmitic acid (4–9%) and stearic acid (1–7%).

The oil can be identified (*BP/EP* test) by the comparison of a thin-layer chromatogram of the sample with that of the pharmacopoeial illustration of the typical oil. Other tests include relative density (*c.* 0.921) and refractive index (*c.* 1.474).

THEOBROMA OIL

Oil of theobroma or cocoa butter may be obtained from the ground kernels of *Theobroma cacao* (Sterculiaceae) by hot expression. The oil is filtered and allowed to set in moulds. Much is refined in Holland. Cocoa butter, as it is commonly termed, consists of the glycerides of stearic, palmitic, arachidic, oleic and other acids. These acids are combined with glycerol partly in the usual way as triglycerides and partly as mixed glycerides in which the glycerol is attached to more than one of the acids. It is the most expensive of the commercial fixed oils and may be adulterated with waxes, stearin (e.g. coconut stearin), animal tallows or vegetable tallows (e.g. from seeds of *Bassia longifolia* and *Stillingia sebifera*). For the character and tests for purity of oil of theobroma, see the pharmacopoeias. Its melting point (31–34°) makes it ideal for the preparation of suppositories.

GERM OILS

The *refined* and *virgin* wheat-germ oils are described in the *BP/EP* and are obtained by cold expression or by other suitable mechanical means from the germ of the wheat grain, *Triticum aestivum* L. The principal fatty acids involved are linoleic (52–59%), palmitic (14–19%), oleic (12–23%) and linolenic (3–10%) with limits for ecosenoic (≯2.0%) and stearic (≯2.0%). Brassicasterol is limited to 0.3% (max) in the sterol fraction. The acid value requirement for the refined oil is low (≯0.9%, or ≯0.3% if the oil is to be used for parenteral purposes) but much higher (≯20.0%) for the virgin oil.

CASTOR OIL (VIRGIN CASTOR OIL)

Castor oil (*cold-drawn castor oil*) is a fixed oil obtained from the seeds of *Ricinus communis* (Euphorbiaceae). The fruit is a three-celled thorny capsule. The castor is a native of India; the principal producing countries are Brazil, India, China, the former Soviet Union and Thailand. There are about 17 varieties, which may be roughly grouped into shrubs and trees producing large seeds, and annual herbs producing smaller seeds. It is mainly the smaller varieties that are now cultivated and these have been developed, by breeding, to give high-yielding seed plants. Mechanical harvesting is now replacing hand-picking.

Characters of seeds.   The seeds show considerable differences in size and colour. They are oval, somewhat compressed, 8–18 mm long and 4–12 mm broad. The testa is very smooth, thin and brittle. The colour may be a more or less uniform grey, brown or black, or may be variously mottled with brown or black. A small, often yellowish, caruncle is usually present at one end, from which runs the raphe to terminate in a slightly raised chalaza at the opposite end of the seed. The testa is easily removed to disclose the papery remains of the nucellus surrounding a large oily endosperm. Within the latter lies the embryo, with two thin, flat cotyledons and a radicle directed towards the caruncle. Castor seeds, if in good condition, have very little odour; taste, somewhat acrid. If the testas are broken, rancidity will develop.

Preparation and characters of oil.   Ninety per cent of the world's castor oil is extracted in Brazil and India. Relatively small amounts of the whole seeds are now exported. The various processes involved in the preparation of castor oil are described in the 8th edition of this book. Briefly, the seeds are deprived of their testas and the kernels cold-expressed in suitable hydraulic presses. The oil is refined by steaming, filtration and bleaching. Cold expression yields about 33% of medicinal oil and further quantities of oil of lower quality may be obtained by other methods.

Medicinal castor oil (virgin castor oil) is a colourless or pale yellow liquid, with a slight odour and faintly acrid taste. For its chemical and physical constants, see the pharmacopoeias. The acid value increases somewhat with age and an initially high value indicates the use of damaged seeds or careless extraction or storage. Castor oil has an extremely high viscosity.

Constituents. Castor seeds contain 46–53% of fixed oil, which consists of the glycosides of ricinoleic, isoricinoleic, stearic and dihydroxystearic acids. The purgative action of the oil is said to be due to free ricinoleic acid and its stereoisomer, which are produced by hydrolysis in the duodenum. These acids have the formula,

$$CH_3[CH_2]_5CH(OH)CH_2CH{=}CH[CH_2]_7COOH$$

For the biogenesis of ricinoleic acid, see Fig. 19.3. Castor oil and the oil from *Ricinus zanzibarinus* are remarkable for their high ricinoleic acid content, which is about 88% and 92% respectively.

The cake left after expression contains extremely poisonous toxins known as ricins, which make it unfit for use as a cattle food. In the body they produce an antitoxin (antiricin). Ricin D is a sugar protein with a strong lethal toxicity; it contains 493 amino acids and 23 sugars. Two other ricins, acidic ricin and basic ricin, have similar properties. Ricin and abrin (see 'Abrus Seeds' below) exhibit antitumour properties. The seeds also contain lipases and a crystalline alkaloid, ricinine, which is not markedly toxic and is structurally related to nicotinamide.

Uses. Castor oil, once widely used as a domestic purgative, is now more restricted to hospital use for administration after food poisoning and as a preliminary to intestinal examination. Owing to the presence of ricin, the seeds have a much more violent action than the oil and are not used as a purgative in the West. Non-ionic surfactants (polyethoxylated castor oils) of variable composition are produced by the reaction of castor oil with ethylene oxide and are used in certain intravenous preparations which contain drugs with low aqueous solubility. The oil and its derivatives find many non-pharmaceutical uses including the manufacture of Turkey Red Oil, soaps, paints, varnishes, plasticizers and lubricants.

The following castor oil derivatives, described as pharmaceutical aids are included in the *BP/EP*:

- *Hydrogenated castor oil.* A fine, almost white to pale yellow powder, practically insoluble in water, m.p. 83–88°C. It contains principally 12-hydroxystearic acid.
- *Polyoxyl castor oil.* A clear yellow viscous liquid or semi-solid, freely soluble in water. Prepared by the reaction of castor oil with ethylene oxide.
- *Hydrogenated polyoxyl castor oil.* Of variable consistency depending on the amount of ethylene oxide/mol.

Allied drugs. *Croton seeds* are obtained from *Croton tiglium* (Euphorbiaceae), a small tree producing similar capsules to those of castor but devoid of spines. The seeds resemble castor seeds in size and shape but have a dull, cinnamon-brown colour and readily lose their caruncles. They contain about 50% of fixed oil which contains croton resin; also 'crotin', a mixture of croton-globulin and croton-albumin comparable with ricin. The oil also contains diesters of the tetracyclic diterpene phorbol (esterifying acid at R^1 and R^2, R^3 = H in the formula below); acids involved are acetic as a short-chain acid, and capric, lauric and palmitic as long-chain acids. These compounds are cocarcinogens and also possess inflammatory and vesicant properties (see 'Diterpenes'). Also present are phorbol-12,13,20-triesters (R^1, R^2 and R^3 are all acyl groups in the formula shown). These are 'cryptic irritants', so called because they are not biologically active as such but become so by removal of the C-20 acyl group by hydrolysis. Rotation locular counter-current chromatography (q.v.) has been used to separate these two groups of esters. A number of the phorbol esters have been tested for anti-HIV-1 activity (S. El-Mekkawy *et al.*, *Phytochemistry*, 2000, **53**, 457). The plant also contains alkaloids. Croton oil should be handled with extreme caution; it is not used in Western medicine, but if taken internally, it acts as a violent cathartic.

Phorbol esters of croton oil

Physic nuts or *Purging nuts* are the seeds of *Jatropha curcas*, another member of the Euphorbiaceae. The seeds are black, oval and 15–20 mm in length. They contain about 40% of fixed oil and a substance comparable with ricin, called curcin. Both seeds and oil are powerful purgatives.

Abrus seeds (prayer beads) are the attractive red and black, but poisonous, seeds of *Abrus precatorius* (Leguminosae). They contain a toxic glycoprotein (abrin) resembling ricin together with another non-toxic peptide having haemagglutinating properties. Various alkaloids (abrine, hyaphorine, precatorine) of the indole type have been reported, also various sterols and lectins. The seeds have been used in folklore medicine in Asia, Africa and S. America to treat many ailments, also to procure abortion and to hasten labour. In India they are employed as an oral contraceptive and as they are remarkably uniform, and each weighs about 1 carat (*c*. 200 mg), have been used traditionally as weights.

EVENING PRIMROSE OIL

The fixed oil obtained by extraction and/or expression from the seeds of *Oenothera* spp. (*O. biennis* L., *O. lamarkiana* L.) Onagraceae contains substantial mounts of esterified γ-linolenic acid (GLA), a C_{18} 6,9,12-triene.

γ-Linolenic acid (GLA)

Arachidonic acid   Prostaglandin E₂ (PGE₂)

19

The principal species cultivated in the UK is *O. biennis* which yields an oil containing 7–9% GLA, although more recent work shows higher yields for the oils of some other species, namely *O. acerviphilla nova* (15.68%), *O. paradoxa* (14.41%) and an ecotype of *O. rubricaulis* (13.75%). Research has involved breeding new varieties for high yields of oil and reducing the lifecycle of the plant from 14 to 7 months (*Pharm. J.*, 1994, **252**, 189).

The sequence for the formation of such acids in the plant via *cis*-linoleic acid has already been indicated in Fig. 19.1. In animal tissues it appears that the prostaglandins are formed from dietary linoleic acid by conversion to GLA which undergoes C_2 addition and further desaturation to give acids such as arachidonic acid, an immediate precursor of some prostaglandins.

The pharmacopoeial tests for the oil are similar to those quoted for borage oil, below.

Beneficial effects of evening primrose oil may well be related to affording a precursor of the prostaglandins for those individuals whose enzymic conversion of linoleic acid to GLA is deficient. The oil is now widely marketed as a dietary supplement, for cosmetic purposes, and more specifically for the treatment of atopic eczema and premenstrual syndrome (prostaglandin E may be depleted in this condition). Further possibilities include its use in diabetic neuropathy and rheumatoid arthritis.

BORAGE OIL

The refined fixed oil expressed from the seeds of *Borago officinalis* L. (starflower), family Boraginaceae contains a higher content of γ-linolenic (GLA) and somewhat less linoleic acid than evening primrose oil. Cultivation of the crop in the UK started some years ago and details of the commercial production of the seed, plant-breeding programme and husbandry are given in a general article by A. Fieldsend, *Biologist*, 1995, **42**, 203.

Principal fatty acids involved in the oil, with *BP/EP* limits, are linoleic (30–41%), γ-linolenic (17–27%), oleic (12–22%), palmitic (9–12%) and smaller percentages of others. The *Pharmacopoeia* also states maximum limits for acid value, peroxide value, non-saponifiable matter, alkaline impurities and brassicasterol.

The oil is used for the same medicinal purposes as evening primrose oil. However, concerning its use for the treatment of atopic eczema, a clinical trial (A. Takwale *et al.*, *Br. Med. J.*, 2003, **327**, 1385) failed to establish any benefit from the high levels of GLA contained in the oil.

Other sources of GLA. A number of other seed oils contain appreciable quantities of GLA, including those of *Ribes nigrum* and *R. rubrum* (the black and red currant) and *Symphytum officinale* (comfrey).

SAW PALMETTO FRUIT

Saw palmetto fruit *BP/EP*, *BHP* is obtained from the palm *Serenoa repens* (Bartram) Small, [*Sabal serrulata* (Michaux) Nichols], family Arecaceae/Palmae, collected when ripe and dried. It is a low, shrubby palm with simple or branched stems usually up to about 3 m in length and bearing palmate leaves divided into many segments and having a petiole edged with sharp needles; hence the common name. The small flowers give rise to globose, one-seeded drupes turning bluish-black when ripe. It is indigenous to the sandy coastal regions of the S.E. states of the US, where it colonizes large areas; commercial supplies come mainly from Florida. The seeds were utilized both as a food and medicinally by the Native Americans.

The dried, dark brown to black fruit is semi-spherical to ovoid, up to 25 mm long, 15 mm wide with a rugged surface formed by shrinkage on drying. The remains of the three-toothed tubular calyx and style may be seen at the distal end, and the scar of the pedicel at the lower end. The hard seed is oval to spherical, measuring some 12 × 8 mm and comprising a thin testa, small perisperm and a larger, horny, pale endosperm and embryo.

A microscopical examination of the powder shows cuticularized, reddish-brown polygonal cells of the epicarp; mesocarpic parenchymatous cells, which are often oil filled or containing crystals of silica; scattered or small groups of sclereids; sclerenchymatous endocarp; and seed characteristics that include pigmented cells of the testa, thickened pitted cells of the endosperm containing fixed oil and aleurone grains.

The drug has an aromatic odour reminiscent of vanilla and a soapy, somewhat acrid, although sweetish, taste.

Constituents. Fatty acids constitute an important feature of the drug. In the mesocarp, originally the fleshy part of the fruit, they occur in the free state, and in the seeds as triacylglycerols. The principal free acids are oleic, lauric, myristic and palmitic acids, with lesser amounts of caproic, caprylic, capric, stearic, linoleic and linolenic acids; for formulae see Tables 19.1, 19.2 and 19.3. The same acids are involved in the fats of the seed endosperm, with oleic and lauric acids most commonly occurring as mixed triacylglycerols (see Fig. 19.7). Fatty acid esters involving propyl and ethyl alcohol (pricipally propyl laurate) are present in small amounts in various extracts.

Other constituents include: flavonoids such as rutin, isoquercitrin (see Fig. 21.15) and others; phytosterols—sitosterol (see Fig. 23.5), its glucosides and esters, and stigmasterol (see Fig. 23.5); immunostimulant polysaccharides involving galactose, arabinose, mannose, rhamnose, glucuronic acid and others; carotenoids; volatile oil.

The *BP/EP* gives a TLC identification test for the powdered drug using β-amyrin and β-sitosterol as reference substances. An assay for total fatty acids, minimum requirement for the dried drug 11.0%, employs gas chromatography of a dimethylformamide extract of the powder; the individual acids separated on the chromatogram are identified by comparison with the chromatogram of a reference solution of the acids mentioned above.

Actions. Most clinical and pharmacological studies on saw palmetto fruits have involved the use of hexane, supercritical CO_2 (see Chapter 17) and ethanol extracts of the drug. Among the activities observed is that of the inhibition of 5α-reductase thus impeding the conversion of testosterone to dehydrotestosterone. The principal use of the drug is for the symptomatic treatment of benign prostatic hyperplasia.

For extended accounts and bibliography on the drug, see E. Bombardelli and P. Morazzoni, *Fitoterapia*, 1997, **68**, 99–113 (58 refs); P. Bradley, *British Herbal Compendium*, 2006, pp. 345–352 (62 refs).

Hydnocarpus oil

This is the fixed oil obtained by cold expression from the fresh ripe seeds of *Hydnocarpus wightiana*, *H. anthelmintica*, *H. heterophylla* and other species of *Hydnocarpus*, and also of *Taraktogenos kurzii*. These plants are found in India, Burma, Siam and Indo-China and belong to the Flacourtiaceae.

The oil of *H. wightiana* contains hydnocarpic acid (about 48%), chaulmoogric acid (about 27%), gorlic and other acids (formulae, see Table 19.4); the structures of several new cyclopentenyl fatty acids have recently been elucidated. These acids do not appear to be formed from straight-chain acids and they accumulate during the last 3–4 months of maturation of the fruit. They are strongly bactericidal towards the leprosy micrococcus, but the oil has now to a large extent been replaced by the ethyl esters and salts of hydnocarpic and chaulmoogric acid. The esterified oil of *H. wightiana* is preferable to that of other species, in that it yields when fractionated almost pure ethyl hydnocarpate. This was included in the *BPC* (1965) but has now been deleted, as more effective remedies are available.

WOOL FAT

Wool fat (*anhydrous lanolin*) is a purified fat-like substance prepared from the wool of the sheep, *Ovis aries* (Bovidae).

Raw wool contains considerable quantities of 'wool grease' or crude lanolin, the potassium salts of fatty acids and earthy matter. Raw lanolin is separated by 'cracking' with sulphuric acid from the washings of the scouring process and purified to fit it for medicinal use. Purification may be done by centrifuging with water and by bleaching.

Wool fat is a pale yellow, tenacious substance with a faint but characteristic odour. It is insoluble in water and a high proportion of water may be incorporated with it by melting (m.p. 36–42°C) and stirring. Soluble in ether and chloroform. Like other waxes, it is not readily saponified by aqueous alkali, but an alcoholic solution of alkali causes saponification. Saponification value 90–105; iodine value 18–32; acid value not more than 1. Hydrous wool fat or lanolin contains 25% water.

The chief constituents of wool fat are cholesterol and isocholesterol, unsaturated monohydric alcohols of the formula $C_{27}H_{45}OH$, both free and combined with lanoceric, lanopalmitic, carnaubic and other fatty acids. Wool fat also contains aliphatic alcohols such as cetyl, ceryl and carnaubyl alcohols. Butylated hydroxytoluene, up to 200 ppm, may be added as an antioxidant.

The pharmacopoeial test for pesticide residues is complex and involves their isolation and subsequent identification. A maximum of 0.05 ppm is permitted for each organochlorine pesticide, 0.5 ppm for each other pesticide and 1ppm for the sum of all pesticides.

Wool Alcohols BP/EP are prepared by the saponification of crude lanolin and the separation of the alcohol fraction. The product consists of steroid and triterpene alcohols, including cholesterol (not less than 30%) and isocholesterol. As for wool fat, an antioxidant may be added.

To test for cholesterol dissolve 0.5 g in 5 ml of chloroform, add 1 ml acetic anhydride and two drops of sulphuric acid; a deep-green colour is produced.

Hydrogenated Wool Fat BP/EP is obtained by the high pressure/high temperature hydrogenation of anhydrous wool fat. It contains a mixture of higher aliphatic alcohols and sterols.

Wool fat is used as an emollient base for creams and ointments.

LARD

Lard (*prepared lard*) is the purified internal fat of the hog, *Sus scrofa* (order Ungulata, Suidae).

For medicinal purposes lard is prepared from the abdominal fat known as 'flare', from which it is obtained by treatment with hot water at a temperature not exceeding 57°C.

Lard is a soft, white fat with a non-rancid odour. Acid value not more than 1.2. Lard has a lower melting point (34–41°C) and a higher iodine value (52–66) than suet. Saponification value 192–198. It should be free from moisture, beef-fat, sesame-seed and cotton-seed oils, alkalis and chlorides.

Lard contains approximately 40% of solid glycerides such as myristin, stearin and palmitin, and 60% of mixed liquid glycerides such as olein. These fractions are somewhat separated by pressure at 0°C and sold as 'stearin' and 'lard oil' respectively. Lard is used as an ointment base but is no longer official in Britain. It is somewhat liable to become rancid, but this may be retarded by benzoination, Siamese benzoin being more effective than the Sumatra variety.

Suet. Suet is the purified internal fat of the abdomen of the sheep, *Ovis aries*. It contains about 50–60% of solid glycerides and melts at about 45°C. It is used as an ointment base in tropical and subtropical countries.

WAXES

YELLOW BEESWAX, WHITE BEESWAX

Beeswax is obtained by melting and purifying the honeycomb of *Apis mellifica* and other bees. The wax is imported from the West Indies, California, Chile, Africa, Madagascar and India. The *EP* and *BP* include separate monographs for the yellow and the white wax.

Preparation. Wax is secreted by worker bees in cells on the ventral surface of the last four segments of their abdomen. The wax passes out through pores in the chitinous plates of the sternum and is used, particularly by the young workers, to form the comb.

Yellow beeswax is prepared, after removal of the honey, by melting the comb under water (residual honey dissolving in the water and solid impurities sinking), straining, and allowing the wax to solidify in suitable moulds.

White beeswax is prepared from the above by treatment with charcoal, potassium permanganate, chromic acid, chlorine, etc., or by the slow bleaching action of light, air and moisture. In the latter method the melted wax is allowed to fall on a revolving cylinder which is kept moist. Ribbon-like strips of wax are thus formed which are exposed on cloths to the action of light and air, being moistened and turned at intervals until the outer surface is bleached. The whole process is repeated at least once, and the wax is finally cast into circular cakes.

Characters. Beeswax is a yellowish-brown or yellowish-white solid. It breaks with a granular fracture and has a characteristic odour. It is insoluble in water and sparingly soluble in cold alcohol, but dissolves in chloroform and in warm fixed and volatile oils (e.g. oil of turpentine).

Constituents. Beeswax is a true wax, consisting of about 80% of myricyl palmitate (myricin), $C_{15}H_{31}COOC_{30}H_{61}$, with possibly a little myricyl stearate. It also contains about 15% of free cerotic acid, $C_{26}H_{53}COOH$, an aromatic substance cerolein, hydrocarbons, lactones, cholesteryl esters and pollen pigments.

Standards. These include a 'drop point' of 61–65° for both the white and yellow wax, acid value, ester value, saponification value and tests for ceresin, paraffin and certain other waxes, and various phenols.

Uses. Beeswax is used in the preparation of plasters, ointments and polishes.

CARNAUBA WAX

Carnauba wax, included in the *BP/EP* (2000) and *USP/NF* (1995), is derived from the leaves of *Copernicia cerifera* (Palmae). It is removed from the leaves by shaking and purified to remove foreign matter.

The wax is hard, light brown to pale yellow in colour and is supplied as a moderately coarse powder, as flakes or irregular lumps; it is usually tasteless with a slight characteristic odour free from rancidity. Esters, chiefly myricyl cerotate, are the principal components, with some free alcohols and other minor constituents. The acid value is low (*BP*, *USP/NF*, 2–7), the saponification value 78–95. It has an iodine value of 7–14. The *BP/EP* includes a TLC test for identity. Carnauba wax is used in pharmacy as a tablet-coating agent and in other industries for the manufacture of candles and leather polish. It has been suggested as a replacement for beeswax in the preparation of phytocosmetics.

20

Carbohydrates

As the name implies, carbohydrates consist of carbon, hydrogen and oxygen with the last two elements usually present in the same proportions as in water. As we have previously noted, carbohydrates are among the first products to arise as a result of photosynthesis. They constitute a large proportion of the plant biomass and are responsible, as cellulose, for the rigid cellular framework and, as starch, for providing an important food reserve. Of special pharmacognostical importance is the fact that sugars unite with a wide variety of other compounds to form glycosides (Chapters 21–25). Mucilages, as found in marshmallow root and psyllium seeds, act as water-retaining vehicles, whereas gums, which are similar in composition and properties, are formed in the plant by injury or stress and usually appear as solidified exudates; both are typically composed of uronic acid and sugar units. The cell walls of the brown seaweeds and the middle lamellae of higher plant tissues contain polysaccharides consisting almost entirely of uronic acid components. All these groups are discussed more fully below, and the drugs and pharmaceutical necessities containing them are listed at the end of the chapter.

SUGARS (SACCHARIDES)

Monosaccharides

These sugars contain from three to nine carbon atoms, but those with five and six carbon atoms (pentoses, $C_5H_{10}O_5$, and hexoses, $C_6H_{12}O_6$) are accumulated in plants in greatest quantity.

The formulae of sugars and other carbohydrates are written in a number of different ways. The structure of glucose as a straight-chain pentahydroxy aldehyde was established by Kiliani in 1886. Emil Fischer, from 1884 onwards, was the most important of the early workers in this field. Their straight-chain formulae are still useful for illustrating the isomerism and stereochemical relationships and, as shown below, can be written in very abbreviated form. Many of the important biological properties of carbohydrates can, however, best be illustrated by ring formulae which show that the same sugar may exist either as a five-membered ring (furanose) or a six-membered ring (pyranose). Glucose has an aldehyde group and is therefore called an aldose or 'aldo' sugar; fructose has a ketone group and is therefore called a ketose. Terms such as 'aldopentose' and 'ketohexose' are self-explanatory. The formulae (Figs. 20.1, 20.2) illustrate these points.

The furanose structure is comparatively unstable but may be stabilized on glycoside formation. The fructose phosphate of the furanose form illustrated in Fig. 20.1 is an intermediate in glycolysis, the anaerobic degradation of hexoses which provides energy for metabolism (see Fig. 18.5). Fructose in nature is always in the furanose form, but when isolated in crystalline form, it has a pyranose structure.

Uronic acids are produced by oxidation of the terminal groups to –COOH (e.g. glucuronic acid from glucose and galacturonic acid from galactose).

Biosynthesis of monosaccharides. Various monosaccharides arise from the photosynthetic cycle (q.v.). D-Fructose-6-phosphate and D-glucose-6-phosphate are universal in their occurrence. Free sugars may accumulate as a result of hydrolysis of the phosphorylated sugars or the latter may be utilized in respiration, converted to sugar nucleotides (e.g. uridine-diphosphoglucose—UDPG) or, by the action of various epimerases, give rise to other monosaccharides (e.g. galactose).

Di-, tri- and tetrasaccharides

These sugars may also be called bioses, trioses and tetroses. They are theoretically derived from two, three or four monosaccharide molecules,

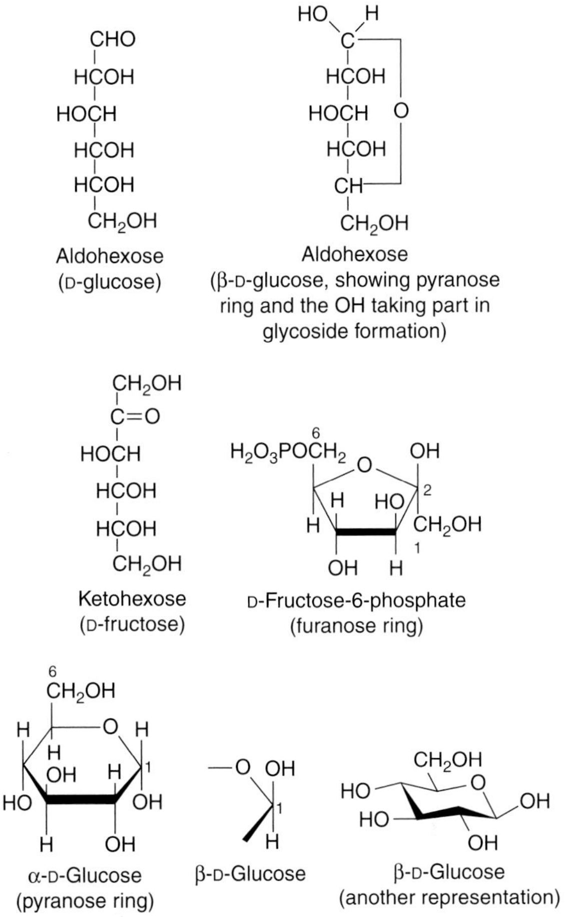

Fig. 20.1
Hexose structures and representation.

respectively, with the elimination of one, two or three molecules of water (Table 20.1). One of the commonest plant disaccharides is sucrose; it is formed in photosynthesis by the reaction of UDPG with fructose-6-phosphate (Fig. 20.3). Control mechanisms for the build-up of sucrose in leaves, and its breakdown for transport to storage organs, are achieved by metabolite effector control of the appropriate enzymes.

The reverse process, hydrolysis, is brought about by suitable enzymes or by boiling with dilute acid. The same sugars may be linked to one another in various ways. Thus, the disaccharides maltose, cellobiose, sophorose and trehalose are all composed of two molecules of glucose joined by α-1,4-, β-1,4-, β-1,2- and α,α-1,1-(non-reducing) linkages, respectively.

POLYSACCHARIDES

By condensation involving sugar phosphates and sugar nucleotides, polysaccharides are derived from monosaccharides in an exactly similar manner to the formation of di-, tri- and tetrasaccharides. The name 'oligo-saccharide' (Greek *oligo*, few) is often applied to saccharides containing from two to 10 units. In polysaccharides the number of sugar units is much larger and the number forming the molecule is often only approximately known. The hydrolysis of polysaccharides, by enzymes or reagents, often results in a succession of cleavages, but the final products are hexoses or pentoses or their derivatives. The term 'polysaccharide' may usefully be taken to include polysaccharide complexes which yield in addition to monosaccharides their sulphate esters, uronic acids or amino sugars.

Table 20.2 indicates the character of some of the polysaccharides.

In addition to the well-established polysaccharide-containing pharmaceutical materials described later in this chapter there is now considerable interest in a number of polysaccharides with other pharmacological activities. These include immuno-modulating, antitumour, anti-inflammatory, anticoagulant, hypoglycaemic and antiviral properties. Specific examples are the glycyrrhizans of *Glycyrrhiza uralensis* and *G. glabra* and the glycans of ginseng and *Eleutherococcus* (q.v.). In general polysaccharides from fungi exhibit antitumour activity,

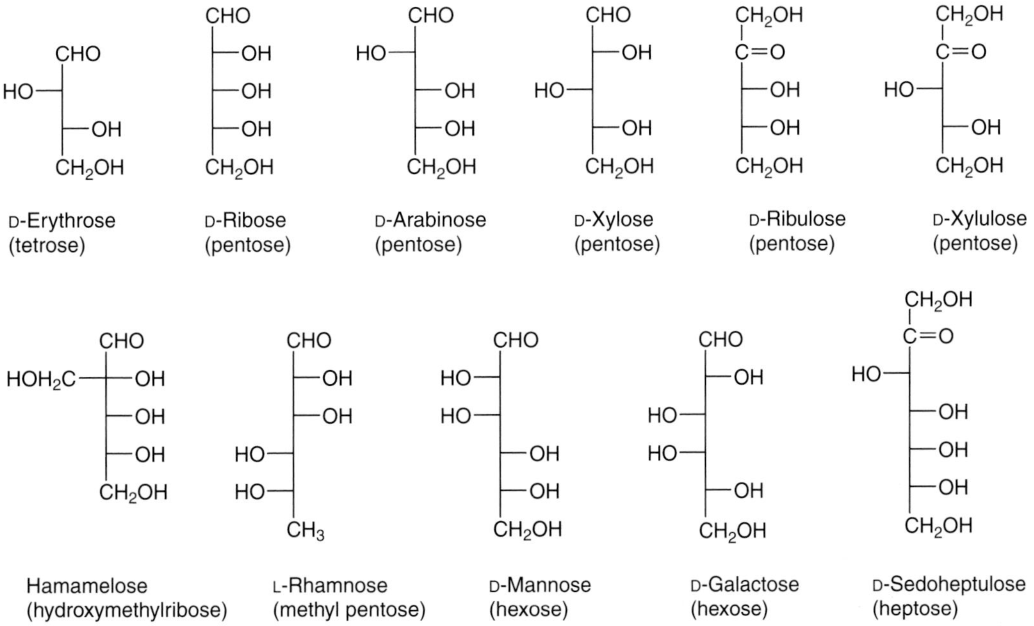

Fig. 20.2
Examples of C_4 to C_7 monosaccharides (Fischer structures).

Table 20.1   Some di-, tri- and tetrasaccharides.

Type	Name	Products of hydrolysis	Occurrence
Di-	Sucrose	Glucose, fructose	Sugar cane, sugar beet, etc.
	Maltose	Glucose, glucose	Enzymic hydrolysis of starch
	Lactose	Glucose, galactose	Milk
	Cellobiose	Glucose, glucose	Enzymic breakdown of cellulose
	Trehalose	Glucose, glucose	Ergot, Rhodophyceae, yeasts
	Sophorose	Glucose, glucose	*Sophora japonica*, hydrolysis of stevioside
	Primeverose	Glucose, xylose	*Filipendula ulmaria*, hydrolysis of spiraein
Tri-	Gentianose	Glucose, glucose, fructose	*Gentiana* spp.
	Melezitose	Glucose, fructose, glucose	Manna from *Larix*
	Planteose	Glucose, fructose, galactose	Seeds of *Psyllium* spp.
	Raffinose	Galactose, glucose, fructose	Many seeds (e.g. cotton-seed)
	Manneotriose	Galactose, galactose, glucose	Manna of ash, *Fraxinus ornus*
	Rhamninose	Rhamnose, rhamnose, galactose	*Rhamnus infectoria*
	Scillatriose	Rhamnose, glucose, glucose	Glycoside of squill
	Other examples of trisaccharides are among the glycosides of *Digitalis* and *Strophanthus* (q.v.)		
Tetra-	Stachyose or manneotetrose	Galactose, galactose, glucose, fructose	Tubers of *Stachys japonica* and manna of *Fraxinus ornus*
	Other examples of tetrasaccharides are among the glycosides of *Digitalis* (q.v.)		

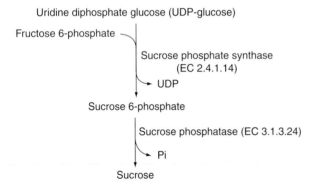

Fig. 20.3
Biosynthesis of sucrose.

those from higher plants are immunostimulatory and the algal polysaccharides, which often contain sulphate, are good anticoagulants.

Tests for carbohydrates
The following are some of the more useful tests for sugars and other carbohydrates.

1. *Reduction of Fehling's solution.* To a heated solution of the substance add drop by drop a mixture of equal parts of Fehling's solution No. 1 and No. 2. In certain cases reduction takes place near the boiling point and is shown by a brick-red precipitate of cuprous oxide. Reducing sugars include all monosaccharides, many disaccharides (e.g. lactose, maltose, cellobiose and gentiobiose). Non-reducing substances include some disaccharides (sucrose and trehalose, the latter a sugar found in some fungi) and polysaccharides. Non-reducing carbohydrates will on boiling with acids be converted into reducing sugars, but students are reminded to neutralize any acid used for hydrolysis before testing with Fehling's solution, or cuprous oxide will fail to precipitate.

2. *Molisch's test.* All carbohydrates give a purple colour when treated with α-naphthol and concentrated sulphuric acid. With a soluble carbohydrate this appears as a ring if the sulphuric acid is gently poured in to form a layer below the aqueous solution. With an insoluble carbohydrate such as cotton-wool (cellulose) the colour will not appear until the acid layer is shaken to bring it in contact with the material.

3. *Osazone formation.* Osazones are sugar derivatives formed by heating a sugar solution with phenylhydrazine hydrochloride, sodium acetate and acetic acid. If the yellow crystals which form are examined under the microscope they are sufficiently characteristic for certain sugars to be identified. It should be noted that glucose and fructose form the same osazone (glucosazone, m.p. 205°C). Before melting points are taken, osazones should be purified by recrystallization from alcohol. Sucrose does not form an osazone, but under the conditions of the above test sufficient hydrolysis takes place for the production of glucosazone.

4. *Resorcinol test for ketones.* This is known as Selivanoff's test. A crystal of resorcinol is added to the solution and warmed on a water-bath with an equal volume of concentrated hydrochloric acid. A rose colour is produced if a ketone is present (e.g. fructose, honey or hydrolysed inulin).

5. *Test for pentoses.* Heat a solution of the substance in a test-tube with an equal volume of hydrochloric acid containing a little phloroglucinol. Formation of a red colour indicates pentoses.

6. *Keller–Kiliani test for deoxysugars.* Deoxysugars are found in cardiac glycosides such as those of *Digitalis* and *Strophanthus* spp. (see Chapter 23). The sugar is dissolved in acetic acid containing a trace of ferric chloride and transferred to the surface of concentrated sulphuric acid. At the junction of the liquids a reddish-brown colour is produced which gradually becomes blue.

7. *Enzyme reactions.* Since certain carbohydrate reactions are only brought about by certain specific enzymes, such enzymes may be used for identification.

8. *Chromatography.* Chromatographic methods are particularly suited to the examination of drug extracts, which may contain a number of carbohydrates often in very small amounts. Not only are they applicable to carbohydrates originally present in the sample (see pharmacopoeial TLC test for honey), but also they may be used to study the products of hydrolysis of polysaccharide complexes such as gums and mucilages. As standards for comparison many pure sugars, uronic acids and other sugar derivatives are commercially available.

Table 20.2   The character of some polysaccharides.

Name	Occurrence and nature
Containing only monosaccharide units	
1. Amylopectin or α-amylose	The main constituent of most starches (over 80%). The molecule has branched chains each consisting of 20–26 α-1,4-linked glucose residues. Several hundred of these chains are linked by α-1,6 glycosidic bonds to neighbouring chains giving a molecule containing some 50 000 glycosyl units. The branching pattern throughout the molecule is not uniform, resulting in some areas that are apparently amorphous (high degree of branching) and others probably crystalline (linear chains predominate with little branching)
2. Amylose or β-amylose	Most starches contain up to 20%, but sometimes absent. Consists essentially of linear chains of α-1,4-linked glucose residues. Several thousand glucose units constitute a chain. It is now recognized that there is a very limited branching (α-1,6-linkages) to the extent of 2–8 branches per molecule
3. Glycogen or animal starch	Important reserve carbohydrate of animal tissues. Molecule resembles that of amylopectin
4. Cellulose	Chief polysaccharide of plant cell walls. Linear chains of β-1,4-linked glucose residues

(Continued)

20

Table 20.2   The character of some polysaccharides. (Cont'd)

5. Inulin

A reserve carbohydrate particularly abundant in the Compositae. Linear chains of up to 50 β-1,2-linked fructofuranose units terminated by a single glucose unit

$n = 35{-}50$

6. Xylans, mannans and galactans

These are often associated with one another and with cellulose. They are difficult to isolate in a pure form. On hydrolysis they yield xylose, mannose and galactose, respectively

7. Hemicelluloses

These polysaccharides occur in the cell wall with cellulose and pectic substances. The nomenclature, dating from 1891, is deceptive because hemicelluloses are not components of cellulose but are formed mainly from hexose and pentose units. Hemicelluloses vary according to source and can be classified as xylans, mannans and galactans according to their principal components

8. Lichenin or lichen starch

A polysaccharide found in lichens. Resembles cellulose but molecule contains about 25% of β-1,3 glucosidic linkages

Polysaccharide complexes containing uronic acid or other units

1. Pectins

These occur in the middle lamellae of cell walls and are abundant in fruits (e.g. apples, oranges) and roots (beets and gentian). The parent substance protopectin is insoluble but is easily converted by restricted hydrolysis into pectinic acids (pectins). Pectins from different sources vary in their complex constitution, the principal components being blocks of D-galacturonic acid residues linked by α-1,4- glycosidic linkages and interspersed with rhamnose units; some of the carboxyl groups are methylated. These molecules are accompanied by small amounts of neutral arabinans (branched polymers of α-1,5-linked L-arabofuranose units) and galactans (largely linear chains of β-1,4- linked D-galactopyranose units)

Repeating units of D-galacturonic acid

2. Algin or alginic acid

Alginic acid is the principal constituent of the cell walls of the brown algae. It was discovered by Stanford in 1880 and is now widely used for the manufacture of alginate salts and fibres (q.v.). The composition varies according to the biological source, thus providing a range of properties which are exploited commercially. It is a heteropolyuronide consisting of chains of β-1,4-linked D-mannuronic acid units interspersed with lengths of α-1,4-linked L-guluronic acid units together with sections in which the two monouronide units are regularly interspersed. In alginic acids from different sources the ratios of the two uronic acids vary from 2:1 to 1:2. The chain length varies with the method of preparation and molecular weight, and viscosity measurements suggest molecules of from 220 to 860 units

β-1,4-linked-D-mannuronic acid units   α-1,4-linked L-guluronic acid units

(Continued)

Table 20.2 The character of some polysaccharides. (Cont'd)

3. Polysaccharides with sulphuric acid esters	Certain algae, including those yielding agar and carrageen, contain a mixture of polysaccharides. Agar, for example, contains a biose formed from D- and L-galactose but also a more complex agaropectin formed from galactose and uronic acid units partly esterified with sulphuric acid. Carrageen has a similar composition
4. Chitin	This is found in some of the lower plants, in insects and in crustaceans. The molecule consists of linear chains of β-1,4-linked N-acetyl-D-glycosamine residues. Its inclusion in the microfibrillar component of the fungal cell wall is analogous to that of the cellulose microfibril

5. Gums and mucilages	Gums such as acacia and tragacanth and mucilages, such as those found in linseed, psyllium seeds and marshmallow root, are found in many plants, where they are usually formed from the cell wall or deposited on it in layers. They are essentially polyuronides consisting of sugar and uronic acid units. Some gums have methoxyl groups (e.g. tragacanth); in others the acidic complex is united with metals (e.g. acacia)

Experimental details and R_f values of sugars in different systems are to be found in standard books on chromatography. The carbohydrate spots obtained after separation are identified by their positions and by reagents. It may be useful to examine them in ultraviolet light. A non-specific reagent for reducing sugars is a freshly prepared ammoniacal silver nitrate solution. More specific reagents giving coloured spots with different sugars include aniline hydrogen phthalate (in water-saturated n-butanol) and naphthoresorcinol (in acetone, water and phosphoric acid). These are applied to the chromatogram with a spray. Although sugars are non-volatile, it is possible by suitable treatment to render them satisfactory for gas chromatography (q.v.)

COMMERCIAL PLANT-DERIVED FIBRES AND PRODUCTS

The biological origin and the structure of plant fibres is discussed in Chapter 42; many have important commercial uses and for a review on their botany, chemistry and processing see McDougall et al., J. Sci. Food, Agric., 1993, **62**, 1.

A number of vegetable fibres have importance in pharmacy, particularly as components of surgical dressings and for the manufacture of artificial fibres and haemostatic dressings. The subject of surgical dressings was, and in many Schools still is, regarded as pharmacognosy-related. However with the more recent advances in the management and concept of wound-healing, many materials of non-vegetable origin are now used which, for an in-depth coverage, bring the topic outside the scope of this book. Described below are the more important primary carbohydrate materials involved.

COTTON, RAW COTTON

Cotton consists of the epidermal trichomes of the seeds of *Gossypium herbaceum* and other cultivated species of *Gossypium* (Malvaceae). The plants are shrubs or small trees which produce three- to five-celled capsules containing numerous seeds. The USA produces about half of the world's cotton, other important sources being Egypt, India and South America. The chief American cottons are derived from *G. barbadense* (Sea Island cotton) and *G. herbaceum* (Upland, Texas or New Orleans cotton).

The hairs of the different species vary in length or 'staple'. The staples of important commercial varieties of cotton are as follows: (1) Sea Island, up to 54.5 mm; (2) Egyptian, 31–38 mm; (3) Brazilian and Peruvian, 29–30 mm; (4) American Upland, about 25.9 mm; (5) Indian, 21.4–29.2 mm.

Preparation. When ripe the bolls are collected, dried and subjected to a ginning process to separate the hairs from the seed. The gin, which may be of a roller or a pneumatic type, is designed to pull the hairs through a narrow space which is too small to allow the seed to pass. In ordinary American or Upland cotton the gin leaves the seeds with a coating of short hairs which have to be removed by a second type of gin known as a 'linter'. These short hairs are used for making the lower grades of cotton wool and rayons. The seeds are used for the preparation of cottonseed oil (q.v.) and cattle cake. Raw cotton contains various impurities, such as immature and broken seeds, fragments of leaf, etc., most of which are removed during the manufacture of yarn.

For spinning very fine yarns Sea Island cotton is used, but for coarser yarns it is possible to use shorter staple cottons. Different machines are used for these two types of yarn, which are known as *combed* and *carded*, respectively. The cotton-combing machine separates all the shorter fibres and a thread is spun consisting of long, well-paralleled, uniform fibres. The short fibres of *comber waste* are used for making the best grades of cotton wool. The carding machine uses fibres which are shorter and less uniform in length, and the absence of combing is shown in the yarn by the irregular arrangement of the fibres, the ends of which often project from the surface.

Microscopy of unbleached cotton. Cotton consists of unicellular hairs the appearance of which has been likened to that of empty, twisted fire-hoses. Their length is up to about 5 cm, diameter 9–24 μm, and the number of twists varies from about 75 cm⁻¹ in the Indian to 150 cm⁻¹

in the Sea Island. Pieces of 'shell' or seed coat, which can often be picked from samples of raw cotton, show hair bases fitting between the thick-walled epidermal cells. The apex is rounded and solid. The cotton hair is cylindrical when young but becomes flattened and twisted as it matures, the large lumen, which contains the remains of protoplasm being much elongated in transverse section. The cellulose wall of the hair is covered with a waxy cuticle which renders it non-absorbent. The cuticle may be stained with ruthenium red. Bleached cotton yarn and absorbent cotton wool (see below) are readily wetted by water.

Tests.   The following tests are applicable to cotton.

1. On ignition, which should be done both by advancing the fibre towards a flame and by heating on porcelain, cotton burns with a flame, gives very little odour or fumes, does not produce a bead, and leaves a small white ash; distinction from acetate rayon, alginate yarn (also wool, silk, nylon).
2. Moisten with N/50 iodine and, when nearly dry, add 80% w/w sulphuric acid. A blue colour is produced; distinction from acetate rayon, alginate yarn, jute, hemp (also wool, silk, nylon).
3. With ammoniacal copper oxide solution, raw cotton dissolves with ballooning, leaving a few fragments of cuticle; absorbent cotton dissolves completely with uniform swelling; distinction from acetate rayon, jute (also wool, nylon).
4. In cold sulphuric acid 80% w/w cotton dissolves; distinction from oxidized cellulose, jute, hemp (also wool).
5. In cold sulphuric acid 60% w/w insoluble; distinction from cellulose wadding and rayons.
6. In warm (40°C) hydrochloric acid *BP* insoluble; distinction from acetate rayon (also silk, nylon).
7. Insoluble in 5% potassium hydroxide solution; distinction from oxidized cellulose (also wool, silk).
8. Treat with cold Shirlastain A for 1 min and wash out; gives shades of blue, lilac or purple; distinction from viscose and acetate rayons, alginate yarn (also wool, silk, nylon).
9. Treat with cold Shirlastain C for 5 min and wash out; raw cotton gives a mauve to reddish-brown colour and absorbent cotton a pink one; distinction from flax, jute, hemp. The Shirlastains may be usefully applied to a small piece of the whole fabric under investigation to indicate the distribution of more than one type of yarn.
10. Gives no red stain with phloroglucinol and hydrochloric acid; distinction from jute, hemp and kapok.
11. Insoluble in formic acid 90% or phenol 90% (w/w); distinction from acetate rayon (also nylon).
12. Insoluble in acetone (distinction from acetate rayon).

ABSORBENT COTTON WOOL, ABSORBENT WOOL

Cotton wool is mainly prepared from linters, card strips, card fly and comber waste. Bales of these short-fibred cotton wastes pass from the yarn manufacturers to the makers of cotton wool. For best-quality cotton wool the comber waste of American and Egyptian cottons is preferred. In this the fibres are reasonably long and twisted and thus suitable for producing a cotton wool having an average staple that will offer appreciable resistance when pulled and not shed a significant quality of dust when shaken gently.

The preparation may be outlined as follows. The comber waste (which arrives in bales) is loosened by machinery and then heated with dilute caustic soda and soda ash solution at a pressure of 1–3 atmospheres for 10–15 h. This removes much of the fatty cuticle and renders the trichome wall absorbent. It is then well washed with water, bleached with dilute sodium hypochlorite solution and treated with very dilute hydrochloric acid. After washing and drying it is in a matted condition and is therefore opened up by machines and then 'scutched'; that is, it is converted into a continuous sheet of fairly even thickness with the fibres loosened ready for the carding machine. The carding machine effects a combing operation and forms a thin continuous film of cotton wool. Several such films are superimposed on one another, interleaved with paper and packaged in rolls.

Tests.   For tests on cotton wool, see under 'Cotton, Raw Cotton'.

Structure of fibre.   Like the cell wall in general, that of cotton consists of a primary and secondary wall. The formation of the former is modified to embrace the enormous longitudinal development of the cell, some thousands of times greater than the width. The microfibrils themselves are unexpandable and are initially laid down in hoops around the fibre, restricting its lateral growth. However, because of their different orientation at the fibre end, longitudinal extension can take place. Owing to the build-up of pressure from successive layers of cellulose the original orientation becomes lost as the fibre matures. Matrix polysaccharides and proteins derived from the Golgi apparatus are also present in the primary wall. The secondary wall, some 5–10 μm thick and consisting almost entirely of pure cellulose, constitutes the main bulk of the mature cotton fibre.

Chemical nature.   Raw cotton consists of cellulose approximately 90% and moisture 7%, the remainder being wax, fat, remains of protoplasm and ash.

Absorbent cotton is a very pure form of cellulose and its chemical and physical properties have been extensively studied. The cellulose molecule is built up of glucose residues united by 1,4-β-glucosidic links (contrast starch). The wall of the cotton fibre, like that of plant cells in general, shows anisotropic properties. When swollen in water, the swelling is in a direction at right angles to the long axis. In the direction of the long axis it shows considerable tensile strength. Examined in polarized light, it shows birefringence, the value of the double refraction depending on the liquid in which the fibre is immersed. This phenomenon, characteristic of mixed bodies with rod-like structural elements, has been termed rodlet-double refraction. Stained with chlor-zinc-iodine and examined microscopically in polarized light (analyser removed), the fibre shows greater absorption when orientated with its long axis parallel to the plane of polarization than when orientated with the long axis at right angles (dichroism). These physical properties suggest that the fibre wall is built up of elongated structural units orientated in some definite manner. The study of the cotton fibre by X-ray analysis has confirmed this and has shown that its cell wall is composed of elongated chain-like molecules (built up of repeating units 1.03 nm long) and orientated in a spiral manner, the spiral making an angle of 30° with the long axis of the fibre. The length of the repeating unit of structure corresponds to that of two glucose residues fully extended. This unit is the 'cellobiose unit', many of which are united in the polysaccharide molecule of cellulose (Table 20.2).

Cellobiose
unit 1.03 nm

The biosynthesis of cellulose in the cotton trichome would appear to involve UDP-glucose originating from sucrose.

Jute

Jute consists of the strands of phloem fibres from the stem bark of *Corchorus capsularis, C. olitorius* and other species of *Corchorus* (Tiliaceae). These are annual plants about 3–4 m high which are cultivated in Bengal, in the delta region of the Ganges and Brahmaputra rivers, and in Assam, Bihar and Orissa.

The fibres are separated from the other plant material by retting and then spun into yarn which can be made up into hessian and sacking. Short fibres left over from the preparation of the yarns and ropes constitute *tow* and in pharmacy the term 'tow' refers to jute, although it can also be applied to hemp and flax. The commercial strands are 1–3 m long and about 30–140 μm in diameter. Each consists of a bundle of phloem fibres composed of lignocellulose. The heavily lignified middle lamella is destroyed by oxidizing agents; a mixture of nitric acid and potassium chlorate may therefore be used to disintegrate the bundles, the individual fibres being then teased out and sketched. Prepared transverse sections should also be examined and compared with those of hemp and flax.

Flax

Flax is prepared from the pericyclic fibres of the stem of *Linum usitatissimum* (Linaceae).

The commercial fibres show fine transverse injuries received during the preparation. Good-quality flax fibre is non-lignified except for the middle lamella. Lignification of the secondary wall, however, takes place as the stem matures, starting at the base, and if the stems are too old before retting, the fibre is coarse and harsh in texture.

Hemp

Hemp is prepared from the pericyclic fibres of the stem of *Cannabis sativa* (Cannabinaceae). The fibre is composed chiefly of cellulose, but some lignification has usually taken place and the percentage of cellulose is lower than in flax.

The fibre ends, in contrast to those of flax, are bluntly rounded. Some of the fibre ends are forked, this bifurcation arising from injuries to the stem. The lumen of the hemp fibre is flattened or oval, in contrast to the small round lumen of flax. Transverse striations seen in commercial fibres arise from beating, the fibres being prepared by partial retting.

Jute, hemp and flax fibres are compared in Table 20.3.

REGENERATED CARBOHYDRATE MATERIAL AND CHEMICALLY MODIFIED FIBRES

Regenerated fibres are those produced from naturally occurring, long-chain molecules which have been isolated, controlled and, if necessary, modified to give a suitable fibre form. The term 'rayon', as in viscose, acetate and cuprammonium rayon, is applied to those derived from the polysaccharide cellulose. The term 'artificial silk' is now out of date. Also in this class is alginate fibre, derived from alginic acid (q.v.).

Viscose (regenerated cellulose, rayon)

This has been developed from a process introduced by three British chemists (Beadle, Bevan and Cross) in 1892, and accounts for the bulk of the world rayon output today. It is also the principal type used in surgical dressings.

The starting material is a cellulose prepared either from coniferous wood, particularly spruce, or scoured and bleached cotton linters. The wood is usually delignified at source (Canada, Scandinavia, etc.) by a process similar to that used for cellulose wadding. It reaches the rayon manufacturers as boards of white pulp, containing 80–90% of cellulose and some hemicellulose (mainly pentosans). The latter, being alkali-soluble, are removed in the first stage of the process, which consists of steeping in sodium hydroxide solution. After most of the excess alkaline liquor has been pressed out, alkali-cellulose (sodium cellulosate) remains. This is dissolved by treatment with carbon disulphide and sodium hydroxide solution to give a viscous (whence the name 'viscose') solution of sodium cellulose xanthate. After 'ripening' and filtering, the solution is forced through a spinneret, a jet with fine nozzles, immersed in a bath which includes dilute sulphuric acid and sodium sulphate, when the cellulose is regenerated as continuous filaments. These are drawn together as a yarn, which is twisted for strength, desulphurized by removing free sulphur with sodium sulphide, bleached, washed, dried and conditioned to a moisture content of 10%.

The viscose yarn may be left as such (i.e. *continuous filament rayon*) for use in such things as blouse fabrics, or it may be cut up to give *staple rayon* ('Fibro') of fixed length from 1 to 8 in. That used in surgical dressings and many other fabrics is made to resemble cotton in dimensions. Suitable spinnerets are used to give a diameter of 15–20 μm and the fibre is cut into lengths usually of 4.8 cm. This staple can be processed on types of spinning and weaving machines used for cotton dressings or it may be left in a loose fibre form as *viscose rayon absorbent wool*.

Table 20.3 Characters of jute, hemp and flax fibres.

	Jute (*Corchorus* spp.)	Hemp (*Cannabis sativa*)	Flax (*Linum usitatissimum*)
Apex	Bluntly pointed or rounded	Mostly blunt and sometimes forked	Sharply pointed
Wall	Without markings; lumen varying in size	Marked striations, cross fissures, and swellings; lumen large and uniform	Thick wall with fine cross lines some intersecting; lumen narrow
Transverse section	Polygonal, sharp angles; lumen oval or circular	Roughly 3- to 6-sided with rounded corners; lumen cleft or branched	5 or 6 straight sides; point-like lumen
Length	0.8–5 mm	35–40 mm	25–30 mm average, but up to 120 mm
Diameter	10–25 μm	16–50 μm	12–30 μm
Phloroglucinol test	Deep red	Slightly red	Colourless or slight pink
Iodine and sulphuric acid	Yellow throughout	Inner wall blue; middle lamella yellow	Blue or violet
Chlor-zinc-iodine	Yellow	Purple to yellow	Purple to yellow

Viscose rayon is a very pure form of cellulose. It yields a trace of ash which contains sulphur. The cellulose molecules of the original natural material, whether wood or cotton, become more separated from one another in the viscose solution than in the vegetable material and in the regenerated fibre are still less closely packed. Radiography has shown that the side-to-side aggregation of the long-chain molecules is different from that in natural celluloses. The size of the molecules is also reduced, wood cellulose having molecules of the order of 9000 glucose residue units, while those of viscose rayon have only about 450.

Viscose rayon gauze and other rayon dressings have the advantage over cotton dressings in that they show no loss of absorbency on storage.

Macroscopical characters. As normally produced, this rayon is a white, highly lustrous fibre (*natural* or *glossy viscose*). Its tensile strength varies from two-thirds to one-and-a-half times that of cotton. When wetted it loses about 60% of its tensile strength, a proportionately greater loss than is found with cotton. Where more than a certain amount of rayon is used in a dressing, the fabric may be required to be rendered water-repellent (e.g. cotton crêpe bandage).

Microscopical characters. The fibres are solid and transparent and 15–20 μm in diameter. They have a slight twist, and show grooves along their length which are principally caused by the spinnerets being immersed in the regenerating solution (compare nylon). The grooves give a characteristic appearance to the transverse section. The ends of the fibres are abrupt and characteristic. The fibres are clearly seen in chloral hydrate solution or in lactophenol, but are almost invisible in cresol (having the same refractive index of 1.53). They appear bright in polarized light with crossed Nicols.

Chemical tests

1. The fibres give the general tests for vegetable and regenerated carbohydrate fibres.
2. On ignition they behave like cotton; distinction from acetate rayon and alginate yarn (also wool, silk, nylon and glass).
3. With N/50 iodine and sulphuric acid, 80%, they give a blue colour similar to that given by cotton; distinction from acetate rayon, alginate yarn, jute, hemp (also wool, silk, nylon).
4. With ammoniacal copper oxide they behave like absorbent cotton; distinction from acetate rayon, jute (also wool, nylon).
5. Cold sulphuric acid, 60% w/w, dissolves the fibre; distinction from cotton, oxidized cellulose, alginate yarn, flax, jute, hemp (also wool).
6. Warm (40°C) Hydrochloric Acid BP does not cause solution; distinction from acetate rayon (also silk, nylon).
7. Boiling potassium hydroxide solution, 5%, insoluble; distinction from oxidized cellulose (also wool, silk).
8. Shirlastain A produces a bright pink; distinction from cotton, oxidized cellulose, acetate, rayon (also wool, silk, nylon).
9. Phloroglucinol and hydrochloric acid produce no red stain; distinction from jute, hemp and kapok.
10. The fibres, like cotton, are insoluble in acetone, formic acid 90% or phenol 90%; distinction from acetate rayon (also nylon).

Delustring and dyeing of fibres. Rayon and other artificial fibres with a natural lustrous appearance may be delustred by addition of the white pigment titanium oxide to the solution (e.g. viscose) or to the melt (e.g. nylon) before extrusion of the filaments. In this way the pigment is evenly distributed inside each filament and delustring is permanent. These fibres may be similarly 'spun-dyed' by addition of

an appropriate dye instead of the titanium oxide. The method results in an exceptional degree of colour fastness.

Matt Viscose (delustrated viscose rayon) is the form normally used in the manufacture of surgical dressings; hence, in general appearance these are very similar to those manufactured from cotton. The individual filaments have the appearance already described, except for the matt white colour and on microscopical examination the pigment particles, which appear black by transmitted light and are scattered throughout the filament. The amount of pigment is controlled by the ash value. Titanium is detected in the ash by dissolving in sulphuric acid, diluting and adding hydrogen peroxide, 3%, when a yellow colour is produced.

Cellulose ethers. These are prepared from purified alkali cellulose derived from cotton linters or delignified wood pulp by the action of caustic soda, as in the initial stages of the production of viscose rayon.

Methylcellulose BP/EP is a whitish, fibrous powder prepared by the action of methyl chloride under pressure on an alkali cellulose, when hydroxyl groups become methylated. A useful grade is that in which two of the three hydroxyl groups of the glucose residue units of the cellulose chain are methylated, and this has the optimum solubility in water. In pharmacy a grade giving a low viscosity is used both to increase the viscosity and to stabilize lotions, suspensions, pastes and some ointments and ophthalmic preparations; one giving a high viscosity is used as a tablet disintegrant. In medicine it is used as a hydrophilic colloid laxative in chronic constipation and can be used in obese persons to curb the appetite, because it gives a feeling of fullness. *Ethylcellulose* is similarly prepared and has like applications.

Carmellose Sodium EP/BP (*sodium carboxymethylcellulose*) is an odourless and tasteless white hygroscopic powder or granules prepared by the action of monochloroacetic acid on alkali cellulose and removal of the byproduct salts. Substitution of hydroxyl groups by carboxymethyl groups occurs over a range depending on the conditions and the cellulose used; there are prescribed limits for the sodium content. It is water-soluble, and a grade giving a medium viscosity contains 0.7 carboxymethyl groups per glucose residue unit. It is insoluble in organic solvents. Its pharmaceutical and medical uses are similar to those of methylcellulose, but as well as being used as a laxative it is a useful antacid.

Carmellose calcium is also official.

Pyroxylin BP (Cellulose nitrate)

Pyroxylin is prepared by the action of nitric and sulphuric acids on wood pulp or cotton linters that have been freed from fatty materials. When dry it is explosive and must be carefully stored, dampened with not less than 25% its weight of isopropyl alcohol or industrial methylated spirits. It is used for making Flexible Collodion BP.

Absorbable haemostatic dressings

The control of bleeding is of vital concern in surgery, and the great disadvantage of the old-type dressing such as a cotton gauze plug is that it has to be removed after bleeding has been checked with a consequent danger of a recurrence of the haemorrhage. Gelatin sponge, oxidized cellulose and alginate dressings overcome this, in that there is no need to remove them after the bleeding has been checked, since they are absorbed by the tissues.

Oxidized cellulose

Oxidized cellulose originated in the USA as a result of the work published by Yackel and Kenyon in 1942. Cotton wool or gauze is treated with nitrogen dioxide until the number of carboxyl groups formed by the oxidation of the primary alcohol groups of the glucose residue units of the cellulose molecules reaches 16–22%. The original cellulose now has glucuronic acid residue units (compare alginic acid) as well as some glucose residue units.

Appearance. Gauze, lint or knitted material, very similar to normal cotton but with an off-white colour, a harsher texture, charred odour and an acid taste. It does not go pasty on chewing. The wool tends to disintegrate on handling. In microscopical appearance the fibres are very similar to those of absorbent cotton.

Tests

1. Does not give the tests for animal fibres and animal source-haemostatics.
2. On ignition it behaves like normal cotton.
3. With iodine and sulphuric acid or ammoniacal copper oxide solution it behaves like absorbent cotton.
4. Slowly soluble in 80% sulphuric acid.
5. Insoluble in warm hydrochloric acid BP.
6. Soluble in the cold in 5% potassium hydroxide solution.
   Complete solubility in aqueous alkali is made the basis of a test for absence of unchanged cotton and foreign particles. The solution in alkali gives with excess acid a white flocculent precipitate (former *BP* test for identity).
7. It reduces Fehling's solution.
8. Shirlastain A gives a pale blue to mauve colour.
9. Shirlastain C gives a brown to olive green.

Uses. It is used as an absorbable haemostatic in many types of surgery, but is incompatible with pencillin, delays bone repair and cannot be sterilized by heat. It has found some application in chromatography.

Alginate fibres

These originated about 1938 in Britain and were further developed during World War II.

The fibres are prepared by a process similar to that for viscose rayon. An aqueous solution of sodium alginate (see this chapter) is pumped through a spinneret immersed in a bath of calcium chloride solution (acidified with hydrochloric acid), when water-insoluble calcium alginate is precipitated as continuous filaments. These are collected, washed and dried. For use in surgical dressings and bacteriological swabs they are reduced to a staple form which may then be processed to a *calcium alginate wool* or a fabric (e.g. *gauze*) in the same manner as used for viscose staple or cotton.

As indicated in Table 20.2, alginic acid is composed of polymers of both mannuronic and guluronic acids. The properties of the two are variable and alginates of different origin have different compositions and properties. This is illustrated by the two commercial haemostatic dressings—Kalostat (BritCair Limited) and Sorbsan (Steriseal—Pharmaplast Limited). The former is derived from the seaweed *Laminaria hyperborea* collected off the Norwegian coast and yields an alginate with a guluronic:mannuronic ratio of 2:1; the latter is prepared from *Laminaria* and *Ascophyllum* species collected off the west coast of Scotland and gives an alginate with a guluronic:mannuronic acid ratio of about 1:2. On a wound surface the α-linkages of the guluronic acid polymer are not easily broken so that fibre strength is retained and a strong gel is formed on contact with the wound exudate. A high ratio of mannuronic acid polymer (β-linkages) yields a product giving a weaker gel and less retention of fibre strength. In practice this means that the Kalostat dressing can be removed from the wound with forceps and Sorbsan is removed by irrigation with, for example, sodium citrate solution.

Calcium alginate fibres of commerce contain substantial traces of substances used to inhibit mould and bacterial growth in the sodium alginate spinning solution. Spinning lubricants such as lauryl or cetyl pyridinium bromide (antibacterial) are also applied to the filaments. These substances must not be used or must be removed in the case of calcium alginate staple for use in, for example, bacteriological swabs.

Before use as an absorbable haemostatic dressing some calcium alginate dressings must be immersed in sodium chloride to give a fibre of the calcium alginate covered by sodium alginate. The degree of conversion is conditioned to give the desired rate of absorption when in use; the greater the proportion of sodium alginate the faster the absorption rate.

Alginate filaments are composed of salts of the long-chain molecules of alginic acid (see Table 20.2) and there is little cross-linking between the chains in the fibre.

Appearance. Fairly lustrous, pale cream-coloured fibres which in microscopical appearance are very similar to those of viscose rayon, being solid grooved rods. The haemostatic dressing ('Calgitex') is almost tasteless and odourless and rather harsh to touch. The gauze is usually a knitted fabric and has little sheen. That with a fast rate of absorption when chewed readily assumes a pasty form somewhat like that of mashed potato. That with a slow rate of absorption remains smoothly coarser in the same time. They do not disintegrate easily on handling. These points and the tests below will serve to distinguish alginate haemostatic dressings from those of oxidized cellulose. First-aid dressings frequently embody an alginate gauze impregnated with a local anaesthetic.

Tests. These refer to calcium alginate fibre or the mixed sodium and calcium salt fibre. They give the general tests for vegetable and regenerated carbohydrate fibres. For distinctions from rayons and oxidized cellulose see earlier.

1. Smoulders in a flame and goes out when removed from flame.
2. With (N/50) iodine and sulphuric acid, a brownish-red colour is produced, the filaments swell and dissolve to leave a strand of insoluble alginic acid.
3. In ammoniacal copper nitrate solution they swell and dissolve.
4. Insoluble in 60% w/w sulphuric acid.
5. Insoluble in warm (40°C) hydrochloric acid BP.
6. Insoluble in boiling 5% KOH (swell and acquire a yellow tint).
7. Soluble in 5% sodium citrate solution.
8. Fibre, 0.1 g, boiled with 5 ml of water remains insoluble but dissolves when 1 ml 20% w/v sodium carbonate solution is added and boiled for 1 min. A white precipitate of calcium carbonate is formed, depending on the proportion of original calcium alginate present. When centrifuged and the clear supernatant acidified, a gelatinous precipitate of alginic acid is produced. The precipitate will give a purple colour after solution in NaOH and addition of an acid solution of ferric sulphate.
9. Shirlastain A gives a reddish-brown colour.
10. Alginate haemostatic fibres are invisible in polarized light with crossed Nicols.

Uses. The alginate absorbable haemostatic dressings are non-toxic and non-irritant. They have advantages over oxidized cellulose, which include selective rate of absorption, sterilization (and resterilization) by autoclaving or dry heat and compatibility with antibiotics such as penicillin. They may be used internally in neurosurgery, endaural and dental surgery to be subsequently absorbed. Externally, they may be used (e.g. for burns or sites from which skin grafts have been taken) to arrest bleeding and form a protective dressing which may be left or later removed in a manner appropriate to the type of dressing employed (see above). Protective films of calcium alginate may also be used by painting the injured surface with sodium alginate solution and then spraying it with calcium chloride solution.

Calcium alginate wool as a swab for pathological work or bacterial examination of such things as food processing equipment and tableware has the great advantage over cotton wool in that it permits release of all the organisms by disintegration and solution of the swab in, for example, Ringer's solution containing sodium hexametaphosphate.

In fabrics the calcium alginate fibres would disintegrate in alkaline solutions (laundering), but this advantage is turned to a commercial virtue by the use of the yarn as a scaffolding thread to support yarns normally too fine to survive the weaving process. The scaffold is removed by an alkaline bath to leave a lightweight fabric.

Cellulose wadding

Cellulose wadding was official in the *BP* 1989. It is prepared from high-grade bleached sulphite wood pulp which is received by the manufacturer in the form of boards about 0.75 m square and 1 mm thick. These are packed in bales containing about 180 kg pulp. The pulp is put in a 'beater', where it is mixed with about 20 times its weight of water and the mixture circulates between a power-driven roll and the bed-plate of the 'beater'. The effect of this is to break up the pulp into separate fibres. When this process is complete, the contents of the beater are mixed with a further quantity of water and then allowed to run in a steady flow on to the 'wire' of the paper machines. This 'wire' is a very fine wire gauze through which water runs, leaving a fine web of fibres on top of the 'wire'. This web is then dried and crêped to give a thin, soft, absorbent sheet. About 30 of these thin sheets are laid together to form cellulose wadding.

When examined microscopically, chemical wood pulps or cellulose wadding show characteristic woody elements, which, however, give no lignin reaction (distinction from mechanical wood pulp). Tracheids with bordered pits and characteristic medullary ray cells are usually observed. The cellulose nature of the walls is shown by the blue colour obtained with iodine followed by 80% sulphuric acid and by their solubility in an ammoniacal solution of copper oxide.

STARCHES

Starch constitutes the principal form of carbohydrate reserve in the green plant and is to be found especially in seeds and underground organs. The green parts of plants exposed to sunlight contain small granules of transitional starch which arise from photosynthesis. During the hours of darkness these are removed to the storage organs. Starch occurs in the form of granules (starch grains) the shape and size of which are characteristic of the species as is also the ratio of the content of the principal constituents, amylose and amylopectin.

A number of starches are recognized for pharmaceutical use. They include maize (*Zea mays* L.), rice (*Oryza sativa* L.), wheat (*Triticum aestivum* L.) and potato (*Solanum tuberosum* L.). Tapioca or cassava starch (*Manihot utilissima*) may be used in place of the above in tropical and subtropical countries.

The more important commercial starches are listed in Table 20.4.

Preparation of starches

Commercial starches, the preparation of which is described below, are not chemically pure and contain small amounts of nitrogenous and inorganic matter.

Table 20.4 Commercial starches.

Family	Plant	Economic product
Cycadaceae	*Zamia floridana*	Florida arrowroot
Gramineae	*Zea mays*	Maize or corn
	Oryza sativa	Rice
	Triticum aestivum	Wheat
	Avena sativa	Oats
	Hordeum sp.	Barley
	Secale cereale	Rye
Palmae	*Metroxylon rumphii*	Sago
Musaceae	*Musa* spp.	Bananas and plantains
Zingiberaceae	*Zingiber officinale*	Ginger
	Curcuma spp.	East Indian arrowroot and turmeric
Cannaceae	*Canna edulis*	Queensland arrowroot or tous les mois
Polygonaceae	*Polygonum fagopyrum*	Buckwheat
Euphorbiaceae	*Manihot utilissima*	Manihot or cassava starch and tapioca
Leguminosae	*Phaseolus vulgaris*	Bean flour
	Ervum lens	Lentil flour
	Pisum sativum	Pea flour
Convolvulaceae	*Ipomoea batatas*	Sweet potato
Solanaceae	*Solanum tuberosum*	Potato

Many patented processes are in use for particular starches, and the procedure adopted depends on the degree of purity desired and the nature of the compounds from which the starch has to be freed. Cereal starches, for example, have to be freed from cell debris, oil, soluble protein matter and the abundant insoluble proteins (glutelins and prolamins) known as 'gluten'. Potato starch, on the other hand, is associated with vegetable tissue, mineral salts and soluble proteins.

Wheat and similar starches were at one time prepared by kneading the ground material in a stream of water, the gluten remaining as a sticky mass, while the starch separated on standing from the milky washings. The following methods are now employed.

Preparation of maize starch.   The grain is first softened by soaking at 50°C for about 2 days in a 0.2% solution of sulphurous acid. This assists disintegration, enabling the embryo or germ to be easily liberated intact and permitting the starch to be readily freed from fibre. During this time lactic acid bacteria are active and metabolize soluble sugars extracted from the maize. The grain, in water, is then distintegrated by attrition mills; these do not break the liberated oil-containing embryos, which, in the older process, were skimmed off. Nowadays the germs are continuously separated from the suspension by liquid cyclones (hydroclones) which operate in batteries of about 12. The germs are used for the preparation of germ oils, which are an important source of vitamins. The remainder of the grain is ground wet and the starch and gluten separated from fibrous material in rotating, slightly inclined stainless steel reels covered with perforated metal sheets. The retained fibre is washed and the total mixture of starch and protein (mill starch) is fractionated into gluten and starch by the use of special starch purification centrifuges; separation depends on the fact that gluten is lighter than starch. In older processes this separation was accomplished by repeated 'tabling', in which the suspension was allowed to flow very slowly through troughs about 40 m long and 0.7 m wide, when the heavier starch was deposited first. The starch suspension from the centrifuge is further purified in other centrifuges and hydroclones, which reduces the protein level.

The subsequent drying process may involve flash dryers or a moving-belt dryer; considerable flexibility in drying time is required to accommodate the various modified starches which are now produced.

Preparation of rice starch. Rice is soaked in successive quantities of 0.4% caustic soda until the material can be easily disintegrated. The softened grain is ground (the compound grains separating into their components), made into a dilute suspension which is repeatedly screened, and the starch separated by standing or by means of a centrifuge. The damp starch is next cut into blocks and dried at 50–60°C for 2 days. The brown outer layer which forms is then scraped from the blocks and drying is continued at a lower temperature for about 14 days, during which time the blocks gradually crack into irregular masses. For pharmaceutical use this 'crystal' starch is powdered.

Preparation of potato starch. The potatoes are washed and reduced to a fine pulp in a rasping machine or in a disintegrator of the hammer-mill type. Much of the cell debris is removed from the pulp by rotary sieves and the milky liquid which passes through the sieve contains starch, soluble proteins and salts, and some cell debris. On standing, the starch separates more rapidly than the other, insoluble, matter and in older processes was purified by techniques resembling the 'tabling' described above; again high-speed centrifugal separators, for use with potato starch (and cassava starch), are now employed for separation and washing. At two or three points during the isolation, sulphur dioxide is added to prevent discoloration of the product by the action of oxidative enzymes. The washed starch is collected, dried to contain about 18% moisture and packaged.

Macroscopical characters. Starch occurs in irregular, angular masses or as a white powder. It is insoluble in cold water but forms a colloidal solution on boiling with about 15 times its weight of water, the solution forming a translucent jelly on cooling. A starch mucilage is coloured deep blue with solution of iodine, the colour disappearing on heating to 93°C but reappearing on cooling. When starches are heated with water, the granules first swell and then undergo gelatinization. The temperatures at which these changes commence and are complete vary with different starches. Starch granules also undergo gelatinization when treated with caustic potash, concentrated solutions of calcium or zinc chlorides, or concentrated solution of chloral hydrate.

Maize starch is neutral, but other commercial starches frequently show an acid (wheat and potato) or alkaline (rice) reaction. The *USP* gives microbial limit tests for *Salmonella* spp. and for *Escherichia coli*.

Microscopical characters. Starches can be identified by microscopical examination. They should be mounted in water or Smith's starch reagent (equal parts of water, glycerin and 50% acetic acid). The size, shape and structure of the starch granules from any particular plant only vary within definite limits, so that it is possible to distinguish between the starches derived from different species. Starch granules may be simple or compound, and the description of a starch granule as 2-, 3-, 4- or 5-compound refers to the number of component granules present in the compound granule. In some cases the compound granule is formed by the aggregation of a large number of simple granules (e.g. rice and cardamoms).

The starting point of formation of the granule in the amyloplast is marked by the hilum, which may be central or eccentric. Granules with an eccentric hilum are usually longer than broad. On drying, fissures often appear in the granule and are seen to originate from the hilum. On microscopical examination, the hilum takes the form of a rounded dot or of a simple, curved or multiple cleft.

The starch granule is built up by the deposition of successive layers around the hilum, and concentric rings or striations are often clearly visible in larger granules, e.g. potato. The striations probably arise from the diurnal deposition of the starch giving variations in refractive index, density and crystallinity. The position and form of the hilum and the presence or absence of well-defined striations are of importance in the characterization of starches.

Some of the more important microscopic characters of the principal starches are set out in Table 20.5 and Figure 20.4.

Table 20.5 Microscopy of starches.

Variety	Form	Small	Medium	Large	Hilum and striations
Maize	Granules from the outer horny endosperm muller-shaped	10	15–25	30	Hilum a central triangular or 2- to 5-stellate cleft. No striations
	Granules from the inner mealy endosperm polyhedral or subspherical	2	10–30	35	
	In commercial starch all the granules are simple				
Wheat	Larger granules lenticular, smaller ones globular. A few compound granules with 2–4 components, which, if separated, are polyhedral	2–9	30–40	45	Hilum a central point, seldom cleft. Concentric but rather faint striations
Rice	Compound granules with an angular outline and from 2 to about 150 components	2	4–6	10	Hilum a central point. No striations
	Component granules polyhedral, with sharp angles				
Potato	Mostly simple granules, hatchet-, wedge-, or mussel-shaped. A few compound granules of 2 or 3 components firmly fused together	2	45–65	110	Hilum in the form of a point; eccentric about 1/3 to 1/4. Concentric striations well-marked; some rings, however, more distinct than others
Tapioca	Mostly simple, subspherical, muller-shaped or round polyhedral	5–10		20–35	Hilum punctate or cleft. Concentric striations

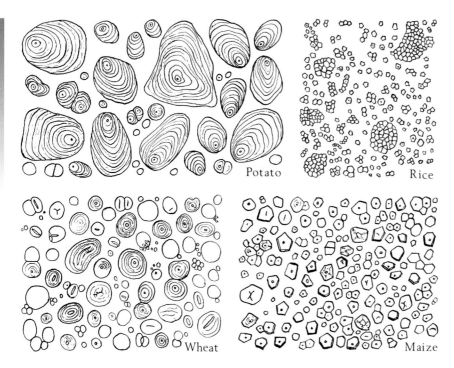

Fig. 20.4
Pharmacopoeial starches. All ×200.

Starch granules show double refraction when examined between crossed Nicols, the granules appearing in the dark field as illuminated objects marked by a dark cross, the bars of which intersect at the hilum.

Starch is required to comply with specified limits for viable microbial contamination including, specifically, *Escherichia coli*.

Chemical composition of starch

Starch granules usually contain two carbohydrates, amylopectin (α-amylose) and amylose (β-amylose); the former constitutes over 80% of most starches. Fractionation of the two components can be achieved by selective precipitation involving the formation of an insoluble complex of amylose with such polar organic substances as butanol or thymol. As indicated in Table 20.2, β-amylose consists essentially of linear chains; these have a helical arrangement with each turn comprising six glucosyl units and giving a diameter of 1.3 nm. Conversely, amylopectin has a branched structure; these differences give the two substances different properties and it is their variation in proportion that contributes towards the distinctive characteristics of a starch from a particular biological source.

Amylose, although water-soluble, gives an unstable solution, which irreversibly precipitates. It is mainly responsible for the deep blue coloration (λ_{max} c.660 nm) given by starch and iodine in which the latter as I_5 becomes trapped as an inclusion complex in the amylose helix. The strong affinity of amylose for iodine means that it will take up to 19% of its weight of iodine and this figure can be used in the determination of amylose in starch. Dilute solutions in water or alkali have an appreciable vicosity and the molecule is extensively degraded by β-amylase to maltose. The course of the hydrolytic reaction may be followed: (1) by treating with iodine and observing the colour changes (starch giving a blue; dextrins purple to reddish-brown; maltose, and glucose, if acid hydrolysis, no colour); (2) by testing portions at intervals with Fehling's solution (the amount of reduction increases with the amounts of sugar formed); or (3) by successive measurements of viscosity (viscosity decreases as hydrolysis proceeds). On the other hand, solutions of amylopectin are relatively stable, the colour given with iodine is purple (λ_{max} c.540 nm), and the iodine-binding is low. β-Amylase can only attack the outer linear chains, not being able to bypass the 1–6 interchain links; as a consequence, amylopectin is hydrolysed to the extent of 50–60% only by the enzyme; complete hydrolysis is achieved by mineral acids and other enzymes.

A very small amount of covalently bound phosphate appears to be a normal component of starch; its exact location within the molecule is uncertain but may represent the phosphorylation of some 1 in 300 glucose molecules. Cereal starches also contain about 1% of lipid which occupies the same helix space as does added iodine.

Biosynthesis of starch. The final stages of the synthesis of starch are associated with amyloplasts—double membrane organelles which develop, like chloroplasts, from protoplasts. Sucrose appears to be the primary substrate which by the mediation of the reversible sucrose synthase and other enzymes is converted to fructose, glucose-1-phosphate and glucose-6-phosphate in the cytosol. The precise pathway involved and the specific substrate which passes into the amyloplast for the final stages of synthesis are a current area of study. One problem is the difficulty of isolating intact amyloplasts for biochemical study. α-Amylase activity in barley has been extensively studied; the endosperm of germinating maize seeds contains four isozymes of α-amylases (α-amylase-1 to -4) and one isozyme of β-amylase (K. B. Subbarao *et al.*, *Phytochemistry*, 1998, **49**, 657). The probable final reactions are indicated in Fig. 20.5. (For a review with 81 refs. see A. M. Smith and K. Denyer, *New Phytologist*, 1992, **122**, 21.)

Mutant varieties. A number of mutant varieties of maize and other crops produce abnormal starch grains some of which have commercial use and possibilities. Thus 'waxy' maize starch contains principally amylopectin producing a tapioca-like starch. It derives its name from the shiny appearance of the broken endosperm. Another mutant, 'amylose extender' is deficient in one of the enzymes responsible for producing the branching of the amylopectin molecule. At least six specific enzyme deficiencies have been identified as associated with abnormal maize starch mutants.

Uses. Starch finds extensive use in dusting powders, in which its absorbent properties are important. In mucilage form it is used as a

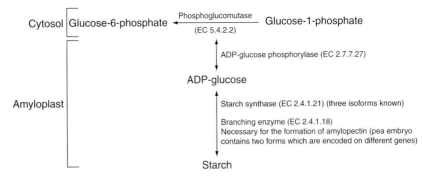

Fig. 20.5
Probable final stages in the biosynthesis of starch.

skin emollient, as a basis for some enemas and as an antidote in the treatment of iodine poisoning. Starch is also used as a tablet disintegrant. For the US food and drinks industry large quantities of maize starch are converted to high-fructose corn syrup by a process involving hydrolysis (glucose producing) and subsequent isomerization. Starch has also provided the plastics industry with a number of new products, including biodegradable polyvinylchloride and polyethylene plastics.

Sterilizable Maize Starch BP is used as a lubricant for surgeons' gloves; it is maize starch subjected to physical and chemical treatments so that it does not gelatinize on exposure to moisture of steam sterilization. Unlike talc, it is completely absorbed by body tissues.

Brazilian arrowroot.   This is the starch obtained from the tubers of the sweet potato, *Ipomoea batatas* (Convolvulaceae). The granules are rounded, polyhedral or muller-shaped, the larger ones being 25–55 μm in diameter.

Portland arrowroot.   The English hedgerow plant, *Arum maculatum* (Araceae) is known by a number of names, including Lords and Ladies, Cuckoo Pint and Wake Robin. The tuberous rootstock is rich in starch and was formerly extracted to give Portland arrowroot. Used for starching Elizabethan ruffs, it was a cause of dermatitis among laundrymaids.

Modified starches

As with cellulose, the starch molecule can be considerably modified by chemical treatments and some of the products have a use in the paper, food, textile, adhesive and other industries. Treatments include acetylation, hydroxyethylation, phosphorylation, inorganic esterification and cross-linking. For pharmaceutical purposes maranta starch (St Vincent Arrowroot), which is no longer commercially available, has been replaced by an ester starch of cassava which has similar properties.

Pregelatinized starch.   This is prepared from maize, rice or potato starch by suitable mechanical rupturing of the grains in the presence of water either with or without heat followed by drying. There are no added materials but the product may be further manipulated to improve flow rate and compressibility properties. It is widely used as a tablet excipient.

Soluble starch.   Soluble starch is prepared by treating commercial potato starch with hydrochloric acid until, after washing, it forms a limpid, almost clear solution in hot water. A soluble starch solution should show little reduction with Fehling's solution and gives a deep blue colour with iodine. On heating with 5% potassium hydroxide solution, it gives a canary-yellow colour; no colour is afforded by ordinary starch and the dextrins give a brown colour when similarly treated.

Commercial dextrins.   High-grade dextrins are prepared by heating starch which has been moistened with a small quantity of dilute nitric

acid and dried, at 110–115°C. The product is known as white dextrin. Inferior dextrins, which have a yellow or brown colour, are prepared by roasting starch at 150–250°C without the addition of acid.

White dextrins may contain up to 15% of soluble starch, the remainder consisting largely of erythrodextrin. Yellow dextrins are more completely hydrolysed and, unlike the white variety, contain appreciable quantities of maltose, which may be detected and estimated by means of Fehling's solution.

FRUCTANS

Fructans are D-fructose polymers each chain being terminated by a single D-glucosyl residue. They are found in nature as oligosaccharides with up to 10 units and as polysaccharides with up to 50 units. The best-known fructan, and the most important pharmaceutically, is inulin, a reserve carbohydrate found in many roots of members of the Compositae and Campanulaceae. The tubers of the Jerusalem artichoke (*Helianthus tuberosus*) and roots of chicory (*Cichorium intybus*) are particularly rich sources. Other fructans are the phleins found in grasses e.g. in *Phleum pratense*, agropyrene in couch grass (q.v.), and sinistrin a component of *Urginea maritima* (q.v.).

Unlike the biosynthesis of starch and cellulose, that of fructan does not originate by the conjugation of identical monosaccharide units but in all cases starts with a molecule of sucrose (glucose + fructose) to which is successively added further molecules of furanofructose. A further distinction from starch biosynthesis is that no monosaccharide nucleotide (cf. glucose adenine diphosphate) is involved in the addition of the fructose units. Various trisaccharides composed of one glucose and two fructose molecules occur in nature and the mode of the linkage of the second fructosyl unit to the sucrose and the extent of the addition of more fructosyl units to the trisaccharide determine the properties of the final polymer. Thus, inulin biosynthesis proceeds via the enzymatic transfer of a fructosyl group from sucrose to another molecule of sucrose giving the trisaccharide 1-ketose and free glucose. A second enzyme (a fructan fructosyl transferase) then mediates the addition of further fructosyl units from other oligomeric fructans. Thus, the final molecule is terminated at one end by a glucosyl unit. However, for the formation of some other fructans different fructosylsucrose trisaccharides are involved and elongation of the polymer chain may occur at either end of the trisaccharide so that the final fructan molecule has a glucosyl residue situated towards the middle of the chain.

INULIN

Inulin *BP/EP* is obtained from the tubers of *Dahlia variabilis*, *Helianthus tuberosus* and other genera of the Compositae; it derives its name from the dahlia, *Inula helenium*, from which it was first isolated in the 19th century. It occurs either in solution in the cell sap (cf. starch granules which are formed in plastids) or in alcohol-preserved material as sphaerocrystalline masses (Fig. 42.1F). It is sparingly soluble in cold water but readily dissolves at around 70°C without gelatinizing. It is neither stained by iodine solution nor hydrolysed by mammalian enzymes.

Chemically inulin consists of a chain of 35–50 1,2-linked fructofuranose units terminated by one glucose unit. The furanose ring systems render the molecules much less rigid than either those of cellulose or starch. In any sample of inulin there is a mixture of molecular species the smaller molecules being probably intermediates in the polymerizing chain.

BP/EP tests include a thin-layer chromatography examination; clarity, colour and specific optical rotation (−36.5° to −40.5°, 2% solution) of solutions and limits for acidity, sulphated ash (0.1%), heavy metals, oxalate etc.

Inulin is not metabolized by the body and is excreted unchanged. As Inulin Injection it is used for the measurement of glomerular filtration rate.

Dandelion root

The root of the dandelion (*Taraxacum officinale*) is an important drug of herbal medicine. Among other constituents it contains up to 40% of carbohydrates, particularly inulin, in the autumn and about 2% inulin in the spring. The fructose content reaches about 18% in the spring. The drug is described in Chapter 29.

ALGAL GELLING AGENTS

The two most important pharmaceutical products in this class are the alginates and agar.

ALGINIC ACID

Large quantities of brown seaweeds are collected from many of the colder waters of the world. Principal producers, approximately in order of quantity, are the USA (California), Norway, Chile, China, Canada (Nova Scotia), Irish Republic, Australia (Tasmania), Iceland, UK (Scotland), South Africa. Some years ago it was reported that the Chinese had developed strains of brown seaweed which would flourish in the warmer East and South China Seas.

The North Atlantic rockweeds (littoral types) (e.g. *Ascophyllum nodosum*) are cut either by hand with sickles or by means of various designs of floating 'combine harvesters'. The remaining world total is mainly storm-cast. After collection, the raw, wet seaweed may either go immediately for processing or be fuel- or sun-dried to 12–17% moisture content, in which form it has an indefinite storage life.

Alginic acid, a hard, horny polysaccharide, was first isolated by the English chemist Stanford (1883) and in Britain was first marketed in 1910; the 1976 estimated world production of alginate was 19 507 tonnes. New methods of extraction are continually being patented but the pattern of Stanford's process is still much followed. The dried milled seaweed is macerated with dilute sodium carbonate solution and the resulting pasty mass diluted with sufficient soft water to make practicable the separation of the insoluble matter by modern super-decanters or continuous-settling devices. Soft water is essential to avoid the precipitation of insoluble alginates. The resulting clear liquor, which contains most of the alginate originally present in the algae, may now be treated in one of two ways: (1) it is poured into dilute sulphuric acid or dilute calcium chloride solution, when the insoluble alginic acid or its salt, calcium alginate, is precipitated as a bulky, heavily hydrated gel, from which liquor is removed by roller- or

expeller-presses. The product obtained looks and handles like wood pulp. By moving the calcium alginate with constant agitation against a stream of hydrochloric acid, the calcium is removed and the highly swollen pulp of alginic acid is roller-pressed and then neutralized with sodium carbonate to give sodium alginate. (2) The clear liquor can be made to precipitate sodium alginate of high purity by the addition of ethyl alcohol directly or after partial evaporation.

Alginic acid *BP/EP* (formula, Table 20.2) is composed of residues of D-mannuronic and L-guluronic acids; the chain length is long and varies (mol. wt. from 35 000 to 1.5×10^6) with the method of isolation and the source of the algae. The degree of polymerization can be varied to meet the properties required. A small proportion of the carbonyls may be neutralized, the pharmacopoeial material having not less than 19.0% and not more than 25.0% carbonyl groups calculated with reference to the dried material. The assay involves back-titration with standardized acid. There are also tests for chlorides, heavy metals, microbial contamination, loss on drying and sulphated ash.

Alginic acid is insoluble in cold water (but swells and absorbs many times its own weight) and slightly soluble in hot water. It is insoluble in most organic solvents. It liberates carbon dioxide from carbonates. With compounds containing ions of alkali metals, or ammonium or magnesium, it reacts to give salts (alginates) which are water-soluble and form viscous solutions typical of hydrophilic colloids. The salts of most other metals are water-insoluble.

The alginates, particularly the sodium salt, have, because of their greater chemical reactivity, certain advantages over agar, starch, pectin, vegetable gums and gelatin. Alginates find applications as stabilizing, thickening, emulsifying, deflocculating, gelling and film- and filament-forming agents in the rubber, paint, textile, dental, food (including ice-cream), cosmetic and pharmaceutical industries. The formulation of creams, ointments, pastes, jellies and tablets are examples in the last-named industry. Alginic acid is also used in tablet and liquid preparations for the control of gastro-oesophageal reflux. Alginate textile fibres and their uses, for example, as absorbable haemostatic dressings have been discussed earlier.

AGAR

Agar (*Japanese Isinglass*) is the dried colloidal concentrate from a decoction of various red algae, particularly species of *Gelidium*, *Pterocladia* (both Gelidaceae, order Gelidiales), and *Gracilaria* (Gracilariaceae, order Gigartinales). Agar is obtained from Japan (*Gelidium amansii*), Korea, South Africa, both Atlantic and Pacific Coasts of the USA, Chile, Spain and Portugal. Some 6500 tonnes are produced annually, of which about one-third originates from Japan. The genus *Gelidium* provides about 35% of the total source material.

Collection and preparation. On the Japanese coast the algae are largely cultivated in special areas, poles being planted in the sea to form supports on which they develop. From time to time the poles are withdrawn and the algae stripped off. Some are also collected from small boats by means of rakes or shovels, or even by diving. The algae are taken ashore and dried; beaten and shaken to remove sand and shells; bleached by watering and exposure to sunlight, the washing also serving to remove salt. They are then boiled with acidulated water for several hours (about 1 part of dry algae to 55 or 60 parts of water), and the mucilaginous decoction filtered, while hot, through linen. On cooling, a jelly is produced which is cut into bars, these being afterwards forced through wire netting to form strips. The manufacture of agar takes place only in winter (November to February), and moisture is removed by successively freezing, thawing and drying at about 35°C. In Japan the algae are collected from May to October.

Characters. Agar occurs in two forms: (1) bundles of somewhat agglutinated, translucent, yellowish-white strips, these being about the thickness of leaf gelatin, 4 mm wide and about 60 cm long; (2) coarse powder or flakes. Agar swells in cold water but only a small fraction dissolves. A 1% solution may be made by boiling and a stiff jelly separates from this on cooling. When Japanese agar is not used, jellies of similar stiffness may be obtained by using 0.7% New Zealand, 1% South African or 2% Australian agar.

A nearly boiling 0.2% solution gives no precipitate with an aqueous solution of tannic acid (distinction from gelatin). Agar also differs from gelatin in that it contains no nitrogen and therefore gives no ammonia when heated with soda lime. When hydrolysed by boiling with dilute acid, galactose and sulphate ions are produced, the former reducing Fehling's solution and the latter precipitating with barium chloride. If agar is ashed and the residue, after treatment with dilute hydrochloric acid, examined microscopically, the silica skeletons of diatoms and sponge spicules will be found. More perfect diatoms can often be isolated by centrifuging a 0.5% solution. The large discoid diatom *Arachnoidiscus*, which is about 0.1–0.3 mm in diameter, species of *Grammatophora* and *Cocconeis*, and sponge spicules are readily discernible in the ash of Japanese agar (see Fig. 20.6). Powdered agar is distinguished from powdered acacia and tragacanth by giving a deep crimson to brown colour with 0.05 M iodine and by staining pink when mounted in a solution of ruthenium red.

Agar *BP/EP* is required to comply with tests for the absence of *Escherichia coli* and *Salmonella*, and general microbial contamination should not exceed a level of 10^3 microorganisms per g^{-1} as determined by a plate count. It has a swelling index (q.v.) of not less than 10 and the determined value must be quoted on the product label.

Constituents. Agar has long been known to yield on hydrolysis D- and L-galactose and sulphate ions. It is now known to be a heterogeneous polysaccharide the two principal constituents of which are agarose and agaropectin. Agarose is a neutral galactose polymer (free from sulphate) which is principally responsible for the gel strength of agar. It consists of alternate residues of 3,6-anhydro-L-galactose and -D-galactose (the disaccharide known as agarobiose). The structure of agaropectin, responsible for the viscosity of agar solutions, is less well established, but it appears to be a sulphonated polysaccharide in which galactose and uronic acid units are partly esterified with sulphuric acid. Pure agarose is commercially available and its gels are recommended for the electrophoresis of, for example, proteins.

Uses. Agar is used in the preparation of culture media, as an emulsifying agent and in the treatment of chronic constipation. Both agar and agarose find extensive use in affinity chromatography (q.v.).

Irish Moss

Chondrus (*Carrageen*) is obtained from the variable red alga *Chondrus crispus* and to some extent from *Gigartina stellata* (Gigartinaceae). Commercial supplies are derived from the north and north-west coast of Ireland, from Brittany and from the Massachusetts coast south of Boston.

Collection and preparation. The algae grow on rocks just below low-water mark, being covered by about 5 or 7 m of water at high tide. In Ireland collection takes place during the autumn; in America, during the summer. The collectors put out in small boats at about half-tide and, after detaching a load of algae from the rocks by means of long rakes, return with them at half-flood. Carrageen is bleached by spreading it on the shore and submitting it for some weeks to the action of sun and dew with about four or five soakings in seawater at suitable intervals. Bleaching by sulphur dioxide has not proved particularly satisfactory. After drying in sheds, the drug is packed in bales weighing up to 300 kg. World production of Irish moss is estimated to be around 20 000 tonnes.

Carrageenan *USP/NF* (1995) is obtained from red seaweeds by extraction with water or aqueous alkali and recovered by alcoholic precipitation, drum drying or by freezing.

Characters. Chondrus when fresh varies in colour from purplish-red to purplish-brown, but the bleached drug is yellowish-white, translucent and horny. It consists of complete, dichotomously branched thalli about 5–15 cm long and of very variable form, some thalli having broad fan-like segments, others having ribbon-like ones. Many samples of Chondrus contain large quantities of the related alga *Gigartina mamillosa*, the mixture being officially sanctioned in many pharmacopoeias. In some districts (e.g. south of Boston) almost pure *Chondrus crispus* may be collected, while in others (e.g. north of Boston) it is almost invariably closely associated with *G. mamillosa*. These algae may be distinguished from one another by the form of their large compound cystocarps, which contain carpospores. Chondrus has oval cystocarps about 2 mm long which are sunk in the thallus, while *G. mamillosa* has peg-like ones about 2–5 mm long, as also has *G. pistillata*. The latter species is rare round the coast of Britain, and its presence would indicate a drug of French origin.

Chondrus is sometimes covered with calcareous matter which effervesces with hydrochloric acid. The drug has a slight odour, and a mucilaginous and saline taste.

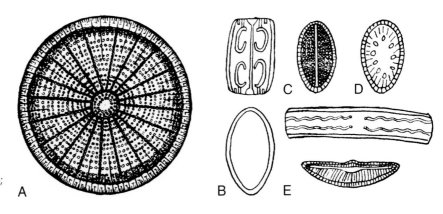

Fig. 20.6
Diatoms associated with Japanese agar. A, *Arachnoidiscus* (diameter 130 μm); B, species of *Grammatophora*; C, *Cocconeis*; D, *Campyloneis*; E, other diatoms.

Chondrus swells in cold water, about 47% slowly dissolving, while on boiling about 75% passes into solution. A 5% decoction forms a jelly on cooling. A cooled 0.3% solution gives no precipitate with solution of tannic acid (distinction from gelatin), and gives no blue colour with iodine (distinction from Iceland moss and absence of starch).

Constituents. The constituents of chondrus resemble those of agar. At least five galactans, known as carrageenans, are present. Three important ones are κ-, ι- and λ-carrageenans, which differ in the amount of 3,6-anhydro-D-galactose they contain and in the number and position of the ester sulphate groups. Like other members of the Gigartinaceae *C. crispus* produces different carrageenans in the two phases of its life cycle; κ-carrageenan predominates in the gametophyte generation and λ-carrageenan in the diploid tetrasporophyte generation (for research on the heterogeneity of both types of plants see B. Matsuhiro and C. C. Urzua, *Phytochemistry*, 1992, **31**, 531). The drug is rich in halogen salts, and, according to Schulzen (1964) the extract differs from that of agar in that it has a higher sulphate and ash content.

Uses. Chondrus is used as an emulsifying agent for cod-liver oil and other oils, as a gelling agent, and as a binder in toothpastes. Its many technical uses involve mainly the food industry.

GUMS AND MUCILAGES

Gums and mucilages have similar constitutions and on hydrolysis yield a mixture of sugars and uronic acids. Gums are considered to be pathological products formed upon injury of the plant or owing to unfavourable conditions, such as drought, by a breakdown of cell walls (extracellular formation; gummosis). Conversely, mucilages are generally normal products of metabolism formed within the cell (intracellular formation) and may represent storage material, a water-storage reservoir or a protection for germinating seeds. They are often found in quantity in the epidermal cells of leaves, e.g. senna, in seed coats (linseed, psyllium etc.), roots (marshmallow) and barks (slippery elm).

TRAGACANTH

The *BP/EP* defines Tragacanth as 'the air-hardened gummy exudate, flowing naturally or obtained by incision, from the trunk and branches of *Astragalus gummifer* Labillardière and certain other species of *Astragalus* from Western Asia'. The genus (Leguminosae) contains some 2000 species and those that yield gum are chiefly thorny shrubs found in the mountainous districts of Anatolia, Syria, Iraq, Iran and the former USSR. So-called Persian tragacanth has been traditionally employed in the UK, with Anatolian tragacanth finding a considerable market on the continent of Europe. The term Persian tragacanth is used by pharmacists to denote the better grades of tragacanth produced in Iran and Turkish Kurdistan.

Formation. The mode of formation of tragacanth is entirely different from that of acacia, the gum exuding immediately after injury and therefore being preformed in the plant, whereas acacia is slowly produced after injury. A section of a tragacanth stem shows that the cell walls of the pith and medullary rays are gradually transformed into gum, the change being termed 'gummosis'. The gum absorbs water and a considerable pressure is set up within the stem. Hanbury, having cut off branches of living plants, stated, 'there immediately exudes from the centre a stream of soft, solid tragacanth, pushing itself out like a worm, to the length of three-quarters of an inch, sometimes in the course of half an hour'.

Botanical sources. The requirement for precise botanical specifications and satisfactory analytical procedures for tragacanth, necessitated by the legal aspects covering its use as a food additive, has rendered the above *BP/EP* definition somewhat inadequate. A survey of the Turkish gum-producing species has indicated that *A. microcephalus* is the principal species employed with smaller amounts of *A. gummifer* and *A. kurdicus* being collected. Also, in an investigation of tragacanth production in Iran in 1957, Gentry (*Econ. Bot.*, 1957, **11**, 40) reported *A. echidnaeformis*, *A. gossypinus* and *A. microcephalus* to be important species. The approximate distribution of a number of gum-producing species found in the areas where tragacanth is collected is shown in Table 20.6.

Collection. Most of the plants from which tragacanth is collected grow at an altitude of 1000–3000 m. The shrubs are very thorny; each of their compound leaves has a stout, sharply pointed rachis which persists after the fall of the leaflets. The mode of collection varies somewhat in different districts, but the following details of collection in the province of Fars are typical.

Gum can be obtained from the plants in their first year but is then said to be of poor quality and unfit for commercial use. The plants are therefore tapped in the second year. The earth is taken away from the base to a depth of 5 cm and the exposed part is incised with a sharp knife having a thin cutting edge. A wedge-shaped piece of wood is used by the collector to force open the incision so that the gum will exude more freely. The wedge is generally left in the cut for some 12–24 h before being withdrawn. The gum exudes and is collected 2 days after the incision. Some of the plants are burned at the top after having had the incision made. The plant then sickens and gives off a greater quantity of gum. However, this practice is not universal, as many plants cannot recover their strength and are killed by the burning. The gum obtained after burning is of lower quality than that obtained by incision only, and is reddish and dirty looking. The crop becomes available in August–September.

Grades. Tragacanth is graded into several qualities by the exporter or middle man. The best grades form the official drug, while the lower grades are used in the food, textile and other industries; their approximate relative values are listed in Table 20.7.

Tragacanth is an expensive commodity; not only has the supply situation increased the price, but also the extra treatment and tests required to meet the *BP/EP* microbial requirements have added to the cost.

Table 20.6   Distribution of gum-yielding *Astragalus* species.

Species	Geographical distribution
A. gummifer	Anatolia and Syria
A. kurdicus	Northern Iraq, Turkey and Syria
A. brachycalyx	Western and S.W. Iran
A. eriostylus	S.W. Iran
A. verus	Western Iran
A. leioclados	Western and central Iran
A. echidnaeformis	Isfahan region of Iran
A. gossypinus	Isfahan region of Iran
A. microcephalus (syn. A. pycnocladus)	Shiraz and Kerman regions of Iran, Turkey
A. adscendens	South western and southern Iran
A. strobiliferus	Eastern Iran
A. heratensis	Khorasan to Afghanistan

Table 20.7 Grades of tragacanth.

Grade		Description	Relative value
Ribbon	No. 1	Fine flat druggists' ribbon	100
	No. 2	White flat druggists' ribbon	93
	No. 3	Light-cream curly ribbon	82
	No. 4	Mid-cream flat ribbon	62
	No. 5	Pinkish mixed ribbon	41
Flake	No. 26	Mid-cream thin flake	38
	No. 27	Amber thick flake	34
	No. 28	Amber-brown thick flake	29
	No. 55	Reddish-brown mixed hoggy flake	26

The ribbon grades are stated to comply with the *BP/EP* requirements; it is principally the flake (26 and down) from Turkey that is available in quantity.

Characters. The official Persian tragacanth occurs in flattened ribbons up to 25 mm long and 12 mm wide. The surface shows a number of ridges which indicates the successive, temporary stoppages of flow from the incision. Fine furrows parallel to the margin of the flake are produced by the uneven edges of the incision. The gum is white or very pale yellowish-white in colour, translucent and horny. It breaks with a short fracture, is odourless and has little taste.

Tragacanth swells into a gelatinous mass when placed in water, but only a small portion dissolves. On the addition of a dilute solution of iodine to a fragment previously soaked in water, relatively few blue points are visible (distinction from Smyrna tragacanth, which contains more starch). With stronger iodine solution the gum acquires a greenish colour (cf. 'Agar').

Constituents. Tragacanth consists of a water-soluble fraction known as tragacanthin and a water-insoluble fraction known as bassorin; they have molecular weights of the order of 840 000. Both are insoluble in alcohol. Tragacanthin and bassorin may be separated by ordinary filtration of an extremely dilute mucilage and the tragacanthin may be estimated by the evaporation of an aliquot portion of the filtrate. Tests show that the best grades of gum contain the least tragacanthin. If the tragacanthin content and moisture content are known, the amount of bassorin may be calculated.

Like other gums, tragacanth is composed of sugar and uronic acid units. Among the products of hydrolysis galacturonic acid, D-galactopyranose, L-arabinofuranose and D-xylopyranose have been identified. C. A. Tischer *et al.*, have reported on the structure of the arabinogalactan fraction (*Carbohydr. Res.*, 2002, **337**, 1647). The *BP/EP* thin-layer chromatography test for identification is based on the products of acid hydrolysis of the gum. Von Fellenberg (1918) pointed out that in the tragacanthin fraction there are no methoxyl groups, but that the bassorin fraction contained about 5.38% methoxyl. Rowson (1937) showed that gums with high methoxyl contents and high bassorin contents gave the most viscous mucilages. Heating or fine powdering produces demethylation with loss of viscosity. Anderson and Bridgeman (*Phytochemistry*, 1985, **24**, 2301) showed that the gum-exudates of the three principal species of Turkish gum-producers are proteinaceous polysaccharides and represent a protein content of about 3–4%, involving 18 amino acids. The relative amino-acid proportions differed in the three gums.

The *BP/EP* includes a test for minimum apparent viscosity of the powdered gum, a *flow time* for gum to be used in the preparation of emulsions, and a microbial limit test, together with compliance tests

for *Escherichia coli* and *Salmonella*. Peroxidase enzymes are usually considered to be absent, but their presence has been detected in commercial samples of genuine drug. The presence of peroxidase enzymes appears to be related to a high starch content; both disappear as gummosis proceeds.

Uses. Tragacanth is used in pharmacy as a suspending agent for insoluble powders, etc., or as a binding agent in pills and tablets. As substitutes become available, its use in the food industry is declining.

Allied drugs

Non-pharmaceutical grades of tragacanth. Large quantities of tragacanth of the lower grades are imported and used in the textile industry and pickle manufacture. The pieces vary in shape and are from a yellow ivory colour to almost black. The lower grades are much contaminated with earth, and their ashes give a strong reaction for iron. The viscosity of mucilages prepared from these grades of tragacanth falls rapidly from the No. 1 to the No. 55, the marked difference in price being fully justified. The lower grades of tragacanth are known as *hog gum* or *hog tragacanth*.

Acacia gum admixed with tragacanth can be detected by TLC of the hydrolysed sample—the presence of rhamnose indicates adulteration.

Chitral gum of Indian commerce is said to be obtained from *Astragalus strobiliferus*.

Sterculia gum (*Karaya gum*) is itself an important article of commerce and is described below. Its presence in tragacanth gum is detected by the gel formation in alcoholic solution and by an acidity test.

Insoluble Shiraz gum is a gum of doubtful botanical origin imported from Iran. When of good quality, it resembles a mixture of bleached and natural Kordofan acacia. It may be distinguished from tragacanth by the fact that it contains no starch and that it gives a reaction for oxidase enzyme.

STERCULIA GUM

Sterculia (*Karaya Gum, Indian Tragacanth, Bassora Tragacanth*) is the dried gummy exudate obtained from the tree *Sterculia urens* (Sterculiaceae). It is produced in India, Pakistan and, to a small extent, in Africa. The gum is of relatively recent introduction, being generally regarded during the early part of the last century as an adulterant and inferior substitute for tragacanth. Now, however, having been shown to be superior to other gums in certain respects, it constitutes an integral part of the gum industry and is official in the *BP*.

Collection and preparation. In central and northern India (Andhra Pradesh, Madhya Pradesh, Rajasthan and Uttar Pradesh) two collections are made each year, before and after the monsoon season: in April–June and in September, respectively. The first collection gives a gum affording the highest viscosity. Blazes, up to about one square foot in area, are made in the larger trees (smaller trees are tapped) and the gum immediately starts to exude; the flow is greatest during the first 24 h and continues for several days. The dried, irregular masses, weighing up to several pounds, are picked off and transported to village centres for purchase by Mumbai merchants. The Indian merchants remove excess bark and roughly sort the gum into two grades; it is further graded in Europe and the USA according to colour and presence of foreign organic matter (mainly bark). It is finally sold as a granulated (crystal), or finely powdered, product.

Unfortunately, in some areas over-production and destructive tapping methods have led to a serious decline in the natural tree population and have necessitated the introduction of 10-year bans on collection.

This has stimulated research on *in vitro* propagation using seedling explants, nodal explants and somatic embryogenesis (S. D. Purohit and A. Dave, *Plant Cell Reports*, 1996, **15**, 704; V. G. Sunnichan *et al.*, *ibid.*, 1998, **17**, 951).

Characters. Good-quality gum occurs in irregular almost colourless, translucent, striated masses weighing up to 25 g or more. Medium grades have a marked pinkish tinge, while the lower grades are very dark and contain a considerable amount of bark. Karaya gum has a marked odour of acetic acid, and when hydrolysed with 5% phosphoric acid, has a volatile acidity (*BP*) of not less than 14% (tragacanth, about 2–3%). According to Janot and Gounard (1938), sterculia has a methoxyl value of 0 (tragacanth 30–40). When boiled with solution of potash, it becomes slightly brownish (tragacanth, canary yellow). Karaya also differs from tragacanth, in that it contains no starch and stains pink with solution of ruthenium red.

In water, sterculia gum has low solubility but swells to many times its original volume. This means that the processing of the gum influences the final product—the coarser granulated grades give a discontinuous grainy dispersion, whereas the fine powder affords an apparently homogeneous dispersion.

Constituents. Partial acid hydrolysis of sterculia yields D-galactose, L-rhamnose, D-galacturonic acid, aldobiouronic acids, an acid trisaccharide and acetic acid; the galacturonic acid and rhamnose units are the branching points within the molecule. Uronic acid residues represent about 37% of the gum.

Uses. The granular grades are used as a bulk laxative, being second only to psyllium seed in use in this respect. The powdered gum is used in lozenges, pastes and denture fixative powders, and it has proved particularly useful as an adhesive for stoma appliances. As a bulk laxative and stimulant it is available, with frangula, as granules.

ACACIA GUM

Acacia (*Gum Arabic*) is a dried gum obtained from the stem and branches of *Acacia senegal* Wild, other species of *Acacia* of African origin and *Acacia seyal* Del. (Leguminosae). *A. senegal* is a tree about 6 m high, which is abundant in the Sudan, particularly in the province of Kordofan, in central Africa and in West Africa. The tree is known in Kordofan as *Hashab* and in Senegambia as *Verek*. The best gum is that produced in Kordofan from tapped trees, but some Senegal and Nigerian gum is of good quality. Apart from 'acacia gardens', wild, self-sown plants are the main source of the gum.

History. Gum was brought from the Gulf of Aden to Egypt in the seventeenth century BC, and in the works of Theophrastus it is spoken of as a product of Upper Egypt. The West African product was imported by the Portuguese in the fifteenth century. Previously, commerce in the Sudan was in the hands of a number of local merchants, but it is now entirely controlled by the 'Gum Arabic Company Ltd', a concessional company set up by the Sudanese Government.

Collection and preparation. Some gum exudes from trees as a result of the cracking of the bark, but the most esteemed, Kordofan variety, is obtained from trees, about 6 years old, tapped in February and March, or earlier, in September after the rains, when the leaves fall. The tapper, with a blow from a small axe, makes a transverse incision in a branch and so twists the axe that the bark is loosened, strips of it being then pulled off above and below the cut. The portion of branch so bared to the cambium measures about 0.5–1.0 m long and 5–7.5 cm wide. This cambium produces new phloem and in about 20–30 days the tears of gum which have formed on the surface may be picked off. The gum is collected in leather bags and is conveyed in sacks to El Obeid and other centres, mostly located along the railway. Here the gum is garbled to free it from sand and vegetable debris, and is sorted. Other acacia gums such as talka gum, the product obtained from *A. seyal* (the talka of the Arabs), are also separated. At one time some of the gum was 'ripened' by exposure to the sun, when it became bleached and dried, developing numerous cracks. During this process, which took 3–4 months, the gum lost about 30% of its weight. Subsequently, this bleached gum became unobtainable.

From El Obeid the drug is sent by rail to Port Sudan, whence large quantities are shipped to London, the USA and other countries. In the London Market Reports three grades are usually quoted, namely handpicked selected (h.p.s.) Kordofan, cleaned Kordofan and talka. Gum arabic is sold in one currency only ($US), so that currency changes also affect the price. The Senegal acacia gum is largely used for pharmaceutical purposes on the Continent and is shipped to Marseilles and Bordeaux. This also occurs in three grades, namely 'gomme du bas du fleuve', 'gomme du haut du fleuve' and 'gomme friable'.

For comments on the impact of the recent Sudan war on the gum arabic industry, see K. Purcell, *HerbalGram*, 2005, **65**, 25; K. Purcell and N. Dennis, *HerbalGram*, 2006, **71**, 24.

Spray-dried acacia, produced by the importers, is becoming of increasing importance and is included as a monograph in the *BP*. In addition to its general usefulness, it has the further advantage of a low viable bacterial count (see below).

Characters. Bleached Kordofan acacia, when available, occurs in rounded or ovoid tears up to about 3 cm diameter, or in angular fragments. The outer surface bears numerous fine cracks which form during the 'ripening' and make the tears opaque. The gum is white or very pale yellow in colour. The tears break rapidly with a somewhat glassy fracture, and much of the drug consists of small pieces. It is odourless and has a bland and mucilaginous taste.

Cleaned and h.p.s. Kordofan gum differs from the above in having fewer cracks which causes it to be more transparent, and in being more yellowish or pinkish in colour. The tears are usually of less uniform size, some being quite small, while others have a diameter of 4 cm or more. The better qualities of Senegal gum closely resemble the Kordofan, but some of the tears are vermiform in shape and, speaking generally, the gum is rather more yellowish in colour.

Tests. Acacia is almost completely soluble in an equal weight of water, solution taking place rather slowly. The solution is slightly acid and becomes more so on keeping, especially if hot water is used to make the solution. It is viscid, but not glairy, and when diluted does not deposit on standing.

A 10% aqueous solution is laevorotatory, gives no precipitate with dilute solution of lead acetate (distinction from tragacanth and agar), gives no colour with solution of iodine (absence of starch and dextrin), and, if of pharmacopoeial quality, gives no reaction for tannin with ferric chloride. A very weak solution precipitates with lead subacetate solution. The mucilage gives a blue colour when treated with solution of benzidine and a few drops of hydrogen peroxide, which indicates the presence of a peroxidase (possible distinction from tragacanth). Because benzidine has carcinogenetic properties, this test is no longer advocated; however, as some pharmaceutical grades of tragacanth have now been shown to contain a peroxidase enzyme system (q.v.), the test has probably less significance than was previously considered. A tincture of guaiacum can also be used to test for the enzyme.

The *BP/EP* thin-layer chromatography test involves fractionation of an acid hydrolysate of the gum and visualization of the separated sugars with anisaldehyde reagent followed by heating.

There are official tests for compliance with limits for microbial contamination (total viable aerobic count, *Escherichia coli* and in the *USP/NF, Salmonella* spp.).

Constituents.   Acacia consists mainly of arabin, the calcium (with traces of magnesium and potassium) salt of arabic acid. Arabic acid may be prepared by acidifying a mucilage with hydrochloric acid and dialysing.

When hydrolysed with dilute sulphuric acid, it yields L-rhamnopyranose, D-galactopyranose, L-arabinofuranose and the aldobionic acid 6-β-D-glucuronosido-D-galactose. This major polysaccharide fraction consists of branched β-(1,3)-linked galactose units with side-chains of arabinose, rhamnose and uronic acids linked through the 1,6-positions. A second component of the gum is a hydroxyproline-rich glycoprotein of high molecular weight; it has a high amino acid composition with a repetitive polypeptide backbone. For further studies on this fraction, see L. J. Goodrum *et al.*, *Phytochemistry*, 2000, **54**, 99.

The glycan composition of the gum is variable, depending on source. Thus that derived from *A. senegal* contains a high proportion of D-galactose relative to L-arabinose, whereas the reverse holds for the gum obtained from *A. seyal*. Also, the latter contains significantly more 4-0-methyl-D-glucuronic acid but less L-rhamnose and unsubstituted D-glucuronic acid than does the gum from *A. senegal*.

Acacia also contains an oxidase enzyme and about 14% of water. It yields about 2.7–4% of ash.

The gum is formed in the cambial region of the plant with gum-containing cysts developing in the inner bark (J.-P. Joseleau and G. Ullmann, *Phytochemistry*, 1990, **29**, 3401).

Hairy root cultures.   These produce a mucilage with a different polysaccharide composition to that of the parent plant.

Uses.   As a general stabilizer in emulsions and as a pharmaceutical necessity in lozenges, etc. Its demulcent properties are employed in various cough, diarrhoea and throat preparations but it is incompatible with readily oxidized materials such as phenols, and the vitamin A of cod-liver oil. It has widespread use in the food, drinks and other industries.

Allied drugs.   *Talka gum* is usually much broken and of very variable composition, some of the tears being almost colourless and others brown.

Ghatti or *Indian gum* is derived from *Anogeissus latifolia* (Combretaceae). It is produced in much the same localities as sterculia gum, and is harvested and prepared in a similar manner. It resembles talka in possessing tears of various colours. Some of the tears are vermiform in shape and their surface shows fewer cracks than even the natural acacia. Aqueous dispersions of the gum have a viscosity intermediate between those of acacia and sterculia gums.

West African Gum Combretum, obtained from *Combretum nigricans*, is not permitted as a food additive but is exploited as an adulterant of gum arabic. Unlike the latter in which the rhamnose and uronic acid units are chain terminal, in gum combretum these moieties are located within the polysaccharides chain. The leaves of this plant contain cytotoxic dammar-3-one pentacyclic triterpene derivatives (G. Simon *et al.*, *Fitoterapia*, 2003, **74**, 339).

Many other gums of the acacia type are occasionally met with in commerce, and many gum exudates of the large genus *Acacia* have been given chemotaxonomic consideration.

GUAR GUM

Guar *BP/EP* is obtained from the ground endosperms of the leguminous plant *Cyamopsis tetragonolobus* (L.) Taub., a species cultivated in India as a fodder crop. The gum is a white or off-white powder which readily forms a mucilage with water. Examined under the microscope the powder, in a glycerol mountant, shows the thick-walled endosperm cells with granular contents.

The principal constituent of the gum is a galactomannan which on hydrolysis gives galactose and mannose; these sugars of the hydrolysate constitute the basis of the pharmacopoeial thin-layer chromatography test for the drug. Other tests refer to the absence of other gums, viscosity, loss on drying, ash and microbial contamination.

Fatty acids, both free and combined as esters, have been reported by GLC-MS analysis.

Guar is available as an oral hypoglycaemic drug; it produces changes in gastric emptying and in the gastrointestinal transition time, which can delay absorption of sugars and oligosaccharides from the gut. Guar also lowers cholesterol levels, possibly by binding bile salts in the gut. However its efficacy in the treatment of diabetes is not considered by all to be fully proven. The gum, with 5–6 times the thickening power of starch, is also used in the food industry.

Guar galactomannan.   *BP/EP* consists of the ground endosperms of *Cyamopsis tetragonolobus* which have been subjected to partial hydrolysis. Tests for identity and purity are given in the *Pharmacopoeia*. It is classed as a pharmaceutical aid.

XANTHAN GUM

This gum is produced artificially by the pure culture fermentation of the bacterium *Xanthomonas campestris* on glucose. It, like cellulose, consists of 1,4-β-glycosidically linked chains of glucose with, additionally, trisaccharide side-chains on alternating anhydroglucose units. These side-chains are composed of two mannose units which encompass a glucuronic acid unit. Pyruvate groups are attached to most of the terminal units with acetyl groups at the C-6 of a number of the mannose moieties next to the glucose chain. The *BP/EP* assay is based on the amount of the pyruvic acid produced by the acid hydrolysis of the gum and should correspond to a content of $\lessgtr 1.5\%$.

Other tests include a limit for 2-propanol (750 ppm as determined by gas chromatography), foreign polysaccharides, a limit of 10^3 bacteria and 10^2 fungi per gram, and a total-ash range of 6.5–16.0% consistent with xanthan gum occurring as the sodium, potassium or calcium salt.

Xanthan gum is used as a pharmaceutical aid, and also finds use in the food and cosmetics industries.

Dextran.   This is another microbial product, produced by species of *Leuconostoc, Klebsiella, Acetobacter* and *Streptococcus*. It is an α-1,6-glucan and is used as a replacement for blood plasma and as an absorbent in biochemical analysis.

PSYLLIUM

(Flea Seed)

The dried, ripe seeds of *Plantago afra* (*P. psyllium*), *P. indica* (*P. arenaria*) and *P. ovata* (Plantaginaceae) are used in medicine. The *US National Formulary* includes all three species under the name 'Plantago Seed'. The *BP/EP* describes the seeds of the first two species under the title 'Psyllium' and the husks of seeds of *P. ovata* are included under 'Ispaghula Husk'. The latter consists of the epidermis and collapsed adjacent layers removed from the ripe seeds.

The seeds of *P. afra* and *P. indica* are known in commerce as Spanish or French psyllium, while those of *P. ovata* are known as blond psyllium, ispaghula, spogel seeds or Indian plantage seeds.

Characters. Some of the more important characters of these seeds are given in Table 20.8.

Constituents. All the seeds contain mucilage in the epidermis of the testa. The seeds may be evaluated by measuring the volume of mucilage produced after shaking the seeds with water and allowing to stand (see *swelling index*, Chapter 16).

Two fractions have been separated from the mucilage; one is soluble in cold water, and the other in hot water giving a highly viscous solution which gels on cooling. On hydrolysis fractions yield D-xylose, L-arabinose and aldobiuronic acid. The seeds also contain fixed oil, aucubin glycoside, various bases, sugars, sterols and protein. The aucubin content differs appreciably in different seed samples and species.

Allied drugs. Wild seeds of *P. ovata* and related species are reported to contain less mucilage than the cultivated variety. *P. asiatica*, a species used in Chinese medicine, contains mucilage the backbone chain of which is composed of β-1,4-linked D-xylopyranose residues having three kinds of branches.

Seeds of *P. major* are reportedly used as a medicinal substitute for *P. ovata*; the seed oil contains an unusual hydroxyolefinic acid. For a review of the traditional uses, chemical constitutents and biological activities of the *P. major* plant see A. B. Samuelsen, *J. Ethnopharm.*, 2000, **71**, 1.

Uses. Plantago seeds are used as demulcents and in the treatment of chronic constipation. Ispaghula husk is used for similar purposes but has a higher swelling factor (40–90).

MARSHMALLOW LEAF

Marshmallow leaf *BP/EP* is the whole, cut or dried leaf of *Althaea officinalis* L. The alternate petiolate leaves, about 7–10 cm long, arise from tall, erect, velvety, stems; the lower leaves are roundish, 3–8 cm across, and the upper ones are narrower and ovate; both are slightly 3–5 lobed, the upper more deeply so, and folded, toothed and covered with a soft velvety down. Microscopically, the powdered drug exhibits numerous long, unicellular trichomes, a few glandular trichomes, anomocytic or paracytic stomata, cluster crystals of calcium oxalate and mucilage-containing parenchymatous cells staining red with ruthenium red solution.

As with marshmallow root, mucilage is the effective constituent, giving the leaves emollient, slightly laxative and antitussive properties. Traditionally, the leaves have been used as a poultice for abcesses. Medicinally, non-specific constituents include flavonoids, e.g. quercetin and kaempferol (see Table 21.5), coumarin and polyphenolic acids.

The leaf is characterized by the pharmacopoeial TLC test, which, with the genuine drug, gives a number of fluorescent zones when viewed in UV light at 365 nm. The swelling index, minimum 12, is higher than that for the root (10).

MARSHMALLOW ROOT

Marshmallow root is derived from *Althaea officinalis* (Malvaceae), a perennial herb which is found wild in moist situations in southern England and Europe. In general appearance it closely resembles the common hollyhock, *Althaea rosea*. The plant has a woody rootstock from which arise numerous roots up to 30 cm in length. The drug is chiefly collected on the Continent from cultivated plants at least 2 years old. The roots are dug up in the autumn, scraped free from cork and dried, either entire or after slicing. The *EP/BP* drug may be peeled or unpeeled, whole or sliced.

The drug occurs in whitish, fibrous pieces about 15–20 cm long and 1–2 cm in diameter, or in small transverse slices. Odour, slight; taste, sweetish and mucilaginous. A transverse section shows a bark about 1–2 mm thick which is separated by a greyish, sinuate cambium from the white, radiate wood. The section shows numerous mucilage cells, the contents of which are coloured a deep yellow by a solution of sodium hydroxide. Structures to be seen in the powdered drug include: variously thickened vessels; fibres; calcium oxalate as cluster crystals 20–25–30–35 μm in diameter; starch granules, mainly single, 3–25 μm in size; thin-walled cork cells.

Marshmallow root contains about 10% of mucilage, the amount being season-dependent; it contains a polysaccharide giving on hydrolysis galactose, rhamnose, galacturonic acid and glucuronic acid. Other components of the mucilage are glucans and an arabinan. The mucilage content of the drug is indicated by the swelling index which, for *BP* purposes should be not less than 10. The upper limit for the total ash of the peeled root is 6.0% and that for the unpeeled 8.0%. Starch, pectin and sugars, and about 2% of asparagine are also present. The latter, which is the amide of aspartic (amino-succinic) acid, is also found in asparagus, potatoes, liquorice, etc.

Marshmallow root, and also the leaves, are used as demulcents, particularly for irritable coughs and throat and gastric inflammation.

MULLEIN FLOWER

Mullein flower *BP/EP* is the dried flower, reduced to the corolla and androecium, of *Verbascum thapsus* L., *V. densiflorum* Bertol. (*V. thapsiforma Schrad.*) and/or *V. phlomoides L.* Family Scrophulariceae.

V. thapsus (great mullein, Aaron's rod, blanket leaf and a number of other synonyms) is common throughout Europe and has long been naturalized in the US from the Atlantic coast west to South Dakota and the south-western states. In general, it is found in waste places, roadsides and on sunny banks. Reaching a height of 2 m, it is a biennial

Table 20.8 Characters of *Psyllium* seeds.

	P. afra	*P. indica*	*P. ovata*
Origin	France, Spain, Cuba	Mediterranean Europe, Egypt	Pakistan, India
Colour	Glossy; deep brown	Dull; blackish-brown	Dull; pinkish grey–brown
Shape	Boat-shaped; outline elongated ovate	Boat-shaped; outline elliptical	Boat-shaped; outline ovate
Length	2.0–3.0 mm	2.0–3.0 mm	1.5–3.5 mm
Weight of 100 seeds	0.09–0.10 g	0.12–0.14 g	0.15–0.19 g
Swelling index	≮10	≮10	≮9; husk, ≮40

terminating in a dense cylindrical spike of yellow flowers. Oval to lanceolate shortly petiolate leaves alternate on the simple stem. The whole plant is blanketed with woolly hairs. *V. densiflorum* (large-flowered mullein), found throughout continental Europe but a rare casual in Britain, differs from the above species in having larger quite flat corollas and decurrent leaves. *V. phlomoides* (orange mullein) is native to central and southern Europe and West Asia. It is an occasional casual in Britain but is widely cultivated as an ornamental. The flowers are yellow to yellow–orange.

A microscopical examination of the yellow to brown or orange powder shows many branched clothing trichomes (see Fig. 42.3), yellow fragments of petals and numerous ovoid pollen grains with a finely pitted exine and three pores.

Constituents. The three species contain the same groups of chemical constituents but with varying proportions and nature of individual compounds. *V. densiflorum* and *V. phlomoides* have been the most intensively studied as these species are the most commonly used on continental Europe. Flavonoids include, among others, apigenin, luteolin, their 7-glucosides and verbascoside. Iridoids include aucubin, catapol and their 6-xylosides (Fig. 20.7). Polysaccharides constitute the important mucilage components of the flowers; a water-soluble acidic arabinogalactan, MW 70 000, has been isolated from commercial material. As a standard for the mucilage content of the drug the *BP* specifies a minimum swelling index of 9 determined on the powdered flowers. A number of saponins have been recorded, including verbascosaponin, the structure of which was finally elucidated in 1992. Other constituents include phenolic acids not specific to mullein.

The *Pharmacopoeia* includes a TLC comparison of an extract of the flowers against reference substances and a test for the presence of iridoids.

Uses. Traditionally for the treatment of bronchial conditions particularly bronchitis and catarrh in which the saponins and mucilage probably act as expectorants and demulcents.

COUCH GRASS RHIZOME

Couch Grass Rhizome *BP/EP, BHP* consists of the washed and dried rhizomes of *Agropyron repens* (L.) Beauv. (*Elymus repens* (L.) Gould),

family Gramineae, sliced or whole with most of the adventitious roots and leaves removed.

The plant, although an invasive and troublesome weed (twitch), has a long history of medicinal use; it was known to Dioscorides and has subsequently been included in many herbals and pharmacopoeias. In Britain it was last included in the *BP* 1914 but was, in 1999, returned as a result of its *EP* status. S.E. Europe (Hungary) supplies most of the commercial material.

Characters. The dried, rigid rhizome is pale yellow, shiny, 2–3 mm thick and usually cut into pieces up to 6 mm in length. It is strongly furrowed longitudinally and, except at the nodes, hollow. The drug is odourless with a slightly sweet taste. Features of the powder include: epidermal cells of two types—one, narrow elongated with wavy and pitted, lignified walls—the second, alternating with the first type, somewhat rounded and unlignified; endodermal cells with U-shaped thickenings; fibres; pitted vessels with annular or spiral thickenings, pitted parenchyma. Calcium oxalate and starch are absent.

Constituents. The rhizomes contain about 10% mucilage and up to 8% of the fructosan polysaccharide triticin. Unlike the inulins (β, 2-1 linkages) the fructosans of the Gramineae, termed *levans*, are fructo-furanose units linked by β,2-6 glycosidic linkages and, as with the inulins, terminated with a sucrose unit. Other constituents are 2–3% of sugar alcohols (mannitol, inositol), 0.01–0.05% volatile oil containing the polyacetylene agropyrene and other volatiles, vanillin and its monoglucoside, phenolic carboxylic acids and silicates.

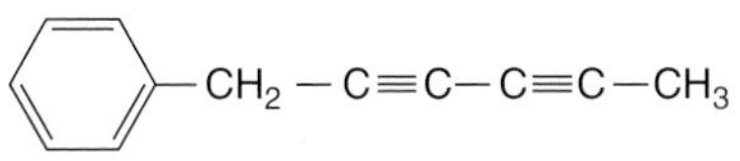

Agropyrene

Tests. The *BP/EP* specifies a water-soluble extractive of ≮25% and foreign matter consisting of greyish-black pieces of rhizome ≮15%. Tests, depending on the presence of starch and thickening of the endodermic cells are given to detect *Cynodon dactylon* (Bermuda grass), found on sandy soils in warmer temperate regions of the world including the shores of S.W. England, and *Imperata cylindrica*, a troublesome weed of subtropical regions.

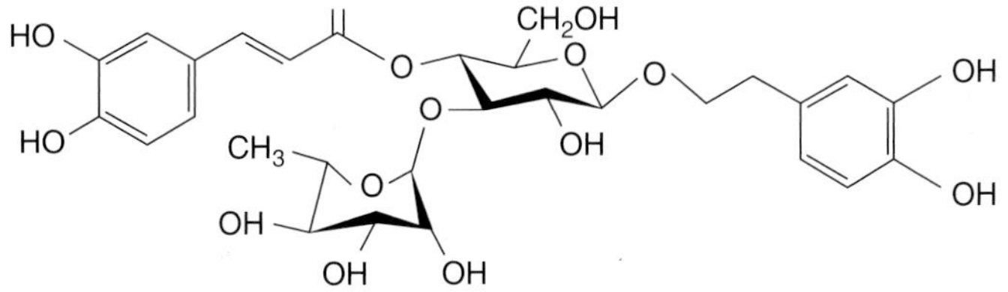

Verbascoside
(Acteoside)

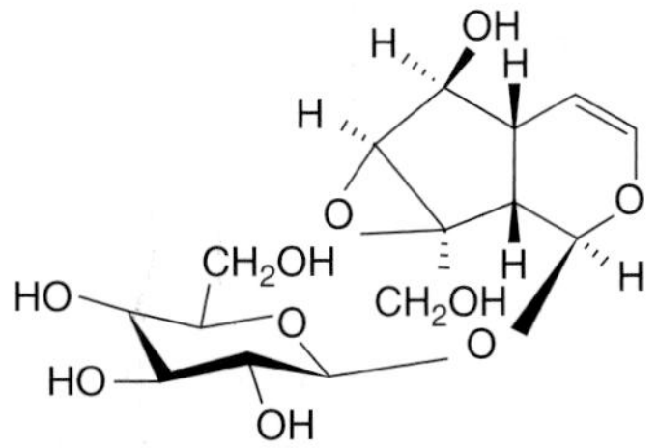

Catapol

Fig. 20.7
Constituents of mullein flowers.

20

Uses. Couchgrass is used as a demulcent and as a diuretic for bladder and kidney complaints, cystitis, gout, etc.

'Aloe vera' products

Aloe vera products are derived from the mucilage located in the parenchymatous cells of the *Aloe vera* leaf and should not be confused with aloes, described in Chapter 21, which originate from the aloetic juice of the pericyclic region. The mucilaginous gel has been used from early times for the treatment of numerous conditions but in recent years its use in the herbal and cosmetic industries has become very big business in the USA, Europe and elsewhere. Raw materials are obtained from plantations in the southern states of the USA, South America and elsewhere. Exaggerated claims have inevitably brought scepticism about the true usefulness of the products which feature as suntan lotions, tonics and food additives.

Research over the last 10 years has, however, largely upheld a number of the therapeutic properties ascribed to the gel. These include the anti-inflammatory properties (wound healing, burn healing, frostbite), gastrointestinal activity (peptic ulcer), antidiabetic activity, anticancer activity (principally animal tests), antifungal activity, antibacterial activity and radiobiological protection. Not all these properties have been unequivocally accepted.

The complex chemistry of the gel makes the attribution of the various activities to specific compounds difficult. Indeed beneficial clinical results for a particular condition may arise from more than one component. Thus wound-healing benefits may derive from the anti-inflammatory, fibroblast-stimulating, antibacterial and hydrophilic properties of the gel.

Some of the conflicting results of tests may be due, in some measure, to the different methods of collecting and subsequent processing of the gel. Thus anthraquinones have been reported as constituents of the gel but their presence may, or may not be, due to some admixture with the aloetic juice from the pericyclic region of the leaf. Also, variations in carbohydrate composition arise due to varietal differences within the species and to seasonal, climatic and soil factors.

Glucomannans constitute a principal component of the gel; some consist of glucose and mannose only or glucose, mannose and glucuronic acid, others are acetylated. Other polysaccharides are galactogalacturans (galactose + galacturonic acid) and galactoglucoarabinomannans. Molecular weights range from 200 000–450 000. An acetylated mannan is available commercially and has a range of reported biological activities. Glycoprotein fractions of the gel which may also influence the immune system have been shown to have proliferation-promoting activity on human and hamster cells *in vitro* (A. Yagi *et al.*, *Planta Medica*, 1997, **63**, 18; 2000, **66**, 180). In a series of papers N. Okamura *et al.* (*Phytochemistry*, 1996, **43**, 495; 1997, **45**, 1511; 1998, **49**, 219) have reported on the isolation of some eleven new chromones. Pectic substances, the triterpenoid lupeol, plant sterols (cholesterol, campestrol, β-sitosterol), possible prostanoids and other organic and inorganic compounds have also been identified in the gel. Five phytosterols which, in animals, show long-term blood-glucose-level control, could be beneficial in the treatment of type 2 diabetes. These were identified as cycloartenol (Fig. 23.1), its 24-methylene derivate, lophenol and its 24-methyl and ethyl derivatives (M. Tanaka *et al.*, *Biol. Pharm. Bull.*, 2006, **29**, 1418).

The intense interest in aloe vera products both from the commercial and scientific viewpoints has made this a topic for very active research. For an extensive review update on the subject (over 300 refs) see T. Reynolds and A. C. Dweck, *J. Ethnopharmacology*, 1999, **68**, 3.

Gels from other species of *Aloe*, e.g. *A. arborescens*, *A. ferox*, have also been examined for their polysaccharide composition.

Quince seeds

Quince seeds are obtained from *Cydonia oblonga* Mill. (Rosaceae), a tree cultivated in South Africa, Central Europe and the Middle East. Iran supplies about 75% of the total world production.

The seeds are separated from the apple- or pear-shaped fruits and dried. They resemble apple pips and frequently adhere together in masses, owing to their surface coating of dried mucilage. The latter is derived from the outer epidermis of the testa. Quince seeds contain about 20% of mucilage, composed of units of arabinose, xylose and uronic acid derivatives, 15% of fixed oil and a small quantity of cyanogenetic glycoside and an enzyme which effects its hydrolysis. The seeds are used as a demulcent, as an emulsifying agent and in the preparation of hair-fixing lotions.

Slippery elm bark

Slippery elm bark is obtained from *Ulmus rubra* Muhlenberg (*Ulmus fulva* Michaux) (Ulmaceae), a tree 15–20 m in height which is widely distributed in the USA and in Canada. In the spring fairly old bark is stripped from the trees. The outer part of the bark is then removed, only the inner part, which forms the commercial drug, being dried. After this has been sawn into convenient lengths, it is bound into bundles with wire.

The drug occurs in broad, flat strips about 50–100 cm in length and from 1 to 4 mm in thickness. A few reddish-brown patches of the imperfectly removed rhytidome may be seen but the remainder consists only of secondary phloem. The outer surface is brownish-yellow and striated, the inner surface yellowish-white and finely ridged. The bark is easily identified by the characteristic, fenugreek-like odour, the strongly fibrous fracture and the fact that it yields mucilage when moistened.

The chief constituent of the bark is mucilage, which is a mixture of two or more polyuronides. The mucilage has demulcent, emollient and nutritive properties. A poultice of the powdered bark is sometimes used.

Other mucilage-containing medicinal plants

Coltsfoot *BHP* 1983 consists of the dried leaves of *Tussilago farfara*, Compositae. It is used (and also the flowers) as a herbal expectorant and contains up to 10% mucilage which on hydrolysis yields a number of sugars and uronic acids. The leaves also contain tannin and a small percentage of pyrrolizidine alkaloids, e.g. senkirkine, which can prove hepatotoxic in sufficient doses. Probably for this reason the herb is no longer included in recent editions of the *BHP*; the German Commission E sets limits for the daily dose of these compounds, as occurring in coltsfoot. Further information on the drug will be found in a review by M. Berry (*Pharm. J.*, 1996, **256**, 234).

For other drugs containing appreciable mucilage see fenugreek seeds and linseed.

MISCELLANEOUS CARBOHYDRATE-CONTAINING DRUGS

HONEY

Honey is a saccharine substance deposited by the hive bee, *Apis mellifera* (order Hymenoptera, Apidae), and other species of *Apis*, in the cells of the honeycomb. Honey is produced in England, but the chief sources of supply are the West Indies, California, Chile, various parts of Africa, Australia and New Zealand.

Collection and preparation. The worker bees, by means of a long, hollow tube formed from the maxillae and labium, take nectar from the flowers they visit and pass it through the oesophagus into the honey-sac or crop. The nectar, which consists largely of sucrose, is mixed with salivary secretion containing the enzyme invertase and while in the honey-sac is hydrolysed into invert sugar. On arrival at the hive the bee brings back the contents of the honey-sac and deposits them in a previously prepared cell of the honeycomb.

The best honey is that derived from flowers such as clover and heather, obtained from hives that have never swarmed, and separated from the cut comb either by draining or by means of a centrifuge. Honey obtained by expression is liable to be contaminated with the wax. The nectar of certain flowers (e.g. of species of *Eucalyptus* or *Banksia*) may give the honey a somewhat unpleasant odour and taste; nectar from *Datura stramonium*, ragworts and *Rhododendron* spp. are known to give poisonous honey.

Appropriate cultivation measures should be in force to prevent the build-up of undue levels of pesticide and herbicide residues in the honey.

Preparation of the honey may involve melting at a moderate temperature, skimming off any impurities that collect on standing and, if necessary, adjusting the water content using refractive index measurement.

Characters.   Honey, when freshly prepared, is a clear, syrupy liquid of a pale yellow or reddish-brown colour. On keeping, it tends to crystallize and become opaque and granular. The odour and taste depend very largely on the flowers used in its preparation.

Constituents and tests.   Honey consists mainly of invert sugar and water. It contains small quantities of sucrose, dextrin, formic acid, volatile oil, wax and pollen grains. Microscopical examination of the latter afford valuable evidence of the source. The most likely adulterants are artificial invert sugar, sucrose and commercial liquid glucose. The tests for purity of the *BP/EP* purified honey should be noted. The limit tests for chloride and sulphate are important, as starch and sucrose may be hydrolysed with acids to give commercial liquid glucose and artificial invert sugar, respectively. Artificial invert sugar contains furfural, which gives a red colour with resorcinol in hydrochloric acid, but this may be formed in genuine honey by prolonged heating or lengthy storage.

The pharmacopoeia limits 5-hydroxymethylfurfural to a maximum of 80 ppm, calculated on dry solids, determined by absorbance measurements at 284 µm; the TLC test identifies glucose and fructose and eliminates excess sucrose. Water content is limited to 20% determined by refractive index measurements (minimum value 1.487). Conductivity (maximum 800 µS. cm⁻¹) and optical rotation (maximum +0.6°) are further standards.

Uses.   Honey is chiefly used in pharmacy as a component of linctuses and cough mixtures and for Oxymel and Squill Oxymel.

FIGS

Fig *BP* is the sun-dried succulent fruits of *Ficus carica* L. (Moraceae). It is widely produced in the Mediterranean countries, particularly Turkey (Smyrna figs), Greece and Spain.

The fruit is produced by the union of the cymose inflorescence to form a hollow, fleshy axis bearing the flowers on its inner surface. The young fruit is rich in latex, but when mature, no latex is found and the fleshy axis contains much sugar. Figs contain about 50% of sugars (chiefly glucose), appreciable quantities of vitamins A and C, smaller amounts of vitamins B and D, and enzymes (protease, lipase and diastase). There is an official requirement for a water-soluble extractive of not less than 60.0%. Figs are used by the *BP* and *BPC* in laxative preparations (e.g. Compound Fig Elixir).

For a review of *Ficus* spp. covering the ethnobotany and potential as anticancer and anti-inflammatory agents see E. P. Lansky *et al.*, *J. Ethnobotany*, 2008, **119**, 195.

FUCUS

Fucus, or bladderwrack, consists of the dried thallus of *Fucus vesiculosus* L., *F. serratus* L. or *Ascophyllum nodosum* Le Jolis., family Fucaceae. The *BP/EP*, under the title Kelp, admits all three species, whereas the *BHP* (1990) monograph is restricted to *F. vesiculosus*. Although the name 'kelp' is often used in connection with *Fucus* spp. it more strictly applies to the larger brown seaweeds of the genera *Laminaria* and *Macrocystis* family, Laminariaceae.

The dried grey to black thallus, sometimes having a whitish coating, is hard and brittle but readily softens in water to become mucilaginous. Depending on the species, air vesicles may, or may not be present.

Bladderwrack contains mucilaginous polysaccharides such as alginic acid, for the extraction of which it may be used (q.v.). It is also rich in trace elements and iodine. The latter is in the form of inorganic salts, bound to protein, and as a constituent of iodo-amino acids such as di-iodotyrosine. Other constituents are polyphenols consisting of phloroglucinol units, sterols and complex lipids.

Note the official limit tests for heavy metals and arsenic, the high total ash value (≯24.0%) (mainly soluble in dilute hydrochloric acid) and loss on drying (≯15.0%). Other standards are the swelling index (≮6.0) and total iodine content (0.03–0.2%) (sodium thiosulphate titration).

Bladderwrack has thyroactive properties and has, in the past, been employed in iodine therapy; however other preparations with a more consistent iodine content are now preferred. Again arising from its iodine content, bladderwrack has been promoted in teas as a slimming agent. In suitable doses it serves as a dietary supplement for trace elements and as a bulk laxative.

CETRARIA

Cetraria or Iceland moss, *Cetraria islandica* (L.) Acharius s.l. (Parmeliaceae), is a foliaceous lichen growing amidst moss and grass in central Europe, Siberia and North America, and on the lower mountain slopes of central Europe and Spain. For medicinal purposes it is usually collected in Scandinavia and central Europe.

The *BP/EP* drug consists of irregularly lobed, leafy thalli, about 5–10 cm long and about 0.5 mm thick. The upper surface is greenish-brown and sometimes covered with reddish points, while the lower surface is pale brown or greyish-green and marked with white, irregular spots. At frequent intervals along the margin of the thallus are minute projections. The dried drug is brittle but becomes cartilaginous on moistening with water. Odour, slight; taste, mucilaginous and bitter. A 5% decoction forms a jelly on cooling, which is stained blue by iodine (distinction from carrageen). It has an official swelling value of ≮4.5 determined on the powdered drug. Sections of the drug reveal the dual nature of the plant, the small rounded cells of the unicellular alga *Cystococcus humicola* being enclosed by the more or less closely woven hyphae of the fungus.

The drug contains carbohydrates, known as lichenin and isolichenin. Lichenin is only soluble in hot water and is not coloured blue by iodine, while isolichenin is soluble in cold water and gives a blue colour with iodine. Both on hydrolysis give glucose. Cetraria also contains a very bitter depsidone, cetraric acid, and other acids such as lichestearic and usnic acids. The latter compound is an antibiotic which may not be unimportant in contributing to the efficacy of Iceland moss as a demulcent for the treatment of cough involving throat irritation. Iceland moss has been used as a bitter tonic and for disguising the taste of nauseous medicines.

20

Prunes

Prunes (Rosaceae) are dried plums derived from *Prunus domestica* L. Of the many cultivated forms, var. *Juliana de Candolle*, which is largely grown in France, produces those commonly used in European medicine. Prunes of excellent quality are also produced in California.

The appearance of prunes requires no description. The pulp contains about 44% of sugars (mainly glucose), malic acid and water. The kernel contains 45% of fixed oil, and small quantities of amygdalin and benzoic acid. Prunes are used in Confection of Senna.

Further reading

Weymouth-Wilson AC 1997 The role of carbohydrates in biologically active natural products. Natural Product Reports 14(2): 99–110

Whistler RL, BeMiller JN (eds) 1993 Industrial gums; polysaccharides and their derivatives, 3rd edn. Academic Press, London, UK

Whistler RL, BeMiller JN 1997 Carbohydrate chemistry for food scientists. Eagan Press, St Paul, Minnesota

21

Phenols and phenolic glycosides

Phenols probably constitute the largest group of plant secondary metabolites. Widespread in Nature, and to be found in most classes of natural compounds having aromatic moieties, they range from simple structures with one aromatic ring to highly complex polymeric substances such as tannins and lignins. Phenols are important constituents of some medicinal plants and in the food industry they are utilized as colouring agents, flavourings, aromatizers and antioxidants. This chapter mainly deals with those phenolic classes of pharmaceutical interest, namely: (1) simple phenolic compounds, (2) tannins, (3) coumarins and their glycosides, (4) anthraquinones and their glycosides, (5) naphthoquinones, (6) flavone and related flavonoid glycosides, (7) anthocyanidins and anthocyanins, (8) lignans and lignin. The biosynthetic origin of some of these compounds involving the shikimic acid pathway is shown in Fig. 21.2. Phenols may also have aromatic rings derived by acetate condensation (Fig. 18.9.).

SIMPLE PHENOLIC COMPOUNDS

Catechol (*o*-dihydroxybenzene) occurs free in kola seeds and in the leaves of *Gaultheria* spp. and its derivatives are the urushiol phenols of the poison oak and poison ivy (q.v.). Derivatives of resorcinol (*m*-dihydroxybenzene) constitute the narcotic principles of cannabis and the glucoside arbutin involves quinol (hydroquinone, *p*-dihydroxybenzene). The taenicidal constituents of male fern, the bitter principles of hops and the lipophilic components of hypericum (q.v.) are phloroglucinol derivatives.

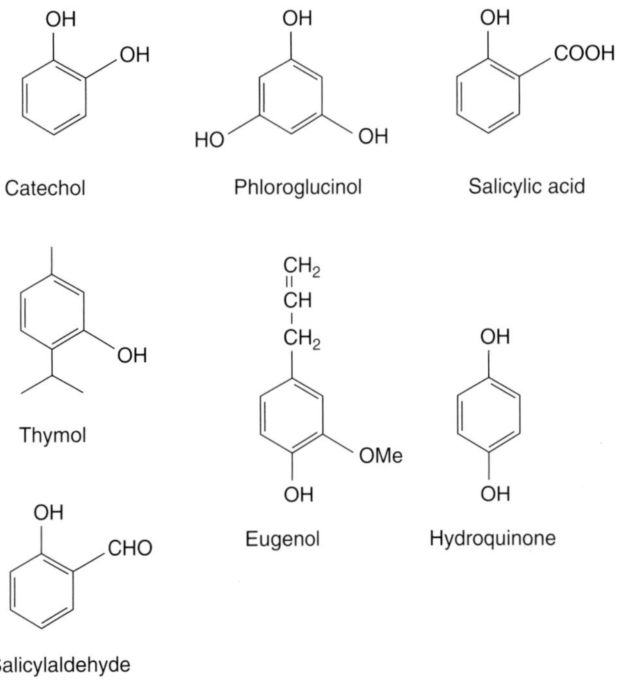

Fig. 21.1
Simple phenolic compounds.

The phenolic compounds in this group often also possess alcoholic, aldehydic and carboxylic acid groups; they include eugenol (a phenolic phenylpropane), vanillin (a phenolic aldehyde) and various phenolic acids, such as salicylic, ferulic and caffeic acids. Glycoside formation is common, and the widely distributed glycoside coniferin and other derivatives of phenolic cinnamic alcohols are precursors of lignin. Some of the best-known simple phenolic glycosides are listed in Table 21.1.

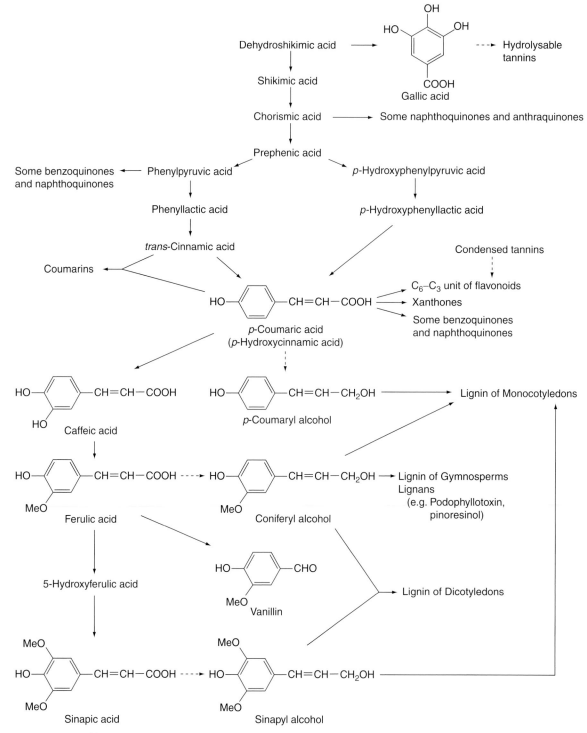

Fig. 21.2
Phenolic compounds originating from shikimic acid (see Fig. 18.8 for details of shikimic acid pathway).

MEADOWSWEET

Meadowsweet *BP/EP*, Filipendula *BHP* 1983 consists of the dried flowering tops of *Filipendula ulmaria* (L.) Maxim. [*Spirea ulmaria* L.], family Rosaceae.

This well-known perennial plant is found in wet meadows, marshes, by rivers, etc. throughout most of Europe, temperate Asia and as an escape in the eastern US and Canada. It is up to 120 cm in height with numerous radical longish petioled leaves. Each leaf is composed of up to five pairs of ovate serrated leaflets. Numerous aromatic cream-coloured flowers form irregular cymose panicles, which are particularly dense on the terminal branches of the leafy stems.

The commercial chopped drug occurs as clumps of broken leaflets dark green on the upper surface, paler and tormentose on the lower. Also brown fragmented flowers, unopened flower buds and small, more or less spirally twisted fruits containing brown seeds. Angular,

Table 21.1 Examples of phenolic glycosides.

Name	Examples of sources	Products of hydrolysis
Salicin	*Salix* and *Populus* spp. *Viburnum prunifolium*	Salicyl alcohol, glucose
Populin (benzoyl-salicin)	*Populus tremula*	Salicyl alcohol, benzoic acid, glucose
Arbutin	Ericaceae and Rosaceae	Hydroquinone, glucose
Phloridzin	Rosaceae, including spp. of *Malus*	Phloretin, glucose
Trilobatin	*Malus, Spiraea*	Phloretin, glucose
Coniferin	Coniferae	Coniferyl alcohol, glucose
Gaultherin	*Gaultheria, Betula* and *Monotropa*	Methyl salicylate, primeverose
Syringin	Particularly in Oleaceae	Methoxyconiferyl alcohol, glucose
Glucovanillin	*Vanilla* spp. and some Gramineae	Vanillin, glucose
Gein	*Geum* spp.	Eugenol, vicianose (glucose + arabinose)
Glucogallin	*Rheum* spp.	Gallic acid, glucose
Hamamelitannin	*Hamamelis virginiana*	Gallic acid (2 mols), hamamelose

greenish-brown longitudinally ridged hollow stems up to 5 mm in diameter constitute a considerable portion of the drug.

Among the complex mixture of structures in the powder the following can be noted: leaves and sepals having lower epidermis with slightly sinuous anticlinal walls, anomocytic stomata and cluster crystals of calcium oxalate up to 40 µm diameter in the mesophyll; papillose epidermis of petals; pollen grains with three pores and a smooth to slightly pitted exine; numerous trichomes, occasionally glandular with a one- to three-celled stalk and multicellular head with brown contents but principally clothing trichomes of various size, often twisted together; vascular tissue of the stem and veins.

Constituents. The *BP/EP* requires a minimum concentration of 0.1% for the steam volatile fraction of Meadowsweet; the flowers have recorded higher values. The major component of the oil (up to *ca* 70%) is salicylaldehyde (Fig. 21.1) together with methyl salicylate, benzaldehyde, benzyl alcohol, and smaller amounts of other components such as vanillin. In 1839, Löwingand and Weidmann, working on meadowsweet, were the first to report salicylic acid as a natural product. Other constituents of the drug are the phenolic glycosides gaultherin (Table 21.1) and spiraein (salicyl alcohol + primerose), various flavonoids, e.g. hyperoside (Fig. 21.18), tannins and mucilage.

The pharmacopoeial TLC test for identity indicates the required presence of methyl salicylate and salicylaldehyde in the test sample. The permitted maximum for stems with a diameter greater than 5 mm is 5% and for foreign matter, 3%.

Action and uses. The *BP/EP* cites meadowsweet as a diuretic; traditionally it has also been used for its anti-inflammatory, astringent and stomachic properties.

Oil of wintergreen

Natural oil of wintergreen was formerly obtained from the leaves of *Gaultheria procumbens* (Ericaceae), but is now distilled from the bark of *Betula lenta* (Betulaceae). Gaultheria oil of the *Indian Pharmacopoeia* is obtained from the fresh plant of *Gaultheria fragrantissima* and contains not less than 98% of esters calculated as methyl salicylate.

WILLOW BARK

Various species of *Salix* which include *S. purpurea* L., (purple willow) *S. daphnoides* Vill. and *S. fragilis* L. (crack willow) are sources of the official drug (*BP/EP, BHP, ESCOP, Complete German Commission E*).

There are about 300 species of *Salix* showing much hybridization and unusual forms. They are distributed in all parts of the North Temperate Zone, the Arctic Zone and the South Temperate Zone. Identification can present difficulties. Species range from tall trees to tiny shrubs. The commercial drug is obtained principally from S.E. Europe but also from Britain and other European countries.

The commercial drug occurs as thin, channelled pieces of varying length, about 1.5 cm wide and 1.5 mm thick. It easily fractures longitudinally and, transversely, shows an inner inconspicuous fibrous fracture. The outer surface is brown, grey or greenish, glossy and smooth or dull and rugged; the inner surface is lightish brown and finely longitudinally striated. The powder is characterized by cork cells, parenchymatous cells containing cluster crystals of calcium oxalate and lignified fibre groups with crystal sheaths of calcium oxalate.

Willow bark is a source of salicin (Table 21.1), a phenolic glycoside now seldom used but generally regarded as the natural forerunner of aspirin. The composition of the glycoside mixture is variable in the bark depending on species, age of bark and time of collection. The latter is usually made in spring when the bark is easily removed from the branches. Other phenolic glycosides are salicortin (an ester of salicin), acetylated salicin (fragilin) and salicortin. Salicin is easy to prepare (see 15th edition of this book) and is a suitable compound with which to introduce students to this class of glycoside.

Flavonoids of the bark (to over 4%) include the 5- and 7-glucosides of naringenin, isoquercitrin and chalcone (see Fig. 21.18). Tannins are of the condensed types (q.v.).

The *BP* requires the dried drug to contain a minimum of 1.5% total salicylic acid derivatives, calculated as salicin. Liquid chromatography with spectrophotometric determination at 270 nm is used for the assay.

Willow is employed as an anti-inflammatory in the treatment of rheumatism, arthritis and muscular pains.

Black haw bark

The root bark of *Viburnum prunifolium* (Caprifoliaceae) was formerly official in most pharmacopoeias, but its use for dysmenorrhoea, threatened abortion and asthma has gradually decreased. It contains about 0.2% of salicin, volatile oil and isovaleric acid, tannin and resin.

HOPS

Hops are the dried strobiles of *Humulus lupulus* L. (Cannabinaceae). Only the pistillate plants are cultivated, large quantities being produced in England (particularly Kent), Germany, Belgium, France, Russia and

California. The strobiles are collected, dried in kilns and pressed into bales known as 'pockets'. They are sometimes exposed to the fumes of burning sulphur, which modifies the sulphur components already in the hops but which is said to stabilize the aroma and colour.

Hops are included in the *EP*, *BP*, *BHP* and in monographs of the *British Herbal Compendium*, ESCOP and German Commission E.

The hop strobiole consists of external and internal sessile bracts which overlap one another and enclose the ovary. Together they form a petiolate greenish-yellow inflorescence 2–5 cm in length. The odour is characteristically aromatic.

On the fruits and bases of the bracts are numerous shining glands. These, when separated, constitute the drug lupulin. The commercial product is generally very impure, owing to the fact that it is obtained by sieving the sweepings of the hop room floors. It occurs as a granular, reddish-brown powder with a characteristic odour and bitter aromatic taste.

The bracts and stipules of the hop contain tannin but the odour and taste of the drug are mainly due to the very complex secretion contained in the lupulin glands. On distillation the fruits yield 0.30–1.0% of an oil composed of well over 100 components and containing terpenes, sesquiterpenes including humulene (Fig. 21.3) and compounds such as 2-methyl-but-3-ene-2-ol and 3-methylbutanoic acid. The two latter, and related substances, increase significantly during processing of the fresh hops. The bitterness is due to crystalline phloroglucinol derivatives known as α-acids (e.g. humulone), β-acids (e.g. lupulone) and also about 10% of resins. 2,3,4-Trithiapentane, *S*-methylthio-2-methylbutanoate, *S*-methylthio-4-methyl-pentanoate and 4,5-epithiocaryophyllene have been isolated from the volatile oil of unsulphurated hops.

There has been considerable recent interest in the wide-ranging biological activities of the constituents of hops. Thus prenylated compounds such as xanthohumol and the recently isolated acylphloroglucinolglucopyranosides have been variously reported to have cytotoxic effects on human cancer cell lines together with antiproliferative, antioxidant and oestrogenic properties. For details, see L. R. Chadwick *et al.*, *J. Nat. Prod.*, 2004, **67**, 2024; G. Bohr *et al.*, *J. Nat. Prod.* 2005, **68**,

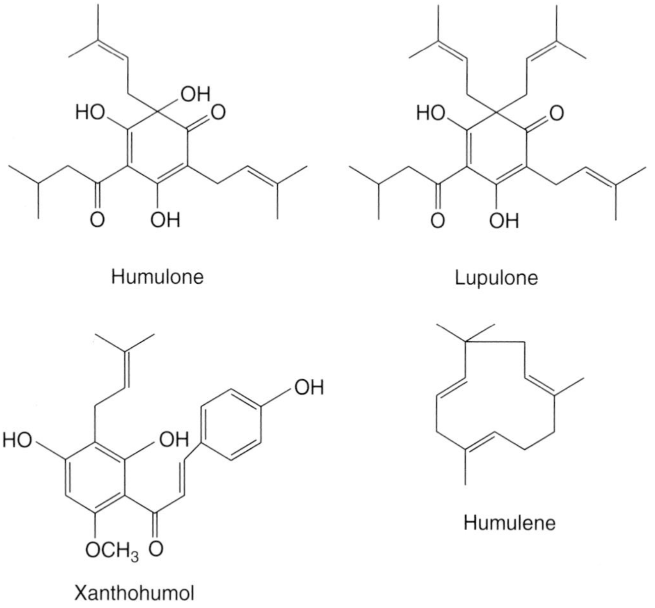

Fig. 21.3
Constituents of hops.

1545. The mildly sedative properties of hops are ascribed, in part, to 2-methyl-3-buten-2-ol; their principal use is as an aromatic bitter in the preparation of beer.

Further reading

Zanoli P, Zavatti M 2008 Pharmacognostic and pharmacological profile of *Humulus lupulus* L. Journal of Ethnopharmacology 116: 383–396

Male fern.   Male fern (*Filix Mas*) consists of the rhizome, frond bases and apical bud of *Dryopteris filix-mas* agg. (Polypodiaceae). The taxonomy of the genus is complicated and the aggregate is composed of a complex of three related species—*D. filix-mas* (L.) Schott. *s. str.*, *D. borrei* Newm. and *D. abbreviata* (Lam and D.-C.) Newm. Other ferns may also be involved in extracts produced globally.

Male fern samples that have not deteriorated in activity due to long storage, etc. should have an internal green colour. The active constituents are an interesting range of phloroglucinol derivatives, which have been thoroughly investigated.

Extracts of male fern were traditionally employed as taenicides, particularly for tape worms, but safer drugs are now available and used in preference.

A full account involving history, characters, constituents and allied drugs is given in the previous edition of this book pp. 214–217.

Kamala

Kamala consists of the trichomes and glands separated from the fruits of *Mallotus philippinensis* (Euphorbiaceae), a tree found in India, Pakistan and the East Indies. It occurs as a dull reddish-brown powder without odour or taste. Under the microscope it is seen to consist of very characteristic globular glands containing red resin, and radiating groups of unicellular curved trichomes. It contains the anthelminthic phloroglucinol derivatives rottlerin and isorottlerin, resins and wax. It is used in India for the treatment of tapeworm infestation; also for treating poultry.

Tar (*Pix Liquida*)

Wood tar is known in commerce as Stockholm tar. It is prepared by the destructive distillation of various trees of the family Pinaceae. In addition to the tar, an aqueous distillate is obtained from which acetic acid, methyl alcohol and acetone are prepared. A residue of wood charcoal remains in the retorts. Wood tar is a blackish semiliquid with a characteristic odour and taste.

The constituents include the following phenols and phenolic ethers: phenol, C_6H_5OH; cresols, $C_6H_4(CH_3)OH$; methyl cresols; catechol or pyrocatechin, $C_6H_4(OH)_2$; guaiacol (methyl catechol) and its homologues. Also the hydrocarbons benzene, toluene (methylbenzene), xylenes (dimethylbenzenes), mesitylene and pseudocumene (trimethylbenzenes), styrene (phenylethylene), naphthalene ($C_{10}H_8$), retene (*m*-methylisopropylphenanthrene), chrysene ($C_{18}H_{12}$) and paraffins.

Pine tar is characterized by the large amount of guaiacol and its homologues which are present. Other tars, such as those of the birch and beech, show considerable differences in composition. Wood tar is acid in reaction, whereas coal tar, which is also official, is alkaline and in light petroleum gives a blue fluorescence. Creosote is obtained from wood tar by distillation. Tar is mainly used externally, in the form of ointment or tar parogen, as a stimulating antiseptic in certain skin diseases.

Wood tar, when shaken with water, gives an aqueous layer that is acid to litmus (cf. coal tar below) (*BP* test for identity).

COAL TAR

Coal tar is prepared by the destructive distillation of bituminous coal; it is a nearly black viscous liquid and when shaken with water gives an aqueous alkaline solution. A petroleum spirit extract has a blue fluorescence enhanced by UV light. The upper ash limit for the *BP* product is 2.0%.

Both coal tar and wood tar are used in the treatment of psoriasis.

VANILLA AND VANILLIN

Vanilla (*Vanilla Pods*) consists of the carefully cured fully grown but unripe fruits of *Vanilla fragrans* (Salis.) Ames (*syn. V. planifolia* Andrews) (Orchidaceae) (Mexican or Bourbon vanilla) and of *V. tahitensis* (Tahiti vanilla). The fruits of other species, such as *V. pompona* (West Indian vanilla), are also used but to a much more limited extent.

Vanilla fragrans is grown, in a semi-wild state, in the woods of eastern Mexico, its natural home. Vanilla is cultivated in Réunion (or Bourbon), Mauritius, Seychelles, Madagascar, Java, Ceylon, Tahiti, Guadeloupe, Martinique and Indonesia. China and India are now major producers and due to oversupply prices have fallen dramatically over the past few years.

History. Vanilla was found in Mexico by the Spaniards, where it was used for flavouring chocolate, a use to which it is still put. It found a place in the *London Pharmacopoeia* of 1721.

Cultivation. Vanilla requires a warm and fairly moist climate. Propagation is simple: cuttings 1–3 m long are attached to trees (e.g. *Casuarina equisetifolia*), where they soon strike roots on the bark. The plant is an epiphyte. It flowers at the end of 2 or 3 years and continues to produce fruit for 30–40 years. The flowers are usually pollinated by women and children, a pointed stick being introduced into one flower after another. Clonal propagation of the vanilla plant has been described together with *in vitro* multiplication using axillary bud explants (P. S. George and G. A. Ravishankar, *Plant Cell Rep.*, 1997, **16**, 490).

Collection and curing. The fruits are collected when the upper part of the pod changes in colour from green to yellow. The characteristic colour and odour of the commercial drug are only developed as a result of enzyme action during the curing. The details of the latter process vary somewhat in different countries, but frequently it consists of slow drying in sheds which are kept at carefully regulated temperatures.

Packing and grading. Before grading, any pods showing a tendency to mould are picked out. The remainder are sorted to size and packed in bundles of 50 pods. Traditionally, these were packed in tin cases or boxes holding about 10–12 kg, soldered up and packed in wooden cases. On arrival in London the tins were opened and the pods were examined. UK supplies now arrive via France or Germany, with some from Madagascar. During storage crystals frequently develop on the surface of the pods.

Characters. Vanilla pods are 15–25 cm long, 8–10 mm diameter and somewhat flattened. The surface is longitudinally wrinkled, dark brown to violet-black in colour, and frequently covered with needle-like crystals of vanillin ('frosted'). The fruits are very pliable and have a very characteristic odour and taste.

Constituents. Green vanilla contains glycosides, namely glucovanillin (vanilloside) and glucovanillic alcohol. During the curing these are acted upon by an oxidizing and a hydrolysing enzyme which occur in all parts of the plant. Glucovanillic alcohol yields on hydrolysis glucose and vanillic alcohol; the latter compound is then by oxidation converted into vanillic aldehyde (vanillin). Glucovanillin, as its name implies, yields on hydrolysis glucose and vanillin (Fig. 21.4).

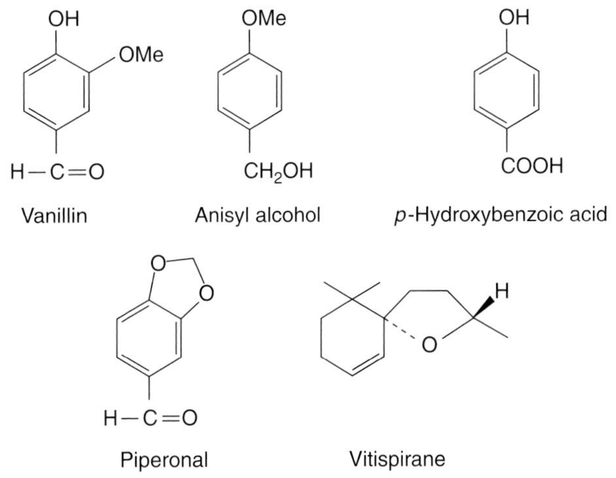

Fig. 21.4
Constituents of vanilla.

The three species given above differ in their relative contents of anisyl alcohol, anisaldehyde (also anisyl ethers and anisic acid esters), piperonal and *p*-hydroxybenzoic acid. These minor components, together with the two diastereoisomeric vitispiranes, add to the flavour of the pods.

Vanillin *BP*/*EP*. Vanillin *BP* is the aldehyde corresponding to methyl-protocatechuic acid and has been synthesized in a number of ways. Large quantities of it are prepared from eugenol isolated from oil of cloves (q.v.) or from guaiacol (methyl catechol). It can also be produced by microbial oxidation of eugenol. In the plant glucovanillin is biosynthesized *via* ferulic acid (see Fig. 21.2). Synthesis begins when elongation of the fruit ceases, which is about 8 months after pollination; before this, other phenolic glycosides predominate.

Adulteration. Extracts of Mexican origin may be adulterated by coumarin, probably arising from the use of tonka beans (q.v.). A capillary GC assay has been described for such products (see R. J. Marles *et al.*, *Economic Bot.*, 1987, **41**, 41).

Uses. Vanilla pods are widely used in confectionery and in perfumery. They have been replaced to some extent, but by no means completely, by synthetic vanillin. About 0.07 parts of vanillin are approximately equivalent to 1 part of the bean, but an essence so prepared fails to represent the odour and flavour of the whole pods.

For a review of natural vanillin, covering biosynthesis, biotechnological production, cell and organ culture and metabolic engineering, see N. J. Walton *et al.*, *Phytochemistry*, 2003, **63**, 505–515.

BEARBERRY LEAVES

(Uva ursi)

Bearberry leaf *EP*/*BP*/*BHP* consists of the dried leaves of *Arctostaphylos uva-ursi*, Ericaceae; ESCOP and German Commission E monographs on the drug are also available.

A. uva-ursi is a small evergreen shrub found in central and northern Europe and in North America. The leaves are dark green to brownish-green, 2–3 cm long, obovate or spathulate, gradually narrowing to a very short petiole, apex obtuse or retuse. They are coriaceous in texture and almost glabrous. The upper surface is shiny and marked with sunken veinlets; the lower surface is lighter and marked with a network of dark veinlets. The drug is odourless but has an astringent and somewhat bitter taste.

Microscopical features include: an upper epidermis of polygonal cells with a thick cuticle; lower epidermis with anomocytic stomata and surrounded by 5–11 subsidiary cells; scars of trichome bases, occasional conical trichomes, crystal fibres.

Bearberry contains the glycosides arbutin (Table 21.1) and methyl-arbutin, about 6–7% of tannin, (+)-catechol, ursone and the flavone derivative quercetin. Some 14 phenolic acid constituents, including gallic and ellagic acids, have been recorded.

The pharmacopoeial drug is required to contain at least 7.0% of hydroquinone derivatives calculated as arbutin. These are assayed by liquid chromatography of an aqueous extract of the leaves with arbutin as a reference and absorbance measurement at 280 nm. The official TLC chromatographic test for identity distinguishes arbutin, gallic acid and hydroquinone. Bearberry is diuretic and astringent and during excretion it exerts an antiseptic action on the urinary tract.

Propolis or bee glue

This is the material with which the honey bee seals cracks and crevices, and varnishes surfaces within the hive. Its composition varies according to geographical source. It is collected by worker bees from the leaf buds and is enriched by wounded plant exudates such as mucilages, gums and resins; bee secretions and enzymes are then mixed in. Like honey, the composition varies according to geographical source.

Propolis has a long history, it being used by the Egyptians in the embalming process (antiputrefactive), by the Greeks and Romans in wound treatment (antiseptic), by the Incas (antipyretic) and by inclusion in the London pharmacopoeias of the 17th century. Today it is used by medical herbalists and has become a popular medicament (S. Castaldo and F. Capasso, *Fitoterapia*, 2002, **73**, S1). It also features in apitherapy—an old tradition that has experienced a recent revival.

Over 160 compounds have been shown to be involved and one analysis gave phenolics (58%), beeswax (24%), flavonoids (6%), terpenes (0.5%), lipids and wax (8%) and bioelements, e.g. Mn, Cu, Zn (0.5%). In temperate regions of Europe the resinous coating of poplar buds (*Populus nigra*, *P. italica*, *P. tremula*) forms a major collection source for the bees and the natural phenolic content of the resin, e.g. esters of caffeic and ferulic acids, vanillin, eugenol, flavonoids, etc., can be used to identify the natural source.

Latterly there have been numerous reports concerning the analysis and biological activity of propolis originating from various regions and especially from Latin American countries. In these areas species of *Araucaria* (Araucariaceae), *Baccharis* (Compositae) and *Clusia* (Guttiferae) have been established as biological sources. In addition to the constituents listed previously, prenylated cinnamic acid and chromane derivatives, diterpenoid acids, lignans and components of the volatile oil have been identified.

Notwithstanding the differences in chemical composition of propolis depending on geographical source, a pronounced antibacterial property is common to all. In temperate regions flavonoid and phenolic esters have been shown to exert bacterial activity. New polyisoprenylated benzophenones have recently been reported as antibacterial agents in propolis of Venezuelan origin (B. Trusheva *et al.*, *Fitoterapia*, 2004, **75**, 683), and similar compounds (propolones) have been found in that of Cuban origin together with garcinelliptone and hyperibone (I. M. Hernández *et al.*, *J. Nat. Prod.*, 2005, **68**, 931). Neoflavonoids with anti-nitric oxide production activity occur in propolis from Nepal (S. Awale *et al.*, *J. Nat. Prod.*, 2005, **68**, 858).

Readers requiring further information on this interesting substance can refer to the references on p. 219 in the 15th edition of this book, and to *Fitoterapia*, Supplement 1, 2002, **73**, S1–S64, devoted entirely to propolis; V. Bankova, *J. Ethnopharmacol.*, 2005, **100**, 114; Y. Lu *et al.*, *Fitoterapia*, 2004, **75**, 267.

CAPSICUM

The *BP/EP* drug (*Chillies*; *Red Peppers*) consists of the dried, ripe fruits of *Capsicum annuum var. minimum* (Miller) Heiser, and small-fruited varieties of *C. frutescens* L. (Solanaceae). In commerce the description given applies to various African commercial varieties (principally from Zimbabwe and Malawi) and these are sold in England as chillies, while the larger but less pungent Bombay and Natal fruits are known as capsicums. Very large *Capsicum* fruits, resembling tomatoes in texture and practically non-pungent, are widely grown in southern Europe as vegetables.

History.   Capsicums appear to be of American origin and were referred to in 1494 by Chanca, a physician who accompanied Columbus on his second voyage to the West Indies. The plants were introduced into India at a very early date, possibly by the Portuguese. 'Ginnie Pepper' was well known in England in 1597 and was grown by Gerarde.

Macroscopical characters.   *African Chillies* are oblong-conical in shape, 12–25 mm long and up to 7 mm wide. The five-toothed calyx and straight pedicel are together about 20–30 mm long. The pericarp is glabrous, shrivelled and orange-red; the Sierra Leone and Zambian chillies usually have a better colour than those from Zanzibar.

Internally the fruits are divided into two cells by a membranous dissepiment to which the seeds were originally attached. The latter, usually about 10–20 in each fruit, are of a flattened reniform shape and are about 3–4 mm long. Like other solanaceous seeds, they have a coiled embryo and oily endosperm. African chillies are very sternutatory and have an intensely pungent taste.

Constituents.   In 1876, Thresh extracted the drug with petroleum, treated the extract with aqueous alkali, and by passing carbon dioxide through the alkaline liquid precipitated crystals of an intensely pungent compound, capsaicin. As may be inferred from the method of preparation, capsaicin is of phenolic nature.

The pungent phenolic fraction of capsicum also contains a proportion of 6,7-dihydrocapsaicin. The capsaicin content of fruits varies appreciably in a range up to 1.5% and is much influenced by environmental conditions and age of the fruit. It occurs principally in the dissepiments of the fruits—for example, entire fruit 0.49, pericarp 0.10, dissepiment 1.79, seed 0.07. The pungency of capsicum is not destroyed by treatment with alkalis (distinction from gingerol, which also contains the vanillyl group) but is destroyed by oxidation with potassium dichromate or permanganate. Chillies also contain ascorbic acid (0.1–0.5%), thiamine, red carotenoids such as capsanthin and capsorubin (see 'Carotenoids') and fixed oil (about 4–16%). They yield about 20–25% of alcoholic extract (capsicin) and about 5% (official limit 10.0%) of ash. Hungarian capsicums or 'Paprika' are derived from a mild race of *C. annuum* and are a convenient source of ascorbic acid. According to Bennett and Kirby, the pungent principle of *C. annuum* is composed of capsaicin 69%, dihydrocapsaicin 22%, nordihydrocapsaicin 7%, homocapsaicin (C_{11} acid) 1% and homodihydrocapsaicin 1%. A number of minor components of this class have been recorded.

In a study of the water-soluble constituents of the fruits of three varieties of *C. annuum*, Izumitani *et al.* (*Chem. Pharm. Bull.*, 1990, **38**, 1299) isolated twelve novel acyclic glycosides (geranyllinalool derivatives) named capsianosides A–F (dimeric esters of acyclic diterpene glycosides) and capsianosides I–V (monomeric compounds of acyclic diterpene glycosides). Further capsianosides have now been reported by J.-H. Lee *et al.*, (*Chem. Pharm. Bull.*, 2006, **54**, 1365). T. Ochi *et al.*, (*J. Nat. Prod.*, 2003, **66**, 1094) record a dimeric capsaicin having almost the same antioxidant activity as capsaicin but with no pungent taste (Fig. 21.5).

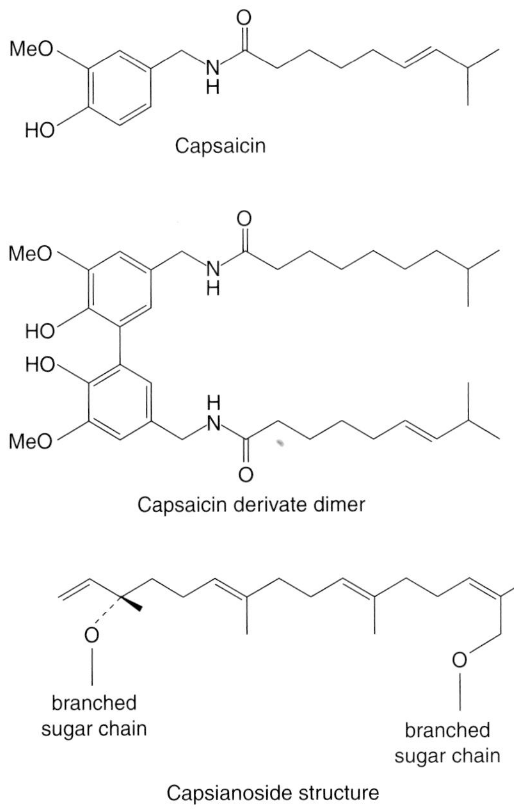

Fig. 21.5
Some constituents of capsicum.

Biogenesis of capsaicin.   Work by Leete and Louden on *C. frutescens* and by Bennett and Kirby on *C. annuum* demonstrated that phenylalanine is incorporated into the C_6–C_1 vanillyl unit of capsaicin, the C-3 of phenylalanine giving the methylene group of the vanillylamine residues; the incorporation probably proceeds via cinnamic, *p*-coumaric, caffeic and protocatechuic acids. Tyrosine did not appear to be a probable precursor. Leete's feeding experiments with [U-^{14}C]-valine gave incorporations consistent with the hypothesis that the C_{10} isodecanoic acid is formed from isobutyryl coenzyme A and three acetate units. More recent work showed that the homo derivatives (C_{11} acid) are formed from leucine and isoleucine.

The ontogenetic formation of capsaicinoids in the fruits of *C. frutescens* involves a prior active accumulation of *p*-coumaroyl, caffeoyl and 3,4-dimethoxycinnamoyl glycosides, 3-*O*-rhamnosylquercetin and 7-*O*-glucosylluteolin. When the fruit ceases to increase in length the amount of these compounds falls and capsaicinoid synthesis commences together with that of the glycosides of vanillic acid and *p*-hydroxybenzaldehyde (see N. Sukrasno and M. M. Yeoman, *Phytochemistry*, 1993, **32**, 839).

Cell cultures.   The biogenetic potential for capsaicin production is reported (1991) as 10 times greater in immobilized cell cultures (alginate entrapment) than in control suspension cultures.

Tests and standards.   The official TLC test for identity establishes the presence of capsaicin and dihydrocapsaicin in the sample. The synthetic equivalent of capsaicin, nonivamide (pelargonyl vanillylamide), a commercial product used as a flavour in the food industry and in medicine as a topical rubifacient, is limited by a liquid chromatographic assay to a maximum of 5% of the total capsaicinoid content.

Liquid chromatography is also used to determine the total capsaicinoid content (minimum 0.4%). A number of colorimetric assays can be used for the quantitative determination of capsaicin (see Table 16.5); the *BPC* 1973 utilized ultraviolet absorption at 248 and 296 nm for the ointment and oleoresin. Foreign matter should not exceed a maximum of 2%; fruits of *C. annuum* L. var. *longum* (Sendtn.) (see 'Bombay capsicums' below) should be absent.

Allied drugs.   *Japanese Chillies* are probably derived from *C. frutescens* and are about 3–4 cm long. They possess about one-quarter of the pungency of the African Chillies, but are now no longer commercially relevant.

Bombay Capsicums are ascribed to *C. annuum* L. The pericarp is thicker and tougher than in the chillies, and the pedicel is frequently bent. They are much less pungent than African chillies.

Natal Capsicums are larger than the Bombay variety, being up to 8 cm long. They have a very bright red, transparent pericarp. They are much less pungent than chillies.

Uses.   Capsicums are used as a condiment under the name of Cayenne pepper. The drug is given internally in atonic dyspepsia and flatulence. It is used externally as a counter-irritant, in the form of ointment, plaster, medicated wool, etc., for the relief of rheumatism, lumbago, etc. Capsaicin creams are available for the relief of pain in osteoarthritis, post-herpetic neuralgia and painful diabetic neuropathy (*Pharm. J.*, 1998, **260**, 692).

Further reading
De AK (ed), Hardman R (series ed) 2003 Medicinal and aromatic plants, Vol 34, Capsicum, the genus *Capsicum*. CRC Press/ Taylor and Francis, Andover, UK. *An overall coverage of the subject, 800 references.*

TANNINS

The term 'tannin' was first applied by Seguin in 1796 to denote substances present in plant extracts which were able to combine with protein of animal hides, prevent their putrefaction and convert them into leather. On this basis a tannin is a substance which is detected qualitatively by a tanning test (the goldbeater's skin test) and is determined quantitatively by its adsorption on standard hide powder. This definition excludes simpler phenolic substances, often present with tannins, such as gallic acid, catechins and chlorogenic acid, although they may under certain conditions give precipitates with gelatin and be partly retained by hide powder. Such substances of relatively low molecular weight are called 'pseudo-tannins'. Most true tannins have molecular weights of from about 1000 to 5000. To be effective for tannage the polyphenol molecule most be neither so large as to be unable to enter the interstices between the collagen fibrils of the animal skin nor so small that it is unable to cross-link between the protein molecules of adjacent fibrils at several points. Many tannins are glycosides. The definition of a tannin as given above is an old, essentially practical one which may be purely fortuitous and, in the light of further research, could prove misleading from the point of view of plant metabolism and plant biochemistry. Indeed, modern authors often treat tannins not as a specific phytochemical group but as examples of polyphenols illustrating particular aspects of gallic acid and flavan-3-ol phytochemistry. The characteristic properties of tannins derive from the accumulation within a moderately sized molecule of a substantial number (1–2 per 100 mol. wt.) of phenolic groups many of which are associated with *o*-dihydroxy and *o*-trihydroxy orientation within a phenyl ring.

The above tannin-protein co-precipitation is important not only in the leather industry but also in relation to the physiological activity of herbal medicines, taste of foodstuffs and beverages, and in the nutritional value of feeds for herbivores. Environmental factors affecting this process have been studied by H. Kawamoto and F. Nakatsubo (*Phytochemistry*, 1997, **46**, 479).

Two main groups of tannins are usually recognized; these are the hydrolysable tannins and the condensed tannins (proanthocyanidins).

Hydrolysable tannins

These may be hydrolysed by acids or enzymes such as tannase. They are formed from several molecules of phenolic acids such as gallic and hexahydroxydiphenic acids which are united by ester linkages to a central glucose molecule. A simple tannin illustrating this point is one derived from a species of sumac (*Rhus*), with a possible structure as shown in Fig. 21.6. Like gallic acid their solutions turn blue with iron salts. They were formerly known as pyrogallol tannins, because on dry distillation gallic acid and similar components are converted into pyrogallol. Two principal types of hydrolysable tannins are gallitannins and ellagitannins which are, respectively, composed of gallic acid and hexahydroxy-diphenic acid units. Ellagic acid (the depside of gallic acid) can arise by lactonization of

hexahydroxydiphenic acid during chemical hydrolysis of the tannin; thus, the term ellagitannin is a misnomer.

Ellagitannins found in plants of medicinal interest, and for which structures have been elucidated include geraniin (Herb Robert and American cranesbill) and tellimagrandins 1 and 2 (Oak bark, Pomegranate and Meadowsweet); Fig. 21.6.

Modern methods of analysis have made considerable advances in the study of tannin chemistry of medicinal plants as evidenced by the work of Okuda on oriental drugs. In 1982 agromoniin, the first of a new class of *oligomeric hydrolysable tannins* was isolated from *Agromonia*. These tannins are composed of two, three or four monomeric units. Something less than 20 of these units including geraniin and tellimagrandins 1 and 2 are known to be involved in the production of over 150 compounds.

As an example, many plants of the Onagraceae e.g. *Oenothera* spp. contain in addition to tellimagrandin, the dimer oenothein B and trimer oenothein A; these macrocyclic ellagitannins are also produced in callus cultures of *O. lacinata* and are of interest for their anticancer and polygalacturonase-inhibiting properties (S. Taniguchi *et al.*, *Phytochemistry*, 1998, **48**, 981).

C-glucosidic ellagitannins are common in a number of families including the Myrtaceae, Hamamelidaceae, Punicaceae and Rosaceae

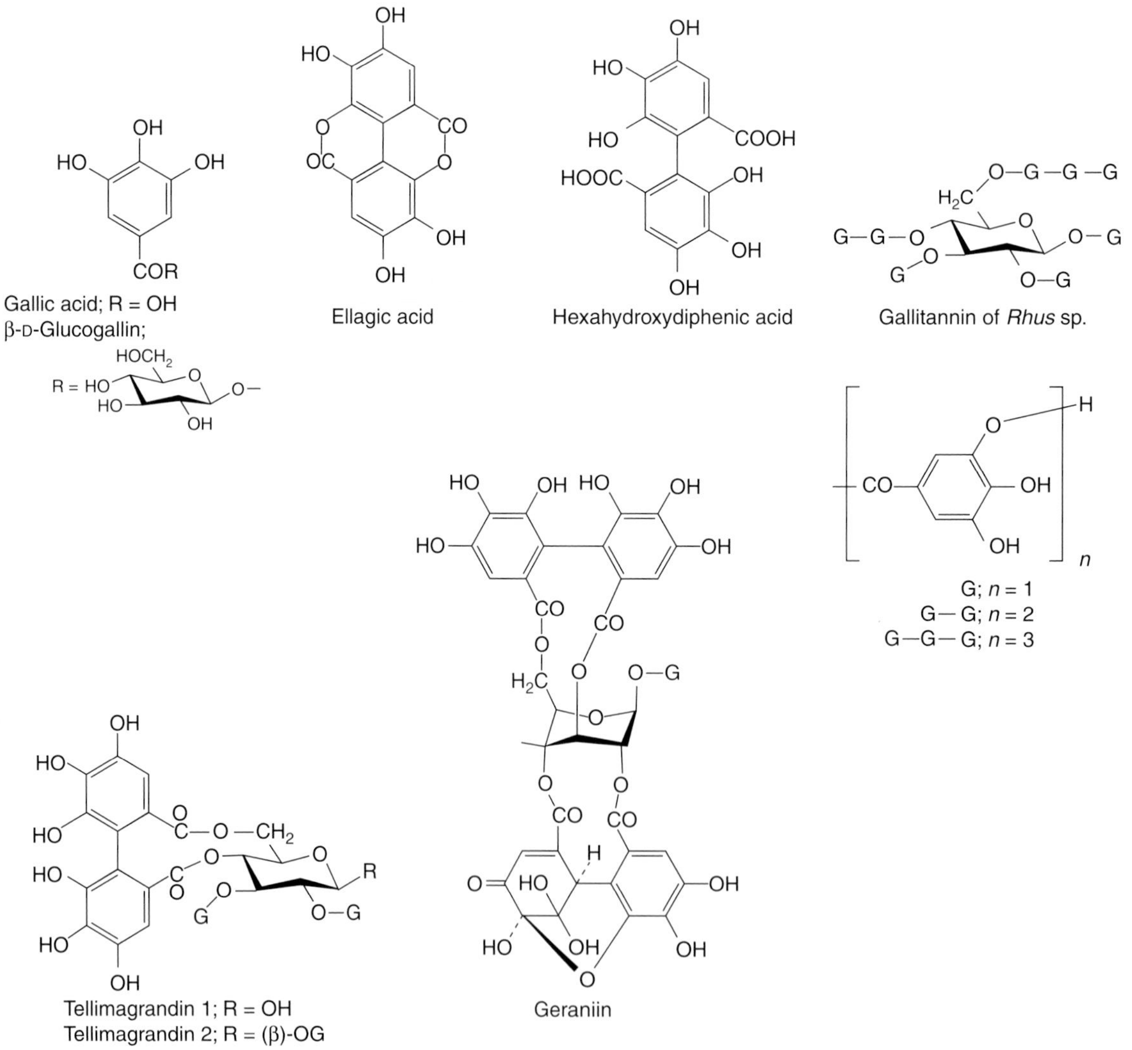

Gallic acid; R = OH
β-D-Glucogallin;
R = [structure shown]

Ellagic acid

Hexahydroxydiphenic acid

Gallitannin of *Rhus* sp.

G; n = 1
G—G; n = 2
G—G—G; n = 3

Tellimagrandin 1; R = OH
Tellimagrandin 2; R = (β)-OG

Geraniin

Fig. 21.6
Examples of hydrolysable tannins and their component acids.

and several have also been recorded as moieties of more than 10 oligomeric ellagitannins.

For an article on the classification of oligomeric hydrolysable tannins and the specificity of their occurrence in plants see Okuda *et al.*, *Phytochemistry*, 1993, **32**, 507.

In a series of enzymatic studies Gross and colleagues indicated the central position of β-D-glucogallin in the early stages of tannin synthesis in *Quercus robur* leaves. This compound appears to act as both donor and acceptor of the galloyl group in the enzymatic formation of 1,6-digalloyl-D-glucose; the responsible enzyme is β-glucogallin: β-glucogallin 6-*O*-galloyl-transferase.

The presumed immediate precursor of the two subclasses of hydrolysable tannins (gallotannins and ellagitannins) is 1,2,3,4,6-pentagalloylglucose, and in a continuation of their enzyme studies the above group have purified (×500) the enzyme responsible for the conversion of the precursor to the gallotannin 3-*O*-digalloyl-1,2,4,6-tetra-*O*-galloyl-β-D-glucose. The source of the enzyme was *Rhus typhina* (staghorn sumac) and its designation is β-glucogallin: 1,2,4,6-pentagalloyl-β-D-glucose galloyl-transferase (R. Niemetz and G. G. Gross, *Phytochemistry*, 1998, **49**, 327).

Examples of drugs containing hydrolysable tannins are:

Gallitannins: rhubarb, cloves, red rose petals, bearberry leaves, Chinese galls, Turkish galls, hamamelis, chestnut and maple.
Ellagitannins: pomegranate rind, pomegranate bark, myrobalans, eucalyptus leaves, kousso, some Australian kinos, chestnut (*Castanea* spp.) and oak bark.

Condensed tannins (proanthocyanidins)

Unlike hydrolysable tannins, these are not readily hydrolysed to simpler molecules and they do not contain a sugar moiety. They are related to the flavonoid pigments and have polymeric flavan-3-ol structures. Catechins, which also occur with the tannins and flavan-3,4-diols (leucoanthocyanidins) are intermediates in the biosynthesis of the polymeric molecules. Stereochemical variations add to the variety of possible structures. Monomeric, dimeric and trimeric forms are illustrated in Fig. 21.7. Work by Japanese phytochemists has exploited modern techniques for separating and determining the structures of these oligomers and polymers including those of cassia bark, *Cassia fistula*, cinchona, *Quercus* and rhubarb.

On treatment with acids or enzymes condensed tannis are converted into red insoluble compounds known as phlobaphenes. Phlobaphenes give the characteristic red colour to many drugs such as red cinchona bark, which contain these phlobatannins and their decomposition products. On dry distillation they yield catechol and these tannins are therefore sometimes called catechol tannins. Like catechol itself, their solutions turn green with ferric chloride.

Some drugs (e.g. tea, hamamelis leaves and hamamelis bark) contain both hydrolysable and condensed tannins. The following are rich in condensed tannins:

1. Barks: cinnamon, wild cherry, cinchona, willow, acacia (wattle, mimosa), oak and hamamelis
2. Roots and rhizomes: krameria (rhatany) and male fern
3. Flowers: lime and hawthorn
4. Seeds: cocoa, guarana, kola and areca
5. Fruits: cranberries, grapes (red wines), hawthorn
6. Leaves: hamamelis, hawthorn and tea, especially green tea
7. Extracts and dried juices: catechu, acacia and mangrove cutches, East Indian kino, butea gum and eucalyptus kino.

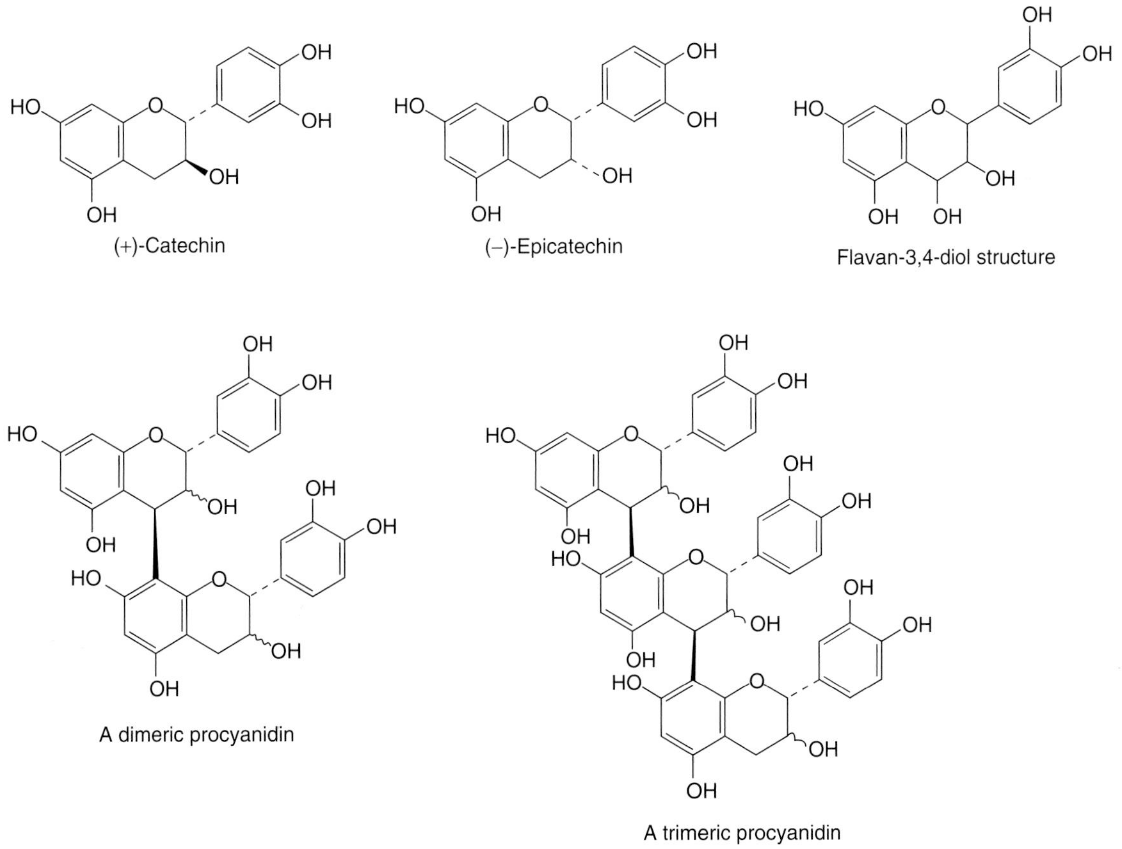

(+)-Catechin

(−)-Epicatechin

Flavan-3,4-diol structure

A dimeric procyanidin

A trimeric procyanidin

Fig. 21.7
Structures associated with condensed tannins.

'Complex tannins'

This term has been applied by Okuda to a newly-discovered group of tannins which are biosynthesized from both a hydrolysable tannin (mostly a *C*-glucoside ellagitannin) and a condensed tannin. The union occurs through a C–C bond between the C-1 of the glucose unit of the ellagitannin and the C-8 or C-6 of the flavan-3-ol derivative. The monomers are also involved in oligomer formation.

To date, complex tannins have not great relevance to mainstream pharmacognosy; monomers have been isolated from the Combretaceae, Fagaceae (*Quercus*, *Castanea*), Myrtaceae, Polygonaceae (*Rheum*) and Theaceae (*Camellia*). It is anticipated that many more compounds of this group will be discovered.

Pseudotannins

As already mentioned, pseudotannins are compounds of lower molecular weight than true tannins and they do not respond to the goldbeater's skin test. Examples:

1. *Gallic acid*: rhubarb and most materials which contain gallitannins
2. *Catechins*: catechu, acacia cutch, many Australian kinos, cocoa, guarana and many other drugs containing condensed tannins
3. *Chlorogenic acid*: maté, coffee (particularly unroasted) and nux vomica (a small quantity only)
4. *Ipecacuanhic acid*: ipecacuanha

Occurrence of tannins. Tannins are of wide occurrence in plants and are usually found in greatest quantity in dead or dying cells. They exert an inhibitory effect on many enzymes due to protein precipitation and, hence, they may contribute a protective function in barks and heartwoods. Commercial tannins, as used in the leather industry, are obtained from quebracho, wattle, chestnut and myrobalans trees. Pharmaceutical tannin is prepared from oak galls (q.v.) and yields glucose and gallic acid on hydrolysis; many commercial samples contain some free gallic acid.

Some plants (clove, cinnamon, etc.) contain tannin in addition to the principal therapeutic constituents. This may complicate extraction or produce incompatibilities with other drugs (many alkaloids, for example, are precipitated by tannins).

Properties and tests. Tannins are soluble in water, dilute alkalis, alcohol, glycerol and acetone, but generally only sparingly soluble in other organic solvents. Solutions precipitate heavy metals, alkaloids, glycosides and gelatin. With ferric salts, gallitannins and ellagitannins give blue-black precipitates and condensed tannins brownish-green ones. If a very dilute ferric chloride solution is gradually added to an aqueous extract of hamamelis leaves (which contains both types of tannin), a blue colour is produced which changes to olive-green as more ferric chloride is added. Other tests are the following.

1. *Goldbeater's skin test*. Soak a small piece of goldbeater's skin in 2% hydrochloric acid; rinse with distilled water and place in the solution to be tested for 5 min. Wash with distilled water and transfer to a 1% solution of ferrous sulphate. A brown or black colour on the skin denotes the presence of tannins. Goldbeater's skin is a membrane prepared from the intestine of the ox and behaves similarly to an untanned hide (a reference sample of hide powder, as used in the *BP* assay of the tannins of Rhatany Root, may be obtained from the European Pharmacopoeia Secretariat, Strasbourg).
2. *Gelatin test*. Solutions of tannins (about 0.5–1%) precipitate a 1% solution of gelatin containing 10% sodium chloride. Gallic acid and other pseudotannins also precipitate gelatin if the solutions are sufficiently concentrated.
3. *Phenazone test*. To about 5 ml of an aqueous extract of the drug add 0.5 g of sodium acid phosphate; warm, cool and filter. To the filtrate add 2% solution of phenazone. All tannins are precipitated, the precipitate being bulky and often coloured.
4. *Test for catechin*. Catechins on heating with acids form phloroglucinol and they can, therefore, be detected by a modification of the well-known test for lignin. Dip a matchstick in the plant extract, dry, moisten with concentrated hydrochloric acid and warm near a flame. The phloroglucinol produced turns the wood pink or red.
5. *Test for chlorogenic acid*. An extract containing chlorogenic acid when treated with aqueous ammonia and exposed to air gradually develops a green colour.

In practice, these tests have to some extent been superseded by the use of TLC, particularly for the identification of crude drugs.

Medicinal and biological properties. Tannin-containing drugs will precipitate protein and have been used traditionally as stypics and internally for the protection of inflamed surfaces of mouth and throat. They act as antidiarrhoeals and have been employed as antidotes in poisoning by heavy metals, alkaloids and glycosides. In Western medicine their use declined after World War II when it was found that absorbed tannic acid can cause severe central necrosis of the liver. Recent studies have concentrated on the antitumour activity of tannins (M. Ken-ichi *et al.*, *Biol. Pharm. Bull.*, 1993, **16**, 379) and it has been shown that, to exhibit a strong activity, ellagitannin monomer units having galloyl groups at the *O*-2 and *O*-3 positions on the glucose core(s), as in the tellimagrandins (Fig. 21.6) are required. Anti-HIV activity has also been demonstrated.

Proanthocyanidins (condensed tannins) are associated with the beneficial effects of various herbs and infusions produced from them. The antitumour activity of green and black tea has been extensively researched in recent years with positive findings. Of the components of tea, epigallocatechin-3-gallate, specifically, has been shown to prevent angiogenesis in mice. Cranberry juice has long been used for reducing bacterial infections of the bladder and these claims have now been supported by a randomized, double-blind, placebo-controlled trial carried out on 153 elderly women (J. Avorn *et al.*, *J. Amer. Med. Assoc.*, 1994, **271**, 751). Fructose has been implicated in this activity but recently, proanthocyanidins prepared from cranberries by reverse-phase and adsorption chromatography were shown to inhibit the adherence of P-fimbriated *E. coli* to uroepithelial-cell surfaces; other *Vaccinium* spp., including blueberries had similar bioactivity, suggesting their contribution to the salutary effects in urinary tract infections (A. Howell *et al.*, *New Engl. J. Med.*, 1998, **339**, 1085).

Further reading

Beecher GR 2004 Proanthocyanidins: biological activities associated with human health. Pharmaceutical Biology 42 (Supplement): 2–20
Waterman PG, Mole S 1994 Analysis of phenolic plant metabolites. Methods in ecology. Blackwell Scientific Publications, Oxford, UK

OAK BARK

Oak bark is the cut and dried bark from the fresh young branches of *Quercus robur* L. (English oak, Common oak), *Q. petraea* Liebl. (Sessile or Durmast oak) and *Q. pubescens* Willd. (Downy oak), family Fagaceae. The three species are recognized by the *BP/EP* and the first two by the *BHP*. The distribution of the species is widespread in Europe and W. Asia. *Q. alba* L. (White oak) is used in the USA.

The commercial bark, obtained principally from E. and S.E. Europe, occurs as channelled pieces, 3–4 mm thick and of various lengths. Younger, thinner pieces have a smooth, greyish-green cork with lenticels, older pieces have a greyish-brown rhytidome and show a fracture, granular in the outer part and fibrous and splintery in the inner part. Conspicuous features of the reddish-brown powder include cork cells, lignified fibres with crystal sheaths of calcium oxalate, pitted sclereids and cluster crystals of calcium oxalate in parenchymatous cells.

Principal constituents are phlobatannins, ellagitannins and gallic acid, a minimum of 3.0% calculated as pyrogallol [$C_6H_3(OH)_3$ (1:2:3)] being specified by the *BP/EP*.

Oak bark is used medicinally for its astringent properties and industrially for tanning and dyeing.

GALLS AND TANNIC ACID

Turkish galls (*Turkey Galls*; *Galla*) are vegetable growths formed on the young twigs of the dyer's oak, *Quercus infectoria* (Fagaceae), as a result of the deposition of the eggs of the gall-wasp *Adleria gallaetinctoriae*.

The dyer's oak is a small tree or shrub about 2 m high which is found in Turkey, Syria, Persia, Cyprus and Greece. Abnormal development of vegetable tissue round the larva is due to an enzyme-containing secretion, produced by the young insect after it has emerged from the egg, which by the rapid conversion of starch into sugar stimulates cell division. As starch disappears from the neighbourhood of the insect, shrinkage occurs and a central cavity is formed in which the insect passes through the larval and pupal stages. Finally, if the galls are not previously collected and dried, the mature insect or imago bores its way out of the gall and escapes. During these changes the colour of the gall passes from a bluish-grey through olive-green to almost white.

Galls are collected by the peasants of Turkey and Syria. After drying they are graded according to colour into three grades, blue, green and white, which are found on the London market.

History. Galls were well known to the ancient writers and Pliny records the use of their infusion as a test for sulphate of iron in verdigris, possibly the earliest mention of an attempt to detect adulteration by chemical means.

Characters. Aleppo galls are globular in shape and from 10 to 25 mm in diameter. They have a short, basal stalk and numerous rounded projections on the surface. Galls are hard and heavy, usually sinking in water. The so-called 'blue' variety are actually of a grey or brownish-grey colour. These, and to a lesser extent the olive-green 'green' galls, are preferred to the 'white' variety, in which the tannin is said to have been partly decomposed. White galls also differ from the other grades in having a circular tunnel through which the insect has emerged. Galls without the opening have insect remains in the small central cavity. Galls have a very astringent taste.

Sections through a gall show a very large outer zone of thin-walled parenchyma, a ring of sclerenchymatous cells, and a small, inner zone of rather thick-walled parenchyma surrounding the central cavity. The parenchymatous tissues contain abundant starch, masses of tannin, rosettes and prisms of calcium oxalate, and the rounded so-called 'lignin bodies', which give a red colour with phloroglucinol and hydrochloric acid.

Constituents. Galls contain 50–70% of the tannin known as gallotannic acid (Tannic Acid *BP/EP*); this is a complex mixture of phenolic acid glycosides varying greatly in composition. It is prepared by fermenting the galls and extracting with water-saturated ether. Galls also contain gallic acid (about 2–4%), ellagic acid, sitosterol, methyl betulate, methyl oleanolate, starch and calcium oxalate. Two new compounds, derivatives of ellagic acid and pentahydroxynaphthalene, isolated from the alcoholic extract of galls have been shown to have nitricoxide- and superoxide-inhibiting activity (H. Hamid *et al.*, *Pharm. Biol.*, 2005, **43**, 317). Nyctanthic, roburic and syringic

acids have more recently been identified and syringic acid has been identified as the CNS-active component of the methanolic extract of galls. (For the isolation of flavonoids of oak galls see M. Ahmed *et al.*, *Fitoterapia*, 1991, **62**, 283.)

Tannic acid is a hydrolysable tannin (see above) yielding gallic acid and glucose and having the minimum complexity of pentadigalloyl glucose. Solutions of tannic acid tend to decompose on keeping with formation of gallic acid, a substance which is also found in many commercial samples of tannic acid. It may be detected by the pink colour produced on the addition of a 5% solution of potassium cyanide.

Allied drugs. Many different kinds of galls are known. They are generally produced on plants, but sometimes on animals. In addition to the large number produced by insects, particularly of the genera *Cynips* and *Aphis*, some are produced by fungi.

Chinese and Japanese galls are of considerable commercial importance. They are produced by an aphis, *Schlectendalia chinensis*, on the petioles of the leaves of *Rhus chinensis* (Anacardiaceae). These galls, which the Chinese call 'wu-pei-tzu', meaning 'five knots', are irregular in shape and partly covered with a grey, velvety down, the removal of which discloses a reddish-brown surface. They break easily and show a large, irregular cavity containing insect remains. They contain 57–77% of tannin and have been valued in China as astringents and styptics for at least 1250 years.

Crowned Aleppo galls are sometimes found in samples of ordinary Aleppo galls. They are about the size of a pea, are stalked, and bear a crown of projections near the apex. The insect producing them is *Cynips polycera*.

Hungarian galls are produced by *Cynips lignicola* on *Quercus robur* growing in former Yugoslavia. They are used in tanning. *English oak galls*, formed by *Adleria kollari* on *Quercus robur*, contain about 15–20% of tannin.

Uses. Galls are used as a source of tannic acid, for tanning and dyeing, and in the manufacture of inks. Tannic acid is used as an astringent and styptic.

HAMAMELIS LEAF

Hamamelis leaf (*witch hazel leaves*) consists of the dried leaves of *Hamamelis virginiana* L. (Hamamelidaceae), a shrub or small tree 2–5 m high, which is widely distributed in Canada and the USA. It is official in the *BP/EP* and is the subject of an ESCOP monograph.

Macroscopical characters. The leaves are shortly petiolate, 7–15 cm long, and broadly oval to ovate in shape; base asymmetrically cordate, apex acute. The lamina is dark brownish-green to green in colour and very papery in texture. The venation is pinnate and the margin crenate or sinuate-dentate. The veins are very conspicuous on the lower surface; they leave the mid-rib at an acute angle and run straight to the margin, where they terminate in a marginal crenation. Odour, slight; taste, astringent and bitter.

The *BP/EP* drug is required to contain not more than 7% of stems and not more than 2% of other foreign matter.

Microscopical characters. The drug has very distinctive microscopical characters. These include characteristic stomata present on the lower surface only; very large lignified idioblasts, crystal cells accompanying the pericyclic fibres, tannin-containing cells and, especially in young leaves, stellate hairs. The calcium oxalate is in monoclinic prisms 10–35 μm long. The stellate hairs (Fig. 42.1H) consist of 4–12 cells united at the base. Each cell is thick-walled and up to 500 μm long.

Constituents. Hamamelis contains gallitannins, ellagitannins, free gallic acid, proanthocyanidins, bitter principles and traces of volatile oil. With ferric chloride solution the gallitannins and the free gallic acid give a blue colour and the ellagitannins, green.

The pharmacopoeia requires the leaves to contain not less than 3.0% tannins; these tannins represent the difference between the total polyphenol content of the leaf and the polyphenol content not absorbed by hide powder. Reagents employed in the assay are Phosphomolyb-dotungstic reagent and sodium carbonate solution with absorbance measurements made at 760 nm; pyrogallol is used as a test solution. The leaves appear to contain no hamamelitannin (see 'Hamamelis Bark', below).

Volatile compounds, although present in small amounts only, have been studied by GC-MS analysis. Some 175 compounds have been distinguished and classified as homologous series of alkanes, alkenes, aliphatic alcohols, related aldehydes, ketones and fatty acid esters; distinctive monoterpenoids were evident (R. Engel *et al.*, *Planta Medica*, 1998, **64**, 251).

A procedure for the identification and assay involving TLC, HPLC, plate densitometry and spectrophotometry for the proanthocyanidins, phenolic acids and flavonoids in leaf extracts has been described (B. Vennat *et al.*, *Pharm. Acta Helv.*, 1992, **67**, 11).

Allied drugs. *Hamamelis bark* occurs in curved or channelled pieces which seldom exceed 10 cm long or 2 cm wide. The bark is silvery grey and smooth, or dark grey and scaly. The inner surface is pinkish and often bears fragments of whitish wood. Sections show a cortex containing prismatic crystals of calcium oxalate, a complete ring of sclerenchymatous cells, and groups of phloem fibres. The bark contains a mixture of hamamelitannin and condensed tannin; the former has recently been demonstrated to be a potent oxygen scavenger (H. Masaki *et al.*, *Phytochemistry*, 1994, **37**, 337). Three separate hamamelitannins, α-, β- and γ-, are now known. The most important, β-hamamelitannin, is formed from two gallic acid molecules and one molecule of the sugar hamamelose. Newer galloylhamameloses and proanthocyanidins have now been identified (C. Haberland and H. Kolodziej, *Planta Medica*, 1994, **60**, 464; C. Hartisch and J. Kolodziej, *Phytochemistry*, 1996, **42**, 191). For the fractionation of those polymeric proanthocyanidins having similar structures but different molecular weights, see A. Dauer *et al.*, *Planta Med.*, 2003, **69**, 89.

Uses. Hamamelis owes its astringent and haemostatic properties to the tannins. Hamamelitannin and the galloylated proanthocyanidins isolated from *H. virginiana* are reported to be potent inhibitors of 5-lipo-oxygenase, supporting the anti-inflammatory action of the drug (C. Hartisch *et al.*, *Planta Medica*, 1997, **63**, 106). The above compounds are presumably not present in Hamamelis Water or Distilled Witch Hazel, which is, however, widely used as an application to sprains, bruises and superficial wounds and as an ingredient of eye lotions. It contains safrole and other volatile components.

TORMENTIL

There are over 300 spp. of *Potentilla* family Rosaceae of which several, including *P. anserina*, (silverweed), *P. reptans* (creeping cinquefoil) and *P. erecta* (common tormentil), find medicinal use. Tormentil *BP/EP* consists of the whole or cut dried rhizome, freed from roots of *P. erecta* (L.) Raeusch. (*P. tormentilla* Stokes). This perennial plant is widely spread throughout central and northern Europe, favouring the acidic soils of marshes, meadows, open woods and hills. Commercial supplies come from East European countries.

Plants are up to 30 cm tall with several loosely pilosed stems bearing leaves consisting of three- to five-toothed finely haired leaflets. Yellow flowers in loose terminal cymes have long pedicels and, unusually for the genus, four petals.

The rhizomes are dark brown on the outer corky layer and white on the inside when freshly broken, but turning red on exposure to the air. The chopped dried drug consists of hard pieces of rhizome with the remains of roots attached. Depressed pale scars from the stems are visible and some remains of stems in the form of fine, branching strands, less than 1 mm in diameter, may also be attached to the rhizome. The fracture is granular, odour faint but not unpleasant and the taste strongly astringent.

Characteristic features of the powder include brown cork cells, parenchymatous tissue containing tannin, sclerenchymatous tissues, vascular elements, starch in conglomerates or as single grains up to about 20 μm in length, and abundant cluster crystals of calcium oxalate up to about 50 μm in diameter.

Constituents. The rhizome contains a mixture of both hydrolysable and condensed tannins (proanthocyanidins). Among the former is agrimoniin, a dimeric ellagitannin found also in *Agrimonia* and *Alchemilla*, and belonging to the same biosynthetic group, ellagic acid and catechol gallates. Other components are flavan-3-ols, the pseudosaponin tormentoside, quinovic acid and various phenylpropanes together with a trace of volatile oil.

Standards. *BP/EP* requirements are a minimum of 7.0% tannins calculated as pyrogallol for the dried rhizome. A maximum of 3% for roots, stems and rhizomes with a black fracture. Other foreign matter limited to 2%. Compliance with a TLC test for identity using catechin as a reference substance.

Uses. As an astringent; internally as an antidiarrhoeic and externally for gargles and inflamed mucous membranes.

HAWTHORN

The leaves, flowers and false fruits are all medicinally useful, the leaves and flowers being used principally for the preparation of infusions, etc. with the fruits employed in the manufacture of prepared medicaments. The dried false fruits of *Crataegus monogyna* and *C. laevigata*, family Rosaceae, together with their hybrids are official in the *EP*, *BP* and *BHP*; similarly the leaf and flower, for which there is also an ESCOP monograph.

The thorny, deciduous trees are native to Europe and have a long medical and ethnobotanical history. Commercial supplies of the dried fruits, required to contain not less than 1.0% procyanidins, originate from Eastern Europe.

Characters. Characteristic of a number of genera of the family Rosaceae, so-called hawthorn berries are false fruits (pomes, and not in the strict botanical sense berries) in which the carpels become adherent to the hollow, fleshy receptacle and the sepals, petals and stamens become situated at the upper end of the fruit. The carpels become stony so that the pome comes rather to resemble a drupe (Ch. 41). The false fruits of *C. monogyna* with one carpel contain a single stony true fruit whereas those of *C. laevigata* with two or three carpels contain two or three fruits.

The dried reddish-brown to dark red fruits have a slight odour and mucilaginous, slightly acid taste; with *C. monogyna* they are up to 10 mm in length and slightly larger for *C. laevigata*. At the upper end of the false fruit are the remains of the five reflexed sepals which surround a shallow depression from the base of which arise stiff lignified tufts of trichomes and the remains of the style (two styles with *C. laevigata*). The base of the fruit may be either attached to a pedicel or show the scar of attachment of the latter.

In addition to the long, lignified, tapering clothing trichomes of the inner surface of the receptacle other microscopical features include: cells of the outer receptacle with red pigmentation; sclereids; calcium oxalate as clusters and in files of cells as prisms; seed fragments showing a mucilaginous testa and embryo cells containing aleurone grains and fixed oil. A more detailed description will be found in the pharmacopoeias.

Constituents. The fruits contain 1–3% oligomeric procyanidins, the structures of which appear to be only partially ascertained together with flavonoids, principally hyperoside about 1%. The leaves in contrast contain less hyperoside and more vitexin rhamnoside.

Thin layer chromatography of a methanolic extract of the drug and fluorescence visualization at 365 nm is used as a test for identity. Procyanidins are evaluated by acid hydrolysis of an alcoholic extract followed by absorbance measurements at 545 nm of the butanol-soluble procyanidins produced.

The leaves and flowers, in contrast to the fruits, contain less hyperoside and more vitexin rhamnoside. In a study of important factors for the use of monitored commercial material, W. Peschel *et al.* (*Fitoterapia*, 2008, **79**, 1) have examined the variability of total flavonoid content of the drug in relation to wild trees, age of cultivation site, sun exposure and harvest time.

Allied species. Adulteration of the readily available product is rare; other species of *Crataegus* may be detected by their having more than three seeds. *C. pinnatifida* fruits are used in Chinese medicine.

Uses. Hawthorn is widely used as a mild cardiac tonic particularly for patients of advancing age. It does not have the toxic effects of *Digitalis* and can usefully be employed before recourse is made to the digitalis cardioactive glycosides.

AGRIMONY

Agrimony *BP/EP*, *BHP* family Rosaceae consists of the dried flowering tops of *Agrimonia eupatoria* L.

This erect, chalk-loving perennial herb is common throughout southern Europe and is indigenous to the British Isles, except for northern Scotland. Related species are found across North America. Hungary and Bulgaria are commercial suppliers of the drug.

The leaves are compound imparipinnate, with four to six opposite pairs of leaflets and a terminal leaflet. Larger leaflets are up to 6 cm in length with coarsely serrate or serrate–dentate margins, usually densely villous and often greyish on the lower surface. The golden flowers, 5–8 mm in diameter, are arranged spirally as terminal spikes. The pendulous fruits, 4–6 mm long, are deeply grooved with small projecting hooked bristles.

Characteristic microscopical features include stiff, thick-walled trichomes (500 μm) often with spiral thickenings and abundant clusters and prisms of calcium oxalate in the leaf mesophyll. Stomata are mainly of the anomocytic, occasionally anisocytic type. Pollen grains are ovoid to subspherical (up to 60 μm × 35 μm) with three pores and a smooth, thin exine.

The *BP* drug is required to contain a minimum of 2.0% tannins, expressed as pyrogallol when assayed by the official 'determination of tannins in herbal drugs'. The TLC test of identification exploits the flavonoid content (rutin and isoquercitroside as test substances). Vitamins, triterpenes, volatile oil have also been reported as components of the drug.

Among other herbal uses, agrimony is employed as a mild astringent, internally and externally, against inflammation of the throat and for gastroenteritis.

ALCHEMILLA

The flowering and aerial parts of the lady's mantle, *Alchemilla xanthochlora* (*A. vulgaris sensu latiore*), family Rosaceae, are described in the *BP/EP* and *BHP* 1996. The plant is widespread in Europe, North America and Asia; commercial supplies are obtained principally from Eastern Europe. In addition to the identification by macroscopic and microscopic characters the pharmacopoeias include thin-layer chromatographic tests providing characteristic fluorescent zones.

The *BP/EP* drug is required to contain not less than 6.0% of tannins expressed as pyrogallol when determined by the official method (cf. Hamamelis and Rhatany). The characterized ellagitannins are pedunculagin and the dimeric alchemillin. Other constituents are flavonoids, quercetin 3-*O*-β-D-glucoside having been isolated as the major flavonoid in leaves of French origin.

Alchemilla acts as an astringent against bleeding and diarrhoea and has a long tradition of use for gynaecological conditions such as menorrhagia.

RHATANY

Rhatany of the *BP* and *EP* (*Krameria*) is the dried root of *Krameria triandra* (Krameriaceae, a small family related to the Leguminosae), a small shrub with decumbent branches about 1 m long. The drug is collected in Bolivia and Peru and is known in commerce as Peruvian rhatany.

The root has a knotty crown several centimetres in diameter and gives off numerous branch roots some of which attain a length of 60 cm. The roots are nearly cylindrical and are covered with a reddish-brown cork, which is scaly except in very young roots. A transverse section shows a reddish-brown bark which occupies about one-third of the radius and encloses a yellowish, finely radiate wood. A small, deeply coloured heartwood is sometimes present in the larger species. The bark readily separates from the wood. The former is astringent but the latter almost tasteless.

The tannins of krameria root (krameria-tannic acid) are entirely of the condensed (proanthocyanidin) type having a 'polymeric' flavin-3-ol structure. In this instance there is a procyanidin:propelargonidin ratio of 35:65 as determined by acid hydrolysis. Astringency of the root is due to compounds with a degree of polymerization of more than five. (For further details see E. Scholz and H. Rimpler, *Planta Med.*, 1989, **55**, 379). A phlobaphene (krameria-red), starch and calcium oxalate are also present. Stahl and Ittel (1981) reported the isolation of two benzofuran derivatives, ratanhiaphenols I and II, from the root. Both compounds are effective u.v. light filters and could be useful in sunprotection preparations. The *BP* and *EP* include an assay for tannins (polyphenols) of not less than 5.0% based on the colour reaction involving alkaline sodium phosphomolybdotungstate (absorbance measured at 760 nm). Polyphenols not adsorbed by hide powder, also determined with the same reagent, are excluded from the calculation.

The drug is used as an astringent and the significant antimicrobial activity of the extract gives rational support for its use in mouth and throat infections.

Ratanhiaphenol I: R^1 = H; R^2 = Me; R^3 = OH
Ratanhiaphenol II: R^1 = Me; R^2 = R^3 = H

Allied species. The roots of several other species are occasionally encountered in commerce, but the Peruvian drug is the only one generally available. *Krameria cystisoides* of Mexican origin has indigenous medicinal uses. It contains over 20 compounds of the lignan, neolignan and norneolignan type. Similar constituents are reported for *K. lanceolata*; see H. Achenbach *et al.*, *Phytochemistry*, 1987, **26**, 1159; 1989, **28**, 1959.

Pomegranate rind

The pomegranate fruit is one of the oldest known to man and has featured in mythology, and as a food and medicine from ancient civilizations of the Middle East to its present wide cultivation in India and surrounding countries, Turkey, southern Europe and California.

Pomegranate rind consists of the dried pericarp of the fruit of *Punica granatum* (Punicaceae). It occurs in thin, curved pieces about 1.5 mm thick, some of which bear the remains of the woody calyx or a scar left by the stalk. The outer surface is brownish-yellow or reddish. The inner surface bears impressions left by the seeds. Pomegranate rind, used in India as a herbal remedy for non-specific diarrhoea, is very astringent and contains about 28% of tannin (ellagitannins) and colouring matters. It should be distinguished from the root bark, which contains alkaloids.

For a discussion of the biochemistry, health effects, commercialization, plant growth and improvement of the pomegranate fruit, see N. P. Seeram *et al.* (eds), R. Hardman (series ed.) 2006 Medicinal and aromatic plants – industrial profiles, Vol 43. Pomegranate. CRC Press, Taylor and Francis Group. Boca Raton, FL., 244 pp.

Aspidosperma barks

The bark of *Aspidosperma quebracho-blanco* (Apocynaceae), which is used as a tanning material, was formerly official in several pharmacopoeias.

Myrobalans

Myrobalans are the dried fruits of *Terminalia chebula* (Combretaceae), a tree common in India. The immature fruits are black, ovoid and about 1–3 cm long. They contain about 20–40% of tannin, β-sitosterol, anthraquinones and a fixed oil containing principally esters of palmitic, oleic and linoleic acids. The tannin and anthraquinone constituents make the drug both astringent and cathartic in action. Microbiological tests support the Indian use of an aqueous extract of the fruit as an anti-caries agent (A. G. Jagtap and S. G. Karkera, *J. Ethnopharmacology*, 1999, **68**, 299).

CATECHU

Gambir or pale catechu of the *BP* 1989; *BP* (Veterinary), 2007 is a dried, aqueous extract prepared from the leaves and young twigs of a climbing shrub, *Uncaria gambir* (Rubiaceae). It must be carefully distinguished from black catechu or cutch. The plant is a native of Malaya and it is largely cultivated for the production of the drug in Indonesia and Malaya for marketing through Singapore.

History. The catechu described by Barbosa (1514) was black catechu or cutch, and the first account of gambir appears to be that of a Dutch trader in 1780. In addition to the cube gambir used in pharmacy, large blocks of the extract are imported for use in dyeing and tanning. Other forms are used in the East for chewing with betel leaf.

Preparation. The preparation of catechu in Johore differs only slightly from the procedure adopted in Indonesia. It consists of extracting the leaves and young twigs with boiling water, evaporating the extract to a pasty consistency and dividing it into cubes, which are then sun-dried. Fuller details of the preparation are given in the 10th edition.

Many different forms of catechu are used in the East, and the drug for the Eastern market frequently has 20–50% of fine rice husks added as the liquid coagulates in the tubs. Such catechu is, of course, unofficial, and contains starch.

Macroscopical characters. Catechu occurs in cubes, which are very friable and may be broken up in transit or, if incompletely dried, may be more or less agglutinated. Of the samples available, those from Indonesia measure 17–22 mm and have a reddish-brown surface, often stamped with a maker's mark, while those from Johore measure 24–29 mm and have a blackish exterior and the faces of the cube are depressed. Internally, both varieties are cinnamon-brown and porous. Odourless; taste, very astringent and at first somewhat bitter, afterwards sweetish.

Microscopical characters. When mounted in water, catechu shows minute, acicular crystals of catechin, many of which are branched and interlacing. They dissolve on warming and a considerable amount of vegetable debris is left. The leaves, particularly the stipules, bear simple, unicellular hairs up to about 350 μm long, with smooth, moderately thick, lignified walls. The twigs have lignified pericyclic fibres, wood fibres, and spiral, annular and pitted vessels. Minute starch grains are commonly present, particularly in the Indonesian drug, but the amount should be strictly limited. Rice husks have been observed in some samples.

Chemical tests

1. *For gambir-fluorescin.* Extract a little of the powdered drug with alcohol and filter. To the filtrate add solution of sodium hydroxide. After shaking, add a few millilitres of light petroleum, shake again and allow to stand. The petroleum spirit layer shows a strong green fluorescence.
2. *For catechin.* This is a modification of the usual test for lignin. Phloroglucinol is formed from catechin and with hydrochloric acid turns a matchstick red.

Constituents. Gambir contains about 7.33% of catechins, 22–50% of catechutannic acid, catechu red, quercitin and gambir-fluorescin.

BP (Vet.) 2007 standards include a loss on drying of not more than 15.0% and a water-insoluble matter of not more than 33.0% with reference to the dried material.

Catechin forms white, acicular crystals which are soluble in hot water and alcohol and give a green colour with ferric salts. Catechutannic acid is an amorphous phlobatannin which appears to be formed from catechin by loss of the elements of water. It readily yields the phlobaphene catechu-red. If the drug is carefully prepared, it will contain a high proportion of catechin and correspondingly smaller amounts of catechutannic acid and catechu-red.

Allied drug. *Cutch* or *black catechu* is an extract prepared from the heartwood of *Acacia catechu* (Leguminosae). Cutch occurs in black, somewhat porous masses. The taste resembles that of gambir. Microscopical examination of the water-soluble residue shows wood fibres and large vessels and sometimes fragments derived from the leaves on which the drug is spread.

Cutch contains 2–12% of catechins, 25–33% of phlobatannin, 20–30% of gummy matter, quercitrin, quercitin, moisture, etc. It yields 2–3% of ash. The catechin (acacatechin) is not identical with that in gambir.

The drug may be distinguished from gambir as it gives no reaction for gambir-fluorescin.

Uses. Catechu is used in medicine as an astringent.

Kinos

The name 'kino' has been applied to a number of dried juices, rich in phlobatannins and formerly used for their astringent properties. They include Malabar kino from *Pterocarpus marsupium* (Leguminosae), butea gum or Bengal kino from *Butea frondosa* (*B. monosperma*) (Leguminosae) and eucalyptus kino or red gum from *Eucalyptus rostrata* (Myrtaceae).

Croton lechleri

The bark of this and related euphorbiaceous trees yield, when slashed, a blood-red sap commonly known in South American folk medicine as Sangre de Grado, Sangre de Drace, or dragon's blood (not to be confused with the dragon's blood obtained from species of *Daemonorops* palms, q.v.). It is used locally for its anti-infective, antitumour and wound-healing properties. Cai *et al.* (*Phytochemistry*, 1991, **30**, 2033; 1993, **32**, 755) have shown proanthocyanidins to be the principal constituents (*c.* 90%) which vary from monomers to heptamers. These polyphenols possess oxygen free-radical scavenging activity and may assist in wound healing (C. Desmarchelier *et al.*, *J. Ethnopharmacology*, 1997, **58**, 103). Minor components isolated are phenols, alcohols, sterols and four diterpenoids, two of the latter being of the clerodane type. An alkaloid, tapsine, has been ascribed as the wound healing constituent; it could also account for the antitumour activity claimed for the latex (Z. Chen *et al.*, *Planta Medica*, 1994, **60**, 541).

Further reading

For various aspects of the chemotaxonomy, chemistry, biosynthesis, enzymology and health factors of tannins and related polyphenols, see
D. Ferreira *et al* (eds) *Phytochemistry* 2005, **66**, 1969–2120, (Pt 1); 2124–2291 (Pt 11)

COUMARINS AND GLYCOSIDES

Derivatives of benzo-α-pyrone such as coumarin (the lactone of *O*-hydroxycinnamic acid), aesculetin, umbelliferone and scopoletin are common in plants both in the free state and as glycosides. Not all are phenolic but they are included here with the phenolic derivatives for convenience. Some 1000 natural coumarins have been isolated. Coumarin itself has been found in about 150 species belonging to over 30 different families, although it is probably present in the undamaged plant as *trans-O*-glucosyloxycinnamic acid. Enzyme activity in the damaged tissue leads to a loss of glucose and a *trans → cis* isomerization followed by ring closure. Coumarin gives a characteristic odour of new-mown hay and occurs in many Leguminosae such as sweet clover, melitot and tonco beans; the latter contain about 1–3% of coumarin. It is also recorded in woodruff, *Asperula odorata* (Rubiaceae) and cassia oil.

In ammoniacal solution these compounds have a blue, blue–green or violet fluorescence, which has long been used as a qualitative test for certain umbelliferous resins such as asafoetida and galbanum. The fluorescence is, of course, more marked if examined in filtered ultra-violet light and is used for the chromatographic visualization of the compounds.

The substitution patterns of some common hydroxy and methoxy coumarins are given in Table 21.2. Structurally more complex coumarins such as the calanolides and inophyllums have received recent attention as potent HIV-1-RT inhibitors (see Chapter 32).

The *furanocoumarins* are closely related to the above and occur particularly in the Rutaceae and Umbellifeare. For example, celery fruits contain rutaretin and its dehydrated derivative apiumetin. Bergapten occurs in bergamot oil and in the Chinese root-drug derived from *Peucedanum decursivum* (Umbelliferae) which also contains the less-common *pyranocoumarins*. Marmesin derivatives (Fig. 13.2) and archangelicin have a reduced furanocoumarin structure consisting of coumarin and a C_5 sub-unit. Other prenylated compounds are the 3-iso-prenylcoumarins, as illustrated by rutamarin of the genus *Ruta*; for recent research on *R. graveolens* see S. D. Srivastava *et al.*, *Fitoterapia*, 1998, **69**, 80. A wide range of biological activities has been demonstrated for these metabolites (see R. H. Galán *et al.*, *Phytochemistry*, 1990, **29**, 2053).

Furanocoumarins are responsible at least in part for the unpredictable and variable effects on drug availability resulting from the consumption of grapefruit juice. Two components of the juice (6', 7'-dihydroxybergamottin and FC26) inactivate cytochrome P450 enzymes (specifically CYP3A4 and CYP3A5) resulting in an increased oral bioavailability of various drugs used to treat cancer, hypertension, heart disease and allergies. However, unnamed constituents of the juice have recently been shown to activate the efflux pump controlling P-glycoprotein-mediated drug transport which secretes absorbed drugs back into the gut. *In vitro* studies have demonstrated reduced absorption of vinblastine, cyclosporin, losartan, digoxin and fexofenadine. The two effects are therefore antagonistic and explain the unpredictable action of grapefruit juice on drug bioavailability. For reports on this research see *The Lancet*, 1999, **353**, 1335; *Pharm. J.*, 1999, **262**, 573; *HerbalGram*, 1998, No. 43, 22.

Table 21.2 Hydroxy and methoxy coumarins.

Compound	Additional groupings	Occurrence
Umbelliferone	HO at 7 (above)	Belladonna and stramonium (Solanaceae): *Daphne mezereum* (Thymeliaceae); *Ferula* species yielding asafoetida and galbanum, and many other Umbelliferae, chicory leaves (Compositae)
Herniarin	CH$_3$O at 7	*Lavandula spica* (Labiatae), *Ruta graveolens* (Umbelliferae) and certain Compositae
Aesculetin	HO at 6, HO at 7	Horse-chestnut (Hippocastanaceae), certain Rosaceae and *Fraxinus* (Oleaceae)
Scopoletin	CH$_3$O at 6, HO at 7	Roots of gelsemium, oat, jalap, scammony, scopolia and belladonna; leaves of tobacco, stramonium, chicory and many others
Fraxin	CH$_3$O at 6, HO at 7, *O*-glucose at 8	*Fraxinus* spp. (Oleaceae)
Chicoriin	CH$_3$O at 6, *O*-glucose at 7	*Cichorium intybus* herb

Ammi species contain furanomethoxycoumarins but are more important for their content of furanobenzo-γ-pyrones (q.v. under 'Flavones').

Bicoumarins are formed from two coumarin moieties and the linkage may occur in a number of ways. Dicoumarol is formed at C3–C3′ through a methylene group and was, in 1941, the first of the series to be isolated. It is a constituent of fermenting hay and is formed by microbial action of coumarin. It is a powerful anticoagulant and haemorrhagic and can cause the death of animals consuming the spoiled fodder.

Further reading

Estévez-Braun A, González RG 1997 Coumarins (1995–1996). Natural Product Reports 14(5): 465–476

Murray RDH 1995 Coumarins (1988–1994). Natural Product Reports 12(5): 477–506

ANGELICA ROOT

The root of the official drug (*BP, EP, BHP*) consists of the rhizome and root of *Angelica archangelica* L. (*A. officinalis* Haffm.) (Umbelliferae), whole or cut and carefully dried. It is required to contain not less than 0.2% of volatile oil. The North American root is derived from *A. atropurpurea* and the Chinese from a number of species under the name *man-mu* or *tangkuei*.

The rhizomes are vertical and up to 5 cm in diameter, greyish-brown or reddish-brown in colour, bearing leaf and stem scars at the apex. Entwined, longitudinally furrowed, roots occur on the lower surface. The fracture is uneven and the transverse surface shows brown spots, indicating secretory cells, situated in the spongy, radiate, off-white bark. Microscopy of the powder shows, among other features, numerous simple starch grains 2–4 μm, yellowish-brown secretory canals, cork cells and lignified reticulately thickened vessels.

Considerable recent work on the genus has resulted in the isolation of a number of furanocoumarins and their glycosides; the formulae of bergapten, angelicin, archangelicin (a diester) and apterin are given in Fig. 21.8, and those of marmesin and psoralen in Fig. 13.2. These compounds are reported to have potent coronary vasodilator effects and are calcium antagonists. Monoterpenes constitute the major components (80–90%) of the volatile oil.

There are official limits for foreign matter, loss on drying (≯10%), total ash (≯10%) and acid-insoluble ash (≯2.0%).

In herbal medicine the root is indicated in the treatment of bronchitis associated with vascular deficiency, and dyspeptic conditions.

MELILOT

Melilot *BP/EP, BHP* 1996 consists of the dried flowering tops of *Melilotus officinalis* (L.) Lam, (common melilot, ribbed melilot, king's clover, yellow sweet clover), family Leguminosae/Papilionaceae. It is found throughout Europe and eastwards to western China, N. America, except the far north, and elsewhere often as a weed of cultivation, probably introduced into Britain, together with other melilots (of which there are three common species), in the 16th century. Habitats include fields, hedgerows and waste places.

Melilot is an erect or decumbent branched biennial up to 100 cm tall. The finely ridged glabrous stems bear alternate stalked trifoliate leaves with two stipules joined to the base of the petiole. The leaflets of the upper leaves are oblong–elliptic, each with acute apex and base, margin entire. The yellow papillionaceous flowers occur in racemes up to 5 cm in length and give rise to almost straight glabrous pods, brown when ripe and transversely rugose. Seeds are wrinkled giving the 'ribbed' of the common name.

Features of the powdered drug include numerous anisocytic stomata with between three and six subsidiary cells on both epidermi; uniseriate covering trichomes composed of two small basal cells and a longer, bent, somewhat warty terminal cell; a few glandular trichomes with a two- to three-celled stalk and biseriate head of four cells; prismatic crystals of calcium oxalate associated with the vascular tissue; papillose epidermal cells of the petals; lignified fibrous anther fragments; spherical–ovoid pollen grains about 25 μm across with three pores and a smooth exine.

Constituents. Coumarin derivatives occur in melilot although coumarin itself is not present to any extent in the living plant. It arises when the plant is crushed, or the dried material treated with water, by the action of a β-gluconidase enzyme specific to *cis-o*-hydroxycinnamic acid glucoside giving first the unstable hydrolytic product coumarinic acid, which then cyclizes to coumarin producing the well-known 'new-mown hay' odour. The *trans*-isomer remains unchanged and is isolated as melilotoside (see F. Bourgoud *et al.*, *Phytochem. Anal.*, 1994, **5**, 127; P. Bradley *British Herbal Compendium*,

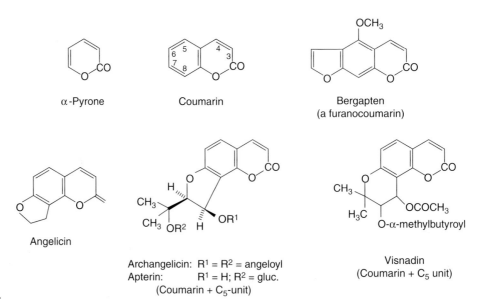

Fig. 21.8
Coumarin and derivatives.

α-Pyrone   Coumarin   Bergapten (a furanocoumarin)

Angelicin

Archangelicin: R¹ = R² = angeloyl
Apterin: R¹ = H; R² = gluc.
(Coumarin + C₅-unit)

Visnadin (Coumarin + C₅ unit)

Dihydro-*o*-coumaric acid
(Melilotic acid)

Melilotoside

Vol. 2, 2006, p. 270). Other acids isolated from melilot include dihydro-*o*-coumaric acid (melilotic acid), caffeic acid and other minor acids. Various oleanene saponins, volatile compounds and flavonoids have also been reported.

The pharmacopoeial TLC identification test for melilot indicates the presence of coumarin and possibly *o*-coumaric acid in the genuine drug. Assay of the coumarin content, minimum 0.3%, involves absorbance measurements at 275 nm on a boiled methanolic extract of the powder.

The various traditional medical uses of the drug have yet to be firmly established by clinical trials.

Tonco seed

Tonco seed or Tonquin beans are the dried seeds of *Dipteryx odorata* Willd. (*Coumarouna odorata* Aubl.) and *Dipteryx oppositifolia* (Leguminosae). The former plant is a native of Guiana and Brazil and is extensively cultivated in Venezuela, while the latter is found in Guiana and northern Brazil. Both are large trees bearing single-seeded fruits about 3–5 cm long.

The fruits are collected when ripe (May and June), they are opened and the seeds are dried in the sun. If sold without further treatment, they are known as 'black' beans. The seeds produced in Venezuela and near its border are larger than those produced in northern Brazil and parts of Guiana. The former, which are more highly valued, are known as 'Angostura' and the latter as 'Para' beans. Large quantities of both Angostura and Para beans are sent to Trinidad, where they are macerated for 24 h in rum and dried in the open air. This treatment causes a crystalline deposit of coumarin to be formed on the testa and the seeds are said to be 'frosted'. Angostura and Para beans thus occur in commerce both black and frosted.

Tonco beans are up to 40 mm long, 10 mm wide and 5 mm thick. They are rounded at one end and bluntly pointed at the other. The surface is black and deeply wrinkled longitudinally, a crystalline encrustation being present in the frosted variety. A transverse section shows a very thin, black testa and two yellowish-brown, planoconvex, oily cotyledons. Odour, very fragrant; taste, aromatic and bitter.

Tonco beans contain 1–3% of coumarin, 25% of fat (containing unsaponifiable sitosterin and stigmasterin) and a larger amount of starch. Ash about 3.5%. Tonco beans are used in tobacco manufacture and in perfumery. Synthetic coumarin has, to some extent, replaced the natural product.

Celery fruit. *Apium; Apii Fructus*

The drug consists of the dried ripe fruits of *Apium graveolens* (Umbelliferae).

The cremocarp is brown, subspherical and about 1–1.5 mm long. The mericarps are mostly separate in the drug and each shows five straight primary ridges. A transverse section is almost pentagonal and shows 6–9 vittae, two on the commissural surface and four to seven in the grooves of the dorsal surface. Odour and taste, aromatic. Celery fruits contain 2–3% of oil consisting of terpenes with smaller quantities of the anhydride of sedanonic acid, the lactone of sedanolic acid and phenols. The fruits also contain a number of coumarins, furanocoumarins and coumarin glycosides.

Celery fruits are official in the *BHP* and have a long-standing use in the treatment of rheumatic diseases; the therapeutic action appears to be potentiated by Taraxacum (q.v.).

ANTHRAQUINONES AND GLYCOSIDES

Long before anything was known of their chemistry, rhubarb, aloes, senna and cascara were recognized as forming a natural group of purgative drugs. Also certain vegetable and animal dyestuffs such as madder and cochineal were of great economic importance before the introduction of synthetic dyestuffs. Later the chemical similarity of these purgative drugs and dyestuffs became apparent, as illustrated by the formulae for emodin (the aglycone of a number of purgative glycosides of *Rhamnus* spp.) and alizarin (the aglycone of a dyestuff of the madder plant).

Emodin

Alizarin

Substances of the anthraquinone type were the first to be recognized, both in the free state and as glycosides. Further work showed that natural products also contained reduced derivatives of the anthraquinones (oxanthrones, anthranols and anthrones) and compounds formed by the union of two anthrone molecules (i.e. the dianthrones).

Because glycosides are often easily hydrolysed, the earlier workers tended to isolate products of hydrolysis rather than the primary glycosides. The following aglycones have long been established: chrysophanol or chrysophanic acid from rhubarb and cascara; aloe-emodin from rhubarb and senna; rhein from rhubarb and senna; emodin or frangula-emodin from rhubarb and cascara. Improved extraction methods, developed by Stoll and his colleagues, led to the isolation of the main senna glycosides, sennosides A and B, in 1941. Since this date many new glycosides including *C*-glycosides and various stereoisomers have been isolated and their structures determined.

In monocotyledons, anthraquinone derivatives are found only in the Liliaceae, in the form of the unusual *C*-glycoside barbaloin. Among dicotyledons they occur in the Rubiaceae, Leguminosae, Polygonaceae, Rhamnaceae, Ericaceae, Euphorbiaceae, Lythraceae, Saxifragaceae, Scrophulariaceae and Verbenaceae. They appear to be absent from the Bryophyta, Pteridophyta and Gymnosperms but occur in certain fungi and lichens. The fungal anthraquinone pigments are nearly all chrysophanol or emodin derivatives.

As indicated in Chapter 18, natural anthraquinones are synthesized either via the acetate–malonate pathway or they are derived from shikimate and mevalonate. The medicinally important purgative anthraquinones are formed by the former route and all have a 1,8-dihydroxy substitution. Conversely, compounds such as alizarin which have one of the rings unsubstituted arise by the second pathway. The relationships between the oxidized and reduced forms of the anthraquinone nucleus are shown in Fig. 21.9.

Modern research indicates that the 1,8-dihydroxyanthraquinone derivatives frequently occur with 1,8-dihydroxynaphthalene glycosides.

Anthraquinones

The derivatives of anthraquinone present in purgative drugs may be dihydroxy phenols such as chrysophanol, trihydroxy phenols such as emodin or tetrahydroxy phenols such as carminic acid. Other groups are often present, for example, methyl in chrysophanol, hydroxymethyl in aloe-emodin and carboxyl in rhein and carminic acid.

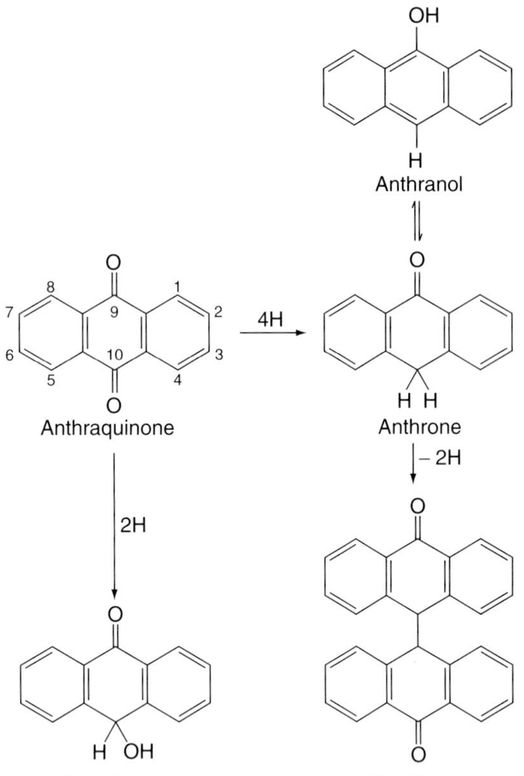

Fig. 21.9
Interrelationship of anthraquinone derivatives.

When such substances occur as glycosides, the sugar may be attached in various positions. See formulae for carminic acid and glucofrangulin. Some examples of anthraquinone derivatives are given in Table 21.3.

Anthraquinone derivatives are often orange-red compounds, which may sometimes be observed *in situ* (e.g. in the medullary rays of rhubarb and cascara). They are usually soluble in hot water or dilute alcohol. Bornträger's test is often used for their detection. The powdered drug is macerated with an immiscible organic solvent, ether is recommended, and after filtration aqueous ammonia or caustic soda is added, when a pink, red or violet colour in the aqueous layer after shaking indicates the presence of free anthraquinone derivatives. If glycosides only are present, the test should be modified by first hydrolysing with alcoholic potassium hydroxide solution or 2 M acid. When alkali is added to powdered drugs or to sections, the red colour produced serves to locate the anthraquinone derivatives in the tissues (e.g. in the medullary rays of cascara bark). If the drug being tested contains either very stable anthraquinone glycosides or reduced derivatives of the anthranol type, Bornträger's test will be negative.

Anthraquinones containing a free carboxylic acid group (e.g. rhein) can be separated from other anthraquinones by extraction from an organic solution with sodium bicarbonate solution.

Anthranols and anthrones

These reduced anthraquinone derivatives occur either free or combined as glycosides. They are isomeric and one may be partially converted to the other in solution. The parent substance, anthrone, is a pale yellow, non-fluorescent substance which is insoluble in alkali; its isomer, anthranol, is brownish-yellow and forms a strongly fluorescent solution in alkali. Anthranol derivatives, such as are found in aloes, have similar properties, and the strong green fluorescence which aloes give in borax or other alkaline solution has long been used as a test for its identification. Anthranols and anthrones are the main constituents of chrysarobin, a mixture of substances prepared by benzene extraction from the material (araroba) found in the trunk cavities of the tree *Andira araroba*. If a little chrysarobin is treated on a white tile with a drop of fuming nitric acid, the anthranols are converted into anthraquinones. A drop of ammonia allowed to mix gradually with the acid liquid produces a violet colour. This modification of Bornträger's test had been used as a test for identity before the underlying chemistry was known.

Oxanthrones

The formula given shows that these are intermediate products between anthraquinones and anthranols. They give anthraquinones on oxidation and Fairbairn's modification of the Bornträger test accomplishes this by means of hydrogen peroxide. An oxanthrone has been reported as a constituent of cascara bark.

Table 21.3 Anthraquinone glycosides and aglycones.

Glycoside	Aglycone	Sugar	OH Groups	Other groups	Occurrence
Ruberythric acid	Alizarin	Primeverose	1,2	–	*Rubia tinctorum*
Rubiadin primeveroside	Rubiadin	Primeverose	1,3	2-methyl	*Rubia tinctorum*
Rubiadin glucoside	Rubiadin	Glucose	1,3	2-methyl	*Rubia tinctorum*
Chrysophanein	Chrysophanol	Glucose	1,8	3-methyl	*Rheum* and *Rumex* spp.
Rheochrysin	Physcion	Glucose	1,8	3-methyl 6-methoxy	*Rheum* spp.
Glucorhein	Rhein	Glucose	1,8	3-carboxylic acid	*Rheum*, *Rumex* and *Cassia* spp.
Gluco aloe-emodin	Aloe-emodin	Glucose	1,8	3-hydroxymethyl	*Rheum* and *Cassia* spp.
Glucochrysaron	Chrysarone	Glucose	1,2,7	6-methyl	*Rheum rhaponticum*
Glucofrangulin A	Emodin	Glucose, rhamnose	1,6,8	3-methyl	*Rhamnus* spp.
Frangulin	Emodin	Rhamnose	1,6,8	3-methyl	*Rhamnus* spp.
Morindin	Morindone	Primeverose	1,5,6	2-methyl	*Morinda* spp. (Rubiaceae)
–	Islandicin	–	1,5,8	6-methyl	*Penicillium islandicum*
Carminic acid	–	Glucose	1,3,4,6	5-carboxylic acid 8-methyl	Cochineal

Aglycone (spanning OH Groups / Other groups)

Dianthrones

These are compounds derived from two anthrone molecules, which may be identical or different; they readily form as a result of mild oxidation of the anthrone or mixed anthrones (e.g. a solution in acetone and presence of atmospheric oxygen). They are important aglycones in species of *Cassia*, *Rheum* and *Rhamnus*; in this group the sennidins, aglycones of the sennosides (see formula), are among the best-known examples. Reidin A, B and C which occur in senna and rhubarb are heterodianthrones, i.e. composed of unlike anthrones, and involve aloe-emodin, rhein, chryophanol or physcion.

It will be noted that two chiral centres (at C-10 and C-10′) are present in the dianthrones, and for a compound having two identical anthrone moieties, e.g. sennidin A, two forms (the 10*S*, 10′*S* and 10*R*, 10′*R*) are possible together with the *meso* form (sennidin B). These compounds also occur in the plant as their 1,1′-diglucosides.

Aloin-type or *C*-glycosides

The aloin obtained from species of *Aloe*, although one of the first glycosides to be isolated, was a problem for investigators for a long time. It is strongly resistant to normal acid hydrolysis but may be oxidized with ferric chloride. A study of its degradation products and infrared spectrum indicated a sugar-like chain and the structure shown, in which the sugar is joined to the aglycone with a direct C–C linkage (a *C*-glycoside). Two aloins (A and B) are known and arise from the chiral centre at C-10; their separation by high-speed countercurrent chromatography (see Chapter 17) has been recently described (C. XueLi *et al.*, *J. Chrom. and Rel. Technol.*, 2007, **30**, 12).

Pharmacological action

The action of the anthraquinone laxatives is restricted to the large bowel; hence their effect is delayed for up to 6 h or longer. The nature of the peristaltic initiation is not known for certain but it has been suggested that the common anthraquinone and anthranol derivatives influence the ion transport across colon cells by inhibition of Cl⁻ channels (J. Hönig *et al.*, *Planta Med.*, 1992, **58** (Suppl. 1), A586).

SENNA LEAF

Senna (*Sennae Folium*) consists of the dried leaflets of *Cassia senna* L. (*C. acutifolia* Delile), which are known in commerce as Alexandrian or Khartoum senna, and of *Cassia angustifolia* Vahl, which are known in commerce as Tinnevelly senna. The senna plants are small shrubs of the family Leguminosae, about 1 m high, with paripinnate compound leaves. *C. senna* is indigenous to tropical Africa and is cultivated in the Sudan (Kordofan, Sennar). *C. angustifolia* is indigenous to Somaliland, Arabia, Sind and the Punjab, and is cultivated in South India (Tinnevelly). The botanical validity for distinguishing between the above two plants has been called in question (Brenan, *Kew Bull.*, 1958, 231), but Fairbairn and Shrestha (*Lloydia*, 1967, **30**, 67) reinvestigated the well-established character differences between the two commercial types (see below) and concluded that the distinction remains valid; any further investigation on the two varieties grown under identical conditions does not appear to have been reported.

History. Senna appears to have been used since the ninth or tenth century, its introduction into medicine being due to the Arabian physicians, who used both the leaves and the pods. It was formerly exported through Alexandria, from where the name of the Sudanese drug is derived.

Collection and preparation. Alexandrian senna is collected mainly in September, from both wild and cultivated plants. The branches bearing leaves and pods are dried in the sun and conveyed to Omdurman. Here the pods and large stalks are first separated by means of sieves (see 'Senna Fruit'). That which has passed through the sieves is then 'tossed' in shallow trays, the leaves working to the surface and heavier stalk fragments and sand to the bottom. The leaves are then graded, partly by means of sieves and partly by hand-picking into (1) whole leaves, (2) whole leaves and half-leaves mixed, and (3) siftings. The whole leaves are those usually sold to the public, while the other grades are used for making galenicals. The drug is packed, somewhat loosely, in bales and sent by rail to Port Sudan, from where it is exported.

Tinnevelly senna is obtained from cultivated plants of *Cassia angustifolia* grown in South India, N.W. Pakistan and Jammu, where the plants are more luxuriant than those found wild in Arabia. It may be grown either on dry land or in wetter conditions as a successor to rice. Being a legume, it usefully adds nitrogen to the soil. Owing to the careful way in which the drug is collected and compressed into bales, few leaflets are usually broken.

Aloin

Sennidin A (10*S*, 10′*S*)   Sennidin A (10*R*, 10′*R*)   Sennidin B (*meso*)

Macroscopical characters. Senna leaflets bear stout petiolules. The lamina has an entire margin, an acute apex, and a more or less asymmetric base. The surfaces are pubescent. Odour, slight but characteristic; taste, mucilaginous, bitterish and unpleasant.

Typical senna leaflets are shown in Fig. 21.10. The main differences between the two varieties are given in Table 21.4.

Microscopical characters. Senna leaflets have an isobilateral structure (see Fig. 41.4). The epidermal cells have straight walls, and many contain mucilage. Both surfaces bear scattered, unicellular, non-lignified warty hairs up to 260 μm long (Fig. 21.10D, G). The stomata have two cells with their long axes parallel to the pore and sometimes a third or fourth subsidiary cell (Fig. 21.10E, F). The mesophyll, consisting of

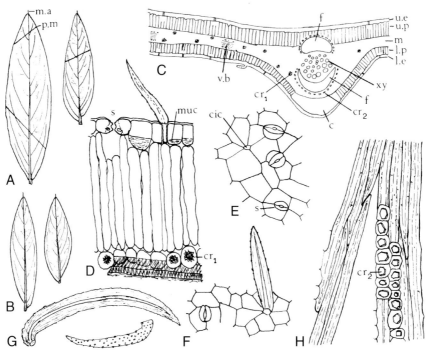

Fig. 21.10
Senna leaflets. A, Indian senna; B, Alexandrian senna (both ×1); C, transverse section of leaflet (×80); D–H, elements of the powder (all ×200); D, leaflet fragment in transverse section; E, F, epidermal fragments in surface view; G, isolated trichomes; H, portion of fibre group with crystal sheath, c, collenchyma; cic, cicatrix; cr₁, cr₂, calcium oxalate crystals of the cluster and prismatic type respectively; f, fibre groups; l.e, lower epidermis; l.p, lower palisade layer; m, mesophyll; muc, mucilage; m.a, mucronate apex; p.m, press mark; s, stoma (paracytic type); u.e, upper epidermis; u.p, upper palisade layer; xy, xylem.

Table 21.4 Comparison of Alexandrian and Indian senna leaves.

Alexandrian senna	Tinnevelly senna
Macroscopical characters	
Seldom exceed 40 mm in length	Seldom exceed 50 mm in length
Greyish-green	Yellowish-green
More asymmetric at base	Less asymmetric at base
Rather more broken and curled at the edges	Seldom broken and usually flat owing to compression
Few press markings	Often shows impressions due to the midvein of other leaflets
Microscopical characters	
Hairs more numerous, the average distance between each being about three epidermal cells	Hairs less numerous, the average distance between each being about six epidermal cells
Most of the stomata have two subsidiary cells only	The stomata having two or three subsidiary cells respectively are in the ratio of about 7:3
Vein-islet number 25–29.5	Vein-islet number 19.5–22.5
Stomatal index 10.0–15.0, usually 12.5	Stomatal index 14.0–20.0, usually 17.5
Chemical tests*	
Ether extract of hydrolysed acid solution of drug gives with methanolic magnesium acetate solution:	The same test:
a pink colour in daylight,	an orange colour in daylight,
a pale greenish-orange in filtered ultraviolet light	a yellowish-green in filtered ultraviolet light
TLC test for distinctive naphthalene derivatives†	
6-Hydroxymusizin glycoside present	Tinnevellin glycoside present

*For full details, see Nandy and Santra, *J. Ind. Pharm. Manuf.,* 1968, **6,** 235.
†See Lemli *et al., Planta Med.,* 1983, **49,** 36.

upper and lower palisade layers and median spongy mesophyll, contains cluster crystals about 15–20 μm in diameter. The midrib is biconvex. Below the midrib bundle is a zone of collenchyma. The midrib bundle and larger veins are almost surrounded by a zone of lignified pericyclic fibres and a sheath of parenchymatous cells containing prisms of calcium oxalate 10–20 μm long (Fig. 21.10 C).

Vein-islet numbers and stomatal indices can be used to distinguish the two species (see Table 21.4) and the *BP/EP* utilizes stomatal index.

Constituents. Since Tutin first isolated aloe-emodin and rhein in 1913, many other compounds based on these two have been obtained. Stoll *et al.* (1941) isolated two active crystalline glycosides, sennoside A and sennoside B. They both hydrolyse to give two molecules of glucose and the aglycones sennidin A and B. Sennidin A is dextro-rotatory and B is its mesoform formed by intramolecular compensation (Fig. 21.12).

The activity of senna was still not fully explained by the isolation of these constituents, and later work, notably by Fairbairn, Friedrich, Friedmann, Lemli and their associates demonstrated the presence of many other (some pharmacologically active) components. These include: sennosides C and D, which are the glycosides of heterodianthrones involving rhein and aloe-emodin; palmidin A (see 'Rhubarb'); aloe-emodin dianthrone-diglycoside, rhein-anthrone-8-glycoside, rhein-8-diglucoside, aloe-emodin-8-glucoside, aloe-emodin-anthrone-diglucoside, possibly rhein-1-glucose, and a primary glycoside having greater potency than sennosides A and B and distinguished from them by the addition of two glucose molecules. A new anthraquinone glycoside, emodin-8-*O*-sophoroside (a diglucoside), has been isolated in 0.0027% yield from dried Indian senna leaves (J. Kinjo *et al.*, *Phytochemistry*, 1994, **37**, 1685).

Two naphthalene glycosides isolated from senna leaves and pods (Lemli *et al.*, *Planta Med.*, 1981, **43**, 11) are 6-hydroxymusizin glucoside and tinnevellin glucoside. The former is found in Alexandrian senna and the latter in Indian senna; this difference has been used as a

6-Hydroxymusizin glucoside:
R¹ = R² = H; R³ = β-D-glucopyranosyl
Tinnevellin glucoside:
R¹ = H; R² = β-D-glucopyranosyl; R³ = Me

distinguishing feature of the commercial varieties, see Table 21.4. Senna also contains the yellow flavonol colouring matters kaempferol (3,4′,5,7-tetrahydroxyflavone), its glucoside (kaempferin) and isorhamnetin; also a sterol and its glucoside, mucilage, calcium oxalate and resin. The structures of water-soluble polysaccharides and a lignan have been reported.

Although senna is not noted for its volatile components, Tutin in his 1913 publication had observed the 'strongly aromatic dark-coloured essential oil'. Over 80 years later W. Schulz *et al.* (*Planta Medica*, 1996, **62**, 540) have again examined the volatiles of senna leaf and recorded (GC-MS) more than 200 components afforded by aqueous distillation. 122 constituents were identified including monoterpenes, phenylpropanes, fatty acids and esters, etc. Hexadecanoic acid was a significant component in addition to many of the more common constituents of volatile oils.

Formation and distribution of anthraquinone derivatives. In young senna seedlings chrysophanol is the first anthraquinone formed, then aloe-emodin appears and finally rhein; this ontogenetic sequence is in keeping with the expected biogenetic order, which involves the successive oxidation of the 3-methyl group of chrysophanol (Table 21.3). In the presence of light glycosylation follows and later the glycosides are translocated to the leaves and flowers. During fruit development the amounts of aloe-emodin glycoside and rhein glycoside fall markedly, and sennosides accumulate in the pericarp.

Lemli and Cuveele (*Planta Med.*, 1978, **34**, 311) considered that fresh leaves of *Cassia senna* contain anthrone glycosides only. By drying between 20 and 50°C these are enzymatically converted to dianthrone forms (sennosides). However, Zenk and coworkers (*Planta Med.*, 1981, **41**, 1) maintained that sennoside formation is not entirely an artefact arising through drying but that these compounds together with the monoanthrones, and their oxidized forms (anthraquinones), are part of a redox system of possible significance to the living cell.

The distribution of sennoside B (determined by Zenk and coworkers by immunoassay) was for a *C. angustifolia* plant (sample dried at 60°C): flowers 4.3%, leaves 2.8%, pericarp 2.4%, stems 0.2%, roots 0.05%. Within the flowers the anthers and filaments contained 7.2%, carpels and ovaries 5.8%, petals 5.2%, sepals 4.7% and flower stalks 3.2%.

Evaluation. It is difficult to remove all fragments of rachis, petiole and stalk from the drug, but the amount of these structures is limited by the *BP* to 3%. In the whole drug the percentage of these is determined by hand-picking and weighing, but with the powdered drug recourse has to be made to quantitative microscopy.

C. senna is cultivated in Russia and the leaves are harvested mechanically; this leads to unavoidable mixture with petioles and stems but, because the active constituents are similar in all parts of the plant, this does not affect the quality of the glycosidal extracts.

Lack of knowledge of the precise active principles of senna coupled with the synergistic action of various compounds hampered the development of a satisfactory chemical assay for the drug. The *BP/EP* determines the total senna leaf glycosides in terms of sennoside B (not less than 2.5%). This involves extraction of the glycosides and free anthraquinones from the leaves, removal of the free aglycones and hydrolysis and oxidation of the remaining sennosides and other glycosides to give rhein and some aloe-emodin, which are then determined spectrophotometrically. Chromatographic tests for the leaf are given in the *BP* and *EP*.

The leaves are officially required to give an acid-insoluble ash of not more than 2.5%.

Allied drugs. *Bombay, Mecca* and *Arabian Sennas* are obtained from wild plants of *C. angustifolia* grown in Arabia. Some of the leaflets are shipped to Port Sudan and are graded like the Alexandrian drug, while some are sent to Bombay and frequently arrive in England with shipments of the Tinnevelly.

The leaflets resemble those of Tinnevelly senna but are somewhat more elongated and narrower, and of a brownish or brownish-green colour. Levin (1929) states that they may be distinguished microscopically from other sennas by their vein islet number.

Dog senna, a variety formerly much esteemed and still used in France, is derived from *Cassia obovata*. The plant is indigenous to Upper Egypt, but was cultivated in Italy in the sixteenth century. The leaves are obovate and quite different in appearance from the official leaflets. When in powder they may be distinguished by the papillose cells of the lower epidermis. Maurin found them to contain 1.0–1.15% of anthraquinone derivatives.

Palthé senna, derived from *Cassia auriculata*, has been found in Indian senna. It may be distinguished by the long hairs, the crimson colour given when boiled with chloral hydrate solution or treated with 80% sulphuric acid and the absence of anthraquinone derivatives. The leaves of other parts of the plant are widely used in Ayurvedic medicine for rheumatism and diabetes. The antioxidant activity of the flowers has been recently demonstrated (L. Pari and M. Latha, *Pharm. Biol.*, 2002, **40**, 512; A. Kumaran and R. J. Karunakaran, *Fitoterapia*, 2007, **78**, 46).

The leaflets of other species of *Cassia* have also been imported, but may be distinguished from the genuine drug by the characters given above.

For Nigeria, the leaves of the local *Cassia podocarpa* have been suggested as a substitute for the official senna; bioassays have given an equivalent activity (A. A. Elujoba and G. O. Iweibo, *Planta Med.*, 1988, **54**, 372).

C. alata produces anthraquinone derivatives and has been used traditionally in Thailand as a laxative. Root cultures have been studied for their anthraquinone-producing properties (N. Chatsiriwej *et al.*, *Pharm. Biol.*, 2006, **44**, 416).

Substitute. *Argel leaves*, which are derived from *Solenostemma arghel* (Asclepiadaceae), were at one time regularly mixed in a definite proportion with Alexandrian senna. The plant occurs in the Sudan, but the leaves are now seldom seen in commerce. If used to adulterate senna powder, it may be distinguished by the two- or three-celled hairs, each of which is surrounded by about five subsidiary cells.

SENNA FRUIT

Senna pods (*Sennae Fructus*) are the dried, ripe fruits of *C. senna* and *C. angustifolia* (Leguminosae), which are known as Alexandrian and Tinnevelly senna pods, respectively. Both have separate monographs in the *BP/EP*.

Collection. The pods are collected with the leaves and dried as described above. After separation from the leaves they are hand-picked into various qualities, the finer being sold in cartons and the inferior ones used for making galenicals.

Characters. The characteristic sizes and shapes of the two varieties are shown in Fig. 21.11. The Tinnevelly pods are longer and narrower than the Alexandrian and the brown area of pericarp surrounding the seeds is greater. The remains of the style are distinct in the Tinnevelly but not in the Alexandrian.

After soaking in water the pods are readily opened and about six wedge-shaped seeds are disclosed, each attached to the dorsal surface of the pod by a thin funicle (Fig. 21.11C). Under a lens the testas of

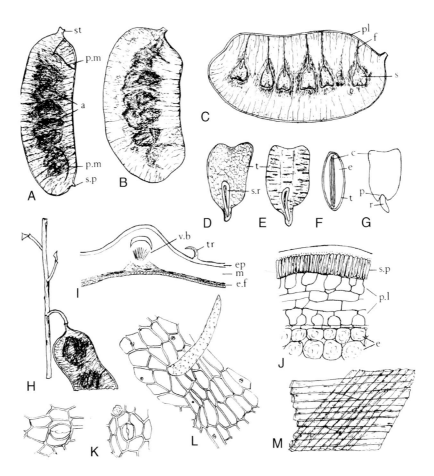

Fig. 21.11
Senna fruits. A, Tinnevelly fruit; B, Alexandrian fruit; C, Alexandrian pod opened to show seeds (all ×1); D, seed of Alexandrian fruit; E, seed of Tinnevelly fruit; F, transverse section of seed; G, isolated embryo with one cotyledon removed (all ×4); H, stem with Tinnevelly fruit attached (×1); I, transverse section of pericarp (×90;) J, transverse section of seed coat; K, fragments of epidermis with stomata; L, fragment of epidermis with trichome; M, fibrous layers from endocarp in surface view (all ×200); a, brown areas of pericarp covering seeds; c, cotyledons; e, endosperm; e.f, fibrous endocarp; ep, epicarp; f, funiculus; m, mesocarp; p, plumule; pl, placenta; p.l, parenchymatous layers of testa; p.m, press marks from other pods; r, radicle; s, seed; st, stalk; s.p, (J) subepidermal palisade; s.p, (A), stylar point; s.r, spathate ridge; tr, trichome; v.b, vascular bundle partially enclosed by fibres.

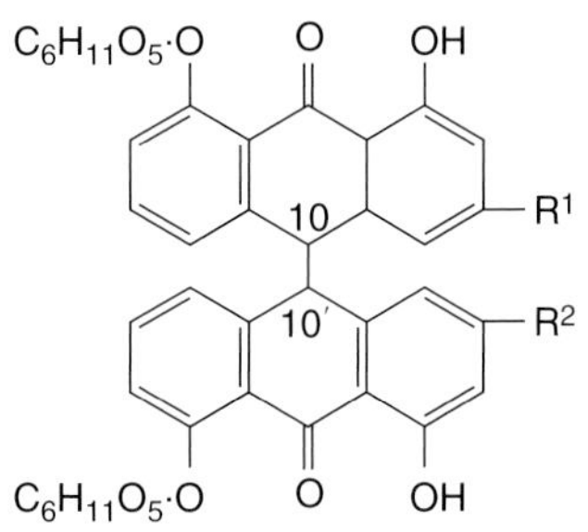

	R¹	R²	10–10′
Sennoside A	COOH	COOH	*trans*
Sennoside B	COOH	COOH	*meso*
Sennoside C	CH$_2$OH	COOH	*trans*
Sennoside D	CH$_2$OH	COOH	*meso*
Aloe-emodin-dianthrone-diglucoside	CH$_2$OH	CH$_2$OH	*trans*
Aloe-emodin-dianthrone-diglucoside	CH$_2$OH	CH$_2$OH	*meso*

Fig. 21.12
Constituents of Senna.

the Tinnevelly show a general reticulation and wavy, transverse ridges, while the Alexandrian show a general reticulation only (Fig. 21.11D, E). The pericarp of the pod bears unicellular hairs and stomata of a type similar to those found on senna leaves; portions of the fibrous layer of the endocarp are very evident in the powder (Fig. 21.11K, L, M).

Constituents. The active constituents of the pods are located in the pericarp; they are similar to those of the leaves, together with sennoside A, which constitutes about 15% of the sennoside mixture. The seeds contain very little sennoside but Zenk's group reported the cotyledons of 3-day-old seedlings to contain amounts equivalent to those in the leaves. Sennoside content varies from about 1.2 to 2.5% in the Tinnevelly (*BP/EP* ≮2.2%) and from about 2.5 to 4.5% in the Alexandrian (*BP/EP* ≮3.4%). C. Terreaux *et al.* (*Planta Medica*, 2002, **68**, 349) have reported the isolation of kaempferol and tinnevellin 8-glucoside from an extract of the Tinnevelly pods together with two new carboxylated benzophenone glucosides. Preparations of the powdered pericarp, e.g. Senna Tablets *BP*, standardized in terms of sennoside B, are now commonly prescribed.

Uses. The use of laxatives is increasing and senna constitutes a useful purgative for either habitual constipation or occasional use. It lacks the astringent after-effect of rhubarb. Despite the availability of a number of synthetics, sennoside preparations remain among the most important pharmaceutical laxatives.

Cassia pods

Cassia pods are the dried ripe fruits of *Cassia fistula* (Leguminosae), a large tree thought to be indigenous to India but now widely cultivated in the tropics. The drug is chiefly obtained from the West Indies (Dominica and Martinique) and Indonesia.

The fruit is a cylindrical indehiscent pod about 25–30 cm long and 20–25 mm diameter. It is dark chocolate brown to black in colour and contains from 25 to 100 oval, reddish-brown seeds separated by membranous dissepiments. In the fresh pods the seeds are completely embedded in black pulp, which, however, gradually dries on the septa. For this reason pods which do not rattle when shaken are usually preferred. The pulp has a prune-like odour and a sweetish taste.

The pulp is dissolved from the crushed fruit by percolation with water. The percolate is strained and evaporated to a soft extract. The most important anthraquinone derivatives of the pulp appear to be rhein and combined sennidin-like compounds. Anthraquinones have been detected in non-differentiating callus cultures. Cassia pulp also contains about 50% of sugars, colouring matter and a trace of volatile oil. The leaves of *C. fistula* contain free and combined rhein, sennidins and sennosides A and B; these compounds exhibit a marked seasonable fluctuation. The heartwood is reported to contain barbaloin and rhein together with a leucoanthocyanidin.

Cassia pulp was formerly used in the form of Confection of Senna. In Ayurvedic medicine the plant is used to treat a variety of ailments. Its antifungal, antibacterial and laxative properties have been established and more recently (T. Bhakta *et al.*, *Pharm. Biol.*, 1998, **36**, 140) its antitussive activity has been demonstrated.

CASCARA BARK

Official cascara sagrada (*Sacred Bark, Chittern Bark*) is the dried bark of *Rhamnus purshianus* DC (*Frangula purshiana* (DC) A. Gray ex J. C. Cooper) (Rhamnaceae). The bark is collected from wild trees, which are 6–18 m high, growing on the Pacific coast of North America (British Columbia, Washington and Oregon). Depleted wild US sources encouraged cultivation of the tree in western Canada, the USA and Kenya but these efforts do not appear to be completely successful.

History. Cascara is a drug of comparatively recent introduction into modern medicine. According to tradition, a cascara, probably *R. californica*, was known to early Mexican and Spanish priests of California; *Rhamnus purshianus*, however, was not described until 1805 and its bark was not introduced into medicine until 1877.

The common, European buckthorn was well known to the Anglo-Saxons; its berries were official in the *London Pharmacopoeia* of 1650.

Collection and storage. The bark is collected from mid-April to the end of August, when it separates readily from the wood. Longitudinal incisions about 5–10 cm apart are first made in the trunk and the bark removed. The tree is then usually felled and the branch bark separated. The pieces are dried in the shade with the cork uppermost. Such material is referred to as 'natural' cascara but commercial supplies are now comminuted to give small even fragments known as 'evenized', 'processed' or 'compact' cascara. During preparation and storage the bark must be protected from rain and damp, or partial extraction of the constituents may occur or the bark may become mouldy. That the bark must be kept for at least 1 year before use is no longer a *BP* requirement but the bark appears to increase in medicinal value and price until it is about 4 years old. Many companies prefer to use bark which has been stored for considerably more than 1 year. To reduce freight and handling charges on the bark, large quantities of the extract are now imported directly.

Macroscopical characters.   The bark occurs in quills, or channelled or nearly flat pieces. All of these forms may attain 20 cm in length and are 1–4 mm thick, the thinner bark being most esteemed. The flat strips from the trunk are usually much wider (up to 10 cm) than the quills or channelled pieces (about 5–20 mm) obtained from the branches.

Cascara (Fig. 21.13A) bears a somewhat patchy, silvery-grey coat of lichens. Pieces bearing moss are also quite common. Between the patches of lichen may be seen a smooth, dark purplish-brown cork marked with lighter-coloured, transversely elongated lenticels. On scraping the cork, no bright purple inner cork is disclosed (distinction from *R. alnus*). The inner surface is dull purplish-brown to

black, striated longitudinally and somewhat corrugated transversely. The fracture is short and granular in the outer part, but somewhat fibrous in the phloem. In the yellowish-brown cortex and phloem lighter groups of sclerenchymatous cells and phloem fibres may be seen with a lens. They may be made more distinct by staining with phloroglucinol and hydrochloric acid. The medullary rays, which tend to curve together in groups, are well seen in sections mounted in potash. Odour, slight but characteristic; taste bitter.

Microscopical characters.   A transverse section of cascara bark (Fig. 21.13B–D) shows a partial coat of whitish lichen, some 10–15 layers of flattened cork cells with reddish-brown contents and a cortex composed of collenchyma, parenchyma and groups of sclereids. The collenchymatous cells show thickened pitted walls and contain chloroplasts filled with starch. Some of the parenchymatous cells also contain chloroplasts and starch; many of them contain a yellow substance coloured violet by alkalis and rosette crystals of calcium oxalate usually 6–10 μm diameter, but occasionally up to 45 μm diameter. The parenchymatous cells abutting on the groups of sclereids contain prisms of calcium oxalate. The sclereids are irregular or ovoid in

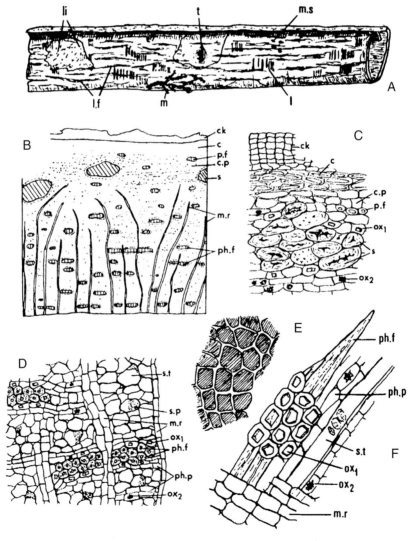

Fig. 21.13
Cascara bark. A, single quill (×0.66); B, general diagram of transverse section of bark (×20); C, transverse section of outer tissues; D, ditto of phloem (both × 200); E, cork cells in surface view; F, fragment of phloem from powder (both × 250); c, collenchyma; ck, cork; c.p, cortical parenchyma; l, lenticel; li, lichen patch; l.f, longitudinal furrows; m, moss; m.r, medullary ray; m.s, mussel scale; ox₁, ox₂, prismatic and cluster crystals of calcium oxalate respectively; p.f, pericyclic fibres; ph.f, phloem fibres; ph.p, phloem parenchyma; s, sclereids; s.p, sieve plate; s.t, sieve tube; t, scar of twig.

shape, are variable in size, and have thick lignified walls sometimes showing stratification and traversed by funnel-shaped pits. A pericycle is not clearly delimited, but the zone immediately outside the phloem in which sclereids and occasional fibres occur is regarded as representing this region. The phloem is composed of zones of tangentially elongated groups of phloem fibres, enclosed in a sheath of parenchymatous cells containing prisms of calcium oxalate which alternate with sieve tubes and phloem parenchyma (Fig. 21.13F). The individual fibres are yellow in colour, are 8–15 μm in diameter, and have thick lignified walls showing stratification and pit canals. The sieve tubes show sieve plates, each with several sieve fields, on the radial walls. The sieve plates are usually covered with a deposit of callus and can be identified after staining with alkaline solution of corallin. The phloem parenchyma resembles that of the cortex, containing plastids, starch, material coloured violet by alkali, and rosettes of calcium oxalate. The medullary rays are 1–5 cells wide and 15–25 cells deep. The medullary ray cells are parenchymatous, somewhat radially elongated and with similar contents to those of the parenchyma; their content of material stained violet by alkali is often high. Fragments of moss leaves and liverworts are usually found in the powder.

Constituents. It has long been recognized that cascara bark stored for at least 1 year gave galenicals which were better tolerated but as effective as those prepared from more recently collected bark. This is presumably due to hydrolysis or other changes during storage. It was also found at an early date that the very bitter taste of cascara is reduced by treating extracts with alkalis, alkaline earths or magnesium oxide. Proprietary extracts of this type became very popular and pharmacopoeias followed the same idea to produce such preparations.

Cascara contains about 6–9% anthracene derivatives which are present both as normal *O*-glycosides and as *C*-glycosides. The following groups of constituents are now manifest.

1. Four primary glycosides or cascarosides A, B, C and D; they contain both *O*- and *C*-glycosidic linkages. Their structures were elucidated in 1974 by Wagner *et al.* as the *C*-10 isomers of the 8-*O*-β-D-glucopyranosides of aloin and chrysophanol. A. Griffini *et al.* (*Planta Med.*, 1992, **58**, Suppl. 1, A593) described the isolation of the pure cascarosides by silica-gel chromatography and HPLC. The complete assignments of ¹H- and ¹³C-NMR signals for these cascarosides were recorded by Manitto *et al.* (*J. Chem. Soc. Perk. Trans I*, 1993, 1577) and the same group (*J. Nat. Prod.*, 1995, **38**, 419) have now isolated two analogous glycosides (cascarosides E and F) derived from emodin (Table 21.3).

Cascarosides of *Rhamnus purshianus*,
Configurations; Cascaroside A = 10β, R = OH; B = 10α, R = OH;
C = 10β, R = H; D = 10α, R = H.

2. Two aloins, barbaloin derived from the aloe-emodin anthrones and chrysaloin derived from chrysophanol anthrone. These *C*-glycosides are probably breakdown products from (1). Also 10-hydroxyaloins A and B (H. W. Rauwaled *et al.*, *Z. Naturforsch*, Teil B, 1991, **46**, 551).

3. A number of *O*-glycosides derived from emodin oxanthrone, aloe-emodin and chrysophanol.
4. Various dianthrones, including those of emodin, aloe-emodin and chrysophanol and the heterodianthrones palmidin A, B and C (see 'Rhubarb'). These dimers are also formed during the preparation and conservation of elixirs and may constitute up to 20% of the total anthracene glycosides (see P. de Witte *et al.*, *Planta Med.*, 1991, **57**, 440).
5. Aloe-emodin, chrysophanol and emodin in the free state.

The primary glycosides are more active than the aloins whereas the free anthraquinones and dimers have little purgative activity. The cascarosides have a sweet and more pleasant taste than the aloins. The *BP/EP* requires the bark to contain not less than 8.0% of hydroxyanthracene glycosides of which not less than 60% consists of cascarosides, calculated as cascaroside A. A two-point spectro-photometric assay is employed with absorbance measurements at 515 nm and 440 nm.

Experiments by Betts and Fairbairn in 1964, although based on a single *fresh* plant, suggested that free anthraquinones are formed by the leaves and that they are stored in the bark mainly as *C*-glycosides, the older bark containing the most *C*-glycosides. *Rhamnus purshianus* cell suspension cultures will produce anthracene derivatives in which the accumulation of these compounds, particularly emodin, is significantly raised by a 12 h light/dark cycle; continuous illumination of the cultures suppresses anthraquinone formation.

Substitutes. Several species of *Rhamnus* have a similar geographical distribution to that of *R. purshianus*. These include *R. alnifolia*, which is too rare to be a likely substitute; *R. crocea*, whose bark bears little resemblance to the official drug, and *R. californica* Esch. The latter is so closely related to *R. purshianus* that some botanists do not divide them into separate species. The plant appears to have a much more southerly distribution than the typical *R. purshianus* and is therefore unlikely to occur in bark of Canadian origin. It has a more uniform coat of lichens and wider medullary rays than the official species, but resembles the latter in having sclerenchymatous cells. The bark of *R. fallax* has been recorded as a cascara substitute. European frangula bark, distinguished by the *BP/EP* TLC test, is described below.

Uses. Cascara is a purgative resembling senna in its action. It is mainly used in the form of liquid extract or elixir or as tablets prepared from a dry extract. It is also used in veterinary work.

FRANGULA BARK

Frangula bark, alder buckthorn, is obtained from *Rhamnus frangula* L. (*Frangula alnus* Mill) (Rhamnaceae), a shrub 3–5 m high and found in Britain and Europe. Commerical supplies are available from Balkan countries and a little from Russia. The plant differs from the common buckthorn, *R. cathartica*, in that it does not possess thorns; it bears dark-purple berries whose medicinal properties have long been accepted. Although much used in England, the demand decreased with the increased popularity of cascara; on the Continent, particularly in France, cascara has not replaced it to the same extent.

The bark, included in the *BP/EP*, is required to contain not less than 7.0% glucofrangulins calculated as glucofrangulin A.

The bark occurs in single or double quills which are usually of smaller size than those of cascara and about 0.5–2 mm thick. It has a purplish cork and transversely elongated, whitish lenticels. On removing the outer cork cells by scraping, a dark crimson inner cork is exposed. The transverse section closely resembles that of cascara but groups of sclerenchymatous cells are absent.

Frangula contains anthraquinone derivatives present mainly in the form of glycosides. The rhamnoside franguloside, or frangulin, was isolated in 1857. This is now known to consist of two isomers, frangulosides A and B, formed by partical hydrolysis of the corresponding rhamnoglucosides, glucofrangulins A and B (Table 21.3). The fresh bark also contains anthranols and anthrones, which are unstable and readily oxidize to the corresponding anthraquinones; Lemli (1965, 1966) detected emodin-dianthrone, palmidin C (see 'Rhubarb'), palmidin C monorhamnoside and emodin-dianthrone monorhamnoside. Wagner *et al.* characterized frangulin B as 6-O-(D-apiofuranosyl)-1,6,8-trihydroxy-3-methylanthraquinone and more recently reported the new glycoside emodin-8-O-β-gentiobioside.

Allied drugs. The common buckthorn, *Rhamnus cathartica*, has a glossy reddish-or greenish-brown cork and does not possess sclereids. It contains frangula-emodin and a glycoside, rhamnicoside, which yields on hydrolysis rhamnicogenol (an anthraquinone derivative), glucose and xylose. Rauwald and Just (*Planta Med.*, 1981, **42**, 244) reported the isolation of the anthraquinone glycoside alaternin; 1,2,6,8-tetrahydroxy-3-methyl-anthraquinone; physcion; chrysophanol; and frangula-emodin. The bark also contains a number of blue-fluorescent substances which in the chromatograms produced by the *BP/EP* tests of identity for Cascara and Frangula serve to distinguish this adulterant. The fluorescent substances have recently been identified as naphtholide glycosides of the sorigenin type, as below.

α-Sorigenin glycoside: R^1 = OCH$_3$ R^2 = glucose
α-Sorigenin-primeveroside: R^1 = OCH$_3$ R^2 = glucose–xylose
β-Sorigenin-primeveroside: R^1 = H R^2 = glucose–xylose

The bark of *R. carniolica* has a dull reddish cork and differs from frangula bark in that it possesses sclerenchymatous cells and has wider medullary rays. In recent years the barks of a number of Turkish species of Rhamnus have been systematically examined for their anthraquinone and flavonoid contents (see M. Koskun, *Int. J. Pharmacognosy*, 1992, **30**, 151 and references cited therein).

RHUBARB

Rhubarb (Chinese Rhubarb) consists of the dried underground parts of *Rheum palmatum* L. (Polygonaceae) or *R. officinale* Baillon or hybrids of these two species, or mixtures of these. The drug appears still to be obtained from both wild and cultivated plants grown on the high plateaux of Asia from Tibet to south-east China. The *BP/EP* drug is required to contain not less than 2.2% of hydroxyanthraquinone derivatives calculated as rhein.

Species and commercial grades. The genus *Rheum* comprises about 50 species, which may be classified into two sections, the first including *R. palmatum* and *R. officinale*, and the second *R. rhaponticum*, *R. undulatum* and *R. emodi*. A systematic study is made unusually difficult by geography and by the tendency of cultivated plants to form hybrids such as *R. palmatum* × *R. undulatum* and *R. palmatum* × *R. emodi*. The exact morphological and chemical characters of such hybrid rhizomes appear not to have been described. Formerly most of the drug was derived from *R. palmatum* L. var. *tanguticum* Maximowicz and *R. officinale* H. Br. and was traditionally known in commerce as Shensi, Canton and high-dried rhubarb. *R. palmatum* and *R. palmatum* var. *tanguticum* now appear to be the chief sources.

The best grade of the present-day drug corresponds to that formerly known as Shensi rhubarb. Another present-day grade is similar to the old Canton. In addition, some inferior drug is exported, much of which fails to give the pink fracture characteristic of good-quality rhubarb.

In practice the grading system is more complex than the above might imply, and currently about a dozen grades of rhubarb are recognized by merchants. The grades commonly listed are: 'flat', 'common round', 'small round', 'extra small round', 'sticks', 'third grade' and lower qualities. The flat and round are further categorized on a percentage basis (e.g. 'flat 90%' or 'common round 80%'), depending on the pinkness and quality of the fracture. However, not all of these grades are necessarily available at any one time. Currently (2000) it is almost impossible to obtain rhubarb from China which meets *BP/EP* requirements for hydroxyanthraquinone derivatives. Demand for the better grades (CR & Flat 80 & 90%) is now almost exclusively for the beverage industry.

History. Chinese rhubarb has a long history. It is mentioned in a herbal of about 2700 BC and subsequently formed an important article of commerce on the Chinese trade routes to Europe. Today it still holds a place in medicine. The first international symposium on the drug was held in Chengde, China in 1990 under the title 'Rhubarb 90'.

Collection and preparation. Provided that the older accounts are still substantially correct, the rhizomes are grown at a high altitude (over 3000 m) dug up in autumn or spring when about 6–10 years old, decorticated and dried. The decorticated rhizomes are when whole roughly cylindrical ('rounds') or if cut longitudinally are in planoconvex pieces ('flats'). Pieces used often to show a hole indicating that they had been threaded on cords for drying.

The drug is exported from Shanghai to Tientsin, often via Hong Kong. The better qualities are packed in tin-lined wooden cases containing either 280 lb or 50 kg, and inferior quality in hessian bags.

Botanical characters of rhizome. The rhizomes of *R. palmatum* and *R. officinale* are similar in structure except for the size and distribution of the abnormal vascular bundles, 'star spots', of the pith. Transverse sections of both, after peeling, show phloem on the outside, cambium, radiate wood and a pith with 'star sports' (Fig. 21.14A, B). In *R. palmatum* the latter are relatively small (about 2.5 mm) and most of them are arranged in a continuous ring; in *R. officinale* the 'star spots' are larger (about 4 mm) and are irregularly scattered.

Macroscopical characters. Despite the large number of commercial grades, it is convenient to describe the various rhubarb types under three headings.

1. *High-grade, Chinghai or Shensi-type.* This drug occurs in rounds or flats weighing up to about 200 g and up to about 15 cm long, although usually smaller. Much of the present-day drug tends to be of small size and may therefore be obtained from younger plants than was formerly the case.

   The drug has a firm texture, non-shrunken appearance and a bright yellow surface showing whitish reticulations. These reticulations are due to the fusiform or lozenge-shaped cut ends of the closely arranged medullary rays (which are reddish-brown) seen against the white background of the phloem parenchyma. In the *palmatum* type the medullary rays are only about 6 cells deep, but in the *officinale* type they may be as much as 200 cells deep. This difference accounts for the fact that the surface of the *officinale* type gives the apperance of parallel red and white lines rather than a reticulation. In both species the appearance of the transverse surface varies according to the depth of peeling, which may extend into the radiate wood or even into the pith.

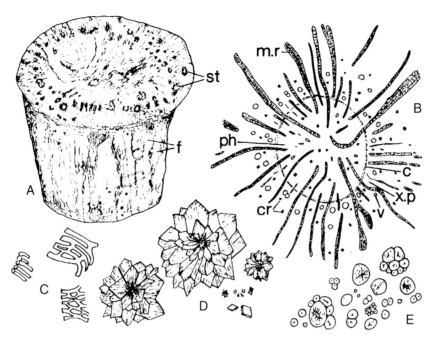

Fig. 21.14
Chinese rhubarb. A, common round (×0.5); B, star spot in transverse section (×20); C–E, fragments of the powder (×200); C, portions of reticulate vessels; D, calcium oxalate crystals; E, starch; c, cambium; cr, crystals; f, facets produced by peeling; m.r, medullary ray; ph, phloem; st, star spot; v, vessel; x.p, xylem parenchyma.

The best rhubarb breaks with a marbled or 'nutmeg' fracture, the freshly broken surface showing a bright pink colour—this is one character used in grading—see above. Such drug gives the bright yellow powder favoured by buyers. Particular attention is paid by the buyer not only to the colour of the fracture, but also to absence of signs of decay or insect attack. Odour, aromatic; taste, bitter and slightly astringent.

2. *Medium-grade or Canton-type.* This has the general characters of the drug described above but has been less carefully prepared. Some pieces are badly trimmed, greyish patches being left on the outer surface. The surface reticulations are less distinct, the fracture granular rather than marbled and the freshly fractured surface of a paler pink colour.

3. *Third grade.* This frequently consists of smaller pieces than in the higher grades. Only a small percentage of the fractured surfaces show a good pink fracture and the remainder a grey, mauve or brown one. These differences are shown in the colour of the powder.

Microscopy of powder.   Powdered rhubarb (Fig. 21.14) is easily identified. It shows abundant calcium oxalate rosettes up to 200 μm in diameter; simple two to five compound starch grains; reticulate vessels and other wood elements which give no reaction for lignin. The yellow contents of the medullary ray cells (anthraquinone derivatives) become reddish-pink with ammonia solution and deep red with caustic alkalis.

Constituents.   As with other anthraquinone-containing drugs, the chemical complexity of rhubarb was not fully appreciated by the earlier research workers. Free anthraquinones were the first substances to be isolated: chrysophanol, aloe-emodin, rhein, emodin and emodin monomethylether or physcion (1844–1905). Glycosides of some of the above were also separated. These substances did not account satisfactorily for the action of the drug, and modern methods of investigation have established the presence of the following types of anthraquinones in rhubarb.

1. Anthraquinones without a carboxyl group (e.g. chrysophanol, aloe-emodin, emodin and physcion). Also their glycosides (e.g. chrysophanein and glucoaloe-emodin). Kopp and coworkers (*Planta Med.*, 1983, **48**, 34 and references cited) isolated a physcion diglucoside and its 8-O-β-D-gentiobioside from *R. palmatum*; other cytotoxic anthraquinone glycosides have recently been isolated including palmatin (1,8-dihydroxy-3-methyl-anthraquinone-1-*O*-β-7D-glucoside; see Kubo *et al.*, *Phytochemistry*, 1992, **31**, 1063 with corrigendum on misspelling of names p. 4399).

2. Anthraquinones with a carboxyl group (e.g. rhein and its glycoside, glucorhein).

3. Anthrones or dianthrones of chrysophanol, or emodin or aloe-emodin, or physcion. The dianthrone glucosides of rhein (sennosides A and B) and the oxalates of these (sennosides E and F), have been isolated (1974) by Japanese workers. Sennosides A and B have been identified in callus cultures of a *R. palmatum* hybrid.

4. Heterodianthrones derived from two different anthrone molecules. For example, palmidin A from aloe-emodin anthrone and emodin anthrone; palmidin B from aloe-emodin anthrone and chrysophanol anthrone; and palmidin C from emodin anthrone and chrysophanol anthrone. Rhein anthrone occurs combined with aloe-emodin anthrone (sennidin C and as sennoside C), chrysophanol anthrone (reidin B) and physcion anthrone (reidin C). These dianthrones may be oxidized into their two components by means of ferric chloride.

In addition to the above purgative compounds, rhubarb contains astringent compounds such as glucogallin, free gallic acid, (–)-epicatechin gallate and catechin. Other derivatives of gallic acid include glycerol gallate, gallic acid glucoside gallates and isolindleyin (a methyl *p*-hydroxyphenylpropionate derivative of a glycogallate). A new class of gallotannins has a sucrose core and chromone glucosides have also been identified (Y. Kashiwada *et al.*, *Phytochemistry*, 1988, **27**, 1469; 1990, **29**, 1007).

Rhubarb also contains starch and calcium oxalate. The total ash is very variable, as the amount of calcium oxalate varies from about 5 to

40%. The acid-insoluble ash should not exceed 1%. The *BP* assay for anthraquinone derivatives is a spectrophotometric method and replaces the former standard for alcohol-soluble extractive.

Ontogenetic production of anthraquinone derivatives. As the drug is collected in autumn, variations in constituents arising from seasonable changes should present no problem. Nevertheless, considerable research has been devoted to this aspect over many years. Work by Lemli and colleagues (1982) indicated that oxidized compounds, the anthraquinones, are the major components of the anthracene mixture in the summer months and the reduced forms, the anthrones, in winter. The conversions occur within a time lapse of about 3 weeks, and just before each, the anthrone diglycoside content increases markedly. Experiments showed that the anthraquinone → anthrone conversion could be artificially induced by decreasing the ambient temperature. Earlier reports by Schmid (1951) suggested that the age of the rhizome also affected the ratio of reduced:oxidized glycosides. Chinese workers have also addressed the problem (*Chem. Abs.*, 1992, **117**, 66652; 66653).

Constituents of rhapontic rhubarb. Rhapontic rhubarb contains a glycoside, rhaponticin, which is a stilbene (diphenylethylene) derivative of the formula

This substance and desoxyrhaponticin (glycoside of 3,5-dihydroxy-4′-methoxystilbene) account for the difference in fluorescence between official and rhapontic rhubarbs. Rhapontic rhubarb does contain anthraquinone derivatives, although these differ from those in the official drug. One is the glucoside glucochrysaron (see Table 21.3).

Chemical tests

1. *Test for anthraquinone derivatives.* A little powder is shaken with 10 ml of ferric chloride solution mixed with 5 ml of hydrochloric acid and heated on a water-bath for 10 min. After filtration and cooling the filtrate is extracted with 10 ml of carbon tetrachloride. The organic layer is separated, washed with 5 ml of water and shaken with 5 ml of dilute solution of ammonia. Official rhubarb gives a rose-pink to cherry-red colour. Rhapontic rhubarb also gives this test.

2. *Test for rhapontic rhubarb.* Macerate 0.5 g of powder with 10 ml of 45% alcohol for 20 min, shaking occasionally. Filter and place one drop of the filtrate on a filter paper. When examined in ultraviolet light, the spot shows no blue colour with official rhubarb but a distinct blue fluorescence if rhapontic rhubarb is present. The colour is intensified by exposure to ammonia vapour. The *BP/EP* test is more specific and employs TLC with ultraviolet light and phosphomolybdic acid spray for visualization of the chromatogram of a methanolic extract with rhaponticin as a standard.

Other rhubarbs

1. *Chinese rhapontic.* This is known commercially as 'Chinese Rhapontica' but has been offered under the names of 'Tai-Hwang' or 'Tze-Hwang' without indication that it is a rhapontic type. It consists of untrimmed pieces sometimes split longitudinally. The transverse surface shows a radiate structure, with concentric rings of paler and darker colour, and a diffuse ring of star spots. The centre may be hollow. The odour, which is sweetish, differs from that of official rhubarb. Rhapontic rhubarb, like the official, gives a positive test for anthraquinone derivatives. When the test for absence of rhapontic rhubarb (see below) is applied, it gives a distinct blue fluorescence, which may be further intensified by exposure to ammonia vapour.

2. *Indian rhubarb.* Indian rhubarb consists of the dried rhizome and roots of *R. australe* (formerly called *R. emodi*) and *R. webbianum*. It is found in Pakistan, Kashmir, Nepal and eastern India and large quantities of the Indian drug have been exported. It occurs in unpeeled or partly peeled pieces, which are barrel-shaped or plano-convex, shrunken and light in weight. Cork cells are present in the powder. The freshly fractured surface is dull orange to yellowish-brown and in ultraviolet light exhibits a deep violet fluorescence.

   A considerable number of the anthraquinone derivatives present in *R. palmatum* have also been reported in Indian rhubarb. L. Krenn *et al.* (*J. Nat. Prod.*, 2003, **66**, 1107; *Chem. Pharm. Bull.*, 2004, 52, 391) have identified a new sulphated anthraquinone glycoside (sulfemodin 8-*O*-β-D-glucoside) together with new 10-hydroxycascarosides C and D and, 10*R*-chrysaloin 1-*O*-β-D-glucopyranoside; some phenolic compounds have antioxidant properties.

3. *English rhubarbs.* Both *R. officinale* and *R. rhaponticum* were formerly grown as drugs but cultivation appears to have ceased. Garden rhubarb for table use is derived from *R. rhaponticum*.

4. *Japanese rhubarb.* A hybrid of *R. coreanum* and *R. palmatum*. It contains anthraquinone derivatives, naphthalene glycosides similar to those illustrated for senna, stilbene glycosides and (+)-catechin.

Uses. Rhubarb is used as a bitter stomachic and in the treatment of diarrhoea, purgation being followed by an astringent effect. The drug is suitable as an occasional aperient but not for the treatment of chronic constipation.

Further reading

Foust CM 1992 Rhubarb—the wondrous drug. Princeton University Press, Princeton, NJ. *This book gives the history of the commerce, botany and medicinal aspects of the drug*

ALOES

Aloes is the solid residue obtained by evaporating the liquid which drains from the transversely cut leaves of various species of *Aloe* (Liliaceae). The juice is usually concentrated by boiling and solidifies on cooling.

The official (*BP, EP, USP*) varieties of aloes are the Cape from South Africa and Kenya, and the Barbados (Curaçao) from the West Indian Islands of Curaçao, Aruba and Bonaire. There are separate pharmacopoeial monographs for each type. Socotrine and Zanzibar varieties are no longer official.

Plants. Of about 180 known species of *Aloe*, the drug is mainly obtained from the following: Cape variety from *Aloe ferox* and its hybrids; Curaçao variety from *Aloe barbadensis*; Socotrine and Zanzibar varieties from *Aloe perryi*. The genus *Aloe* includes herbs, shrubs and trees, bearing spikes of white, yellow or red flowers. *Aloe ferox* is an example of the arborescent type and *A. barbadensis* of the herbaceous type. Aloe leaves are fleshy, are strongly cuticularized and are usually prickly at the margins.

It has been suggested that if natural stocks of *A. ferox* became exhausted then *A. classenii* and *A. turkanensis* would be preferable for cultivation because chemical races would not be a problem and their production of sideshoots would make vegetative propagation easier. However, some problems have arisen concerning the commerce in the

African aloes because the Washington Conference of the Convention on International Trade in Endangered Species (CITES) placed all species of *Aloe*, with the exception of *A. vera* (a cultivar of *A. barbadensis*), on the protected list.

Leaf structure.   Transverse sections of an *Aloe* leaf usually show the following zones: (1) a strongly cuticularized epidermis with numerous stomata on both surfaces; (2) a region of parenchyma containing chlorophyll, starch and occasional bundles of needles of calcium oxalate; (3) a central region which frequently occupies about three-fifths of the diameter of the leaf, consisting of large, mucilage-containing parenchymatous cells; (4) a double row of vascular bundles which lie at the junction of the two previous zones and have a well-marked pericycle and endodermis. The aloetic juice from which the drug is prepared is contained in the large, pericyclic cells and sometimes in the adjacent parenchyma. When the leaves are cut, the aloetic juice flows out. No pressure should be applied or the aloes will be contaminated with mucilage. The mucilage, contained in zone 3 as above is used in the cosmetic and herbal industries in 'aloe vera' preparations (see Chapter 19).

History.   According to legend, Socotrine aloes was known to the Greeks as early as the fourth century BC; the Greek colonists were sent to the island by Alexander the Great solely to preserve and cultivate the aloe plant. The drug was apparently known in England in the tenth century, and from the seventeenth century records of the East India Company it would appear that they frequently purchased the whole stock of aloes of the 'King of Socotra'. Socotrine and Zanzibar aloe were for many years the only official aloes, but they have now been replaced by the Cape and Curaçao varieties. Cape aloes was first exported about 1780 and became official in Britain in 1932. Barbados aloes was produced from about 1650 and lapsed about the beginning of the present century. The production of Curaçao (also called Barbados) aloes was started by the Dutch in the Islands of Curaçao, Aruba and Bonaire about 1817; recently aloes of similar type has been exported from nearby Venezuela.

Preparation and characters of Cape aloes.   Cape aloes is prepared from wild plants of *A. ferox* and its hybrids. The leaves are cut transversely near the base and about 200 of them are arranged round a shallow hole in the ground, which is lined with plastic sheeting or more traditionally a piece of canvas or a goatskin. The leaves are arranged so that the cut ends overlap and drain freely into the canvas. After about 6 h all the juice has been collected and it is transferred to a drum or paraffin tin in which it is boiled for about 4 h on an open fire. The product is poured while hot into tins, each holding 25 kg, where it solidifies. For export the tins are placed in cases holding either two, four or eight tins.

The drug occurs in dark-brown or greenish-brown, glassy masses. Thin fragments have a deep olive colour and are semitransparent. The powder is greenish-yellow, and when pieces of the drug have rubbed against one another, patches of powder are found on the surface. The drug has a very characteristic, sour odour (the so-called rhubarb or apple-tart odour), which is particularly noticeable if one breathes on the drug before smelling. Taste, nauseous and bitter. The powder when examined under the microscope in lactophenol is usually amorphous.

Preparation and characters of Barbados (Curaçao) aloes.   Curaçao aloes is produced from cultivated plants of *A. barbadensis*. The cut leaves are stacked in V-shaped troughs arranged on a slope so that the juice flows from a hole at one end of the trough into a collecting vessel. When sufficient juice has been collected, it is evaporated in a copper vessel. The temperature used is generally lower than in the case of Cape aloes and the product is, therefore, usually opaque, although some which is semi-transparent may be produced and is known in commerce as 'Capey Barbados'. Originally Barbados and Curaçao aloes were packed in gourds, now seen only in museums. The present-day drug is exported in cases each holding about 58.5 kg.

Typical Barbados aloes varies in colour from yellowish-brown to chocolate-brown, but poorer qualities that have been overheated may be almost black. The drug is opaque and breaks with a waxy fracture. The semi-transparent 'Capey Barbados' becomes more opaque on keeping. Curaçao has a nauseous and bitter taste and a characteristic odour recalling iodoform. Mounted in lactophenol, it shows small acicular crystals.

Substitutes and adulterants.   Socotrine and Zanzibar aloes are now rare in the British market, and Natal aloes from *A. candelabrum* is no longer imported. Socotrine is yellowish-brown to blackish-brown, opaque and breaks with a porous fracture. Zanzibar is similar but has a waxy fracture and may be packed with leaves or skins (so-called 'monkey-skin aloes'). All may be distinguished from official aloes by chemical tests.

Chemical tests

1. General. For the following tests boil 1 g of drug with 100 ml of water, add a little kieselguhr and filter. Use separate portions of the filtrate for the following tests.
   (1) *Borax reaction.* To 5 ml of solution of aloes add 0.2 g of borax and heat until dissolved. Pour a few drops of the liquid into a test-tube nearly full of water. A green fluorescence is produced the origin of which is discussed below.
   (2) *Bromine test.* To 2 ml of solution of aloes add 2 ml of freshly prepared solution of bromine. A pale yellow precipitate of tetrabromaloin is produced. This test is not specific for aloes.

2. Special.
   (1) *Nitric acid test.* To 5 ml of solution of aloes add 2 ml of nitric acid. Cape aloes gives a brownish colour rapidly changing to green; Barbados a deep brownish-red; Socotrine a pale brownish-yellow; Zanzibar a yellowish-brown colour. Nitric acid may be applied direct to the powdered drugs with similar results.
   (2) *Nitrous acid test.* To an aqueous solution of aloes add a few small crystals of sodium nitrite and a little acetic acid. A rich pink to carmine is given by Barbados and a lesser pink by Cape; Socotrine and Zanzibar show little change in colour.
   (3) *Klunge's isobarbaloin test.* To 20 ml of an aqueous 1 in 200 solution of aloes add a drop of saturated copper sulphate solution, following by 1 g of sodium chloride and 10 ml of alcohol 90%. With Barbados aloes a wine-red colour is developed, which persists for at least 12 h. With Cape aloes a lesser coloration may develop, which, however, rapidly fades to yellow. Zanzibar and Socotrine aloes give no colour. The appearance of the red colour may be hastened by warming.
   (4) *Modified Bornträger's test.* As mentioned under 'Constituents', small quantities of aloe-emodin may occur in aloes, but the amounts are usually too small for them to form the basis of a reliable test. Therefore, a modified Bornträger's test which employs ferric chloride and dilute hydrochloric acid to bring about *oxidative hydrolysis*, can be used. The anthraquinones liberated are extracted with carbon tetrachloride and give a rose-pink to cherry-red colour when their solution is shaken with dilute ammonia.

A chromatographic test is included in the *BP/EP* together with assays for hydroxyanthracene derivatives. Of the latter Barbados aloes should contain not less than 28% and Cape aloes not less than 18% calculated as barbaloin.

Constituents. Aloes contain *C*-glycosides and resins. The crystalline glycosides known as 'aloin' were first prepared by T. and H. Smith of Edinburgh, UK, from Barbados aloes in 1851; Aloin (*BP*, 1988) contains not less than 70% anhydrous barbaloin. The main crystalline glycoside, barbaloin, is found in all the commercial varieties (Leger, 1907). Leger showed that on heating to about 160°C barbaloin is partly converted into amorphous β-barbaloin. This substance is said to be absent from the Barbados variety, but present to the extent of about 8% in the Cape.

Barbaloin is a *C*-glycoside—a 10-glucopyranosyl derivative of aloe-emodin-anthrone. Unlike *O*-glycosides, it is not hydrolysed by heating with dilute acids or alkalis. It can, however, be decomposed by *oxidative hydrolysis*, with reagents such as ferric chloride, when it yields glucose, aloe-emodin anthrone and a little aloe-emodin. It will be seen from the formula of barbaloin that stereoisomerism is possible at C-10; in 1979 both isomers were obtained by HPLC of a methanolic extract of *Aloe ferox* and in 1980 Auterhoff *et al.* separated commercial aloin into its stereoisomers. The absolute configuration of the two aloins was independently elucidated by Rauwald *et al.* (*Angew. Chem., Int. Ed. Engl.*, 1989, **28**, 1528) and Manitto *et al.* (*J. Chem. Soc., Perk. Trans. 1*, 1990, 1297); aloin A is (10*S*)-barbaloin and aloin B the (10*R*)-epimer (Fig. 21.15). The two are interconvertible via the corresponding anthranol form. All varieties of aloes give a strong greenish fluorescence with borax, a characteristic of anthranols, which are readily formed from anthrones by isomeric change. This has long been used as a general test for aloes.

Small quantities of aloe-emodin are sometimes present in aloes, and Cape aloes also contains aloinosides A and B, which are *O*-glycosides of barbaloin; aloinoside B has rhamnose attached via an oxymethyl group at C-3. In *A. barbadensis* free and esterified 7-hydroxyaloins A and B are characteristic 10-*C*-glucosyl-anthrones. These compounds are responsible for the violet-purple colours given in various specific tests for Barbados aloes (see H. W. Rauwald *et al.*, *Planta Med.*, 1991, **57**, Suppl. 2, A129).

The resin of aloes, reputed to have a purgative action, has been periodically investigated from the end of the nineteenth century onwards. In South African spp. (e.g. *A. ferox*) aloesin (now often referred to as aloeresin B) was identified in 1970 by Haynes *et al.*, and was the first *C*-glucosyl-chromone to be described. Other 5-methylchromones isolated from Cape aloes include aloeresin A and C which are *p*-coumaroyl derivatives linked via a hydroxyl of the glucose. Two non-glucosylated 5-methylchromones present in smaller amounts than the aloesins were reported in 1997. A glycosidic 6-phenylpyran-2-one derivative (aloenin A) was isolated and characterized from *A. arborescens* leaves in 1974 by Japanese workers. Aloenin B has now been obtained from Kenya aloes (see formulae). (For research on these and related constituents see G. Speranza *et al.*, *Phytochemistry*, 1993, **33**, 175; *J. Nat. Prod.*, 1992, **55**, 723; 1993, **56**, 1089; 1997, **60**, 692. Two aloesol derivatives (Fig. 21.14) have been isolated: 8-*C*-β-D-glucopyranosyl-7-*O*-methyl-(R)-aloesol (L. Duri *et al.*, *Fitoterapia*, 2004, **75**, 520) from a commercial sample (Kenya) and the 10*S* diastereoisomer from *A. vera* (N. Okamura *et al.*, *Phytochemistry*, 1996, **43**, 495).

Three new naphtho[2,3-*c*]furan derivatives have recently been isolated from a commercial sample of Cape aloes (J. Koyama *et al.*, *Phytochemistry*, 1994, **37**, 1147).

As with other anthraquinone-producing plants, in *Aloe* species the content of anthraquinones is subject to seasonal variation, and these compounds are implicated in the active metabolism of the plant. McCarthy and coworkers in South Africa have shown that the anthraquinone derivatives are confined to the leaf juices and that aloin reaches a maximum concentration in the dried leaf juices of *A. ferox* and *A. marlothi* in the summer (24.1% in November) and is lowest in winter (14.8% in July).

Uses. Aloes is employed as purgative. It is seldom prescribed alone, and its activity is increased when it is administered with small quantities of soap or alkaline salts, while carminatives moderate its tendency to cause griping. It is an ingredient of Compound Benzoin Tincture (Friars' Balsam).

There appears to be little variation of the major constituents of the leaf exudate of *A. ferox* depending on geographical location of the plant but selection of high-yielding strains giving a high production of aloin (25%) is recommended for commercial cultivation (B.-E. van Wyk *et al.*, *Planta Medica*, 1995, **61**, 250).

'Aloe vera' products See Chapter 20.

Further reading

Reynolds T (ed), Hardman R (series ed) 2004 Medicinal and aromatic plants – industrial profiles, Vol 38. Aloes – the genus Aloe. CRC Press, Taylor and Francis Group, Boca Raton, FL, 408 pp.

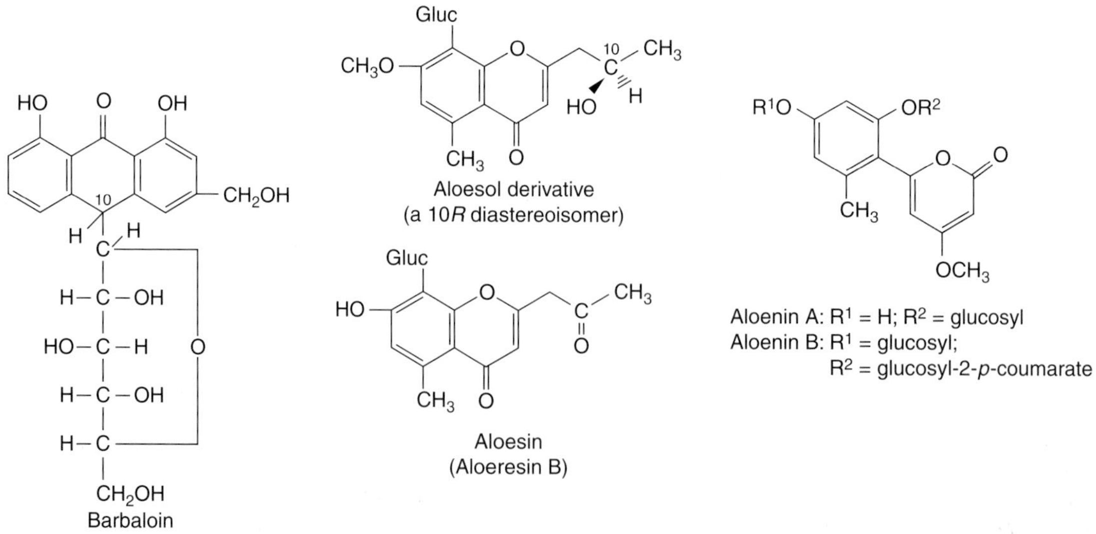

Fig. 21.15
Constituents of aloes

Aloesol derivative (a 10*R* diastereoisomer)

Aloesin (Aloeresin B)

Barbaloin

Aloenin A: R¹ = H; R² = glucosyl
Aloenin B: R¹ = glucosyl; R² = glucosyl-2-*p*-coumarate

Chrysarobin

Chrysarobin is a mixture of substances obtained from araroba or Goa powder by extraction with hot benzene. Araroba is extracted from cavities in the trunk of *Andira araroba* (Leguminosae). Chrysarobin contains chrysophanol anthranol, the corresponding anthrone and other similar constituents; it gives a strong green fluorescence in alkaline solution. Chrysarobin was formerly much used for skin diseases and is still occasionally prescribed.

Madder

The root of *Rubia tinctorum* (Rubiaceae) was formerly grown in large quantities as a dyestuff, but has been almost completely replaced by synthetic dyes. It contains several anthraquinone glycosides, the chief of which, ruberythric acid (Table 21.3) yields on hydrolysis alizarin and primeverose. Twenty compounds have been isolated from the roots and their mutagenicity studied (Y. Kawasaki *et al.*, *Chem. Pharm. Bull.*, 1992, **40**, 1504), and three hydroxymethylanthraquinone glycosides have been described (N. A. El-Emary and E. Y. Backheet, *Phytochemistry*, 1998, **49**, 277).

HYPERICUM—ST JOHN'S WORT

Hypericum consists of the dried aerial parts of *Hypericum perforatum*, family Hypericaceae (Clusiaceae) gathered usually at the time of flowering or shortly before. Commercial extracts are standardized on their naphthodianthrone content, expressed as hypericin.

The plant is abundant throughout Europe in grassland, woodlands and hedges, extending to the Himalayas and Central and Russian Asia, except in Arctic regions. It was introduced into N.E. America and Australia at an early stage of colonization where it has since become a noxious weed. It is a herbaceous perennial, usually forming a colony with a spreading root system. The bright yellow flowers are in handsome terminal corymbs.

History. The plant was known in ancient Greece for its medicinal attributes and since the Middle Ages has been used for its anti-inflammatory and healing properties. It also became highly regarded for the treatment of mental illness. The generic name derives from the Greek *hyper*—above, and *icon* (eikon)—picture, referring to the ancient practice of hanging the plant above religious pictures to ward off evil spirits. The common name St John's wort is attributed to the fact, among others, that it comes into flower around St John's Day (June 24th).

The drug is now included in the *BP/EP*, a number of European pharmacopoeias, the *British Herbal Pharmacopoeia*, the *American Herbal Pharmacopoeia*, and as monographs for the German Commission E and ESCOP.

Collection. Collection is from wild and cultivated plants and increased demand has meant that farmers in the US and Australia who battled to eradicate it as a weed now harvest it as a viable crop. Care should be taken during collecting as contact photosensitivity has been reported. Drying at 70° for 10 hours is recommended.

Macroscopy. The drug consists of green leaf fragments and stems, unopened buds and yellow flowers. Oil glands are visible in the leaves as transparent areas, hence the specific name *perforatum*, and as small black dots on the lower surface. The opposite, sessile leaves are 1.5–4.0 cm in length, elliptical to ovate in outline, glabrous with an entire margin. Pieces of hollow stem are cylindrical with two faint ribs on either side.

The odour is distinct and the taste slightly sweet and astringent.

Microscopy. The upper epidermal cells of the leaf are sinuous in outline with beaded anticlinal walls; the lower epidermis possesses anomocytic and paracytic stomata. The mesophyll has large hypericin-containing oil glands, some with red contents, and these are also found in the petals and sepals. Pollen grains are ellipsoidal, 20–25 μm in diameter, with three pores and a smooth exine. Trichomes and calcium oxalate are absent.

In an innovative study, Rapisarda *et al.* (*Pharm. Biol.*, 2003, **41**, 1) have used scanning electron microscopy and image analysis involving size and shape parameters of leaf epidermal cells to provide a quantitative morphological analysis of the three Italian *Hypericum* spp.— *H. perforatum* L., *H. hircinum* L. and *H. perfoliatum*. The markers obtained provided key factors for the identification and selection of these species and their hybrids.

Constituents. Hypericum contains a variety of constituents with biological activity.

Anthraquinones. Principally hypericin and pseudohypericin; also iso-hypericin and emodin-anthrone. The *BP/EP* requires not less than 0.08% of total hypericins expressed as hypericin calculated with reference to the dried drug. The extracted hypericins are assayed by absorption measurement at 590 nm.

Prenylated phloroglucinol derivatives. Hyperforin (2.0–4.5%), adhyperforin and furohyperforin (L. Verotta *et al.*, *J. Nat. Prod.*, 1999, **62**, 770), the latter at concentrations of about five per cent of the hyperforin content. These phloroglucinols constitute the principal components of the lipophilic extract of the plant and are considered to be the most important active constituents regarding antibiotic and antidepressant properties. Unfortunately, they are very prone to oxidative transformations and a number of such degradation products have been identified, see L. Verotta *et al.*, *J. Nat. Prod.*, 2000, **63**, 412; V. Vajs *et al.*, *Fitoterapia*, 2003, **74**, 439. For an article, with many

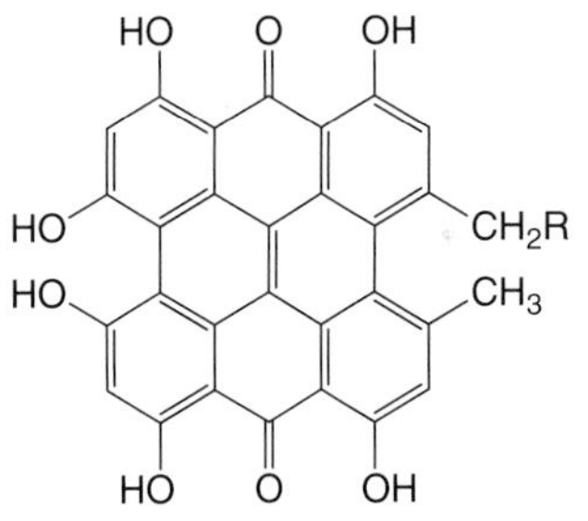

Hypericin, R = H
Pseudohypericin, R = OH

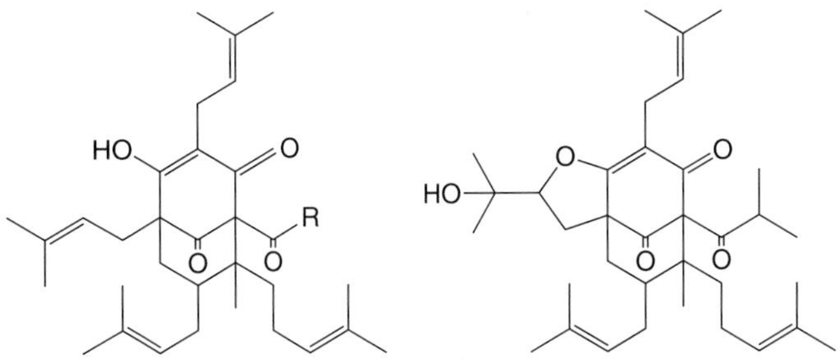

Hyperforin, R = CH(CH₃)₂
Adhyperforin, R = CH(CH₃)CH₂CH₃

Furohyperforin

Fig. 21.16
Hypericins and phloroglucinols of hypericum.

21

references, on the wide-ranging aspects of hyperforin, see L. Beerhues, *Phytochemistry*, 2006, **67**, 2201.

The involvement of branched-chain amino acids in the biosynthesis of hyperforin and adhyperforin has been demonstrated with shoot cultures of *H. perforatum*: L-[U-^{13}C$_5$] valine and L-[U-^{13}C$_6$] isoleucine, when fed to the shoots, were incorporated respectively into the side-chains of hyperforin and adhyperforin. Production of the former was not increased by the administration of unlabelled L-valine, whereas the latter was enhanced by the feeding of the unlabelled L-isoleucine (K. Karppinen *et al.*, *Phytochemistry*, 2007, **68**, 1038). Two phloroglucinols, hyperfirin and adhyperfirin, previously reported to be precursors of hyperforin and adhyperforin, respectively, have now been detected in the plant (E. C. Tatsis *et al.*, *Phytochemistry*, 2007, **68**, 383).

Flavonoids. These include flavonols such as kaempferol, luteolin and quercetin, the flavanol glycosides quercitrin, isoquercitrin and hyperoside. The biflavonoid amentoflavone (Fig. 21.18) is confined principally to the flowers (A. Umek *et al.*, *Planta Medica*, 1999, **65**, 388).

Selected formulae for the above are shown in Figs 21.16 and 21.18.

Volatile oil. Up to 0.35% consisting principally of saturated hydrocarbons including alkanes and alkanols in the range C$_{16}$–C$_{29}$.

Other constituents. Many other components of hypericum have been reported including various plant acids (caffeic, chlorogenic, etc.), amino acids, vitamin C, tannins and carotenoids.

Many reports have appeared concerning the distribution of the above constituents in different organs of the plant and generally on a weight for weight basis it is the flowers, particularly the petals, that possess the highest concentrations. According to an Australian report (I. A. Southwell *et al.*, *Phytochemistry*, 1991, **30**, 475) it is the narrow-leaved varieties, both in Europe and Australia, that possess a relatively high proportion of oil glands and give a higher yield of hypericin compared with the broad-leaved forms. Hypericin concentrations determined on twelve samples of herb collected throughout Oregon varied widely (0.01–0.38%) (G. H. Constantine and J. Karchesy, *Pharm. Biol.*, 1998, **36**, 365). B. Buter *et al.* (*Planta Medica*, 1998, **64**, 431) have suggested that a key factor for successful future field production will rest in the selection of genetically superior strains giving increased secondary metabolite production, together with improvements in agro-technological methods. In this connection R. J. Percifield *et al.* (*Planta Medica*, 2007, **73**, 1525), studying 50 *Hypericum* accessions, have demonstrated the value of amplified fragment-length polymorphism analysis for the characterization of closely related samples.

Cell culture of *Hypericum* spp. and their chemotypes has proved extremely variable in naphthadianthrone yields with pseudohypericin production exceeding that of hypericin (T. Kartnig *et al.*, *Planta Medica*, 1996, **62**, 51). Flavonoids, completely different to those of the intact plant and including the new compound 6-C-prenylluteolin, have been identified in callus cultures of *H. perforatum* (A. P. C. Dias *et al.*, *Phytochemistry*, 1998, **48**, 1165).

Other *Hypericum* spp. The genus contains some 400 spp.; most of the more common ones have lower or nil hypericin contents and are often distinguishable in the dried condition by the nature of the ridges on the stem. *H. maculatum* (Imperate St John's wort) is similar in constituents to *H. perforatum* but contains less; it may be distinguished by the slightly quadrangular stem and larger leaves. *H. hirsutum*, *H. tetrapterum* and *H. montana* are other common European species.

The essential oils of two Turkish species (*H. hyssopifolium* and *H. lysimachioides*) are rich in sesquiterpene hydrocarbons, but unlike some other species investigated, poor in monoterpene hydrocarbons. Caryophyllene oxide is a major component. Both oils possess antimicrobial activities (Z. Toker *et al.*, *Fitoterapia*, 2006, **77**, 57). Eight species from S. Brazil showed no detectable amounts of hypericin

or pseudohypericin (A. Ferraz *et al.*, *Pharm. Biol.*, 2002, **40**, 294). *H. chinense* finds use in Japanese folk medicine for the treatment of female disorders. It contains acyl phloroglucinols and spirolactones; six new xanthones have been reported (N. Tanaka and Y. Takaishi, *Chem. Pharm. Bull.*, 2007, **55**, 19).

Action and uses. An explosion in the popularity of St John's wort related to its unregulated availability for the treatment of mild to moderate depression. In the USA, for the first eight months of 1999, it ranked second to ginkgo as the best-selling product of the herbal mainstream market, with retail sales valued at over 78 million (M. Blumenthal, *HerbalGram*, 1999, **47**, 64). In Germany, it represented 25% of all antidepressant prescriptions. It was described as 'nature's Prozac', without the disadvantageous side-effects of the latter. However, a cautionary warning was struck by two reports (S. Piscitelli *et al.*, *Lancet*, 2000, **355**, 547; F. Ruschitzka *et al.*, *Lancet*, 548). In the first, St John's wort was observed to lower plasma concentrations of the protease inhibitor indinavir. In the second report, heart transplant rejection, as a result of the lowering of ciclosporin plasma concentrations below therapeutic levels, followed St John's wort therapy. It has subsequently transpired that St John's wort will adversely affect the performance of a number of common drugs by causing their rapid elimination from the body, either by enhanced metabolism or as a result of increased action of the drug transporter *P*-glycoprotein. Among common drugs so affected are anticoagulants such as warfarin, digoxin, tricyclic antidepressant agents, simvastatin and others.

In the UK, there are currently (2007) no specific restrictions on the sale of St John's wort as a herbal preparation but it is recommended that professional advice be sought if it is to be taken in conjunction with other medicines.

Further reading

Ernst E (ed), Hardman R (series ed) 2003 Medicinal and aromatic plants – industrial profiles, Vol 31. Hypercium: The genus *Hypericum*. CRC Press, Taylor and Francis Group, Boca Raton, FL

COCHINEAL

Cochineal is an important colourant and indicator and consists of the dried female insects, *Dactylopius coccus*, containing eggs and larvae. It contains about 10% of carminic acid which is a *C*-glycoside anthraquinone derivative (Table 21.3). The insects are described in detail in Chapter 33.

NAPHTHOQUINONES AND GLYCOSIDES

The nature of these compounds was indicated earlier; they are produced by higher plants, fungi and actinomycetes and exhibit a broad range of biological actions including fungicidal, antibacterial, insecticidal, phytotoxic, cytostatic and anticarcinogenic. In plants they commonly occur in the reduced and glycosidic forms as illustrated by the 4β-D-glucoside of α-hydrojuglone, a constituent of walnut tree leaves (*Juglans regia*, Juglandaceae).

On extraction and work-up, or in the soil, the compounds are oxidatively converted to the coloured naphthoquinone. In some heart-woods, e.g. *Diospyros* spp. (Ebenaceae) napthoquinones occur as monomers, complex dimers and trimers. In addition to timber usage (ebony) many species of *Diospyros* are used world-wide in the traditional medicine of countries where they grow. S. Ganapaty *et al.* (*Phytochemistry*, 2006, **67**, 1950) have reported on the antiprotozoal properties of various naphthoquinones, *viz* two naphthaldehydes, diospyrin, 8′-hydroxydiospyrin and plumbagin isolated from the roots of *D. assimilis*. *Plumbago zeylanica* (Plumbaginaceae) grows throughout tropical Africa and Asia and the root is used in Indian medicine; it contains juglone in addition to pentacyclic triterpenes.

4β-D-Glucoside of α-hydrojuglone   Juglone

Lawsone   Plumbagin

Naphthoquinones have been shown to be biosynthesized via a variety of pathways including acetate and malonate (plumbagin of *Plumbago* spp.), shikimate/succinyl CoA combined pathway (lawsone) and shikimate/mevalonate combined pathway (alkannin).

Henna

Henna consists of the dried leaves of *Lawsonia inermis* (Lythraceae), a shrub cultivated in north Africa including Egypt, India and Ceylon. The leaves are greenish-brown to brown and about 2.5–5 cm long. The apex is mucronate, the margin entire and revolute, and venation pinnate. Henna contains a colouring matter, lawsone (a hydroxynaphthoquinone), various phenolic glycosides, coumarins, xanthones, quinoids, β-sitosterol glucoside, flavonoids including luteolin and its 7-*O*-glucoside, fats, resin and henna-tannin. (For a report on new glucosides see Y. Takeda and M. O. Fatope, *J. Nat. Prod.*, 1988, **51**, 725.) Henna is commonly used as a dye for the hair, and wool washed in a dilute solution of ammonia and boiled in a decoction of the drug should be dyed Titian red.

The astringent stem-bark of *L. inermis* is traditionally used in India for the treatment of jaundice, enlargement of the liver and spleen, and for various skin diseases. Isoplumbagin, exhibiting significant anti-inflammatory activity, has been isolated from the bark in 0.05% yield (M. Ali and M. R. Grever, *Fitoterapia*, 1998, **69**, 181). For a recent report on the hepatoprotective activity of the bark see S. Ahmed *et al.*, *J. Ethnopharmacology*, 2000, **69**, 157.

Lithospermums

The genus *Lithospermum* (60 spp.) (Boraginaceae) contains plants with hormonal activity. The seeds of the European *L. officinale* (gromwell) were formerly official in several pharmacopoeias.

The reported constituents of the herb are shikonin, a naphthoquinone derivative; scyllitol, a cyclitol; a cyanoglucoside-lithospermocide; caffeic, chlorogenic and ellagic acids; and catechin-type tannins. Shikonin, the enantiomer of alkannin (found in Anchusa Root, see below) is also a constituent of *L. erythrorhizon* root and is produced for the cosmetic and pharmaceutical industries in Japan by cell culture of the plant. Among the many publications on this subject, Tani *et al.* (*Phytochemistry*, 1992, **31**, 690) reported on the structure of an endogenously produced oligogalacturonide necessary for the induction of shikonin biosynthesis in the culture. For investigations relating to the biosynthesis of shikonin from p-hydroxybenzoic acid and geranyl pyrophosphate in *L. erythrorhizon* see T. Okamoto *et al.*, *Phytochemistry*, 1995, **38**, 83.

In the Far East, preparations of the purple roots have long been used for the treatment of burns, inflammations, wounds and ulcers. In Europe, alkanna root has been similarly employed and it has now been shown in laboratory tests that shikonin and alkannin have no significant difference in anti-inflammatory activity. The occurrence of these naphthoquinones is of interest, since similar compounds occur in the related families Rubiaceae (*Galium*, *Rubia*), Verbenaceae and Bignoniaceae. *Lithospermum arvense* is used as an oral contraceptive in Central Europe, as it suppresses the oestrus cycle. The North American *Lithospermum ruderale* has similar hormonal activity.

Alkanna root

Alkanet or Anchusae Radix is the dried root of *Alkanna tinctoria* (Boraginaceae), a herb found in Hungary, southern Europe and Turkey. It consists of reddish-purple roots about 10–15 cm long and 1–2 cm diameter near the crown. The surface is deeply fissured and readily exfoliates. Attached to the crown are the remains of leaves having whitish, bristly hairs. Alkanna is used for colouring oils and tars and in the form of a tincture for the microscopical detection of oils and fats. The pigments are naphthoquinone derivatives of the formulae below.

Alkannin itself may be an artefact arising from various esters. Most of the pigment compounds produced in cell culture appear to give alkannin on KOH hydrolysis (TLC, R_f values) and root cultures give pigments identical to those extracted from normal roots (G. Mita *et al.*, *Plant Cell Rep.*, 1994, **13**, 406).

Other members of the Boraginaceae—for example, *Macrotomia cephalotes* (Syrian Alkanet)—produce similar red naphthoquinones.

CHROMONES AND XANTHONES

These compounds are structural derivatives of benzo-γ-pyrone and although not of great pharmaceutical importance a few compounds are worthy of mention.

Chromones are isomeric with the coumarins. A simple derivative is eugenin (Fig. 21.17) found in the clove plant, *Syzygium aromaticum*. More complex are the furanochromones, the active constituents of the fruits of *Ammi visnaga* (q.v.).

Xanthones are found mainly in the Gentianaceae and Guttiferae, otherwise scattered sporadically throughout the plant kingdom as in the Moraceae and Polygalaceae. The characteristic oxygenation pattern of these compounds derived from higher plants indicated that they were of mixed shikimate–acetate origin whereas xanthones derived from fungi show a characteristic acetate derivation. An important step in their biosynthesis appears to be the oxidative coupling of hydroxylated benzophenones. Simple oxygenated derivatives, such as gentisin which contributes to the yellow colour of fermented Gentian Root (q.v.), are found in both the Gentianaceae and Guttiferae. More highly oxygenated compounds and *O*-glycosylxanthones are found in the former family whereas prenylated xanthones, several of which have antimicrobial properties,

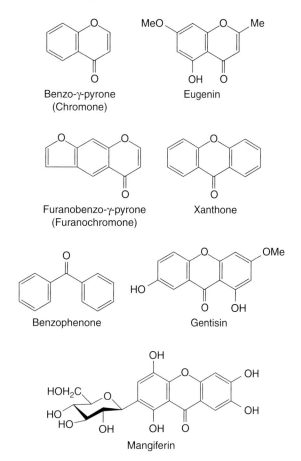

Fig. 21.17
Chromones and xanthones.

are widely distributed in the latter. For studies on the antifungal xanthones from the roots of *Marila laxiflora*, Guttiferae, see J.-R. Ioset, *Pharm. Biol.*, 1998, **36**, 103. The *C*-glycosyl xanthone mangiferin (Fig. 21.17) is found in several species of *Hypericum* and in *Cratoxylem pruniflorum* and Chiretta (*Swertia chirata*). Mangiferin has anti-inflammatory, antihepatotoxic and antiviral properties. In contrast to its CNS-stimulant properties other xanthones exhibit CNS depressive properties in rats and mice.

The mycotoxin pigments of *Claviceps purpurea* (ergot) are complex xanthones called secalonic acids. They contribute, with the ergot alkaloids, to the toxic properties of the whole drug.

Further reading

Bennett GJ, Lee H-H 1989 Xanthones from Guttiferae. Phytochemistry 28(4): 967–998. *165 refs*
Peres V, Nagem TJ 1997 Trioxygenated naturally occurring xanthones. Phytochemistry 44(2): 191–214. *Review with 262 refs and 181 listed compounds including 55 fungal and lichen metabolites*

FLAVONE AND RELATED FLAVONOID GLYCOSIDES

The flavonoids which occur both in the free state and as glycosides are the largest group of naturally occurring phenols. More than 2000 of these compounds are now known, with nearly 500 occurring in the free state. They are formed from three acetate units and a phenylpropane unit as has already been outlined (Fig. 18.11) and are typed according to the state of oxygenation of the C₃ unit, i.e. C-2,3,4 (see

Fig. 21.18 and Table 21.5). Examples given in this section all have a γ-pyrone moiety with the exception of the chalcones, which although not strictly flavonoids are biosynthetically related. The anthocyanins are described later.

The flavones and their close relations are often yellow (Latin *flavus*, yellow). They are widely distributed in nature but are more common in the higher plants and in young tissues, where they occur in the cell sap. They have been used extensively as chemotaxonomic markers and are abundant in the Polygonaceae, Rutaceae, Leguminosae, Umbelliferae and Compositae (see Table 21.5).

They occur both in the free state and as glycosides; most are *O*-glycosides but a considerable number of flavonoid *C*-glycosides are known. Dimeric compounds with, for example, a 5′-8-carbon–carbon linkage are also known (biflavonoids). The glycosides are generally soluble in water and alcohol, but insoluble in organic solvents; the genins are only sparingly soluble in water but are soluble in ether. Flavonoids dissolve in alkalis, giving yellow solutions which on the addition of acid become colourless.

Although the original high hopes for the therapeutic usefulness of flavonoids were not immediately realized, recent researches have demonstrated their involvement in the medicinal action of drugs such as liquorice root, Roman chamomile and gingko. It is very probable that a number of herbal remedies, whose constituents are as yet unknown, will be shown to contain active flavonoids. Of the 84 drugs described in the *BHP*, Vol 1, 1991, some 36 contain flavonoids but not necessarily as the active constituents. A number of flavonoid-containing herbs have now been included in the *BP/EP*, examples are Birch Leaf, Calendula Flower, Elder Flower, Horsetail, Lime Flower, Motherwort and Passiflora. The group is known for its anti-inflammatory and antiallergic effects, for antithrombitic and vasoprotective properties, for inhibition of tumour promotion and as a protective for the gastric mucosa. Some of these pharmacological properties can be explained on the basis of antioxidant activity as has recently been shown for tiliroside (see Lime Flower) and the related gnaphaliine isolated from the aerial parts of *Helichrysum italicum* (G. R. Schinella *et al.*, *Fitoterapia*, 2007, **78**, 1). Many flavonoid-containing plants are diuretic (e.g. buchu and broom) or antispasmodic (e.g. liquorice and parsley). Some flavonoids have antitumour, antibacterial or antifungal properties. E.-A. Bae *et al.* (*Planta Medica*, 1999, **65**, 442) have recently investigated the *in vitro* anti-*Helicobacter pylori* activity of a number of flavonoids (hesperidin, hesperetin, naringin, naringenin, diosmin, diosmetin) and suggest that even if not potent inhibitors of, they may contribute to the prevention of gastritis. Others, e.g. fustic (from the wood of *Morus tinctoria*) and sumac (leaves of *Rhus* spp.) are colouring and tannin materials.

Pure flavone, which is colourless, occurs on the surface of some species of *Primula*. As shown in Table 21.5, many flavones are phenolic or methoxyl derivatives and form sap-soluble glycosides. The intensity of their yellow colour increases with the number of hydroxyl groups and with increase of pH.

Isoflavonoids. Isoflavones are found in the heartwood of species of *Prunus* and in species of *Iris*, and are particularly abundant in the Leguminosae (e.g. in dyer's broom, *Genista tinctoria*). The latter contains genistin (not to be confused with the gentisin of gentian), the 7-glucoside of genistein. Rotenone contained in the roots of *Derris* and *Lonchocarpus* species (see Chapter 40) is an isoflavonoid in which the 2,3 double bond of an isoflavone is reduced.

Phyto-oestrogens. Isoflavones, along with coumestans (also flavonoids) and lignans (q.v.), belong to a class of substances known as non-steroidal phyto-oestrogens. Both structurally and functionally they are similar to oestradiol (see Fig. 23.4) and related sex hormones

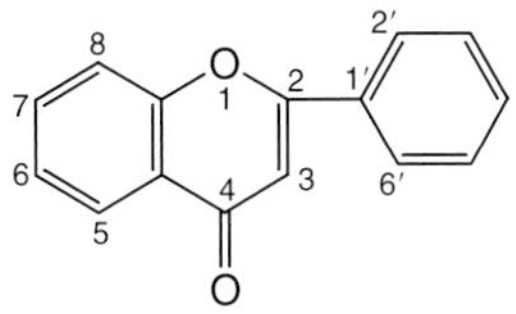

Flavone
(2-phenyl-γ-chromone)

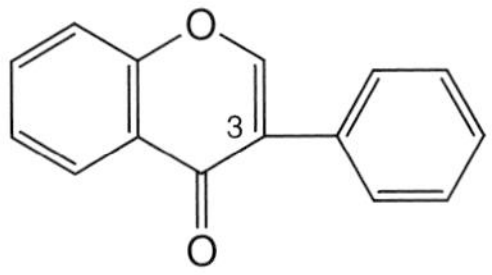

Isoflavone
(3-phenyl-γ-chromone)

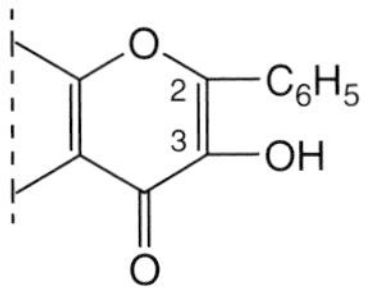

Flavonol

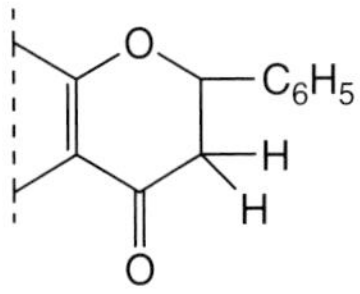

Flavanone

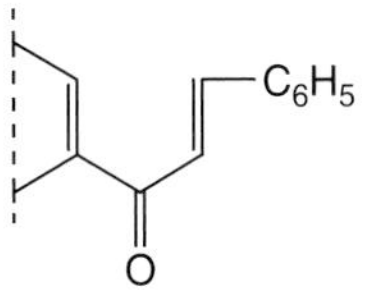

Chalcone

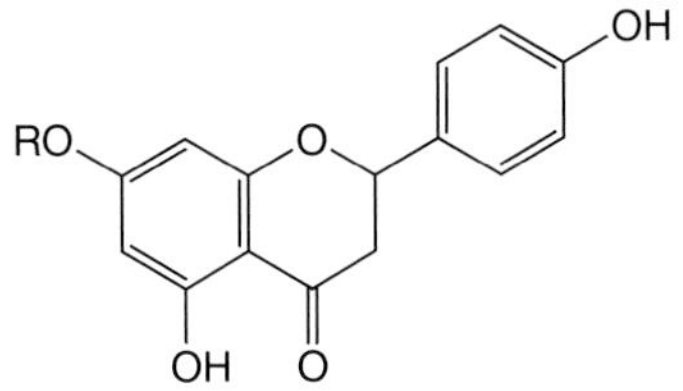

Naringenin; R = H
Naringin; R = rhamno-glucosyl
(Flavanones)

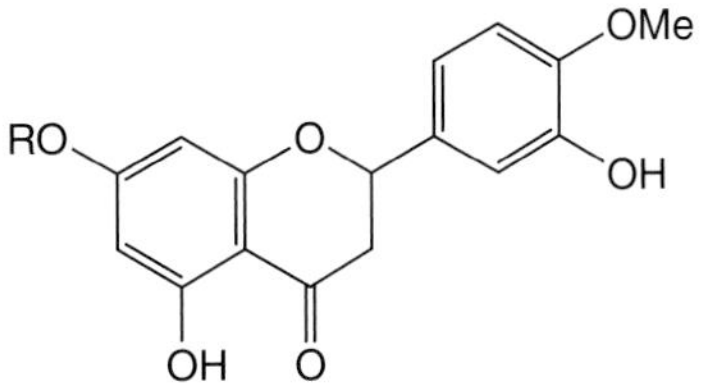

Hesperetin; R = H
Hesperidin; R = rhamno-glucosyl
(Flavanones)

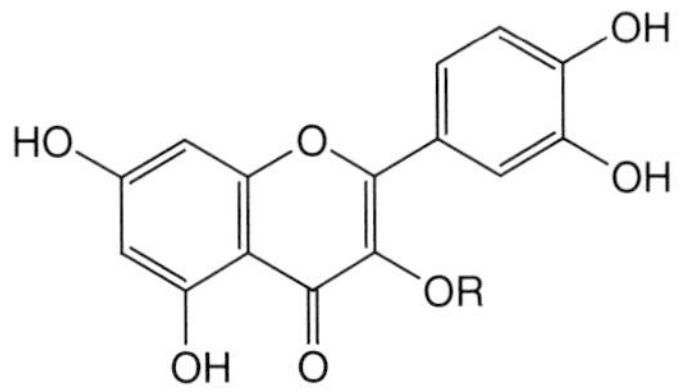

Quercetin; R = H
Hyperoside; R = galactosyl
Isoquercitrin; R = glucosyl
Rutin; R = rhamno-glucosyl
(Flavonols)

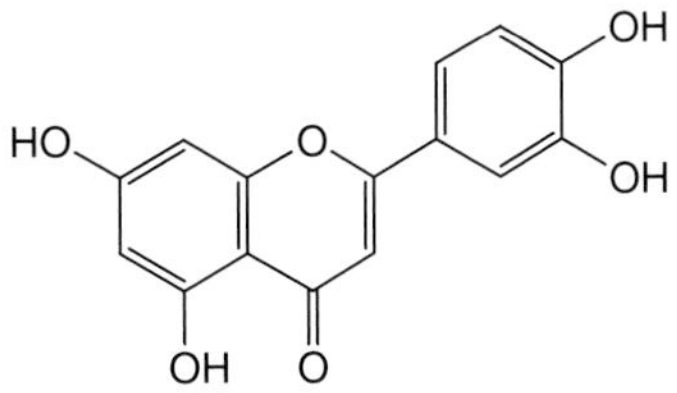

Luteolin
(Flavone)

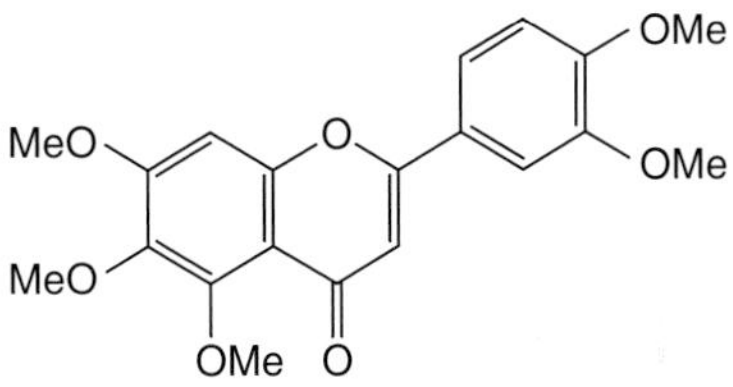

Sinensetin
(Flavone)

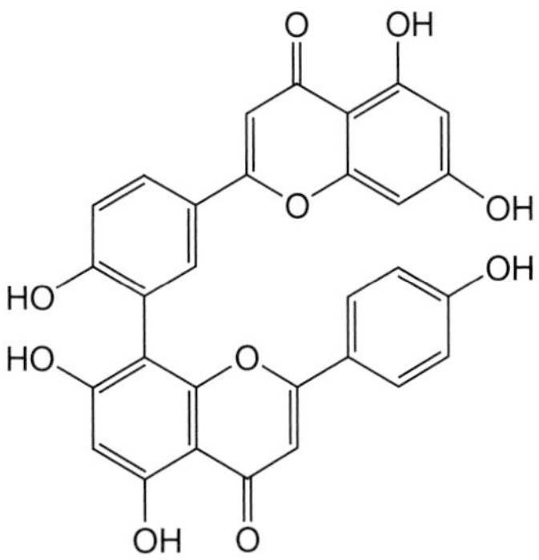

Amentoflavone

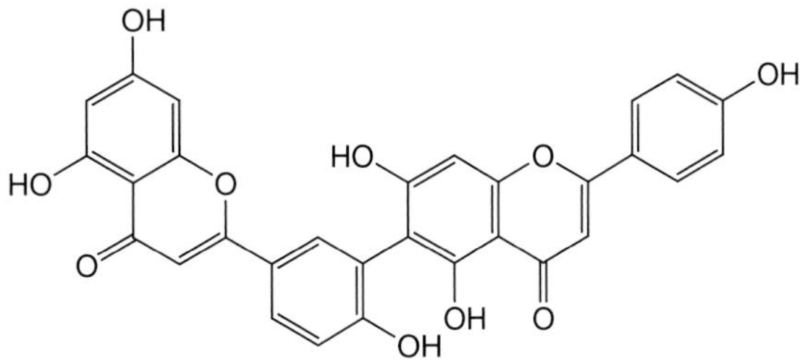

Robustaflavone

(Biflavonols)

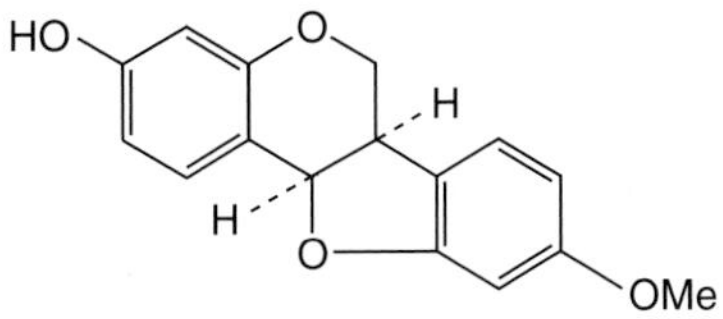

Medicarpin—a pterocarpan
(isoflavone derivative)

Fig. 21.18
Structural types of flavonoids, aglycones and glycosides.

and exert weak oestrogenic effects. They are present in certain foods and herbal remedies and are well-documented as producing infertility in animals as, for example, clover disease in sheep grazing on clovers containing a high phyto-oestrogen content.

Studies provoking much medical and general press attention have centred on the role of phyto-oestrogens as dietary constituents having positive effects in the prevention of cancer, heart disease and post-menopausal symptoms.

Foods containing appreciable quantities of isoflavones are soya beans, soy products and other legume crops; they are also present in the herbs Red Clover Flower *BHP* (*Trifolium pratense*) and broomtops (*Cytisus scoparius*). In the plant they occur free or in the glycosidic form, in the latter case being hydrolysed by colonic bacteria to give the active aglycone; genistein and daidzein are the principal examples, the latter being formed from formononetin (Table 21.5). As plant nutraceuticals, these compounds are more fully discussed in Chapter 32.

A new class of non-steroidal phyto-oestrogens are the prenylated flavonoids. Many of these compounds are known and this activity has been described for 8-isopentenylnaringenin.

Biflavonoids. The first biflavonoid to be isolated was gingetin, in 1929. Now more than 100 are known with a variety of biological activities being reported. Amentoflavone is of wide distribution, e.g. species of *Ginkgo*, *Hypericum*, *Rhus* and together with robustaflavone has been shown to have activity against influenza A virus, HSV-1 and HSV-2 viruses (Y.-M. Lin *et al.*, *Planta Medica*, 1999, **65**, 120).

Further reading

Andersen M and Markham KR 2006 Flavonoids, chemistry biochemistry and application. CRC Press/Taylor and Francis, Boca Raton, FL., xiv, 1237

Cos P *et al*. 2003 Phytoestrogens and recent developments. Planta Medica 69 (7): 589–599

Gross M 2004 Flavonoids and cardiovascular disease. Pharmaceutical Biology 42 (Supplement): 121–135

Neuhouser ML 2004 Flavonoids and cancer prevention: what is the evidence in humans? Pharmaceutical Biology 42 (Supplement): 36–45

Pietta P-G 2000 Flavonoids as antioxidants. Journal of Natural Products 63(7): 1035–1042

AGNUS CASTUS FRUIT

The *BP/EP*, *BHP* drug consists of the whole, ripe, dried fruit of *Vitex agnus castus* L., family Verbenaceae. Synonyms include Chaste tree, Chaste

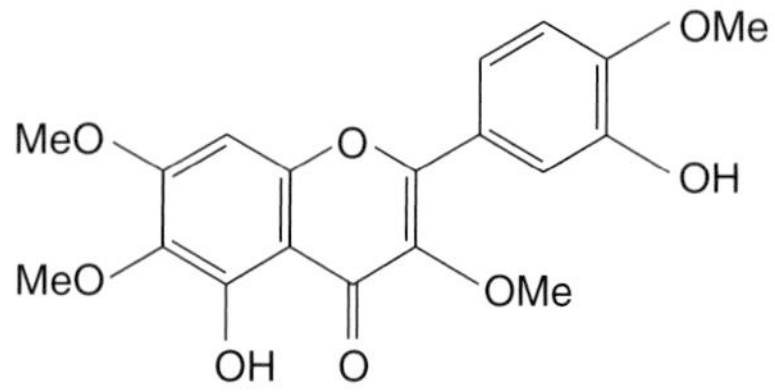

Casticin
(Flavonoid)

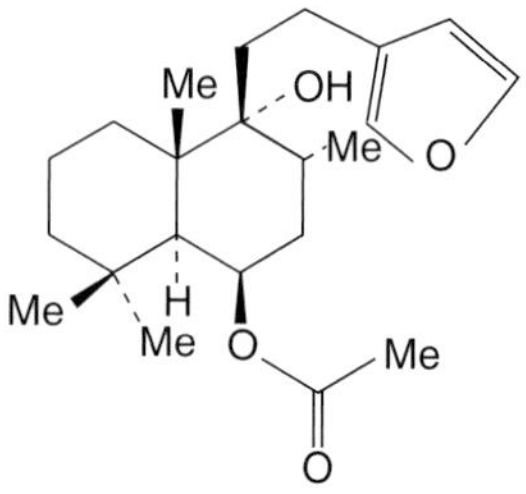

Rotundifuran
(Labdane-type diterpenoid)

Fig. 21.19
Constituents of agnus castus.

berry and Monk's pepper, alluding to its association with chastity. The plant is a shrub or small tree found in the Mediterranean regions of southern Europe; Morocco and Albania are important commercial suppliers.

The small dark berries are collected from the wild in autumn and dried. As such, they are blackish-brown in colour with a diameter of up to 5 mm, quadrilocular and four-seeded. A persistent toothed calyx covers up to three-quarters of the fruit. Features of the powder include covering and glandular trichomes from the calyx and numerous diverse fragments from the pericarp and seeds—all detailed in the official monographs.

Extensive studies on the phytochemistry have involved flavonoids (of which the *BP* specifies a minimum content of 0.08% calculated as casticin), also vitexin, penduletin and kaempferol; diterpenes including rotundifuran (Fig. 21.19) and vitexilactone; and various iridoids including aucubin (Fig. 24.1). The latter is used as a reference in the

Table 21.5 Flavonoid types and examples.

Type	Compound	Nature	Occurrence
Flavone	Chrysin	Dihydroxy 5,7	*Prunus, Populus* (heartwood and Balm of Gilead Bud)
Flavone	Butin	Trihydroxy 7,3',4'	*Butea monosperma* seeds (antifertility activity)
Flavone	Apigenin	Trihydroxy 5,7,4'	Parsley, Roman chamomile flower
Flavone	Luteolin	Tetrahydroxy 5,7,3',4'	*Reseda luteola* and as glycosides in celery, peppermint, wild carrot etc.
Flavone	Fisetin	Tetrahydroxy 3,7,3',4'	Yellow cedar wood and the dyestuff sumac
Flavonol	Quercetin	Pentahydroxy 3,5,7,3',4'	As the rhamnoglucoside rutin and as many other glycosides
Flavonol	Kaempferol	Tetrahydroxy 3,5,7,4'	Senna
Flavonone	Eriodictyol	Tetrahydroxy 5,7,3',4'	Yerba santa (Hydrophyllaceae)
Flavonone	Liquiritigenin	Dihydroxy 7,4'	Liquorice
Chalcones	Unstable isomers of flavonones		Family Rutaceae and liquorice
Xanthone	Gentisin	1,7-Dihydroxy-3-methoxy	*Gentiana* and *Swertia* spp.
Isoflavone	Formononetin	Dihydroxy 7,4'	Cimicifuga rhizome, red clover flower
	Genistein	Trihydroxy 5,7,4'	Red clover flower, as glucoside in *Genista*
Biflavone	Amentoflavone	Hexahydroxy 2× (5,7,4')	Ginkgo, hypericum, *Rhus* spp.

TLC test of identity and casticin is assayed by liquid chromatography. Volatile oil (*ca* 0.5%) consists mainly of mono- and sesquiterpenes.

The drug has a long history of use in various menstrual problems and in deficient lactation. In 2001 it was recommended as a therapeutic option for premenstrual syndrome where no cause could be identified (R. Schellenberg *et al.*, *Br. Med. J.*, 2001, **322**, 134) and further supported in 2006 by research demonstrating its activation of the μ-opiate receptor (D. E. Webster *et al.*, *J. Ethnopharmacol*, 2006, **106**, 216).

Allied drug. Vitex negundo fruits are used in Asian medicine and can be distinguished from the *BP* drug by larger fruits.

BIRCH LEAF

Birch leaf has been included in several European pharmacopoeias for many years. The *BP/EP* drug consists of the dried whole or broken leaves of *Betula pendula* Roth. and/or *B. pubescens* Ehrh. and hybrids, family Betulaceae, containing not less than 1.5% of flavonoids calculated as hyperoside. *B. pendula* (silver birch) is common throughout Europe and *B. pubescens* (downy or white birch) is Eurasian in origin. Commercial supplies derive largely from Eastern Europe, China and the former USSR.

Leaves from *B. pendula* are 2.5–6.0 cm in length and 2–5 cm wide, glabrous, green on the upper surface, lighter green on the lower; in shape rhomboidal, triangular or ovoid in outline with a broadly tapering or cuneate base attached to a long petiole. The margin is biserrate, the apex long and acuminate. Larger veins are pinnate with an overall reticulation.

B. pubescens has similar, somewhat smaller, more rounded and often slightly pubescent leaves. The apex is neither long nor acuminate and the marginal teeth are smaller and less obviously apically directed than with *B. pendula*.

The microscopical characteristics of both species are similar, the lower epidermi having, in surface view, straight-walled cells and numerous anomocytic stomata with four to eight subsidiary cells. Calcium oxalate crystals occur as clusters in the mesophyll cells and as crystal fibres near the larger veins. Peltate sessile glands situated in shallow depressions are numerous on both surfaces. *B. pubescens* possesses unlignified unicellular thick-walled covering trichomes 80–**100**–**200**–600 μm in length.

The flavonoid compositions of both *B. pendula* and *B. pubescens* are similar with total flavonoids (about 3%) including hyperoside (up to 0.8%), quercitrin (up to 0.14%), myricetin galactoside (up to 0.37%) and other glycosides of quercetin (e.g. the arabinoside avicularin), kaempferol and myricetin. For a detailed analysis of 14 batches of *B. pendula* and three batches of *B. pubescens* see A. Carnat *et al.*, *Ann. Pharm. Franc.*, 1996, **54**, 231. This group also found the flavonoid level of older leaves of *B. pendula* to be lower than that of young leaves. The small proportion (0.1%) of essential oil contains sesquiterpene oxides. Other constituents of the leaves are (+)-catechin, monoterpene glycosides, triterpene alcohols and esters of the dammarene type. The mineral content (*c.* 4%) is particularly rich in potassium.

The official assay involves an acid hydrolysis of the powdered sample followed by extraction of the flavonoids, and their determination by absorption measurements at 425 nm.

Preparations of the leaf are used as an irrigant of the urinary tract, especially in cases of inflammation and renal gravel. Birch leaf is also an antirheumatic and has been employed to treat gout; as an astringent it is used as a mouthwash.

Birch bark has found traditional use in medicine for the topical treatment of skin diseases; it contains proanthocyanidins and considerable amounts of triterpenoid derivatives of the lupane (betulin, betulinic acid, lupeol) and oleane (oleanolic acid) types. Recently, M. Laszczyk *et al.* (*Planta Medica*, 2006, **72** 1353) have described the isolation and the physical, chemical and pharmacological properties of a gel extract from the outer bark containing triterpenes which can be applied topically to the skin; its cytotoxic properties were demonstrated experimentally. Betulinic acid is a potential agent for the treatment of human melanoma.

CALENDULA FLOWER

Source. Calendula flower derives from the marigold *Calendula officinalis* L., family Compositae, and is not to be confused with 'marigold' referring to *Tagetes* spp. The *EP* and *BP* specify the whole or cut, dried, and fully opened flowers detached from the receptacle and obtained from cultivated varieties. The *BHP* allows also the whole composite flowers which includes the involucre of bracts.

C. officinalis is a native of Central, Eastern and Southern Europe and commercial supplies are obtained largely from Eastern Europe and Egypt.

Characters. Detailed descriptions for the ligulate florets and the composite flower heads will be found in the *BP* and *BHP* respectively. Diagnostic features are the morphology of the ligulate and tubular florets, various biseriate clothing and glandular trichomes (see e.g. Fig. 42.4), pollen grains with a spiny exine, and corolla fragments with yellow oil-droplets, calcium oxalate and fairly large anomocytic stomata.

Constituents. Flavonoids, triterpenoids, essential oil and polysaccharides are the principal constituents of calendula flowers. All groups have been shown to exhibit pharmacological activity and serve to illustrate the difficulty of devising an assay which represents the true therapeutic activity of the drug. The *EP* and *BP* determine the flavonoid content, expressed as hyperoside (not less than 0.4%), utilizing the same method as for Birch Leaf. Other assays based on triterpenoid assessment have been described.

The flavonoid mixture involves quercetin and isorhamnetin derivatives. Triterpenoid saponins (calendulosides A–F, see Table 23.5) are glycosides based on oleanolic acid-3-*O*-β-D-glucuronide and are present in variable proportions (2–10%) depending on time of harvesting and chemotype. The roots are a richer source than the flowers. These saponins have haemolytic and anti-inflammatory activity. Polysaccharides include a rhamnoarabinogalactan (M_r 15 000; rhamnose 24.8%, arabinose 34.2%, galactose 41.0%) and two arabinogalactans with M_r's of 25 000 and 35 000 (J. Varljen *et al.*, *Phytochemistry*, 1989, **28**, 2379). Antitumour and phagocytosis stimulation properties have been reported for the polysaccharide fraction. At least 15 compounds have been identified in the essential oil.

Other constituents of the flowers are triterpene alcohols (e.g. α- and β-amyrin, calenduladiol, etc.), sesquiterpenes and carotenoids.

Uses. Calendula is used internally for the alleviation of gastrointestinal disorders and externally, as an ointment or lotion, for the treatment of minor wounds and rashes.

ELDER FLOWER

Elder flower consists of the dried flowers of *Sambucus nigra* L., family Caprifoliaceae. This shrub or small tree is native throughout Europe and Western and Central Asia; commercial supplies of the flowers come principally from Eastern Europe, small quantities are collected in the UK.

Characters. The elder inflorescence consists of small regular flowers arranged in compound umbel-like cymes; calyx superior,

21

5-toothed; corolla flat, rotate, deeply 5-lobed, creamy white with 5 stamens inserted in the tube; anthers yellow. The flowers have a slightly bitter taste and a sweet, not altogether agreeable odour.

The microscopical characters of the corolla include numerous small oil globules and an upper epidermis with cells having slightly thickened, beaded walls and a striated cuticle. Epidermal cells of the calyx also have striated walls and those at the basal end exhibit unicellular marginal teeth. Calcium oxalate is seen as idioblasts of sandy crystals. There are numerous pollen grains about 30 μm in diameter (as measured in a chloral hydrate mountant) with a faintly pitted exine and three germinal pores and furrows.

Constituents. The drug contains a small proportion (up to c. 0.2%) of a semi-solid volatile oil consisting of free acids, principally palmitic acid, and C_{14}–C_{31} n-alkanes. By 1985 over 80 components had been identified in the oil.

Flavonoids (up to 3.0%) are predominantly flavonols and their glycosides: rutin predominates with smaller quantities of isoquercetrin, astragalin and hyperoside together with the aglycones quercetin and kaempferol.

Other constituents are triterpenes (α- and β-amyrin principally as esters of fatty acids), triterpene acids (ursolic, oleanolic and 20β-hydroxyursolic acids), various other plant acids (chlorogenic, p-coumaric, caffeic and ferulic acids, (Fig. 19.5), and their β-glucosides), sterols, mucilage, tannin and traces of sambunigrin (Table 25.1).

Standards. There are BP/EP limits for discoloured, brown flowers (15%) and for fragments of coarse pedicels and other foreign matter (8%). Thin-layer chromatography is employed as a test for identity with further modification to detect adulteration with Sambucus ebulus. Flavonoids, calculated as isoquercetrin are determined by absorbance measurements at 425 nm.

Allied species. Sambucus ebulus (danewort) is a perennial, foetid glabrous herb with a creeping rhizome and upright little-branched stems. It occurs throughout Europe and apart from habit, is distinguished from S. nigra by obvious ovate stipules. S. canadensis, American elder, is a somewhat smaller tree than S. nigra and is widely spread throughout North America; it is used similarly to S. nigra.

Uses. Elder flowers are administered principally as an infusion or herbal tea for the treatment of feverish conditions and the common cold; it acts as a diaphoretic but the mechanism and constituents involved are unclear. The flowers also have diuretic properties.

It may be noted that the sialic acid-binding lectin present in elder stem-bark extracts finds considerable current use in certain biochemical procedures.

HORSETAIL

Equisetum BHP 1996, Horsetail BP/EP consists of the dried sterile aerial parts of Equisetum arvense L. (common horsetail). The plant is found throughout Europe, common in Britain, central China and parts of N. America, preferring the moist sandy or loamy soil of hedgebanks, fields or waste places. Classed within the Pteridophyta (p. 21) it is a flowerless perennial, 20–80 cm in height producing in the spring chlorophyll-free jointed stems each terminating in a sporangia-producing cone. Apparent in the summer are jointed green stems with grooved, toothed sheaths at the nodes together with whorls of many-jointed, spreading branches. It is these sterile structures that constitute the medicinal drug.

Macroscopically, the drug consists of broken green stems and branches, the larger pieces being up to 80 cm in length and 5 cm in diameter. The surface is rough to the touch and the fracture short, exposing a large central cavity. The internodes of the main stem have up to 15 vertical grooves and at the nodes a sheath with as many triangular lanceolate teeth as grooves on the internodes. The branches are solid, again with internodes, the lowest of which on each branch is longer than the sheath with which it is associated.

Diagnostic features of the powder include: characteristic epidermis with paracytic stomata overlapped by the two adjacent subsidiary cells; two-celled non-lignified protuberances on the ridged areas; large-celled parenchyma with many lacunae; non-lignified fibres up to 1 mm long with narrow lumens; small spirally or annularly thickened lignified vessels.

Constituents. Various flavonoids occur in horsetail to the extent of 1.0%, the BP/EP requiring a content of at least 0.3% total flavonoids expressed as isoquercitroside. A major component is quercetin 3-glucoside, also luteolin glycosides in some samples (Fig. 21.18). Chemical races of horsetail involve flavonoids, see M. Veit et al., Planta Medica, 1989, **55**, 214. Horsetail also contains a naturally high mineral content, with silicic acid and silicates comprising about 8% of the drug; also present are potassium and aluminium chlorides, all contributing to a high ash value for the drug for which, unusually for crude drugs, the pharmacopoeia sets a minimum, as well as higher limit, viz: total ash within 12–27%, acid-insoluble ash within 3–15%. Alkaloids are usually absent or present in small amounts, but see below for poisonous adulterants. Phenolic acids, saponins and phytosterols are among other reported constituents.

Uses. At one time the high siliceous mineral content of horsetail rendered it useful for the abrasive cleaning of copper and bare wooden objects. Traditionally, it has been used medicinally for its diuretic, haemostatic and astringent properties in particular for genitourinary complaints and externally to assist wound healing.

Allied species. A number of Equisetum spp. grow in similar damp localities to that of E. arvense, including E. sylvaticum the wood horsetail, E. palustre the marsh horsetail and E. fluviatile the water horsetail and might be mistaken or substituted for the genuine drug. As these are known to cause animal poisoning due to the alkaloids, e.g. palustrine and saporins, which have been reported, correct identification of the drug is essential. This is addressed by the pharmacopoeial macroscopic and microscopic descriptions of the drug, briefly covered above, and the TLC test for 'Other Equisetum species and hybrids'.

JAVA TEA

Java tea BP/EP, BHP consists of the dried leaves and tops of stems of Orthosiphon stamineus Benth. (O. aristatus Miq., O. spicatus Bak.), family Labiatae/Laminiaceae.

The plant is a perennial shrub up to 1 m in height with a four-angled stem bearing pointed leaves and lilac-coloured flowers arranged in whorls with four very long blue–violet stamens. It is native to S.E. Asia and Australia. Commercial supplies come from plants cultivated in Indonesia; the leaves and tips are collected shortly before flowering.

Characters. The shortly petiolate leaves are 2–7 cm long with pointed apex, cuneate base, coarsely serrate margin, deep green to yellowish-green upper surface, greenish-grey lower surfaces and, often pigmented pinnate venation.

Microscopical characteristics include wavy-walled, slightly beaded epidermal cells, diacytic stomata more numerous on the lower surface, laminaceous glandular trichomes having in contrast to many other species only four secretory cells, multicellular uniseriate conical clothing trichomes often with reddish contents. The stems afford considerable non-specific vascular tissue.

Constituents. Flavonoids as represented by sinensetin (Fig. 21.18) and various derivatives; diterpenes as illustrated by orthosiphols A–J and other highly oxygenated diterpenes (see S. Awale *et al.*, *Chem. Pharm. Bull.*, 2003, **51**, 268); various benzochromenes, including methylripariochromene A in variable amounts and others; volatile oil up to 0.7% and containing β-caryophyllene and its oxide, α-humulene, β-elemene, etc.; caffeic acid and its derivatives, particularly rosmarinic acid; phytosterols such as β-sitosterol; and inorganic salts, particularly potassium at around 3.0%.

The *BP/EP* requires a minimum content of 0.05% sinensetin for the drug determined by liquid chromatography using sinensetin as the reference compound.

Uses. Traditional uses in Europe invoke the diuretic properties of the drug for the treatment of urinary and kidney problems; in S.E. Asia it is used for the treatment of diabetes and hypertension.

LIME FLOWER

Lime Flower *BP/EP* consists of the dried inflorescences of *Tilia cordata* Miller (small-leaved lime), *T. platyphyllos* Scop. (broad-leaved lime), *T. × vulgaris* Heyne or a mixture of these, family Tiliaceae. The trees are native throughout Europe and extensively planted. Commercial supplies of the flowers come from China, the Balkans, Turkey and Hungary, the latter exporting (1997) over 100 tonnes.

The inflorescences consist of pendulous long-peduncled cymes consisting of yellowish-green flowers, the peduncles being adnated to almost glabrous, strap-shaped bracts for about half their lengths. Each flower has five petals, five sepals, numerous stamens forming five groups, and a five-lobed stigma. The odour is faintly aromatic and the taste sweet and mucilaginous.

Features of the microscopy are the mucilaginous cells of the sepals and petals; small clusters of calcium oxalate crystals throughout the parenchymatous tissues; oval to slightly triangular pollen grains, 30–40 μm in diameter and having three germinal pores and a finely granulated exine; other general features of the sepals and petals.

The flavonoid constituents comprise quercetin glycosides (rutin, hyperoside, quercitrin, etc.) and kaempferol glycosides (tiliroside, astragalin). Mucilage, present chiefly in the bracts consists largely of galactomannans, and a small proportion of volatile oil (*c.* 0.02–0.1%) containing farnesol, farnesyl acetate, geraniol and eugenol gives the drug its characteristic faint odour, more pronounced with the fresh flowers. Phenolic acids and proanthocyanidins are also present.

| kaempferol | glucose | *p*-coumaric acid |

Tiliroside

The official upper limit for foreign matter in Lime Flower is 2.0% with observations for the absence of *T. americana* (basswood) and *T. tomentosa* based on flower structure. No assay is given but methods have been published in the German literature.

As with most herbal remedies lime flowers have a multiplicity of applications. In action they are diaphoretic, antispasmodic and expectorant and as such are used, often in conjunction with other herbs, as a nerve tonic, for the treatment of catarrh and indigestion, and for the alleviation of headaches.

MOTHERWORT

The dried aerial parts of *Leonurus cardiaca* L. family Labiatae/Lamiaceae constitute the drug Motherwort *BP/EP*, Leonurus *BHP* 1983 (common name lion's tail). The herb is collected during the flowering period.

L. cardiaca is native to Siberia and found generally throughout Europe from Scandinavia to the N. Mediterranean countries; it is rare in Britain, occurring on waste land, in hedges, ditches etc., and has become naturalized in N. America. A perennial herb 60–150 cm in height, it has square stems and alternate leaves. The lower and middle leaves are distinctly divided into five to seven pointed, dentate lobes, whereas the upper leaves are three-lobed, dark green on the upper surface with few trichomes, paler green and felted on the lower surface. Labiate flowers occur in well-separated whorls in the axils of the upper leaves, the general form giving rise to the generic and one of the common names of the plant (see above). The pubescent flower is white or pink, often spotted on the lower lip of the corolla; the angled calyx has five teeth the two lower ones being sharply recurved.

The microscopic features of the green powder are characteristic of the family and include: straight-walled cells of the upper epidermis with striated cuticles, the lower epidermis with anisocytic stomata, glandular trichomes with short unicellular stalks and multicellular heads, numerous covering trichomes occasionally up to 1500 μm in length, vascular tissue of stems and veins, small clusters and single crystals of calcium oxalate.

For the dried drug the *BP/EP* limits brown or yellow leaves to 2% and other foreign matter to 2%.

Constituents. Apart from the earlier isolation of stachydrine (formula, see Fig. 26.2), it was in the period 1970–1985 that the major constituents of motherwort were elucidated; these include flavonoids, iridoids, terpenoids and tannins.

Flavonoids include hyperoside, kaemferol-3-D-glucoside, quercitrin and rutin (for formulae of these see Fig. 21.18 and Table 21.5). Iridoids include leonuride (see Fig. 24.1), ajugol and others. Minor alkaloids in addition to the major alkaloid stachydrine include the stereoisomers of its 4-hydroxy derivative (turicin) and betonicine (see formula under 'Yarrow'). Diterpenes of the labdane type include leocardin and a diterpene similar to marrubiin (q.v.). For the structural determination of three new labdane diterpenes see K. Vijai *et al.*, *Planta Medica*, 2008, **74**, 1288.

The *BP/EP* requires a minimum flavonoid content for the drug of 0.2% expressed as hyperoside and assayed by absorbance measurements at 425 nm on a hydrolysed extract.

Traditional uses. For nervous tension and menstrual problems. There is some pharmacological support for its use as a uterotonic and for cardiovascular disorders.

OLIVE LEAVES

The olive (*Olea europaea* L., family Oleaceae), best known medicinally for its expressed oil (q.v.), is also used in continental Europe for

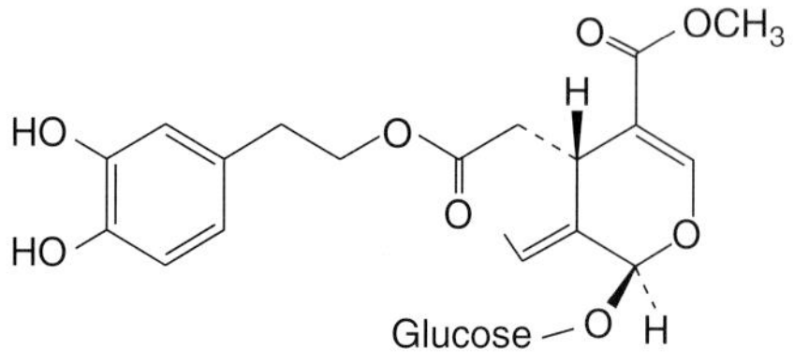

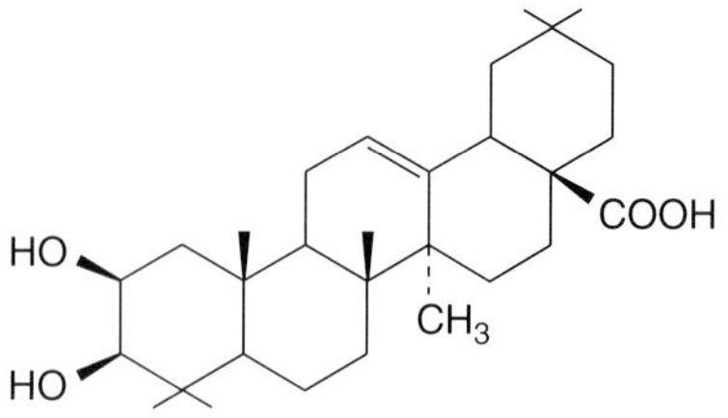

Fig. 21.20
Constituents of olive leaves.

Oleuropein

Maslinic acid

the antiseptic, astringent and sedative properties of the leaves. It can be employed both internally and externally.

The dried, leathery leaves, 30–50 mm long and 10–15 mm wide are elliptic, oblong or lanceolate in shape. The apex is mucronate, base shortly petiolate and tapering; margin entire and somewhat recurved. The upper surface is dark green, the lower paler due to a covering of silvery trichomes.

Microscopy of the powder shows thick walled polygonal epidermal cells with small anomocytic stomata on the lower surface together with large peltate trichomes, often broken. Sclereids are apparent.

Flavonols, including rutin (Fig. 21.18) and oleuropein are the principal components. Both compounds are used in the *BP/EP* TLC test for identity and there is a minimum requirement of 5.0% for oleuropein determined by liquid chromatography using a standard solution of it as reference. The pentacyclic triterpenoid maslinic acid occurs in the petioles and has various biological activities; it may offer advantages in the resistance to oxidative stress in animals (Montilla M. P. *et al.*, *Planta Med.*, 2003, **69**, 472).

Triterpene acids have been isolated from plant-cell suspension cultures; they include six ursane-type acids and two oleane-type acids (oleanolic and maslinic) with the ursane-type predominant (H. Saimaru *et al.*, *Chem. Pharm. Bull.*, 2007, **55**, 784).

Olive leaves are used as an infusion for their tranquillizing effect in nervous tension and for their antiseptic, astringent and febrifuge properties.

PASSIFLORA

Passiflora (Passion Flower) consists of the dried aerial parts of *Passiflora incarnata* L. collected during the flowering and fruiting period. The drug is described in the *BP*, *EP*, *BHP*, the *British Herbal Compendium*, Vol. 1 and in an *ESCOP* monograph; it is also official in the French, German and Swiss pharmacopoeias. The genus is native to South America and species are widely cultivated as ornamentals. *P. incarnata* is imported from the USA, India and to some extent from the West Indies.

By the nature of its definition, the macroscopical and microscopical characteristics of the drug are numerous and for these the reader should consult one of the sources mentioned above.

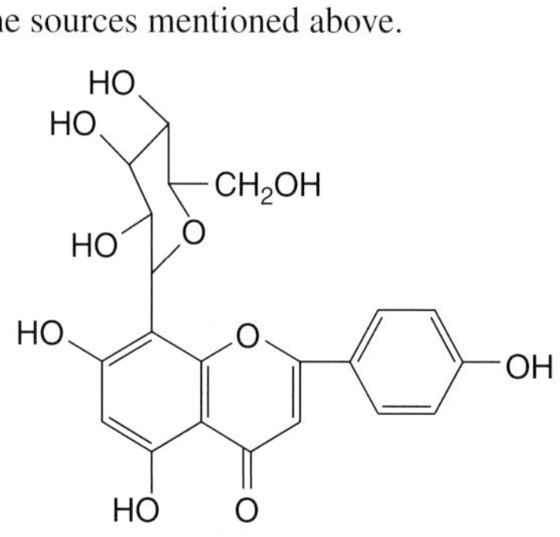

Vitexin

Constituents of the genus include flavonoids, mainly *C*-glycosides of apigenin and luteolin such as vitexin, isovitexin, orientin, iso-orientin and their 2″-β-D-glucosides. The *BP* drug is required to contain not less than 1.5% total flavonoids calculated as vitexin (measurement at 401 nm) after treatment of a dry extract with methanol in glacial acetic acid followed by boric acid and oxalic acid in anhydrous formic acid. Other constituents include traces of volatile oil, cyanogenetic glycosides and possibly traces of alkaloids of the harman type. Species other than *D. incarnata* (*P. coerulea*, *P. edulis*) are eliminated by thin-layer chromatography.

Passiflora has sedative actions; it is a popular ingredient of herbal preparations designed to counteract sleeplessness, restlessness and irritability.

For a review update covering all aspects of the drug (over 200 refs). see K. Dhawan *et al.*, *J. Ethnopharmacol.*, 2004, **94**, 1–23.

SPINY RESTHARROW ROOT

Spiny restharrow, *Ononis spinosa* L., family Leguminosae/Papilionaceae (syn. Restharrow, Cammock, Stayplough) is widely distributed throughout most of Europe except for the mountainous regions and the extreme north, also western Asia and North Africa; in England it is less common than the related species *O. repens* (Common restharrow). The plant is cultivated in Europe for medicinal purposes and harvested in the autumn. It is principally the roots that are used for medicinal purposes.

The dried drug consists of brown, longitudinally grooved roots, somewhat flattened and twisted and showing in transverse section a distinct radial arrangement of the xylem vascular tissue. The fracture is short and fibrous. Microscopical features include rounded starch grains and vascular tissue having vessels with small bordered pits.

Constituents. Isoflavones include the pterocarpan medicarpin (Fig. 21.18) (also a constituent of lucerne), homopterocarpin-7-*O*-glucoside and trifolirhizin (maackianin-7-*O*-glucoside); possibly the isoflavone formonoetin and its 7-*O*-glucoside. Tannins, lectins and triterpenoids, including α-onocerin (α-onoceradiendiol) have also been recorded. Volatile oil (0.02–0.29%), occurring in the entire plant, gives the drug a somewhat unpleasant odour and contains principally anethole, carvone and menthol; among other constituents are methone, camphor and estragole.

The *BP/EP* identification of the drug includes a TLC test.

Uses. The roots are traditionally used for their diuretic, antilithic and anti-inflammatory properties in the treatment of infections of the urinary tract and in removal of kidney and bladder stones.

Hesperidin and rutin

Although flavonoid preparations such as hesperidin and rutin are used in medicine, they do not appear to have justified the high hopes which followed the work of Szent–Györgyi in 1935 on the 'citrin' (sometimes known as vitamin P) of paprika and lemon peel. Citrus and other fruits have long been included in the human diet and, in addition to ascorbic acid and other compounds, provide flavonoids which decrease capillary fragility and are therefore employed in cases of hypertension and radiation injuries. The substance formerly known as 'citrin' is now known to be a mixture of the rhamnoglucosides of eriodictyol (a tetrahydroxyflavone) and methyl eriodictyol (hesperetin). Among the commercially available products of this type are some produced by the citrus industry containing hesperidin. A similar glycoside, rutin, (Fig. 21.18) the rhamnoglucoside of quercetin, is found in many plants, and commercial supplies are made from tobacco residues, *Sophora* and *Eucalyptus* spp. or buckwheat (*Fagopyrum esculentum*), which yields about 3–4%. Hairy root cultures of *F. esculentum* are reported to give a higher flavonol production than normal root cultures (F. Trotin *et al.*, *Phytochemistry*, 1993, **32**, 929). The flowers of *Sambucus nigra* (elder) have long been used in domestic and veterinary medicine, particularly in the form of ointment. They contain *p*-coumaric acid, rutin and kaempferol.

Rutin occurs as a yellow crystalline powder, soluble in alkali but only slightly soluble in water. Rutin on hydrolysis yields quercetin, rhamnose and glucose, while hesperidin yields hesperetin (or methyl eriodictyol), rhamnose and glucose.

BUCKWHEAT HERB

The drug consists of the dried aerial parts of *Fagopyrum esculentum* Moench, family Polygonaceae, collected when the plant is flowering and prior to fruiting.

Fagopyrum esculentum originated in Central Asia and by the Middle Ages was being cultivated in Europe as a source of grain and green fodder. It has been cultivated in the UK and is now found wild on wasteground as an escape. The fresh plant contains a photosensitizing agent, which, if consumed by animals exposed to sunlight, can cause them damage.

The plant is a little-branched, glabrous herb often with reddish stems and producing a cymose paniculate inflorescence with pink or white flowers. Dark green leaves, paler on the lower surface, are broadly triangular in outline, cordate–saggitate and acuminate. Features of the powder include anomocytic stomata, epidermal papilla-like projections over the veins, numerous calcium oxalate cluster crystals up to 100 μm and small prismatic crystals, vascular tissue of leaf and stem, spherical pollen grains and corolla fragments.

Rutin (see above) is the most important therapeutic constituent of the herb and the *BP/EP* requires a minimum content of 4.0% determined by liquid chromatography with absorbance measurements at 350 nm.

Buckwheat is used in the treatment of various circulatory disorders, including varicose veins, chilblains and retinal bleeding.

Silybin and silymarin

A number of flavonolignans—for example, silybin and silymarin (a 1,4-dioxan produced by the oxidative combination of taxifolin and coniferyl alcohol)—have antihepatotoxic properties, and extracts of plants containing them—for example, *Silybum marianum* (*Carduus marianus*), Compositae—are widely used in Germany for the treatment of liver ailments. The fruits of *S. marianum* contain silybin, silydianin and silychristin. For further details and structure of silybin see Chapter 29.

Visnaga

The drug consists of the dried ripe fruits of *Ammi visnaga* (Umbelliferae), an annual plant about 1–1.5 m high. It grows in the Middle East and is collected, particularly in Egypt. The greyish-brown

mericarps are usually separate but are sometimes attached to the carpophore. Each mericarp is broadly ovoid and about 0.5 mm long. It has five prominent primary ridges and six vittae. Odour, slightly aromatic; taste, very bitter.

Khellin, the most important active constituent, is crystalline and has been synthesized. It is 2-methyl-5,8-dimethoxyfuranochrome. It occurs to the extent of about 1%, the highest concentration being reported in the immature fruits, and is accompanied by two other crystalline compounds, visnagin (about 0.1%) and khellol glucoside (about 0.3%). The fruits contain a minute amount (less than 0.03%) of volatile oil. Contrary to previous ideas that khellin and visnagin are located in the vittae, Franchi *et al.* (*Int. J. Crude Drugs. Res.*, 1987, **25**, 137) have shown that, for fruits collected in Southern Tuscany, the furanochromones are present in the large secretory canals of the primary ribs and in the endosperm.

Khellin: R¹ = OCH₃, R² = H
Visnagin: R¹ = R² = H
Khellol glucoside: R¹ = H, R² = *O*-Glucoside

The drug has long been used in Egypt. Khellin, which is now commercially available in tablets and injection, is a potent coronary vasodilator. It has been employed in the treatment of angina pectoris and bronchial asthma, but its use appears to be limited by undesirable side-reactions.

ANTHOCYANIDINS AND GLYCOSIDES

Anthocyanidins are flavonoids structurally related to the flavones. Their glycosides are known as anthocyanins. These names are derived from the Greek *antho*-, flower, and *kyanos*, blue. They are sap pigments and the actual colour of the plant organ is determined by the pH of the sap. For example, the blue colour of the cornflower and the red of roses is due to the same glycosides and both of these plants on hydrolysis with hydrochloric acid yield cyanidin hydrochloride.

Anthocyanidin structure

Cyanidin chloride

Table 21.6 gives a few examples of these numerous and very widely distributed compounds. The most common anthocyanidin, cyanidin, occurs in about 80% of permanently pigmented leaves, 69% of fruits and 50% of flowers. Cyanidin is followed in order of frequency by delphinidin and pelargonidin.

21

Table 21.6 Common anthocyanidins.

Anthocyanidin	R	R′	Occurrence of glycosides
Pelargonidin	H	H	Flowers of *Pelargonium* (Geraniaceae) and pomegranate
Cyanidin	OH	H	Cornflowers, red poppies, *Rosa* spp., cocoa and cherries
Peonidin	OCH$_3$	H	Peony (Ranunculaceae)
Delphinidin	OH	OH	*Delphinium* and *Viola* spp.
Petunidin	OH	OCH$_3$	*Petunia* spp. (Solanaceae)
Malvidin	OCH$_3$	OCH$_3$	*Malva* spp., purple grades

Anthocyanidins are precipitated from aqueous solutions as lead salts or as picrates. After hydrolysis with 20% hydrochloric acid, anthocyanidin hydrochlorides, being only slightly soluble, often crystallize out. Chromatographic methods are widely used for the separation and identification of both the aglycones and sugars.

The sugar components are usually attached in the 3- or (more rarely) 5-position. It may be noted that in flavone glycosides the attachment is usually in the 7-position. They may be monosaccharides (glucose, galactose, rhamnose or arabinose); disaccharides (e.g. the rhamnoglucoside of *Antirrhinum* spp.); or trisaccharides (e.g. the 5-glucoside-3-rutinoside of certain Solanaceae such as *Atropa* and *Solanum*). Diglucosides, in which separate glucose molecules are attached in both the 3- and 5-positions, are common (e.g. *Campanula* and *Dahlia* spp.).

Despite their considerable biological importance the anthocyanidins are of little pharmaceutical significance as such, but as previously considered they constitute the monomers of the polymeric condensed tannins (q.v.).

For a review covering the analysis and biological activities of anthocyanins, see J.-M. Kong *et al.*, *Phytochemistry*, 2003, **64**, 923–933.

BILBERRY FRUIT

Bilberry (*Vaccinium myrtillus* L., family Vacciniaceae/Ericaceae) also known as blaeberry, whortleberry and huckleberry, is distributed throughout Europe, N. Asia and N. America including Canada. It grows on the acid soils of mountainous regions, heaths and moorlands and is found in most, particularly northern, regions of the British Isles. The plant is a glabrous, deciduous shrub up to 60 cm tall with creeping rhizomes and numerous erect stems and branches. It bears ovate, bright green leaves, 1–3 cm in length, pitcher-shaped greenish-pink flowers and globose berries about 8 mm in diameter, blue–black when ripe with a glaucous bloom. The quadri- or quinque-locular mesocarp of the fruit contains many ovoid, small, brown seeds. The edible sweet-tasting berries are collected from July to September. Both leaves and fruits were recognized in the Middle Ages for their medicinal value and separate monographs for fresh and dried fruits are now included in the *BP/EP*.

Constituents of the fruits. Anthocyanins, particularly glucosides and galactosides of cyanidin, peonidin, delphinidin, petunidin and malvidin (Table 21.6) are responsible for the final colour of the berries. These pigments increase in quantity during ripening whereas that of the polyphenols (−)-epicatechin, (+)-catechin and dimeric proanthocyanidins (Fig. 21.7) decrease. Other constituents include a number of common phenolic acids, vitamin C and volatile compounds. Over 100 volatiles have been identified, the principal ones that afford

the characteristic odour of the berries being *trans*-2-hexenal, ethyl 3-methylbutyrate and ethyl 2-methylbutyrate.

For the dried fruits, the *BP/EP* specifies a minimum tannin content of 1.0% expressed as pyrogallol and for the fresh fruits a minimum of 0.30% anthocyanins expressed as cyanidin-3-glucoside chloride. The latter is determined by absorption measurements at 528 nm on an acidified aqueous extract of the dried fresh berries. The loss on drying of the fresh berries is 80–90%.

Frozen fresh berries should be stored at or below −18°C. It is important to inspect the dried drug for insect and mouldiness.

Uses and actions. Bilberry has many traditional medicinal uses, a number of which have been supported by fairly extensive pharmacological research. For detailed references, the reader should consult J. Barnes *et al.*, *Herbal Medicines*, 2nd edn. 2002, p. 73, The Pharmaceutical Press, London. See also P. Morazzoni *et al.*, *Fitoterapia*, 1996, **66**, 3 for an overall review of bilberry.

STILBENES

Two stilbenes of pharmacognostical interest are rhaponticin and resveratrol. The former is a glycosidal constituent of rhapontic rhubarb (q.v.) and due to its fluorescence in u.v. light has long been used to detect adulteration of the official rhubarb. Resveratrol is a constituent of species of *Arachis*, *Cassia*, *Eucalyptus*, *Polygonum* and *Veratrum*. Recent interest has centred on its occurrence in grape preparations including red wine, and its therapeutic properties as an antioxidant, anti-inflammatory, anti-PAF and anticancer agent. It may also reduce the risk of coronary heart disease (J. S. Soleas *et al.*, *Clinical Biochemistry*, 1997, **30**, 91). As a constituent of 'darakchasava', it has long featured in Indian medicine (B. Paul *et al.*, *J. Ethnopharmacology*, 1999, **68**, 71).

Pinosylvin, a natural stilbene of the heartwood of *Pinus* spp. is related to, and has similar antibacterial properties to, resveratrol. S. K. Lee *et al.*, *Fitoterapia*, 2005, **76**, 258.

Stilbenes are biosynthesized from hydroxycinnamic acids and acetate.

For further discussion, see Chapter 32: The plant nutraceuticals.

Resveratrol, R = OH
Pinosylvin, R = H

LIGNANS AND LIGNIN

Lignans are dimeric compounds formed essentially by the union of two molecules of a phenylpropene derivative. At one time it was thought that these compounds were early intermediates in the formation of lignin but it is now recognized that they are offshoots of the principal lignin biosynthetic pathway. Unlike lignin they are optically active compounds and probably arise by stereospecific, reductive coupling between the middle carbons of the side-chain of the monomer. Some 300 lignans have been isolated and categorized into a number of groups according to structural features. Important pharmaceutical examples are the lignans of *Podophyllum* spp. (q.v.) which appear to be formed from two molecules of coniferyl alcohol or the corresponding acid with subsequent modification; apparently, a sinapic acid derivative, as might be expected by the inspection of the podophyllotoxin molecule, is not involved.

Some medicinal plants which contain lignans and which illustrate some of the structural types of this class of compound are given in Table 21.7. The lignans cited are not, however, necessarily the therapeutically active constituents of the plant.

Neolignans are also derived from the same units as lignans but the C_6–C_3 moieties are linked head to tail or head to head and not through the β–β' carbons. They occur in the heart-woods of trees of the Magnoliaceae, Lauraceae and Piperaceae. *Magnolia officinalis* and *M. obovata* are used in Chinese medicine. Magnolol, a neolignan isolated from the bark, has the following reported activities: CNS depressant and muscle relaxant, antiplatelet, antimicrobial, antitumour, anticancer, insecticidal, etc. (S. D. Sarker, *Fitoterapia*, 1997, **63**, 3).

Lignin is an important polymeric substance, $(C_6$–$C_3)_n$, laid down in a matrix of cellulose microfibrils to strengthen certain cell walls. It is an essential component of most woody tissues and involves vessels, tracheids, fibres and sclereids.

Lignins from different biological sources vary in composition, depending on the particular monomeric units of which they are composed (see Fig. 21.2). Variations in lignin constitution also arise as a result of random condensations of the appropriate alcohols with mesomeric free radicals formed from them by the action of a laccase-type (oxidase) enzyme. As there is no template for this non-enzymic condensation the lignin molecules formed vary in structure and so it is not possible to isolate lignin as a compound of defined composition.

The diagnostic value of lignin in crude drug analysis is covered in Chapter 42.

Further reading

Ward RD 1999 Lignans, neolignans and related compounds. Natural Product Reports 16(1): 75–96

Magnolol

Table 21.7 Occurrence of lignans in medicinal plants.

Species	Lignans	Notes
Guaiacum officinale, *G. sanctum* Source of Guaiacum Resin	α-Guaiaconic acid	A furano-type lignan. See 'Guaiacum resin' for other details. (+)-Neo-olivil of similar structure is the principal lignan of *Urtica dioica*
Myristica fragrans (Nutmeg)	Macelignan	A dibenzylbutane-type lignan
Piper cubeba (Tailed pepper)	(−)-Cubebin	A tetrahydrofuran-type lignan. Fruits contain c. 2% of (−)-cubebin together with related compounds

(Continued)

Table 21.7 Occurrence of lignans in medicinal plants. (Cont'd)

Species	Lignans	Notes
Podophyllum spp.	Podophyllotoxin	This aryltetralin-type lignan and other related compounds are the principal active constituents of *Podophyllum* root and rhizome (see Chapter 27). Also found in linseed, q.v.
Schisandra chinensis	Wuweizisu C	A dibenzocyclooctadiene-type lignan. This and other lignans of the same class have antihepatotoxic activity—see Chapter 29. Similar compounds are found in Korean Red Ginseng, q.v.
Silybum marianum *Urtica dioica* (Stinging nettle) *Viscum album* (Mistletoe) *Eleutherococcus senticosus* (*Acanthopanax senticosus*)	Silybin and others Neo-olivil derivatives Eleutheroside E [(−)-syringaresinoldiglucoside]	*Flavonolignans* (see Chapter 29) Tetrahydrofuran-type lignans A tetrahydrofurofuran-type lignan. Occurs in a number of plants together with related compounds including eleutheroside D, the diastereoisomer
Zanthoxylum clava-herculis (Prickly ash bark)	(+)-Asarinin	A tetrahydrofurofuran-type lignan. Occurs in prickly ash bark together with alkaloids, coumarins, amides, resins etc. Plants of this genus used in Western, Indian and Chinese herbal medicine

22

Volatile oils and resins

VOLATILE OILS

Volatile or essential oils, as their name implies, are volatile in steam. They differ entirely in both chemical and physical properties from fixed oils. With the exception of oils such as oil of bitter almonds, which are produced by the hydrolysis of glycosides, these oils are contained largely as such in the plant. They are secreted in oil cells, in secretion ducts or cavities or in glandular hairs (see Chapter 42). They are frequently associated with other substances such as gums and resins and themselves tend to resinify on exposure to air.

Production and uses of volatile oils

Large quantities of volatile oil are produced annually; as examples, for lemon oil, eucalyptus oil, clove leaf oil and peppermint oil world production annually runs into several thousand metric tons each.

Although the production of major oils is highly organized, a number of developing countries have volatile oil-rich flora not fully utilized or cultivated and the United Nations Industrial Development Organisation has taken steps to inform on the setting-up of rural based small-scale essential oil industries (see 'Further reading'). India and China now produce large quantities of oil for export.

Volatile oils are used for their therapeutic action, for flavouring (e.g. oil of lemon), in perfumery (e.g. oil of rose) or as starting materials for the synthesis of other compounds (e.g. oil of turpentine). For therapeutic purposes they are administered as inhalations (e.g. eucalyptus oil), orally (e.g. peppermint oil), as gargles and mouthwashes (e.g. thymol) and transdermally (many essential oils including those of lavender, rosemary and bergamot are employed in the practice of aromatherapy.

Those oils with a high phenol content, e.g. clove and thyme, have antiseptic properties, whereas others are used as carminatives. Oils showing antispasmodic activity, and much used in popular medicine, are those of *Melissa officinalis, Rosmarinus officinalis, Mentha piperita, Matricaria chamomilla, Foeniculum vulgare, Carum carvi* and *Citrus aurantium*. The antispasmodic activity of some of these oils has also been demonstrated experimentally. The constituents of many volatile oils are stated to interfere with respiration and electron transport in a variety of bacteria, hence accounting for their use in food preservation and in cosmetic preparations.

Composition of volatile oils

With the exception of oils derived from glycosides (e.g. bitter almond oil and mustard oil) volatile oils are generally mixtures of hydrocarbons and oxygenated compounds derived from these hydrocarbons. In some oils (e.g. oil of turpentine) the hydrocarbons predominate and only limited amounts of oxygenated constituents are present; in others (e.g. oil of cloves) the bulk of the oil consists of oxygenated compounds. The odour and taste of volatile oils is mainly determined by these oxygenated constituents, which are to some extent soluble in water (note orange-flower water, rose water, etc.) but more soluble in alcohol (note tinctures or essences of lemon, etc.). Many oils are terpenoid in origin; a smaller number such as those of cinnamon and clove contain principally aromatic (benzene) derivatives mixed with the terpenes. A few compounds (e.g. thymol, carvacrol), although aromatic in structure, are terpenoid in origin.

Evaluation. Various pharmacopoeial procedures are given for the evaluation of volatile oils. Odour and taste are obviously important in the preliminary examination; however oils should not be tasted neat but only after dilution with a sugar solution in ethanol as prescribed in the *BP*. Physical measurements including optical rotation, relative density and refractive index are regularly employed for identification and

α-Cadinene   Diterpene skeleton   Abietic acid

assessment of purity; similarly thin-layer chromatograms. Capillary gas chromatographic profiles are used to determine the proportions of individual components of certain oils. Advances in gas chromatography have now made possible the ready determination of the chirality of particular components of volatile oils thus detecting adulteration with synthetic material or unwanted other oils; examples of its use are carvone in caraway oil, linalol in coriander oil and linalol and linalyl acetate in neroli oil. The ketone and aldehyde contents of oils such as caraway and lemon respectively are determined by reaction with hydroxylamine hydrochloride (oxime formation) and titration of the liberated acid. Other general tests described in the *BP* include examination for fixed and resinified oils (residue after evaporation), foreign esters (conversion to a crystalline deposit) and presence of water (turbidity of a carbon disulphide solution).

There have been a number of recent problems (1999) with the occurrence of tetrachloromethane in essential oils, particularly spearmint oil. This is probably not due to deliberate adulteration (the adulterant is present at low ppm levels) but a consequence of cleaning the drums before use with offending solvent and inefficient removal of it before filling the drums. Unfortunately on detection it renders the oil useless, as in food tetrachloromethane is prohibited.

The volatile oil content of crude drugs is commonly determined by distillation (Chapter 16).

Biogenesis. The origin of metabolites with phenylpropane and terpenoid structures has been discussed in Chapter 18. In medicinal essential oils the number of the former is limited but for the monoterpenes which arise at the geranyl pyrophosphate (GPP) level of terpenoid synthesis there are numerous examples. Analyses show that these oils commonly contain 40–80 monoterpenoids, many in relatively small proportion. A major constituent of one oil may be a minor one in another.

Three groups of monoterpenoid structures are involved: (1) acyclic or linear; (2) monocyclic; and (3) bicyclic. In the plant they are sequentially derived from limonene in this order as illustrated in Fig. 22.1. Relatively few enzymes, termed cyclases, appear to determine the skeletal class (e.g. menthanes, pinanes, thujanes etc.) and it is possible that these serve as rate-limiting enzymes. However, regulatory factors for the control of synthesis operate not only at the biosynthetic enzyme level *per se* but in a hierarchical manner up to the whole-organism level.

Because of the *trans* geometry of the double bond at the C-2 of GPP, direct cyclization to limonene is not possible and for *Mentha* spp. it has been shown that (−)-limonene synthase located within the oil glands catalyses the isomerization of GPP to enzyme-bound (+)-3S-linalyl pyrophosphate with subsequent cyclization to (−)-limonene. However, many enzymatic steps are involved in the subsequent modifications and interconversions of these monoterpenes. Some components of volatile oils are sesquiterpenes ($C_{15}H_{24}$) (q.v.) and they include cadinene, zingiberene (structure, Fig. 18.17) and caryophyllene. The formulae of some of the more common constituents of pharmaceutical volatile oils are given in Fig. 22.2.

It is increasingly evident that some monoterpenes and other components of volatile oils also occur in plants in the glycosidic form. Thus, geraniol, nerol and citronellol occur as glycosides in the petals of *Rosa dilecta*, thymol and carvacrol as glucosides and galactosides in *Thymus vulgaris* and eugenol, benzyl alcohol, β-phenylethyl alcohol, nerol, geraniol and geranic acid as glucosides in *Melissa officinalis*. It is considered that these glucosides of monoterpenols and of 2-phenylethanol are translocated from leaves to flowers as aroma precursors.

Table 22.1 may be used to compare the compositions of important volatile oils. The classification is arbitrary, since an oil may contain a number of compounds all about equally important but belonging to different chemical classes. The substance used for classification is not necessarily the one present in greatest amount. Thus, nutmeg is classified

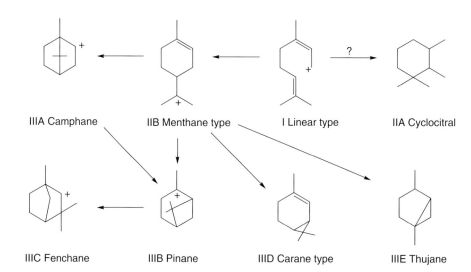

Fig. 22.1
Possible biogenetic relationships between some monoterpene types.

IIIA Camphane   IIB Menthane type   I Linear type   IIA Cyclocitral

IIIC Fenchane   IIIB Pinane   IIID Carane type   IIIE Thujane

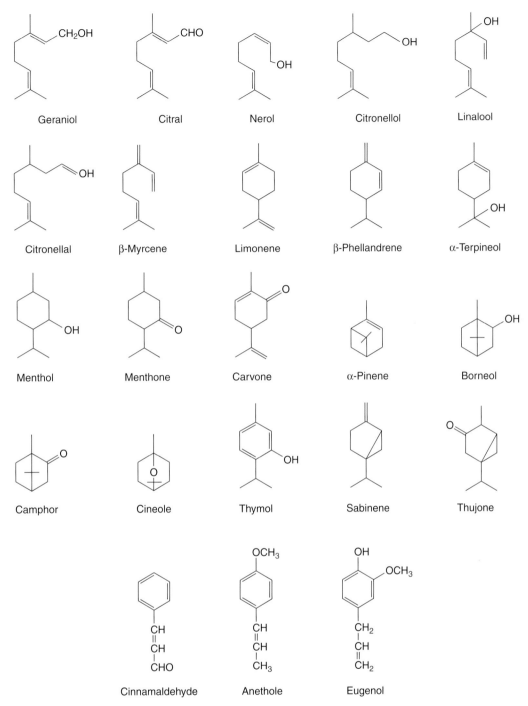

Fig. 22.2
Some components of pharmaceutical oils.

on its myristicin and lemon on citral, although these constituents form only a small percentage of these oils.

C$_{20}$ or diterpenoid compounds include such resin acids as (+)- and (−)-pimaric acid and their isomer, the abietic acid of pine resin. The abietane acids have antimicrobial, antiulcer and cardiovascular properties (for a review covering some 56 acids over the period 1967–92 see A. S. Feliciano *et al.*, *Planta Med.*, 1993, **59**, 485). Many diterpenoids (e.g. vitamin A and gibberellic acid) do not belong to the volatile oil–resin group. Similarly, only a small proportion of triterpenoid compounds (C$_{30}$) are found as resin constituents (e.g. in *Euphorbia resinifera*).

Preparation of volatile oils

All the official volatile oils are extracted by distillation with the exception of oil of lemon and oil of cade. The distillation of volatile oils by means of water or steam has long been practised, but modern plants possess many advantages over the older stills, in which charring and undesirable decomposition of the oil often took place. Modern volatile oil stills contain the raw material on perforated trays or in perforated baskets. The still contains water at the base which is heated by steam coils, and free steam under pressure may also be passed in. Tough material such as barks, seeds and roots may be comminuted to

Table 22.1 Composition of volatile oils.

Name	Botanical name	Important constituents
Terpenes or sesquiterpenes		
Tea-tree	*Melaleuca alternifolia*	Cyclic monoterpenes
Turpentine	*Pinus* spp.	Terpenes (pinenes, camphene)
Juniper	*Juniperus communis*	Terpenes (pinene, camphene); sesquiterpene (cadinene); alcohols
Cade (Juniper Tar Oil)	*Juniperus oxycedrus*	Sesquiterpenes (cadinene); phenols (guaiacol, cresol)
Alcohols		
Coriander	*Coriandrum sativum*	Linalol (65–80% alcohols); terpenes
Otto of rose	*Rosa* spp.	Geraniol, citronellol (70–75% alcohols); esters
Geranium	*Pelargonium* spp.	Geraniol; citronellol; esters
Indian or Turkish geranium (Palmarosa)	*Cymbopogon* spp.	Geraniol (85–90%)
Sandalwood	*Santalum album*	Santalols (sesquiterpene alcohols), esters, aldehydes
Esters and alcohols		
Bergamot	*Citrus bergamia*	Linalyl acetate, linalol
Lavender	*Lavandula officinalis*	Linalol; linalyl acetate (much); ethyl-pentyl ketone
Rosemary	*Rosmarinus officinalis*	Borneol and linalol (10–18%); bornyl acetate, etc. (2–5%); terpenes; cineole
Pumilio pine	*Pinus mugo* var. *pumilio*	Bornyl acetate (about 10%); terpenes; sesquiterpenes
Peppermint	*Mentha piperita*	Menthol (about 45%); menthyl acetate (4–9%)
Aldehydes		
Cinnamon bark	*Cinnamomum verum* Presl.	Cinnamaic aldehyde (60–75%); eugenol; terpenes
Cassia	*Cinnamomum cassia*	Cinnamic aldehyde (80%)
Lemon	*Citrus limon*	Citral (over 3.5%); limonene (about 90%)
Lemon grass	*Cymbopogon* spp.	Citral and citronellal (75–85%); terpenes
'Citron-scented' eucalyptus	*Eucalyptus citriodora*	Citronellal (about 70%)
Ketones		
Spearmint	*Mentha spicata* and *M. cardiaca*	Carvone (55–70%); limonene, esters
Caraway	*Carum carvi*	Carvone (60%); limonene, etc.
Dill	*Anethum graveolens*	Carvone (50%); limonene, etc.
Sage	*Salvia officinalis*	Thujone (about 50%); camphor; cineole etc.
Wormwood	*Artemisia absinthium*	Thujone (up to 35%); thujyl alcohol; azulenes
Phenols		
Cinnamon leaf	*Cinnamomum verum* Presl.	Eugenol (up to 80%)
Clove	*Syzygium aromaticum* (L.) Merr & L. M. Perry	Eugenol (85–90%); acetyl eugenol, methylpentyl ketone, vanillin
Thyme	*Thymus vulgaris*	Thymol (20–30%)
Horsemint	*Monarda punctata*	Thymol (about 60%)
Ajowan	*Trachyspermum ammi*	Thymol (4–55%)
Ethers		
Anise and Star-anise	*Pimpinella anisum* and *Illicium verum*	Anethole (80–90%); chavicol methyl ether, etc.
Fennel	*Foeniculum vulgare*	Anethole (60%); fenchone, a ketone (20%)
Eucalyptus	*Eucalyptus globulus*	Cineole (over 70%); terpenes, etc.
Cajuput	*Melaleuca* spp.	Cineole (50–60%); terpenes, alcohols and esters
Camphor	*Cinnamomum camphora*	After removal of the ketone camphor contains safrole; terpenes, etc.
Parsley	*Petroselinum sativum*	Apiole (dimethoxysafrole)
Indian dill	*Peucedanum soja*	Dill-apiole (dimethoxysafrole)
Nutmeg	*Myristica fragrans*	Myristicin (methoxysafrole) up to 4%; terpenes (60–85%); alcohols, phenols
Peroxides		
Chenopodium	*Chenopodium ambrosioides* var. *anthelmintica*	Ascaridole (60–77%), an unsaturated terpene peroxide
Non-terpenoid and derived from glycosides		
Mustard	*Brassica* spp.	Glucosinolates
Wintergreen	*Gaultheria procumbens*	Methyl salicylate
Bitter almond	*Prunus communis* var. *amara*	Benzaldehyde and HCN (from amygdalin)

facilitate extraction but flowers are usually placed in the still without further treatment as soon as possible after collection. Distillation is frequently performed in the field.

The distillate, which consists of a mixture of oil and water, is condensed and collected in a suitable receiver which is usually a Florentine flask or a large glass jar with one outlet near the base and another near the top. The distillate separates into two layers, the oil being withdrawn through the upper outlet and the water from the lower outlet, or vice versa in the case of oils, such as oil of cloves, which are heavier than water. The oil-saturated aqueous layer may be returned to the still or may form an article of commerce, as in the case of rose water and orange-flower water.

Certain oils (e.g. oil of cajuput, oil of caraway, oil of turpentine and oil of Australian sandalwood) are rectified. Rectification usually takes the form of a second distillation in steam, which frees the oil from resinous and other impurities. Light and atmospheric oxygen appear to have an adverse effect on most volatile oils and the official directions with regard to storage should be rigidly followed. The distillation of oil of chenopodium must be done as rapidly as possible, as the chief constituent, ascaridole, gradually decomposes on boiling with water.

Extraction of oils used in perfumery. Certain oils used in perfumery, such as oil of rose, are prepared by steam distillation as described above but many of the flower perfumes require other treatment. An important centre for the extraction of flower oils is Grasse, in the south of France. Here the oils are extracted by *enfleurage*, by digestion in melted fats, by pneumatic methods or by means of solvents. In the *enfleurage* process glass plates are covered with a thin layer of fixed oil or fat upon which the fresh flowers are spread. The volatile oil gradually passes into the fat and the exhausted flowers are removed and replaced by a fresh supply. Formerly the flowers had to be picked off by hand but this is now done mechanically. Only a small percentage of the flowers, which resist the action of the machine, require removal by the fingers or by means of a vacuum cleaner. The pneumatic method, which is similar in principles to the *enfleurage* process, involves the passage of a current of warm air through the flowers. The air, laden with suspended volatile oil, is then passed through a spray of melted fat in which the volatile oil is absorbed. In the digestion process the flowers are gently heated in melted fat until exhausted, when they are strained out and the perfume-containing fat is allowed to cool. It will be seen that in each of the above processes the volatile oil has now been obtained in a fatty base. The volatile oil is obtained from this by three successive extractions with alcohol. The alcoholic solutions may be put on the market as flower perfumes or the oil may be obtained in a pure form by recovery of the alcohol. Solvent extraction is based on the Soxhlet principle (see Chapter 16).

Further reading
De Silva KT 1995 A manual on the essential oil industry. UNIDO, Vienna

Oil of rose
Oil of rose (*Otto* or *Attar of Rose, Oleum Rosae*) is a volatile oil obtained by distillation from the fresh flowers of *Rosa damascena, R. gallica, R. alba* and *R. centifolia* (Rosaceae). It is included in the *USP/NF*, 1995. The chief producing countries are Bulgaria, Turkey and Morocco but smaller quantities are prepared elsewhere.

The oil is prepared in copper alembic stills by the peasants or in large factories under careful scientific control. Some 3000 parts of flowers yield only one part of oil. The oil is very expensive and very liable to adulteration. The 'peasant distilled' oil usually fetches a lower price than that produced in the larger works.

The oil is a pale yellow semisolid. The portion which is solid at ordinary temperatures forms about 15–20% and consists of odourless stearoptene containing principally saturated aliphatic hydrocarbons (C_{14}–C_{23} normal paraffins). The liquid portion forms a clear solution with 70% alcohol. It consists of the alcohols geraniol, citronellol, nerol and 2-phenylethanol with smaller quantities of esters and other odorous principles. Although the alcohols form about 70–75% of the oil, the odour is so modified by the other constituents, such as sulphur containing compounds, that no artificial mixture of the known constituents can be made to reproduce the odour of the natural oil. Phenylalanine has been shown to act as a precursor of the 2-phenylethanol; acetate and mevalonate are incorporated into the terpene alcohols. A citronellyl disaccharide glycoside has been identified as an aroma precursor of citronellol in flowers of *R. damascena* var. *bulgaria* (N. Oka et al., *Phytochemistry*, 1998, **47**, 1527). Among a number of lines of callus derived from the leaf-bud of *R. damascena* a few have been shown to produce 2-phenylethanol.

From *Rosa rugosa* var. *plena* growing in central China some 108 compounds have been identified in the flower oil; these include citronellol (60%), geraniol (8.6%), nerol (2.8%), citronellyl acetate (2.7%) and *E,E*-farnesol (2.5%). For a review see Y. Hashidoko, *Phytochemistry*, 1996, **43**, 535.

Oil of rose is of great importance in perfumery (for a fuller account of its history and utilization see Widrlechner, *Econ. Bot.*, 1981, **35**, 42).

PEPPERMINT LEAF AND PEPPERMINT OIL

Peppermint Leaf as defined in the *BP* and *EP* is the dried leaves of *Mentha × piperita* L. (Labiatae). It is required to contain not less than 1.2% of volatile oil. The oil is obtained from the same plant by steam distillation using the flowering tops. The European and American oil appears to be derived to a large extent from the two varieties *M. piperita* var. *vulgaris* Sole ('black mint') and *M. piperita* var. *officinalis* Sole ('white mint').

Mentha × piperita is, as implied by the written botanical name, a hybrid species from the two parents, *M. spicata* ($2n = 36$ or 48) and *M. aquatica* ($2n = 96$). *M. × piperita* strains commonly have a somatic number of 72, a smaller proportion 66, but other figures have also been reported.

Macroscopical characters. All the mints have square stems and creeping rhizomes. The flowers are arranged in verticillasters and have the floral formula K(5),C(5),A4,G(2). The black mint, which is the one most commonly cultivated in England, has purple stems and dark green petiolate leaves which are tinged with purple. The leaf blades are 3–9 cm long and have a grooved petiole up to 1 cm long. They have a pinnate venation with lateral veins leaving the midrib at about a 45° angle, acuminate apex and sharply dentate margin. Glandular trichomes can be seen as bright yellowish points when the lower surface is examined with a hand lens. The leaves are broader than those of *M. spicata* (spearmint), but narrower than those of *M. aquatica* (water mint). The small, purple flowers appear in late summer.

Microscopical characters. The microscopy of peppermint leaves is typical of the family, showing numerous diacytic stomata on the lower surface (Fig. 42.2G), three- to eight-celled clothing trichomes with a striated cuticle (Fig. 42.4C), and two types of glandular trichome, one with a unicellular base and small single-celled head and the other with a multicellular head characteristic of the family (Fig. 42.5E). Calcium oxalate is absent.

There is a 5% limit of stems over 1 mm in diameter for the official leaves, and as mints are very susceptible to most diseases, there is a 10% limit of leaves infected by *Puccinia menthae*.

Of commercial importance has been the development by mutation breeding at the A. M. Todd Co. of a strain of Mitcham peppermint resistant to the wilt disease *Verticillium albo-duram* var. *menthae*. The strain retains the Mitcham cultivar organoleptic characteristics and gives a good oil production in verticillium-prone soils where cultivation with the ordinary varieties is impossible.

OIL OF PEPPERMINT

The oil of the *BP* (1993) was required to contain 4.5–10% of esters calculated as menthyl acetate, not less than 44% of free alcohols calculated as menthol and 15–32% of ketones calculated as menthone. However, these chemical evaluations are now replaced by a capillary GC profile; limits for individual compounds are limonene 1.0–5.0%, cineole 3.5–14.0%, menthone 14–32%, menthofuran 1.0–9.0%, isomenthone 1.5–10.0%, menthylacetate 2.8–10.0%, menthol 30.0–55.0%, pulegone ≯4.0%, carvone ≯1.0%. The ratio of the cineole to limonene contents exceeds 2.

Small quantities of the sesquiterpene viridoflorol form a useful identification characteristic of the oil. A basic fraction of the oil contains a number of pyridine derivatives such as 2-acetyl-4-isopropyl pyridine which has a powerful grass-like minty odour. High-resolution GC has been used to identify over 85 components of the oil.

As with other cultivated Labiatae, the oil composition of *M. × piperita* is greatly influenced by genetic factors and seasonal variations (see relevant chapters). The task of elucidating the nature of the genetic control for the formation of various constituents has been rendered difficult by the hybrid and polyploid nature of the genus. Much progress in this area was achieved by M. J. Murray, a mint breeder with the A. M. Todd Company, Kalamazoo, Michigan. His collection of over 600 accessions of mint species, which has continued to be researched and added to, now forms the basis of the collection of the USDA-ARS-National Clonal Germplasm Repository in Cornvallis, Oregon.

Biogenesis of peppermint monoterpenoids. The biosynthetic isoprenoid origin of monoterpenes was mentioned at the beginning of this chapter. As the essential oils of the Labiatae are synthesized in the cells of the glandular trichomes, techniques such as cell and root culture are of little value as experimental tools. However, new procedures, using gentle abrasion of leaf surfaces with glass beads, have been developed for isolating in high purity and excellent yield, peltate glandular trichomes of peppermint which retain their biosynthetic activity.

Developmental changes in the oil composition of the leaves include the disappearance of limonene, the accumulation of 1,8-cineole, the conversion of menthone to menthol and the acetylation of menthol. All these processes begin at the distal extremity of the leaf and shift progressively to the leaf base (B. Voirin and C. Bayer, *Phytochemistry*, 1996, **43**, 573).

A proposed pathway for the formation of monoterpenes in peppermint is given in Fig. 22.3. A number of enzymes involved in the reactions have been characterized. The hydrolase system involving (−)-limonene-3-hydroxylase in the formation of the alcohol (−)-*trans*-isopiperitenol is cytochrome-P450-dependent and is associated with the oil gland microsomal fraction. The remaining steps are catalysed by operationally soluble enzymes of the oil cells. It will be noted that (+)-pulegone is a branching point for the formation of menthol stereoisomers.

Japanese peppermint oil is derived from *Mentha canadensis* var. *piperascens*; it contains 70–90% menthol, for the extraction of which it is largely used. The commercial dementholized Japanese oil contains approximately the same amount of menthol and its esters as the American oil.

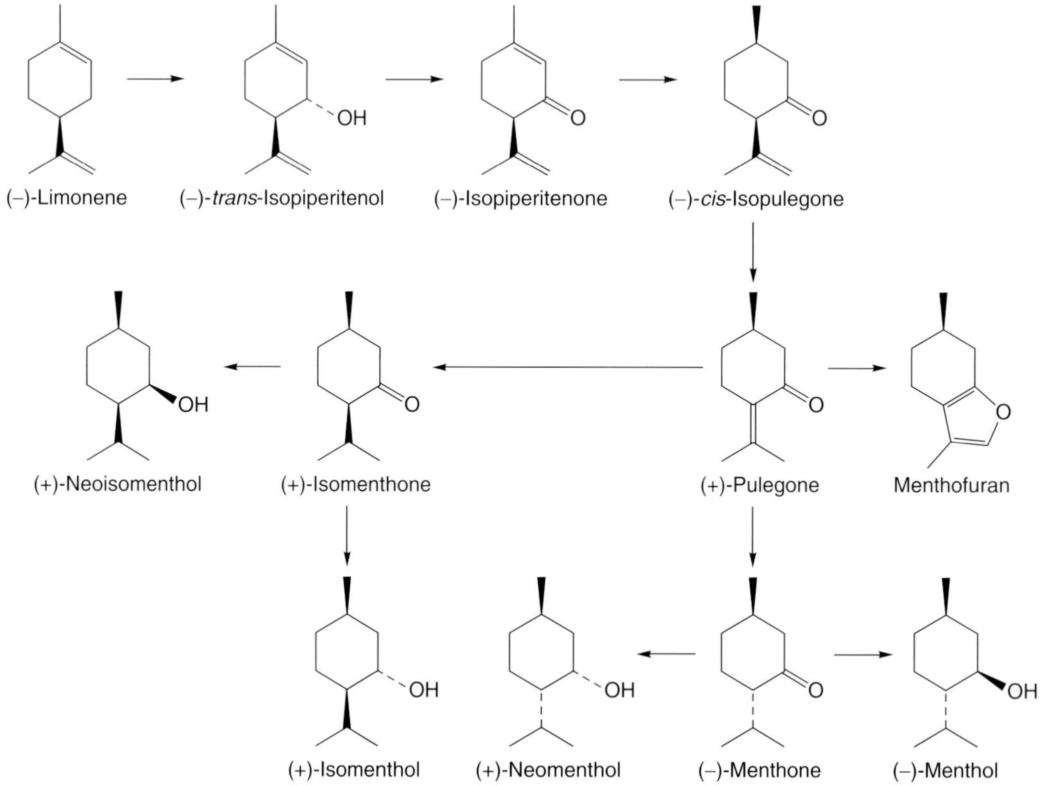

Fig. 22.3
A possible biogenetic scheme for some monoterpenoids of *Mentha × piperita*.

(−)-Limonene   (−)-*trans*-Isopiperitenol   (−)-Isopiperitenone   (−)-*cis*-Isopulegone

(+)-Neoisomenthol   (+)-Isomenthone   (+)-Pulegone   Menthofuran

(+)-Isomenthol   (+)-Neomenthol   (−)-Menthone   (−)-Menthol

DEMENTHOLIZED MINT OIL *BP*

This is cited as the volatile oil from *Mentha arvensis* var. *piperascens* from which the menthol has been partially removed. The two commercial oils, Brazilian and Chinese, differ somewhat in their ranges of ester and alcohol contents; standards are given for each. For both, the cineole:limonene ratio, as determined by GC, is less than unity.

SPEARMINT OIL

Spearmint or ordinary garden mint consists of the dried leaf and flowering top of *Mentha spicata* L. (*M. viridis* Linn.) and *Mentha × cardiaca* (Labiatae). The *BP* oil is prepared by steam distillation and should contain not less than 55% of carvone, 2–25% limonene with upper limits for a number of other constituents as determined by gas chromatography. The commercial oil was originally produced in North America but the industry has now largely transferred to India.

Characters. Mint has more or less crumpled, opposite, ovate-lanceolate leaves, 3–7 cm long. The apex is acute or acuminate, and the margin unequally serrate. The leaves differ from those of peppermint in that they are almost sessile and have a bright green colour free from purple.

Constituents. Oil of spearmint contains (−)-carvone, (−)-limonene, phellandrene and esters. As with *M. × piperita* limonene is the precursor of the monoterpenoids and in this case the action of a (−)-limonene-6-hydroxylase predominates to give the alcohol (−)-*trans*-carveol which is oxidized to carvone (Fig. 22.4). Dihydrocarvone is formed later in the season and is absent from plantlets produced by shoot-tip culture. Again like peppermint, oil production is influenced by the age of plant, time of collection, chemical varieties and hybridization.

Further reading
Lawrence BM (ed), Hardman R (series ed) 2007 Medicinal and aromatic plants – industrial profiles, Vol 44, Mint: The genus *Mentha*. CRC Press, Boca Raton, FL

SAGE LEAF

The official drug consists of whole or cut leaves of *Salvia officinalis* (Labiatae) containing not less than 1.5% (whole leaf) or 1.0% (cut leaf) of essential oil which is determined by steam distillation. The plant is indigenous to Mediterranean areas but is now cultivated world-wide, principally for its use as a culinary herb.

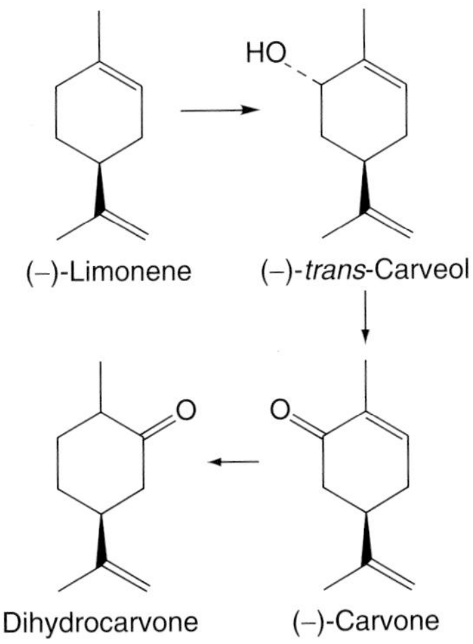

Macroscopical characters. The petiolate oblong-lanceolate leaves are up to 10 cm length and 2 cm in breadth, greenish-grey on the upper surface and tomentose on the lower with a markedly reticulate venation. The leaf apex is rounded, the base rounded or cordate and the margin crenulate. The odour and taste are characteristically pungent.

Microscopical characters. The upper epidermal cells have beaded anticlinal walls, the lower ones are thin-walled and sinuous; both epidermi possess diacytic stomata. Glandular trichomes of the typical labiate type occur on both surfaces with rarer uniseriate glandular trichomes having a double- or single-celled head. Clothing trichomes are numerous, particularly on the lower surface, composed of a short thickened basal cell with articulated and bent terminal cells. A few single-celled warty-walled trichomes are present. The long protective trichomes serve to distinguish *S. officinalis* from *S. sclarea* and *S. pratensis* (M. Then *et al.*, *Acta Pharm. Hung.*, 1998, **63**, 163).

Constituents. The volatile oil of sage contains about 50% of α- and β-thujone together with cineole, borneol and other constituents (Fig. 22.2). Varieties and other species of sage contain differing amounts of thujone.

Non-volatile components of the leaf include diterpenes, phenolic glycosides based on caffeic and *p*-hydroxybenzoic acids (for recent isolations see M. Wang *et al.*, *J. Nat. Prod.*, 1999, **62**, 454), and tannins.

Action and uses. Sage as an infusion is used as a mouthwash and gargle for its antiseptic and astringent action. Recent attention has focused on the cholinergic activity of the drug and its possible role in the treatment of Alzheimer's disease and memory loss. It is interesting to note that long before recent advances in the understanding of the neurobiology of Alzheimer's disease, plant materials including sage and balm (*Melissa officinalis*) were recommended in old reference books as possessing memory-improving properties (see E. K. Perry *et al.*, *J. Pharm. Pharmacol.*, 1999, **51**, 527). The phenolic glycosides of sage together with those of *Melissa officinalis* and *Lavandula angustifolia* possess antioxidant properties (J. Hohmann *et al.*, *Planta Medica*, 1999, **65**, 576).

THREE-LOBED SAGE LEAF

Three-lobed sage leaf *BP/EP* also known as Greek sage, consists of the whole or cut, dried leaves of *Salvia fructicosa* Mill. (*S. triloba* L. fill) containing not less than 1.8% essential oil in the whole drug and not less than 1.2% in the cut drug. The leaves have a grey–green upper surface and conspicuously downy underside. They are somewhat larger (8–50 mm in length, 4–20 mm in width) than those of common sage and are considerably more pubescent. The clothing trichomes and odour (spicy and similar to that of eucalyptus oil) constitute features of the powder, which otherwise resembles *S. officinalis*.

An alcoholic extract of the drug subjected to TLC is used by the *BP* to detect the presence of cineole and the almost complete absence of thujone in the sample.

SAGE OIL

Sage oils are produced commercially by steam distillation from a number of *Salvia* species but the oil composition is not uniform, as illustrated by the three species considered here. For this reason, the *BP/EP* specifies one species, *S. sclarea* L., the clary sage, as the source

(−)-Limonene   (−)-*trans*-Carveol

Dihydrocarvone   (−)-Carvone

Fig. 22.4
Biosynthetic pathway for major constituents of spearmint oil.

22

of the official oil. The plant is a native of Mediterranean regions and had been introduced into England by the the 14th century.

The pharmacopoeia specifies the acceptable concentration limits for constituents of the oil as follows: α- and β-thujone (less than 0.2%), linalol (6.5–24.0%), linalyl acetate (50–80%); α-terpineol (less than 5.0%), germacrene-D (1.0–12%) and sclareol (0.4–2.6%).

The oil is widely used for flavouring and perfumery purposes.

ROSEMARY LEAF

Rosemary leaf *BP/EP*, *BHP* is the whole dried leaf of *Rosmarinus officinalis* L., family Labiatae. The plant is native to Mediterranean regions and is widely cultivated elsewhere in herb gardens and as an aromatic ornamental. Many horticultural varieties varying in habit and flower colour exist. Commercial supplies of the leaf come principally from Spain, Morocco and Tunisia.

R. officinalis is an aromatic evergreen shrub, variable in its form, but mostly with stems reaching a height of over 1 m. The bilobed corollas of the flowers are pale to dark blue and occur clustered in spikes at the ends of the branches; they are larger than those of either lavender or the mints. The leathery, opposite leaves are up to 4 cm long and up to 4 mm wide with entire strongly recurved margins and prominent midribs. The upper surfaces are green, the lower ones grey and somewhat woolly due to numerous branched trichomes. Typical labiate hairs contain the volatile oil, of which the *BP* specifies a minimum content of 1.2% calculated on the anhydrous drug.

Constituents. The compositon of the essential oil is considered under 'Rosemary Oil', below. Hydroxycinnamic acids include caffeic acid and a dimer rosmarinic acid (a characteristic metabolite of the subfamily Saturejoidae to which *Rosmarinus* belongs). For the dried leaf, the *BP* sets a minimum requirement of 3.0% for total hydroxycinnamic acids expressed as rosmarinic acid.

In recent years, a large number of phenolic abietane diterpenoids have been recorded for the leaves including the potent antioxidant carnosic acid together with its degradation products carnosol, rosmanol, epirosmanol and 7-methylepirosmanol. For new recently isolated diterpenes, see A. A. Mahmoud *et al.*, *Phytochemistry*, 2005, **66**, 1685; C. L. Cantrell *et al.*, *J. Nat. Prod.*, 2005, **68**, 98. Triterpenes include the alcohols α- and β-amyrin, ursolic acid and oleanolic acid.

In vitro cell cultures of rosemary have been produced which biosynthesise carnosic acid, carnosol and rosmarinic acid (A. Kuhlmann and C. Rohl, *Pharm. Biol.*, 2006, **44**, 401).

Uses. Rosemary leaves have many traditional uses based on their antibacterial, carminative and spasmolytic actions.

Further reading

Petersen M, Simmonds MSJ 2003 Molecules of interest. Rosmarinic acid. Phytochemistry 62: 121–125. *Includes discovery (1958), derivatives, distribution, chemistry, biological activity*

ROSEMARY OIL

Rosemary oil is steam distilled from the flowering aerial parts of *Rosmarinus officinalis* L. The fresh material yields about 1–2% of a colourless to pale yellow volatile oil with a very characteristic odour. It contains 0.8–6% of esters and 8–20% of alcohols. The principal constituents are 1,8-cineole, borneol, camphor, bornyl acetate and monoterpene hydrocarbons, principally α-pinene and camphene. Many minor components have been identified. Chemical races (G. Flamini *et al.*, *J. Agric. Food Chem.*, 2002, **50**, 1512) and geographical variants concerning the proportions of constituents in the oils are known. The *BP/EP* accordingly gives the limits for the percentage content of 12 constituents for oils of the Spanish type and for those of the Moroccan and Tunisian type. These are determined by gas chromatography.

The oil is frequently used in aromatherapy, in the perfumery industry and for the preparation of spirits and liniments for medical use; it has antibacterial and antispasmodic properties.

LEMON BALM

Lemon balm *BP/EP* consists of the dried leaf of *Melissa officinalis* L. family Labiatae/Lamiaceae; Balm leaf *BHP* 1990 is from the same source but also includes the flowering tops. The plant is a perennial herb native to southern and eastern Mediterranean regions but now widely grown in gardens for its aroma or for culinary purposes and cultivated commercially in Eastern Europe and Spain.

The leaves are opposite on a hairy quadangular stem; flowering branches arise in the axils of the lower leaves and flowers in clusters at the upper ends of the stems. The two-lipped corollas are initially white, changing later to pale blue or pink; the calyx is toothed with long spreading hairs. Leaf blades are 3–7 cm in length, longly petiolate on the lower parts of stems but shortly so on the upper parts, margins are deeply crenate or serrate, veins are prominent on the lower pale-green surface. Microscopical features are characteristic of the Lamiaceae and include eight-celled glandular trichomes, clothing trichomes and diacytic stomata on the lower epidermis.

Lemon balm yields only a small quantity of volatile oil (0.06–0.4%), which none the less gives the plant, when crushed, its strong lemon-like odour. Principal components of the oil are the aldehydes citral (composed of the isomers geranial and neral) and citronellal. Other components in smaller proportions are citronellol, nerol and

Carnosic acid   Carnosol   Rosmarinic acid

the sesquiterpene β-caryophyllene; in all, over 70 constituents have been reported. Due to the low yield of oil from the plant, lemon balm oil is subject to adulteration with lemon-grass oil (*Cymbopogon citratus*), lemon-scented verbena oil (*Aloysia triphylla*) or various citrus products.

The *BP/EP* drug is assayed on its total content ($\leqslant$4.0%) of hydroxycinnamic acid derivatives expressed as rosmarinic acid (p. 270); these are mainly structurally related to caffeic acid. Other constituents are flavonoids, principally luteolin glycosides (Table 21.5).

For over 2000 years lemon balm has been used for medicinal and culinary purposes. It is used traditionally for its sedative, spasmolytic and antibacterial properties; more recently it has been investigated by a number of researchers for its topical use in the treatment of Herpes labialis.

THYME

A number of *Thymus* species have been used traditionally for their medicinal and culinary properties. Under the above heading, the *BP/EP* recognizes the leaves and flowers separated from the dried aerial parts of *T. vulgaris* L. and *T. zygis* L., family Labiatae, or mixtures of the two. The former is the garden thyme or common thyme, native to Mediterranean regions, and possibly introduced into Britain by the Romans; the latter is also known as Spanish thyme.

Both species have similar morphological and microscopical characteristics and can be difficult to distinguish in the dried state. Stems above 15 mm in length and over 1 mm in diameter are limited to 10% by the pharmacopoeia. The grey–green leaves are slightly hairy on the upper surface and densely so on the lower surface, up to 12 mm long, and 3 mm wide, opposite, sessile and ovate to lanceolate in shape with slightly rolled edges. Under the microscope, both species show on the lower surface volatile oil-containing glandular trichomes typical of the Labiatae and numerous warty-walled clothing trichomes. The characteristic elbow-shaped trichomes of *T. vulgaris* are illustrated in Fig. 42.4. Numerous thick bundles of fibres are apparent in the powder of *T. zygis*.

Constituents. The volatile oil composition of thyme can vary enormously and various chemotypes have been recorded, particularly regarding thymol and carvacrol. The official drug is required to contain not less than 1.2% volatile oil, of which not less than 40% consists of thymol and carvacrol. It is these phenols that are largely responsible for the antiseptic, antitussive and expectorant properties of the drug. Other common variables of the oil are cymene (10–24%) and γ-terpinene (4–18%). Two extreme variations recorded are an almost complete lack of thymol and carvacrol in *T. vulgaris* and an oil containing 74% thymol from *T. zygis*.

A number of monoterpenoid glycosides occur in the leaves, particularly glucosides and galactosides of thymol and terpineol; seven new such constituents have recently been described (J. Katajima *et al.*, *Phytochemistry*, 2004, **65**, 3279; *Chem. Pharm. Bull.*, 2004, **52**, 1013). Flavones, highly oxygenated flavones, flavanones and dihydroflavonals may be responsible for the spasmolytic effect of the leaves, and the biphenyls reported in 1989 may have deodorant properties. Other constituents include rosmarinic acid (see 'Rosemary') up to 2.6%, various acids, tannins and resins. Rosmarinic acid and 3′-*O*-(8″-Z-caffeoyl) rosmarinic acid have been reported as the most important radical scavengers of the leaves (A. Dapkevicins *et al.*, *J. Nat. Prod.*, 2002, **65**(6), 892).

THYME OIL

Thyme Oil *BP/EP* is obtained by steam distillation from the *fresh* flowering aerial parts of *Thymus vulgaris* L., *T. zygis* Loefl. *ex* L., or a mixture of both species. The oil therefore resembles that obtained from the official drug described above but reflects any changes that occur during drying and storage. The oil may vary in colour from yellow to dark reddish-brown; it has an aromatic spicy odour suggesting that of thymol.

As with the whole drug, the constituents are subject to variation due to geographic and genetic factors. The *BP* therefore requires a gas chromatographic profile and provides limits for the proportions of major constituents, which are: β-myrcene (1–3%), γ-terpinene (5–10%), *p*-cymene (15–28%), linalol (4.0–6.5%), terpinen-4-ol (0.2–2.5%), thymol (36–55%) and carvacrol (1.0 and 4.0%).

WILD THYME

The *BP/EP* drug is defined as the whole or cut, dried, flowering aerial parts of *Thymus serpyllum* L.s.l. It is required to contain a minimum of 0.3% essential oil (dried drug).

The species is an extremely variable aggregate, differing in its forms and chemical constituents both locally and across its wider geographical distribution. It grows on heaths, dry grasslands, dunes and in rocky environments extending from coasts to the lower mountain slopes of central and northern Europe, including the UK.

Wild thyme is used both medicinally and as a flavour in a similar manner to the common thyme, but is less powerful in its actions. The principal constituents are again thymol and carvacrol, which, however, vary appreciably according to source; some chemotypes contain neither of these phenolic compounds. For quality control, the *BP/EP* relies on the minimum oil content (as above) and TLC to indicate the presence of thymol and carvacrol and to give an indication of their respective concentrations.

For those essential oils having a low phenol content, major constituents have been variously reported as cineole, β-caryophyllene, neerolidol, myrcene, geranyl acetate and linalyl acetate. Other constituents of the drug (flavonoids, various acids, triterpenes) again resemble those of garden thyme.

The drug has been used traditionally for the treatment of respiratory infections, gastrointestinal problems and skin conditions requiring an antiseptic.

For an elaboration of the chemical constituents, pharmacological actions, therapeutics and research references concerning the thymes, see P. Bradley, 2006, *British Herbal Compendium*, Vol. 2, pp. 369–375; 389–392. British Herbal Medical Association, Bournemouth, UK. For a complete overview of all aspects of the genus, see Stahl-Biskup, E. (ed.), Hardman, R. (series ed.) 2002 Thyme: the genus *Thymus*. Taylor and Francis, New York. 230 pp., *956 references.*

OREGANO

There is a large number of marjorams, and various varieties are cultivated extensively for ornamental and culinary purposes. Two medicinally used species described in the *BP/EP* are *Origanum onites* L. (syn. *Majoram onites*) the pot marjoram or Greek oregano, and *O. vulgare* L. subsp. *hirtum* (Link) Ietsw., a subspecies of the wild marjoram, or oregano, family Labiatae. The dried leaves and flowers are separated from the stems; a mixture of both species may be used. Both have a strong, thyme-like odour. Both appear similar in the dried state but the leaves of *O. onites* are yellowish–green whereas those of *O. vulgare* are more distinctly green. In the powdered form, both show typical laminaceous characteristics.

In view of the diverse nature of the genus, with many varieties of the above and the fact that other plants may be sold commercially under the name 'oregano', the characteristics of the oil are important. The *BP/EP* requires a minimum of 2.5% oil in the drug and a minimum 1.5% carvacol and thymol. Other constituents of the oil include caryophyllene, β-bisabolene, cymene, linalool and borneol. Plants grown near the Mediterranean coast are stated to be the most fragrant of all. Tannins, sterols, flavonoids and resin have been reported in the drug. A reddish dye can be obtained from the aerial parts of *O. vulgare*.

Uses. Although in Britain oregano is not used medicinally to any extent, its thymol content gives it strong antiseptic properties. Traditionally its uses include the treatment of digestive disorders, pharnygeal infections and mild fevers.

Further reading

Kintzios SE (ed), Hardman R (series ed) 2002 Oregano: the genus *Origanum* and *Lippia*. Taylor and Francis, New York, 277 pp. *839 references*

LAVENDER FLOWER

The general term 'lavender' applies to a number of species and numerous hybrids and varieties of the genus *Lavandula*, plants used from classical times for their aromatic and medicinal properties. The generic name derives from the Latin *lavare*, referring to the use of lavender by the Romans as a bath perfume. The numerous cultivated varieties vary in their flower colour (blue through purple to white), habit, foliage and, importantly, their oil composition as indicated under 'Lavender Oil' below; many are hybrids and do not breed true.

Lavender flower *BP/EP* 2007, *BHP* 1983 consists of the dried flowers of *L. angustifolia* P.Mill. (*L. officinalis* Chaix). It is required (*BP*) to contain a minimum volatile oil content of 1.3% expressed on a dry weight basis.

The flowers, up to 5 mm in length, are packed closely together in verticillasters on a quadrangular stem forming a compact terminal spike. Each verticillaster consists of six to ten shortly stalked flowers. In the fresh condition, oily glandular trichomes can be discerned among the numerous covering trichomes on the surface of the five-lobed calyx. The blue corolla is bilabiate with an upper bifid lip and a lower three-lobed lip.

Microscopical features of the powder include fragments of the calyx and corolla with numerous associated glandular and clothing trichomes; prismatic crystals of calcium oxalate in cells of the calyx; pollen grains up to about 35 μm in diameter with six pores and six pitted lines radiating from the poles; vascular tissue from the pedicel.

Gas chromatographic analysis of the oil isolated in the volatile oil determination above is employed by the *BP/EP* to establish the absence in the sample of species and varieties other than *L. angustifolia*. The chromatogram obtained is compared with that of a reference solution containing five compounds expected to be found in the oil of a genuine sample; the peak for camphor should not exceed 1% of the total area of the peaks thus excluding camphoraceous species such as *L. latifolia*.

Uses. Although it is the volatile oil of lavender that is principally used for medicinal purposes the *BHP* 1983 cites flatulent dyspepsia, colic and depressive headache as indications for use of the flowers.

It may be used in combination with other drugs such as rosemary, valerian, meadow-sweet and others.

LAVENDER OIL

The botanical source of lavender oil is *Lavandula angustifolia* Miller (*Lavandula officinalis* Chaix), family Labiatae. Originally (*BP* 1980) oil from this species was referred to as 'foreign oil' to distinguish it from that of *L. intermedia* Loisel, which was termed 'English oil'. The latter has a much finer fragrance than the Continental oil and there were separate pharmacopoeial standards for the two oils. Unfortunately the straggly habit of the English lavender does not lend itself to mechanical harvesting and oil produced commercially is now of the Continental type. France, once the principal producer, has been superseded by Bulgaria, with smaller quantities of oil coming from the former USSR, Australia and other countries.

Lavender oil types. The taxonomy of the lavenders is confusing and Continental oils differ among themselves owing to the fact that a number of different species, varieties and hybrids are distilled. The true lavender, *L. officinalis*, yields the best oil when grown at a fairly high altitude, the variety growing under these conditions being known as 'petite lavande'. At a lower altitude the 'lavande moyenne' yields a somewhat less esteemed oil. 'Grande lavande', *L. latifolia* Villers (*L. spica* DC), yields a much coarser oil, which is sold as oil of spike. The above plant readily hybridizes with *L. officinalis* yielding a plant known as 'grosse lavande' or 'lavandin', the oil of which is intermediate in character between that of the parent forms. According to Tucker (*Baileya*, 1981, **21**, 131), of the many names applied to this hybrid species, the correct one is *L. × intermedia* Emeric ex Loiseleur. As hybrids the plants do not breed true and are normally propagated vegetatively; a simple efficient method for the *in vitro* shoot regeneration from the leaves has offered possibilities for future breeding (S. Dronne *et al.*, *Plant Cell Reports*, 1999, **18**, 429). The lavandin oil market is controlled by the French with Spain the principal producer.

The evergreen plant flowers from July to September and the fresh flowering spikes yield about 0.5% of volatile oil. The amount varies according to variety, season and method of distillation; modern steam stills give a rather larger yield than those in which the flowers are boiled with water. Genuine Continental lavender oil normally contains over 35% of esters. Oil of spike, which is largely used in cheap perfumery, contains little ester but a high proportion of free alcohols (about 23–41% calculated as borneol); 30 components have been identified. The nature of the alcohols also varies from a mixture of linalol and geraniol in the best lavender oil to borneol in oil of spike. Hybrids are of intermediate character (e.g. 'lavandin oil') and contain about 6–9% of esters and about 35% of alcohols. An analysis of the Spanish oil (J. de Pascual Teresa, *Planta Medica*, 1989, **55**, 398) enabled the identification of 50 compounds, the principal ones being 1:8-cineole, linalol and camphor; in contrast to the oil of *L. angustifolia*, linalyl acetate was not present.

A GC profile together with prescribed percentage ranges of 10 components of the pharmaceutical oil is given in the *BP/EP*; linalol (20–45%) and linalyl acetate (25–46%) are the principal constituents with a maximum limit for camphor of 1.2%. Chiral chromatography is used to determine the chiral purity of the linalol and linalyl acetate contents.

As with other Labiatae, *Lavandula* cell cultures do not produce essential oil and for *L. vera* rosmarinic acid is the principal phenolic component together with caffeic acid and traces of others. An enol ester of caffeic acid is a blue pigment also found in cell cultures (see E. Kovatcheva *et al.*, *Phytochemistry*, 1996, **43**, 1243).

Species of *Lavandula* other than the above are also cultivated. *L. stoechas* has a markedly different odour and of its 51 volatile components, fenchone, pinocaryl acetate, camphor, eucalyptol and myrthenol predominate. Large producers are Spain and France. Oil from wild plants growing in the Algiers region of Algeria contained as significant constituents fenchone (31.6%), camphor (22.4%), *p*-cymene (6.5%) lavandulyl acetate (3.0%) and α-pinene (1.0%). Fifty-four components amounting to *ca* 73% of the oil were identified (T. Dob *et al.*, *Pharm Biol.*, 2006; **44**, 60).

Uses. Lavender oil is principally used in the toiletry and perfumery industries and occasionally in ointments, etc., to mask disagreeable odours. It is employed pharmaceutically in the antiarthropod preparation Gamma Benzene Hexachloride Application. Lavender flowers are included in the *BHP* and are indicated for the treatment of flatulent dyspepsia and topically, as the oil, for rheumatic pain. The oil is extensively used in aromatherapy (q.v.).

CARAWAY FRUIT

Caraway (*Caraway Fruit*) consists of the dried, ripe fruits of *Carum carvi* (Umbelliferae), a biennial herb about 1 m high. It occurs both wild and cultivated in central and northern Europe (The Netherlands, Denmark, Germany, Russia, Finland, Poland, Hungary and Britain) and in Egypt, Morocco, Australia and China.

History. Caraway fruits were known to the Arabian physicians and probably came into use in Europe in the thirteenth century.

Macroscopical characters. The commercial drug (Fig. 22.5) usually consists of mericarps separated from the pedicels. The fruits are slightly curved, brown and glabrous, about 4–7 mm long, 1–2.3 mm wide and tapered at both ends; they are crowned with a stylopod often with style and stigma attached. Each mericarp shows five almost equal sides, five narrow primary ridges, and, when cut transversely, four dorsal and two commissural vittae. They have a characteristic aromatic odour and taste.

Microscopical characters. A transverse section of a caraway mericarp (Fig. 22.5) shows five primary ridges, in each of which is a vascular strand with associated pitted sclerenchyma and having a single secretory canal at the outer margin of each. The six vittae which appear somewhat flattened and elliptical in transverse section may attain a width of 350 μm; they extend from the base of the fruit to the base of the stylopod. They are lined with small, dark reddish-brown cells and contain a pale yellow or colourless oleoresin (Fig. 22.5B, C). The raphe lies on the inner side of the endosperm, which is non-grooved. Occupying the majority of the transverse section is the endosperm, with thickened cellulose walls (having also deposits of a β-(1,4)-mannan as a reserve polysaccharide) and containing fixed oil and aleurone grains having one or two microrosettes of calcium oxalate. The embryo, which is situated near the apex of the mericarp, will only be seen in sections passing through that region.

More detailed examination shows that the outer epidermis of the pericarp is glabrous (cf. aniseed) and has a striated cuticle (cf. fennel). The mesocarp consists of more or less collapsed parenchyma and lacks the reticulated cells of fennel. The endodermis (or inner epidermis of the pericarp) (Fig. 22.5F) consists of a single layer of elongated cells, arranged more or less parallel to one another and not showing the 'parquetry' arrangement of coriander.

Constituents. Caraway contains 3–7% of volatile oils (*BP* not less than 3.0%), 8–20% of fixed oil, proteins, calcium oxalate, colouring matter and resin.

Uses. Large quantities of caraway fruits are used for culinary purposes. The fruits and oil are used in medicine for flavouring and as carminatives. The carminative and antispasmodic properties have been experimentally verified.

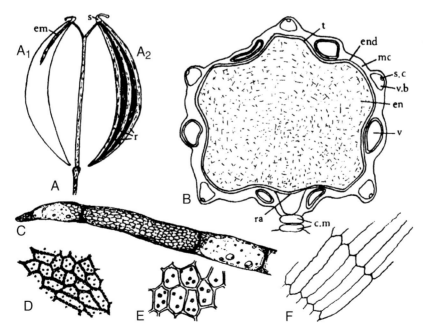

Fig. 22.5
Caraway. A, mericarps showing attachments to carpophore; A₁, mericarp sectioned longitudinally to show position of embryo; A₂, mericarp side view (×8). B, transverse section of mericarp (×50); C, portion of vitta isolated by alkali maceration (×25); D, screids of mesocarp; E, endosperm cells with micro-rosette crystals of calcium oxalate; F, endocarp layer in surface view (all ×200). c.m, commissural meristeles; em, embryo; en, endosperm; end, endocarp; mc, mesocarp; r, three of five primary ridges; ra, position of raphe; s, stylopod; s.c, secretory canal; t, testa; v, vitta; v.b, vascular bundle with associated finely pitted sclerenchyma.

Further reading

Nemeth E (ed), Hardman R (series ed) 1998 Medicinal and aromatic plants—industrial profiles, Vol. 7. Caraway: the genus *Carum*. Harwood Academic, Amsterdam. *529 references*

CARAWAY OIL

The volatile oil (Caraway Oil *BP/EP*) consists largely of the ketone carvone and the terpene limonene (formulae, Fig. 22.4) with small quantities of dihydrocarvone, carveol and dihydrocarveol. As there is a demand for pure carvone, there is a considerable amount of decarvonized oil available for adulteration.

Official tests include a TLC examination to ascertain the presence of carvone and carveol and the measurement of optical rotation (+65° to +81°), refractive index (1.484–1.490) and acid value (maximum 1.0). The proportions of individual components are required to fall within certain limits as determined by gas chromatography: limonene (30–45%), carvone (50–65%), β-myrcene (0.1–1.0%) with maximum limits for *trans*-dihydrocarvone and *trans*-carveol (both 2.5%). The gas chromatographic chirality assay limits (−)-carvone to 1.0%.

DILL AND DILL OIL

Dill (*Dill Fruit*) consists of the dried, ripe fruits of *Anethum graveolens* (Umbelliferae), a small annual indigenous to southern Europe. It is cultivated in Central and Eastern Europe and Egypt. Dill was known to Dioskurides and was employed in England in Anglo-Saxon times.

Macroscopical characters. The drug usually consists of separate, broadly oval mericarps, about 4 mm long and 2–3 mm broad. The fruits are very much compressed dorsally, the two central ridges being prolonged into membranous wings, while the dorsal ones are inconspicuous. The fruits have an aromatic odour and taste similar to those of caraway.

Microscopical characters. Each mericarp has four vittae on the dorsal surface and two on the commissural. The outer epidermis has a striated cuticle (distinction from fennel), and the mesocarp contains lignified, reticulate parenchyma (distinction from caraway). The endosperm is much flattened but otherwise resembles that of caraway.

Constituents. The volatile oil (Dill Oil *BP/EP*) resembles oil of caraway in containing carvone and limonene. The European fruits yield about 3–4% of volatile oil, which should contain from 43 to 63% of carvone; the carvone content is determined by reaction with hydroxylamine hydrochloride (oxime formation) and titration of the liberated acid. Other constituents reported for the oil include *trans*- and *cis*-dihydrocarvone, *trans*- and *cis*-carveol, limonene, D- and L-dihydrocarveol, α- and γ-terpinene, α-phellandrene and others. Chemical types based on the proportion of carvone present, and the presence or absence of dillapiole and myristicin have been distinguished.

Monoterpene glycosides have been isolated from the water-soluble fraction of the fruits.

For further details on constituents, see T. Ishikawa *et al.*, *Chem. Pharm. Bull.*, 2002, **50**, 501; M. Kosar *et al.*, *Pharm. Biol.*, 2005, **41**, 491.

Uses. Like caraway, dill is used as a carminative and flavour; it is much used in infant's gripe water.

Allied drug. *Indian Dill*, derived from a variety of *A. graveolens* consists of whole cremocarps which bear pedicels and are narrower and less compressed than the European drug. Indian dill oil contains dillapiole and less carvone.

CORIANDER AND CORIANDER OIL

Coriander (*Coriander Fruit*) of the *BP* is the dried, nearly ripe fruit of *Coriandrum sativum* (Umbelliferae), an annual about 0.7 m high with white or pinkish flowers. It is indigenous to Italy, but is widely cultivated in The Netherlands, Central and Eastern Europe, the Mediterranean (Morocco, Malta, Egypt), China, India and Bangladesh. Coriander is mentioned in the papyrus of Ebers (*c*. 1550 BC), and in the writings of Cato and Pliny. It was well known in England before the Norman Conquest. Ukraine is the major producer of oil and controls the world price on a supply and demand basis; in one large factory continuous distillation has replaced the batch process.

Macroscopical characters. The drug (Fig. 22.6A) usually consists of the whole cremocarps, which, when ripe, are about 2.3–4.3 mm diameter and straw-yellow. Each consists of two hemispherical mericarps united by their margins. Considerable variation exists in coriander. The Indian variety is oval, but the more widely distributed spherical varieties vary in size from the Ukrainian 2.3–3.7 mm to the Moroccan 4.0–4.3 mm. The apex bears two divergent styles. The 10 primary ridges are wavy and inconspicuous; alternating with these are eight more prominent, straight, secondary ridges. The fruits have an aromatic odour and a spicy taste. They are somewhat liable to insect attacks.

Microscopical characters. A transverse section of a fully ripe fruit shows only two mature vittae in each mericarp, both on the commissural surface (Fig. 22.6B). The numerous vittae present in the immature fruit on the dorsal surface of each mericarp gradually join and are eventually compressed into slits. The outer part of the pericarp, which possesses stomata and prisms of calcium oxalate, is more or less completely thrown off. Within the vittae-bearing region of the mesocarp a thick layer of sclerenchyma is formed, which consists of pitted, fusiform cells. These sclerenchymatous fibres tend in the outer layers to be longitudinally directed and in the inner layers to be tangentially directed. In the region of the primary ridges more of the fibres are longitudinally directed; in the secondary ridges nearly all are tangentially directed. Traversing the band of sclerenchyma and corresponding in position to the primary ridges are small vascular strands composed of a small group of spiral vessels. The mesocarp within the sclerenchymatous band is composed of irregular polygonal cells with lignified walls. The inner epidermis of the pericarp is composed of 'parquetry' cells, which in the powder are often seen united to the cells of the inner mesocarp. The testa is composed of brown flattened cells. The endosperm is curved and consists of parenchymatous cells containing fixed oil and aleurone grains. The latter contain rosettes of calcium oxalate 3–10 mm diameter (see Fig. 22.6 C–F).

Constituents. Coriander fruits contain up to 1.8% of volatile oil according to origin (*BP/EP* standard not less than 0.2%). The distilled oil (Coriander Oil *BP/EP*) contains 65–70% of (+)-linalool (coriandrol), depending on the source, and smaller amounts of α-pinene, γ-terpinene, limonene and *p*-cymene together with various non-linalool alcohols and esters. Some 40 constituents have been identified. The *BP/EP* uses GC for the evaluation of the oil with linalool and geraniol as internal standards; there is also a test for chiral purity ((R)-linalool, maximum 14%). Other constituents isolated from the fruits include flavonoids, coumarins, isocoumarins, phthalides and phenolic acids. T. Ishikawa *et al.* (*Chem. Pharm. Bull.*, 2003, **51**, 32) obtained 33 compounds from the water-soluble fraction of a methanolic extract of the fruits; new constituents included monoterpenoids, monoterpenoid glycosides, monoterpenoid glucoside sulphates and aromatic compound glycosides. The high content of fats (16–28%) and protein (11–17%) in the fruits make distillation residues suitable for animal feed. The fruits yield 5–7% of ash.

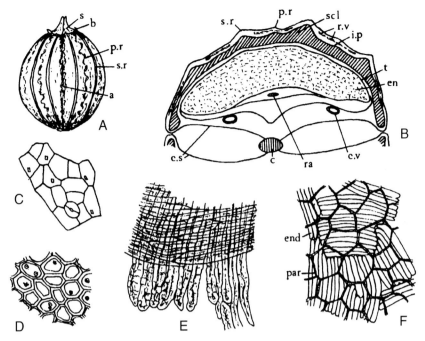

Fig. 22.6
Coriander. A, Whole fruit (×8); B, transverse section of fruit (×16); C, fragment of epicarp in surface view with stoma and small prismatic crystals of calcium oxalate; D, endosperm cells with microrosette crystals of calcium oxalate; E, layers of sclerenchyma from the mesocarp; F, lignified parenchyma of the mesocarp and underlying endodermis showing 'parquetry' arrangement (all ×200). a, line of attachment of mericarps; b, sepal; c, carpophore, c.s, commissural surfaces; c.v, commissural vitta; en, endosperm; end, endodermis; par, lignified parenchyma of mesocarp; p.r, primary ridge; ra, raphe; r.v, remains of dorsal vittae; s, stylopod; scl, sclerenchyma; s.r, secondary ridge; t, testa.

The unripe plant has an unpleasant, mousy odour, which is also present in oil distilled from unripe fruits (mainly aldehydes such as *n*-decanal contained in peripheral vittae). Marked changes occur in volatile oil composition during ontogenesis; the peripheral vittae flatten and lose their oil, all of which is then produced by the commissural vittae. During ordinary storage of the fruits, the oil composition undergoes considerable alteration.

Uses.   Very large quantities of the spice are produced in many countries for domestic purposes, such as for use in curries. In the former USSR linalool is isolated from the oil as starting material for other derivatives. Pharmaceutically coriander and its oils are used as a flavouring agent and carminative.

ANISEED AND ANISEED OIL

Aniseed (*Anise Fruit*) of the *BP* and *EP* consists of the dried, ripe fruits of *Pimpinella anisum* (Umbelliferae), an annual plant indigenous to the Levant but widely cultivated both in Europe (Spain, Germany, Italy, Russia, Bulgaria), Egypt and America (Chile, Mexico). Anise is mentioned in the writings of Theophrastus, Dioskurides and Pliny. It was cultivated in Germany in the ninth century. Spain and Egypt are the principal producers of the oil.

Macroscopical characters.   The drug (Fig. 22.7A) consists of greyish-brown, pear-shaped, somewhat compressed cremocarps, which are usually attached to pedicels 2–12 mm in length. The cremocarps are

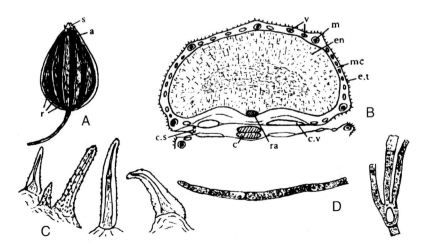

Fig. 22.7
Aniseed. A, Side view of cremocarp showing line of attachment to the two mericarps (×8); B, transverse section of mericarp (×25); C, covering trichomes of epicarp (×200); D, branched and unbranched vittae isolated by alkali maceration (×25). a, Line of attachment of mericarps; c, carpophore; c.s, commissural surfaces; c.v, commissural vitta; en, endosperm; e.t, epicarp bearing trichomes; m, meristele; mc, mesocarp; r, three of five primary ridges of one mericarp; ra, raphe; s, stylopod; v, vittae.

3–6 mm long and 2–3 mm broad. The Spanish (Alicante) and Italian are distinguished by their large size and light colour, while the German and 'Russian' are smaller, more ovoid and darker. Each mericarp has five somewhat wavy ridges and is slightly pubescent on the dorsal surface. They have an aromatic odour and a sweet, aromatic taste.

Microscopical characters. Microscopical examination shows that the epidermis bears numerous papillae and unicellular hairs. On the dorsal surface of each mericarp are from 15 to 45 branched vittae. A small amount of vascular tissue and reticulated parenchyma is present. The endosperm is slightly concave on the commissural surface and contains protein and fixed oil (see Fig. 22.7B–D).

Constituents. Anise fruits yield 2–3% of volatile oil (*BP/EP* ≮ 2.0%), which is almost identical with that obtained from star-anise fruits. A number of water-soluble constituents have been isolated from the fruits including various glucosides, see E. Fujimatu *et al.*, *Phytochemistry*, 2003, **63** (5).

Aniseed Oil. *BP/EP* tests and standards for the oil include: TLC identification of anethole and anisaldehyde; maximum limit of 0.1% for fenchone and 0.01% for foeniculin; *trans*-anethole 87–94%; estragole 0.5–5.0%, anisaldehyde 1.0–1.4% and linalol <1.5% determined by gas chromatography.

STAR ANISE FRUIT AND OIL

The star-anise *Illicium verum* Hook, f., family Illiciaceae, is an evergreen tree about 4–5 m in height, indigenous to the south-west provinces of China. The fruits are collected and the oil distilled locally in China and Vietnam.

The fruits consist of eight (rarely seven or nine) one-seeded follicles. Each follicle is about 12–17 mm long. The pericarp is reddish-brown, woody and only slightly wrinkled. Each carpel has, as a rule, partly dehisced to expose the seed. The latter has a brittle, shining testa and an oily kernel. The beak of each carpel is not turned upwards and the fruit stalk, which is about 3 cm long, is curved (distinction from *I. religiosum*). The oil, which is present in both seed and pericarp, gives the drug an aromatic odour and spicy taste.

The genuine fruits of *I. verum* should yield a minimum of 7.0% volatile oil containing not less than 86.0% of *trans*-anethole. More recently, they have been employed for the extraction of shikimic acid (see Fig. 19.5), which is the starting material for the synthesis of the antiviral drug Tamiflu (Roche). As a consequence, the plant is in some danger of over-exploitation and other sources of the acid are being investigated (q.v.).

Bastard star-anise or *shikimi fruits* occur in Eastern commerce and are occasionally exported. They are derived from *I. religiosum* (*I. anisatum*), a species cultivated near the Buddhist temples in Japan and also on the mainland. The carpels are equal in number to those of *I. verum* but are smaller, are much wrinkled and have a curved-up apex. The stalk is shorter than the genuine fruit, and straight. These fruits, which contain shikimic acid, are poisonous, as they contain an amorphous toxic substance sikimitoxin, and a crystalline toxic substance sikimin. New phenylpropanoid glycosides have been recently reported (Z.-H. Jiang *et al.*, *Chem. Pharm. Bull.*, 1999, **47**, 421). In recent years, Japanese workers have isolated a number of novel sesquiterpene lactones (anisatin-like compounds) from the pericarps of various *Illicium* species including *I. verum*; a number of these compounds are convulsants. T. Nakamura *et al.* (*Chem. Pharm. Bull.*, 1996, **44**, 1908) describe the isolation of three sesquiterpenoid compounds (veranistans, A,B,C) which are neurotoxins. For additional isolations, see J.-M. Huang *et al.*, *Chem. Pharm. Bull.*, 2000, **48**, 657.

Star anise oil

The essential oil should contain 87–94% *trans*-anethole, 0.5–5.0% of estragole and smaller amounts of anisaldehyde (0.1–0.5%) and

foeniculin (0.1–3.0%); other minor components include chavicol methyl ether (an isomeride of anethole), *p*-methoxyphenylacetone, safrole and other minor components. The oil is, for all ordinary purposes, indistinguishable from that of *P. anisum* but differences in the gas chromatographic profiles can be seen. The oil is liable to atmospheric oxidation and both anisic aldehyde and anisic acid are normally present. This change is said to diminish the tendency of the oil to solidify, which it normally does on cooling to about 15°C. In the past, the oil was imported in lead containers and some pharmacopoeias give a limit test for heavy metals.

Both aniseed oil and star anise oil are used as flavouring agents and as carminatives. Anethole (a colourless crystalline solid m.p. 21°C) may be prepared from the oil or manufactured synthetically.

BITTER FENNEL AND SWEET FENNEL

Bitter Fennel consists of the dried ripe fruits of *Foeniculum vulgare*, subsp. *vulgare*, var. *vulgare* (Umbelliferae). It is cultivated in many parts of Europe and much is imported from India, China and Egypt. The commercial drug consists partly of whole cremocarps and partly of isolated mericarps. Bitter fennel, now little used in British medicine, is more fully described in the 11th edition of this book. The drug has, however, been re-introduced into the *BP* on account of its *EP* status.

The fruits contain 1–4% of volatile oil with higher yields recorded.

The principal constituents of bitter fennel oil, with *BP/EP* prescribed limits, are fenchone (12–25%), *trans*-anethole (55–75%) together with anisaldehyde (maximum 2.0%) and estragole (methyl chavicol) (maximum 5.0%). Minor components include limonene and other monoterpene hydrocarbons.

Anethole is derived via the shikimic acid pathway and fenchone (a bicyclic monoterpene) is formed from fenchol by the action of a dehydrogenase. Other components of the fruits include flavonoids, coumarins and glycosides. The latter, which may have a biogenetic relationship with the volatile oil constituents, have been actively investigated by Japanese workers. Thus M. Ono *et al.* (*Chem. Pharm. Bull.*, 1995, **43**, 868; 1996, **44**, 337) describe a number of monoterpene glycosides based on 1,8-cineole and *cis*-miyabenol C which they have termed foeniculosides I–IX. J. Kitajima, T. Ishikawa and co-workers in nine studies on the water-soluble glycosides and sugars of fennel fruit (*Chem. Pharm. Bull.*, 1998, **46**, 1587, 1591, 1599, 1603, 1643, 1738; 1999, **47**, 805, 988) have recorded alkyl-, erythro-anethol-, *p*-hydroxyphenylpropylene glycol-, fenchane-, menthane-, aromatic (phenylpropane etc)- and 1,8-cineole-type glycosides. It is of further interest that of the cineole-type glycosides

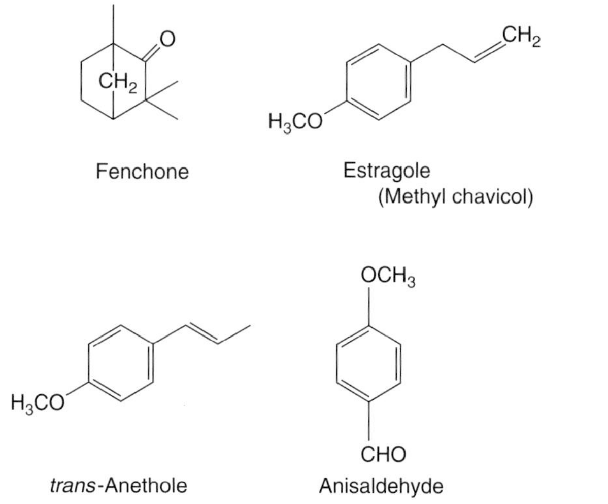

Fig. 22.8
Constituents of fennel oils.

one had previously been isolated from *Cunila spicata* (Lamiaceae), a plant used in Brazilian traditional medicine, one from the peel and flower buds of *Citrus unshiu* and two were biotransformation products from a *Eucalyptus* cell suspension culture following administration of 1,8-cineole. Annual world production of the oil is less than 5 tonnes.

Fennel and its volatile oil are used as an aromatic and carminative.

Sweet Fennel is derived from *F. vulgare*, subsp. *vulgare*, var. *dulce* and is also included in the *BP/EP*. The fruits resemble those of the bitter variety but have a sweet taste and lower volatile oil content (not less than 2.0%) of different quantitative composition. Not less than 80% of the oil is required to be anethole, not more than 7.5% fenchone, and not more than 10% estragole.

Further reading

Jodral MM (ed), Hardman R (series ed) 2004 Medicinal and aromatic plants – industrial profiles, Vol 40. Illicium, Pimpinella and Foeniculum. CRC Press, Boca Raton, FL, 256 pp.

Cumin

Cumin consists of the dried ripe fruits of *Cuminum cyminum* (Umbelliferae), a small, annual plant indigenous to Egypt. It is widely cultivated and UK supplies are obtained from Sicily, Malta, Mogadore and India. Spain and Egypt are the major cumin oil producers.

Cumin fruits are about 6 mm long and resemble caraway at first glance. The mericarps, however, are straighter than those of caraway and are densely covered with short, bristly hairs. Whole cremocarps attached to short pedicels occur, as well as isolated mericarps. Each mericarp has four dorsal vittae and two commissural ones. The odour and taste are coarser than those of caraway.

Cumin yields 2.5–4.0% of volatile oil. This contains 25–35% of aldehydes (cuminic aldehyde), pinene and α-terpinol.

As with other umbelliferous fruits the water-soluble constituents of cumin have been recently investigated. Compounds isolated include flavonoid glycosides such as the 7-*O*-β-D-glycopyranosides of apigenin and luteolin, some 16 monoterpenoid glycosides and new sesquiterpenoid glucosides, e.g. cuminosides A and B (T. Ishikawa *et al.*, *Chem. Pharm. Bull.*, 2002, **50**, 1471; T. Takayanagi *et al.*, *Phytochemistry*, 2003, **63**, 479).

Cumin was one of the commonest spices in the Middle Ages. It is employed in Indian medicine (for a study of its activity see S. C. Jain *et al.*, *Fitoterapia*, 1992, **63**, 291).

TURPENTINE OIL

Pharmaceutical turpentine oil is obtained by distillation and rectification from the oleoresin produced by various species of *Pinus*. The unrectified oil is the turpentine of commerce. The resin remaining in the still is the source of colophony (q.v. under 'Resins').

Rectification of the commercial oil consists of treatment with aqueous alkali to remove traces of phenols, cresols, resin acids etc. and possible redistillation.

The genus *Pinus* is widely distributed and many countries have considerable reserves of pine forest. The principal species employed are (1) *Pinus palustris* (longleaf pine) and *P. elliottii* (slash pine) in the S. and S.E. United States; (2) *P. pinaster* (*P. maritima*) in France, Italy, Portugal and Spain; (3) *P. halepensis* in Greece and Spain; (4) *P. roxburghii* (*P. longifolia*) in India and Pakistan; (5) *P. massoniana* and *P. tabuliformis* in China; (6) *P. carribaea* var. *hondurensis* and *P. oocarpa* in Central America and (7) *P. radiata* in New Zealand.

The collection of the oleoresin is very labour-intensive and for this reason output in the USA has declined considerably. Principal world producers are now Portugal and China; other contributors, in addition to the USA, include Spain, Greece, Morocco, France, India, the former USSR, Honduras and Poland. Many other countries produce smaller quantities for their own use. It is considered that about 250 000 trees are required to sustain a small commercial processing plant.

Oil of turpentine is a colourless liquid with a characteristic odour and a pungent taste. It is soluble in alcohol, ether, chloroform and glacial acetic acid. Oil of turpentine is optically active, but the rotation varies not only with the species of pine from which it has been obtained, but also

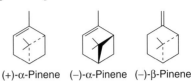

(+)-α-Pinene   (–)-α-Pinene   (–)-β-Pinene

in samples taken from the same tree at different periods. Samples taken from the same tree at different times have given rotations varying from –7° 27′ to +18° 18′ in the case of *Pinus palustris*, and –28° 26′ to +1° 23′ in the case of *Pinus heterophylla*. The French oils from *Pinus pinaster* are strongly laevorotatory (–20° to –38°). Over forty components have been identified in French turpentine oil derived from *P. pinaster*.

Oil of turpentine consists chiefly of the terpenes (+)- and (–)-α-pinene, (–)-β-pinene and camphene. These tend to undergo atmospheric oxidation, with the formation of complex resinous substances, the removal of which is accomplished by the process of rectification mentioned above. The varying optical rotations of differing turpentines are mainly due to the varying proportions of the (+)- and (–)-α-pinenes present; (–)-β-pinene is found in almost all *Pinus* spp. in a high state of optical purity and typically occurs with the predominantly (+)-α-pinene. These two isomers have opposite absolute configurations. Other components of the oil which find industrial uses are β-phellandrene, δ-3-carene (a major component of Indian and 'Russian' turpentines), limonene, *p*-cymene, longifoline and estragol.

Oil of turpentine is now rarely given internally. Externally it is used as a counterirritant and rubefacient. For inhalation, terebene is usually preferred. *Terebene* is prepared from oil of turpentine by the action of cold sulphuric acid, which converts the pinene into the optically inactive (±)- limonene (dipentene). Now, most turpentine is processed to give its various constituents which find use in the manufacture of fragrances, flavours, vitamins, insecticides, etc.

PINUS PINASTER TYPE TURPENTINE OIL

This oil, official in the European and British Pharmacopoeias 2007, is obtained by steam distillation of the oleoresin from *Pinus pinaster* Aiton and rectified. The French oils from this species are strongly laevorotatory (limits –40° to –28°), *cf*. Oil of Turpentine *BP*. The principal constituents and official limits are α-pinene (70–85%), β-pinene (11–20%) and limonene (1–7%). Other components in small amounts are camphene, car-3-ene, β-myrcene, longifolene, β-caryophyllene and caryophyllene oxide. Over 40 compounds have been reported in *P. pinaster* oil.

Standards relevant to the quality of turpentine oils are refractive index, relative density, residue on evaporation, optical rotation, acid value and peroxide value. Tests for fixed oils and resinified oil together with solubility in alcohol are also important.

Turpentine oils are used medicinally for their rubefacient acitivity.

Canada turpentine

Canada turpentine, or 'Canada balsam' as it is often incorrectly called, is an oleoresin obtained from the stem of *Abies balsamea* (Pinaceae), the balsam fir. It is collected in eastern Canada and in the State of Maine in the USA. The oleoresin in the bark occurs in schizogenous ducts and large cavities. As the cavities fill with secretion, blister-like swellings develop on the trunk, and it is from these that the oleoresin is collected.

Canada turpentine when fresh is a pale-yellow liquid with a slight, greenish fluorescence and is of honey-like consistency. It has a pleasant, terebinthinate odour and a somewhat bitter and acrid taste. On exposure to air, Canada turpentine becomes more viscous and finally forms a glass-like varnish, a property which rendered it suitable as a microscopic mountant and as a cement for lenses. It contains volatile oil (23–24%) and a number of terpenoid acids.

Pumilio pine oil

A distillation of the fresh leaves of the pumilio pine, *Pinus mugo* var. *pumilio* (Pinaceae) yields the *BP* (1980) oil. It is produced in Eastern Europe.

The oil has an agreeable odour and contains principally terpenes and sesquiterpenes, with up to 10% bornyl acetate (*BP* 1980 limits 4–10% of ester). It may be distinguished from other similar oils by the above ester content and its weight per millilitre value. It is used as a decongestant inhalant, in the preparation of compound thymol glycerin, and as a constituent of zinc undecenoate dusting-powder.

Savin tops

These are the young shoots of *Juniperus sabina* (Cupressaceae), an evergreen shrub about 2–6 m high. It grows wild in the mountains of Austria, Switzerland, Italy, France and Spain. The leaves are imbricated, sessile, more or less adnate to the stem and usually opposite and decussate. The shape and size of the leaves differ very considerably on different parts of the plant. Each leaf has a depression on its dorsal surface, below which is a large oil gland in the mesophyll. This oil gland is oval in young leaves but more elongated in old ones. Savin contains a volatile oil (1–3%) which is a powerful irritant both internally and externally. It contains the terpene alcohol sabinol and its acetate. Other constituents are podophyllotoxin (0.2%), coumarins and savinin. Many diterpenoids with various skeletal structures have been reported among the non-volatile constituents of a hexane fraction of the berries of this plant. (For reports see A. San Feliciano *et al.*, *Phytochemistry*, 1991, **30**, 695; *Fitoterapia*, 1991, **62**, 435.)

Oil of cade

Oil of cade is obtained by the destructive distillation of the woody portions of *Juniperus oxycedrus* (Cupressaceae). It is prepared in Portugal, Spain and former Yugoslavia.

The distillate is allowed to stand for at least 15–20 days when a layer constituting oil of cade may be separated.

Oil of cade is a reddish-brown or blackish, oily liquid. Odour, empyreumatic; taste, aromatic, bitter and acrid. The chief constituents are sesquiterpenes (e.g. cadinene) and phenolic compounds (guaiacol, ethyl guaiacol and cresol).

The oil composition of the leaves of *J. oxycedrus* resembles that of *J. communis* (below). The oil is of variable composition; based on geographical location, subspecies and varieties, T. Dob *et al.*, (*Pharm. Biol.*, 2006, **1**, 1) suggest a classification of the oil based on four chemotypes: α-pinene, limonene, sabinene and *trans*-pinocarveol.

Oil of cade has been used for veterinary purposes for centuries, and has been prescribed for skin diseases.

JUNIPER BERRIES AND OIL

Juniper berries are the dried ripe fruits of *Juniperus communis* (Cupressaceae), an evergreen shrub or small tree. They are collected in former Yugoslavia, Italy, Hungary, Poland, Thuringia, Sweden and other countries. Generally speaking, the berries from the more southern countries contain the most oil.

In Tuscany the collection of the berries is very much a family industry. Bushes are beaten to remove the ripe fruits and the product is roughly cleaned before drying. Importers may further remove extraneous material by a winnowing process involving warm air. Any green berries are removed and the remaining fruits graded.

The female cones consist of scales arranged in whorls of three. The berry-like fruit takes 2 years to ripen, eventually becoming a deep purple colour and having a bluish-grey bloom. On drying, the berries become somewhat darker and shrivel slightly. They are about 3–10 mm in diameter. The apex shows a triradiate mark and depression indicating the sutures of the three fleshy scales. At the base there are usually six, small, pointed bracts arranged in two whorls, but occasionally three or four such whorls are found.

A transverse section of the fruit shows a thin outer skin or epicarp, a yellowish-brown, pulpy mesocarp and three seeds. The seeds lie close together in the centre of the fruit and are hard and woody. Partly embedded in the hard testa of each seed are large oleoresin glands. These usually number from four to eight on the outer side of the seed, and one or two on the inner. The drug has a pleasant, somewhat terebinthinate odour, and a sweetish taste.

The main constituents are volatile oil (about 0.5–1.5%), invert sugar (about 33%) and resin; the *BP/EP* specifies a minimum essential oil content of 1.0% with reference to the anhydrous drug.

The aerial parts of this species and its varieties have been examined for water-soluble constituents resulting in the isolation of various phenylpropanoid, neolignan and flavonoid glycosides. Megastigmane glycosides and a new monoterpene glucoside have recently been reported (T. Nakanishi *et al.*, *Chem. Pharm. Biol.*, 2005, **53**, 783). For a phytochemical and genetic survey of the species, see N. Filipowicz *et al.*, *Planta Med.*, 2006, **72**, 850.

Juniper berries are used for the preparation of oil of juniper and in making certain varieties of gin. The oil has diuretic and antiseptic properties. It has been reported that commercial oils vary in composition and prolonged intake of some may cause kidney damage. These side-effects are correlated with a high terpene hydrocarbon content and a low proportion of terpinen-4-ol.

Oil of Juniper *BP/EP*

This is obtained from the non-fermented berry cones of *Juniperus communis* L. by steam distillation. The oil contains over 60 constituents, although over 100 compounds have been detected in oil from wild berries collected in Greece. Principal components and official limits are α-pinene (20–50%), β-myrcene (1–35%), limonene (2–12%), β-pinene (1–12%), terpinen-4-ol (0.5–10%), sabinene (less than 20%) and β-caryophyllene (less than 7.0%). Other components not quantitatively specified are cadinene, camphene and various alcohols and esters.

The above figures demonstrate the possible variable composition of Juniper oil. For commercial oils in general this variation can be great and, as reported by P. Bradley (*BHPC*, Vol. 2, 2006), such oils are rarely prepared from a uniform source and may involve the distillate from fermented berries after their use in the manufacture of gin or the use of unripe berries, needles and wood of the plant.

Juniper oil is traditionally used for its diuretic, carminative and antirheumatic properties. Side-effects of some oils have been attributed to a relatively high proportion of terpene hydrocarbons and a low proportion of terpinen-4-ol.

BITTER ORANGE PEEL

Bitter orange peel is the dried outer part of the pericarp of the ripe or nearly ripe fruit known as the bitter, Seville or Bigarade orange. In botanical characteristics the tree is not unlike the sweet orange and both are regarded as subspecies or varieties of *Citrus aurantium* L. (Rutaceae).

These are named, respectively, *C. aurantium* var. *amara*-L. and *C. aurantium* var. *sinensis* L. (*C. sinensis* (L.) Osbeck.). The bitter orange is not as widely cultivated as the sweet orange and European supplies come from southern Spain (Seville and Malaga), Sicily (Messina and Palermo), Tripoli via Malta and the West Indies. The dried bitter peel is official in the *BP/EP*.

History. The bitter orange tree appears to have been introduced from northern India into eastern Africa, Arabia and Syria, whence it was brought to Europe by either the Arabs or Crusaders about AD 1200. The sweet orange was not known in Europe until the fifteenth century and appears to be of Chinese origin.

Collection and preparation. Orange peel may be prepared in the Mediterranean countries or in England. The peel should be removed with as little of white 'zest' as possible. Hand-cut, English dried peel is most esteemed. The peel may be removed in four 'quarters', or in a spiral band. It is also found in thin strips, similar to those found in marmalade, cut by machines. The so-called Maltese is of this type, which is known as 'gelatin-cut'. Fine slicing causes the rupture of a large number of oil glands and some loss in aroma.

Characters. The colour of the dried peel is somewhat variable, but frequently reddish-brown in the spiral form and greenish-brown in the 'quarters'. The other surface is rugged, being somewhat raised over the oil glands, which are clearly seen in sections with the naked eye. The inner surface bears a small amount of white 'zest'. Fragrant odour; aromatic and very bitter taste.

Microscopic examination shows a small-celled epidermis with characteristic stomata; parenchyma containing prismatic crystals of calcium oxalate 20–45 mm long, or sphaerocrystalline masses of hesperidin; small anastomosing vascular bundles; and large oil-filled cavities usually arranged in two irregular rows.

Constituents. Dried bitter orange peel contains not less than 2.0% of volatile oil, vitamin C and the flavonoid glycosides hesperidin and neohesperidin. The latter, present to the extent of 5–14% in the unripe peel, gradually disappears on ripening.

Citrus glycosides and limonoids. *Citrus* fruits contain a large number of flavanone glycosides. The best-known of these, hesperidin (see Fig. 21.18), was first isolated in 1828. It is present in oranges, both bitter and sweet, and in lemons. See also 'Flavone and Related Flavonoid Glycosides' and 'Hesperidin and Rutin'. An isomer of hesperidin, neohesperidin, is present in certain samples of Seville oranges. Naringin, present in some Seville oranges, is the chief flavonoid constituent of the grapefruit. Coniferin (Table 21.1) has been reported in *C. sinensis* and may add to the effects of limonin and naringin.

The bioproduction of neohesperidin and naringin in callus cultures of *C. aurantium* has been demonstrated (J. A. del Río *et al.*, *Plant Cell Rep.*, 1992, **11**, 592).

Uses. Bitter orange peel is used as a flavouring agent and as a bitter tonic. Hesperidin in the soluble form as in the fresh fruit functions as vitamin P.

Sweet orange peel

The peel of the sweet orange is thinner than that of the bitter, more yellowish in colour and less rough, and the taste, though pungent and aromatic, lacks the extreme bitterness of the Seville peel. As studied in Valencia orange peel, the colour originates from a complex mixture of carbonyl carotenoids, the principal components being violeoxanthin (9-*cis*-violaxanthin), di-*cis*-violaxanthin and all-*trans*-violaxanthin, together with a number of other carotenoids.

ORANGE OILS

The volatile oil from the orange may be extracted by methods other than by distillation (see 'Lemon Oils' for details of methods). That from the bitter orange is known as *Essence de Bigarde* and that from the sweet orange is called *Essence de Portugal*. The latter is official in the *BP/EP* and is obtained by mechanical expression of the fresh peel; although chemically almost identical with the bitter orange oil, it does not have the bitter taste or odour of the latter. These oils contain the terpene (+)-limonene and smaller quantities of citral, citronellal, methyl anthranilate, etc. In 1988, 62 components from the steam-distilled oil of Libyan fresh orange peel were identified. Sixteen of the identified compounds had not previously been reported as orange volatiles (A. J. MacLeod *et al.*, *Phytochemistry*, 1988, **27**, 2185). Brazil and the USA are the largest producers of sweet orange oil.

Terpeneless orange oil

By removing about 95% of the terpenes by vacuum distillation a terpeneless oil of orange may be obtained. One part of the terpeneless oil is equivalent to about 15 parts of the sweet orange oil. The *BP/EP* oil is required to contain not less than 18% of aldehydes calculated as decanal.

BITTER ORANGE FLOWER OIL

This oil, also known as **Oil of Neroli**, official in the *BP/EP* is prepared by steam distillation from fresh flowers of the bitter orange. An alcoholic solution of the oil has a violet-blue fluorescence arising from the small content (0.1–1.0%) of methyl anthranilate which is also responsible for the characteristic odour of the oil. Other constituents, with *BP/EP* permitted ranges, are *trans*-nerolidol (1.0–5.0%), geranylacetate (1.0–5.0%), α-terpineol (2.0–5.5%), linalyl acetate (2.0–15.0%), linalol (28.0–44.0%), limonene (9.0–18.0%), β-pinene (7.0–17.0%). There is a TLC test for the absence of bergapten, present should the oil be adulterated with that from the bitter peel.

In Britain the oil was traditionally used for the making of concentrated orange-flower water, syrup of orange flowers and Cologne spirit. It is used in aromatherapy.

Naringin

Limonin

22

LEMON PEEL

Lemon peel (*Limonis Cortex*) is obtained from the fruit of *Citrus limon* (L.) Burm. f. (Rutaceae), a small tree, 3–5 m high, cultivated in the countries bordering the Mediterranean and elsewhere (see 'Lemon Oils'). The lemon is of Indian origin and appears to have been unknown in Europe until the twelfth century. Numerous varieties and hybrids (particularly with *C. medica* Risso) are cultivated. Dried lemon peel is official in the *BP/EP*.

Collection and preparation. Lemons are collected in January, August and November, before their green colour changes to yellow. They are exported in cases containing from 200 to 360 fruits. The smaller fruits, which would not have a ready sale, are used in the preparation of oil of lemon. The peel is removed with a sharp knife in the form of a spiral band.

Characters. Dried lemon peel occurs in spiral bands up to 2 cm wide and 2–3 mm thick. Some pieces bear the apex of the fruit, which has a nipple-like appearance. The outer surface is rough and yellow; the inner surface is pulpy and white. Odour, strong and characteristic; taste, aromatic and bitter. The anatomical structure closely resembles that of orange peel (q.v.).

Constituents. Dried lemon peel contains not less than 2.5% of volatile oil (see below), vitamin C, hesperidin and other flavanone glycosides, mucilage and calcium oxalate. Lemon peel is mainly used for flavouring purposes.

LEMON OILS

Lemons are widely cultivated and the volatile oil is prepared around the Mediterranean, North and South America, in Australia and in parts of Africa. Lemon and other *Citrus* oils are best extracted by means other than distillation. The definition of pharmaceutical lemon oil given in the *British Pharmacopoeia* states that it is obtained by suitable mechanical means, without the aid of heat, from the fresh peel of *C. limon* (L.) Burm. f.

Once the oil has been separated from the peel, it can be distilled without deterioration in quality, and some expressed oil of lemon is fractionally distilled to make terpeneless oil of lemon (q.v.). Distillation direct from the peel is quite different, and, although much oil is prepared from the peel by steam distillation, this is inferior and does not comply with the definition given above. Distilled oil of lemon is cheaper than that prepared by expression and large quantities of it are made and used for non-pharmaceutical purposes.

History. Both expressed and distilled oils of lemon were sold in Paris as early as 1692. The sponge process as used in Sicily was described by Barrett in 1892. Machines were first introduced for oil of lemon production in 1920 and by 1930 about half the Italian oil was produced by their aid. New machines are being frequently introduced, and although some hand-expressed oil is still made (e.g. for eau de cologne, which requires the highest quality), pharmaceutical oil is now machine made.

Preparation. Oil of lemon is only one of several products made from lemons. In addition to dried peel, much lemon peel is candied with sugar. The pulp of the fruit yields on expression lemon juice, which may be canned or used for the preparation of citric acid and citrates. Pulp residues are used for pectin manufacture and as cattle food.

The following processes are used for the production of oil:

Hand methods. As these are no longer applicable to pharmaceutical oils they will not be described here and the reader is referred to earlier editions of this book for accounts of the *spugna* or sponge process, the *scorzetta* process, and the *écuelle à piquer* process.

Machine processes. The quality of machine-produced oil is rather inferior to the best hand-pressed. The machines are designed to set free the oil by puncture, rasping or cutting and by imitating the gentle squeezing action of the sponge method. The superiority of sponge-pressed oil appears to be due to the fact that there is virtually no contact between the oil and the inner white part of the peel (*albedo*). Deterioration in odour results from enzyme action in the finely divided albedo and is likely to be most pronounced when the machines penetrate deeply into the peel and when the resulting finely divided albedo and the water used for spraying are in contact with the oil for any length of time.

For the reasons given above, mincing of the whole fruit or peel followed by expression is unsatisfactory. Machines such as the *pelatric* which abrade the fruit surface are rather better, because they give less admixture of oil and albedo. The *sfumatrice machines* (squeezing machines) as first introduced, imitate more closely the hand method, since they exert a gentle pressing action on the peel passing on a stainless-steel band against stationary protrusions. Spray water is used to remove the oil, which is separated by a centrifuge. The *new sfumatrice* machines are a modification of the above in which fine knives cut into the outer peel (*flavido*), but partly also in the *albedo*. After treatment in these the peel shows 'almost invisible criss-cross cuts'. The newest machines extract the oil more completely than the older ones and therefore give a substantially higher yield.

Distilled oil. Although not official, some lemon oil is produced by distillation, mainly from the residues of the expression processes. It fetches a much lower price than either 'hand-pressed' or 'machine-made' oil.

Constituents. Lemon oil contains terpenes (about 94% mainly (+)-limonene), sesquiterpenes, aldehydes (citral, about 3.4–3.6%, and citronellal) and esters (about 1% geranyl acetate). Limonene (see Fig. 22.2) is a liquid, b.p. 175°C. Citral (see Fig. 22.2) or geranial, a liquid, b.p. 230°C, is the aldehyde corresponding to the alcohol geraniol. Lemon oil shows a marked tendency to resinify and should be protected from the action of air and light as much as possible. It has been shown by the use of GC and TLC that the oil obtained directly from the oil glands of the rind by capillary insertion differs from the fresh and stored commercial oils in composition. Principal reactions which cause these changes are oxidations of monoterpenes, aldehydes and esters, peroxide formation, polymerizations and isomerizations (e.g. limonene → α-terpinene).

Adulteration. Oil of lemon was at one time frequently adulterated with oil of turpentine, but analysts now have to contend with more scientific methods of adulteration. These include the addition of terpenes obtained in the preparation of 'terpeneless oil of lemon' and the addition of the cheaper distilled oil of lemon. The value of the oil is judged to some extent on the citral content, but a normal citral content alone is not a sure indication of purity, since citral may be added from a cheaper source such as oil of lemon-grass, which contains 75–85% of this aldehyde. It will be gathered that a careful examination of the oil by both physical and chemical methods is necessary, as exemplified by the standards and tests given in the *BP*.

Uses. Oil of lemon is used for flavouring and in perfumery.

Terpeneless lemon oil

Terpeneless Lemon Oil of the *BP* is prepared by concentrating lemon oil *in vacuo* until most of the terpenes have been removed, or by solvent partition. The concentrate is the terpeneless oil, which has a citral content of 40–50%. Terpeneless lemon oil is equivalent in flavour to about 10–15 times its volume of lemon oil; Lemon Spirit *BP* is a 10% solution in ethanol (96%) and it is also an ingredient of Compound Orange Spirit *BP*.

Buchu leaf

The name 'buchu' is applied to the leaves of several species of *Barosma* (*Agathosma*) (Rutaceae) grown in South Africa. The leaf, official in the *BHP*, is obtained from *Barosma betulina* (Thunb). Bartl. & Wendl. and known in English commerce as 'short' or 'round' buchu. The leaves of *Barosma crenulata* (oval buchu) and *B. serratifolia* (long buchu) are also used.

The leaves of *B. betulina*, *B. crenulata* and *B. serratifolia* are all small, shortly petiolate, green to greenish-yellow in colour, and supplied with numerous oil glands which are readily visible on holding them to the light.

Round or *short buchu* consists of the leaves and a small percentage of the stems, fruits and flowers of *Barosma betulina*. The leaves are 12–20 mm long and 4–25 mm broad. They are rhomboid-obovate in shape, with a blunt and recurved apex. The margin is dentate in the upper two-thirds of the leaf and serrate towards the base. A large oil gland is situated at the base of each marginal indentation and at the apex, while numerous smaller ones are scattered throughout the lamina. The leaves when dry are brittle and coriaceous, but on moistening become cartilaginous or mucilaginous. Odour and taste, strong and characteristic. Reddish-brown fragments of stems, up to about 5 cm, brown fruits with five carpels and flowers with five whitish petals are usually present, but an excessive amount of these must be regarded as an adulteration.

Oval buchu is obtained from *Barosma crenulata* Hooker. The leaves, which are accompanied by a certain amount of stem, are 15–30 mm long and 7–10 mm broad. The shape is more or less oval; the apex is blunt but not recurved and possesses a terminal oil gland; marginal serration very minute. (For a report see E. Wollenweber and E. H. Graven, *Fitoterapia*, 1992, **62**, 86.)

Long buchu is obtained from *Barosma serratifolia* Willd. The leaves are 12–40 mm long and 4–10 mm broad, and linear lanceolate in shape; the apex is truncate and possesses a terminal oil gland; the margin is serrate.

Buchu leaves contain volatile oil, diosmin (see Fig. 42.1B), mucilage, resin and calcium oxalate. In addition to the principal components pulegone, menthone, isomenthone and limonene the oil, in which over 120 components have been identified, contains diosphenol or buchu camphor to which the diuretic activity of the drug has been ascribed. The characteristic odour of the oil has been ascribed to sulphur compounds and *p*-menthane-8-thio-3-one has been characterized; it is present in quantities of up to 0.5% of the oil and is probably derived from (−)-pulegone. Buchu is still occasionally used as a diuretic and urinary antiseptic and is considered effective by herbal practitioners. For a recent review see A. Moola and A. M. Viljoen, *J. Ethnopharm.*, 2008, **119**, 413.

NUTMEG AND NUTMEG OIL

Nutmegs are the dried kernels of the seeds of *Myristica fragrans* (Myristicaceae), an evergreen tree about 10–20 m high, indigenous to the Molucca Islands. The plant is now widely cultivated not only in Indonesia and Malaysia (Molucca Islands, Sumatra, Java and Penang), but also in Ceylon and the West Indies (Grenada). Current world demand for nutmegs stands at about 10 000 tonnes per annum of which about 75% originates from Indonesia and 15% from Grenada.

History. Nutmegs and mace appear to have been first introduced into the Levant by the Arabs in the middle of the twelfth century and by the end of that century were found in northern Europe. The native country of the nutmeg (the Molucca or Spice Islands) was known to Arabian writers of the thirteenth century, and the Banda Islands, a group of the Moluccas where the plant is very abundant, were discovered by the Portuguese in 1512. The Portuguese, after holding the spice trade for about a century, lost it to the Dutch, who maintained a complete monopoly by destroying the trees in neighbouring islands and preventing the export of living seeds. The ordinary drying process destroys the vitality of the seeds, but they were also soaked in milk of lime for many weeks and were seldom sold until they were several years old. The Spice Islands were occupied by the English for a few years (1796–1802), during which period the opportunity was taken to start cultivation in Penang and Sumatra. Until the trees so planted reached maturity the effect of the Dutch restriction was still felt, and in 1806 the import price of mace in London was as high as £10 kg^{-1}.

Cultivation of the spice was subsequently introduced to the West Indies and during the Second World War production of nutmegs in Grenada was expanded enormously. In 1955 a hurricane destroyed 90% of the trees but the industry has now recovered and nutmegs remain the island's main commodity export.

Cultivation, collection and preparation. Nutmeg trees can be grown from fresh seed sown in the shell. The seeds germinate in about 5 weeks, and when the young plants are about 6 months old, they are transplanted to the fields. When the sex can be determined (5–8 years), the male trees are reduced to about 10% of the total. This method leads to irregularly spaced trees in the plantation and now in Grenada vegetative propagation of the female trees is performed by *marcotting* or *air layering*. In this, female shoots are split but not detached, and by the use of hormone powder and suitable packing of the wound, are induced to root. This takes 4–18 months after which the rooted shoots are detached and brought on before planting out. A success rate of over 40% for rooting is now obtainable. Another technique which has been used to increase the number of female trees is the employment of approach grafts. The trees bear fruit from their eighth or ninth year and continue to fruit well for about 20–30 years. The peach-like fruit splits when ripe, exposing the seed with its lobed, red arillus. The plant fruits almost continuously and two or three crops are collected annually. In the East the fruits are collected by hand or by means of a hooked stick, but in Grenada the fruits are allowed to fall to the ground. The orange-yellow pericarp which is about 12.5 mm thick, is usually removed on the spot. Later the arillus is picked off and constitutes, when dried, mace. From mature plantations the annual yield per acre is about 250–500 kg of nutmeg and about 50–100 kg of mace. The nutmegs are dried in the shells, the procedure differing according to local conditions but usually taking about 3–6 weeks. In Malaya sun-drying is used to some extent, but the seeds require adequate cover at night or in wet weather. Large quantities are dried in ovens and in brick buildings. In the latter the seeds are placed on trays over low charcoal fires, being turned and gradually moved nearer to the fires during the process. When drying is completed, the kernel rattles within the brittle testa, which constitutes about one-quarter of the weight of the seed. The testa is cracked by means of a wooden truncheon, mallet or special machine, and the nutmeg extracted. However, machines are liable to cause bruises, and cracking by hand is preferable. The liming of nutmegs to reduce insect attack is now less commonly practised than in the past. After cracking, the nutmegs are now usually graded abroad into sizes represented by numbers per unit weight. Elongated nutmegs, which fetch a lower price, and small or damaged ones are kept separate. Nutmegs are exported in barrels or cases containing about 50 kg.

Macroscopical characters. Nutmegs are broadly oval in outline, 2–3 cm long and about 2 cm broad. If not heavily limed, the surface is of a brown or greyish-brown colour and is reticulately furrowed. At one end is a light-coloured patch with brown lines radiating from the hilum, which is surrounded by a raised ring. From this an ill-defined furrow (imprint of the raphe) runs to the chalaza, at the opposite end of the kernel, where there is a small dark depression. Odour, strong and aromatic; taste, pungent and slightly bitter.

A longitudinal section (Fig. 22.9C) has a lustrous, marbled appearance. The outer tissue, which consists of dark brown perisperm, penetrates the light brown endosperm, the infoldings branching and giving rise to the marbled appearance. The perisperm possesses fibrovascular bundles, the position of which is indicated by the reticulate furrows found on the outer surface.

Microscopical characters. The outer perisperm cells are radially flattened and have brownish contents, insoluble in potassium hydroxide or chloral hydrate. A few of the cells contain prismatic or disc-shaped crystals, thought to consist of potassium acid tartrate. The inner perisperm shows numerous extensive lamellae, corresponding to the furrows on the surface, and penetrating into the endosperm. These lamellae are composed of parenchymatous cells with thin brown walls and of oval oil cells, and show in their outer part vascular strands composed of lignified spiral vessels. The endosperm is composed of parenchymatous cells, with thin brown cell walls, and containing simple or 2–10 compound starch grains (individual grains up to 22 μm in diameter, globular or irregular in shape, with sometimes a slit-like hilum); aleurone grains, the larger of which show a well-defined crystalloid; and feathery crystals of fat. A few tannin cells, containing tannin and starch, occur scattered in the endosperm.

Allied drugs. *Papua nutmegs* are derived from *M. argentea*, a tree grown in New Guinea. They are often taken to Macassar and enter commerce as Macassar, Papua, long or wild nutmegs. They have a uniform, scurfy surface, little odour and a disagreeable taste.

Bombay nutmegs are derived from *M. malabarica*, grown in India. They are very long and narrow and lack the characteristic aroma of the genuine drug.

Mace. Common mace or Banda mace consists of the dried arillus or arillode of *M. fragrans*. This, when fresh, is of a bright red colour and is removed either by the finger or a knife. When removed entire, it forms 'double blade' mace, but if in two pieces, it is known as 'single blade' mace. After flattening by treading under the feet or pressing between boards the mace is slowly dried. The volatile oil of mace resembles that of nutmeg, the major phenolic compounds isolated being dehydrodiisoeugenol and 5'-methoxydehydrodiisoeugenol, both of which have a significant antibacterial action. In recent years a series of lignans and neolignans has been isolated from mace; see Table 21.7 for the formula of macelignan.

Bombay mace is a regular article of commerce, although almost valueless as a spice. It is dark red in colour, is lacking in aroma and yields about 30% of extractive to light petroleum (genuine mace yields about 3.5%). Papua mace is distinguished by its shape, dull brownish surface, lack of aroma and acrid taste.

Constituents. Nutmegs yield 5–15% of volatile oil and also contain 30–40% fat, phytosterin, starch, amylodextrin, colouring matter and a saponin. They yield about 3% of total ash and about 0.2% of acid-insoluble ash. The psychotropic properties of nutmeg are discussed under 'Hallucinogens'.

Uses. Nutmegs, maces, and their oils are largely used for flavouring and as carminatives. In traditional Indian medicine an aqueous extract of nutmeg is used for the treatment of infantile diarrhoea.

NUTMEG OIL

Nutmeg oil is distilled from the kernels imported into Europe and the USA, and is produced in Indonesia (about 120 tons annually), Sri Lanka (30 tons) and India (5 tons). It contains (*BP/EP* limits as determined by gas chromatography), α-pinene (15–26%), β-pinene (13–18%), sabinine (14–29%), myristicin (5–12%), limonene (2–7%), γ-terpinene (2–6%), terpinen-4-ol (2–6%), car-3-ene (0.5–2%), safrole (2.5% maximum). Other minor constituents include elemicin and isoelemicin, eugenol, methyleugenol, methoxyeugenol, methylisoeugenol and isoeugenol.

There are differences in optical rotation, refractive index, weight per millilitre and solubility in alcohol between the West Indian and East Indian oils. Myristicin (formula Chapter 39), is 4-allyl-6-methoxy-1,2-methylenedioxybenzene. It is crystalline and, owing to its high boiling point, is mainly found in the last portions of the distillate. Myristicin is toxic to human beings and large doses of nutmeg or its oil may cause convulsions. Workers in Canada and Japan have isolated a considerable

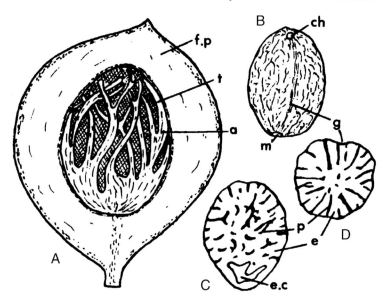

Fig. 22.9
Myristica fragrans. A, Fruit with half of the pericarp removed; B, nutmeg (dried kernel); C, longitudinal section nutmeg; D, transverse section nutmeg (all × 1). a, Aril (mace); ch, chalaza; e, endosperm; e.c, cavity left by embryo; f.p, fleshy pericarp; g, groove marking line of raphe; m, micropyle region; p, perisperm; t, testa.

number of dimeric phenyl-propanoids from the seed; the units include isoeugenol, elemicin and myristicin. Similar dimeric compounds, shown to cause significant changes in hepatic enzyme systems, have been isolated from mace oil (W. S. Woo et al., *Phytochemistry*, 1987, **26**, 1542).

Calamus

Calamus or sweet flag consists of the rhizome of *Acorus calamus* (Araceae), which occurs in commerce both peeled and unpeeled. The perennial plant is common on the banks of streams. Originating in Asia, it is now widely distributed in Asia, Europe and North America. The subcylindrical rhizome is up to 20 cm long and 2 cm diameter; longitudinally furrowed on the upper surface and with conspicuous root scars on the lower surface.

Calamus contains 2–4% of volatile oil containing a number of sesquiterpenes and asarone, a compound related to myristicin (see 'Nutmeg and Nutmeg Oil'). Calamus has been official in many pharmacopoeias, and although still used in some regions, is now mainly used as a source of calamus oil, which is employed in perfumery. The composition of the oil from $2n$, $3n$ and $4n$ varieties differs and the β-asarone content increases with ploidy. As the phenylpropane derivatives have been shown to be carcinogenic in animal tests, Keller and Stahl (*Planta Med.*, 1983, **47**, 71; 1985, p. 6) recommend the selection of races for pharmaceutical use. The oil from the rhizome of the American $2n$ race contains no β-asarone but consists of shyobunones and acorones, which are also components of the pharmaceutically used oils. GC-MS studies combined with gene sequencing have also been employed for the identification of a $2n$ β-asarone-free race (C. M. Bertea et al., *Phytochemistry*, 2005, **66**, 507).

Asarone

2,6-Di-epi-shyobunone
(Main constituent of
diploid calamus oil)

Acorone

Chemotypes of *A. calamus* having differences in essential oil composition have been DNA profiled (N. Sugimoto et al., *Biol. Pharm. Bull.*, 1999, **22**, 481).

A number of sesquiterpenes based on the cadinane, acorane and eudesmane skeletons have been isolated from *A. calamus* and some of these are strong germination inhibitors of lettuce seeds. Such secondary metabolites are called allelochemicals, well-known examples being the nagilactones of *Podocarpus nagi* (K. Nawamaki and M. Kuroyanagi, *Phytochemistry*, 1996, **43**, 1175).

For details of the main constituents of calamus and the acetylcholinesterase inhibitory activity of the oil, see P. K. Mukhergee et al., *Planta Medica*, 2007, **73**, 191.

Further reading

Mukherjee PK, Kumar V, Mal M, Houghton PJ 2007 *Acorus calamus*: scientific validation of Ayurvedic tradition from natural resources. Pharmaceutical Biology 45(8): 651–666. *A review (ca 130 refs) exploring the various constituents and pharmacological activities of the drug*

Motley TJ 1994 Ethnobotany of sweet flag (*Acorus calamus*). Economic Botany 48(4): 397–412. *A comprehensive review with over 160 references*

CINNAMON AND CINNAMON OIL

The *BP/EP* states that 'cinnamon is the dried bark of the shoots grown on cut stock of *Cinnamomum zeylanicum* Blume, freed from the outer cork and underlying parenchyma.' However, Kostermans (see *Bibliographia Lauracearum*, 1964) indicates the plant to be more correctly named *C. verum* Presl. (Lauraceae), of which there are two varieties, better called subspecies, one (var. *subcordata* Nees) with ovate, subcordate leaves, the other (var. *vulgare* Nees, now properly called var. *verum*) with oblong or elliptic leaves pointed at both ends; both produce a good drug. Many other 'varieties' (about 23) have been described and exist wild in Sri Lanka and southern India; most of these, however, on current taxonomic grounds, represent other species. The tree is also cultivated in the Seychelles, Madagascar, Martinique, Cayenne, Jamaica and Brazil. Ceylon cinnamon is the commonest variety on the English market, but good-quality Seychelles drug, which closely resembles the product from Sri Lanka, is also available.

The British and Americans do not give the same meaning to the words 'cinnamon' and 'oil of cinnamon'. In Britain cinnamon and oil of cinnamon are derived as above. In the USA, however, 'Cinnamon NF' is Saigon cinnamon and 'Oil of Cinnamon NF' is the oil which British call Cassia Oil, which is derived from Cassia bark (q.v.).

History. Cassia bark was known to the Chinese in 2700 BC but it is not until the thirteenth century that any reference is found to the collection of cinnamon in Ceylon. Ceylon was occupied by the Portuguese in 1536, the Dutch in 1656, and the English East India Company in 1796. Cinnamon cultivation was started by the Dutch in 1770 and they exercised a strict monopoly comparable with their monopoly of nutmegs. This was continued until the monopoly of the English East India Company was abolished in 1833.

Cultivation, collection and preparation. In Sri Lanka about 26 000 acres are devoted to cinnamon plantations. Most of the plantations are small and are situated in the southern or western provinces. Sri Lanka and the Seychelles both export large quantities of cinnamon leaf oil.

The production of the characteristic compound quills of the inner bark is a multistage process and was fully described and illustrated in earlier editions of this book. Briefly, the cinnamon plants are grown from seed and coppiced almost to the ground when 2 or 3 years old. About five or six shoots are allowed to grow from the stump and are kept vertical by pruning. After about 18 months of growth, and when some 3 m long and 2 cm diameter, shoots are harvested, trimmed and, following a few hours 'fermentation', they have the bark removed with a non-ferrous knife. The peeled bark is then stretched over a suitable stick and the outer cork and cortex scraped off with a curved scraper. Individual pieces of scraped bark are then placed one inside the other and built up to a length of about 42 in (c. 106 cm). The compound quills are dried on wooden frames in the open air without exposure to direct sunlight and then finally sorted into grades and made into compact bales of about 45 kg.

The traditional grades of cinnamon are designated: 00000, 0000, 000, 00, 0, 1, 2, 3, 4, quillings, featherings, chips. Most commercial material corresponds to Nos. 1–4 grades. Quillings and featherings consist of small pieces, the latter often containing some outer bark; they are used for grinding and for oil distillation. Chips consist mainly of outer pieces of bark, and the oil derived from them has a lower specific gravity and a lower aldehyde content than that from the inner bark.

Macroscopical characters. Cinnamon is imported in large bundles about 1 m in length. Retailers generally receive their supplies in shorter lengths known as 'cigar lengths'. The drug consists of single or double compound quills about 6–10 mm diameter and of varying length (Fig. 22.10). In the different grades the thickness of each piece of bark varies considerably, but in good-quality cinnamon it is usually not more than about 0.5 mm, while the number of pieces of bark forming the compound quill varies from about 10 to 40. The external surface of each piece is yellowish-brown and shows longitudinal shining, wavy lines (pericyclic fibres) and occasional scars and holes (indicating the positions of leaves or twigs). The inner surface is somewhat darker and longitudinally striated. The bark breaks with a short, splintery fracture. Odour is fragrant; taste, warm, sweet and aromatic.

Microscopical characters. Transverse sections of cinnamon (Fig. 22.10) show under the microscope a complete absence of epidermis and cork. Shrivelled remains of cortex occur in patches. The outer limit of the bark is marked by a pericycle composed of a continuous ring of three to four layers of sclereids with small groups of pericyclic fibres embedded in it at intervals. The latter produce the lighter-coloured, wavy, longitudinal lines on the outside of the commercial bark. The sclereids (Fig. 22.10) have thickened lignified walls, showing well-defined pit-canals. The thickening on the outer walls is often less pronounced than on the radial and inner tangential walls. The lumen is clearly visible and sometimes contains starch. The pericyclic fibres range from 1000 to 2500 µm long and have strongly thickened lignified walls showing stratification and pit-canals. Primary phloem cannot be distinguished. The secondary phloem is composed of phloem parenchyma containing oil and mucilage cells; phloem fibres; and medullary rays. The sieve-tube tissue, embedded in the phloem parenchyma, is often obliterated. The phloem parenchyma is composed of thin-walled cells, with yellowish-brown walls, and contains starch in compound and simple grains, the latter not exceeding 10 µm diameter (those of *Cinnamomum cassia* often exceed this figure) and numerous acicular crystals of calcium oxalate about 5–8 µm long. Some of the phloem parenchyma cells contain tannin. The secretion cells, containing volatile oil or mucilage, are two or three times the diameter of the phloem fibres, and are axially elongated. The phloem fibres, which occur isolated or in tangential rows, are more abundant towards the inner part of the bark. They are usually less than 30 µm in diameter (those of *C. cassia* measure 30–40 µm in diameter) and have a length of 200–600 µm. The thick lignified walls show stratification. The secondary phloem is divided up by the radial medullary rays, which are uni- or biseriate near the cambium but become broader towards the outside by tangential growth of the cells. The rays are 7–14 cells high. The medullary ray cells are radially elongated, thin-walled with yellow–brown cell contents containing numerous acicular crystals of calcium oxalate. For illustrations of the powdered elements, see Fig. 22.10.

Constituents. Cinnamon contains volatile oil (*BP/EP* not less than 1.2%), phlobatannins (which have been little investigated compared with those of cassia) mucilage, calcium oxalate and starch.

CINNAMON OIL

Oil of cinnamon contains about 60–75% w/w of *trans*-cinnamic aldehyde, $C_6H_5CH=CHCHO$. Genuine oils also contain 4–10% of phenols (chiefly eugenol), hydrocarbons (pinene, phellandrene and caryophyllene), and small quantities of ketones, alcohols and esters; GLC shows the presence of many compounds and limits for specific constituents are given in the *Pharmacopoeia*. Oil distilled from fresh bark samples collected in Ghana by Angmor *et al.* (*Planta Med.*, 1979, **35**, 342) contained a high proportion of cinnamyl acetate, but by a protracted preparation of the drug which simulated the commercial preparation this ester was largely converted into aldehyde. Phenylalanine has been shown to be a precursor of both cinnamic aldehyde and eugenol in the

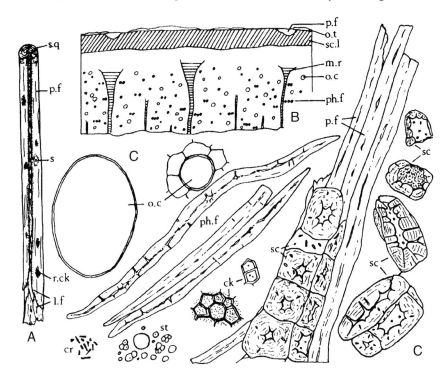

Fig. 22.10
Cinnamon. A, Compound double quill (× 0.5); B, transverse section (×50); C, elements of the powder (×200). ck, Cork cells; cr, acicular crystals of calcium oxalate; l.f, laminated fracture of compound quill; m.r, medullary ray; o.c, oil cells; o.t, remains of outer tissues; p.f, pericyclic fibres; ph.f, phloem fibres; r.ck, residual patches of cork; s, scar of twig; sc, sclereids; sc.l, sclereid layer of pericycle; s.q, transverse surface of compound quill; st, starch granules.

living plant, but the metabolic interrelationships between the aromatic compounds appear complex.

The oil is liable to adulteration with cinnamon leaf oil and with oil of cassia. Oil of cassia contains about 80–95% of aldehydes and a similar test with ferric chloride gives a brown colour. Oil from the root-bark contains much camphor and other monoterpenes but negligible phenylpropanes.

Allied drugs. *Cayenne cinnamon* consists of the bark of cultivated plants of *Cinnamomum zeylanicum* grown in French Guiana, Brazil and some of the islands of the West Indies. It is generally obtained from older branches than the Ceylon drug and appears to be inferior to it in quality. It is not used to any extent in Britain.

C. loureirii is commercially important in Vietnam and grows in the mountainous districts of Annam. The plant, which is closely related to *C. cassia* is also found in China and Japan. It resembles cassia bark more closely than cinnamon, and occurs in quills up to 30 cm long, 4 cm wide and 0.5–7.0 mm thick. The outer surface is greyish-brown, warty and ridged. The odour is coarser than that of Ceylon cinnamon and the taste sweeter.

Uses. Cinnamon is used as a flavouring agent and mild astringent. The oil has carminative properties and is a powerful germicide.

CEYLON CINNAMON LEAF OIL

The oil is obtained by steam distillation of the leaves of *Cinnamomum verum* J. S. Presl. It is a commercial article, and some twenty times the amount of the bark oil is produced. It contains 70–95% of eugenol (*BP/EP* limits 70–85%) giving the oil a clove-like odour. An alcoholic solution of the oil gives with ferric chloride solution a blue colour; other components of the oil, which are limited individually within the range 1.0–7% and determined by gas chromatography, are cineole, linalol, β-caryophyllene, safrole, *trans*-cinnamic aldehyde, cinnamyl acetate, eugenol and coumarin. Other standard specifications are relative density, refractive index and optical rotation.

The high eugenol content gives the oil antiseptic and anaesthetic properties; it is mainly employed for the extraction of eugenol and in the cosmetic industry in carnation-type perfumes.

Cassia, Chinese cinnamon or cassia lignea

Various barks have been imported under the name of 'cassia'. That known in the London market as Chinese cassia lignea is derived from *C. cassia* Blume, a tree cultivated in the south-eastern provinces of China (Jiangxi and Guangdong). When about 6 years old, the bark is removed from the older branches, the twigs and leaves being used for distillation. The cork and cortex are partly removed by planing, the bark tied into bundles and exported in boxes, via Guangzhou and Hong Kong.

Cassia bark occurs in channelled pieces or single quills up to 40 cm long, 1–2 cm wide and 1–3 mm thick. The outer surface is darker than that of Ceylon cinnamon and, owing to careless planing, shows patches of grey cork. The odour is coarser than that of cinnamon and the taste more astringent.

Transverse sections resemble cinnamon as far as the inner part of the bark is concerned, except that the starch grains and phloem fibres are somewhat larger. However, the utility of the fibre size for distinguishing the two barks has been questioned owing to the limited sample numbers used in the original investigation. Outside the sclerenchymatous ring is the cortex and cork layer.

Cassia bark has been reported to contain about 10% mucilage, whereas Ceylon and Seychelles cinnamon samples contained 1.6–2.9%. TLC tests have also been used for distinguishing the barks. Such

distinctions could well arise from the fact that the Ceylon cinnamon is an inner bark, whereas with cassia bark outer cortex and cork are present.

Cassia yields 1–2% of volatile oil which, when pure, contains no eugenol but rarely less than 85% of cinnamic aldehyde; other components are cinnamyl acetate, phenylpropyl acetate and numerous trace constituents. 2′-Hydroxycinnamaldehyde has recently been isolated from the stem bark (B.-M. Kwon *et al.*, *Planta Medica*, 1996, **62**, 183). The oil is included in the *USP/NF* under the name of Cinnamon Oil and is required to contain not less than 80% by volume of aldehydes. Large quantities of oil are distilled from the leaves and twigs as well as from the bark. Although inferior in flavour to the oil of *C. zeylanicum*, it is cheaper and is described in many pharmacopoeias.

Considerable advances in the chemistry of the non-volatile components of cassia bark have been made by Japanese researchers and have demonstrated the pharmacological activities of these substances. In a number of papers Nohara *et al.* (see *Phytochemistry*, 1985, **24**, 1849 and references therein) have reported the isolation of a series of diterpenes from a fraction of the bark showing antiallergic activity. Aqueous extracts have been shown to have antiulcerogenic activity (T. Akira *et al.*, *Planta Med.*, 1986, p. 440).

In 1986 Morimonto *et al.* characterized a number of compounds of the tannin complex (*Chem. Pharm. Bull.*, **34**, 633, 643) as below. Three flavan-3-ol glucosides were identified as (–epicatechin 3-*O*-, 8-*C*- and 6-*C*-β-D-glucopyranosides respectively. Three oligomeric procyanidins (named cinnamatannins A₂, A₃, A₄) were tetra-, penta- and hexameric compounds respectively, consisting exclusively of (–)-epicatechin units linked linearly through C-4–C-8 bonds (see formula). Free (–)-epicatechin and procyanidins were present, the latter occurring also in dimeric form and as *C*-glucosides.

up to six (–)-epicatechin units

Cinnamatannins of cassia bark

An arabinoxylan which activates the reticuloendothelial system was described in 1989; this neutral polysaccharide, named cinnaman AX, contains L-arabinose and D-xylose in the respective molar ratio of 4:3. Other pharmacologically similarly-acting polysaccharides have been reported in *Panax* and *Saposhnikovia*.

Callus and suspension cultures of *Cinnamomum cassia* produce large amounts of condensed tannins; the precursors (–)-epicatechin and-procyanidins B2, B4 and C1 have been isolated from callus cultures (see K. Yazaki and T. Okuda, *Phytochemistry*, 1990, **29**, 1559).

Cassia bark is an important drug of Oriental medicine.

Cassia 'buds', perhaps inappropriately named, are the dried immature fruits of *C. cassia*. They yield about 20% of volatile oil having a cinnamaldehyde content of around 80%.

Java or Indonesian cinnamon is derived from *C. burmanii* Blume, and is used in Holland. The tree is found in Sumatra, through Java to Timor. It may be distinguished from ordinary cinnamon when in powder by the presence of tabular crystals of calcium oxalate. The oil contains about 75% of cinnamic aldehyde.

Oliver bark or *black sassafras* is obtained from the so-called Brisbane 'white sassafras' tree, *C. oliveri*, a native of Queensland. It is used locally as a cinnamon substitute. The bark is easily distinguished from the drugs mentioned above. It occurs in flat strips about 20 cm long, 4 cm wide and 1 cm thick. The outer surface is brownish and warty, and bears patches of greyish cork. It yields about 1–2.4% of volatile oil.

Further reading

Ravindran PN *et al* (eds), Hardman R (series ed) 2004 Medicinal and aromatic plants – industrial profiles, Vol. 36 Cinnamon and cassia: the genus *Cinnamonum*. CRC Press, Boca Raton, FL 384 pp.

TEA-TREE OIL

The clear, colourless to pale-yellow oil is obtained by distillation from the leaves and terminal branches of *Melaleuca alternifolia* (Maiden and Betch) Cheel, family Myrtaceae, and other species of *Melaleuca* including *M. linariifolia* Smith and *M. dissitiflora* F. Mueller. These species are closely related to *M. leucadendron* (q.v.) and occur wild in New South Wales, Australia, where they constitute a well-known article of traditional aboriginal medicine.

Cyclic monoterpenes constitute the principal components of the oil, for which the *BP/EP* sets specified limits: terpinen-4-ol (30.0% minimum), γ-terpinene (10–28%), *p*-cymene (0.5–12.0%), α-terpinene (5–13%), cineole (less than 15.0%), other components generally present in smaller amounts for which limits are given include α-pinene, sabinene, limonene, terpinolene, aromadendrene and α-terpineol. These compounds are determined by gas chromatography using a reference solution for calculation. Other pharmacopoeial tests are relative density, refractive index, optical rotation and TLC.

In recent years the popularity of tea-tree preparations has increased enormously to include antiseptic creams for skin treatment, inhalations and pastilles for throat infections. A recent report (D. V. Henley *et al.*, *New Engl. J. Med.*, 2007, **356**, 479) records that natural lavender and tea-tree oils in moisturisers can cause breast enlargement in prepubertal boys. Laboratory tests on breast cells have shown that the oils activate the female oestrogen receptor and suppress male hormones.

Further reading

Southwell I, Lowe R (eds), Hardman R (series ed) 1999 Medicinal and aromatic plants—industrial profiles, Vol. 9. Tea tree: the genus *Melaleuca*. Harwood Academic, Amsterdam. *589 references*

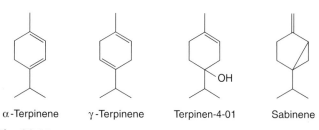

α-Terpinene   γ-Terpinene   Terpinen-4-01   Sabinene

Fig. 22.11
Some monoterpenoids of tea-tree oil; for others see Fig. 22.2.

NATURAL CAMPHOR

Natural camphor is a white, dextrorotatory ketone, $C_{10}H_{16}O$ (see Fig. 18.17), obtained from the wood of *Cinnamomum camphora* (Lauraceae), a tree which is widely grown in Taiwan, Japan and south China; it is also produced commercially in India and Georgia. Synthetic camphor, which is optically inactive, is prepared from turpentine and would probably have completely replaced the natural product had it not been for other important byproducts of the industry. Monographs for both the natural and synthetic camphor are included in the *BP/EP*.

Preparation.   The best yield of camphor is obtained from old trees. The wood is cut into chips and treated with steam, when a solid sublimate of camphor and liquid volatile oil pass into the receiver. The volatile oil is treated to yield more camphor and much of the residual camphor oil is used as a source of safrole. The impure camphor is treated with lime and charcoal and resublimed into large chambers. It collects in the form of 'flowers of camphor', which can be made into the familiar blocks by hydraulic pressure. Camphor can also be prepared from suitable leaves of the tree and their use is helping to reduce the complete destruction of camphor tree forests.

Synthetic camphor is largely prepared from American turpentine. By the action of hydrogen chloride the pinene is converted into bornyl chloride which, on treatment with sodium acetate, yields isobornyl acetate. Hydrolysis of this is to isoborneol and subsequent oxidation gives camphor.

Tests for identity and purity of natural camphor are important to eliminate synthetic racemic material, excess camphor oil, and camphors from inappropriate natural sources. These tests include melting point (175–179°C), specific optical rotation (+40.0 to +43.0), acidity and limit of halogens (particularly chlorides arising from the synthesis of racemic camphor), gas chromatographic detection of extraneous material arising from the synthesis of camphor and other sources including α- and β-pinene, cineole, fenchone, fenchol and borneol.

Characters.   Camphor occurs in small, colourless crystals or in transparent fibrous blocks. It has a characteristic odour and a pungent, aromatic taste, which is followed by a sensation of cold. It volatilizes at ordinary temperatures, forming an encrustation on the walls of the vessel in which it is kept.

Camphor oil (see above) contains, in addition to camphor, safrole, borneol, heliotropin, vanillin and terpineol, a number of sesquiterpene alcohols. Oil of Pakistan origin has been shown to contain 25 monoterpenoids, and four chemotypes with respect to oil composition have been recorded for Vietnamese material.

Allied drugs.   Borneo camphor, obtained from *Dryobalanops aromatica* (Dipterocarpaceae), and Ngai camphor, obtained from *Blumea balsamifera* (Compositae), are used in China and Japan. In California laevorotatory camphor is produced from species of *Artemisia* (Compositae).

Uses.   Camphor is used externally as a rubefacient, and internally as a mild antiseptic and carminative. It finds many non-pharmaceutical uses. Large quantities were once used in the manufacture of celluloid.

Canella bark

Canella bark is the dried rossed bark of *Canella alba* (*C. winterana*) (Canellaceae), a small tree growing in the Bahamas and Florida. It occurs in quills or channelled pieces up to 5 cm long and 5 mm thick. It contains about 1% of volatile oil and as a condiment goes under the names of 'white cinnamon' or 'wild cinnamon'. The oil contains monoterpenes, eugenol and myristicin.

Canellal

3-Methoxy-4,5-methylene-
dioxycinnamaldehyde

In 1978 a novel antimicrobial sesquiterpene dialdehyde (canellal) was reported from the bark and more recently 3-methoxy-4,5-methylenedioxy-cinnamaldehyde. Cannellal also has insect antifeedant, antifungal and cytoxic properties. For work on the isolation of drimane sesquiterpenes and other compounds, see D. Kioy *et al.*, *J. Nat. Prod.*, 1989, **52**, 174; 1990, **53**, 1372 and M. S. Al-Said *et al.*, *Phytochemistry*, 1990, **29**, 975.

Oil of Cajuput

Oil of Cajuput is a volatile oil distilled from the fresh leaves of *Melaleuca leucadendron* L. and other species of *Melaleuca* (Myrtaeceae) and rectified by steam distillation. The plants are evergreen shrubs or trees found in the East Indies and Australia. Most of the oil is produced in the islands of Bouru and Banda. It has a pleasant, camphoraceous odour and a bitter aromatic taste. It contains about 50–60% of cineole, terpineol and its acetate, terpenes and sesquiterpenes.

Medicinally, the oil is used both internally and externally as a stimulant and for the treatment of various parasitic conditions. It finds considerable use in India and the Far East.

Pimento or allspice

Pimento (*Jamaica* or *Clove Pepper*) is the dried nearly ripe fruit of *Pimenta dioica* (Myrtaceae), an evergreen tree grown in the West Indies (Jamaica, Cuba, Trinidad etc.) and central America.

The fruits are collected before they are quite ripe, as they otherwise lose much of their aroma and become filled with a sweet pulp; they are normally sun-dried but artificial drying has been recommended.

The pimento flower and fruit closely resemble those of the clove. The biocular ovary, however, develops two seeds, whereas only one is produced in the clove. Pimento fruits are globular and 4–7 mm in diameter. At the apex of the fruit are four small calyx teeth surrounding a short style (cf. clove fruit, Fig. 22.12). The pericarp is reddish-brown, rough and woody, and about 1 mm thick. Sections show numerous oil glands in the pericarp. Each of the two loculi contains a single planoconvex seed. Pimento has a characteristic aromatic odour and taste.

Pimento fruits yield about 3–4.5% of volatile oil which, estimated for eugenol by the method used for oil of cloves, shows a phenol content of 65–80%. The oil also contains cineole, (−)-phellandrene and caryophyllene; in all some 44 compounds have been identified.

CLOVE AND CLOVE OIL

Cloves are the dried flower buds of *Syzygium aromaticum* (*Eugenia caryophyllus*) (Myrtaceae), a tree 10–20 m high which is indigenous to the Molucca or Clove Islands. It is cultivated in Zanzibar and in the neighbouring island of Pemba, which together, for many years, produced more than three-quarters of the world's supply of cloves. However, the industry has deteriorated in these areas and the principal producers are now Madagascar, Indonesia and Brazil. Smaller quantities are grown in Sri Lanka and Tanzania.

History. Cloves were used in China as early as 266 BC and by the fourth century they were known in Europe, although very expensive.

The Spice Islands were occupied by the Portuguese at the beginning of the sixteenth century, but they were expelled by the Dutch in 1605. As in the case of nutmegs, the Dutch made every effort to secure a monopoly, destroying all the trees in their native islands (Ternate, Tidor, Mortir, Makiyan and Bachian) and cultivating them only in a group of small islands, of which Amboyna is the largest. In 1770, however, the French succeeded in introducing clove trees into Mauritius, and cultivation was afterwards taken up in Sumatra (1803), Penang, Cayenne, Madagascar, Zanzibar (1818), Pemba and elsewhere.

Collection and preparation. The flower buds are collected when their lower part turns from green to crimson. In Zanzibar and Pemba collection takes place twice yearly, between August and December. The inflorescences are collected from movable platforms. The cloves are dried in the open air on mats and separated from their peduncles, the latter forming a separate article of commerce known as 'clove stalks' (Fig. 22.12D). If left too long on the tree, the buds open and the petals fall, leaving 'blown cloves'; later the fruits (Fig. 22.12C) known as 'mother cloves' are produced. A small proportion of these, usually at a stage intermediate between that of a clove and a fully ripe fruit, are frequently found in the drug. Cloves are imported in bales covered with matting made from strips of coconut leaves.

Macroscopical characters. Cloves are 10–17.5 mm long (cf. A and B in Fig. 22.12). The Penang and Amboyna varieties are the largest and plumpest and are most esteemed, but they are in such demand in the East that relatively small quantities of them reach Europe; they are used principally for the making of pomanders. The Zanzibar variety, however, is of good quality, although smaller and leaner than the Penang and of a blackish-brown rather than a reddish-brown colour.

The 'stalk' of the clove consists of a cylindrical hypanthium or swelling of the torus, above which is a bilocular ovary containing numerous ovules attached to axile placentae. The 'head' consists of four slightly projecting calyx teeth; four membranous, imbricated petals, and numerous incurved stamens around a large style (Fig. 22.12E).

Cloves have a strong, fragrant and spicy odour and a pungent, aromatic taste. When indented with the fingernail, they readily exude oil. Cloves sink in freshly boiled and cooled water (distinction from cloves which have been exhausted of volatile oil).

Microscopical characters. The hypanthium, in the region below the ovary, shows in transverse section (Fig. 22.12) a heavy cuticularized epidermis in which occur stomata, slightly raised above the surface and showing well-defined substomatal spaces. Within this is a zone of roughly radially arranged parenchymatous cells containing numerous schizolysigenous oil glands arranged in two or three more or less intermixed layers. The oil glands are ellipsoidal in shape, with the long axis radial, and show an epithelium composed of two or three layers of flattened cells. The contents of the oil glands are soluble in alcohol and are blackened by treatment with alcoholic ferric chloride or osmic acid. The ground mass of parenchyma also gives the blackening with ferric chloride. Cluster crystals of calcium oxalate (5–25 μm in diameter) occur in many of the parenchymatous cells. Within the oil gland layer is a zone of cells with somewhat thickened walls, embedding a ring of bicollateral vascular bundles. The ground tissue of this zone contains cluster crystals of calcium oxalate. The meristeles are enclosed in an incomplete ring of lignified fibres; the xylem is composed of 3–5 lignified spiral vessels. Within the ring of vascular bundles is a zone of aerenchyma composed of air spaces separated by lamellae one cell thick, which supports the central columella. The ground tissue of the columella is parenchymatous and is particularly rich in calcium oxalate clusters. In the outer region of the columella is a ring of some 17 small vascular bundles.

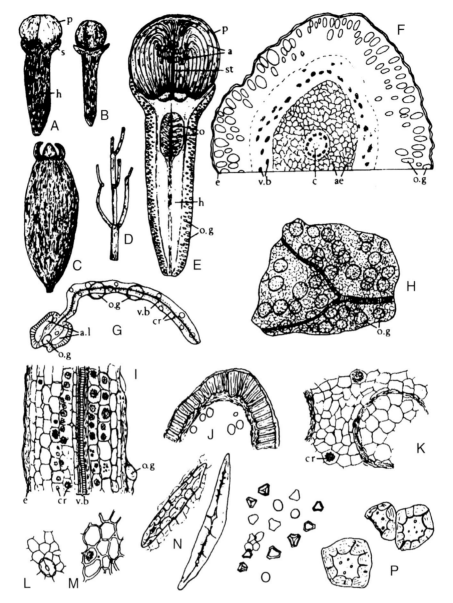

Fig. 22.12
Syzygium aromaticum. A, Penang clove; B, Zanzibar clove; C, fruit (mother clove), (all ×2); D, clove stalk (×1); E, clove cut longitudinally (×5); F, transverse section of hypanthium; G, portion of anther (both ×15); H, surface view of petal (×50); I–P, elements of powdered clove (all ×200); I, portion of anther filament; J, fibrous wall of anther lobe and immature pollen; K, fragment of hypanthium showing portions of oil glands; L, epidermal cells and stoma of hypanthium; M, parenchyma of hypanthium; N, phloem fibres; O, pollen grains; P, sclereids from clove stalk. a, Stamens; ae, aerenchyma; a.l, anther lobes; c, columella; cr, cluster crystal of calcium oxalate; e, epidermis; h, hypanthium; o, ovules; o.g, oil gland; p, imbricated petal; s, sepal; st, style; v.b, vascular bundle.

The hypanthium, in the region of the ovary, shows epidermis, oil gland layer and ring of bicollateral bundles. Within this is a zone of cells with very strongly thickened cellulose walls, limited internally by an inner epidermis forming the wall of the ovary. The dissepiment of the ovary is parenchymatous; the placentae are rich in cluster crystals and contain vascular bundles. If sections of the hypanthium are mounted in a concentrated solution of potassium hydroxide, acicular and radiately aggregate crystals separate, owing to the presence of the phenol eugenol in the oil.

The sepals and petals have a simplified leaf structure. The mesophyll parenchyma contains calcium oxalate and embeds numerous oil glands. The epidermis of the sepals shows stomata. The epidermis of the petals is devoid of stomata and is composed of very irregular cells.

The stamens are composed of filament, connective and anther. The filament shows an epidermis of longitudinal elongated cells, a ground mass of parenchyma embedding numerous oil glands and a single vascular strand enclosed in a sheath of crystal cells. The vascular strand is continuous into the connective, which is terminated by an oil gland. The fibrous layer of the anther wall is composed of cells showing spiral bands of lignified thickening. The pollen grains are triangular in outline and 15–20 μm diameter. The style and stigma yield similar characters to those of the filament. See Fig. 22.12 for the illustrated characters of the powder.

Starch, prisms of calcium oxalate and lignified sclereids are absent from a powder consisting of the flower buds only. Clove stalks contain lignified sclereids (Fig. 22.12P) and reticulately thickened xylem vessels. Clove fruits ('anthophylli', 'mother cloves') contain starch. As there is a permissible pharmacopoeial limit (not more than 6%) for these structures in the drug, a few sclereids and starch grains may therefore be found in the powder. There are also limits for deteriorated cloves (≯2.0%) and other foreign matter (≯0.5%).

Constituents. Cloves contain about 14–21% of volatile oil (see below), 10–13% of tannin, various triterpene acids and esters, and glycosides of the following: aliphatic and monoterpenoid alcohols, eugenol, isoeugenol, farnesol, nerolidol, sitosterol, stigmasterol and campestrol.

Uses. Cloves are used as a stimulant aromatic, as a spice and for the preparation of the volatile oil. The sesquiterpenes of clove have been cited as potential anticarcinogenic compounds.

Clove oil

Oil distilled in Britain and the US usually requires no purification, but oil distilled abroad (e.g. in Madagascar) is, when imported, usually wet and discoloured by the presence of metallic salts. The latter type of oil is always rectified and may be sold with different eugenol contents. Oil of cloves is a colourless or pale yellow liquid, which is slightly heavier than water (relative density 1.047–1.060). It is soluble in from one to two volumes of alcohol (70%).

Clove oil contains 84–95% of phenols (eugenol with about 3% of acetyleugenol), sesquiterpenes (α- and β-caryophyllenes) and small quantities of esters, ketones and alcohols. Some 28 compounds have been reported in the oil and this rather low number, compared with many other oils, is due to the lack of monoterpene derivatives. The phenols can be estimated by absorption with solution of potassium hydroxide in a graduated flask, as described in the *BP* (1989). The current *BP/EP* employs GC using internal standards for the determination of eugenol (limits 75–88%), β-caryophyllene (5–14%), acetyl eugenol (4–15%) and other components. Those oils which have a relatively low phenol content are known in commerce as 'opt' and are the ones mainly used in pharmacy, while the 'strong' oils are used in the manufacture of vanillin.

β-Caryophyllene

Oil of clove, like other essential oils, should be stored in well-filled, airtight containers, protected from light and heat. It is used as a flavouring agent, stimulant, aromatic and antiseptic.

Clove stem oil is produced in Tanzania and in Madagascar; it is used mainly in the flavouring and perfumery industries. *Clove leaf oil* is distilled in Madagascar, Tanzania and in Indonesia, and is used for the isolation of eugenol.

EUCALYPTUS LEAF

Eucalyptus leaf of the *EP* and *BP* consists of whole or cut dried leaves of the older branches of *Eucalyptus globulus* Labill. Eucalyptus trees possess two kinds of leaves, those on young plants being cordate and sessile whereas those on mature trees which constitute the official drug are petiolate and scimitar-shaped. The dried leaves are greyish-brown in colour, coriaceous in texture and have lateral veins which anastomose near the margin. Secretory oil glands are visible in leaves held to the light. Microscopy shows epidermal cells with thick cuticle, anisocytic stomata, together with mesophyll having schizogenous oil glands and prisms and cluster crystals of calcium oxalate.

The leaves are required to contain not less than 2.0% v/w of essential oil and have limits of 3% for dark and brown leaves, 5% for stems and 2% for other foreign matter. Other significant components of the leaves are phloroglucinol-sesquiterpene coupled compounds named macrocarpals, which show antibacterial activity against oral pathogenic microorganisms and inhibition of glycosyltransferase activity. Such substances could have potential in the maintenance of oral hygiene. For further details see K. Osawa and H. Yasuda, *J. Nat. Prod.*, 1996, **59**, 823.

EUCALYPTUS OIL

Oil of eucalyptus is distilled from the fresh leaves of various species of *Eucalyptus* (Myrtaceae) and rectified. Eucalyptus oils are produced in Portugal, South Africa, Spain, China, Brazil, Australia, India and Paraguay.

Only a certain number of species produce oils suitable for medicinal use. The chief requirements are a high cineole content and the absence of appreciable quantities of phellandrene and aldehydes (for formulae see Fig. 22.2). Suitable oils are derived from *E. polybractea*, *E. smithii*, *E. globulus* and *E. australiana*. In the case of the latter species the oil used in pharmacy is that collected during the first hour of the distillation, that which passes over subsequently being used for mineral separation. 'Citron-scented' eucalyptus oil, which is derived from *E. citriodora*, is used in perfumery and contains a high proportion of the aldehyde citronellal.

Characters. Oil of eucalyptus is a colourless or pale yellow liquid. It has an aromatic and camphoraceous odour; a pungent, camphoraceous taste, which is followed by a sensation of cold. It is required to contain not less than 70.0% of cineole. 1,8-Cineole and *o*-cresol form a solid complex and the crystallizing temperature of this forms the basis for the official assay of the oil. The *Pharmacopoeia* also includes a TLC identification test, and tests which limit the content of aldehydes and phellandrene; these eliminate oils containing citronellal and the so-called industrial eucalyptus oils.

Uses. Eucalyptus oil is much used for alleviating the symptoms of nasopharyngeal infections, for treating coughs and as a decongestant. It is taken internally in the form of mixtures, inhalations, lozenges and pastilles and applied externally as ointments and liniments.

Further reading
Boland DJ, Brophy JJ, House APN (eds) 1991 Eucalyptus leaf oils: use, chemistry, distillation and marketing. ACIAR/CSIRO Inkata Press, Melbourne, Australia

GINGER

Ginger (*Zingiber*) is the scraped or unscraped rhizome of *Zingiber officinale* (Zingiberaceae). The *BP* drug is known in commerce as 'unbleached ginger'. *Z. officinale*, a reed-like plant, is grown in many parts of the world, including Jamaica, China, India and Africa. Jamaica ginger, once the traditional pharmaceutical ginger, has been largely replaced by other sources.

History. Ginger has been cultivated in India from the earliest times; the plant is unknown in the wild state. The spice was used by the Greeks and Romans, and was a common article of European commerce in the Middle Ages. It was well known in England in the eleventh century. Ginger was introduced into Jamaica and other West Indian islands by the Spaniards, and a considerable quantity of the drug was sent from the West Indies to Spain as early as 1547.

Cultivation and preparation. Ginger grows well at subtropical temperatures where the rainfall is at least 1.98 m per annum. As the plant is sterile, it is grown by vegetative means. Selected pieces of rhizome ('seed pieces' or 'setts') each bearing a bud are planted in holes or trenches during March or April, preferably in a well-drained clayey loam. The procedures resemble potato cultivation. Mulching or manuring is necessary as the plant rapidly exhausts the soil of nutrients. When the stems wither, about December or January, the rhizomes are ready for collection. For the scraped drug, after removal of soil the rhizomes are killed by boiling water. They are then carefully peeled, thoroughly washed and then dried in the sun on mats or barbecues. During drying they are turned from time to time and protected during any damp weather. This first drying usually takes about 5 or 6 days. To obtain a whiter product the ginger is again moistened and dried for a further two days, when it is ready for export. It should not be limed.

With some gingers little or no cork is removed ('coated' or 'unscraped' gingers) and these grades are now also included in the *BP/EP*; these are sometimes whitened by dusting with calcium carbonate or lime but are eliminated by the *BP* ash value (not more than 6.0%).

Macroscopical characters. The dried scraped drug (Fig. 22.13) shows little resemblance to the fresh rhizome, owing to loss in weight and shrinkage. It occurs in sympodially branched pieces known as 'hands' or 'races'. These are 7–15 cm long, 1–1.5 cm broad and laterally compressed. The branches arise obliquely from the rhizome, are about 1–3 cm long and terminate in depressed scars or in undeveloped buds. The outer surface is buff-coloured and longitudinally striated or fibrous; it shows no sign of cork. The drug breaks with a short fracture, the fibres of the fibrovascular bundles often projecting from the broken surface. It has an agreeable aromatic odour and a pungent taste.

In transverse section a lens shows the cortex, a dark line (the pericycle and endodermis, the latter without starch) and the stele with numerous scattered fibrovascular bundles. Similar bundles also occur in the cortex. The bundles appear as greyish points, the smaller yellowish points which can also be seen being secretion cells.

The unscraped rhizome resembles the above in structure but is more or less covered by brownish layers of cork with conspicuous ridges; the cork readily exfoliates from the lateral surfaces but persists between the branches.

Microscopical characters. The unpeeled rhizome, in transverse section (Fig. 22.13C), shows a zone of cork tissue, differentiated into an outer zone of irregularly arranged cells produced by suberization of

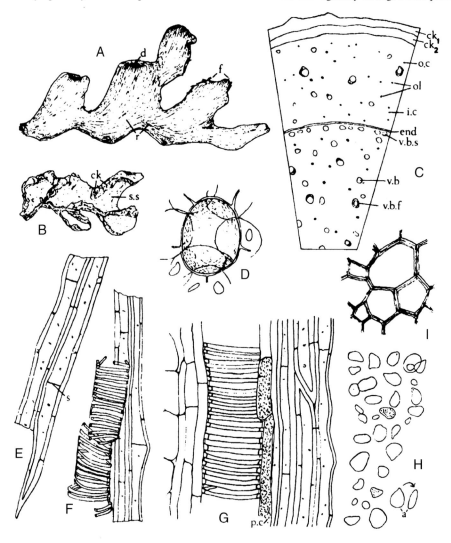

Fig. 22.13
Ginger. A, Peeled Jamaican rhizome; B, partially peeled African root (both ×0.75); C, diagrammatic transverse section of unpeeled rhizome (×15); D, oleoresin cell with adjacent parenchyma; E, portions of septate fibres; F, G, portions of septate fibres with attached vessels; H, starch; I, cork cells in surface view from unpeeled drug (all ×200). a, Starch granule, side- and end-aspects; ck, cork; ck₁, irregularly arranged cells of outer cork; ck₂, radially arranged cork cells; d, depressed scar; end, endodermis; f, projecting fibres; i.c, inner cortex; ol, oleoresin cells; o.c, flattened cells of outer cortex; p.c, pigment cell; r, ridges produced by vascular bundles; s, septum; s.s, scraped surface; v.b, vascular bundle; v.f.b, vascular bundle with fibrous sheath; v.b.s, ring of small vascular bundles.

the cortical cells without division and an inner zone of cells arranged in radial rows and produced by tangential division of the cortical cells. No cork cambium is differentiated. Within the cork is a broad cortex, differentiated into an outer zone of flattened parenchyma and an inner zone of normal parenchyma. The cortical cells contain abundant starch grains. These are almost entirely simple, ovoid or sack-shaped, are 5–15–30–60 μm long and have a markedly eccentric hilum (Fig. 22.13H). Scattered in the cortex are numerous oil cells, with suberized walls enclosing yellow–brown oleoresin. The inner cortical zone usually contains about three rings of collateral, closed vascular bundles. The larger bundles are enclosed in a sheath of septate, non-lignified fibres. Each vascular bundle contains phloem, showing well-marked sieve-tubes and a xylem composed of 1–14 vessels with annular, spiral or reticulate thickening. These vessels do not give a marked lignin reaction with phloroglucinol and hydrochloric acid. Axially elongated secretion cells with dark contents occasionally accompany the vessels. The inner limit of the cortex is marked by a single-layered endodermis free from starch. The outermost layer of the stele is marked by a single-layered pericycle. The vascular bundles of the stele resemble those of the cortex, and are, except for a ring of small bundles immediately within the pericycle, scattered as is typical of monocotyledonous stems. The ground mass of the stele is composed of parenchyma resembling the cortical parenchyma and containing much starch, and numerous oil cells. Cork cells are absent from the scraped drug. (For illustrations of the above features see Fig. 22.13D–H.)

Constituents. Ginger contains about 1–2% of volatile oil (*BP/EP* ≮1.5%); for the assay, liquid paraffin (10 drops) or other antifoaming agent may be added to the distillation flask. The rhizomes also contain 5–8% of resinous matter, starch and mucilage. Oil of ginger, to which the drug mainly owes its aroma, contains a mixture of over 50 constituents, consisting of monoterpenes (β-phellandrene, (+)-camphene, cineole, citral and borneol), sesquiterpene hydrocarbons (zingiberene, β-bisabolene, (*E,E*)-α-farnesene, β-sesquiphellandrene and *ar*-curcumene) and the sesquiterpene alcohol zingiberol. Over 50 volatile constituents of fresh organically grown ginger (fresh Chinese white and Japanese yellow varieties) have been recorded (S. D. Jolad *et al.*, *Phytochemistry*, 2004, **65**, 1937).

The pungency of ginger is due to gingerol, an oily liquid consisting of homologous phenols. The principal one of these is [6]-gingerol (i.e. where *n* = 4). It is formed in the plant from phenylalanine, malonate and hexanoate (see Denniff *et al.*, *J. Chem. Soc. Perkin*, *I*, 1980, 2637).

Smaller amounts of gingerols with other chain-lengths are also present. Similarly, [6]-gingerdiol is accompanied by four analogues which were isolated as minor components of the rhizome by Kikuzaki *et al.* from the less-polar fractions of the dichloromethane extracts (*Phytochemistry*, 1992, **31**, 1783). The same group also characterized (*Phytochemistry*, 1991, **30**, 3647; 1996, **43**, 273) a number of diaryl-heptanoids and a further seven have since been reported from Chinese *Z. officinalis* (J. Ma *et al.*, *Phytochemistry*, 2004, **65**, 1137). These diarylheptanoids are similar to the curcuminoids present in greater quantity in turmeric (q.v.). A number of diarylheptanones – gingerenones A, B, C and isogingerenone B have been investigated by Endo and colleagues (*Phytochemistry*, 1990, **29**, 797). Other minor components are methylgingediol, gingediacetates, methylgingediacetates and a C_{20}-dialdehyde.

The pungency of gingerol is destroyed by boiling with 2% potassium hydroxide. Boiling with baryta water decomposes it with formation of a phenolic ketone called zingerone and aliphatic aldehydes (mainly normal heptaldehyde). Zingerone also occurs in the rhizome and, like gingerol, is pungent but possesses in addition a sweet odour. Its pungency is destroyed by prolonged contact with 5% sodium hydroxide. Shogaols, components

of the oil, represent compounds formed by loss of water from the gingerols and were not thought to be present in the fresh rhizome. However, T.-S. Wu *et al.* (*Phytochemistry*, 1998, **48**, 1889) have now isolated three new dehydroshogaols from fresh roots purchased from a market in Taiwan. For formulae of ginger constituents see Figure 22.14.

Varieties. The plant which yields the official ginger is grown in many tropical countries, including India (Cochin, Calicut and Bengal), Africa (Nigeria, Sierra Leone), China, the East Indies, Cochin China, Australia and Florida. The chief varieties in English commerce are the Chinese, Nigerian, Cochin and African.

A number of commercial varieties of root, oleoresin and essential oil are available, seemingly derived from *Z. officinale*; whether these arise from different chemical races, from differences in cultivation and harvesting techniques or from different climatic conditions is not clear. They vary considerably in sensory characters. Australian oils are characterized by a 'lemon, citrus-like' odour. Oil from Fiji has a high citral content and a relatively high content of 1,8-cineole similar to Japanese oil.

Nigerian ginger. The best Nigerian closely resembles the Jamaica drug, but can be distinguished from it in the whole condition by its somewhat darker colour, its smaller size and that it is rather less deeply scraped. Nigerian ginger has a more pungent taste and rather less aroma than Jamaican. It yields less volatile oil (about 0.7–1%).

Cochin ginger. This is grown in southern India and is imported via Bombay or Madras. It occurs in both coated and scraped forms. The coated variety bears on the upper and lower surfaces a wrinkled reddish-grey cork which readily exfoliates. The lateral surfaces are without cork but are decidedly darker than the surface of the Jamaican drug. Pieces may be found of almost exactly the same size and shape as the Jamaican, but on the whole the pieces are smaller and the branches somewhat thicker. Cochin ginger is more starchy and breaks with a shorter fracture than the official; it is equally pungent but less agreeably aromatic. *Calicut ginger* closely resembles the Cochin, but the latter is usually regarded as the better grade.

Chinese ginger. This is produced in large quantity as various grades; it is sliced as opposed to split and the peeled drug is reported to be of Jamaican quality. It is often the principal variety available in the UK.

African ginger. This is typically smaller and darker than the Cochin. It is 'coated', a brown cork extending over a greater area than in the Cochin. The relatively small exposed portions of cortex on the lateral sides are grey to blackish in colour. It lacks the fine aroma of the Jamaica drug, although exceeding it in pungency. *Bombay ginger* resembles the African.

Allied drugs. *Japanese ginger* is derived from *Z. mioga*. The volatile oil which it contains differs in physical properties from that of the official species and gives the drug a bergamot-like odour. The taste is less pungent than that of *Z. officinale* and the starch grains are compound and less eccentric.

Preserved ginger consists of young undried rhizomes which are preserved by boiling in syrup. The West Indian variety is made from the official plant, but that from China is said to be obtained from the greater galangal, *Alpinia galanga* (Zingiberaceae).

Galangal rhizome, now little used in England although employed on the Continent, is derived from the lesser galangal, *A. officinarum*.

Adulteration. Most of the likely vegetable adulterants can be detected by a routine microscopical examination. Powdered ginger may have been prepared from 'wormy' drug, and so attention should be paid to the absence of insect fragments.

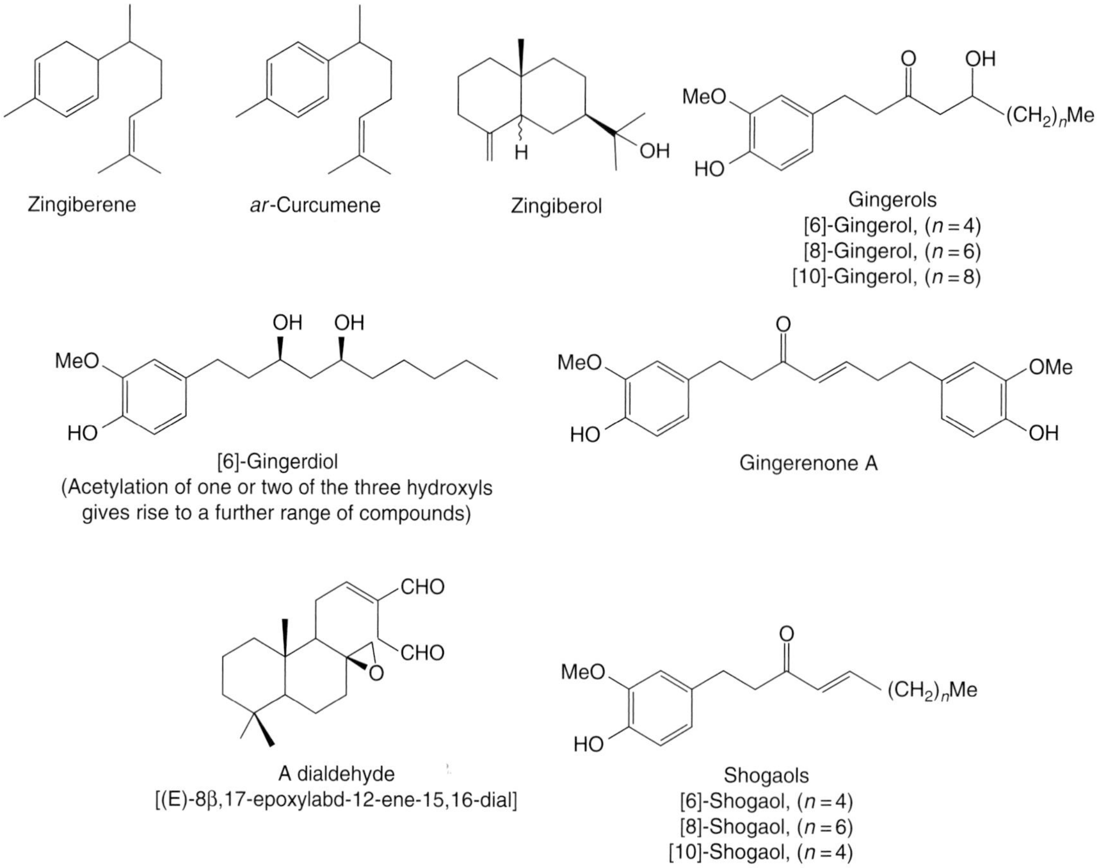

Fig. 22.14
Constituents of ginger.

Adulteration may also take the form of the addition of 'spent ginger' which has been exhausted in the preparation of essence. This may be detected by the official standards for alcohol-soluble extractive, water-soluble extractive, total ash and water-soluble ash.

Exhausted ginger and, more particularly, ginger galenicals may have their pungency increased by the addition of capsicum or grains of paradise. The suspected liquid, or a tincture prepared from the suspected powder, is heated in a water-bath with caustic alkali. The liquid is then evaporated, and the residue acidified with hydrochloric acid and shaken with ether. Some of the ethereal solution evaporated on a watch-glass gives a residue which is not markedly pungent to taste. This test depends on the fact that gingerol is more readily decomposed by alkalis than are capsaicin or paradol.

Uses and actions. Ginger is used as a carminative and stimulant. A US study by Mowrey and Clayson (*Lancet*, 1982, **1**, 655) indicated that powdered ginger may be a more effective antiemetic than dimen-hydrinate (Dramamine). The authors suggested that it may ameliorate the effects of motion sickness in the gastrointestinal tract itself, in contrast to antihistamines, which act centrally. Other reports claim that ginger is effective in the control of excessive and uncontrolled vomiting occurring in the first trimester of pregnancy and that it might provide a cheap antiemetic adjunct to cancer therapy (S. S. Sharma *et al.*, *J. Ethnopharmacology*, 1997, **57**, 93).

A considerable number of pharmacological studies involving the digestive, central nervous and cardiovascular systems have been reported for the isolated constituents of ginger. These activities include the potent inhibitory actions of the gingerols against prostaglandin synthetase which correspond with the anti-inflammatory and anti-platelet aggregation properties of the drug. These compounds, together with [6]-shogaol, also produce enhanced gastrointestinal activity with effects on bile secretion. The C_{20}-dial mentioned previously has a cholesterol-biosynthesis inhibitory activity in animal preparations and is assumed to be a HMG-CoA reductase inhibitor (M. Tanabe *et al.*, *Chem. Pharm. Bull.*, 1993, **41**, 710). The sesquiterpene hydrocarbons have also been associated with the antiulcer activity of the drug. A strong antibacterial and antifungal action has been demonstrated for a number of the rhizome constituents.

Further reading

Ravindran PN *et al* (eds), Hardman R (series ed) 2005 Medicinal and aromatic plants – industrial profiles, Vol 41. Ginger: the genus *Zingiber*. CRC Press, Boca Raton, FL. 520 pp.

Turmeric

Turmeric (*Curcuma*) is the dried rhizome of *Curcuma longa* (Zingiberaceae), cultivated in India, West Pakistan, China and Malaya. It contains constituents similar to those of ginger and is described in Chapter 29 under 'Antihepatotoxic Drugs'.

For a review of the principal pharmacological activities of turmeric (anti-inflammatory, hepatoprotective, antimicrobial, wound healing, anti-cancer, antitumour, antiviral) see R. C. Srimal, *Fitoterapia*, 1997, **68**, 483.

A radioprotective effect ascribed to free radical scavenging and electron/hydrogen donation has been demonstrated in mice (D. Choudhary *et al.*, *J. Ethnopharmacology*, 1999, **64**, 1) and an assay-guided fractionation of an ethanolic extract has furnished three DPPH free-radical scavenging diaryheptanoids: curcumin, demethoxycurcumin and bisdemethoxycurcumin (DPPH = 1,1-diphenyl-2-picrylhydrazyl). See E. K. Song *et al.*, *Planta Med.*, 2001, **67**, 876.

Further reading

Ravindran PN *et al* (eds) Hardman R (series ed) 2007 Medicinal and aromatic plants – industrial profiles, Vol 45, Turmeric: the genus *Curcuma*. CRC Press, Taylor and Francis Group, Boca Raton, FL

CARDAMOM FRUIT AND CARDAMOM OIL

Cardamom consists of the dried, nearly ripe fruits of *Elettaria cardamomum* Maton var. *minuscula* Burkill (Zingiberaceae). The seeds, the part used medicinally and as a spice, are directed to be kept in the fruits until required for use. This prevents loss of volatile oil and helps one to distinguish the fruits from those of *E. cardamomum* var. *major* (unofficial long wild native cardamoms) and from the fruits of other genera of the same family. However, to cut costs on transport much seed is now imported in sealed tins. Cardamom is expensive, its price among other common spices being exceeded only by those of saffron and vanilla.

Principal producers are Sri Lanka, southern India and Guatemala.

History. Cardamoms are mentioned in the early Sanskrit writings of Susruta, but it is difficult to say with any certainty when they first appeared in Europe. Immense quantities are still used in Hindu festivals. Both *Amomum* and *Cardamomum* appear in a list of Indian spices liable to duty at Alexandria, about AD 176–180. The Portuguese navigator Barbosa (1514) appears to have been the first to mention the source of our official drug as the Malabar coast.

Production, collection and preparation. Although wild plants are found in India and Sri Lanka, cardamoms are mainly obtained from cultivated plants. Propagation is by seedlings or vegetatively but the latter gives problems owing to possible infection by mosaic or katte virus. The plant is reed-like, 4 m or more high, and bears long leaves arising from the rhizome. As the capsular fruits on the same raceme ripen at different times and it is important to collect them when nearly ripe

and before they split to shed their seeds, it is best to cut off each fruit at the correct stage with a pair of short-bladed scissors. Pickers can, by this method, collect about 5 kg of fruit per day, although collecting all the fruits on one raceme together is naturally quicker. In Sri Lanka and India flowering and fruiting continues for practically the whole year but most of the crop is collected from October to December.

The fruits are dried slowly, either outdoors or in a curing house. Too-rapid drying is to be avoided, as it causes the fruits to split and shed their seeds. Sometimes the capsules are remoistened and further exposed to the sun but this sun-bleaching, although improving the appearance, also increases the number of split fruits. Bleaching may also be done by placing trays of the fruit over burning sulphur. Bleached fruits appear to have become less common and there is now an increased proportion of the unbleached Alleppy and Ceylon greens. The green curing procedure is also used in Guatemala and it has been claimed that enhanced colour retention is obtained by soaking the fruits for 10 min in 2% sodium carbonate solution before drying.

The capsules have the remains of the calyx at the apex and a stalk at the base. These may be removed either by hand-clipping or by machines. The fruits are then graded by means of sieves into 'longs', 'mediums', 'shorts' and 'tiny'. If they have been sulphur-bleached, they are aired in the open before being packed for export.

Macroscopical characters. The cardamom fruit is an inferior, ovoid or oblong capsule, about 1–2 cm long. The size, shape and surface vary in the different commercial varieties and grades (see below). The apex is shortly beaked and may show floral remains, while the base is rounded and shows the remains of the stalk. Internally the capsule is three-celled, a double row of seeds attached to axial placentas occurring in each cell. In good samples the seeds form about 70% of the total weight. The seeds in each loculus are tightly pressed together and usually separate in a single mass.

Each seed is about 4 mm long and 3 mm broad and somewhat angular. The colour varies from a dark reddish-brown in fully ripe seeds to a much paler colour in the unripe ones. The testa is transversely wrinkled and is covered by a membranous aril. A groove on one side of the seed indicates the position of the raphe and a depression at one end of the hilum. Cardamom seeds have a strongly aromatic odour and a pleasantly aromatic, although somewhat pungent, taste.

Seeds cut longitudinally and transversely and stained with iodine show the aril, testa, perisperm (containing starch) and the endosperm and embryo (both free from starch), as illustrated in Fig. 22.15.

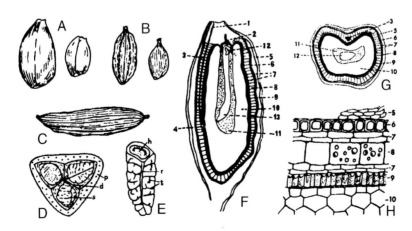

Fig. 22.15
Cardamom fruits and seeds. A, Mysore; B, Alleppy green; C, long, wild native (all × 1); D, transverse section of fruit (×1.5); E, whole seed (about × 4); F, longitudinal section of seed; G, transverse section of seed; H, arrangement of cells in transverse section of seed coat. d, Dissepiment of fruit; p, pericarp; r, raphe; s, seed; t, wrinkled testa; 1, funicle; 2, operculum or embryonic cap; 3, raphe; 4, chalaza; 5, arillus; 6, epidermis of testa; 7, parenchyma layers of the testa; 8, oil cell layer; 9, sclerenchymatous layer of testa; 10, perisperm; 11, endosperm; 12, embryo; 13, haustorium.

22

Varieties. *Mysore* fruits have a cream or pale buff colour and a nearly smooth surface. *Malabar* are usually smaller and have a rather darker and less smooth pericarp. *Mangalore* resemble the Malabar but are usually more globular and have a rougher pericarp; they occur both bleached and semi-bleached. *Alleppy* fruits are narrower than the above varieties, have a markedly striated pericarp and vary in colour from greenish-buff to green. *Ceylon greens* resemble Alleppy, but are generally greener and more elongated. The seeds of the above varieties are almost indistinguishable from one another, and also from the seeds of the *long wild native* cardamom (see below under 'Allied drugs'.)

Microscopical characters. Sections of the seed (Fig. 22.15) show a very thin membranous arillus, enveloping the seed and composed of several layers of collapsed cells, yellow in colour and containing oil. The brownish testa is composed of the following layers. (1) An outer epidermis consisting of a single layer of cells rectangular in transverse section, longitudinally elongated and with prosenchymatous end walls in surface view; light yellow in colour and having slightly thick end walls. (2) A single or double layer of parenchymatous cells, elongated at right angles to the long axis of the overlying epidermal cells (see Fig. 22.15H). (3) A single layer of large parenchymatous cells containing volatile oil; in the region of the raphe there are two layers of oil cells separated by the raphe meristele. (4) Several layers of small flattened parenchymatous cells, their structure often partially obliterated. (5) An inner epidermis of sclerenchymatous cells, radially elongated, with anticlinal and inner walls very strongly thickened and reddish-brown in colour. Lumen bowl-shaped and containing a module of silica (see Fig. 22.15H). The operculum or embryonic cap is composed of two or three layers of these sclerenchymatous cells, continuous with those of the inner epidermis. The micropyle is a narrow canal passing through the operculum. Within the testa is a well-developed perisperm composed of parenchymatous cells packed with minute globular starch grains, 4 μm diameter and containing in the centre of each cell a small prismatic crystal of calcium oxalate. The perisperm encloses the endosperm and embryo, both composed of thin-walled cells rich in protein.

Cardamom pericarps or husks which have been used for the adulteration of powdered drugs may be identified in the form of powder by the pitted fibres and spiral vessels of the fibrovascular bundles and by the abundant, empty parenchymatous cells.

Constituents. Samples of cardamom seed yield 2.8–6.2% (*BP* not less than 4.0%) of volatile oil and also contain abundant starch (up to 50.0%), fixed oil (1–10%) and calcium oxalate.

Cardamom oil. The oil is distilled in relatively limited quantities in Sri Lanka, India and Guatemala with an estimated global production of some 4 tonnes in 1984. The oil contains a high proportion of terpinyl acetate and cineole and smaller quantities of other monoterpenes, including alcohols and esters. Over 40 compounds have been identified in the oils of *Elettaria* species. The *BP* requires an ester value of 90–156 and an optical rotation of +20° to +40°. The loss of oil from seeds kept in the pericarp is small but a loss of 30% in 8 months takes place when the seeds are separated from the fruits. Gas chromatography has shown oils from different varieties of cardamom to have qualitatively the same composition, but variations in the proportions of individual components are evident.

Allied drugs. The *long wild native cardamoms* of Sri Lanka (Fig. 22.15C) are derived from *E. cardamomum* var. *major* Thwaites. They are much more elongated than the official variety, sometimes attaining

a length of about 4 cm. The pericarps are dark brown and coarsely striated. The oil distilled from them is used in liqueurs.

'*Amomum*', of the *Indian Pharmaceutical Codex*, consists of the ripe or nearly ripe seeds of *Amomum aromaticum* or *A. subulatum*. The former, obtained from Bengal and Assam, is known as Bengal Cardamom; the latter, obtained from Nepal, Bengal, Sikkim and Assam, as Nepal or Greater Cardamom.

No other similar drugs, unless we include grains of paradise (see below), are imported in any quantity or with any regularity; the following is a list of allied species the seeds of which somewhat resemble those of the true cardamom: *A. cardamomum*, the round or cluster cardamom of Siam and Java; *A. xanthioides*, the bastard or wild Siamese cardamom; *A. maximum*, a Javanese plant; *Aframomum korarima*, the Korarima or Abyssinian cardamom; *A. mala*, the East African cardamom; *A. hanburii* and *A. daniellii*, Cameroon cardamoms; *A. angustifolium*, Madagascar cardamom; *Costus speciosus*, Chinese cardamom. The antiplasmodial activity of *A. zambesiacum* seeds has been investigated and five new labdane diterpenoids and five known ones isolated (M. Kenmogne *et al.*, *Phytochemistry*, 2006, **67**, 433).

Uses. The principal uses of cardamom are as a flavouring agent in curries and cake. Large quantities are used in Scandinavia and Germany and, with a large proportion of Asiatics in the population, consumption has increased in Britain. Some is used in the manufacture of liqueurs and a relatively small amount in pharmacy, chiefly in the form of Compound Tincture of Cardamom.

Biological activities demonstrated for cardamom include antimicrobial, anti-inflammatory, analgesic, antispasmodic and, recently, gastroprotective (A. Jamal *et al.*, *J. Ethnopharmacol.*, 2006, **103**, 149).

Grains of paradise

This spice, also known as Guinea grains or melegueta pepper, has been an article of commerce from very early times. It consists of the seeds of the West African reed-like herb *Aframomum melegueta* (Zingiberaceae), which has many of the characters of cardamom (q.v.).

The seeds are hard, reddish-brown, about 3 mm long and of a flattened pyramidal shape. The testa is papillose. Internally the structure resembles that of a cardamom seed. They have an aromatic odour and a pungent taste. The aroma is due to about 0.5% of volatile oil which contains principally β-caryophyllene, α-humulene and their epoxides. The pungency arises from paradol, a substance related to gingerol, and from small quantities of shogaol and gingerol. For the detection of paradol in ginger galenicals, see 'Ginger'. The essential oils from the seeds of *A. melegueta* and other *Aframomum* spp. from the Cameroon have been analysed by GC-MS (C. Menut *et al.*, *Flavour Fragrance J.*, 1991, **6**, 183). The seeds are used in alcoholic liquors and to some extent in veterinary medicine. Excessive consumption of the seeds can lead to ocular toxicity (S. A. Igwe *et al.*, *J. Ethnopharmacology*, 1999, **65**, 203).

CHAMOMILE FLOWERS

Roman Chamomile Flowers are the expanded flower-heads of *Chamaemelum nobile* (L.) All (*Anthemis nobilis* L.) (Compositae), collected from cultivated plants and dried. Chamomiles are cultivated in the south of England and in Belgium, France, Germany, Hungary, Poland, former Yugoslavia, Bulgaria, Egypt and Argentina. As a result of long cultivation most of the tubular florets present in the wild plant have become ligulate, and it is these 'double' or 'semi-double' flower-heads which form the commercial drug. They are included in the *BP/EP*.

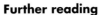
History. Owing to the large number of similar composite plants, it has proved impossible to trace the drug in classical writings. The double variety was certainly known in the eighteenth century.

Collection. The flowers are collected in dry weather and carefully dried. The crop is often damaged by wet weather and the discoloured flowers then obtained fetch a much lower price than those having a good colour.

Characters. Each dried flower-head (Fig. 22.16A) is hemispherical and about 12–20 mm in diameter (the *BP* imposes a 3% limit on small or blemished heads). The florets are of a white to pale buff colour, the outer ones hiding the involucre of bracts. A few hermaphrodite, tubular florets are usually found near the apex of the solid receptacle (see Fig. 22.16B). A transition between the typical tubular florets and typical ligulate ones is often seen. The ligulate florets show three teeth (or occasionally two), the centre one being most developed. There are four principal veins. The corolla is contracted near its base into a tube from which a bifid style projects. The ovary is inferior and devoid of pappus. Each floret arises in the axil of a thin membranous bract or palea which has a blunt apex. At the base of the receptacle is an involucre consisting of two or three rows of oblong bracts which have membranous margins.

Chamomiles have a strong, aromatic odour and a bitter taste. The *BP/EP* includes a TLC test for identity and requires the drug to contain not less than 0.7% of volatile oil and not more than 10.0% water.

Constituents. Chamomiles contain 0.4–1.0% of volatile oil which is blue when freshly distilled owing to the presence of azulene. Other components of the oil are *n*-butyl angelate (principal), iso-amyl angelate, 3-phenylpropyl isobutyrate, tridecanal, pentadecanal and terpenes. Chamomiles also contain sesquiterpene lactones of the germacranolide type, hydroperoxides, dihydroxycinnamic acid and apigenin (a trihydroxy flavone) and luteolin both free and as glucosides. (For the isolation of other constituents see A. Carnat *et al.*, *Fitoterapia*, 2004, **75**, 32.

Uses. Considerable quantities of chamomiles are used in domestic medicine in the form of an infusion (for dyspepsia, etc.) or poultice or in shampoo powders. For the production of volatile oil, the entire aerial parts are usually used.

Further reading

Franke R and Schilcher H (eds), Hardman R (series ed) 2005 Medicinal and aromatic plants Vol 42. Chamomile: industrial profiles. CRC Press, Boca Raton, FL. 288 pp.

MATRICARIA FLOWERS

Matricaria flowers (German or Hungarian chamomile flowers) are the dried flower-heads of *Matricaria recutita* L. (*Chamomilla recutita* (L.) Rausch.) (Compositae). The plant is a native to and is cultivated in southern and eastern Europe; Argentina and Egypt are also producers. It is official in the *EP* and described in the *BP*.

The capitulum when spread out, is 10–17 mm in diameter and consists of a receptacle, an involucre, 12–20 marginal ligulate florets and numerous central tubular florets. Unlike chamomile flowers, matricaria possesses a hollow receptacle which is devoid of paleae (see Fig. 22.16C–E). Broken flowers are limited to 25%. The drug has a pleasant aromatic odour.

Constituents. The flower-heads are required to contain not less than 0.4% of a blue volatile oil; this consists mainly of the sesquiterpenes α-bisabolol, chamazulene and farnesene. Chamazulene itself does not occur in the plant but is formed from a sesquiterpene lactone (matricin) during steam distillation.

Flavones and coumarins (e.g. herniarin) are present and the dried ligulate florets contain 7–9% of apigenin glucosides (the 7-glucoside and a mixture of acetates as determined by ^{13}C-NMR analysis) and 0.3–0.5% free apigenin, which may arise by post-harvest hydrolysis of the glucosides. In this respect, V. Švehlíková *et al.* (*Phytochemistry*, 2004, **65**, 2323) have studied the isolation, identification and stability of apigenin-7-*O*-glucoside in the white florets.

A number of chemotypes depending on the proportions of bisabolol, bisabolol oxides and farnesene in the oil have been described. Most Turkish varieties of *M. chamomilla* yield yellow oils containing no chamazulene; 2*n* and 4*n* races have been studied for their respective coumarin variations (A. Pastirová *et al.*, *Pharm. Biol.*, 2005, **43**, 205). For an article listing the many known constituents of matricaria flowers see A. Ahmad and L. N. Nisra, *Int. J. Pharmacognosy*, 1997, **35**, 121.

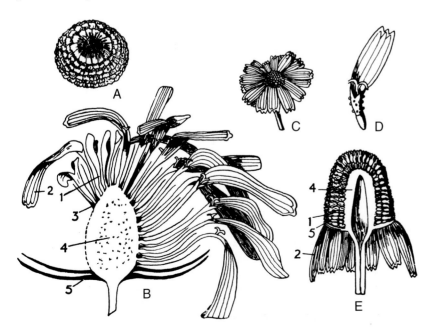

Fig. 22.16
A, Cultivated Roman chamomile; B, the same cut longitudinally; C, German chamomile; D, a ligulate floret of same; E, German chamomile cut longitudinally. 1, Tubular floret; 2, ligulate floret; 3, palea; 4, receptacle; 5, bract of involucre. (B after Greenish, remainder after Gilg.)

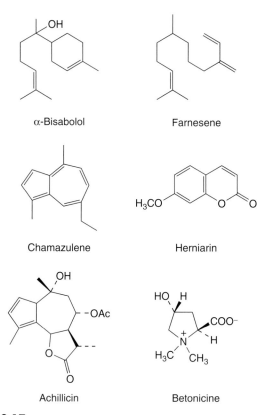

Fig. 22.17
Constituents of matricaria flowers.

Uses. Matricaria flowers are mainly used on the Continent of Europe and in the USA for their anti-inflammatory and spasmolytic properties. The ulcer-protective properties of German chamomile have been ascribed to bisabolol-type constituents, on which considerable pharmacological work has been reported. Four optically active isomers of bisabolol are possible; extracts for pharmaceutical use should be prepared only from clearly defined types containing the active constituents.

Allied drug. *Tanacetum parthenium* (L.) Schultz-Bip.; *Chrysanthemum parthenium* (L.) Bernh., or *feverfew flowers* may be single or double. The receptacle is flatter than that of the Roman chamomile and may or may not bear paleae. If the latter are present, they are acute and less membranous than those of the chamomile. The whole flowering tops are usually sold. Feverfew herb yields 0.07–0.4% of volatile oil. It is used in herbal medicine; for details concerning its content of sesquiterpene lactones see Chapter 24.

MATRICARIA OIL

Matricaria oil is that steam-distilled from the fresh or dried flower heads or flowering tops of *Matricaria recutita* L. Resulting from the chemotypes mentioned above two types of oil are described in the pharmacopoeia—one rich in bisabolol oxides and the other rich in (−)-α-bisabolol. These compounds, together with chamazulene, are determined by gas chromatography.

These oils are blue in colour and have a characteristic odour.

YARROW

Yarrow (millefolium, milfoil) is described in the *BP/EP*, *BHP* and a number of continental pharmacopoeias. It is also the subject of German

Commission E and ESCOP monographs. The drug consists of the dried flowering tops of *Achillea millefolium* L. (Compositae), an extremely diverse aggregate species with varying chromosome numbers and differences in oil composition. The *British Herbal Compendium*, Vol. 1, 1992 points out that work reported under '*Achilleum millefolium*' may refer to *A. millefolium* sensu stricto or any number of other species which have been more recently and narrowly defined.

Yarrow is native to Europe and Western Asia but is now widespread in most temperate regions including N. America; commercial supplies come largely from south-eastern Europe, although it is also collected in other European countries including the UK.

Characters. The flowers occur in characteristically dense terminal corymbs about 3–5 cm in diameter and composed of capitula 3–5 cm in diameter. Each capitulum possesses an involucre of bracts, usually with five white to reddish ligulate ray florets, and 3–20 tubular disk florets. The fruits are achenes. The powdered material contains numerous elements, not only from the flower but also from stems and leaves. These include the typical Compositae pollen grains, leaf epidermis with anomocytic stomata and glandular and clothing trichomes again typical of the Compositae. Fuller details are given in the *BP* and *EP*.

Constituents. The pharmacopoeia requires an essential oil content of not less than 0.2% and not less than 0.002% of proazulenes calculated as chamazulene (Fig. 22.17). The tetraploid form of the plant (*A. millefolium* L., ssp. *collina* Becker) appears the most suitable as it produces considerable chamazulene as a component of the oil whereas the widespread hexaploid species (*A. millefolium* L., ssp. *millefolium*) lacks this guaianolide sesquiterpene. Germacranolide- and eudesmanolide-type sesquiterpenes are also constituents of the oil together with caryophyllene, sabinene, α- and β-pinene, borneol, bornyl acetate, camphor and small quantities of thujone. The proazulenes are determined by measurement of the absorbance (608 nm) of the oil (in xylene) obtained by distillation from the herb.

Other isolates from yarrow include sesquiterpene lactones (achillin, achillicin, etc.), flavonoids (apigenin, luteolin, quercetin and their 7-*O*-glycosides), alkaloids (betonicine, stachydrine, trigonelline) and various acetylenes, coumarins, triterpenes, sterols and plant acids.

V. K. Agnihotri *et al.* (*Planta Med.*, 2005, **71**, 280) studied plants from two different high-altitude (1600 m) populations propagated under uniform environmental conditions at a lower altitude (300 m); the populations represented two ecotypes, a 1:8-cineole type and a borneol type, which differed in oil content and in composition of mono- and sesqui-terpenes.

Uses. Yarrow is used, as is chamomile and matricaria, to treat various skin conditions and digestive disorders. Its pharmacological actions can arise from various groups of compounds—anti-inflammatory (chamazulene and prochamazulenes, apigenin, salicyclic acid), haemostatic (betonicine), spasmolytic (flavonoids).

Further reading

Chandler RF, Hooper SN, Harvey HJ 1982 Ethnobotany and phytochemistry of yarrow, *Achillea millefolium*, Compositae. Economic Botany 36: 203–223
Hofmann L, Fritz D, Nitz S, Kollmannberger H, Drawert F 1992 Essential oil composition of three polyploids in the *Achillea millefolium* 'complex'. Phytochemistry 31: 537–542

WORMWOOD

Wormwood is essentially the dried leaves and flowering tops of *Artemisia absinthium* L., Compositae, widely distributed in Europe and the New World and recorded as a household remedy from biblical times. It is now included in the *EP*, *BP*, *BHP* 1983 and a number of European pharmacopoeias. There are official requirements for its volatile oil content and bitterness. The principal producers are the former USSR, Bulgaria, former Yugoslavia, Hungary and Poland; it is also cultivated in the USA and elsewhere.

Absinthin

Artabsinolide C
Artabsinolide A = 2-ketone
Artabsinolide B = 4-epimer, 2-ketone

The plant is a subshrub with deeply dissected leaves. The insignificant globose flowers form loose panicles and consist mainly of tubular florets and a few yellow ray florets. The leaves and grooved stems are covered with silky hairs.

Characteristic features of the microscopy are the T-shaped trichomes (see Fig. 42.3I) on both leaf epidermi; these have uniseriate stalks of up to three cells and long tapering unicellular heads. There are numerous unicellular long, twisted trichomes and secretory trichomes with biseriate two-celled stalks and heads of two to four cells. The stomata are of the anomyocytic type. Numerous spherical pollen grains, 30 µm in diameter with three pores and a spiny exine, are seen in the powdered drug.

The drug has an aromatic odour and is intensely bitter. The active constituents are the bitter substances and essential oil. Bitter substances (0.15–0.4%) consist of sesquiterpene lactones, principally the dimeric guaianolide absinthin (0.20–0.28%), artabsin, artabsinolides A, B, and C and others. They are evaluated in the *BP* by the organoleptic test for 'bitterness value' using a quinine hydrochloride solution for comparison. The essential oil (*BP* requirement not less than 0.2%) is variable in composition according to geographical source and chemotype with any one of *p*-thujone, *trans*-sabinyl acetate, *cis*-epoxyocimene and chrysanthenyl acetate forming over 40% of the mixture; also present are other sesquiterpenes and monoterpenes.

Over the years many medicinal properties have been ascribed to wormwood. It is considered of value for promoting the appetite, for its strengthening effect in the treatment of colds and influenza, for gall bladder and menstrual problems and for the expulsion of round worms. Thujone is toxic, making the cultivation of low-thujune chemotypes desirable. The herb is also used in the making of liqueurs.

LOVAGE

Lovage is the whole or cut dried rhizome and root of *Levisticum officinale* (*Ligusticum levisticum*), family Umbelliferae. The official drug should contain not less than 0.4% essential oil for the whole drug and not less than 0.3% for that in the cut condition calculated with reference to the anhydrous drug.

3-Butylphthalide   Ligusticum lactone   Ligustilide

The plant is native to southern Europe, western Asia and the Orient but has for a long time been cultivated elsewhere; it is produced commercially in the Balkans, Germany, Holland, Poland and the USA.

In habit, lovage is a tall, aromatic perennial herb with bipinnate, cauline leaves coarsely toothed at the apex and greenish-yellow flowers. The rhizomes and roots are obtained from plants 2 to 3 years old and when split, cut and dried are in pieces up to 5 cm in diameter for the rhizomes and up to 25 cm in length for the roots. Externally the drug is greyish-brown in colour and longitudinally furrowed; a transverse section of the roots shows a thick yellowish-white bark separated from a brownish-yellow radiate wood by a dark line. Oil-containing structures are visible in the outer regions of the transverse section. Microscopic characters of the powdered drug include polygonal or rounded cork cells as seen in surface view, considerable parenchyma, reticulately thickened vessels, fragments of secretory cells and single and compound starch granules.

The drug contains up to 1.0% of volatile oil, the characteristic odoriferous components being alkyl phthalides of which 3-butylphthalide (*c*. 32%), ligustilide (*c*. 24%) and ligusticum lactone are principal components. Terpenes include α- and β-pinene, α- and β-phellandrene, α- and β-terpinene, camphene, myrcene, etc. Other constituents are various coumarins and plant acids. The *BP* includes a TLC examination as a test for identity and for the absence of angelica root.

Lovage has been used for centuries as a herbal remedy. It has carminative, diuretic and antimicrobial properties making it useful for the treatment of dyspepsia, cystitis and as a mouthwash for tonsillitis. Herbalists usually prescribe it in admixture with other drugs.

Tansy

Tansy (*Tanacetum vulgare* (L.); *Chrysanthemum vulgare* (L.) Bernh.) (Compositae) is used as an anthelminthic in herbal medicine but its poisonous properties are well appreciated. The herb contains about 0.2–0.6% volatile oil containing around 70% of thujone. Many sesquiterpene lactones have been isolated from the flowers and herb together with flavones. Numerous chemical races, originating from different geographical areas, are known and involve both the oil constituents and the sesquiterpenes. (For a series of reports involving three other species of *Tanacetum* see O. O. Thomas, *Fitoterapia*, 1989, **60**, 138, 231, 329 and references cited therein. With regard to the anti-inflammatory properties of the herb, C. A. Williams *et al.* (*Phytochemistry*, 1999, **51**, 417) have compared the flavonoids of *T. vulgare* and feverfew, and revised some flavonoid formulae.)

Sandalwood oil

Sandalwood oil is obtained from the heartwood of *Santalum album* (Santalaceae), an evergreen tree 8–12 m in height which is widely distributed in India and the Malay Archipelago.

Supplies are mainly derived from Indonesia and southern India where the trees are systematically cultivated and the cutting is controlled. The volatile oil is contained in all the elements of the wood, medullary ray cells, vessels, wood fibres and wood parenchyma. The oil contains about 90–97% of sesquiterpene alcohols, distinguished for purpose of analysis as 'santalol'. This consists of α-santalol (b.p. 300–301°C) and β-santalol (b.p. 170–171°C). The hydrocarbon fraction contains about nine components.

C. G. Jones *et al.* (*Phytochemistry*, 2006, **67**, 2463) have discussed the biosynthesis of sandalwood oil sesquiterpenes chemotaxonomically with respect to the co-occurrence patterns of the four types studied: (1) α- and β-santalenes and bergamotene, (2) γ- and β-curcumene, (3) β-bisabolene and α-bisabol, and (4) four unidentified sesquiterpenes.

Recent reports suggest that the oil is being adulterated with polyethylene glycols. The oil is now mainly used in perfumery; a possible chemoprotective action on liver carcinogenesis in mice has been demonstrated (S. Banerjee *et al.*, *Cancer Lett.*, 1993, **68**, 105). Bioassay-guided fractionations coupled with NMR structural determinations have shown that of eleven sesquiterpenes, (Z)-α-santalol and (Z)-β-santalol have strong anti-*Helicobacter pylori* activities against a clarithromycin resistant strain. (T. Ochi *et al.*, *J. Nat. Prod.*, 2005, **68**, 819).

Australian sandalwood oil is prepared by distillation and rectification from the wood of *Eucarya spicata*, a small tree growing in Western Australia. It contains sesquiterpene alcohols.

RESINS, GUM-RESINS AND SIMILAR SUBSTANCES

The term 'resin' is applied to more or less solid, amorphous products of complex chemical nature. On heating they soften and finally melt. They are insoluble in water and usually insoluble in petroleum spirit but dissolve more or less completely in alcohol, chloroform and ether. Chemically, resins are complex mixtures of resin acids, resin alcohols (resinols), resin phenols (resinotannols), esters and chemically inert compounds known as resenes. The chemical structures of many of these compounds have now been elucidated.

Resins, as described above, are often associated with volatile oils (oleoresins), with gums (gum-resins) or with oil and gum (oleo-gum-resins). However, no hard and fast distinction can be made between these groups, as products such as mastic and ammoniacum, which are usually considered as a resin and a gum-resin, respectively, both contain volatile oil. Resins may also be combined in a glycosidal manner with sugars, as in the Convolvulaceae.

The term 'balsam' is often wrongly applied to oleoresins such as Canada turpentine and copaiba, and should be reserved for such substances as balsam of Peru, balsam of Tolu and storax, which contain a high proportion of aromatic balsamic acids (see Chapter 19). These balsams, if containing free acids, are partially soluble in hot water, owing to the solubility of benzoic and cinnamic acids, while the aromatic esters and resins are insoluble. Benzoin is perhaps best described as a balsamic resin.

The above products are usually contained in schizogenous or schizolysigenous ducts or cavities. They are often preformed in the plant (i.e. they are normally physiological products), but the yield is usually increased by injury (e.g. in the case of *Pinus*). Many products (e.g. benzoin and balsam of Tolu) are not formed by the plant until it has been injured: that is, they are of pathological origin. The gums which are often associated with resins and volatile oils usually resemble acacia gum in chemical nature and in the fact that they are often accompanied by oxidase enzymes. While resins are usually produced in ducts or cavities, they may be found in other positions—for example, in the resin cells of bloodroot, in the elements of the heartwood of guaiacum, in the external glands of Indian hemp, in the internal glands of male fern or in the glands on the surface of the lac insect.

MYRRH

Myrrh (*Arabian* or *Somali Myrrh*) is an oleo-gum resin, obtained from the stem of various species of *Commiphora* (Burseraceae), growing in north-east Africa and Arabia. British texts have traditionally given the principal source as *C. molmol* but Tucker (*Econ. Bot.*, 1986, **40**, 425) states that the chief source today is *C. myrrha*. The *EP* and *BP* definition cites *Commiphora molmol* Engler and/or other species of *Commiphora*. Two other species, *C. abyssinica* and *C. schimperi*, both of which may attain a height of 10 m, grow in Arabia and Abyssinia. The drug is chiefly collected in Somaliland and Ethiopia.

History.   Products of the myrrh type were well known to the ancients under the names of *bola*, *bal* or *bol*. The drug is still known to the Indian traders as 'heerabol', while the Somalis call it 'mulmul' or 'ogo'. The name 'myrrh' is probably derived from the Arabic and Hebrew word *mur*, which means bitter. Many references occur in the Old Testament, but the product was apparently that derived from *C. erthyaea* var. *glabrescens*, which is known to the Somalis as 'habbak hadi', and commercially as perfumed bdellium or bissabol.

Guban myrrh, which is produced from the trees of the Somali coast area known as the Guban, is rather oily and is regarded as inferior to the more powdery 'ogo' produced further inland.

Collection.   Almost all members of the Burseraceae possess in the phloem oleoresin canals, which are formed schizogenously and may afterwards unite with one another to form schizolysigenous cavities. This occurs in the species *Commiphora*. Much of the secretion is obtained by spontaneous exudation from the cracks and fissures which commonly form in the bark, and some is obtained from incisions made by the Somalis. The yellowish-white, viscous fluid soon hardens in the great heat to reddish-brown masses, which are collected by the Somalis. As bdelliums and gums are collected at the same time, these frequently find their way into the drug and have subsequently to be picked out.

Characters.   Myrrh occurs in somewhat irregular tears or masses weighing up to about 250 g. The surface is reddish-brown or reddish-yellow in colour and powdery. The drug fractures and powders readily, the freshly exposed surface being of a rich brown colour and oily. Whitish marks are sometimes seen and thin splinters are translucent. Myrrh has an aromatic odour and an aromatic, bitter and acrid taste.

Myrrh forms a yellowish emulsion when triturated with water. When extracted with alcohol (90%), as in the preparation of Tincture of Myrrh, a whitish mass of gum and impurities remains. The *BP* alcohol-insoluble matter should not exceed 70%. Lump myrrh usually yields not more than 5% of ash, but the commercial powdered drug frequently yields more. It may be distinguished from perfumed bdellium and similar products by allowing an ethereal extract of the drug to evaporate to dryness and passing the vapour of bromine over the resinous film produced. A violet colour is given by genuine myrrh but not by bdellium. TLC and visualization with ultraviolet light at 365 nm is used by the *BP* as an identification test and also to establish the absence of *C. mukul*, an inferior bdellium product.

Constituents.   Myrrh contains 7–17% of volatile oil, 25–40% of resin, 57–61% of 'gum' and some 3–4% of impurities.

The volatile oil contains terpenes, sesquiterpenes, esters, cuminic aldehyde and eugenol. The sesquiterpene fraction (Fig. 22.18) contains furanosesquiterpenes including furanogermacranes, furanoguaianes and furanoeudesmanes (N. Zhu *et al.*, *J. Nat. Prod.*, 2001, **64**, 1460). Furaneudesma-1,3-diene and curzarene have morphine-like properties and act on the CNS opioid receptors; furanodiene-6-one and methoxy furanoguaia-9-ene-8-one show antibacterial and antifungal activity against standard strains of pathogenic species (P. Dolara *et al.*, *Nature*, 1996, **379**, 29; *Planta Medica*, 2000, **66**, 356). The oil, which is distilled outside the countries of origin, readily resinifies and then gives a violet colour with bromine.

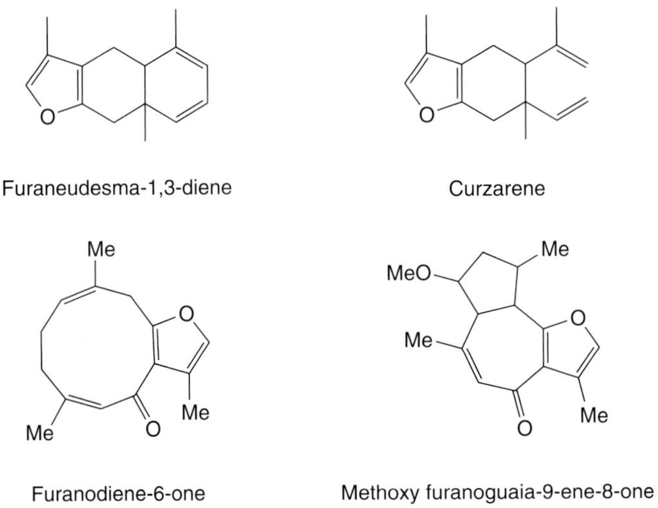

Furaneudesma-1,3-diene

Curzarene

Furanodiene-6-one

Methoxy furanoguaia-9-ene-8-one

Fig. 22.18
Constituents of myrrh.

The chemistry of the resins is complex and not fully elucidated. The larger ether-soluble portion contains α-, β- and γ-commiphoric acids, the esters of another resin acid and two phenolic resins. The smaller ether-insoluble fraction contains α- and β-heerabomyrrholic acids. The crude alcohol-insoluble matter ('gum') contains about 18% of protein and 64% of carbohydrate containing galactose, arabinose and glucuronic acid. This gum is associated with an oxidase enzyme.

Allied drugs. Four different varieties of 'bdellium' were recognized by Holmes. Of these, *perfumed* or *scented bdellium* or *bissabol* is probably derived from *C. erythaea* var. *glabrescens*. It resembles soft myrrh in appearance but is easily distinguished from it by the more aromatic odour and by the fact that it does not give a violet colour with the bromine test. *Hotai bdellium* or *gum hotai* is opaque and odourless; it contains a saponin and is used for washing the hair. The resin of *C. confusa* collected in Kenya contains dammarane triterpenoids, as does *C. kua* (L. O. A. Manguro *et al.*, *Chem. Pharm. Bull.*, 2003, **51**, 479, 483).

Uses. Myrrh is used in incense and perfumes. Like many other resins, it has local stimulant and antiseptic properties. It is chiefly employed in medicine in the form of a mouth-wash or gargle for its astringent effect on mucous membranes. A number of its traditional and historic uses have received experimental support.

Olibanum

Olibanum (*Frankincense*) is an oleo-gum-resin obtained by incision from the bark of *Boswellia carterii, B. frereana* and other species of *Boswellia* (Burseraceae), small trees indigenous to north-eastern Africa and Arabia. The drug occurs in more or less ovoid tears, 5–25 mm long, which are sometimes stuck together. The surface is dusty and of a yellowish, bluish or greenish tint. Fracture, brittle; inner surface, waxy and semitranslucent. Odour is characteristic, especially when burned; taste, slightly bitter. The drug contains 3–8% of volatile oil consisting of numerous terpenes (e.g. *p*-cymene) and sesquiterpenes, about 60–70% of resin, and 27–35% of gum. In 1956 the gum was found to contain two polysaccharides; one consisting of units of galactose and arabinose and the other of galactose and galacturonic acid. Modern methods of analysis have allowed the taxonomic identity of diverse frankincense products to be determined; examples are incense mixtures, traditional medicines and archaeological specimens (S. Hamm *et al.*, *Phytochemistry*, 2005, **66**, 1399).

Olibanum is used in incense and fumigating preparations. Formerly, it was considered a stimulant and has been used in China for the treatment of leprosy. With animal models, Duwiejua *et al.* (*Planta Medica*, 1993, **59**, 12) have reported a positive anti-inflammatory activity for the drug.

Asafoetida

Asafoetida is an oleo-gum-resin obtained by incision from the living rhizome and root of *Ferula foetida* Regel, *F. rubricaulis* Boiss., and other species of *Ferula* (Umbelliferae), plants about 3 m in height. The drug is collected in Iran, Pakistan and Afghanistan.

Collection and preparation. The collection of asafoetida involves removal of the stem and the cutting of successive slices from the vertical rootstock. After each slice is removed, oleo-gum-resin exudes and, when sufficiently hardened, is collected. The product is packed in tin-lined cases for export.

Characters. Asafoetida occurs in two principal forms.
Tears. These are rounded or flattened and about 5–30 mm diameter. They are greyish-white, dull yellow or reddish-brown in colour, some specimens acquiring the latter colour with age, while others remain greyish or yellowish.
Mass. This consists of similar tears to those described above agglutinated into masses and usually mixed with fruits, fragments of root, earth and other impurities. Mass asafoetida is the commonest commercial form.

Asafoetida has a strong, alliaceous odour and a bitter, acrid and alliaceous taste. It should yield not more than 50% of matter insoluble in alcohol (90%) and not more than 15% of ash.

Constituents. Asafoetida consists of volatile oil, resin, gum and impurities. The oil has a particularly evil smell and contains sulphur compounds of the formulae $C_7H_{14}S_2$, $C_{16}H_{20}S_2$, $C_8H_{16}S_2$, $C_{10}H_{18}S_2$, $C_7H_{14}S_3$, and $C_8H_{16}S_3$; some of these show pesticidal activity. The flavour is largely due to *R*-2-butyl-1-propenyl disulphide (a mixture of *E* and *Z* isomers), 1-(1-methylthiopropenyl)-1-propenyl disulphide and 2-butyl-3-methylthioallyl disulphide (both as mixtures of diastereoisomers). The drug also contains a complex mixture of sesquiterpene umbelliferyl ethers mostly with a monocyclic or bicyclic terpenoid moiety; more recently (G. Appendino *et al.*, *Phytochemistry*, 1994, **35**, 183) three new sesquiterpene coumarin ethers have been isolated. Also present are asaresinol ferulate and free ferulic acid. For selected formulae see Fig. 22.19. The drug contains no free umbelliferone (distinction from galbanum). However, on boiling it with hydrochloric acid and filtering into ammonia, a blue fluorescence is produced owing to the formation of umbelliferone. Ferulic acid is closely related to umbellic acid and umbelliferone (both of which occur in galbanum).

Allied drugs. Galbanum and ammoniacum are oleo-gum-resins obtained, respectively, from *Ferula galbaniflua* and *Dorema ammoniacum*. Galbanum contains, besides umbelliferone, a number of umbelliferone ethers; also gum and up to 30% of volatile oil containing numerous mono- and sesquiterpenes, azulenes and sulphur-containing esters. Ammoniacum, listed in the *BHP*, contains free salicylic acid but no umbelliferone. The major phenolic constituent is ammoresinol; Appendino *et al.* (*Helv. Chim. Acta*, 1991, **74**, 495) isolated an epimeric mixture of prenylated chromandiones termed ammodoremin. The volatile oil (*c.* 0.5%) contains various terpenoids

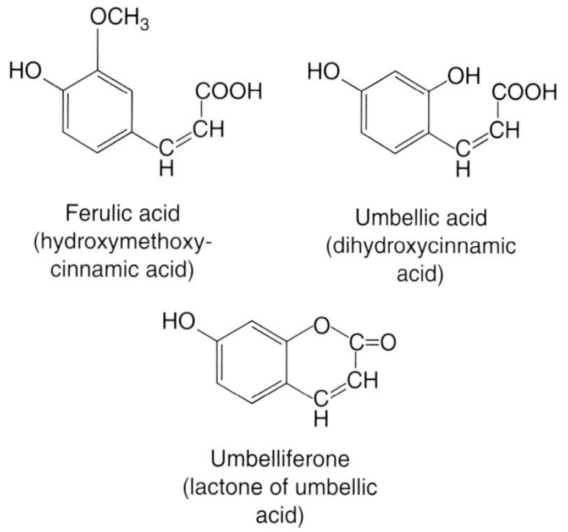

Fig. 22.19
Constituents of asafoetida.

with ferulene as the major component. The demonstration of the broad spectrum and antimicrobial activity of ammoniacum has supported its traditional use for chest infections (M. Rajani *et al.*, *Pharm. Biol.*, 2002, **40**, 534).

Uses. Asafoetida is included in the *BHP* (Vol. 1, 1990) and is employed for the carminative and expectorant properties of the volatile oil fraction. It is an ingredient of certain sauces.

Damiana

Damiana consists of the dried leaves of *Turnera diffusa* var. *aphrodisiaca* (Turneraceae), and probably other species of *Turnera*. The drug is collected in Bolivia and Mexico. The leaves are yellowish-green to green in colour, broadly lanceolate, shortly petiolate, and 10–25 cm long; margin with 3–6 teeth on each side; veins pinnate and prominent on the lower surface. The drug usually contains some of the reddish-brown, cylindrical twigs, flowers and spherical fruits. Damiana has an aromatic odour and taste. It contains 0.5–1.0% of volatile oil, from which thymol, α-copaene, δ-cadinene and calamenene have been isolated; in addition, a brown amorphous substance, damianin, resins and gum.

It would appear that in Mexico the wild populations of the plant are threatened by over-collection, and cultivation is recommended using micropropagation, the latter having now been shown to be a commercial feasibility (L. Alcaraz-Meléndez *et al.*, *Plant Cell Rep.*, 1994, **13**, 679.)

Damiana is traditionally used in Mexico and Southern USA to revive libido where subconscious causative factors are involved. Elixir of Damiana and Saw Palmetto or other admixtures are used as an aphrodisiac for men.

For a review of the genus *Turnera* (*93 references*), see S. Kumar *et al.*, *Pharm. Biol.*, 2005, **43**, 383.

Copaiba

Copaiba is an oleoresin obtained from the trunks of various species of *Copaifera* (Leguminosae) and contains at least 24 sesquiterpene hydrocarbons and a number of diterpenes. It was formerly used as a urinary antiseptic but has now been almost completely replaced by antibiotics and other drugs.

Eriodictyon leaf

Eriodictyon or Yerba Santa consists of the dried leaf of *Eriodictyon californicum* (Hydrophyllaceae), a low evergreen shrub of the hills and mountains of California and northern Mexico.

The leaves usually occur in fragments; when entire, they are lanceolate, 5–15 cm long and 1–3 cm wide. The apex is acute; the base slightly tapering into a short petiole. The margin is irregularly serrate or crenate-dentate. The upper surface is yellowish-brown to greenish-brown and covered with a glistening resin. The lower surface is greenish-grey to yellowish-grey, conspicuously reticulate, with greenish-yellow or brown veins, and minutely tomentose (cottony) between the reticulations. The leaves are thick and brittle. They have an aromatic odour and a balsamic bitter taste, which becomes sweetish and slightly acrid.

Eriodictyon contains volatile oil, resin, eriodictyol (see 'Hesperidin' and 'Eriodictyol'), homoeriodictyol, chrysoeriodictyol, xanthoeriodictyol, eriodonol, eriodictyonic acid and ericolin.

Yerba Santa is employed in the USA for the preparation of a fluid extract and Aromatic Eriodictyon Syrup, which is used to mask the taste of bitter and otherwise disagreeable medicines, particularly quinine. American Indians smoked or chewed the leaves as a cure for asthma. Some herbalists consider it an excellent expectorant. Externally it can be used for the treatment of bruises, insect bites, etc.

Gamboge

Gamboge is a gum-resin obtained from *Garcinia hanburii* (Guttiferae), a tree indigenous to South-East Asia.

Gamboge is a typical gum-resin, and when triturated with water, it forms a yellow emulsion. Good gamboge contains 70–80% of resin (gambogic acid) and 15–20% of water-soluble gum with which is associated an oxidase enzyme. Gamboge acts as a purgative but is now little used in human medicine. It is used as a pigment. For a report on its bioactivity, see A. Panthong *et al.*, *J. Ethnopharmacol.*, 2007, **111**, 335.

MASTIC

Mastic is a resin or, more correctly, an oleoresin containing little oil, obtained from various cultivated varieties of *Pistacia lentiscus* L. (Anacardiaceae); the *BP/EP* specifies var. *latifolius* Coss; another quoted in the literature is var. *chia* from the Greek island of Chios, which is the principal exporter.

The plant is an evergreen shrub and tapping is limited by law to the period 15 July–15 October. The base of the shrub is cleared of weeds, flattened and covered with a special white soil to receive some of the flow. The stem and larger branches are then wounded by means of a gouge-like instrument which makes an incision about 2 cm long and 3 mm deep. Each plant is tapped repeatedly for about 5 or 6 weeks, receiving in all about 200–300 wounds. A special tool is used for removing the tears which harden on the plant and the flat plates of mastic which collect on the ground. These are graded by the collector and regraded, washed and dried in a central depot before being exported in wooden boxes. Chios exports about 250 000 kg annually.

Mastic occurs in yellow or greenish-yellow rounded or pear-shaped tears about 3 mm diameter. The shape of the tears is sufficient to distinguish them from those of sandarac. The tears are brittle but become plastic when chewed. Odour, slightly balsamic; taste, mildly terebinthinate.

The resin component of mastic is a complex mixture. It contains tri-, tetra- and penta-cyclic triterpene acids and alcohols (for a report see F.-J. Marner *et al.*, *Phytochemistry*, 1991, **30**, 3790). About 2% of volatile oil is also present, the pharmacopoeial minimum being 1%; over 60 compounds have been reported from mastic and up to 250 recorded in plant oils. The principal components appear to be the monoterpene hydrocarbons α-pinene, β-myrcene and camphene. Four neutral novel triterpenoids and ten triterpenoid acids have now been characterized, see V. P. Papageorgiou *et al.*, *J. Chromat. A*, 1997,

769, 263. The acid value of about 50 (*BP*, 1980, not more than 70) distinguishes it from East Indian or Bombay mastic, which has an acid value of more than 100.

Mastic is used in the preparation of Compound Mastic Paint and as a microscopical mountant. In Greece and the Middle East mastic has been used for centuries as a protective agent for the stomach, and investigations at the University of Nottingham Medical School indicated success in the treatment of gastric ulcers. Research has shown that mastic will kill *Helicobacter pylori* at concentrations of 0.06 mg/ml (see F. U. Huwez *et al.*, *New Engl. J. Med.*, 1998, 339, 1946). Further studies were planned with patient volunteers infected with *H. pylori* (*Pharm. J.*, 2000, **264**, 459).

Sandarac

Sandarac is a resin obtained from the stem of *Tetraclinis articulata* (Cupressaceae), a tree 6–12 m high, which is found in North and North-west Africa and in Spain.

Sandarac occurs in small tears about 0.5–1.5 cm in length. These usually have an elongated, stalactic or cylindrical shape, globular or pear-shaped tears being relatively rare. The surface is covered with a yellowish dust, but the interior is more or less transparent, and if the tears are held up to the light, small insects can frequently be seen embedded in them. The drug is easily powdered and when chewed remains gritty, showing no tendency to form a plastic mass (distinction from mastic). The drug has a faint, terebinthinate odour, and a somewhat bitter taste.

Sandarac resin consists of sandarocopimaric acid (inactive pimaric acid), sandaracinic acid, sandaracinolic acid and sandaracoresene. The drug also contains a bitter principle and 0.26–1.3% of volatile oil.

Grindelia herb

Grindelia or gum plant consists of the dried leaves and flowering tops of *Grindelia camporum* (*G. robusta*), *G. humilis* and *G. squarrosa* (Compositae), collected in south-western USA. The plants are herbaceous with cylindrical stems, sessile or amplexicaul leaves, and resinous flower-heads each surrounded by an involucre of linear-lanceolate bracts. Odour, balsamic; taste, aromatic and bitter.

In the wild 2*n* and 4*n* forms occur and selection of the latter for cultivation should produce higher yields of resin (J. L. McLaughlin *et al.*, *Econ. Bot.*, 1986, **40**, 155).

Grindelia contains about 20% of resin, which contains a large number of labdane diterpene acids termed grindelanes and methyl esters (see B. A. Timmermann *et al.*, *Phytochemistry*, 1985, **24**, 1031; M. Adinolfi *et al.*, *ibid.*, 1988, **27**, 1878). The plants yield about 0.2% of a volatile oil containing over 100 components. Oil composition from the different species varies quantitatively with bornyl acetate and α-pinene the major components of the monoterpenoid fraction (see G. Kaltenbach *et al.*, *Planta Medica*, 1991, **57**, (Suppl. 2), A82). For a report on the oil content, and its antioxidant activity, of plants raised experimentally in Central Italy, see D. Fraternale *et al.*, *Fitoterapia*, 2007, **78**, 443.

The herb has been used for the treatment of bronchitis and asthma, but is now mainly employed in the form of a lotion for dermatitis produced by the poison ivy, *Rhus toxicodendron* (Anacardiaceae). Some grindelanes have been shown to have antifeeding deterrent activity towards aphids.

Guaiacum resin

Guaiacum resin is obtained from the heartwood of *Guaiacum officinale* and *G. sanctum* (Zygophyllaceae), small evergreen trees found in the dry coastal regions of tropical America. *Guaiacum officinale* is found on the coast of Venezuela and Colombia and in the West Indies, while *G. sanctum* occurs in Cuba, Haiti, the Bahamas and Florida. Little is now found in commerce.

Guaiacum resin occurs in large blocks or rounded tears about 2–3 cm diameter. The freshly fractured surface is brown and glassy. The powder is greyish but becomes green on exposure. Taste, somewhat acrid; odour, when warmed, aromatic. When free from woody debris, guaiacum is soluble in alcohol, chloroform and solutions of alkalis. An alcoholic solution gives a deep blue colour (guaiac-blue) on the addition of oxidizing agents such as ferric chloride. This colour is destroyed by reducing agents. Colophony, the most likely adulterant, may be detected by the cupric acetate test.

Some of the main resinous constituents are lignans. These are phenolic compounds having a C_{18} structure formed from two C_6–C_3 units (Table 21.7). Guaiaretic acid, which forms about 10% of guaiacum resin, is a diaryl butane.

The flowers, fruit and bark of the tree contain triterpenoid and nortriterpenoid saponins.

For use as a reagent the resin as extracted from the wood by means of chloroform is said to be the most sensitive. An alcoholic solution is used for the detection of blood stains, cyanogenetic glycosides, oxidase and peroxidase enzymes.

Guaiacum resin, included in the *BHP* (Vol. 1, 1990) is indicated for the treatment of chronic rheumatic conditions. It is a permitted food additive in the USA and in Europe.

COLOPHONY

Colophony (rosin) is the resin remaining in the still after removal of the volatile turpentine oil from the oleoresin of species of *Pinus* (see Turpentine Oil). Generally, the resin obtained from trees during their first year of tapping is of a lighter colour than that obtained subsequently. Traditionally, some 17 grades of rosin have been recognized, extending from the almost black wood rosin (B&F grades) through paler colours to the window glass (WG), water white (WW) and extra white (X) grades. For a detailed account of the oleoresin collection (cup and gutter method) and preparation of the rosin, see the 15th edition of this book.

Characters. The colophony described in the *BP/EP* occurs in translucent glassy masses of a pale yellow or amber colour. It is brittle and easily powdered. It fuses gradually at about 100°C, and at a higher temperature burns with a smoky flame, leaving not more than about 0.1% of ash. Colophony is insoluble in water but soluble in alcohol, ether, benzene and carbon disulphide.

Chemical tests
1. Dissolve about 0.1 g of powdered resin in 10 ml of acetic anhydride. Add one drop of sulphuric acid on a glass rod. Care should be taken to see that the apparatus used is dry, that the solution is cold and that concentrated sulphuric acid is used. On adding the acid a purple colour, rapidly changing to violet, is produced.
2. Shake a little powdered colophony with light petroleum and filter. Old samples of resin are usually much less soluble in this solvent than fresh ones. Shake the solution with about twice its volume of dilute solution of copper acetate. The petroleum layer becomes emerald-green in colour, a change which is due to the formation of the copper salt of abietic acid.

Constituents. Colophony contains resin acids (about 90%), neutral inert substances formerly known as resenes and esters of fatty acids.

The exact composition varies with biological source, preparation, age and method of storage.

The resin acids are isomeric diterpene acids. It will be noted that colophony has a high acid value of 150–180.

Before distillation the resin contains large amounts of (+)- and (−)-pimaric acids. During distillation the (+)-pimaric acid is stable but the (−)-pimaric acid undergoes isomeric change into abietic acid, the major constituent of the commercial resin (see formula, p. 264). On heating at 300°C abietic acid undergoes further molecular rearrangement to produce some neo-abietic acid. The commercial 'abietic acid' is prepared by digesting colophony with weak alcohol.

The abietane acids have been considerably investigated over recent years; they are obtained chiefly from colophony but are also present in other conifers of the Araucariaceae, Cupressaceae, Pinaceae and Podocarpaceae. Their activities are mainly antimicrobial, antiulcer and cardiovascular; some have filmogenic, surfactant and antifeedant properties.

Uses.   The amount of colophony used in pharmacy for the preparation of zinc oxide and other adhesive plasters, ointments, etc., is relatively small. Much rosin is artificially modified by hydrogenation or polymerization; products involving its use include paper size, adhesives, printing inks, rubber, linoleum, thermoplastic floor tiles and surface coatings.

Further reading

Keeling CI, Bohlman J 2006 Diterpene resin acids in conifers. Phytochemistry 67(22): 2415–2423. *A review focusing on recent discoveries in the chemistry, biosynthesis, molecular biology, regulation and biology. Many refs*

Ipomoea

Ipomoea (*Orizaba Jalap, Mexican Scammony Root*) is the dried root of *Ipomoea orizabensis* (Convolvulaceae), a convolvulaceous twining plant with a fusiform root about 60 cm long. The drug is collected in the Mexican State of Orizaba and is exported from Vera Cruz.

Orizaba was originally imported as a substitute or adulterant of jalap or its resin ('jalapin'). However, the resin is more soluble in ether than is jalap resin and more closely resembles that obtained from the root of *Convolvulus scammonia*, which was the original source of scammony resin.

Whole roots of ipomoea are rarely imported, and the drug usually consists of transverse or oblique slices about 3–10 cm wide and 2–4 cm thick.

The outer surface is covered with a greyish-brown, wrinkled cork. The transverse surface is greyish or brownish and shows about 3–6 concentric rings of fibrovascular bundles. The parenchymatous tissue of both bark and stele resembles that of jalap in containing starch and calcium oxalate. Like jalap, the section shows numerous scattered secretion cells with resinous contents. Odour, slight; taste, faintly acrid.

Ipomoea, when extracted with alcohol (90%), yields about 10–20% of a complex resinous mixture, of which about 65% is soluble in ether. The chief constituents of ipomoea resin are the methyl pentosides and other glycosides of jalapinolic acid and its methyl ester; these are the orizabins. Also isolated are the scammonins, the structures of which are indicated below. For details of these resin glycosides see B. Hernández-Carlos *et al.*, *J. Nat. Prod.*, 1999, **62**, 1096. Also present are sitosterol and other phytosterol glycosides.

Ipomoea is mainly used for the preparation of ipomoea resin. It resembles jalap in medicinal properties.

Jalap

Jalap consists of the dried tubercles or tuberous roots of *Ipomoea purga*, a large, twining plant indigenous to Mexico. Most of the drug is imported from eastern Mexico under the name of 'Mexican' or 'Vera Cruz' jalap. Convolvulaceous tubers with purgative properties were brought to Spain about 1565.

The traditional system of production in Central Vera Cruz has been described by A. Linajes *et al.* (*Econ. Bot.*, 1994, **48**, 84). Scarification of seeds prior to sowing is the secret of obtaining a 95% germination rate in 8 days. The productive period extends from July to February and the harvested tubers are smoke-dried in small wooden sheds using unseasoned *Liquidamber macrophylla* wood for fuel. During this process there is a weight loss of 50–75%. This method gives a product more resistant to fungal and insect attack than does simple drying. The yield is 2.4–3.0 tons of fresh root/hectare which can be increased, as in India, to 4.8 tons/hectare by the use of cow manure.

Jalap tubercles are fusiform, napiform or irregularly oblong in shape, and 3–5 cm long. They are extremely hard and heavy. The surface is covered with a dark brown, wrinkled cork, which is marked with lighter-coloured, transverse lenticels. The larger pieces may bear gashes, which have been made to facilitate drying. The tubercles may be softened for cutting by prolonged soaking in water. Cut transversely they show a greyish interior, a complete cambium ring fairly close to the outside and within it numerous irregular dark lines. The drug has a slight, smoky odour; the taste is at first sweetish, afterwards acrid. A description of the microscopy of jalap was given in the 11th edition.

Jalap contains 9–18% of resin contained in secretion cells and giving a yellow stain with iodine water. It may be extracted from the powdered drug with boiling alcohol (90%). On pouring a concentrated tincture into water, the resin is precipitated and may be collected, washed and dried. The complexity of these convolvulaceous resins has prevented, until recently, their isolation in a pure form and they have been studied by investigating the products of their hydrolysis (short-chain volatile fatty acids, hydroxy fatty acids and sugars). The main constituent of jalap resin is convolvulin, a substance with some 18 hydroxyl groups esterified with valeric, tiglic and exogonic acids. Exogonic acid is 3,6-6,9-dioxidodecanoic acid. (For its stereochemical structure see E. N. Lawson *et al.*, *J. Org. Chem.*, 1992, **57**, 353).

Exogonic acid

Jalap is a powerful hydragogue cathartic and was formerly extensively used either as standardized powder, as Jalap Resin or as Jalapin. The latter is the decolorized ether-insoluble portion of Jalap Resin.

Recently, using modern techniques, Japanese researchers have carried forward the investigation of those convolvulaceous species which are of relevance to the oriental market. Examples are given below.

Brazilian Jalap Rhizome

This is derived from *Ipomoea operculata* and constitutes a substitute for Mexican jalap. In a series of papers Ono and colleagues (see *Chem. Pharm. Bull.*, 1992, **40**, 1400 and references cited therein) characterized 18 operculins (ether-soluble resin glycosides). These resemble the other known jalapins in that they are monomers with similar intramolecular macrocyclic ester structures in the glycosidic acid moieties. However, their component acids (*n*-decanoic and *n*-dodecanoic acids) are characteristically different from those of previously known resin glycosides (isobutyric, 2-methylbutyric and tiglic acids), see 'Jalap' above. On alkaline hydrolysis a particular operculin will give a characteristic operculinic acid along with *n*-decanoic and *n*-dodecanoic acids. Operculinic acid E, for example, is 11S-jalapinolic acid 11-*O*-α-L-rhamnopyranosyl-

(1→2)-β-D-glucopyranoside. The formula for 11S-jalapinolic acid (common to all operculinic acids) is given below:

11S-Jalapinolic acid

Ipomoea batatus. This species, the sweet potato, is widely cultivated as a food but it has also traditional (Brazilian) medicinal uses and a number of pharmacological claims have been made for it. In 1979 Kawasaki *et al.* reported the roots to contain a mixture of hexa-, hepta- and octa-decylferulates; Noda *et al.* (*Chem. Pharm. Bull.*, 1992, **40**, 3163) isolated five new ether-soluble resin glycosides called simonins I–V. The arrangement of the acids in relation to the carbohydrate moieties of the molecule is illustrated by simonin I.

Simonin I

Similar compounds (stoloniferins) have been recorded in *Ipomoea stolonifera* (N. Noda *et al.*, *Phytochemistry*, 1998, **48**, 837).

The roots of *Convolvulus scammonia* (*vide supra*) contain ether-soluble resin glycosides called scammonins; they possess a glycosidic acid, e.g. scammonic acid A, and have an intramolecular macrocyclic ester structure involving various sugars (see H. Kogetsu *et al.*, *Phytochemistry*, 1991, **30**, 957).

VOLATILE OILS IN AROMATHERAPY

Aromatherapy is based primarily on the use of volatile oils, either singly or in admixture. They are administered in baths (drops of oil are added to the water and vigorously mixed), in compresses, in massage and as inhalations. For compress and massage usage the volatile oils are mixed with a suitable carrier (e.g. the fixed oils of apricot kernel, evening primrose, starflower, sweet almond to cite but a few) and for inhalation vaporizers and burners are available in addition to the traditional steam inhalation or use of the handkerchief or tissue.

A number of the oils used in aromatherapy have already been mentioned and include those from benzoin, black pepper, German chamomile, cinnamon leaf, clove, eucalyptus, fennel, frankincense, ginger, juniper berry, lavender, lemon, myrrh, neroli, orange, peppermint, pine, rose, sandalwood, spearmint, tea-tree and thyme. Others are listed below, citing: Botanical source; Geographical origin (but not necessarily the sole); Parts of the plant from which the oil is extracted; Extraction process; and Principal constituents. It must be remembered that volatile oils can contain over 100 constituents, most in very small amounts, and the principal components might not be those giving the oil its unique characteristics.

Basil. *Ocimum basilicum*, Labiatae; Egypt; Leaves and flowering tops; Distillation; Linalool, cineole, methyl chavicol.

Bergamot. *Citrus bergamia*, Rutaceae; Sicily; Peel; Expression; Linalyl acetate, linalool, limonene.

Cedarwood. *Cedrus atlantica*, Pinaceae; Morocco; Wood chips and shavings; Distillation; α-Cedrene, atlantone, atlantol.

Citronella. *Cymbopogon nardus*, Graminae; Sri Lanka; Grass leaves; Distillation; Geranyl acetate, citronellol, citronellal.

Clary sage. *Salvia sclarea*, Labiatae; Hungary; Leaves and flowering tops; Distillation; Linalyl acetate, linalool.

Cypress. *Cupressus sempervirens*, Cupressaceae; France; Tree needles and cones; Distillation; Pinene, carene, terpinolene, camphene.

Grapefruit. *Citrus paradisi*, Rutaceae; USA; Peel; Expression; Limonene.

Jasmine. *Jasminum officinale*, Oleaceae; India; Flowers; Solvent extraction; Benzyl acetate, linalyl acetate, benzyl alcohol, linalool.

Lemongrass. *Cymbopogon citratus*, Gramineae; India; Grass leaves; Distillation; Citral, geraniol, linalool.

Lime. *Citrus medica*, Rutaceae; Peru; Fruit; Distillation; Citral, limonene, linalool, camphene, sabinene.

Mandarin. *Citrus reticulata*, Rutaceae; Spain; Fruit peel; Expression; Limonene, terpenene, myrcene.

Marjoram (Sweet). Origanum majorana, Labiateae; Egypt; Dried leaves and flowering tops; Distillation; Terpinene, terpineol, myrcene, ocimene, sabinene, cymene, geranyl acetate.

Melissa. *Melissa officinalis*, Labiatae; Cultivated UK; Flowering tops; Distillation; Citral.

Myrtle. *Myrtus communis*, Myrtaceae; Morocco; Leaves and twigs; Distillation; Limonene, linalool, geraniol, myrtenol.

Palmarosa. *Cymbopogon martini*, Gramineae; Comoros; Grass leaves; Distillation; Geraniol, linalool, geranyl acetate.

Patchouli. *Pogostemon patchouli*, Labiatae; Indonesia, India, Europe, USA; Dried leaves; Distillation; Patchoulol, pogostol.

Petitgrain. *Citrus aurantium*, Rutaceae; Paraguay, France; Leaves and twigs; Distillation; Linalyl acetate, linalool.

Pine. *Pinus sylvestris*, Pinaceae; Austria; Pine needles; Distillation; Terpenes, sesquiterpenes, bornyl acetate.

Ravensara. *Ravensara aromatica*, Lauraceae; Madagascar; Leaves; Distillation; Estragole, pinene, caryophyllene.

Rose Absolute. *Rosa centifolia*, Rosaceae; Morocco; Fresh flowers; Solvent extraction; Similar constituents to Rose otto.

Rose Otto. *Rosa damascena*, Rosaceae; Bulgaria; Fresh flowers; Distillation; Citronellol, geraniol, 2-phenylethanol, nerol.

Vetiver. *Vetiveria zizanioides*, Gramineae; Indonesia, Reunion; Grass roots; Distillation; Alcohols, ketones.

Ylang Ylang. *Cananga odorata* var. *genuina*, Annonaceae; Madagascar, Reunion; Fresh flowers; Steam distillation; Acetates of geranyl and benzyl alcohols, linalool, caryophyllene.

Further reading
Lis-Balchin M 2006 Aromatherapy science, a guide for healthcare professionals. Pharmaceutical Press, London

23

Saponins, cardioactive drugs and other steroids

Plant materials containing saponins have long been used in many parts of the world for their detergent properties. For example, in Europe the root of *Saponaria officinalis* (Caryophyllaceae) and in South America the bark of *Quillaja saponaria* (Rosaceae). Such plants contain a high percentage of glycosides known as saponins (Latin *sapo*, soap) which are characterized by their property of producing a frothing aqueous solution. They also have haemolytic properties, and when injected into the blood stream, are highly toxic. The fact that a plant contains haemolytic substances is not proof that it contains saponins, and in the species examined by Wall (1961) only about half of those containing haemolytic substances actually contained saponins. When taken by mouth, saponins are comparatively harmless. Sarsaparilla, for example, is rich in saponins but is widely used in the preparation of non-alcoholic beverages.

Saponins have a high molecular weight and a high polarity and their isolation in a state of purity presents some difficulties. Often they occur as complex mixtures with the components differing only slightly from one another in the nature of the sugars present, or in the structure of the aglycone. Various chromatographic techniques have been employed for their isolation. As glycosides they are hydrolysed by acids to give an aglycone (sapogenin) and various sugars and related uronic acids. According to the structure of the aglycone or sapogenin, two kinds of saponin are recognized—the steroidal (commonly tetracyclic triterpenoids) and the pentacyclic triterpenoid types (see formulae below). Both of these have a glycosidal linkage at C-3 and have a common biogenetic origin via mevalonic acid and isoprenoid units.

Steroid skeleton   Pentacyclic triterpenoid skeleton

A distinct subgroup of the steroidal saponins is that of the steroidal alkaloids which characterize many members of the Solanaceae. They possess a heterocyclic nitrogen-containing ring, giving the compounds basic properties (as an example see solasodine, Fig. 23.5).

STEROIDAL SAPONINS

The steroidal saponins are less widely distributed in nature than the pentacyclic triterpenoid type. Phytochemical surveys have shown their presence in many monocotyledonous families, particularly the Dioscoreaceae (e.g. *Dioscorea* spp.), Agavaceae (e.g. *Agave* and *Yucca* spp.) and Smilacaceae (*Smilax* spp.). In the dicotyledons the occurrence of diosgenin in fenugreek (Leguminosae) and of steroidal alkaloids in *Solanum* (Solanaceae) is of potential importance. Some species of *Strophanthus* and *Digitalis* contain both steroidal saponins and cardiac glycosides (q.v.). Examples of saponins and their constituent sugars are given in Table 23.1.

Steroidal saponins are of great pharmaceutical importance because of their relationship to compounds such as the sex hormones, cortisone, diuretic steroids, vitamin D and the cardiac glycosides. Some are used as starting materials for the synthesis of these compounds. Diosgenin is the principal sapogenin used by industry but most yams, from which it is isolated, contain a mixture of sapogenins in the glycosidic form.

Table 23.1 Examples of steroidal saponins.

Steroidal saponin	Sugar components	Occurrence
Sarsaponin (Parillin)	3 glucose, 1 rhamnose	*Smilax* spp.
Digitonin	2 glucose, 2 galactose, 1 xylose	Seeds of *Digitalis purpurea* and *D. lanata*
Gitonin	1 glucose, 2 galactose, 1 xylose	Seeds and leaves of *D. purpurea* and seeds of *D. lanata*
Dioscin	1 glucose, 2 rhamnose	*Dioscorea* spp.

As with cardiac glycosides, the stereochemistry of the molecule is of some importance, although not so much so for cortisone manufacture. Natural sapogenins differ only in their configuration at carbon atoms 3, 5 and 25, and in the spirostane series the orientation at C-22 need not be specified (cf. steroidal alkaloids). Mixtures of the C-25 epimers—for example, diosgenin (Δ^5,25α-spirosten-3β-ol) and yamogenin (Δ^5,25β-spirosten-3β-ol)—are of normal occurrence and their ratio, one to the other, is dependent upon factors such as morphological part and stage of development of the plant. In some instances in the plant, the side-chain which forms ring F of the sapogenin is kept open by glycoside formation as in the bisdesmosidic saponin sarsaparilloside of *Smilax aristolochiaefolia*.

BIOGENESIS OF STEROIDAL SAPONINS

Steroidal saponins arise via the mevalonic acid pathway; the preliminary stages have been discussed in Chapter 18. A scheme for the subsequent cyclization of squalene to give cholesterol is illustrated in Fig. 23.1. Cholesterol, the wide distribution of which in plants has only relatively recently been shown, can be incorporated into a number of C_{27} sapogenins without side-chain cleavage (Fig. 23.2), although it is not necessarily an obligatory precursor. Extensive investigations involving whole plants, homogenates and cell cultures have been performed to elucidate these detailed pathways, including the origin of the 25-epimers (e.g. diosgenin and yamogenin).

As early as 1947 Marker and Lopez had postulated that steroidal saponins exist in plants in a form where the side-chain is held open by glycoside formation. However, direct evidence for the natural occurrence

of these compounds was not forthcoming for another 20 years. It has been shown that such open-chain saponins are, like the more common ones, formed from cholesterol. In *Dioscorea* homogenates one such compound has been converted to dioscin (a diosgenin glycoside) (Fig. 23.3).

NATURAL STEROIDS FOR THE PRODUCTION OF PHARMACEUTICALS

Although *total* synthesis of some medicinal steroids is employed commercially, there is also a great demand for natural products which will serve as starting materials for their *partial* synthesis.

As indicated in Fig. 23.4, which illustrates the range of steroids required medicinally, cortisone and its derivatives are 11-oxosteroids, whereas the sex hormones, including the oral contraceptives, and the diuretic steroids have no oxygen substitution in the C-ring. Fig. 23.5 shows some of the more important natural derivatives which are available in sufficient quantity for synthetic purposes. Hecogenin with C-ring substitution provides a practical starting material for the synthesis of the corticosteroids, whereas diosgenin is suitable for the manufacture of oral contraceptives and the sex hormones. Diosgenin, however, can also be used for corticosteroid synthesis by the employment, at a suitable stage in the synthesis, of a microbiological fermentation to introduce oxygen into the 11α-position of the pregnene nucleus.

Efforts are constantly being made to discover new high-yielding strains of plants and to assure a regular supply of raw material by the cultivation of good-quality plants. Hardman in a review on steroids (*Planta Med.*, 1987, **53**, 233) recorded that, annually, the American *Chemical Abstracts* contained some 3000 references pertinent to plant steroids or related compounds. Some of the better-known examples of steroidal sapogenins and their sources are given in Table 23.2. (For a review, tabulating over 200 sapogenins, see A. V. Patel *et al.*, *Fitoterapia*, 1987, **58**, 67.)

Dioscorea species

Tubers of many of the dioscoreas (yams) have long been used for food, as they are rich in starch. In addition to starch, some species contain steroidal saponins, others alkaloids. From a suitable source the sapogenins are isolated by acid hydrolysis of the saponin. Previous fermentation of the material for some 4–10 days often gives a better yield. The water-insoluble sapogenin is then extracted with a suitable

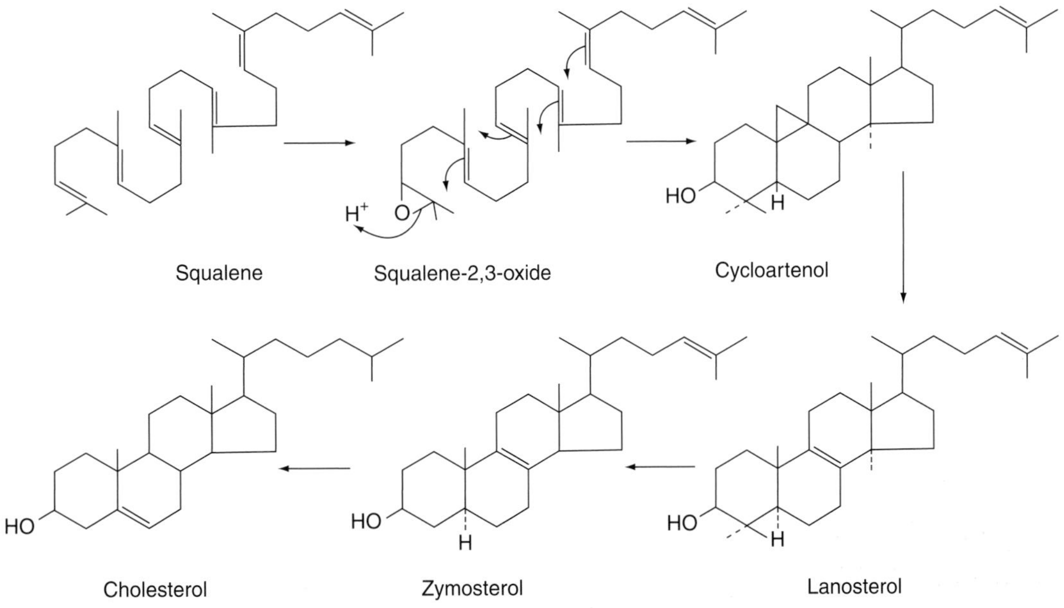

Fig. 23.1
Possible route for the formation of cholesterol in higher plants and algae.

Squalene   Squalene-2,3-oxide   Cycloartenol

Cholesterol   Zymosterol   Lanosterol

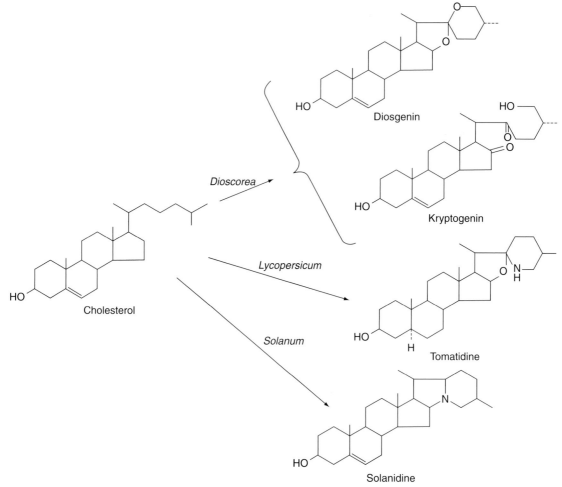

Fig. 23.2
Some plant metabolites of cholesterol.

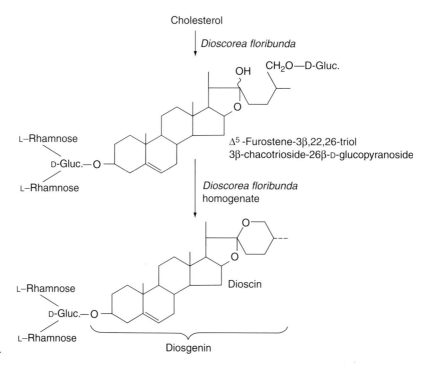

Fig. 23.3
Formation and metabolism of an
open-chain saponin in *Dioscorea*.

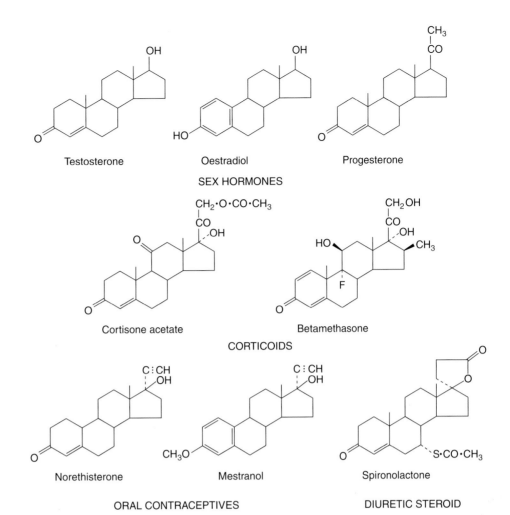

Fig. 23.4
Examples of structures of therapeutically active steroids.

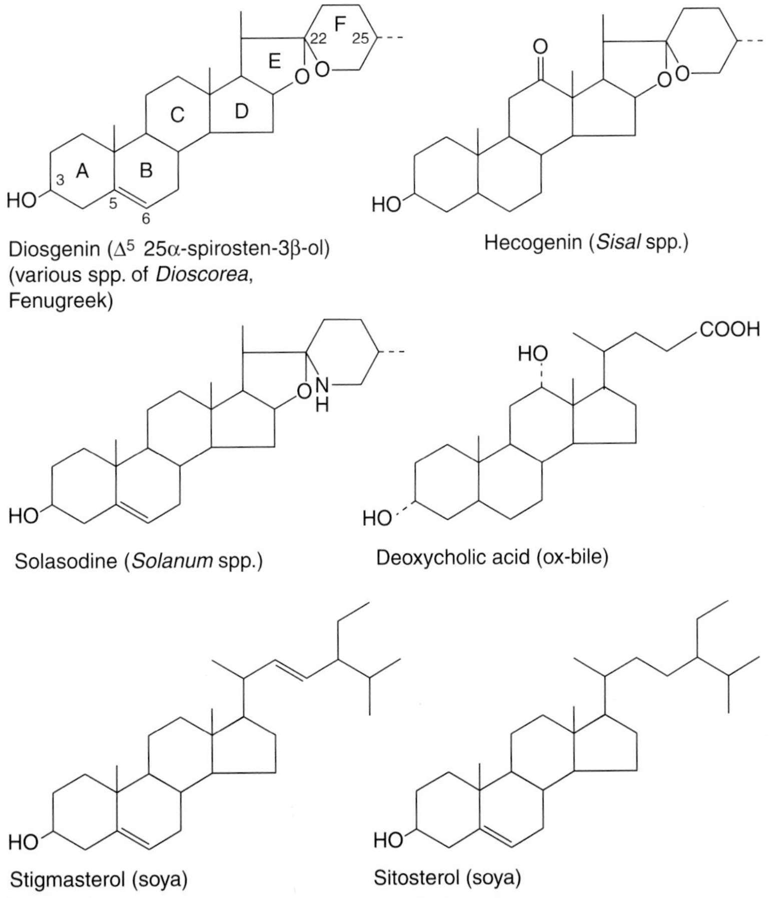

Testosterone   Oestradiol   Progesterone

SEX HORMONES

Cortisone acetate   Betamethasone

CORTICOIDS

Norethisterone   Mestranol   Spironolactone

ORAL CONTRACEPTIVES   DIURETIC STEROID

Fig. 23.5
Some naturally occurring steroids.

Diosgenin (Δ⁵ 25α-spirosten-3β-ol)
(various spp. of *Dioscorea*,
Fenugreek)

Hecogenin (*Sisal* spp.)

Solasodine (*Solanum* spp.)

Deoxycholic acid (ox-bile)

Stigmasterol (soya)

Sitosterol (soya)

23

Table 23.2 Some steroidal sapogenins and their sources.

Sapogenin	Species	Location
Diosgenin	*Dioscorea sylvatica*	Transvaal and Natal
	D. mexicana and *D. composita*	Mexico and Central America
	D. collettii, D. pathaica and *D. nipponica*	China
	D. floribunda	Guatemala and cultivated in India
	D. deltoidea and *D. prazeri*	India
	D. tokoro	Japan
	Costus speciosus	India
	Kallstroemia pubescens	Tropical America; introduced into West Brazil
	Trillium spp.	North America
	Trigonella foenum-graecum	India, Egypt, Morocco
Hecogenin	*Agave sisalana*	Subtropical America and cultivated in Kenya for sisal and saponin
	A. rigida	Mexico
	Hechtia texensis	Central America
Sarsapogenin	*Yucca* spp., *Smilax* spp.	Central America
Sarmentogenin	*Strophanthus* spp.	Africa

organic solvent. Both wild and cultivated plants are used. Cultivation requires attention to correct soil and drainage, support for the vines and freedom from weeds, virus, fungus and insect attack. According to the species, the tubers reach maturity in 3–5 years and on average, yield 1–8% of total sapogenin.

Until 1970 diosgenin isolated from the Mexican yam was the sole source for steroidal contraceptive manufacture. With the nationalization of the Mexican industry, however, prices were increased to such an extent that manufacturers switched to hecogenin for corticosteroids, to other sources of diosgenin and to the use of the steroidal alkaloids of *Solanum* species. Total synthesis also became economically feasible and is now much used. More recently, the economics of steroid production have again changed in that China is now exporting large quantities of diosgenin; it is of high quality, being free of the 25β-isomer yamogenin, although this is of no commercial significance, and is reasonably priced. Three of the many *Dioscorea* spp. found in China and used commercially are given in Table 23.2; the tubers of these yield 2% of diosgenin, with the average content of diosgenin for the main areas of production (Yunnan Province and south of the Yangtze River) being 1%.

Sisal

Hecogenin is obtained commercially as the acetate in about 0.01% yield from sisal leaves (*Agave sisalana*). In East Africa, from leaf 'waste' stripped from the leaves during removal of the fibre, a hecogenin-containing 'sisal concentrate' is produced. From this the 'juice' is separated and allowed to ferment for 7 days. The sludge produced contains about 80% of the hecogenin originally present in the leaves; steam at 1380 kPa pressure is employed to complete the hydrolysis of the original glycosides. By filtration and drying a concentrate containing about 12% hecogenin and varying amounts of other sapogenins is produced. This crude material is shipped for further processing and cortisone manufacture. Hecogenin is also produced in Israel

and China. A number of new steroidal saponins have been isolated from the dried fermented residues of Chinese *A. sisalana* forma Dong No. 1 (see Yi Ding *et al., Chem. Pharm. Bull.*, 1993, **41**, 557).

A survey of 34 species of *Agave* by Blunden and colleagues in 1978 showed that the extracts of most yielded steroidal sapogenins. Previously it had been shown that certain commercial samples of crude sapogenins from *A. sisalana* also contained the dihydroxy steroid rockogenin, sometimes in appreciable quantity; this compound appears to be an artefact formed during processing and should be avoided. A dihydroxyspirostane, barbourgenin, has been described (G. Blunden *et al., J. Nat. Prod.*, 1986, **49**, 687). *Agave* hybrids with a high hecogenin content and relatively free of tigogenin, with which it is usually associated, have been developed. Gbolade *et al.* (*Fitoterapia*, 1992, **63**, 45) reported on factors (season, geographical location) affecting steroidal sapogenin levels in Nigerian *Agave* and *Furcraea* species.

Another genus of the Agavaceae which has been systematically studied for the presence of steroidal compounds is *Cordyline* in which many sapogenins, including 1,3-dihydroxysapogenins, have been detected.

FENUGREEK

Although included in this section as a potential industrial source of diosgenin, the seeds of *Trigonella foenum-graecum* L. (Leguminosae) are also described in the *BP* and *EP*. However their principal current use is as a spice; India, Morocco and Egypt among others being important producers.

The very hard seeds have a strong characteristic odour and are irregularly rhomboidal and oblong or square in outline. They are somewhat flattened and are divided into two unequal parts by a groove in the widest surfaces. Their shape and size, and position of the embryo and hilum are shown in Fig. 23.6. The *BP/EP* describes the seeds as brown to reddish-brown but in commerce olive-green or yellow-brown samples are often

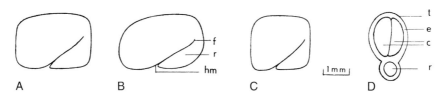

Fig. 23.6
Commercial fenugreek seed. A, Morocco, Israel; B, Ethiopia; C, India, Pakistan; D, transverse section of a seed. c, Cotyledons; e, endosperm; f, furrow; hm, hilum and micropyle region; r, radicle; t, testa. (After Fazli and Hardman, *Trop. Sci.*, 1968 **10**, 66.)

encountered. Microscopically the testa and hypodermis are characteristic and the mucilage-containing endosperm enables the swelling index (q.v.) of the seeds (not less than six) to be used as a test of purity.

Fenugreek contains the simple pyridine-type alkaloid trigonelline; this base, also reported in garden peas, hemp seed, coffee and many other products was first isolated and described by Jahns in 1885. Today it serves as the reference substance for the *BP/EP* TLC identification test for the drug. Pharmaceutical manufacturing interest lies in a number of steroidal sapogenins, particularly diosgenin which is contained in the oily embryo. Fazli and Hardman investigated a number of commercial samples of seed as possible commercial sources of diosgenin (see reference in Fig. 23.6) and reported contents of 0.8–2.2% expressed on a moisture-free basis. In 1986, Gupta and colleagues isolated a series of furostanol glycosides (F-ring opened) named trigofoenocides A–G. In a series of papers, further furostanol glycosides designated trigoneosides Ia, Ib–XIIa have been reported in Egyptian seeds (T. Murakami *et al.*, *Chem. Pharm. Bull.*, 2000, **48**, 994). As with dioscoreas, the yield of diosgenin is increased by fermentation of the seeds prior to acid hydrolysis. Although the diosgenin yield is lower than that of the dioscoreas, fenugreek is an annual plant which will also give fixed oil, mucilage, flavouring extracts and high-protein fodder as side-products. A number of Hardman's registered varieties have been subjected to field trials in the UK. However, as long as other cheap sources of diosgenin are available commercially, fenugreek must be regarded as a fall-back source for this sapogenin.

A non-essential amino acid, 4-hydroxyisoleucine, first identified by Fowden *et al.* in 1973, constitutes up to 80% of the free amino acid composition of fenugreek seeds and has been shown to possess insulin-stimulating properties both *in vitro* and *in vivo* (C. Haefelé *et al.*, *Phytochemistry*, 1997, **44**, 563). Some 39 components of the volatile oil fraction have been identified.

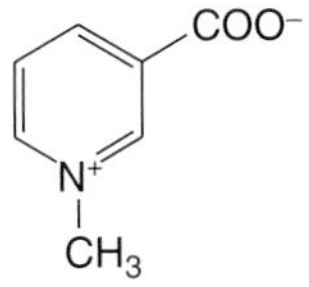

Trigonelline

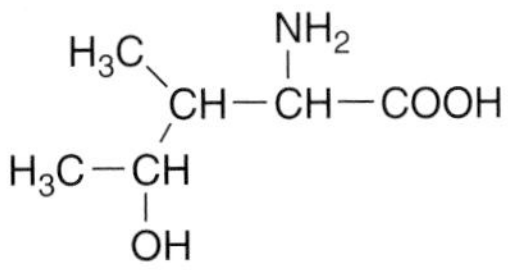

4-Hydroxyisoleucine

Based on mucilage content, the *BP/EP* sets a swelling index of not less than 6.0 for the powdered seeds.

In addition to its use as a spice and potential source of diosgenin fenugreek is widely employed in traditional systems of medicine. Its antidiabetic, cholesterol-lowering, anti-inflammatory, antipyretic, antiulcer and anticancer properties have been demonstrated.

Further reading

Petropoulos GJ (ed), Hardman R (series ed) 2002 Fenugreek: The genus *Trigonella*. CRC Press, Taylor and Francis Group, Boca Raton, FL, 200 pp. *646 refs*

Solanum species

This large genus (over 1000 spp.) is noted for the production of C_{27} steroidal alkaloids in many species. Some of these alkaloids are the nitrogen analogues of the C_{27} sapogenins (e.g. solasodine and diosgenin:

Fig. 23.5). Another series of C_{27} compounds contain a tertiary nitrogen in a condensed ring system (e.g. solanidine; Fig. 23.2). These compounds can also be employed in the partial synthesis of steroidal drugs, and a number of companies have devoted considerable attention to commercial production. Species so exploited are *Solanum laciniatum, S. khasianum* (a nearly spineless variety has been produced) and *S. aviculare*; trials on the production of *S. marginatum* have been conducted in South America. Zenk and colleagues have assayed over 250 spp. of *Solanum* for solasodine. A number of new glycosides have been isolated from *S. dulcamara* leaves and include two based on tigogenin and two on soladulcidine.

The steroidal alkaloids were reviewed in 1993 by Atta-ur-Rahman and M. I. Choudhary (*Methods in Plant Biochemistry* (ed. P. G. Waterman) Vol. 8. Academic Press, London, p. 451).

Soya bean sterols

The soya (soy, soja) plant, *Glycine max* (*G. soya*) (Leguminosae) is extensively cultivated for its seeds, which are rich in oil and protein. The seeds also contain appreciable quantities of the phytosterols stigmasterol and sitosterol (Fig. 23.5). Although not sapogenins, they are included here because they are now used extensively for steroid synthesis. They are obtained as byproducts of soap-making, being components of the unsaponifiable matter of the fixed oil. Pure stigmasterol, with its unsaturated side-chain is amenable to chemical conversion to suitable starting materials and can replace diosgenin. But it was more recently that sitosterol, the saturated side-chain of which could not be removed chemically without ring fragmentation, became commercially useful as the result of the discovery of a suitable microbiological side-chain removal. Both phytosterols are now processed by microorganisms. Similar phytosterols are found in other products—for example, cotton-seed oil, tall-oil (from the wood-pulp industry) and sugarcane wax.

For details of the soya isoflavones and their dietary importance, see Chapter 32: *The plant nutraceuticals*.

Sarsaparilla root

Sarsaparilla consists of the dried roots and sometimes also of the rhizomes of species of *Smilax* (Liliaceae, modern authors, Smilacaceae). The determination of the exact geographic and botanical sources of the numerous varieties which have from time to time been imported has been a matter of some difficulty (see Table 23.3).

The plants produce numerous roots, 3 m or so long, which are attached to a short rhizome. The roots are cut, sufficient, however, remaining in the ground for the plant to resume its growth. Sometimes

Table 23.3 Varieties of sarsaparilla.

Variety and geographic source	Synonyms	Botanical source
Mexican (Southern Mexico, Guatemala, British Honduras)	Vera Cruz or Grey	*Smilax aristolochiaefolia*
Honduras (Guatemala, British Honduras, Honduras, cultivated in Jamaica)	Brown	*S. regelii*
Ecuadorian and Peruvian	Guayaquil	*S. febrifuga*
Central American	Costa Rica or 'Jamaican'	Undetermined spp.

the rhizomes as well as the roots are collected. After drying in the sun the drug is made into bundles and the bundles into bales.

Sarsaparilla is imported in large bales bound with wire. Each bale usually contains numerous bundles of approximately uniform size. These consist of long roots, with or without pieces of rhizome and aerial stems. The commercial varieties (Table 23.4) differ from one another in colour, ridges and furrows; in the presence or absence of rhizome and aerial stems; in the relative proportions of cortex, wood and pith, as seen in transverse section; in their microscopical structure. The drug is nearly odourless but has a somewhat sweetish and acrid taste. Owing to the presence of saponins, aqueous extractives froth readily.

Much chemical work has been done on sarsaparillas without proper botanical identification of the material. Different species contain one or more steroidal saponins. Two isomeric genins are known: smilagenin and sarsasapogenin. These differ only in their configuration at C-25 and correspond to the reduced forms of diosgenin and yamogenin respectively. The principal crystalline glycoside of *Smilax aristolochiaefolia* is parillin (sarsasaponin, sarsasaponoside); it was first isolated from a sample of Jamaica sarsaparilla in 1913 by Power and Salway. On hydrolysis it gives sarsasapogenin, three molecules of glucose and one of rhamnose. Sarsaparilloside, contained in the same species, is a bisdesmosidic saponin (i.e. it possesses two distinct glycosyl groupings, in this case at C-3 and C-26) and represents the parillin molecule with an opened F-ring stabilized by glucosylation.

Uses. Sarsaparilla formerly enjoyed a high reputation in the treatment of syphilis, rheumatism and certain skin diseases. It is included in the *BHP* (1960) where it is indicated in the treatment of psoriasis and eczema, and for rheumatism and rheumatoid arthritis. Its action would appear to arise from the steroid content of the roots. Sarsaparilla is widely used as a vehicle, and large quantities are employed in the manufacture of non-alcoholic drinks. The genins are used in the partial synthesis of cortisone and other steroids.

Black Cohosh

Black Cohosh, Cimicifuga *BHP* 1983, is the dried rhizome and roots of *Actea racemosa* L. syn. *Cimicifuga racemosa* [L.], Nutt., family Ranunculaceae. This perennial plant is native to Canada and the northern American states and was well-known to the native Americans of these areas. The drug contains substances with endocrine activity and extracts have been widely employed in herbal medicine to treat menopausal and other female disorders, as well as various rheumatic conditions. However, in the 1990s doubts arose over its safety following reports concerning its hepatotoxicity; restrictions on its use have now been applied in a number of countries.

The rhizomes contain a number of triterpenoid glycosides, including actein, 23-epi-26-deoxyactein and cimiracemoside C. Cimicifugoside

M and cimifugin can specifically serve as indicators for species identification (K. He *et al.*, *Planta Med.*, 2002, **66**, 635). Phenyl propanoside esters are also present including cimiracemates A–D together with ferulic acid, isoferulic acid and methyl caffeate (S.-N. Chen *et al.*, *Phytochemistry*, 2002, **61**, 609). For other reports, see M. Nishida *et al.*, *Chem. Pharm. Bull.*, 2003, **51**, 1215; H. Yoshitsu *et al.*, *Chem. Pharm. Bull.*, 2006, **54**, 1322.

Actein

Cimiracemate A

BUTCHER'S BROOM

Butcher's broom, *Ruscus aculeatus* L. family Liliaceae, is a perennial, rigid, dark green much-branched bush, 2–3 feet in height. The leaf-like structures, twisted at the base and terminating in a sharp point, are actually cladodes—flattened stems or internodes that resemble and function as leaves. Small white flowers that arise in the axils of scarious bracts are followed by red berries, which appear situated on the surface of the cladodes.

The species is found in woods and dry places, extending across southern Europe to the Caucasus, and northward to Belgium. It is common in some southern areas of England.

The *BP/EP* drug consists of the dried, whole or broken roots and rhizomes of the plant. These are collected in autumn and dried to give yellow, knotty pieces of rhizome up to 10 cm in length, showing stem scars on the upper surface and roots and root-scars on the lower surface. A very hard, central cylinder can easily be removed from the outer layer.

Microscopical characteristics, as seen in the powder, include cells with thickened beaded walls with large oval pits, thin-walled

Table 23.4 Macroscopical characters of sarsaparilla.

	Mexican	Honduras	Ecuadorian	Central American
Bundles	Up to 65 m long. Rhizomes and stems up to 10%	50–75 cm long. Roots only	About 50 cm long. Rhizomes and stems up to 10%	About 45 cm long. Roots only
Diameter of roots	3.5–6 mm	2–5.5 mm	2–6 mm	1–4.5 mm
Colour	Greyish-reddish- or yellowish-brown	Reddish-brown to dark brown	Reddish-brown to purplish	Reddish-brown to yellowish brown
Hypodermal and endodermal cells	Horse-shoe thickening	Uniform thickening	Variable. Sometimes not uniform thickening	Uniform thickening

parenchyma containing calcium oxalate, thick-walled fibres, and small vessels.

The rhizomes of this plant contain saponins related to those of *Dioscorea*; thus, one sapogenin is 1β-hydroxydiosgenin (ruscogenin). The plant glycosides involve up to three sugars attached at the C-1 hydroxyl with glucose terminating an uncyclized side-chain at C-26 (for detailed structures see Bombardelli *et al.*, *Fitoterapia*, 1972, **43**, 3). In a series of publications on *Ruscus aculeatus* M. Yoshikawa *et al.* have described many more saponins of both the spirostanol and furostanol series and recently, a new saponin which is unique in having a diglucoside unit at C-23 of the spirostanol skeleton (*Phytochemistry*, 1999, **51**, 689). Both the alcoholic extract of the roots and the ruscogenins themselves have anti-inflammatory activity, produce diminished capillary permeability and exert a vasoconstrictor effect in the peripheral blood vessels. On the continent of Europe ointments and suppositories containing the active constituents are available for the treatment of conditions responding to the above effects.

The *BP/EP* TLC test for identity uses stigmasterol and ruscogenins as reference substances and a vanillin reagent for their visualization. A minimum of 1.0% total sapogenins, expressed as ruscogenins (mixture of neoruscogenin and ruscogenin) is specified; liquid chromatography is used for the assay.

Allied species. Various ruscogenins and a major new saponin have been detected in the rhizomes of *Ruscus colchicus* and *R. hypoglossum* (E. de Combarieu *et al.*, *Fitoterapia*, 2002, **73**, 583; 2003, **74**, 423, corrigendum).

ELEUTHEROCOCCUS

The drug Siberian Ginseng (*BP/EP, BHP*) consists of the dried, whole or cut organs of *Eleutherococcus senticosus* Maxim. [*Acanthopanax senticosus* (Rupr. et Maxim.) Harms], family Araliaceae. The plant is native to China and is now cultivated there and in Russia, Japan and Korea.

Characters. The pale brown, uneven rhizomes, up to 4 cm in diameter, bear the scars of aerial stems and on the lower surface are roots and root scars. The fracture is fibrous and the internal surface light brown to pale yellow. The cylindrical roots are of variable length, up to about 1 cm in diameter, knotty and somewhat branched. When dry the bark is not easily removed from the underlying xylem; commercially it may be removed at harvest and both wood and bark used. Features of the powder include lignified fibres, reticulate and border-pitted vessels, parenchymatous cells containing cluster crystals of calcium oxalate and secretory canals with brown contents. Odour faintly aromatic; taste bitter and persistent.

Constituents. The rhizomes and roots contain a number of constituents termed eleutherocides (A to G; M). These, however, are not all of the same chemical group but include the phenyl propane glycosides eleutheroside B (syringin) and its aglycone sinapyl alcohol; also the lignans (−)-syringaresinol diglucoside (E) and its stereoisomer (D) (formulae Table 21.7), together with caffeic acid and its ethyl ester, chlorogenic acid and coniferaldehyde. Coumarins include coumarin, isofraxidin 7-glucoside (B₁) and sesamin (B₄). A group of heteroglycans (eleutherans A to G) have been studied for their hypoglycaemic activity. Other constituents include hedera-saponin (M), daucosterol (A) and volatile oil, about 0.8%.

The *BP/EP* requires a minimum content of 0.8% for the sum of eleutheroside B and eleutheroside E determined by liquid chromatography using UV spectrophotometric absorption at 220 nm and measurement of peak areas. These eleutherosides are also characterized by the TLC test for identity.

DNA analysis has been used to authenticate Japanese and Chinese commercial samples of the drug (T. Maruyama *et al.*, *Planta Medica*, 2008, **74**, 787).

Uses. Eleutherococcus has been used in Chinese medicine since antiquity for the treatment of rheumatoid complaints and for its revitalization properties. For many years, its adaptogenic qualities have been utilized in former USSR countries and now in W. Europe it is employed as a tonic in states of fatigue.

Further reading
Davydov M, Krikorian AD 2000 *Eleutherococcus senticosus* (Rupr. and Maxim.) (Araliaceae) as an adaptogen: a closer look. J. Ethnopharmacology 72: 345–393. *An extensive discussion including chemical constituents, numerous formulae, over 200 refs*

GINSENG

For some 2000 years the roots of *Panax ginseng* C. A. Meyer (Araliaceae) have held an honoured place in Chinese medicine. Today it is a product of world-wide usage. Production is principally confined to China, Korea and Siberia, although it is cultivated commercially on a small scale in Holland, England, Germany and France (Champagne district).

The most expensive ginseng is that derived from Korean root. The plant, about 50 cm tall with a crown of dark green verticillate leaves and small green flowers giving rise to clusters of bright red berries, is cultivated under thatched covers and harvested when 6 years old. Sun-drying of the root, after removal of the outer layers, produces white ginseng, whereas the red ginseng is obtained by first steaming the root, followed by artificial drying and then sun-drying. Rootlets are numerous on the lower surface of white ginseng but normally absent from red ginseng. The roots are graded and packed. Nineteenth-century descriptions record the care then taken with the preparation, silk, cotton and paper wrappings being used according to the quality of the drug; the wrapped roots were finally stored in containers with quicklime. Small roots are processed separately and form a separate article of commerce. The *BP/EP* recognizes both red and white ginseng.

The scraping of the roots before drying would appear to be disadvantageous because histochemical tests and GLC analysis show the active saponins to be located outside the root cambium.

Constituents. *P. ginseng* roots have been thoroughly studied by modern methods of analysis and, of the many compounds isolated, the medicinal activity appears to reside largely in a number of dammarane-type saponins termed ginsenosides by Japanese workers and panaxosides by Russian workers. These two series of compounds, all now generally termed ginsenosides, are glycosides respectively derived from the diol 20(S)-protopanaxadiol and the triol 20(S)-protopanaxatriol. Examples of the former are ginsenosides R_{b1}, R_{b2} and R_{b4} and of the latter ginsenosides (panaxosides) R_e, R_f, R_{g1}, R_{g2} (see Fig. 23.7). Acid hydrolysis of these saponins involves ring closure of the aglycone giving either panaxadiol or panaxatriol (Fig. 23.7). Some 30 ginsenosides have been named, although not all fit into the above scheme, e.g. ginsenoside R_o is an oleanolic acid derivative. Glucose is the principal sugar involved with some input of arabinose and rhamnose.

The *BP/EP* specifies a minimum of 0.40% for the sum of ginsenosides R_{g1} and R_{b1}; this is determined by liquid chromatography of a methanolic extract using a reference solution containing the two ginsenosides to he assayed, with absorption measurements at 203 nm. TLC is used as a test for identity and to exclude substitution with *P. quinquifolium*, which contains no ginsenoside Rf.

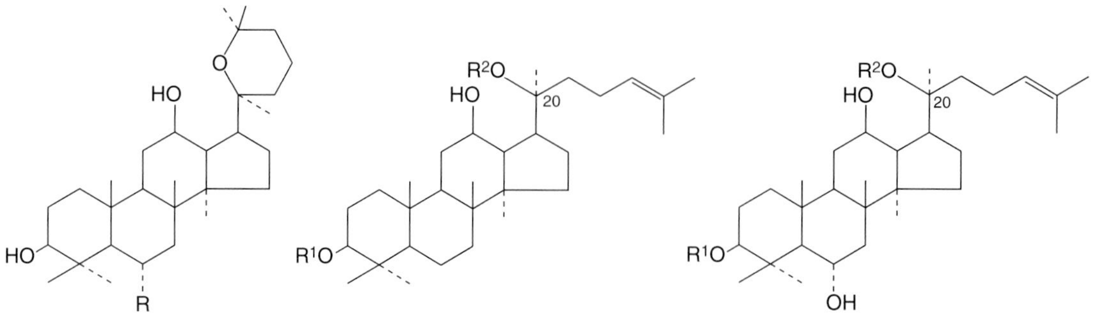

Panaxadiol, R = H
Panaxatriol, R = OH

20(S)-Protopanaxadiol,
$R^1 = R^2 = H$

Ginsenoside Rb1,
R^1 = Gluc (1–2) gluc
R^2 = Gluc (1–6) gluc

20(S)-Protopanaxatriol,
$R^1 = R^2 = H$

Ginsenoside Rg1,
$R^1 = R^2$ = gluc.

Fig. 23.7
Steroids associated with ginseng.

Two other groups of compounds present in the root which have known therapeutic activity are high molecular weight polysaccharides (glycans) and acetylenic compounds. The glycans of *P. ginseng* have been named panaxans (A–U); panaxans A and B have been shown to be constituted mainly of α-(1 $\rightarrow$ 6) linked D-glucopyranose units with C-3 branching and a small component of peptide. (For the isolation of other polysaccharides termed ginsenans see M. Tomoda *et al.*, *Biol. Pharm. Bull.*, 1993, **16**, 1087.) Those glycans tested have hypoglycaemic, antiulcer and immunological properties. One acidic polysaccharide MW 150000, originally isolated in 1993, and composed of 3.7% protein, 47.1% hexoses and 43.1% galacturonic acid, has antineoplastic immuno-stimulant properties.

A considerable number of mainly C_{17}, but also C_{14}, polyacetylenic alcohols have been isolated from the roots in recent years and are typified by panaxynol and panaxydol (Fig. 23.8). These compounds have been shown to have antitumour properties and Japanese patents exist for their isolation and derivatization. The cytotoxic activity of the C_{17}-polyacetylenes against leukaemia cells has been shown to be almost 20 times greater than that for the C_{14}-compounds (Y. Fujimoto *et al.*, *Phytochemistry*, 1992, **31**, 3499). K. Hirakura *et al.* have characterized a series of polyacetylenes named ginsenoynes A–K (see *Phytochemistry*, 1992, **31**, 899 and references cited therein) and subsequently (*ibid.*, 1994, **35**, 963) three new linoleoylated polyacetylenes.

Other constituents include sesquiterpenes (panacene, β-elemene, panasinsanol A and B, ginsenol, etc.) to be found in the volatile oil (0.05–0.1%), together with various monoterpenes and monoterpene alcohols. Three minor sesquiterpenes recently identified are panaxene, panaginsene and ginsinsene (R. Richter *et al.*, *Phytochemistry*, 2005, **66**, 2706). Lignans of the dibenzocyclooctadiene type have been isolated from Korean Red Ginseng (Fig. 23.8). Minor components isolated from ginseng roots include sterols, vitamins of the D group, flavonoids and amino acids.

Uses. In Asia the drug is held in esteem for the treatment of anaemia, diabetes, gastritis, sexual impotence and the many conditions arising from the onset of old age. In the West, too, it has in recent years become an extremely popular remedy particularly for the improvement of stamina, concentration, resistance to stress and to disease; in this sense the action of the drug is described as 'adaptogenic'.

Many 'ginseng' products are available as OTC products either for oral administration or as cosmetic preparations. In the US mainstream market for herbal sales, for the first eight months of 1999 ginseng stood at third place, with retail sales valued at over $60 million. Ginseng is included in the *BHP* (1996) and 29 references covering its constituents and actions are given in the *British Herbal Compendium*, Vol. 1 (1992).

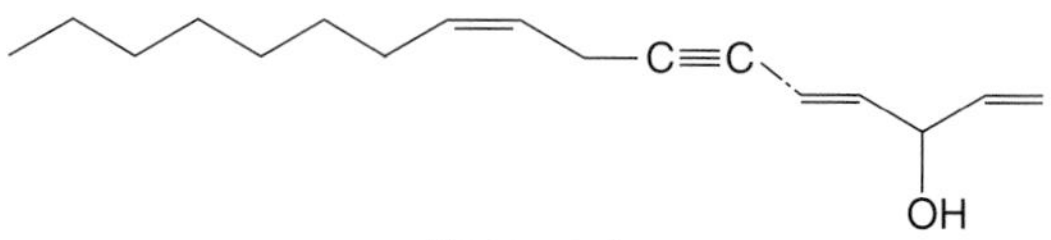

Panaxynol

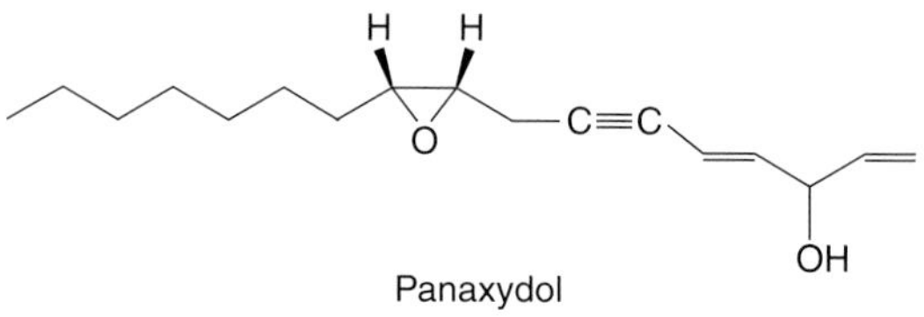

Panaxydol

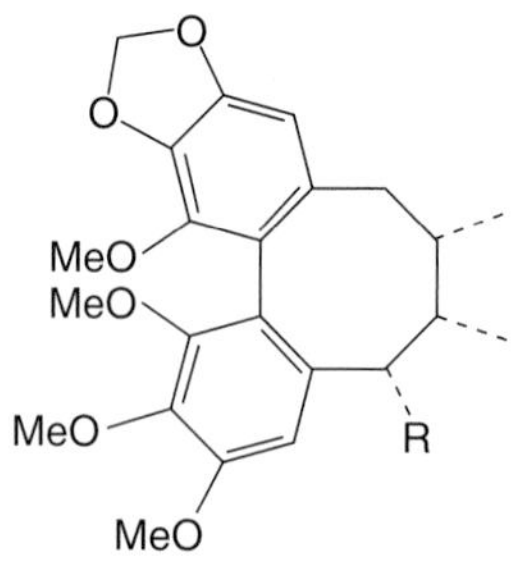

Gomisin N; R = H
Gomisin A; R = OH

Fig. 23.8
Acetylenes and lignans of ginseng.

Allied species. *Panax quinquefolium* root is one of the major drugs of US foreign trade. It is produced in the eastern USA and Canada, 90% of the US cultivated drug coming from north-central Wisconsin. Some of the ginsenosides of this species are the same as those of the Chinese and Korean drug; others appear to differ. In addition to 14 known dammarane-type saponins, M. Yoshikawa *et al.* (*Chem. Pharm. Bull.*, 1998, **46**, 647) identified a further five new compounds designated quinquenosides I–V. D. Don *et al.* (*Chem. Pharm. Bull.*, 2006, **54**, 751) have reported on a new dammarane-type saponin, ginsenoside R_{g8}, together with other known ginsenosides. In 1997, Kitanaka *et al.* showed the hybrid *P. ginseng* × *P. quinquefolium* to be superior to either parent in production of ginsenosides. However, as the plant is sterile, root cultures were established and these showed a comparable ginsenoside production to the field grown material (D. Washida *et al.*, *Phytochemistry*, 1998, **49**, 2331).

Panax pseudoginseng ssp. *himalaicus* var. *augustifolius* (Himalayan ginseng). The roots contain active saponins and ginsenosides R$_0$ and R$_{b1}$; chikusetsusaponins IVa and VI have been recorded. Shukla and Thakur (*Phytochemistry*, 1990, **29**, 239) characterized pseudoginsenoside-RI$_2$ which consists of oleanolic acid, phthalic acid, glucuronic acid and xylose moieties arranged as below:

Oleanolic acid $\xrightarrow{(3\rightarrow1)}$ glucuronic acid $\xrightarrow{(2\rightarrow1)}$ xylose

Oleanolic acid $\xrightarrow{(3\rightarrow1)}$ glucuronic acid $\xrightarrow{(2\rightarrow1)}$ xylose $\searrow$ phthalic acid

Panax notoginseng roots (Sanchi-ginseng) contain dammarane saponins, identical or similar to those of ginseng. M. Yoshikawa *et al.* (*Chem. Pharm. Bull.*, 1997, **45**, 1039; 1056) have isolated, in addition to 14 known saponins, nine new dammarane-type oligoglycosides named notoginsenosides A–J. The roots also contain a polysaccharide (sanchinan-A) having a branched structure with a galactose backbone and side-chains containing arabinose and galactose; this glycan contains a small amount of protein and possesses reticuloendothelial activating properties (K. Ohtani *et al.*, *Planta Med.*, 1987, **53**, 16).

Panax japonicum and *P. japonicum* var. *major* contain chikusetsusaponins, ginsenosides and glycans.

Panax vietnamensis (Vietnamese ginseng). The roots are a secret remedy of the Sedang ethnic minority and contain a number of known and new ginsenosides (N. M. Duc *et al.*, *Chem. Pharm. Bull.*, 1993, **41**, 2010; 1994, **42**, 115, 634).

Further reading

Court WE (ed), Hardman R (series ed) 2000 Medicinal and aromatic plants—industrial profiles, Vol 15. Ginseng: the genus *Panax*. Harwood Academic, Amsterdam

PENTACYCLIC TRITERPENOID SAPONINS

Unlike the steroidal saponins, the pentacyclic triterpenoid saponins are rare in monocotyledons. They are abundant in many dicotyledonous families, particularly the Caryophyllaceae, Sapindaceae, Polygalaceae and Sapotaceae. Among the many other dicotyledonous families in which they have been found are the Phytolaccaceae, Chenopodiaceae, Ranunculaceae, Berberidaceae, Papaveraceae, Linaceae, Zygophyllaceae, Rutaceae, Myrtaceae, Cucurbitaceae, Araliaceae, Umbelliferae, Primulaceae, Oleaceae, Lobeliaceae, Campanulaceae, Rubiaceae and Compositae. Altogether some 80 families are involved.

In these saponins the sapogenin is attached to a chain of sugar or uronic acid units, or both, often in the 3-position, as in the examples above. Biosynthesis, as with the steroids, involves ring-closure of squalene and is illustrated in Fig. 23.9.

Triterpenoid saponins may be classified into three groups represented by α-amyrin, β-amyrin and lupeol.

The related triterpenoid acids are formed from these by replacement of a methyl group by a carboxyl group in positions 4, 17 or 20 (Fig. 23.10).

Plant materials often contain these saponins in considerable amounts. Thus, primula root contains about 5–10%; liquorice root about 2–12% of glycyrrhizic acid (and a correspondingly larger amount of glycyrrhizin, the potassium calcium salt); quillaia bark up to about 10% of the mixture known as 'commercial saponin'; the seeds of the horsechestnut up to 13% of aescin. As some plants contain more than one saponin and purification is often difficult, the structures of even some of the well-known saponins given in Table 23.5 have only recently been established. Oleanolic acid also occurs as a saponin in sugar beet, thyme, *Guaiacum* spp. (also in the nor-form), and in the free state in olive leaves and clove buds.

Further reading

Tan N, Zhou J, Zhao S 1999 Advances in structural elucidation of glucuronide oleane-type triterpene carboxylic acid 3,28-*O*-bisdesmosides (1962–1997). Phytochemistry 52(2): 153–192

LIQUORICE ROOT

The pharmacopoeial drug is now defined as the dried unpeeled or peeled, whole or cut root and stolons of *Glyrrhiza glabra* L. and/or of *G. inflata* Bat. and/or *G. uralensis* Fisch. Varieties of *G. glabra* traditionally yielding the commercial drug are:

1. *Glycyrrhiza glabra* var. *typica* Reg. et Herd., a plant about 1.5 m high bearing typical papilionaceous flowers of a purplish-blue colour. The underground portion consists of long roots and thin rhizomes or stolons. The principal root divides just below the crown into several branches which penetrate the soil to a depth of 1 m or more. A considerable number of stolons are also given off, which attain a length of 2 m but run nearer the surface than the roots. The plant is grown in Spain, Italy, England, France, Germany and the USA.

2. *G. glabra* L. var. *glandulifera* Wald. et Kit. is abundant in the wild state in Galicia and central and southern Russia. The underground portion consists of a large rootstock, which bears numerous long roots but no stolons.

3. *G. glabra* var. β-*violacea* Boiss. yields the 'Persian' liquorice, which is collected in Iran and Iraq in the valleys of the Tigris and Euphrates; it bears violet flowers.

Much commercial extract is now obtained from the other species cited above.

Primula-saponin = L-rhamnose, D-glucose-D-galactose $\big\rangle$ D-glucuronic acid-*O*-3-primulagenin

Glycyrrhizic acid = D-glucuronic acid-D-glucuronic acid-*O*-3-glycyrrhetinic acid

α-Amyrin   β-Amyrin   Lupeol

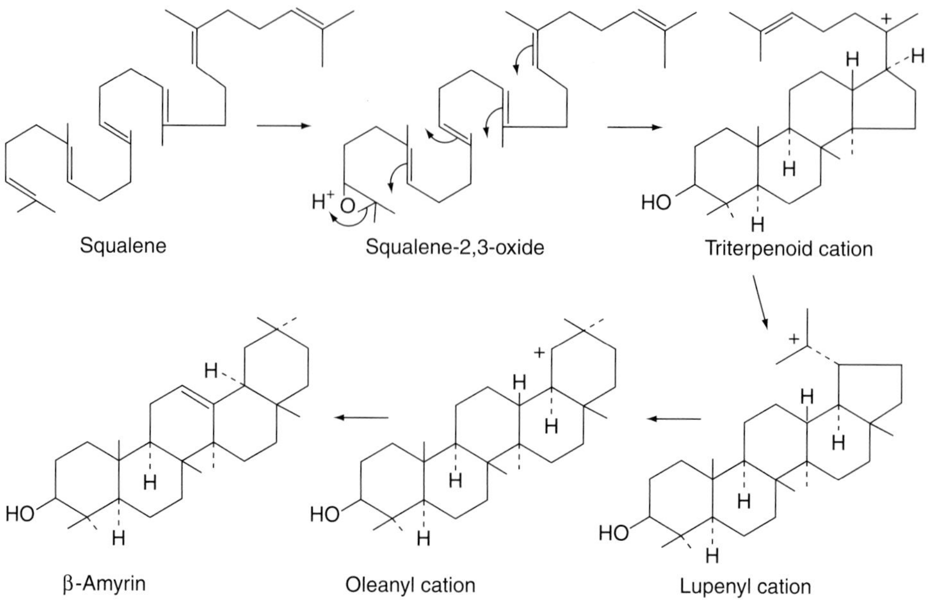

Fig. 23.9
Biosynthetic pathway of triterpenoids.

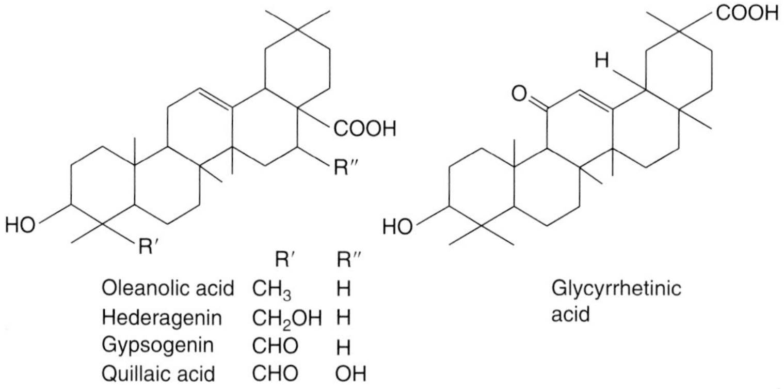

Fig. 23.10
Some triterpenoid acids of saponins.

	R′	R″
Oleanolic acid	CH₃	H
Hederagenin	CH₂OH	H
Gypsogenin	CHO	H
Quillaic acid	CHO	OH

Table 23.5 Pentacyclic triterpenoid saponins.

Saponin	Genin	Sugar components	Occurrence
Aescin	Aescigenin	2 glucose, 1 glucuronic acid (1 tiglic acid)	*Aesculus hippocastanum*
Aralin	Aralidin	2 arabinose, 1 glucuronic acid	*Aralia japonica*
Calendulasaponin A	Oleanolic acid	2 glucose, 1 galactose, 1 glucuronic acid	*Calendula officinalis*
Glycyrrhizic acid	Glycyrrhetinic acid	2 glucuronic acid	*Glycyrrhiza* spp.
Guaianin	Noroleanolic acid	1 rhamnose, 1 glucose, 1 arabinose	*Guaiacum* spp.
Gypsophilasaponin	Gypsogenin	1 galactose, 1 xylose, 1 arabinose, 1 fucose, 1 rhamnose	*Gypsophila* spp. and other Caryophyllaceae
Hederacoside A (hederin)	Hederagenin	1 glucose, 1 arabinose	*Hedera helix* (ivy) and other Araliaceae and Sapindaceae
Symphytoxide A	Hederagenin	1 arabinose, 2 glucose	*Symphytum officinale* roots
Primula-saponin	Primulagenin	1 rhamnose, 1 glucose, 1 galactose, glucuronic acid	*Primula* spp.
Quillaja-saponin	Quillaic acid (hydroxygypsogenin)	Glucuronic acid, 6 sugars and acyl moieties	*Quillaia saponaria*
Saikosaponin a	Saikogenin F	1 glucose, 1 fructose	*Bupleurum* spp.

History. Liquorice is referred to by Theophrastus. The Roman writers referred to it as *Radix dulcis*, but it does not appear to have been cultivated in Italy until about the thirteenth century. Its cultivation in England, now commercially ceased, has been traced back as far as the sixteenth century.

Cultivation and collection. In western Europe liquorice is cultivated, but the 'Russian' and 'Persian' drugs are obtained from wild plants. In China, large-scale cultivation is replacing collection from the wild. The plants usually grow well in deep, sandy but fertile soil, near streams. They are usually propagated by replanting young pieces of stolon but may be grown from seed. The underground organs are developed to a sufficient extent by the end of the third or fourth year, when they are dug up and washed. Some are peeled and cut up into short lengths before drying, but much is now used unpeeled. The drug is imported in bales. In southern Italy and the Levant a large proportion of the crop is made into stick or block liquorice. This is prepared by the process of decoction, the liquid being subsequently clarified and evaporated to the consistency of soft extract. The latter is made into blocks or sticks, stamped with the maker's name (e.g. Solazzi), dried, and exported in cases, which often contain bay laurel leaves. Chinese blocks weighing 5 kg each are available.

Macroscopical characters. The Spanish and Italian drugs are derived from the variety *typica*. They are sold as 'Spanish' liquorice irrespective of their exact geographical source. Typical '*Spanish*' liquorice occurs in straight pieces from 14 to 20 cm or more in length and from 5 to 20 mm in diameter. If unpeeled, they have a dark, reddish-brown cork, and the runners, which are more numerous than the roots, bear buds. The peeled drug has a yellow, fibrous exterior. Fracture, fibrous; odour, faint, but characteristic; taste, sweet and almost free from bitterness.

Unpeeled 'Russian' liquorice occurs in somewhat tapering pieces up to 30 cm long and 5 cm in diameter. It is of less regular appearance than the Spanish and consists of rootstock and roots. The surface is covered with a somewhat scaly, purplish cork. The pieces of rootstock often bear buds and have a pith, but the roots may be distinguished from the stolons of the Spanish drug by the absence of buds. Fracture, very fibrous, the strands of fibres tending to separate from one another. This variety is sometimes peeled. The taste is sweet but usually not entirely free from bitterness or acridity. 'Persian' liquorice from Iran closely resembles the Russian variety and is generally unpeeled. Anatolian or Turkish liquorice may be peeled or unpeeled and some pieces may have a diameter of up to 8 cm.

Much commercial liquorice root currently available in Britain is of Chinese origin. It is imported in bundles of stolons each bundle being about 15 cm long, 15 cm diameter, and bound with wire. The bundles are packed in plaited wood containers. Generally, the stolons have a smaller diameter than the European drug.

Microscopical characters. Both roots and runners show secondary thickening—the absence of a medulla in the root and its tetrarch structure (Fig. 41.8A–C) serving to distinguish the sections. The epidermis and most of the cortex are absent, being thrown off by the development of cork. The outer surface of the unpeeled drug is bounded by some 10 rows of narrow cork cells. Within the cork is a phelloderm or secondary cortex composed of parenchymatous cells, some of which may become collenchymatous. These cells contain simple starch grains about 10 μm diameter; a few contain prisms of calcium oxalate. The secondary phloem is composed of alternating zones of groups of fibres and sieve tissue. The phloem fibres are very thick-walled, are lignified and occur in cylindrical bundles surrounded by a sheath of parenchymatous cells each of which contains a single prism of calcium oxalate 10–35 μm in length. The sieve-tube tissue suffers partial obliteration but remains functional in the cambial region. The cambium is an incomplete line composed of about three layers of flattened cells. The secondary xylem is composed of large vessels, wood fibres and wood parenchyma. The vessels are 80–200 μm in diameter and show reticulate or pitted walls. The pits are slit-like bordered pits.

The vessels occur singly in small groups and alternate with bundles of wood fibres resembling the phloem fibres in form and in being enclosed in a sheath of parenchyma containing calcium oxalate. The parenchyma of the xylem has lignified pitted walls. The secondary tissues are divided by radial medullary rays 3–5 cells wide in the xylem and funnel-shaped in the phloem. These rays are up to 100 cells high (Fig. 23.11).

The characters of *G. uralensis* are more fully discussed in the next monograph.

Constituents. Since 1990 considerable research has been published on the constituents of liquorice mainly by Japanese workers in whose country the drug, imported from China, is an important traditional medicine. Unfortunately, the Chinese commercial drug, as investigated, may be derived from a number of species, e.g. *Glycyrrhiza uralensis*, *G. inflata* and *G. glabra*, so that it is not always possible to assign particular reported constituents to a specific source.

Liquorice owes most of its sweet taste to glycyrrhizin, the potassium and calcium salts of glycyrrhizinic acid. Glycyrrhizinic acid is the diglucopyranosiduronic acid of glycyrrhetic (glycyrrhetinic) acid, which has a triterpenoid structure (Fig. 23.12). Other hydroxy- and deoxy-triterpenoid acids related to glycyrrhetic acid have been isolated; the C-20 epimer of glycyrrhetic acid is named liquiritic acid.

The yellow colour of liquorice is due to flavonoids, which received further considerable study when in 1978 the antigastric effect of flavonoid-rich fractions was recognized. They include liquiritin, isoliquiritin (a chalcone, which occurs as a glycoside), liquiritigenin, isoliquiritigenin (chalcone form) and other compounds. Isoliquiritigenin is reported to be an aldose-reductase inhibitor and may be effective in preventing diabetic complications. Rhamnoliquiritin was isolated from the roots in 1968. Many flavonoids and isoprenoid-substituted flavonoids from *G. glabra* of various origins have since been reported. These include the pyrano-isoflavan, glabridin (Fig. 23.12) and, more recently, two minor isoflavones, glabriso flavone A and B, and glabrocoumarone (Fig. 23.12) (T. Kinoshita *et al.*, *Chem. Pharm. Bull.*, 2005, **53**, 847). Various 2-methylisoflavones have been isolated from indigenous Indian roots together with an unusual coumarin (liqcoumarin), 6-acetyl-5-hydroxy-4-methyl-coumarin. An examination of liquorice from five countries has shown the flavonoid content to be geographically consistent, varying only in the relative proportions of constituents. Japanese traditional (kampo) extracts prepared by boiling show a high content of flavonoid aglycones which may be pharmacologically more active than the parent glycosides.

Other active constituents of liquorice are polysaccharides with a pronounced activity on the reticuloendothelial system. Research on these, at first devoted to *G. uralensis*, has been extended to *G. glabra* var. *glandulifera* from which glycyrrhizan GA has been characterized as the representative polysaccharide with immunological activity (K. Takada *et al.*, *Chem. Pharm. Bull.*, 1992, **40**, 2487). It has an estimated mass of 85 000 with a core structure which includes a backbone chain of β-1,3-linked D-galactose residues 60% of the units carrying side chains (composed of β-1,3- and β-1,6-linked D-galactosyl residues) at position 6.

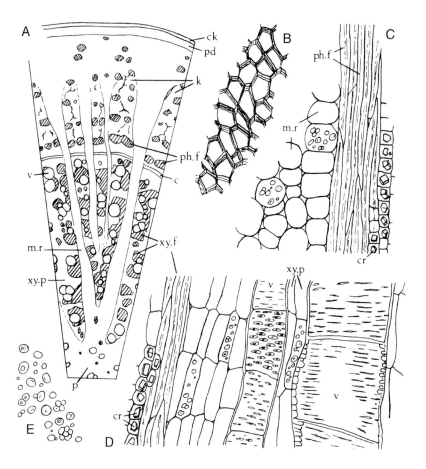

Fig. 23.11
Glycyrrhiza glabra. A, Transverse section of stolon (×25);
B, fragment of cork layer from powder, in surface view;
C, portion of longitudinal section through phloem;
D, longitudinal section of wood; E, starch granules
(all ×200). c, Cambial zone; ck, cork layer; cr,
calcium oxalate crystals; k, non-functional sieve tissue
(keratenchyma); m.r, medullary ray; p, pith; pd,
phelloderm; ph.f, phloem fibres; v, vessel; xy. f, xylem
fibres; xy. p, xylem parenchyma.

The roots also contain about 5–15% of sugars (glucose, sucrose); about 1–2% of asparagine (amide of aspartic or aminosuccinic acid); 0.04–0.06% volatile compounds; β-sitosterol; starch; protein; bitter principles (glycyramarin). The latter are particularly abundant in the outer tissues and are therefore largely removed in the peeled variety of liquorice.

Published analytical figures for the amount of glycyrrhizin in liquorice vary considerably. These differences are due partly to different analytical methods and partly to actual variations in the percentages present in different commercial varieties and samples; 6–13% is the usual range. Glycyrrhizin is confined mainly to the roots but falls rapidly in concentration in organs above soil level. In a field study on *G. glabra* growing in Uzbekistan, H. Hayashi *et al.*, (*Chem. Pharm. Bull.*, 2003, **51**, 1338) found that, based on the relative occurrence of rutin and isoquercetin, the populations could be divided into two distinct types.

Cell cultures. Suspension cell cultures of liquorice do not appear to produce either glycyrrhizin or glycyrrhetic acid but soyasaponins I and II, the amounts depending on culture strain and influence of plant hormones. The principal isoflavonoid produced is formononetin (C. Arias-Castro *et al.*, *Plant Cell Tissue and Org. Cult.*, 1993, **34**, 63). Glycyrrhetic acid added to the cell culture undergoes a different mode of glycosylation to that normally occurring in the roots.

From hairy root cultures, initiated by *Agrobacterium rhizogenes*, two new prenylated flavonoids (licoagrochalcone A and licoagrocarpin) together with eight known flavonoids, have been isolated (Y. Asada *et al.*, *Phytochemistry*, 1998, **47**, 389).

Allied drug. Other species which have been investigated, some of which find domestic use, include *G. aspera*, *G. echinata*, *G. hirsuta*,

G. inflata, *G. macedonia*, *G. pallidiflora* and *G. yunnanensis*. (For research papers on these species see K. Ohtani *et al.*, *Phytochemistry*, 1994, **36**, 139; T. Fukai *et al.*, *ibid.*, 1994, **36**, 233.)

Standardization. The *BP/EP* requires a minimum content of 4.0% glycyrrhizic acid determined by liquid chromatography using monoammonium glycyrrhizate as a reference and absorption measurements at 254 nm. The total ash should not exceed 10.0% (unpeeled drug) or 6.0% (peeled drug) and the ash insoluble in hydrochloric acid similarly 2.0% (unpeeled drug), 0.5% (peeled drug).

Action and uses. Liquorice has long been employed in pharmacy as a flavouring agent, demulcent and mild expectorant. Gibson (*Lloydia*, 1978, **41**, 348) in a summary of the uses of liquorice from 2100 BC, pointed out that many of the early claims for a broad spectrum of uses for this drug appear to be borne out by modern pharmacological research; a view that has been further substantiated during the last decade. The recognition of the deoxycorticosterone effects of liquorice extracts and glycyrrhetinic acid has led to its use for the treatment of rheumatoid arthritis, Addison's disease and various inflammatory conditions. Interestingly, the flavonoid component of the root, which possesses antimicrobial properties, also exerts spasmolytic and antiulcerogenic activity. A Japanese patent (*Chem. Abs.*, 1992, **117**, 55948) describes the formulation of a liquiritin cream as beneficial, with no adverse effects, for the removal of skin stains in patients with chloasma, senile melanoderma, etc.

Unlike cortisone, liquorice may give symptomatic relief from peptic ulcer pain. It has been reported that glycyrrhizin gel can act as a useful vehicle for various drugs used topically; not only are the anti-inflammatory and antiviral effects relevant but also glycyrrhizin enhances skin penetration by the drug. Excessive consumption of

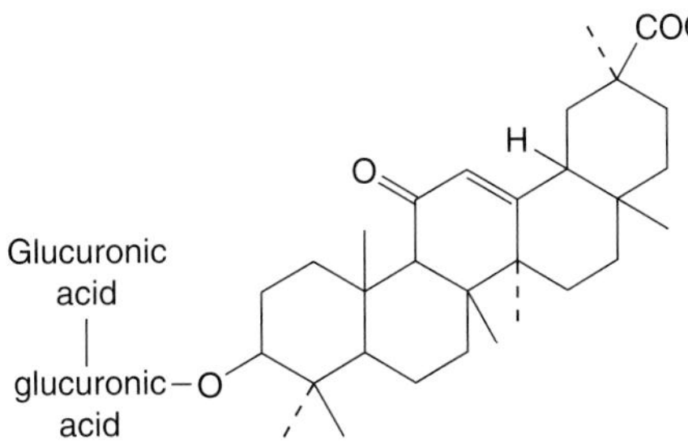

Glycyrrhizinic acid
(Glycyrrhizin = mixture of calcium and sodium salts
of glycyrrhizinic acid)

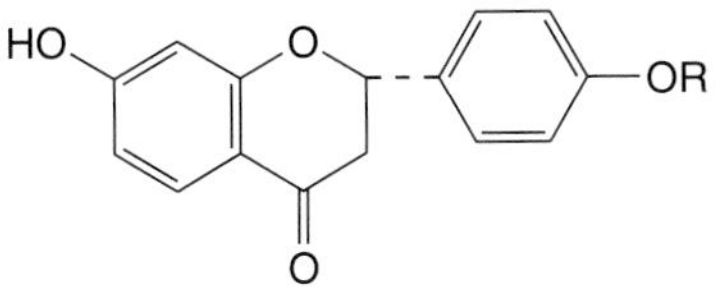

Liquiritin; R = Glucosyl
Liquiritigenin; R = H

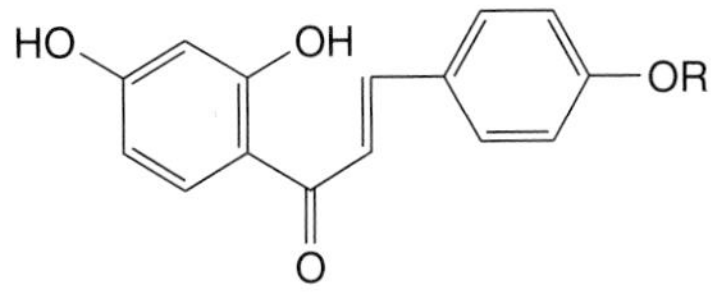

Isoliquiritin; R = Glucosyl
Isoliquiritigenin; R = H

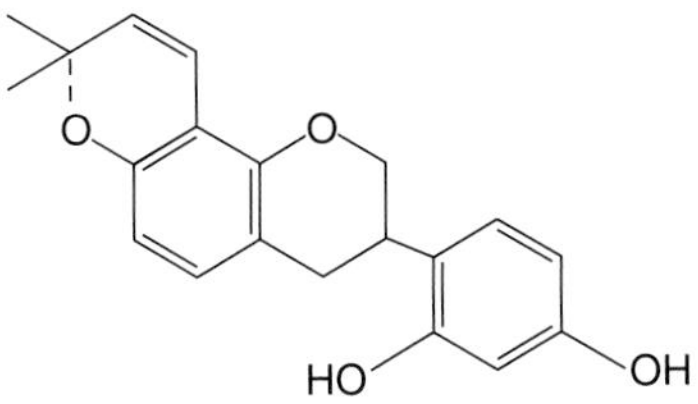

Glabridin

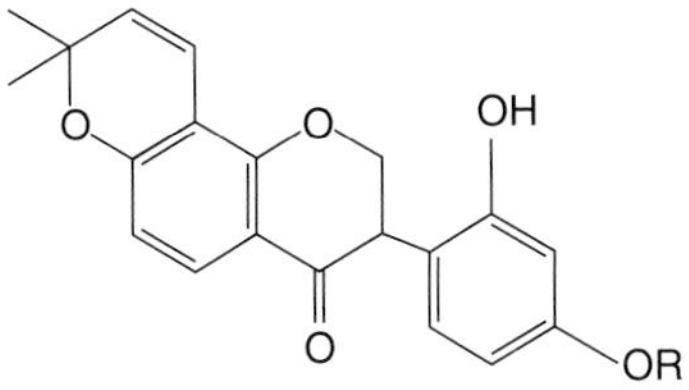

R = H; Glabroisoflavone A
R = CH$_3$; Glabroisoflavone B

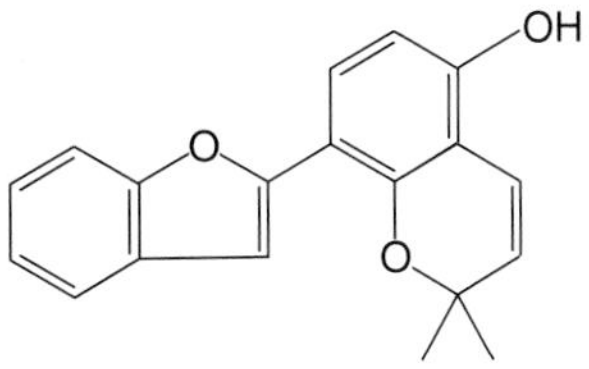

Glabrocoumarone

Fig. 23.12
Some constituents of liquorice root.

liquorice leads to hypertension and hypokalaemic alkosis; the hospitalization of an individual taking 200 g liquorice daily was reported in 1998. Most of the liquorice imported is used in the tobacco trade and in confectionery.

Further reading

Fiore C *et al* 2005 A history of the therapeutic use of liquorice in Europe. J Ethnopharmacology 99(3): 317–324
Hostettmann K, Marston A 1995 Saponins. Cambridge University Press, Cambridge

LIQUORICE ROOT FOR USE IN TRADITIONAL CHINESE MEDICINE

The *BP* 2007 included the above as a monograph involving the dried unpeeled roots and rhizomes of *Glycyrrhiza uralensis* Fisch., *G. inflata* Bat. or *G. glabra* L.

Unlike Liquorice Root *BP/EP*, the commercial drug consists of the roots and rhizomes sliced transversely or longitudinally giving irregularly circular to ovoid pieces up to about 3 mm thick. The outer surface is dark reddish-brown and longitudinally wrinkled. The general microscopical features of the powder resemble those for *G. glabra*.

G. uralensis, Manchurian liquorice, as present in a commercial sample bears a chocolate-brown, exfoliating cork and differs from *G. glabra* in internal structure, the medullary rays being curved and lacunae being present in the wood. It appears to contain about as much glycyrrhizin as the other varieties, together with a number of new oleane-type triterpene oligosaccharides called licorice saponins (I. Kitagawa *et al.*, *Chem. Pharm. Bull.*, 1993, **41**, 1567). Only traces of sugars are present and it gives an unpleasantly pungent extract. As with *G. glabra*, the yellow colouring matter contains the flavonoid glycoside liquiritin, a glycoside involving liquiritigenin, apiose and glucose, and a new chalcone oligoglycoside isoliquiritin apioside. Like *G. glabra*, *G. uralensis* contains polysaccharides showing immunological activities; glycyrrhizan UA is composed of L-arabinose, D-galactose, L-rhamnose and D-galacturonic acid.

As the supply of wild plants of *G. uralensis* is practically exhausted there is now large scale cultivation of the drug in the Inner Mongolian area of China. A new biflavonoid named lichobichalcone and twelve known flavonoids from the cultivated roots have been reported (H. Bal *et al.*, *Chem. Pharm. Bull.*, 2003, **51**, 1095).

Actions. In common with *G. glabra*, many pharmacological activities have been cited for *G. uralensis*; these include: antihepatotoxic, antimutagenic, antimicrobial, antitumour and antiulcer. Glycyrrhisoflavone and glyasperin C have been reported as tyrosinase inhibitors (H. J. Kim *et al.*, *Planta Medica*, 2005, **71**, 785).

PRIMULA ROOT

Primula root *BP/EP* consists of the dried rhizome and root of *Primula veris* (L.) (cowslip) or *P. elatior* Hill. (oxlip), Primulaceae. These species occur wild throughout Europe with Bulgaria and Turkey the principal commercial sources. British herbal medicine has however traditionally used the leaves, flowers and roots of *P. vulgaris* (the common primrose).

The greyish-brown drug may be whole or cut with pieces of rhizome up to 5 cm in length and bearing the remains of stems and leaves together with numerous roots. Microscopical features include parenchymatous cells, reticulately thickened vessels and simple and compound starch granules. *P. elatior* is differentiated by the possession of groups of pitted sclereids.

Constituents include a mixture of triterpenoid saponins of the oleane type (5–10%) and phenolic glycosides such as primulaverin (primulaveroside). The latter, by enzyme hydrolysis during the drying process, forms the disaccharide primeverose and methyl 5-methoxysalicylate, the latter being responsible for the odour of the drug.

The pharmacopoeia includes a chromatographic test to detect *Vincetoxicum hirundinaria*, Aesclepiadaceae, a poisonous plant with similar-looking roots to those of *Primula* spp. The substitute also differs microscopically in its vascular structure and possesses numerous calcium oxalate crystals.

Primula root, like senega, is used as an expectorant for the treatment of bronchial conditions.

QUILLAIA BARK

Quillaia bark (*Soap Bark, Panama Wood, Quillaia*) is the dried inner bark of *Quillaja saponaria* Molina and of other species of *Quillaja* (Rosaceae). *Quillaja saponaria* is a tree about 18 m high found in Chile, Peru and Bolivia. It has been introduced into India and California. The generic name is derived from the Chilean word *quillean*, to wash, from the use made of the bark.

Macroscopical characters. Quillaia bark occurs in flat strips about 1 m long, 20 cm broad and 3–10 mm thick. It consists almost entirely

of phloem, the outer region in which successive cork cambia develop having been more or less completely removed. A few, reddish- or blackish-brown patches of rhytidome adhere to the outer surface, which is otherwise of a brownish-white colour and reticulated. The rhytidome consists of dead portions of secondary phloem enclosed by secondary cork layers. The inner surface is yellowish-white and fairly smooth. The bark breaks with a splintery fracture and is inclined to laminate (between the zones of hard and soft phloem). Large crystals of calcium oxalate may be seen with the naked eye. The powdered drug is very sternutatory and produces an abundant froth when shaken with water. Taste, acrid and astringent.

Microscopical characters. A transverse section of quillaia bark has a chequered appearance which is caused by the crossing of the medullary rays by alternating bands of lignified and non-lignified phloem. The medullary rays are usually 2–4 cells wide. The phloem fibres are tortuous and often accompanied by small groups of rectangular sclereids. The parenchyma contains numerous starch grains up to 20 μm diameter and single prisms of calcium oxalate up to 20 μm long.

Constituents. The bark contains a mixture of saponins which on hydrolysis yield the principal sapogenin quillaic acid (hydroxygypsogenin) and gypsogenin (Fig. 23.10) together with sugars, uronic acids and acyl moieties. It is little wonder that the constitution of quillaia saponin proved difficult to unravel by classical procedures as it has now been shown to contain at least 60 different saponins (D. C. van Setten *et al.*, *Anal. Chem.*, 1998, **70**, 4401). Di- and tri-saccharides are attached at C-3 and various complex oligosaccharides at C-28, the fucosyl moiety of which may be substituted with C_9-aliphatic acids or an *O*-acetyl group (S. Guo *et al.*, *Phytochemistry*, 2000, **53**, 861; **54**, 615). A typical structure is shown below.

Quillaia contains about 10% of saponins, *BP* ethanol (45%)-soluble extractive not less than 22.0%, and also sugars, starch and calcium oxalate.

Uses. Quillaia is used as an emulsifying agent, particularly for tars and volatile oils.

SENEGA ROOT

Senega of the *BP* and *EP* consists of the dried root crown and root of *Polygala senega* L. (Polygalaceae) or of closely related species of *Polygala* or a mixture of these. A variety found in N. America and now cultivated in Japan is *P. senega* var. *latifolia* Torr. et Gray, a robust perennial herb some 20–30 cm tall. Formerly abundant in eastern Canada and eastern USA it is now collected further westward.

Component of quillaia saponin

History. Senega was used by the North American Indians as a snakebite remedy. It was employed by Tennent in 1734 for pleurisy and pneumonia, and its value was made known in London in 1738.

Macroscopical characters. Senega occurs in pieces 5–10 cm long and 2–12 mm diameter. The lower part is yellowish but the crown is somewhat darker. The latter is knotty and bears numerous, often purplish buds and the remains of aerial stems, which should not exceed about 2%. The tapering and often curved root frequently divides into two or more branches. Some, but by no means all, of the pieces bear a keel or ridge in the form of a rapidly descending spiral. The drug frequently has a marked odour of methyl salicylate. Taste, at first sweet, afterwards acrid. The saponins present cause the drug to have sternutatory properties and to froth when shaken with water.

Transverse sections of different senega roots, or the same root cut at different levels, have widely different appearances. Some have a normal bark, which occupies nearly half the radius, and a uniform central wood with narrow medullary rays. In others, however, an abnormal local development of phloem gives rise to the keel, while one or more exceptionally wide, V-shaped, medullary rays give a very characteristic appearance to the wood. This is well seen in sections stained with phloroglucinol and hydrochloric acid.

For illustrations, see the 14th edition of this book, p. 309.

Constituents. Senega contains 6–12% of triterpenoid saponins. Earlier work based on the hydrolysis of the crude saponin mixture (senegin) produced a variety of products but during the 1970s Japanese workers characterized a number of individual saponins based on the aglycone presenegenin with glucose at C-3 and a number of sugars and a cinnamic acid derivative forming a branched chain at C-28; the units comprising the principal glycoside seneginin II are shown in Fig. 23.13. It is interesting to note the involvement of fucose, a deoxy sugar also found in certain cardioactive glycosides (Fig. 23.15) and in the saikosaponins (q.v.).

A number of oligosaccharide multi-esters have recently been identified in the roots (see H. Saitoh *et al.*, *Chem. Pharm. Bull.*, 1993, **41**, 1127, 2125) and named senegoses A–I. They appear to be di-and tetra-saccharides involving glucose and fructose esterified with acetic, benzoic, and *trans-* and *cis-*ferulic acids. A further series, senegoses J–O, are pentasaccharides (*Idem., ibid.*, 1994, **42**, 641). These compounds are structurally similar to the tenuifolioses previously isolated by the same group of workers from *P. tenuifolia* (*vide infra*).

Allied species and substitutes. *P. tenuifolia* is used in China and Japan as an expectorant, tonic and sedative. It contains constituents similar to those of *P. senega*, including saponins, xanthones, phenolic glycosides (tenuifolisides A–D) and oligosaccharides (tenuifolioses A–F), see Y. Ikeya *et al.*, *Chem. Pharm. Bull.*, 1994, **42**, 2305). The bark, also used medicinally in China, Korea and Japan, has sedative, expectorant and anti-inflammatory properties. A number new phenones, tenuiphenones A–D, have recently been reported (Y. Jiang and P. Tu, *Chem. Pharm. Bull.*, 2005, **53**, 1164).

Tenuiphenone A

Many new triterpene saponins of *P. japonica* and *P. fallax* named polygalasaponins have been reported. The aglycone of a number of these saponins is bayogenin (Fig. 23.13). For recent new isolations, see H. Wang *et al.*, *Chem. Pharm. Bull.*, 2006, **54**, 1739; W. D. Zhang *et al.*, *Fitoterapia*, 2006, **77**, 336.

Southern or *White senega* is collected in the southern USA from *P. alba* and *P. boykini*. The roots are smaller than those of *P. senega* and have a normal wood.

Uses. Senega is used as a stimulant expectorant in chronic bronchitis. It is often prescribed with other expectorants such as ipecacuanha and ammonium carbonate.

EUROPEAN GOLDENROD

It is necessary to distinguish between two commercial sources of goldenrod used in medicine: one is native to Europe and Asia and the other involves two species of *Solidago* native to N. America, which are now naturalized and cultivated in Europe. Although generally similar in morphological form and constituents, there is variation between the two sources and the *BP/EP* includes them in separate monographs.

European Goldenrod *BP/EP*, Goldenrod *BHP* 1996 consists of the whole or cut, dried flowering aerial parts of *Solidago virgaurea* L. It is common in Britain, preferring dry woods and grassland, rocky areas, dunes, etc. The species is polymorphic with many named varieties.

A perennial herb, it is up to 1 m in height with stems, often reddish-brown at the base, somewhat branched and leafy. The lower leaves are up to 10 cm in length, obovate to lanceolate, toothed and narrowing at the base to a winged petiole. The stem leaves are alternate becoming progressively smaller, entire, inconspicuously toothed, sessile to amplexicaul, glabrous or slightly pubescent. The short-stalked yellow flowerheads are arranged around the stem in a terminal raceme or panicle. The involucre of greenish-yellow imbricate bracts is arranged in two to four rows; each capitulum possesses six to twelve ray florets and many tubular florets, both yellow. The fruits are brown, ribbed achenes 2–4 mm in length.

Features observable in the powdered drug include epidermal leaf fragments with striated cuticle and anomocytic stomata, various uniseriate clothing trichomes with some having an extended pennant-like terminal cell, glandular trichomes, cluster crystals of calcium oxalate, pappus hairs; compositae pollen grains.

Constituents. The principal constituents of European goldenrod are oleane-type saponins based on polygalacic acid-3-glucoside (Fig. 23.13). Four such compounds, subsequently designated virgaureasaponins B, C, D and E were 3, 28-bisdesmosidic glycosides involving glucose, rhamnose, xylose and fucose with acylation of the fucose with a chain of two or three β-hydroxybutyric acid moieties (G. Bader *et al.*, *Planta Med.*, 1995, **61**, 158); see Fig. 23.13 and *cf* Senega. Compounds B and C were identical with solidagosaponins XIV and XVIII belonging to a series of saponins (solidagosaponins I–XXIX) isolated from fresh plants of the Asian variety of *S. virgaurea* (Y. Inose *et al.*, *Chem. Pharm. Bull.*, 1991, **39**, 2037; 1992, **40**, 946; T. Miyase *et al.*, *Chem. Pharm. Bull.*, 1994, **42**, 617).

A number of flavonoids have been identified in the drug including chlorogenic acid and rutin, which are characterized in the pharmacopoeial TLC test; no quercitrin is evident, distinguishing this species from *S. gigantea* and *S. canadensis*. Other flavonoids include kaempferol, hyperoside and isoquercitrin. The presence of a diglucoside, leiocarposide (0.4–0.8%) is a further distinction from the above two species. Caffeic acid derivatives and phenolic acids in small amount are also present.

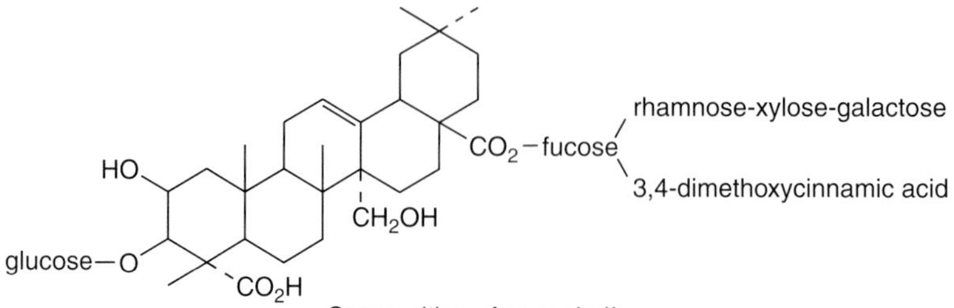

rhamnose-xylose-galactose

CO_2—fucose

3,4-dimethoxycinnamic acid

Composition of senegin II
(*Polygala senega*)

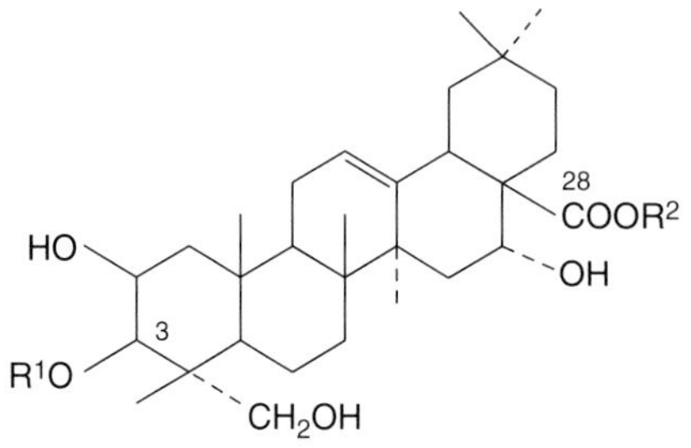

$COOR^2$

Polygalacic acid: R^1 = H, R^2 = H

Virgaureasaponins: R^1 = glucose, R^2 = fucose

rhamnose-xylose-rhamnose

β-hydroxybutyric acid
(×2 or ×3)

(*Solidago virgaurea*)

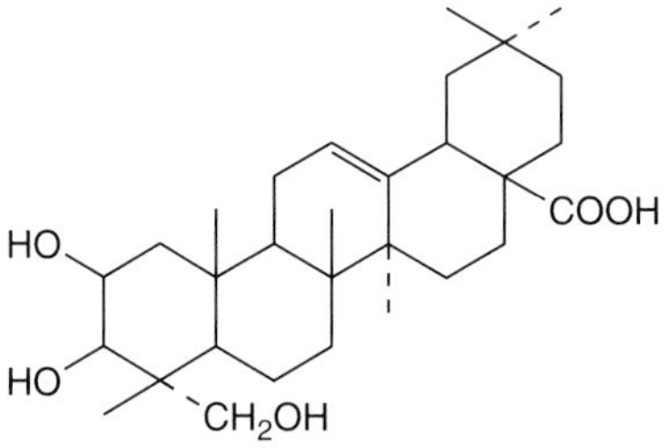

Bayogenin
(*Polygala japonica, P. fallax*)

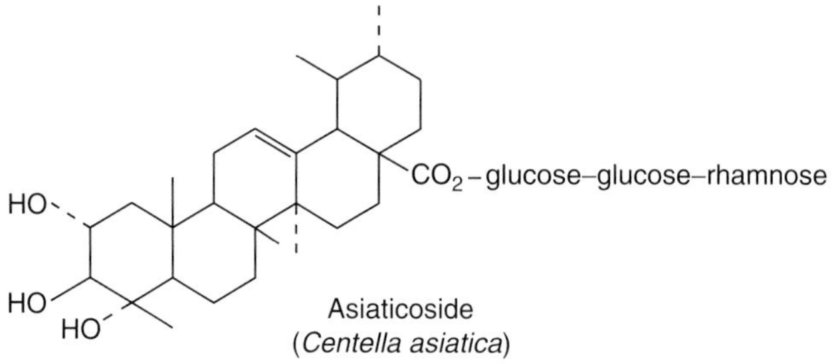

CO_2—glucose–glucose–rhamnose

Asiaticoside
(*Centella asiatica*)

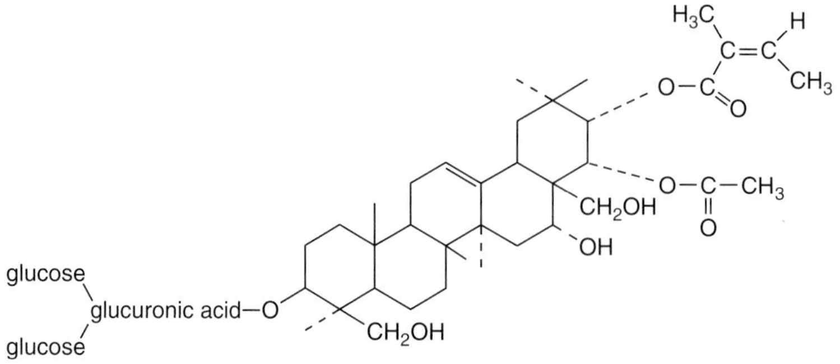

glucose

glucuronic acid—O

glucose

Fig. 23.13
Triterpenoids of *Polygala, Solidago
Centella* and *Hippocastanum.*

Component of 'aescin'
(*Aesculus hippocastanum*)

Uses. Used principally in traditional medicine for the treatment of urinary tract infections; also for catarrh and whooping cough and externally for the treatment of insect bites, wounds, etc.

GOLDENROD

Goldenrod *BP/EP* consists of the whole or cut, dried, flowering parts of *Solidago gigantea* Ait or *S. canadensis* L., their varieties or hybrids and/or mixtures of these. Family Compositae.

These species are two of some 100 spp. of *Solidago* native to America and were introduced into Europe as ornamentals, being much larger and showier than the native *S. virgaurea*; as garden escapes they have become naturalized along streams, rivers, lakes and waste places.

S. canadensis (*S. altissima*), tall goldenrod, is a native of eastern N. America. It is a vigorous erect plant 1–2.5 m with a spread of about 1 m. The stems are pubescent throughout with lanceolate, sharply pointed, three-veined leaves, roughish above, pubescent below. Broadly plumose heads of yellow flowers form a large pyrimidal panicle from August to November making for an attractive autumn border plant.

S. gigantea (*S. serotina*) resembles the above but below 1 m the stems are glabrous and the flowers are larger in compact erect corymbose panicles.

The pharmacopoeial description relates to both species and their hybrids. In the powder the absence of multicellular trichomes with a bent-over terminal cell should be noted, cf. European goldenrod.

Constituents. As with European goldenrod, bidesmosidic saponins are present in both *S. gigantea* and *S. canadensis*. Bayogenin (Fig. 23.13) is the aglycone common to both. The *canadensis* and *gigantia* saponins differ from one another in the length and structure of the saccharide chains, particularly in those units bonded to the C-3 position of bayogenin. Unlike *S. virgaurea*, there is no acylation of the sugar chains. Eight such saponins were isolated from *S. canadensis* and four from *S. gigantea* (M. Sovova *et al.*, *Ceska Slov. Farm.*, 1999, **48**, 113; *Chem. Abs.*, 1999, **131**, 240355 m).

Other constituents of *S. canadensis* include sesquiterpenes, di- and tri-terpenes and a very low content (1 mg/kg) of a new phenolic diglucoside related to that found in *S. virgaurea* (J. S. Zhang *et al.*, *Fitoterapia*, 2007, **78**, 69). Two new quercetin and kaempferol glycosides have recently been reported (B. Wu *et al.*, *Chem. Pharm. Bull.*, 2007, **55**, 815).

In common with European goldenrod the drug is assayed for its flavonoid content, a minimum of 2.5% flavonoids, expressed as hyperoside (dried drug), being required by the *BP/EP*. This high value may reflect the large proportion of flowers in collections of these plants. Quercitrin, chlorogenic acid and rutin are detected in the official TLC test (quercitrin is absent in the same test involving *S. virgaurea*).

Uses. In European phytotherapy for much the same purposes as European goldenrod—urolithiasis, cystitis, rheumatism and as an antiphlogistic.

Saikosaponins

This group of oleanene saponins occurs in the roots of *Bupleurum falcatum* (Umbelliferae), a drug long-used in Chinese medicine for the treatment of hepato-biliary disorders and known to possess anti-inflammatory properties. For a fuller description and formulae see Chapter 29.

Horse chestnut seed

Horse chestnut seeds and the tree *Aesculus hippocastanum* (Hippocastanaceae) need no description; native to western Asia the species is now widely distributed over the world as an ornamental.

Medicinally the seeds have long been used for their saponin content, the principal component being aescin (in recent publications termed 'escin') which occurs in concentrations of up to 20% in the dried seeds. As with a number of these well-known triterpenoid saponins it is only recently that it has been possible to elucidate completely their chemical structures and, as with other crude saponins, aescin itself has been shown to be a mixture of many closely related compounds. Acid hydrolysis of the aescin complex gives the saponin aescigenin and the sugars glucose, xylose, galactose and glucuronic acid together with esterifying acetic, butyric, isobutyric, angelic and tiglic acids. From 1996–1998 M. Yoshikawa *et al.* described nine new such acylated polyhydroxyoleane triterpene oligoglycosides (escins Ia, Ib, IIa, etc.) together with three isoescins (*Chem. Pharm. Bull.*, 1998, **46**, 1764). As an example of one such structure see Fig. 23.13.

The seeds also contain flavones (quercitin, kaempferol and their glycosyl derivatives, Fig. 23.13), coumarins and tannins.

Extracts of horse chestnut have been traditionally employed both in the West and East for the treatment of peripheral vascular disorders including haemorrhoids, varicose veins, leg ulcers and bruises. OTC products are now available, their efficacy supported by a number of scientific reports. Thus some of the escins are anti-inflammatory, inhibiting the activity of lysosomal enzymes that damage capillary walls; coumarins cause a thinning of the blood, so much so that horse chestnut is contraindicated with anticoagulants such as warfarin; tannins tone the blood vessel walls and flavonoids are anti-inflammatory.

Further reading
Bombardelli E, Morazzoni P, Griffini A 1996 *Aesculus hippocastanum* L. Fitoterapia 67(6): 483–511. *A review with 143 references*

CENTELLA

Centella (Indian pennywort, gotu kola, Indian water navelwort, tiger grass) consists of the dried fragmented aerial parts of *Centella asiatica* (L.) Urban, family Umbelliferae syn. *Hydrocotyle asiatica*. It is typically found in moist situations throughout the pantropics including Pakistan, India, S.E. Asia and Africa. It has important traditional uses in India and Africa for the treatment of leprosy, and in the former for meditation purposes under the name *brahmi*.

The plant resembles the European marsh pennywort as a creeping perennial with kidney-shaped leaves, grouped at the stem nodes, up to 5 cm broad with small pink flowers giving fruits in umbels of two to four bicarpellate schizocarps.

The drug consists of a grey–green, compressed mass involving stems, leaves, flowers and fruits. Microscopical examination shows polygonal leaf epidermal cells with a striated cuticle, paracytic stomata and long, often twisted unicellular trichomes on the petiole epidermis. Also prisms of calcium oxalate crystals, bundles of septate fibres and fragments of the fruit with a parquetry arrangement of some cells.

Constituents. As an important Ayurvedic drug, Centella has been investigated over a long period of time and numerous constituents have been recorded. Among the most active are triterpenoid saponins, principally asiaticoside (Fig. 23.13), together with brahmoside, brahminoside, centelloside and medecasside, based on corresponding terpinic acids that also occur in the free state.

A minimal content of volatile oil consists principally of sesquiterpenes. O. A. Oyedej and A. J. Afolayan (*Pharm. Bull.*, 2005, **43**, 249), in a comparison of the Japanese oil with that from plants grown in S. Africa, have identified by GC-MS some 40 constituents, the chief of which are α-humulene (21.06%), β-carophyllene, myrcene, germacrene B and bicyclogermacrene. Samples varied in composition and showed broad-spectrum antibacterial activity.

Among other constituents of centella are flavonoids (quercetin, kaempferol, etc.) phytosterols, amino acids and a bitter principle, vallerin.

Uses. The *BHP* (1983) lists centella as a mild diuretic, antirheumatic, dermatological agent and peripheral vasodilator; topically as vulnerary. As such, it is used for rheumatic conditions and as a skin tonic in wound healing. Employed for indolent wounds it is also included in medicinal creams and some cosmetic preparations. These uses have largely been supported by pharmacological data.

IVY

Ivy does not feature strongly in British herbal medicine but, with a considerable number of other European drugs, it is now included in the *BP* as a result of its *EP* status. The drug consists of the whole or cut aerial leaves of *Hedera helix* L. family Araliaceae collected in the spring. This familiar climber and creeper is widely distributed throughout Europe and Asia. Non-flowering shoots produce alternate palmate three- to five-lobed leaves with conspicuous pale veins; leaves of the flowering shoots are often larger, ovate or rhombic and entire. Microscopical features include: epidermal cells with wavy anticlinal walls, occasionally anisocytic but mainly anomocytic stomata on the lower epidermis, mucilage cells of the mesophyll and cluster crystals of calcium oxalate about 40 μm in diameter.

Important constituents of ivy are saponins involving the pentacyclic triterpenoid genins hederagenin, bayogenin and oleanolic acid. Examples are given in Fig. 23.14; see also F. Delmas *et al.*, *Planta Medica*, 2000, **66**, 343. Other constituents are flavonoids (rutin, quercetin), caffeic acid derivatives (chlorogenic, rosmarinic acid, etc.), sterols, polyacetylenes and volatile oil.

The *BP/EP* TLC test for identity indicates the presence of α-hederin and heteracoside C; a minimum concentration of 3.0% heteracoside C determined using liquid chromatography is specified.

Ivy-leaf extracts have been traditionally used as an expectorant for the treatment of various chest conditions, such as bronchitis and whooping cough; also for gout and rheumatic pains. Like most saponins, those of ivy are toxic in excess causing diarrhoea, vomiting and allergy. Externally, ivy is used cosmetically and for a variety of skin conditions. Molluscidal, antibacterial and antileishmanial properties have been reported for the saponins.

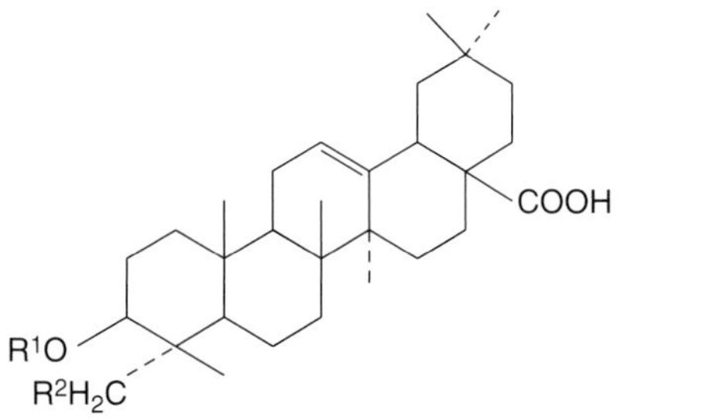

	R¹	R²
α-Hederin	Ara 2–1 Rha	OH
β-Hederin	Ara 2–1 Rha	H
Hederacolchiside A₁	Ara [Glc 4–1] 2–1 Rha	H

Fig. 23.14
Saponins of Ivy.

CARDIOACTIVE DRUGS

A considerable number of plants scattered throughout the plant kingdom contain C_{23} or C_{24} steroidal glycosides which exert on the failing heart a slowing and strengthening effect. In Western medicine it is the glycosides of various *Digitalis* species that are extensively employed. The introduction of the foxglove (*D. purpurea*) into British medicine for treatment of dropsy by the Birmingham physician and botanist William Withering, in 1785, constitutes one of the fascinating stories of medicine. It was not realized at that time, however, that dropsy could be the result of a heart condition. Before the introduction of digitalis it was treated by the oral administration of dried and powdered toad-skins; later investigations were to show that this treatment too, did not lack a pharmacological basis. The action of the digitalis glycosides on the heart is discussed in Chapter 6.

The heart-arresting properties of these glycosides also render them most effective as arrow poisons and a number of tropical plants are better-known in this respect than for their medicinal use.

Distribution in nature

In plants cardiac glycosides appear to be confined to the Angiosperms. Cardenolides (see below) are the more common and are particularly abundant in the Apocynaceae and Asclepiadaceae, but are also found in some Liliaceae (e.g. *Convallaria*), and in the Ranunculaceae, Moraceae, Cruciferae, Sterculiaceae, Euphorbiaceae, Tiliaceae, Celastraceae, Leguminosae and Scrophulariaceae. The bufanolides occur in some Liliaceae (e.g. *Urginea*) and in some Ranunculaceae (e.g. *Helleborus*). In toad venoms the genins are partly free and partly conjugated with suberylarginine.

Some of the main genera containing cardiac glycosides are as follows: Apocynaceae: *Adenium*, *Acokanthera*, *Strophanthus*, *Apocynum*, *Cerbera*, *Tanghinia*, *Thevetia*, *Nerium*, *Carissa* and *Urechites*; Asclepiadaceae: *Gomphocarpus*, *Calotropis*, *Pachycarpus*, *Asclepias*, *Xysmalobium*, *Cryptostegia*, *Menabea* and *Periploca*; Liliaceae: *Urginea*, *Bowiea*, *Convallaria*, *Ornithogalum* and *Rohdea*; Ranunculaceae: *Adonis* and *Helleborus*; Moraceae: *Antiaris*, *Antiaropsis*, *Naucleopsis*, *Maquira* and *Castilla*; Cruciferae: *Erysimum* and *Cheiranthus*; Sterculiaceae: *Mansonia*; Tiliaceae; seeds of *Corchorus* spp.; Celastraceae: *Euonymus* and *Lophopetalum*; Leguminosae: *Coronilla*; and Scrophulariaceae. In the latter family cardiac glycosides have been found only in the genus *Digitalis* if we include in this the plant which some botanists call *Digitalis canareniensis* and others place in the genus *Isoplexis*.

Structure of glycosides

Two types of genin may be distinguished according to whether there is a five-or six-membered lactone ring. These types are known respectively as cardenolides (e.g. digitoxigenin) and bufanolides or bufadienolides (e.g. scillarenin). The following formulae indicate their structure and ring numbering:

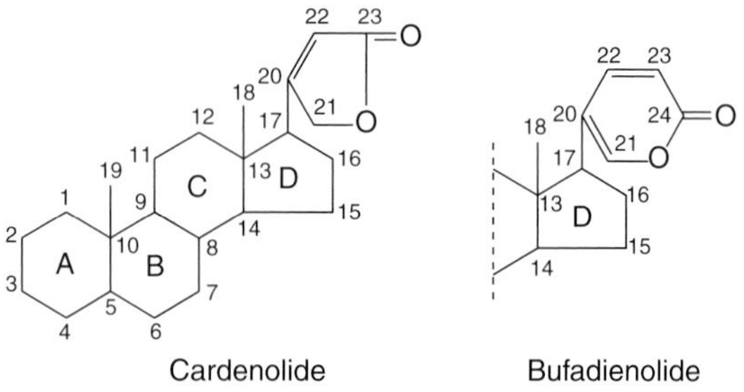

Cardenolide   Bufadienolide

Substitution patterns for some typical genins are given in Table 23.6.

The sugar moieties, attached to the aglycone by a C-3,β-linkage, are composed of up to four sugar units which may include glucose or

Table 23.6 Genins of some cardioactive glycosides.

Genins	Carbon ring numbering							
	1	3	5	10	11	12	14	16
Cardenolides								
Digitoxigenin		OH		CH$_3$			OH	
Gitoxigenin		OH		CH$_3$			OH	OH
Gitaloxigenin		OH		CH$_3$			OH	OCHO
Digoxigenin		OH		CH$_3$		OH	OH	
Diginatigenin		OH		CH$_3$		OH	OH	OH
Strophanthidin		OH	OH	CHO			OH	
Ouabagenin	OH	OH	OH	CH$_2$OH	OH		OH	
Dienolides								
Scillaridin A*		OH		CH$_3$			OH	
Scilliphaeosidin*		OH		CH$_3$		OH	OH	
Hellebrigenin		OH	OH	CHO			OH	

*Double bond at C4–C5

rhamnose together with other deoxy-sugars whose natural occurrence is, to date, known only in association with cardiac glycosides. A number of the deoxy-sugars are 2,6-dideoxyhexoses (e.g. digitoxose) or their 3-*O*-methyl ethers (e.g. cymarose). In addition to rhamnose and fucose, a number of other 6-deoxyhexose derivatives have more recently been discovered together with 2-*O*-methyl and 2-*O*-acetyl sugars. In the case of fucose, the D-form is known only in cardiac glycosides, whereas the L-form is widely distributed in nature. Cardiac glycosides involving cyclic sugars are known in *Calotropis* spp. and probably occur in other members of the Asclepiadaceae.

A characteristic arrangement of the carbohydrate side-chain at C-3 is: aglycone-(characteristic cardiacglycoside sugars, or rhamnose)$_x$-(glucose)$_y$; *X* and *Y* may = 0 and there are some modifications of this general pattern. Some examples of the sugars found in these glycosides are given in Fig. 23.15.

Biogenesis of cardiac glycosides

Aglycones of the cardiac glycosides are derived from mevalonic acid but the final molecules arise from a condensation of a C$_{21}$ steroid with a C$_2$ unit (the source of C-22 and C-23). Bufadienolides are condensation products of a C$_{21}$ steroid and a C$_3$ unit (Fig. 23.16).

Progesterone, which is formed with cardiac glycosides, in *Digitalis lanata* as a result of feeding pregnenolone, is itself a precursor of the cardiac glycosides. Work, involving *Strophanthus kombé*, on the intermediates between progesterone and the cardenolides affords evidence consistent with the pathway: progesterone → 5β-pregnanolone → 5β-hydroxypregnanolone → cardenolides (Fig. 23.17). Similar transformations have also been demonstrated in *Digitalis purpurea* cultures but alternative pathways exist depending on whether hydroxylation of the nucleus occurs before or after the essential acetate condensation for the butenolide ring formation. Indeed, work involving some nine enzymes has helped to demonstrate that cardenolide genins arise as a result of a complex interlinking multi-dimensional system of pathways rather than by a single route leading directly to the end product.

As is evident from Fig. 23.17, a key enzyme in the biosynthesis of cardiac glycosides is progesterone 5β-reductase. Such an enzyme is also involved in the production of animal steroids so it is of interest to note that I. Gavidia *et al.* (*Phytochemistry*, 2007, **68**, 853) have shown that with *Digitalis purpurea* this enzyme is not homologous with the

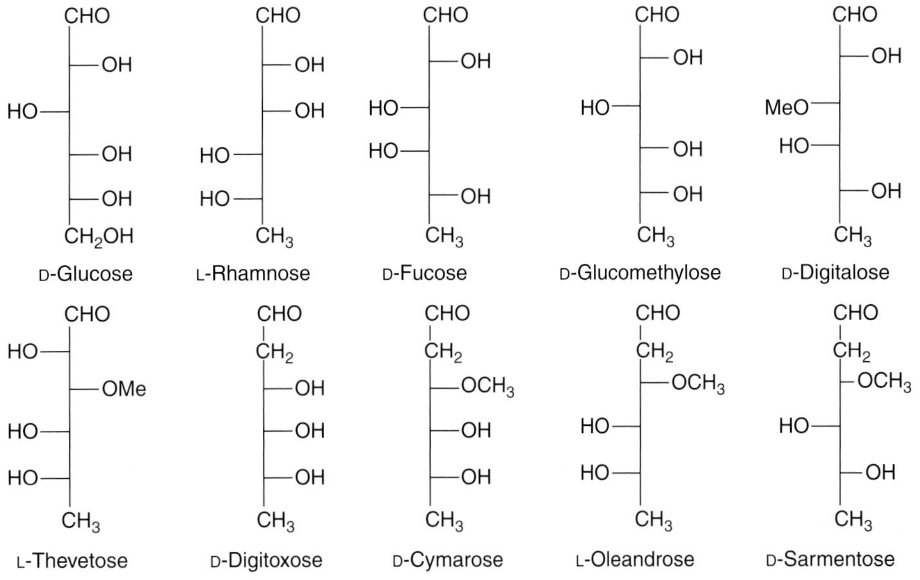

Fig. 23.15
Some examples of sugars found in cardiac glycosides (Fischer representation).

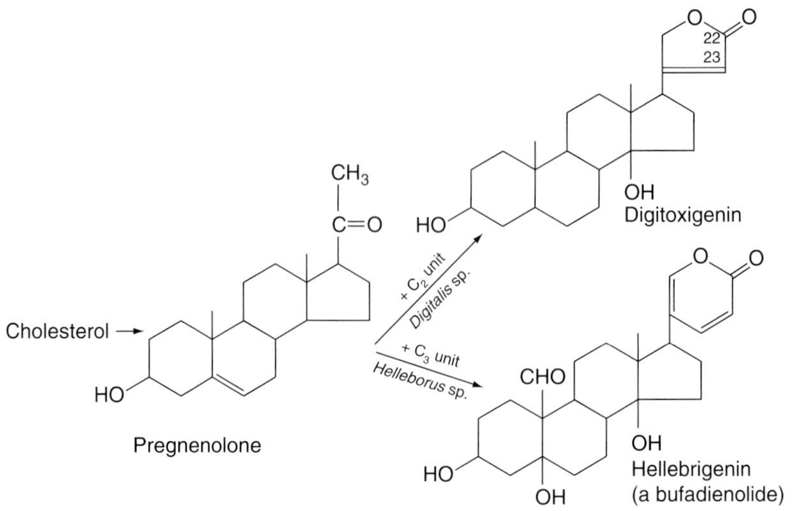

Fig. 23.16
Formation of aglycones of cardiac glycosides
from a C_{21} steroid.

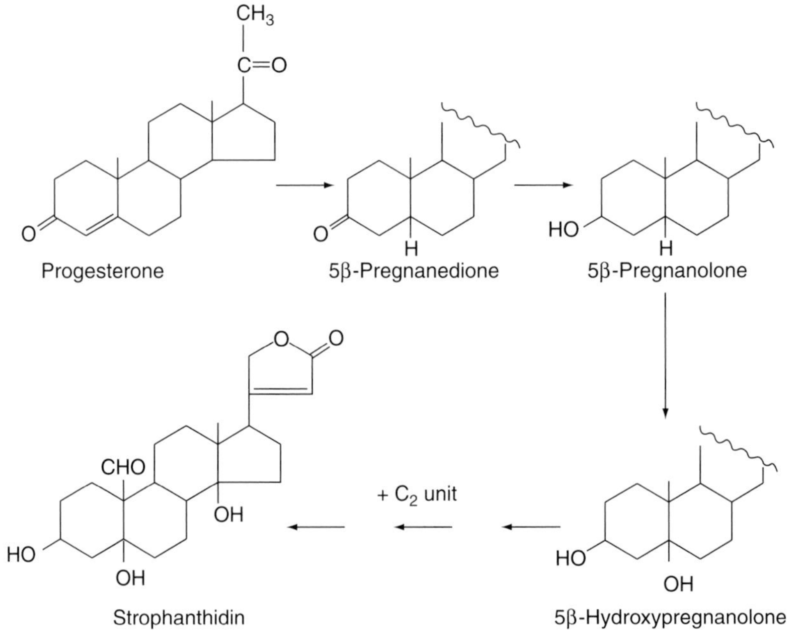

Fig. 23.17
Suggested intermediates in the metabolism
of progesterone to cardiac glycosides.

corresponding enzyme in animals, suggesting that the steroid pathway evolved independently in plants and animals. Apparently, a similar situation occurs with 3β-hydroxy-Δ5-steroid dehydrogenase, an enzyme preceding the above in the cardenolide pathway.

Biogenetic studies involving the side-chain indicate that glucose is the most effective precursor of digitoxose and of the sugar side-chain of the *Nerium oleander* glycosides. Some ten enzymes have now been shown to be involved in the sugar side-chain biosynthesis in *Digitalis* species.

Tests and assays

The tests and assays available for cardioactive medicinals depend on biological activity, reactions of the sugar side-chain of the glycosides, and properties of the butenolide side-chain. Traditionally, the *BP* employed a biological assay for Digitalis (and formerly Strophanthus) on the basis that, compared with chemical and physical assays, it offered the best indication of the combined activity of the complex mixture of glycosides present. Now no biological assays are included for cardioactive drugs.

For digitalis leaves, the *EP* and *BP* utilize the red-violet colour (λ_{max} 540 nm) produced by the interaction of cardenolides and 3,5-dinitrobenzoic acid. Other colour reactions based on the butenolide moiety are the red-orange (λ_{max} 495 nm) given with an alkaline sodium picrate reagent (*EP* assay for digitoxin and digoxin), the red colour with xanthydrol reagent (*EP* test for digitalis leaf) and the red colour (λ_{max} about 470 nm) produced with sodium dinitroprusside. In the ultraviolet region the butenolide side-chain exhibits λ_{max} 217 nm and with purified substances, for example the eluted glycoside zones produced by TLC which contain little extraneous material, this can be used for rapid evaluation. These spectroscopic tests do not, in themselves, distinguish between glycosides and their corresponding aglycones.

A colour test specific for the digitoxose moiety is the Keller–Kiliani test; for details see 'Digitalis Leaf'. The test is employed by the *EP* for the identification of digitoxin and digoxin and by the *BP* as an assay for digoxin injection and tablets (λ_{max} 590 nm).

The separation and determination of individual glycosides by TLC, electrophoresis and GLC (derivatized glycosides) has received much attention over the years.

CARDENOLIDES

Of the cardioactive glycosides, those of the cardenolide group (Table 23.6) are the most important medicinally. Synthesis of these compounds has presented obvious difficulties but in recent years a large number of synthetic monosides have been prepared; one of these, a mannoside of strophanthidin, has proved extremely potent. All the medicinal preparations are derived from natural sources.

DIGITALIS LEAF

Digitalis (*Purple Foxglove Leaves*) consists of the dried leaves of *Digitalis purpurea* L. (Scrophulariaceae). It is required to contain not less than 0.3% of total cardenolides calculated as digitoxin.

History. Foxglove leaves appear to have been used externally by the Welsh 'Physicians of Myddfai' but the plant had no name in Greek or Latin until named digitalis by Fuchs (1542). The poisonous nature of the leaves was well known, and the drug was recommended by Parkinson in 1640; it was introduced into the *London Pharmacopoeia* of 1650. William Withering published his work on the clinical use of foxglove in 1785. For further reading, of largely historical interest, see J. K. Aronson (1985), *An Account of the Foxglove and its Medical Uses 1785–1985*, Oxford, Oxford University Press. Groves and Bisset have reviewed the topical use of *Digitalis* prior to William Withering pointing out the evidence for effective transdermal passage of the glycosides (*J. Ethnopharmacol.*, 1991, **35**, 99).

Plant. The foxglove is a biennial or perennial herb which is very common in the UK and most of Europe, including some Mediterranean regions of Italy, and is naturalized in North America. It is produced commercially in Holland and Eastern Europe. In the first year the plant forms a rosette of leaves and in the second year an aerial stem about 1–1.5 m in height. The inflorescence is a raceme of bell-shaped flowers of the floral formula K(5), C(5), A4 didynamous, G(2). The common wild form of the plant has a purple corolla about 4 cm long, the ventral side of which is whitish but bears deep purple eyespots on its inner surface. Many horticultural varieties exist, but these are of low therapeutic potency. The fruit is a bilocular capsule which contains numerous seeds attached to axile placentae.

Digitalis grows readily from seed. In the wild state it is usually found in semi-shady positions. It grows well in sandy soil, provided that a certain amount of manganese is present, this element being apparently essential and is always to be found in the ash.

Collection. Either first- or second-year leaves are permitted by the pharmacopoeias.

There has been a long-standing general belief that the pharmacological activity of leaves increases during the course of a day to reach a maximum in the early afternoon. Biological assays have given some support to this supposition and variations involving individual glycosides have also been reported.

After collection the leaves should be dried as rapidly as possible at a temperature of about 60°C and subsequently stored in airtight containers protected from light. Their moisture content should not be more than about 6%.

Macroscopical characters. Digitalis leaves (Fig. 23.18) are usually ovate-lanceolate to broadly ovate in shape, petiolate and about 10–30 cm long and 4–10 cm wide. The dried leaves are of a dark greyish-green colour. The lamina is decurrent at the base; apex subacute. The margin is crenate or dentate and most of the teeth show a large water pore. Both surfaces are hairy, particularly the lower, and a fringe of fine hairs is found on the margin. The veins are depressed on the upper surface but very prominent on the lower. The main veins leave the midrib at an acute angle, afterwards branching and anastomosing repeatedly. The drug has no marked odour, but a distinctly bitter taste.

Microscopical characters. A transverse section of a foxglove leaf shows a typical bifacial structure and a midrib strongly convex on the lower surface (Fig. 23.18). Stomata and hairs are present on both surfaces, but are more numerous on the lower one. Calcium oxalate is absent. The palisade tissue is interrupted at the midrib. A zone of collenchyma underlies both epidermi in the midrib region. The crescent-shaped midrib bundle is enclosed in an endodermis one or two cells thick developed as a starch sheath. The pericycle is parenchymatous above and collenchymatous below. Sclerenchymatous fibres are absent.

Surface preparations (Fig. 23.18C, D) show that the upper epidermis consists of polygonal, relatively straight-walled cells, and bears both clothing and glandular hairs. The cells of the lower epidermis are wavy, and the stomata and hairs much more numerous than on the upper surface of the leaf. The stomata are small and slightly raised above the surrounding cells. The clothing hairs are uniseriate, two- to seven-celled, bluntly pointed, smooth or finely warty, with cells often collapsed alternatively at right angles (Fig. 23.18). The glandular hairs have a unicellular or occasionally a short uniseriate pedicel, with a unicellular or bicellular terminal gland (Fig. 23.18E). The cuticle of the hairs and epidermal cells may be stained red with a solution of Sudan Red in glycerin.

Prepared digitalis. This was a standardized powder of the *BP* (1989); it was adjusted to strength with weaker powdered digitalis or with powdered grass.

Constituents The chemistry of digitalis has engaged the attention of many workers since about 1820. Important progress was made by Nativelle (1868), Kiliani (1891), Stoll (1938) and Haack *et al.* (1956).

The primary (tetra) glycosides (purpurea glycoside A, purpurea glycoside B and glucogitaloxin) all possess at C-3 of the genin a linear chain of three digitoxose sugar moieties terminated by glucose. Purpurea glycosides A and B, first characterized by A. Stoll in 1938, constitute the principal active constituents of the fresh leaves. On drying, enzyme degradation takes place with the loss of the terminal glucose to give digitoxin, gitoxin and gitaloxin, respectively. Digitoxin and gitoxin are therefore the main active components of the dried drug. Poor storage conditions will lead to further hydrolysis and complete loss of activity. The gitaloxigenin series with its formyl group at C-16 is less stable than the other two series and was not discovered until 1956; the glycosides of this series are claimed to have similar or greater activities than those of the digitoxigenin group. The aglycones digitoxigenin and gitoxigenin are produced by acid hydrolysis of the respective glycosides but they are not found in quantity in the fresh or dried leaves. The aglycones, the formulae of which are shown in Fig. 23.19 are formed in the plant via the acetate-mevalonate pathway as already indicated in Fig. 23.16.

Other glycosides, present in small proportions, and involving the same genins contain digitalose and glucose; they exist as mono- and diglycosides. In this group verodoxin is claimed to have a toxicity of three times that of gitaloxin. These series are listed in Table 23.7. In 1961 small yields of yet other glycosides were reported from digitalis and include those with an acetylated side-chain (see Table 23.8).

Over the years much attention has been given to the variation of glycoside content in digitalis both throughout the 2-year life cycle and during the

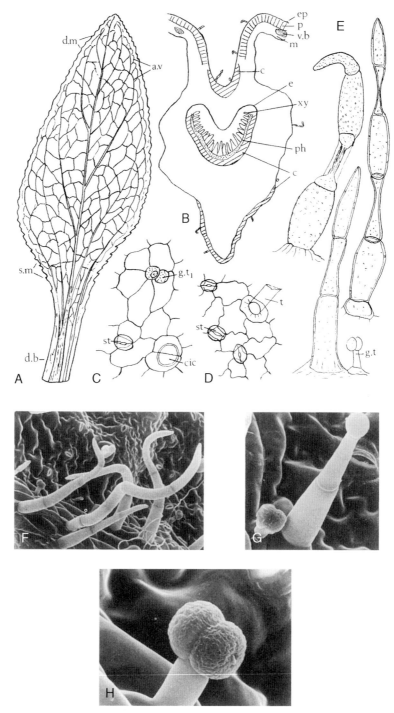

Fig. 23.18
Digitalis purpurea leaf. A, First-year leaf (×0.25); B, transverse section midrib of first-year leaf (×15); C, upper epidermis; D, lower epidermis; E, trichomes (all ×200); F–H, scanning electron micrographs: F, lower surface or leaf and G, H ditto showing glandular trichomes. a.v, Anastomosing veins; c, collenchyma, cic, cicatrix; d.b, decurrent base; d.m, dentate margin; e, endodermis; ep, epidermis; g.t, glandular trichome; g.t₁, ditto surface view; m, mesophyll; p, palisade; ph, phloem; s.m, serrate margin; st, stoma; t, trichome base; xy, xylem. (Photos: Lorraine Seed and R. Worsley.)

course of a single day. General conclusions are not easily drawn, because of the apparently contradictory results obtained by different workers. These contradictions probably arise from the different methods of assay employed, the different environmental conditions of the plants studied, and the possible use of different chemical races. It is generally agreed that first-year leaves collected July–August have the highest content of total glycosides and that after a fall during the winter months, another peak, but not as high as the first-year one, is reached at the time of flowering.

For plants of Belgian origin, Lemli showed, in 1961, by chromatographic analysis that digitalinum verum and glucoverodoxin are formed first in the young leaves and then cease to accumulate further. At this stage small amounts only of purpurea glycoside B and glucogitaloxin are present but these steadily increase, finally to reach 40% of the total glycosides. Purpurea glycoside A is formed last and eventually becomes the major component at 50% of the total glycoside mixture.

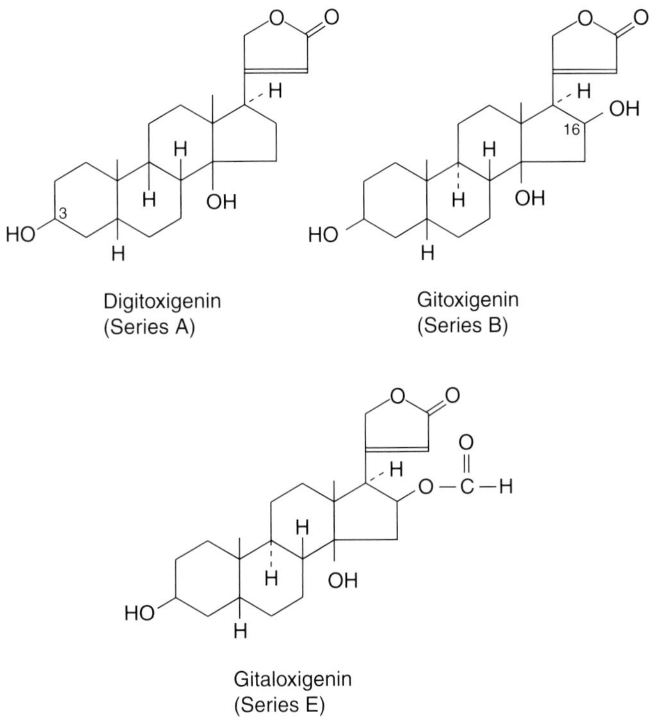

Digitoxigenin
(Series A)

Gitoxigenin
(Series B)

Gitaloxigenin
(Series E)

Fig. 23.19
Aglycones of *Digitalis purpurea* cardioactive glycosides.

Chemical races with respect to glycosides derived from digitoxin and gitoxin have been identified.

Digitalis purpurea leaves also contain anthraquinone derivatives, which include: 1-methoxy-2-methylanthraquinone, 3-methoxy-2-methylanthraquinone, digitolutein (3-methylalizarin-1-methylether), 3-methylalizarin, 1,4,8-trihydroxy-2-methyl-anthraquinone, etc. Saponins have also been isolated from the leaves, the sapogenins being produced more readily than cardenolides towards the end of the growing season. A number of leaf flavonoids have been described.

Keller–Kiliani test for digitoxose. Boil 1 g of powdered digitalis leaf with 10 ml of 70% alcohol for 2–3 min, filter; to 5 ml of filtrate add 10 ml of water and 0.5 ml of strong solution of lead acetate; shake and filter. Shake the filtrate with 5 ml of chloroform, allow to separate, pipette off the chloroform and remove the solvent by gentle evaporation in a porcelain dish. Dissolve the cooled residue in 3 ml of glacial acetic acid containing two drops of 5% ferric chloride solution. Carefully transfer this solution to the surface of 2 ml of concentrated sulphuric acid; a reddish-brown layer forms at the junction of the two liquids and the upper layer slowly becomes bluish-green, darkening with standing.

Digitalis seeds. The seeds of *D. purpurea* contain different glycosides from those of the leaves. When extracted and standardized, they are known as 'Digitalin' (Digitalinum Purum Germanicum or amorphous Digitalin). This consists of the physiologically active 'digitalinum verum', with other water-soluble glycosides, including the saponins digitonin and gitonin.

Allied drugs. *Digitalis thapsi* is found in Spain and Italy. The leaves have a crenate margin and decurrent lamina. The leaves are characterized by the absence of non-glandular hairs, the presence of glandular hairs of two types, some consisting of a bicellular gland and unicellular stalk, others having a unicellular gland and a three- to four-celled stalk, the presence of a striated cuticle, pericyclic fibres and small prisms of calcium oxalate. The vein-islet number is higher than the other *Digitalis* species, varying from 8.5 to 16. *D. lutea* has a potency similar to those of *D. purpurea* and *D. ferruginia* and is cultivated in the former USSR. *D. ferruginea* ssp. *ferruginea* is the most widespread of the nine *Digitalis* spp. which grow in Turkey. For a report on the isolation of phenylethanoid glycosides from the aerial parts see Ihsan Çalis *et al.*, *Chem. Pharm. Bull.*, 1999, **47**, 1305.

Adulterants. The characters described above, particularly the margin, venation and trichomes, distinguish the official leaves from all the adulterants which have been recorded. For example, mullein leaves (*Verbascum thapsus*) are densely covered with large branched woolly hairs (see Fig. 42.4I). Other possible adulterants are comfrey (*Symphytum officinale*; see Fig. 42.3G), primrose (*Primula vulgaris*; see Fig. 42.5G, H), elecampane (*Inula helenium*), ploughman's spikenard (*Inula conyza*) and nettle (*Urtica dioica*).

Uses. Digitalis preparations are mainly used for their action on cardiac muscle (see Chapter 6).

Table 23.7   Aglycone and sugar components of digitalis leaves.

Sugar components (attached at C-3)	Aglycone		
	Digitoxigenin (Series A)	Gitoxigenin (Series B)	Gitaloxigenin (Series E)
Glucose–(digitoxose)₃–	Purpurea glycoside A	Purpurea glycoside B	Glucogitaloxin
(Digitoxose)₃–	Digitoxin	Gitoxin	Gitaloxin
Glucose–digitalose–	Gluco–odoroside H	Digitalinum verum	Glucoverodoxin
Digitalose–	Odoroside H	Strospeside	Verodoxin

Table 23.8   Acetylated side-chain glycosides of *Digitalis purpurea*.

Glycoside	Aglycone	Sugar moieties
Acetyl glucogitoroside	Gitoxigenin	Glucose–acetyldigitoxose–
Acetyl digitalinum verum	Gitoxigenin	Glucose–acetyldigitalose–
Purlanoside A	Digitoxigenin	Glucose–(digitoxose)₂–acetyldigitoxose–
Purlanoside B	Gitoxigenin	Glucose–(digitoxose)₂–acetyldigitoxose–

23

Further reading

Aronson JK 1985 An account of the foxglove and its medical uses 1785–1985. Oxford University Press, Oxford

Groves MJ, Bisset NG 1991 A note on the use of *Digitalis* prior to William Withering. Journal of Ethnopharmacology 35: 99–103

DIGITALIS LANATA LEAF

The plant, *Digitalis lanata* (Scrophulariaceae), the leaves of which are used as a source of the glycosides digoxin and lanatoside C, is a perennial or biennial herb about 1 m high, indigenous to central and south-eastern Europe. It is also cultivated in Holland, Ecuador and the USA. Some 1000 tonnes of plant material are required annually to meet world demand.

Characters. The leaves are sessile, linear-lanceolate to oblong-lanceolate and up to about 30 cm long and 4 cm broad. The margin is entire, the apex is acuminate and the veins leave the midrib at a very acute angle. The distinctive microscopical characters are the beaded anticlinal walls of the epidermal cells, the 10–14-celled non-glandular trichomes which are confined almost exclusively to the margin of the leaf, and the glandular hairs found on both surfaces; some have bicellular heads and unicellular stalks, while others have unicellular heads and 3–10-celled, uniseriate stalks. As in *D. purpurea*, pericyclic fibres and calcium oxalate are absent.

Constituents. First isolated by Stoll in 1933, the primary glycosides resemble those of *D. purpurea* but are acetylated at the digitoxose moiety next to the terminal glucose. This confers crystalline properties on the compounds, making them more amenable to isolation. Partial hydrolysis of the glycosides occurs during the drying and storage of leaves, and deacetylation will produce products the same as in *D. purpurea*. In addition to the above series of glycosides, two others, involving digoxigenin and diginatigenin (Table 23.6 and Fig. 23.20), are found in the leaves.

The principal glycosides of *D. lanata* leaves are listed in Table 23.9. In a series of papers by D. Krüger and colleagues (*Planta Med.*, 1984, **50**, 267 and references cited therein) nine other glycosides based on digitoxigenin and digoxigenin are described; two sugars involved, not listed in Table 23.9, are xylose and 2,6-dideoxyglucose.

Using radioimmunoassay techniques (q.v.), Weiler and Westerkamp have been able to assay many thousands of individual plants and by selection have obtained races yielding 2–4 times the quantity

Digoxigenin (Series C)   Diginatigenin (Series D)

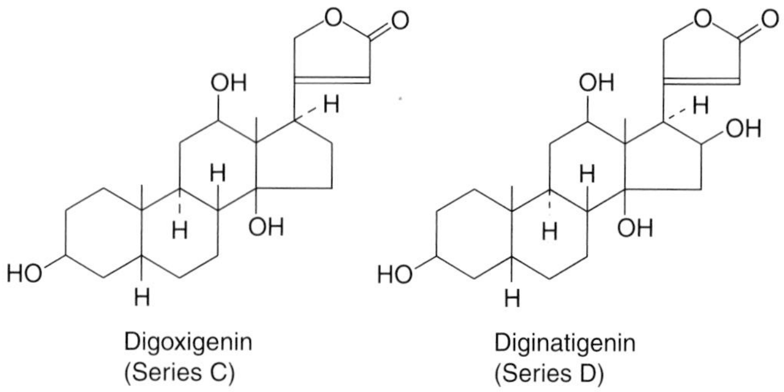

Fig. 23.20
Aglycones of *Digitalis lanata* cardioactive glycosides. See Fig. 23.19 for those also found in *D. purpurea*.

of digoxin found in normal mixed populations (see Chapter 14 for further details). Lehtola *et al.* (1981) found that digoxigenin glycoside levels do not appear to be influenced by collection date (June 28–September 9) or by time of collection (a.m. or p.m.). However, total glycoside levels are higher in first-year leaves but the important medicinal glycosides (e.g. lanatoside C) attain their highest levels in the second-year plants. Rather similar results have been recorded for a Brazilian cultivar (F. C. Braga *et al.*, *Phytochemistry*, 1997, **45**, 473). The primary glycosides appear to be stored exclusively in the vacuoles of cells.

Anthraquinone derivatives, similar to those found in *D. purpurea*, have been recorded in the leaves and a number of flavonoid glycosides characterized.

Cell and organ culture. Both cell and hairy root cultures of *D. lanata* have proved disappointing as a source of cardioactive glycosides. Green tissues appear to be a requisite and green hairy roots produced by light exposure give a 600-fold increase in cardenolide accumulation over roots cultivated in the dark. Luckner and colleagues have studied the development and cardenolide formation of somatic embryos; they established the optimum conditions for the regeneration of shoots from shoot tips and the subsequent adaptation of the regenerated *D. lanata* plants to open ground (*Planta Med.*, 1990, **56**, 53; 175).

Table 23.9 Some cardioactive glycosides of *Digitalis lanata* leaves.

Glycoside	Aglycone	Sugar moieties
Lanatoside A	Digitoxigenin	Glucose–acetyldigitoxose–(digitoxose)$_2$–
Acetyldigitoxin	Digitoxigenin	Acetyldigitoxose–(digitoxose)$_2$–
Digitoxin	Digitoxigenin	(Digitoxose)$_3$–
Glucoevatromonoside	Digitoxigenin	Glucose–digitoxose–
Digitoxigenin-*O*-glucosyl-6-deoxyglucoside	Digitoxigenin	Glucose–glucomethylose–
Glucodigifucoside	Digitoxigenin	Glucose–fucose–
Lanatoside B	Gitoxigenin	Glucose–acetyldigitoxose-(digitoxose)$_2$–
Glucogitoroside	Gitoxigenin	Glucose–digitoxose–
Digitalinum verum	Gitoxigenin	Glucose–digitalose–
Lanatoside C	Digoxigenin	Glucose–acetyldigitoxose-(digitoxose)$_2$–
Acetyldigoxin	Digoxigenin	Acetyldigitoxose–(digitoxose)$_2$–
Deacetyl-lanatoside C	Digoxigenin	Glucose–(digitoxose)$_3$–
Digoxin	Digoxigenin	(Digitoxose)$_3$–
Digoxigenin–glucosyl–bis–digitoxoside	Digoxigenin	Glucose–(digitoxose)$_2$–
Lanatoside D	Diginatigenin	Glucose–acetyldigitoxose-(digitoxose)$_2$–
Lanatoside E	Gitaloxigenin	Glucose–acetyldigitoxose-(digitoxose)$_2$–
Glucolanadoxin	Gitaloxigenin	Glucose–digitoxose–
Glucoverodoxin	Gitaloxigenin	Glucose–digitalose–

Uses The leaves are used almost exclusively for the preparation of the lanatosides and digoxin. Over the past decades digoxin has become the most widely used drug in the treatment of congestive heart failure. In long-term treatments patients require about 1 mg day^{-1} and the world-wide use of the drug now amounts to several thousand kilograms per year.

Proprietary preparations of the lanatoside complex, lanatoside C and lanatoside A are available in various countries but the glycoside from *D. lanata* most widely used is digoxin. Acting similarly to digitalis leaf, digoxin is more rapidly absorbed from the gastrointestinal tract than are the purpurea glycosides, which renders it of value for rapid digitalization in the treatment of atrial fibrillation and congestive heart failure. Lanatoside C is less well absorbed than digitoxin but it is less cumulative and for rapid digitalization the deacetyl derivative is preferable.

CARDIAC GLYCOSIDES OF THE APOCYNACEAE

At least a dozen genera of the Apocynaceae are known to contain cardioactive glycosides. Although all parts of the appropriate plants contain the glycosides, the latter often become concentrated in particular structures (e.g. seeds, barks, etc.). Extracts of a number are used as arrow poisons.

Strophanthus

Seeds of East African *Strophanthus kombé* were formerly official in the *BP* and a tincture prepared from them was used similarly to digitalis. The principal glycosides are K-strophanthoside, K-strophanthin-β and cymarin, all based on the genin strophanthidin (Table 23.6). Many minor glycosides have also been isolated. The seeds also contain about 30% of fixed oil, the bases trigonelline and choline, resin and mucilage.

For a full description of the seeds of this and other species, see earlier editions.

Strophanthus gratus seeds contain 4–8% of ouabain (G-strophanthin), a rhamnose glycoside more stable than those present in other species. It can be isolated in a pure crystalline form, and has been used as a standard in biological assays and for the preparation of ouabain injections. Ouabain is also the principal glycoside of the wood of the African *Acokanthera schimperi* (*A. ouabaio*). For the structure of the aglycone see Table 23.6.

Strophanthus sarmentosus seeds yield a number of glycosides with sarmentogenin as the aglycone. See also Chapter 14 for other information on these seeds.

The oleander glycosides

Nerium oleander, the oleander plant, and related species contain glycosides having a similar action to that of digitalis. Of Mediterranean origin, this evergreen flowering tree is widely cultivated in Japan and other countries as a garden and roadside ornamental.

The principal constituents of the leaves are oleandrin and digitalinum verum. Oleandrin is the monoside, comprising oleandrigenin (16-acetylgitoxigenin) and L-oleandrose. Other components are interesting, as they demonstrate modification of the cardiac activity with change of structure. Thus, the uzarigenin glycosides have a *trans*-fusion of the A/B rings at C-5 (uzarigenin = 5α-digitoxigenin) and have a lowered activity. And the adynerigenin and presumably also the Δ^{16}-dehydroadynerigenin glycosides involving diginose and digitalose are inactive. Adynerigenin is digitoxigenin in which the 14-OH group has been replaced with an 8,14-ββ-epoxy group.

The leaves also contain gitoxigenin and digitoxigenin glycosides. A new glycoside, neridiginoside, has recently been obtained by activity directed isolation using the CNS depressant effect of a methanolic extract of the leaves on mice; it is the 3β-*O*-(D-diginosyl)-glycoside of a 5β,14β-cardenolide. Three other known constituents nerizoside, neritaloside and odoroside-H were also obtained (S. Begum *et al.*, *Phytochemistry*, 1999, **50**, 435 and references cited therein). For the isolation of three new triterpenes, see L. Fu *et al.*, *J. Nat. Prod.*, 2005, **68**, 198. From the bark and twigs, new pregnanes in addition to the known neridienone have been described and their anti-inflammatory and cytotoxic properties studied (L. Bai *et al.*, *J. Nat. Prod.*, 2007, **70**, 14).

Two glycosides isolated from *N. odorum*, in addition to others, are oleandrigenin-β-D-glucosyl-β-D-diginoside and gentiobiosyloleandrin.

The seeds of *Thevetia peruviana* (*T. neriifolia*) the yellow oleander, are a rich source of the glycoside thevetin A, which by partial hydrolysis and the loss of two glucose units yields peruvoside, the therapeutic cardioactive properties of which are well-known. Peruvoside consists of L-thevetose linked to the aglycone cannogenin. Thevetin has found use in continental Europe, and is considered particularly useful in cases of mild myocardial insufficiency and where digitalis intolerance exists.

Oleander ingestion causes many cases of poisoning world-wide; in 1994, 303 cases were reported in Texas, and in Australia during 1972–8 it was responsible for 27% of paediatric plant poisonings. Fatal cases have been reported elsewhere and in Sri Lanka the use of the

Adynerigenin

Cannogenin

Neridiginoside

Neridienone

seeds in suicide attempts, particularly among teenagers, poses a problem (see M. Eddleston *et al.*, *Lancet*, 2000, **355**, 967 and references cited therein).

MISCELLANEOUS SOURCES

Plants which contain medicinally useful cardenolides have been obtained from other families (Asclepiadaceae, Cruciferae, Euphorbiaceae, Liliaceae, Moraceae, Leguminosae, Ranunculaceae, Sterculiaceae).

Convallaria

The lily of the valley, *Convallaria majalis* (Liliaceae) is much used on the continent of Europe and in herbal medicine for its cardioactive properties which are similar to those of digitalis but much less cumulative. Either the aerial parts, collected when the flowers are beginning to open, or the rhizomes and roots, are used.

The principal glycoside is convallatoxin which on hydrolysis gives strophanthidin (Fig. 23.17) and (−)-rhamnose. The plant contains many minor cardenolides, about 40 glycosides associated with nine different aglycones having been identified. Sugars not recorded elsewhere for cardiac glycosides are allose and the disaccharide rhamnosido-6-deoxyallose. (For the isolation of novel cardenolides see V. K. Saxena *et al.*, *J. Nat. Prod.*, 1992, **55**, 39.)

The glycosides appear to be formed in the leaves and a turnover apparently takes place towards the end of the vegetative period. Bioconversions which lead to the formation of minor glycosides have been studied, along with the utilization of digitoxigenin and digitoxin by the plant for production of convallatoxin.

Convalloside, a glycoside of the seeds, when acted on by strophanthobiase yields convallatoxin and D-glucose. A number of flavonoid glycosides are also present in the leaves, and the roots contain a saponin, convallamaroside, which is a 22-hydroxyfuranostanol saponin with three independent sugar chains at C-1, C-3 and C-7.

Japanese lily of the valley, *Convallaria keiskei*, contains glycosides of convallagenin.

The dried aerial roots of *Adonis vernalis* (Ranunculaceae) contain more than 30 cardenolides, acting similarly to those of strophanthus; cymarin is the major constituent. (See B. Kopp *et al.*, *Phytochemistry*, 1992, **31**, 3195.)

The aerial parts of *Erysimum canescens* and other species of *Erysimum* (Cruciferae) are used in the former USSR, and contain glycosides based on strophanthidin. Erysimin, for instance, gives on hydrolysis strophanthidin and digitoxose. Another drug, used in Russia similarly to digitalis, is derived from the bark of the silk-vine *Periploca graeca* (Asclepiadaceae). Its principal glycoside, periplocin, affords on hydrolysis glucose, cymarose and periplogenin.

BUFADIENOLIDES

The bufadienolides (Table 23.6) are less widely distributed in nature than are the cardenolides; they are found in some Liliaceae and Ranunculaceae, and in the toad venoms the genins are partly free and partly combined with suberyl arginine. Therapeutically they find little use as cardioactive drugs because of their low therapeutic index and their production of side-effects. However squill (q.v.) has a time-honoured place as an expectorant and has been widely used in the treatment of cough.

In a review (see 'Further reading') Krenn and Kopp have listed 267 bufadienolides for the period 1967–1995 found in six plant families—Crassulaceae, Hycinthaceae (Liliaceae), Iridaceae, Melianthaceae, Ranunculaceae and Santalaceae—and in animals in the Bufonidae, Cilucridae and Lampyridae.

SQUILL

Squill *BP* consists of the dried sliced bulbs of *Drimia maritima* (L.) Stearn [*Urginea maritima* (L.) Baker], Liliaceae collected after the plant has flowered and from which the membranous outer scales have been removed. *D. maritima* occurs wild as an aggregate of at least six species of varying chromosome number, not all giving a bulb with an acceptable glycoside content. *D. maritima* (L.) Baker *sens. str.* is hexaploid and is a variety from which the commercial drug can be obtained and which has recently been the most studied. It is known in commerce as white squill. That grown in the Mediterranean area (Italy, Malta) is now almost unobtainable and the principal source is Indian squill (see below). Red squill, which is also derived from a variety of *U. maritima*, is collected in Algiers and Cyprus, and differs from the white in containing red anthocyanin pigment and the glycoside scilliroside.

Collection and preparation The bulbs are collected in August, a month in which the plant has finished flowering and is without aerial leaves. After the dry outer scales have been removed, the bulbs are cut transversely into thin slices. These are dried in the sun or by stove heat, when they lose about 80% of their weight. The dried slices are packed in bags (containing about 50 kg) or in barrels.

History. Squill was well known to the early Greek physicians and to the Egyptians. A vinegar of squills was known to Dioskurides and an oxymel of squills to the Arabian physicians.

Macroscopical characters. Squill bulbs are pear-shaped and about 15–30 cm diameter. Whole bulbs are rarely imported because they tend to start growing unless stored in a refrigerator.

The dried drug occurs in yellowish-white, translucent strips about 0.5–5 cm in length and tapering at both ends. The drug is brittle when perfectly dry, but it readily absorbs moisture and becomes tough and flexible. The hygroscopic nature is particularly noticeable in the powdered drug, which, if carelessly stored, tends to cake into solid masses and develop mould. It should be stored in an atmosphere free from moisture. Odour, slight; taste, bitter and acrid.

Microscopical characters. Under the microscope squill shows abundant large polygonal parenchymatous cells of the mesophyll, many of which contain mucilage, surrounding a bundle of many raphides of calcium oxalate (see Fig. 42.9G). The individual crystals are 50–**250–500**–900 μm long and 1–6 μm diameter. The mucilage sheath is stained by corallin soda. Very occasional small, rounded, starch grains, about 10 μm diameter, are present in the mesophyll cells. The epidermis is composed of rectangular cuticularized cells, in surface view polygonal and usually axially elongated. Stomata are absent or very rare on the adaxial surface; a few are constantly present on the abaxial surface. They are anomocytic, circular in outline, with wide guard cells. The mesophyll is traversed by numerous small vascular bundles, which account for the presence in the powdered drug of occasional small spiral and annular xylem vessels.

Constituents. Pure glycosides were not isolated until in 1923 Stoll separated a crystalline glycoside, scillaren A, and an amorphous mixture of glycosides, scillaren B. Scillaren A, the most important constituent of squill, is readily hydrolysed by an enzyme scillarenase or by acids as shown at top of p. 331.

Small quantities of glucoscillaren A (a triglycoside) also occur in the bulb. Other glycosides with 12α- and 12β-OH substitution have similar sugar side-chains at C-3. Other minor glycosides and the isolation of new bufadienolides are described by B. Kopp and L. Krenn (*Phytochemistry*, 1996, **42**, 513; *J. Nat. Prod.*, 1996, **59**, 612). *D. maritima* collected

Enzymic hydrolysis → Proscillaridin A + Glucose

Acid | hydrolysis

Scillaridin A + Rhamnose

Acid hydrolysis → Scillaridin A + Scillabiose
(Scillarenin)   (Glucose + Rhamnose)

Scillaren A

in Egypt is markedly different in chemical constitution to bulbs of *U. aphylla* from Greece and Turkey, and *U. numidica* from Tunisia.

Many flavonoids have been detected in extracts of the bulb of *U. maritima*; they include quercetin derivatives and kaempferol polyglycosides together with *C*-glycosides such as vitexin and isovitexin. The drug also contains sinistrin, a fructan resembling inulin; it is composed largely of β-D-fructofuranosyl residues. M. Iizuka *et al.* have recorded 33 compounds isolated from the squill bulb—ten were new natural compounds, nine were bufadienolides and one was a lignan (*Chem. Pharm. Bull.*, 2001, **49**, 282). Idioblasts (see above) contain calcium oxalate crystals embedded in mucilage consisting mainly of glucogalactans. Anthocyanins are present in small amount.

Tests.   The *BP* specifies an ethanol (90%) extractive of not less than 68.0%, an acid-insoluble ash limit of not more than 1.5%, mucilage staining red with alkaline corallin solution and no purple stain with 0.01-M iodine solution.

Action and uses.   The glycosides are poorly absorbed from the gastrointestinal tract, they are of short-action duration and they are not cumulative. In small doses the drug promotes mild gastric irritation causing a reflex secretion from the bronchioles. It is for this expectorant action that it is widely used; in larger doses it causes vomiting.

Red squill
See 'Rodenticides', Chapter 40.

INDIAN SQUILL OR URGINEA

This consists of the dried, usually longitudinally sliced, bulb of *Drimia indica* (Roxb.) J. P. Jessop [*Urginea indica* (Roxb.) Kunth.]. The drug is used in India and has now been reintroduced into the *BP* and is described in the *BHP*. It occurs in curved pieces of a slightly darker colour than the European squill, which it closely resembles. The strips are sometimes united in groups of about four to eight to a portion of the axis, such pieces being seldom found in the European drug. Also in contrast to the latter, the mucilage of the mesophyll cells stains red with alkaline corallin solution and reddish-purple with iodine solution.

The constituents appear to be similar to those of white squill.

Uses.   Indian squill has a digitalis-like action on the heart and in small doses is used as an expectorant in the same way as European squill.

Black hellebore rhizome
Black hellebore rhizome is obtained from *Helleborus niger* (Ranunculaceae), a perennial herb indigenous to Central Europe. It contains three crystalline cardiac glycosides: helleborin, helleborein

and hellebrin. Of these, the last two have a digitalis-like action, hellebrin being approximately 20 times more powerful than helleborein. The aglycone hellebrigenin (Fig. 23.16) is the bufadienolide analogue of strophanthidin. The drug which has abortifacient as well as cardiotonic properties is considered dangerous and is now obsolete in ordinary medicine.

Further reading
Krenn L, Kopp B 1998 Bufadienolides from animal and plant sources. Phytochemistry 48(1): 1–29
Steyn PS, van Heerden FR 1998 Bufadienolides of plant and animal origin. Natural Product Reports 15(4): 397–414

OTHER STEROIDS

There are few other types of steroidal compounds in addition to those already discussed that have, at the moment, any pharmaceutical significance.

The phytosterols (e.g. stigmasterol and sitosterol) have been mentioned in connection with steroid synthesis, and the role of cholesterol in the biosynthesis of other steroids has been noted (Figs 23.2, 23.16). Steroidal alkaloids in which the nitrogen may be either cyclic or noncyclic are considered in Chapter 26.

WITHANOLIDES

This class of steroidal lactones involves an ergostane-type framework in which C–22 and C–26 are appropriately oxidized to form a δ-lactone ring.

Chemists had long been interested in the constituents of *Withania somnifera* (Solanaceae), an Indian plant well-known in traditional medicine, and in 1968 Israeli workers determined the structure of a constituent lactone (withaferin A) of the plant; since then many more compounds of this now large class, have been characterized. They are subdivided into nine groups: withanolides, withaphysalins, physalins, nicandrenones, jaborols, ixocarpalactones, perulactones, acnistins and miscellaneous withasteroids (see M. Leopoldina *et al.*, *Planta Medica*, 2004, **70**, 551).

In addition to their potential pharmacological value as sedatives, hypnotics, antiseptics and antimitotics, some withanolides are cell differentiation inducers—compounds of a new type of antitumour agent (M. Kuroyanagi *et al.*, *Chem. Pharm. Bull.*, 1999, **47**, 1646). Withanolides have proved of interest because of their occurrence as chemical races of *Withania* and because of their structural variation in hybrids of different races (q.v.). Other genera of the family in which they occur include *Acnistus*, *Datura*, *Deprea*, *Hyoscyamus*, *Iochroma*, *Jaborosa*, *Lycium*, *Nicandra*, *Physalis* and *Solandra*.

Withanolide skeleton

Withaferin A

The first report of a withanolide from the Labiatae concerns the characterization of a new compound, ajugin, from *Ajuga parviflora* whole plants (P. M. Khan *et al.*, *Phytochemistry*, 1999, **51**, 669). Previously the steroidal lactone, ajugalactone, had been isolated from *A. decumbens*; this compound has an α,β-unsaturated carbonyl group and inhibits insect metamorphosis (contrast the ecdysones below). A number of other species have been used by various cultures to treat a variety of ailments. There are rare reports of withanolides of the Taccaceae and Leguminosae.

The isolation of new withanolides continues to be an active area of research.

Ajugalactone

Ecdysones. The ecdysis of insects relates to the moults which larvae undergo during their transformation into an adult, a process controlled by complex hormonal mechanisms. Ecdysones, or insect-moulting hormones, are substances which stimulate these changes, and one example is ecdysone itself, which was first isolated from silk-worm pupae.

Only a few such compounds have been isolated from arthropods, but in plants they occur in much greater variety and abundance. Ecdysterone (20-hydroxyecdysone) is also an example of one which has been obtained from both plant and insect sources; whether a plant–insect relationship exists with regard to this substance and whether such compounds have a function in the plant is at present not known. It is perhaps

significant, however, that insects do not themselves biosynthesize steroids *de novo* and rely on plant materials for suitable precursors.

In the plant, cholesterol is a precursor of insect-moulting hormones, and in one morphological group of *Helleborus* they are formed together with bufadienolides (q.v.) and saponins.

Cucurbitacins. These tetracyclic triterpenoids are of interest because of their cytotoxic and antitumour properties. They occur in the Cucurbitaceae and other families such as the Euphorbiaceae and Cruciferae. Cucurbitacin A was isolated in 1953 and its structure determined in 1963. They may occur in the glucosidic form and are hydrolysed by the enzyme elaterase. The formulae of two examples are given below.

Cucurbitacin E (elaterin); R = CH₃CO
Cucurbitacin I (elaterin B); R = H

Cycloartanes. As was indicated previously (see Fig. 23.1) the ring closure of squalene 2,3-oxide yields cycloartenol as an intermediate in plant sterol biosynthesis. However, these phytosterols are also found in the free state in a wide range of plants; medicinal examples include the neem and olive plants, *Euphorbia* spp., *Hypericum*, the woody nightshade and a number of members of the Cucurbitaceae. The formula of one such compound is given below.

Ecdysterone

Cycloartenone

24

Miscellaneous isoprenoids

In addition to the groups of compounds considered in Chapters 22 and 23, there exists in nature a tremendous range of other isoprenoids, some of which have become of increasing interest as medicinal agents. There are also those plant metabolites of 'mixed' biogenetic origin which contain an isoprenoid moiety (e.g. some indole alkaloids, the cannabinoids and chlorophylls) and these are considered in other appropriate chapters.

MONOTERPENES

As illustrated in Figures 18.18 and 18.19, the monoterpenes are derived from the C_{10} geranyl pyrophosphate and constitute important components of volatile oils. Other examples are given below. Monoterpenoid compounds are reviewed regularly in *Natural Product Reports* (for coverage of the 1990 literature see D. H. Grayson, *ibid.*, 1994, **11**, 225).

IRIDOIDS

The iridoids are cyclopentan-[c]-pyran monoterpenoids and constitute a group of which the number of known members is constantly increasing. The name derives from *Iridomyrmex*, a genus of ants which produces these compounds as a defensive secretion. In a series of reviews covering the years up to December 1989 several hundred iridoids, classified originally into 10 groups, have been listed. Junior (*Planta Med.*, 1990, **56**, 1) has reviewed (146 refs) the isolation and structure elucidation of these compounds. Most occur as glycosides; some occur free and as bis compounds. There are many seco-iridoids, see secologanin, in which the pyran ring is open, and in a few the pyran ring oxygen is replaced by nitrogen, Fig. 24.1.

For a review covering new naturally occurring iridoids reported during 1994–2005, see B. Dinda *et al.*, *Chem. Pharm. Bull.*, 2007, **54**, 159–222; for Part 2 covering the identification of 158 new plant seco-iridoids from 1994 to 2005 and the bioactivity of the two groups, see B. Dinda *et al.*, *Chem. Pharm. Bull.*, 2007, **55**, 689–728.

Of pharmaceutical significance is their presence in Valerian, Gentian and Harpagophytum and the involvement of loganin (Chapter 26) as a precursor of the non-indole portion of some alkaloids.

GENTIAN

Gentian (Gentian Root *BP, EP, BHP*) consists of the dried fermented rhizomes and roots of the yellow gentian, *Gentiana lutea* L. (Gentianaceae), a perennial herb about 1 m high found in the mountainous districts of central and southern Europe and Turkey. Important districts for its collection are the Pyrenees, the Jura and Vosges Mountains, the Black Forest, former Yugoslavia and the Carpathians.

As it is now a protected plant in some areas, attempts are being made to cultivate it in some EU countries (France, Italy, Germany); for this, the initial selection of plant material is of vital importance.

History. Gentian, possibly not derived from the species now official, was known to Dioskurides and Pliny. The drug was commonly employed during the Middle Ages.

Collection and preparation. When the plants are 2–5 years old, the turf is carefully stripped around each and the rhizomes and roots are dug up. This usually takes place from May to October, collection in the autumn being more difficult on account of the hardness of the soil, although possibly preferable from the medicinal point of view. There is no UK demand for 'white' or unfermented gentian, the commercial

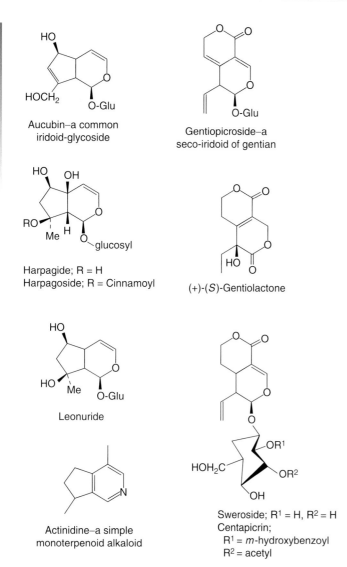

Fig. 24.1
Examples of iridoids.

Aucubin–a common iridoid-glycoside

Gentiopicroside–a seco-iridoid of gentian

Harpagide; R = H
Harpagoside; R = Cinnamoyl

(+)-(*S*)-Gentiolactone

Leonuride

Actinidine–a simple monoterpenoid alkaloid

Sweroside; R¹ = H, R² = H
Centapicrin;
R¹ = *m*-hydroxybenzoyl
R² = acetyl

drug consisting of 'red' or fermented gentian. The method of preparing this varies somewhat in different districts. Usually, the drug is made into heaps, which are allowed to lie on the hillside for some time and may even be covered with earth. After it is washed and cut into suitable lengths the drug is dried, first in the open air and then in sheds. Prepared in this way the drug becomes much darker in colour, loses some of its bitterness and acquires a very distinctive odour.

Macroscopical characters. The plant has a cylindrical rhizome which may attain a diameter of 4 cm and give off roots more than 1 m in length. The crown bears 1–4 aerial stems. The fresh root is whitish and fleshy internally and practically odourless.

The commercial drug consists of simple or branched, cylindrical pieces up to 20 cm long and 1–3 cm diameter. The outer surface is covered with a yellowish-brown cork. The rhizomes are usually of larger diameter than the roots and frequently bear one or more apical buds and encircling leaf scars. On drying, the rhizomes wrinkle transversely, whereas the roots wrinkle longitudinally. The drug is brittle when perfectly dry, but readily absorbs moisture from the air and becomes very tough. It has a characteristic odour and a sweet taste, which later becomes bitter.

Microscopical characters. A transverse section shows an orange–brown bark separated by a darker cambium line from the porous, very indistinctly radiate wood. Only the rhizomes show a pith. More detailed examination shows about 4–6 rows of thin-walled cork cells between which and the cambium is a somewhat thick-walled phelloderm and wide zone of brown, thin-walled parenchyma containing oil globules and minute needles of calcium oxalate. Small groups of soft phloem are seen but phloem fibres are absent.

Examination of the wood and pith shows abundant parenchyma having similar cell contents to those of the bark. The vessels occur either isolated or in small groups and show mainly reticulate or scalariform thickening; a few spiral and annular vessels occur. Groups of soft phloem ('phloem islands', 'interxylary phloem') occur in the xylem. The drug contains very little starch and no sclerenchymatous cells or fibres.

Allied drugs. The roots of other species of *Gentiana* (e.g. *G. purpurea*, *G. pannonica* and *G. punctata*) have been imported. They appear to have similar medicinal properties to the official drug but are usually of smaller size. In India the roots of *G. kurroa* and *Picrorhiza kurroa* are used as gentian substitutes under the name of 'kathi roots'. *G. kurroa*, however is now considered to be a threatened species and shoot multiplication and root formation in *in vitro* cultures have been studied for its possible propagation. Similarly, work in Japan has focused on the mass production of *G. triflora* plants by the cultivation of tissue segments in artificial media in the presence of growth hormones. The *BP/EP* includes a TLC test to differentiate between the official drug and related species.

Adulterants. Adulteration, probably due to careless collection, sometimes occurs. The rhizomes of *Rumex alpinus*, which give the test for anthraquinone derivatives, have been reported; also a dangerous but easily detected admixture with the rhizomes of *Veratrum album*.

Constituents. Gentian contains bitter glycosides, alkaloids, yellow colouring matters, sugars, pectin and fixed oil.

The seco-iridoid *gentiopicroside* (also known as gentiopicrin and gentiamarin; formula see Fig. 24.1) is the principal constituent and was isolated from fresh gentian root in 1862. It occurs to the extent of about 2% and on hydrolysis yields a lactone (gentiogenin) and glucose. A biphenolic acid ester of gentiopicroside, amarogentin, which occurs in small amount (0.025 to 0.05%) has a bitterness value some 5000 times greater than that of gentiopicroside and is therefore an important constituent of the root; other bitters isolated are sweroside and swertiamarin. The isoprenoid gentiolactone has been separated into its enantiomers (Fig. 24.1) by HPLC involving a chiral column (R. Kakuda *et al.*, *Chem. Pharm. Bull.*, 2003, **51**, 885) and the same group of workers (J. Toriumi *et al.*, *Chem. Pharm. Bull.*, 2003, **51**, 89) has reported on new triterpenes in addition to α-amyrin, β-amyrin and lupeol.

The yellow colour of fermented gentian root is due to xanthones (Chapter 21) and includes gentisin (also known as gentiamarin) (Fig. 21.16), isogentisin and gentioside (a 3β-primeverosidoisogentisin). Gentian also contains *gentisic acid* (2,5-dihydroxybenzoic acid) and about 0.03% of the alkaloids gentianine and gentialutine, which may be artefacts of the preparation process.

The bitter principles of *G. lutea* and *G. purpurea* have been assayed by HPLC and separated preparatively by overpressure layer chromatography. The official *BP bitterness value* of the root should be not less than 10 000 when determined by comparison with quinine (200 000).

Gentian is rich in sugars, which include the trisaccharide *gentianose*, the disaccharides *gentiobiose* and *sucrose*. During the fermentation process these are partially hydrolysed into glucose and fructose. If fermentation is allowed to proceed too far, the hexose sugars are converted into alcohol and carbon dioxide. Gentian should yield 33–40% of water-soluble extractive (*BP* not less than 33%), but highly fermented root yields much less.

For references to the chemical composition and to the seasonal variations in the content of secondary metabolites, in the aerial parts of *G. lutea*, see N. Menković *et al.*, *Planta Medica*, 2000, **66**, 178.

Three monoamine oxidase inhibitors have been located in the bark (H. Haraguchi *et al.*, *Phytochemistry*, 2004, **65**, 2255).

Uses. Gentian is used as a bitter tonic. In traditional medicine it has been employed to treat various gastrointestinal conditions, as an anti-inflammatory and wound-healing agent. It is also reported to have choleretic, antioxidative, hepatoprotective and antifungal activities (see A. Mathew *et al.*, *Pharm. Biol.*, 2004, **42**, 8).

CENTAURY

Centaury (*BP/EP, BHP*), family Gentianaceae consists of the dried flowering aerial parts of *Centaureum erythraea* Rafn, including *C. majus* and *C. suffruticosum*.

The biennial plant, some 30 cm in height, is widely distributed throughout Europe, N. America, N. Africa and W. Asia; it is exported from Morocco, Bulgaria and Hungary.

As seen in the dried drug, the hollow stems are yellowish-green with distinct ribs; the sessile leaves, 1–5 cm long, are light green in colour, obovate or spathulate in outline with an entire margin and an obtuse apex; the inflorescence consists of a tubular five-toothed calyx and a joined five-lobed, white-pinkish corolla, five stamens and a cylindrical ovary having parietal placentation and several small brown seeds.

Features of the above are seen in the powder and include fragments of leaf having sinuous epidermal cells with striated cuticles and prisms, occasionally clusters, of calcium oxalate in the mesophyll cells; pollen grains are about 25–30 μm in diameter with three pores and a pitted exine.

The drug has a very bitter taste due to small amounts of seco-iridoid glycosides. Compounds characterized include centapicrin, swertiamarin, sweroside and gentiopicroside. The *BP* TLC test for identity uses a swertiamarin/rutin test solution. Other constituents include flavonoids (up to 0.4%), methylated xanthone derivatives, traces of pyridine and actinidine alkaloids (Fig. 24.1), triterpenoids and various acids.

Centaury is employed as a bitter, stimulating the appetite and increasing the secretion of bile and gastric juice.

BOGBEAN LEAF

Bogbean Leaf *BP/EP, BHP* is the dried, entire or fragmented leaf of *Menyanthes trifoliata* L., family Menyanthaceae. It is a perennial glabrous aquatic or bog plant up to 30 cm in height with leaves and flowers raised above the surface of the water. It grows widely throughout Europe, northern Morocco and N. America. Commercial supplies come largely from central Europe.

The trifoliate leaves have petioles (7–20 cm) with a long, sheathing base. The leaflets are obovate or elliptic with an entire or sometimes sinuous margin and spathulate base. The taste is very bitter and persistent.

Microscopical features include thin-walled sinuous epidermal cells with anomocytic stomata, cuticular striations and characteristic aerenchyma in the leaf lamina and petiole.

The constituents include: the bitter seco-iridoid glycosides menthiafolin and loganin; flavonoids (hyperin, kaempferol, quercetin, rutin

and trifolioside); small amounts of tannin; triterpenes including the betulinic acid derivative menyanthoside which is the principal saponin of the rhizome; phenol-carboxylic acids; coumarins.

Menthiafolin

Loganin is used as a reference in the *BP* TLC examination and a minimum of 3000 is specified for the bitterness test.

Bogbean leaf is used for its bitter and diuretic properties and for the treatment of various rheumatic conditions.

PLANTAIN

Three common European plantains are *Plantago major* L. (common plantain), *P. media* L. (hoary plantain) and *P. lanceolata* L.s.l. (ribort plantain, ribwort). They are distributed generally throughout Europe and temperate Asia and have become naturalized in the US and elsewhere; they are common weeds of lawns and cultivated ground. The dried leaves of *P. major* collected at the time of flowering are included in the *BHP* 1983 and the leaves and scape of *P. lanceolata* in the *BP/EP* (the scape is the leafless ridged pedicel bearing the terminal spike.

The leaves of *P. major* are 10–30 cm in length, ovate or elliptic, entire or irregularly toothed with the blade abruptly contracting into the long petiole. In the dried drug the leaves are brittle and often folded. *P. lanceolata* has strongly ribbed, ovate to lanceolate leaves up to 30 cm in length and 4 cm wide with the blade gradually narrowing into the petiole which is about half as long as the blade. The leaf margin is distinctly toothed. The deeply furrowed five- to seven-ribbed scape usually exceeds the leaves in length and terminates in a characteristic spike of bracts and small white flowers, the long stamens of which in the fresh plant are particularly conspicuous.

Both species have similar microscopical features and these, particularly the clothing and glandular trichomes, are fully described in the pharmacopoeias.

Constituents. The constituents appear similar for both species and include the iridoid aucubin and derivatives (Fig. 24.1), flavonoids, e.g. apigenin and luteolin (see Table 21.5), sugars, mucilage and various organic acids. The *BP/EP* requires a minimum of 1.5% of total *o*-dihydroxycinnamic acid derivatives expressed as acteoside and detects contamination of the drug with *Digitalis lanata* leaves by TLC.

Uses. Traditional uses of plantain depend on its stated expectorant, diuretic and antihaemorrhagic properties.

VALERIAN ROOT

Valerian consists of the rhizome, stolons and roots of *Valeriana officinalis* L.s.l. (Valerianaceae), collected in the autumn and dried at a temperature below 40°C. The plant is a perennial about 1–2 m high. It is obtained from wild and cultivated plants in The Netherlands, Belgium,

France, Germany, eastern Europe and Japan. It is also cultivated in the USA. Polyploidy occurs in *V. officinalis* and there are diploid, tetraploid and octoploid types. British valerian is usually octoploid and central European usually tetraploid.

Cultivation, collection and preparation. Valerian-growing in England has now ceased. Much drug is still produced in Europe, particularly in Holland; trials carried out in 1971–74 at Poznán on light soil showed that propagation by sowing seed, as distinct from the more laborious planting of seedlings, is fully justified.

History. The word '*Valeriana*' is first met with in writings of the ninth and tenth centuries. The drug is mentioned in Anglo-Saxon works of the eleventh century, and was much esteemed not only for its medicinal properties, but also as a spice and perfume. Spikenard ointment, which was used by the Romans and has long been used in the East, was prepared from young shoots of *Nardostachys jatamansi*.

Macroscopical characters. The drug consists of yellowish-brown rhizomes, stolons and roots. The rhizomes are erect, 2–4 cm long and 1–2.5 cm wide, and may be entire or sliced. The roots, which are up to 10 cm long and 2 mm diameter, are more or less matted and broken. In some samples of the drug they almost completely envelop the rhizome, while in others they are mainly separated from it. The drug breaks with a short and horny fracture and is whitish or yellowish internally. The development of the characteristic odour during drying and storage results from a breakdown of the unstable valepotriates and the hydrolysis of esters of the oil to give isovaleric acid as a product, see below. The taste is camphoraceous and slightly bitter.

Microscopical characters. A transverse section of the rhizome shows a thin periderm, a large parenchymatous cortex which is rich in starch and an endodermis containing globules of volatile oil. Within a ring of collateral vascular bundles lies a large pith containing scattered groups of sclerenchymatous cells.

A transverse section of a root shows an epidermis bearing papillae and root hairs, and an exodermis containing globules of oil. The cortex and pith, the latter well-developed in old roots, contain starch. The starch is present mainly in compound grains with two to four components, measuring 3–20 μm diameter.

Constituents. The drug yields about 0.5–1.0% of volatile oil. This contains esters (bornyl isovalerate, bornyl acetate (*c.* 13.0%), bornyl formate, eugenyl isovalerate, isoeugenyl isovalerate), alcohols, eugenol, terpenes and sesquiterpenes (e.g. valerenal, *c.* 12%). The latter comprise various acids, esters, alcohols and a ketone (faurinone) some of which are illustrated in the formulae shown (Fig. 24.2).

Also present in the drug are epoxy-iridoid esters called valepotriates: for example valtrate, didrovaltrate, acevaltrate, and isovaleroyloxyhydroxydidrovaltrate (see formulae).

Valerian also contains alkaloids (0.05–0.1% in the dried root); no structures have been assigned to those (e.g. chatinine and valerine) described in the older literature. Two quaternary alkaloids with a monoterpene structure and which are not identical with those previously isolated have been reported; they are similar to skytanthine and related alkaloids, which occur in widely separated families.

Seasonal variations in the constituents of valerian raised in the Netherlands have been reported. Thus the accumulation of valerenic acid and its derivatives together with valepotriates reached a maximum

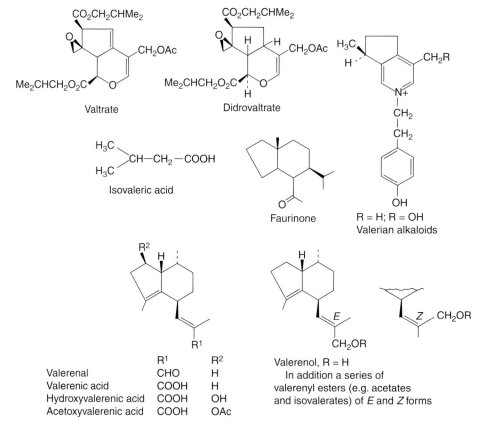

Fig. 24.2
Some constituents of valerian.

in February to March whereas the volatile oil remained essentially constant during the period of study. Strains producing 0.9% essential oil and a high content of valerenic acid and derivatives (0.5%) were recognizable (R. Bos *et al.*, *Planta Medica*, 1998, **64**, 143). For the clinical significance of such strains see 'Action and uses'.

Thirteen valepotriates have been identified in the suspension root culture of *V. officinalis*; root differentiation promotes production. A new iridoid diester, not present in untransformed roots, has been reported in hairy root cultures of var. *sambucifolia* which also produce various kessane derivatives, tentatively identified as kessyl alcohol and acetate. (F. Grünicher *et al.*, *Phytochemistry*, 1995, **38**, 103; **40**, 142).

Quality control. The pharmacopoeia requires a minimum volatile oil content of 0.5% for the whole drug and 0.3% for the cut drug. There is a minimum requirement for sesquiterpenic acids of 0.17% calculated as valerenic acid and maximum values for total ash (12.0%) and ash insoluble in hydrochloric acid (5.0%). Stem bases are limited to 5.0%.

Allied drugs. *Indian valerian*, which is official in the *Indian Pharmacopoeia*, consists of the dried rhizome and roots of *Valeriana wallichii*. It is collected in the Himalayas. The drug consists of yellowish-brown rhizomes, 4–8 cm long and up to 1 cm thick, and a very variable amount of roots up to 7 cm long and 1–2 mm thick. The rhizomes are unbranched and somewhat flattened dorsiventrally. The upper surface bears leaf scars and the lower surface roots or root scars. The rhizome breaks with a short fracture, and the horny interior shows a small dark bark, a well-marked cambium, about 12–15 light-coloured xylem bundles and a dark pith and medullary rays. The odour is valerianaceous and the taste bitter and camphoraceous. The drug contains valepotriates and about 0.3–1.0% of volatile oil containing esters of isovalerenic and formic acids.

Centranthus ruber root (Valerianaceae) also contains a number of the valepotriates of valerian.

Japanese valerian or *kesso* is obtained from *Valeriana angustifolia*. It yields as much as 8% of volatile oil, which is, however, not identical with the oil in the European drug.

Action and uses. Valerian is used as a carminative, and as an antispasmodic in hysteria and other nervous disorders. It is often prescribed with bromides or other sedatives. Considerable quantities of valerian are used by the perfumery industry.

Previously, one problem with valerian preparations was their unreliability of action and this undoubtedly arose from both the unstable nature of the active constituents and the genetic variability of the plant material. The situation was not helped by the lack of success in ascetaining the identity of the sedative components. The volatile oil did not appear to account for the entire action of the drug and the alkaloids were also ruled out in this respect. Subsequent characterization and demonstration of activity in the group of compounds termed valepotriates in the late 1960s and early 1970s appeared in part to resolve the situation and interest turned to these compounds. Nevertheless, it had previously been demonstrated that two sesquiterpene components of the oil, valerenic acid and valeranone, were physiologically active. Further, a related species *Nardostachys jatamansi*, which is used in Asia for the treatment of nervous diseases, was shown to contain valeranone but lacked valepotriates. In 1978 the pharmacological properties of valeranone were confirmed and Japanese workers concluded that the sedative properties of Japanese valerian could be ascribed to this group of compounds. When, therefore, reports on the cytotoxicity of valtrate and didrovaltrate appeared

in 1981 and 1982 (although no side-effects of oral administration of valerian in man have been reported), attention switched to races and species of valerian, as well as selective preparations of the drug, which lacked these compounds.

Further reading

Houghton PJ (ed), Hardman R (series ed) 1997 Medicinal and aromatic plants—industrial profiles, Vol 1. Valerian—the genus *Valeriana*. Harwood Academic, Netherlands

DEVIL'S CLAW (HARPAGOPHYTUM)

Devil's claw *BP/EP* consists of the cut and dried tuberous secondary roots of *Harpagophytum procumbens* D.C. and/or *H. zeyheri* L. Decne. It contains not less than 1.2% harpagoside calculated with reference to the dried drug.

The plant, which derives its name from the characteristic structure of the fruit, is native to Southern and Eastern Africa and is largely obtained from Namibia, with lesser amounts from S. Africa and Botswana. In 2002, at the height of the drug's popularity, exports from S. Africa amounted to some 1018 tonnes of dried tubers, representing millions of plants. To avoid extinction of the plant, a proposal was made to add it to the CITES list but in deference to the effect on the economy of rural areas this was withdrawn and efforts were initiated to develop microprogation techniques to solve the problem. For a full review, see 'Further reading'.

Description. The drug consists of mainly transverse, often fan-shaped slices of the tuberous root with a reddish-brown to dark brown, longitudinally wrinkled, cork. Seen in transverse section the vascular bundles are arranged in radial rows. It is odourless but has a very bitter taste.

Microscopical features of the root include thin-walled yellowish-brown cork cells, thin-walled cells of cortical parenchyma which may contain reddish-brown contents, needles and crystals of calcium oxalate together with the vascular elements. Starch grains are absent.

Constituents. The roots contain iridoid glycosides, flavonoids, various phenolic acids, triterpenes including oleanic and ursolic acids, a quinone (harpagoquinone) and a high concentration of sugars consisting principally of the trisaccharide stachyose (Table 20.1). The principal glycosides are harpagide and its cinnamoyl ester (Fig. 24.1) together with the epoxyiridoid glycoside procumbide. 6-Acetylacteoside and 2,6-diacetylacteoside have been isolated from commercial roots (N. M. Munkombwe, *Phytochemistry*, 2003, **62**, 1231).

The *BP/EP* includes a TLC test for identification using a solution of harpagoside as reference and a liquid chromatographic assay with methyl cinnamate as an internal standard. The total ash should not exceed 10.0% and the loss on drying not more than 12.0%.

Action and uses. Devil's claw has a wide reputation for the treatment of rheumatic disease and although the therapeutic contributions of the various constituents have not been unambiguously established, animal tests indicate that the iridoids are involved in the anti-inflammatory and analgesic effects.

Further reading

Stewart KM, Cole D 2005 The commercial harvest of devil's claw (*Harpagophytum* spp.) in southern Africa: the devil's in the details. J Ethnopharmacology 100 (1–2): 225–236

24

SESQUITERPENES

Sesquiterpenes are biogenetically derived from farnesyl pyrophosphate (Figs 18.18 and 18.19) and in structure may be linear, monocyclic or bicyclic. They constitute a very large group of secondary metabolites, some having been shown to be 'stress compounds' (q.v.) formed as a result of disease or injury. For many years their presence in certain volatile oils and resins has been recognized.

SESQUITERPENE LACTONES

Over 6000 compounds of this group are known and continue to constitute an active area of research. They are particularly characteristic of the Compositae but also occur sporadically in other families. Not only have they proved of interest from chemical and chemotaxonomic viewpoints, but also many possess antitumour, antileukaemic, cytotoxic and antimicrobial activities. They can be responsible for skin allergies in humans and they also act as insect-feeding deterrents.

Germacranolides   Guaianolides

Eudesmanolides   Xanthanolides

Chemically, the compounds can be classified according to their carbocyclic skeletons; thus, from the germacranolides can be derived the guaianolides, pseudoguaianolides, eudesmanolides, eremophilanolides, xanthanolides, etc. A structural feature of all these compounds, which appears to be associated with much of the biological activity, is the α,β-unsaturated-γ-lactone. As examples see the entries below on 'Santonica Flowers', 'Feverfew', 'Chicory' and 'Arnica'. Other Compositae which are herbal remedies and contain sesquiterpene lactones are *Taraxacum officinale* (dandelion), *Artemisia absinthium*, *Cichorium* spp., *Bidens* spp. and *Eupatorium* spp.

Sesquiterpene lactones of the Umbelliferae are interesting in that the usual skeletal types (germacranolides, guaianolides, etc.) are found but all differ in their stereochemistry from the analogous compounds of the Compositae. It is therefore possible that although the biosynthetic steps in the two families form two parallel series of compounds, the conformation of the *trans,trans*-farnesyl diphosphate precursor is different in the two cases.

ARNICA FLOWERS

The drug consists of whole or partially broken dried flower-heads of *Arnica montana* L. (Compositae), a perennial herb with a creeping rhizome. The principal producers are the former Yugoslavia, Spain, Italy and Switzerland where it grows on the lower mountain slopes.

Characters. The receptacle, if present, is about 8 mm in diameter and is slightly convex. It bears pits, corresponding to the position of the flowers, in each of which is a stiff bristle. The involucre consists of two rows of dark-green, hairy, lanceolate bracts about 1 cm in length.

The pistillate, ligulate florets are about 3 cm long. Each consists of a yellow corolla having three teeth and seven to twelve veins, a style and stigma, and a pubescent, dark-brown achene 5 to 7 mm long. The latter is pubescent and glandular and is surmounted by a large, white pappus consisting of very characteristic, barbed bristles. The disc florets resemble the ligulate ones but have a tubular corolla and are hermaphrodite. When examined microscopically, numerous spiny pollen grains and the form of the hairs are seen. Odour, slight but agreeable; taste, bitter and acrid.

R = H (helenalin), and various lower fatty acid groups (see text)

R = H (11,13 dihydrohelenalin), and various lower fatty acid groups (see text)

Constituents. The flowers contain volatile oil (0.5–1.0%), a range of methylated flavones and sesquiterpene lactones of the pseudoguaianolide type which include esters involving acetic acid and various C_4 and C_5 acids (e.g. isobutyric, 2-methyl butyric, isovaleric, and tiglic acids). The principal active constituents (antirheumatic, antiarthritic, antihyperlipidaemic, respiratory analeptic) are esters of helenalin and 11,13-dihydrohelenalin. The former is characteristic of Eastern European flowers and the latter of Spanish flowers. Other constituents include diterpenes and pyrrolizidine alkaloids (tussilagine and isotussilagine).

J. A. Douglas *et al.* (*Planta Medica*, 2004, **70**, 166) have studied variations in the sesquiterpene lactone levels throughout the flower-heads; highest levels were recorded for the disc florets (0.872%), lower levels for the ray florets (0.712%) with the flower receptacles (0.354%) and stems (0.028%) the lowest. The total steroidal lactone levels for the drug rose as the flowers matured.

Quality control. The *BP/EP* 2000 tests include thin-layer chromatography to exclude *Calendula officinalis* and a liquid chromatography assay to determine total lactone sesquiterpenes (not less than 0.40% expressed as helenalin tiglate).

Allied Drug. *Arnica rhizome* consists of the dried rhizome and roots of *Arnica montana*. The rhizome is dark brown in colour, about 2 to 10 cm long, and 2 to 6 mm in diameter. It bears numerous wiry roots and cataphyllary leaves. The transverse section shows a yellowish bark containing oleoresin ducts, a ring of wedge-shaped vascular bundles, and a large pith. The constituents are similar to those of the flowers. About 10 per cent of inulin is also present, but starch is absent.

Uses. Arnica has astringent properties; tinctures and infusions of the dried flower-heads and rhizomes have both been long used as a domestic remedy for the treatment of sprains and bruises. However, neither should be applied to broken skin and treatment should be discontinued should dermatitis develop. In some countries, the use of the drug is subject to legal restrictions.

An arnica gel product was the first 'traditional herbal medicine' to be granted registration in the UK under new regulations introduced by the Medicines and Healthcare products Regulatory Agency (*Pharm. J.*, 2006, **277**, 566).

FEVERFEW

Feverfew, *Tanacetum parthenium* (L.) Schultz Bip. [*Chrysanthemum parthenium* (L.) Bernh.] family Asteraceae/Compositae has a long history as a medicinal plant. It is probably native in S.E. Europe, Asia Minor and the Caucasus but is now established throughout Europe and in N. and S. America, where it is found on roadsides and waste areas.

The plant is a strongly aromatic herb with erect, branching, somewhat downy, stems reaching a height of up to 60 cm. The leaves are pinnate with ovate or oblong segments, pinnatifid and toothed; yellowish-green and pubescent to subglabrous. The numerous flowerheads, 12–22 mm in diameter are long-stalked and form broad terminal corymbs. The involucre is hemispherical with pubescent bracts, white ray florets and yellow disc florets. The fruits are achenes.

Features of the powdered drug include portions of leaf epidermis having a striated cuticle and anomocytic stomata, vascular tissue from the stems and veins, numerous large uniseriate covering trichomes, glandular trichomes, portions of the florets and typical Compositae pollen grains.

Some commercial samples of the drug may be devoid of flowers.

Constituents. In common with many other Compositae, feverfew is phytochemically characterized by the production of sesquiterpene lactones, which can be classified as indicated above. Germacranolides include parthenolide, 3β-hydroxyparthenolide, costunolide, 3β-hydroxycostunolide and others. Chrysanthemin A (canin) and chrysanthemin B are stereoisomers of the guaianolide group, and magnoliolide and others are eudesmanolides. Other constituents are a small amount (up to about 0.07%) of volatile oil containing monoterpenes and sesquiterpenes, tannins and flavonoids.

Feverfew is standardized on its parthenolide content and the *BP/EP* requires a minimum of 0.2% with reference to the dried drug. The assay involves liquid chromatography of a methanolic extract of the drug using parthenolide as reference compound and absorbance measurements at 220 nm. The assay is particularly important as commercial products vary enormously in parthenolide content, some having none at all. This may be due to chemical races known to exist for the species or to confusion in nomenclature, particularly in the US, where the term 'feverfew' may be applied to species other than *T. parthenium*.

Parthenolide   Picrotoxinin

Uses. Feverfew has long been used for the treatment of fever, arthritis, migraine, menstrual problems and other disorders. More recently,

it attracted much popular and scientific interest resulting from favourable reports concerning its use for the prophylactic treatment of migraine headaches.

Chicory

Chicory (*Cichorium intybus*, family Compositae) is indigenous to Europe and is now widespread in northern states of the USA, Canada and parts of Asia; it is widely cultivated. The plant prefers calcareous soils and is easily recognized by its bright blue flowers borne on stiffly erect grooved stems with coriaceous dark-green toothed leaves. In Europe and the USA the root is a traditional herbal remedy and in India the seeds and flowers are also used.

As with some other species of the Compositae the dried roots contain a high proportion (up to 58%) of inulin (q.v.) together with sugars. The coumarins chicoriin, esculetin, esculin, umbelliferone and scopoletin (see Table 21.2) are found in the leaves. Chicory roots also contain various sesquiterpene lactones and glycosides (M. Sato *et al.*, *Chem. Pharm. Bull.*, 1988, **36**, 2423); examples from the 13 isolated compounds include cichorioside A (eudesmane type), 8-deoxylactucin (guaiane type) and picriside B (germacrane type). Lactucin and lactucopicrin show antimalarial activity (T. A. Bischoff *et al.*, *J. Ethnopharmacology*, 2004, **95**, 455),

Decoctions of the root are used as a diuretic and to treat liver ailments; the root is also cited as a tonic and laxative. Extracts of the root and root callus culture have been pharmacologically tested, with positive results, for their antihepatotoxic properties. The roasted roots are well-known for their use in coffee mixtures and as a coffee substitute.

The roots of the culinary *Cichorium endivia* (endive) contain the same constituents as those of *C. intybus*.

Fish berries

Fish berries or cocculus indicus consists of the dried fruits of *Anamirta cocculus* (Menispermaceae), a climbing shrub found in south-eastern Asia (particularly the Malabar coast of India) and the East Indies.

As in the other members of the Menispermaceae, the dorsal side of the fruit grows more rapidly than the ventral, with the result that the fruit becomes reniform and the base and apex both lie on the concave side. The pericarp is rough and woody and the cup-shaped seed consists of an oily endosperm surrounding the embryo, which lies with its radicle pointing towards the apex of the fruit. The two cotyledons occupy separate slit-like cavities in the endosperm. The drug has no odour; the pericarp is tasteless, but the seed is intensely bitter.

The seed contains about 1.5% of a bitter, crystalline, highly toxic substance, 'picrotoxin'. This consists of equimolecular proportions of picrotoxinin, $C_{15}H_{16}O_6$, and picrotin, $C_{15}H_{18}O_7$. Picrotoxinin (see formula) is a highly oxygenated sesquiterpene derivative. The seeds also contain about 50% of fat.

Picrotoxin has been official. It is used intravenously in poisoning by barbiturates and other narcotics. Very small quantities of the fruits are sufficient to stupefy fish.

Orris

Orris rhizome is obtained from three species of *Iris* (Iridaceae), namely *I. florentina*, found in northern Italy, *Iris germanica* found in northern Italy, France, central Europe, Morocco and northern India, and *Iris pallida*, found in Italy (Florence and Lucca) and eastern France. The chief varieties in English commerce are known as Florentine and Veronese. Orris is also produced in Morocco.

Orris root has been used in perfumery from Greek and Roman times. The plants are dug up in August and September, and the peeled

24

rhizomes are dried in the sun for about 5 days either on matting (Florentine) or threaded on cords (Veronese). When dry they are stored for about 3 years in order to develop their full aroma.

Mogadore orris is usually inferior to the European, the rhizome being smaller, darker and less fragrant.

Orris rhizome contains volatile oil which contains irone (see formula below), a substance having an odour of violets. An isomeric substance, ionone, is used as a synthetic violet perfume. Orris also contains starch, calcium oxalate, iridin (a flavone related to rutin), isoflavones, and β-sitosterol and its glycosides.

Powdered orris root is used in dusting powders, while the oil is used in perfumery not only for its delicate odour, but also as a fixative for artificial violet perfumes.

Santonica flowers

Wormseed consists of the dried unexpanded flower-heads of *Artemisia cina* and other santonin-containing species of *Artemisia* (Compositae). *A. cina* is a small plant abundant in Turkestan, where a factory for the extraction of santonin exists at Chimkent. Santonin is prepared from *Artemisia* species found wild in the Kurran valley in Pakistan, and cultivation in this area has been successfully commenced.

The chief anthelminthic constituent of the drug is the sesquiterpene lactone santonin. It has the structure given below. Wormseed also contains a little volatile oil and a second, crystalline lactone, artemisin, closely related to santonin. The amount of santonin present varies considerably not only in the different species and hybrids, but also at different seasons of the year; Russian workers have reported diurnal variations.

In use wormseed has been replaced by santonin, which is very efficient in its action on roundworms. It has less effect on thread worms and none whatever on *Taenia*.

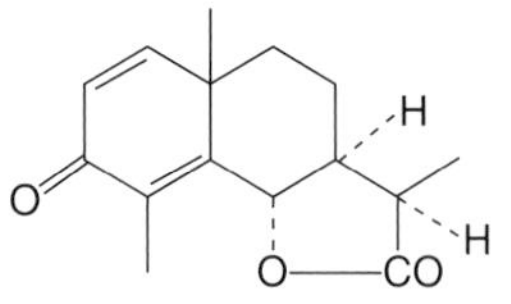

α - Santonin 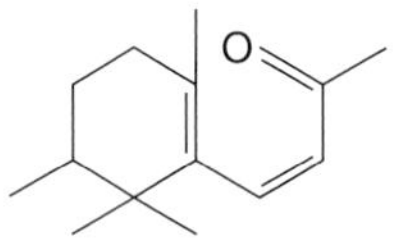   β - Irone

Artemisinin

This unusual sesquiterpene lactone possesses an endoperoxide moiety and is a component of the Chinese antimalarial drug Qinghaosu. It has been successful in treating cases of chloroquine-resistant *Plasmodium falciparum* and particularly cerebral malaria. The increased demand for the drug has led to a supply problem, accompanied by a vast increase in price, giving the WHO concern that the African campaign against malaria would be put in jeopardy. Production of the plant source (sweet Annie) is being increased and it is hoped that a new semi-synthetic bioequivalent artemisinin will lower the cost of treatment (see K. Purcell, *HerbalGram*, 2006, **69**, 24).

Artemisinin (Fig. 24.3) occurs in the herb *Artemisia annua* along with smaller amounts of other cadinane-type sesquiterpenes; by 1993 around 16 of these compounds had been isolated from the plant. Various studies on the accumulation of artemisinin during the development of the plant have been reported; some indicate the highest content before flowering, others at full flowering (see J. F. S. Ferreira *et al.*, *Planta Med.*, 1995, **61**, 167). K.-L. Chan *et al.* (*Phytochemistry*, 1997, **46**, 1209–14) report that artemisinin as isolated from *A. annua* is polymorphic in form. Previously regarded as orthorhombic, the crystals may also be triclinic with the latter possessing a higher dissolution rate.

Callus cultures of *Artemisia annua* have been reported to produce scopoletin and a triglyceride but no artemisinin. However, shoots differentiated from the callus were comparable with the whole plant (G. D. Brown, *J. Nat. Prod.*, 1994, **57**, 975). A suggested pathway for the biosynthesis of artemisinin involves the conversion of a germacranolide to a cadinane-type compound (structure p. 264) and thence through a series of intermediates including artemisinic acid and artemisitene, two sesquiterpenes which have also been isolated from the plant. The structure, biosynthesis and functions of artemisinin have been reviewed (90 refs) by S. Bharel *et al.* (*Fitoterapia*, 1996, **67**, 387).

Further reading

Efferth T 2007 Antiplasmodial and antitumor activity of artemisinin—from bench to bedside. Planta Medica 73(4): 299–309. *See also Chapter 28*

Gossypol

Hemigossypol and related aldehydes together with the dimeric gossypol (Fig. 24.3) are sesquiterpene stress compounds found in the subepidermal glands, immature flower buds and seed kernels of the cotton plant (*Gossypium* spp.). Gossypol was first isolated in 1899, its structure was established in the 1930s and later confirmed by synthesis and spectroscopy.

In addition to having insecticidal and various pharmacological properties, gossypol is of considerable pharmaceutical interest in that in humans it functions as a male antifertility agent. In China it was tested experimentally as a contraceptive with 12 000 men. Work is in progress to reduce possible side-effects and to find alternative systems of delivery. Chinese workers also claim the drug to be active in the therapy of menorrhagia, leiomyoma and endometriosis. Endometrial atrophy occurred in all cases (67 women) and complete recovery of the endometrium was observed within 6 months of the cessation of gossypol treatment.

Inspection of the structural formula of gossypol reveals no chiral centre for the molecule. However, it acquires chirality by the restricted rotation of the bond connecting the two naphthyl moieties and so a pair of atropisomers exist. The compound isolated from the cotton plant was racemic, and this was used in the Chinese clinical trial above;

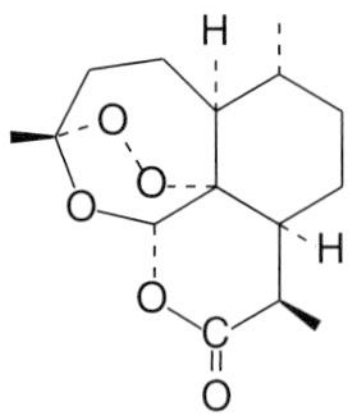

Fig. 24.3
Cadinane-type sesquiterpenes of *Artemisia* and *Gossypium*.

Artemisinin

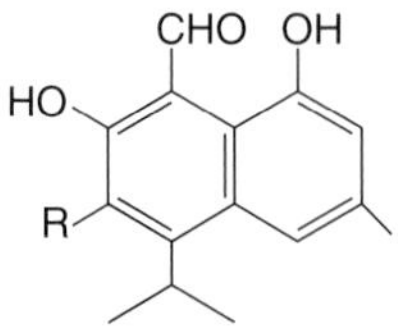

Hemigossypol, R = OH
6-Methoxyhemigossypol, R = OMe
6-Deoxyhemigossypol, R = H

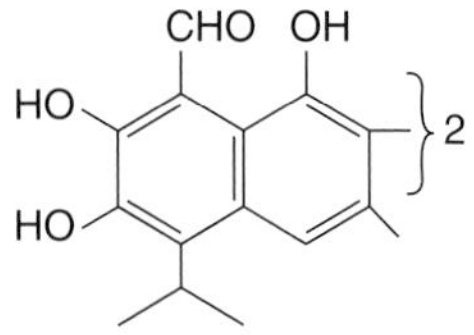

Gossypol

in 1987 the (−)-isomer was shown to be the pharmacologically active principle. By using modern quantitative enantiomorphic separation techniques Cass *et al.* (*Phytochemistry*, 1991, **30**, 2655) have shown that the gossypol enantiomer ratio appears to be species related. Thus, an excess of (+)-gossypol was found in the seeds of each variety tested of *Gossypium arboreum*, *G. herbaceum* (Asiatic cotton) and *G. hirsutum* (Upland cotton) whereas (−)-gossypol was in excess in each variety of *G. barbadense* (Egyptian, Tanguis or Pima cotton). Concordant findings have also been reported by other workers (J. W. Jaroszewski *et al.*, *Planta Med.*, 1992, **58**, 454).

DITERPENOIDS

The origin of the C$_{20}$ diterpenoids, involving the mevalonate pathway, was indicated earlier in Fig. 18.2. The group comprises a structurally diverse range involving hundreds of compounds which may be acyclic or possess 1–5 ring systems. They may also be of mixed origin as illustrated by the diterpenoid alkaloids of *Taxus* and *Aconitum*.

Diterpenoids constitute the active constituents of a number of medicinal plants and are of current interest for their potential as future drugs, either, as isolated from the plant, or as modified derivatives. They include such resin acids as (+)- and (−)-pimaric acid, their isomers, and abietic acid of pine resin. Different stereochemical configurations having the same skeletal structure are also seen in the tetracyclic kaurane and *ent*-kaurane groups (Fig. 24.4); the latter includes the sweetening agent stevioside (Chapter 33) and the gibberellins. The cytotoxic activity of a number of natural and synthetic *ent*-kauranes has been studied (S. Rosselli *et al.*, *J. Nat. Prod.*, 2007, **70**, 347).

The gibberellins, first obtained from fungi of the genus *Gibberella* but also found in higher plants, are diterpenoid acids which have a marked effect on growth of seedlings; they are considered in Chapter 12. Phytol, C$_{20}$H$_{39}$OH, an unsaturated alcohol, is a component of the chlorophyll molecule. Vitamin K$_1$, an antihaemorrhagic compound, first discovered in plants in 1929, is also a phytol derivative. Vitamin A, a diterpenoid, is referred to below under 'Carotenes'. Furanoditerpenes constitute the bitter principles of calumba root (q.v.). *Teucrium chamaedrys*, wall germander, and *T. scorodonia*, wood sage, family Labiatae, are both used in herbal medicine as diaphoretics and antirheumatics. Besides containing small amounts of volatile oil, flavonoids and tannins, both herbs produce diterpenes of the neoclerodane type. Other diterpenoid derivatives include some of the alkaloids of species of *Aconitum* (q.v.), *Daphne*, *Delphinium*, *Garrya*, *Taxus* and *Tripterygium*. Some diterpenes from *Kalmia latifolia* (Ericaceae) have antifeedant properties with respect to the gypsy moth.

Forskolin (coleonol; Fig. 24.4) a diterpene isolated by Indian workers from *Coleus forskohlii* (Labiatae) is the last compound to be formed in the biogenetic sequence of the polyoxygenated diterpenes. Many chemical races of the plant have been revealed and studies on artificial propagation are in progress as, in India, the species is fast becoming extinct owing to large-scale indiscriminate collection. For a pharmacognostical evaluation of the root, see S. K. Srivastava *et al.*, *Pharm. Biol.*, 2002, **40**, 129. Preparations of *Coleus* species have long been used in Hindu and Ayurvedic traditional medicine particularly for the treatment of heart diseases, abdominal colic, etc. Forskolin has been demonstrated to have hypotensive, spasmolytic, cardiotonic and platelet aggregation inhibitory activity; because of its unique adenylate cyclase stimulant activity it is considered a promising drug for the

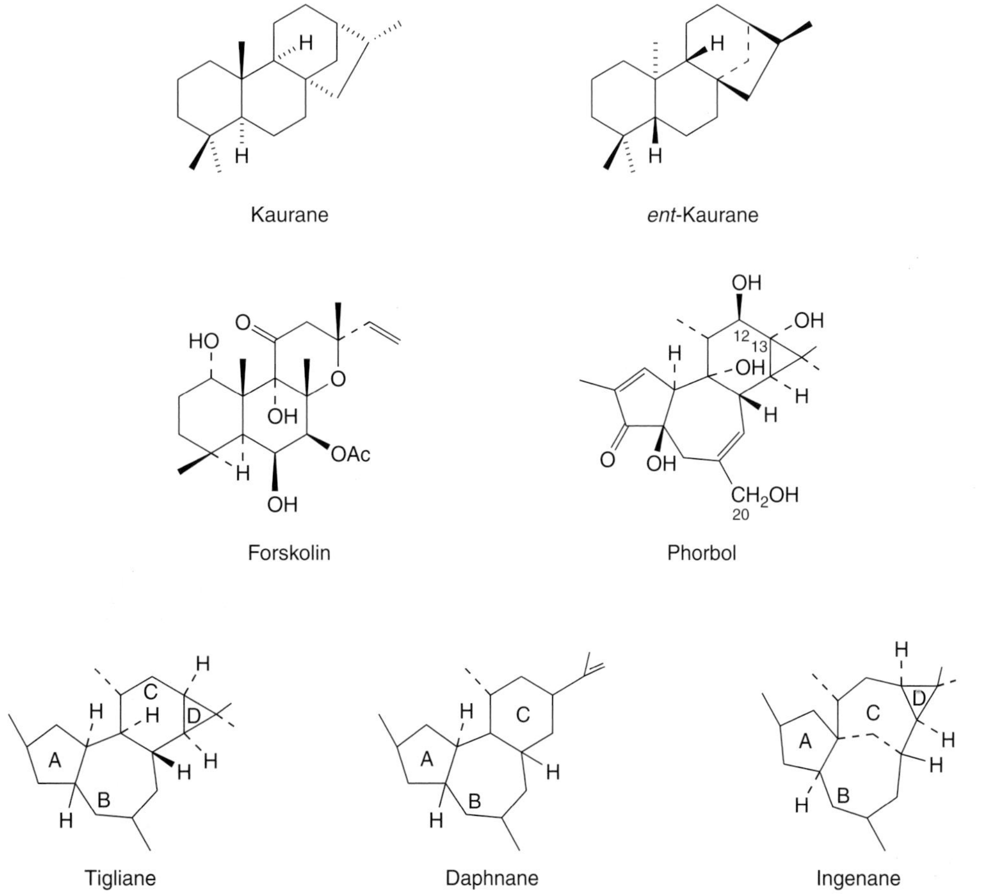

Fig. 24.4
Diterpenoid hydrocarbons and oxygenated compounds (see text).

Kaurane   *ent*-Kaurane

Forskolin   Phorbol

Tigliane   Daphnane   Ingenane

24

treatment of glaucoma, congestive cardiomyopathy and asthma (see R. A. Vishwakarma *et al.*, *Planta Med.*, 1988, **54**, 471.)

The diterpenes of the Euphorbiaceae, e.g. esters of phorbol (Fig. 24.4), and related compounds of other families not only have medicinal potential but are also proving to be useful pharmacological tools; they are described below.

Other drugs containing diterpenes, described in Chapter 21, are agnus castus (rotundifuran and vitexilactone), Java tea (orthosiphols, etc., isopimarone-type diterpenes) and motherwort (labdane-type diterpenes).

Tiglianes, Daphnanes and Ingenanes. These three related groups of diterpenoid compounds (Fig. 24.4) are found in the Euphorbiaceae (e.g. *Croton tiglium* q.v., *Euphorbia* spp.) and the Thymelaeaceae (e.g. *Daphne*, *Lasiosiphon*, *Pimelea* and *Gnidia* spp.). Biologically, they produce intense inflammation on application to the skin and have both tumour-promoting and antitumour activity. Of particular interest are the esters of phorbol (a tigliane derivative). It is the 12,13-diester, 12-*O*-tetradecanoyl-phorbol-13-acetate, which has been most extensively used in pharmacological investigations although *Croton tiglium* contains some 10 others. As pharmacological tools they are valuable in that they substitute for diacylglycerol in the activation of the phosphorylating enzyme protein kinase C; the shape of the molecules, with their long-chain ester groupings, seems to match the side-chains on the natural second messenger, diacylglycerol. The 12,13,20-triesters of phorbol are termed 'cryptic irritants' because they do not exhibit pro-inflammatory activity on mammalian skin unless the C-20 acyl group is removed by hydrolysis.

Further reading

Baloglu E, Kingston D S 1999 The taxane diterpenoids. Journal of Natural Products 62(10): 1448–1472. *Review with 71 references. 350 Taxane diterpenoids classified with information on plant sources, structures, actions, etc.*

Ginkgo

The leaves of ginkgo are obtained from the dioeceous tree *Ginkgo biloba* (Maidenhair-tree) (Ginkgoaceae), the only extant species of an otherwise fossil family of the pre-Ice Age flora. As the specific name implies the leaves are bilobed, each lobe being triangular in outline with a fine radiating, fan-like venation. The leaf is glabrous, petiolate and has an entire margin. The drupe-like fruits possess a bad-smelling pulp and contain seeds with an edible kernel.

Native to China and Japan but cultivated ornamentally in many temperate regions, the tree has a long medicinal history being recorded as early as 2800 BC in the Chinese literature; traditional Chinese medicine uses mainly seed preparations. It is only relatively recently that the drug has received much attention in the West, where in the USA, for the first 8 months of 1999, ginkgo held its place as top of the herbal mainstream market with retail sales valued at over $100 million (M. Blumenthal, *Herbalgram*, 1999 (No. 47), p. 64). In Europe it was estimated in 1993 to have an annual turnover of about $500 million (O. Sticher, *Planta Medica*, 1993, **59**, 2). Standardized extracts prepared in France and Germany are much used in Europe for the treatment of circulatory diseases resulting from advancing age. The leaves are official in the *BHP* 1996 and the *BP/EP*.

Constituents. From among the many groups of compounds isolated from ginkgo it is the diterpene lactones and flavonoids which have been shown to possess therapeutic activity.

Five diterpene lactones (ginkgolides A, B, C, J, M) have been characterized; these have a cage structure involving a tertiary butyl group and six 5-membered rings including a spiro-nonane system, a tetrahydrofuran moiety and three lactonic groups (Fig. 24.5). These compounds are platelet-activating factor (PAF) antagonists (see Chapter 6) and as they do not react with any other known receptor their effect is very specific. Related to the above, and also possessing a tertiary butyl group, is the sesquiterpene bilobalide; no PAF-antagonist activity has been demonstrated for this compound.

Some 33 flavonoids have now been isolated from the leaves and involve mono-, di- and tri-glycosides of kaempferol, quercetin, myricetin and isorhamnetin derivatives. The tree also synthesizes a number of biflavonoids based on amentoflavone; there has been recent interest in these compounds arising from their antilipoperoxidant, antinecrotic and radical-scavenging properties.

Ginkgolic acids are urushiol-type alkylphenols and occur in quantity in the seed coat and to a much lesser extent in the leaves. They are most noticeably observed in poison ivy (Chapter 39) and are associated with allergic responses, particularly dermatitis. For this reason in 1997 the German Government Commission E limited the ginkgolic acid content of standardized extracts to 5 ppm. Other potentially toxic alkylphenols are the cardanols and cardols (Fig. 24.5). The albumen of the seed also contains neurotoxic 4′-*O*-methylpyridoxine (ginkgotoxin) and this has been shown by A. Arenz *et al.* (*Planta Medica*, 1996, **62**, 548) to be present also in the leaves, but in concentrations too low to exert any significant ill-effects in medicines and foods.

Bioproduction. Various investigators have reported considerable fluctuations of terpene concentration in leaves throughout the year, with a maximum in early autumn. With the flavonoids there is a higher concentration of flavonol glycosides in spring leaves and of biflavones in autumn leaves. The age of the tree is an important factor in determining the terpene content of the leaves; those leaves from young trees (10 yr) are the richest source whereas the content is dramatically lowered in leaves of old trees (100–120 yr).

Work by D. J. Carrier *et al.* (*Phytochemistry*, 1998, **48**, 89) has suggested that terpene trilactone (bilobalide + ginkgolides) synthesis might occur in actively growing tissues such as terminal buds. Ginkgolide B can be produced in cultured cells derived from ginkgo leaves and attempts to maximize yields by optimization of the cultural conditions have been reported (M. H. Jeon *et al.*, *Plant Cell Reports*, 1995, **14**, 501). Whereas terpene production is low in cell cultures, isolated *in vitro* root cultures accumulate terpenes in concentrations of the same order as those found in the leaves of young trees (J.-P. Balz *et al.*, *Planta Medica*, 1999, **65**, 620).

Evaluation. Commercial extracts are usually standardized for flavonoid glycosides and triterpene lactones together with a limit for ginkgolic acid. Although the marketing of pure ginkgolides has not yet proved feasible there are a number of reported laboratory separations and assays utilizing GC-MS, HPLC-MS, HPLC-RI. N. Fuzzati *et al.* describe a new HPLC-UV method, not requiring enrichment procedures, for the quantification of ginkgolic acid in extracts (*Fitoterapia*, 2003, **75**, 247). For the crude drug, the *BP/EP* requires a 0.5% content of flavonoids calculated as flavone glycosides; these are assayed by the liquid chromatography of a hydrolysed acetone extract and spectrophotometric measurements at 370 nm.

Uses. Ginkgo has a traditional use as an antiasthmatic, bronchodilator, and for the treatment of chilblains. Extracts of the leaf containing selected constituents are used especially for improving peripheral and cerebral circulation in those elderly with symptoms of loss of short-term memory, hearing and concentration; it is also claimed that vertigo, headaches, anxiety and apathy are alleviated and positive results have been obtained in trials involving the treatment of dementia and Alzheimer's disease (see 'Further reading').

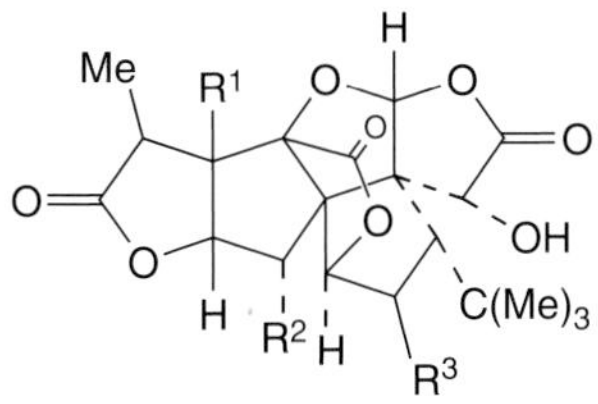

Ginkgolide structures

	R^1	R^2	R^3
Ginkgolide A:	OH	H	H
Ginkgolide B:	OH	OH	H
Ginkgolide C:	OH	OH	OH
Ginkgolide J:	OH	H	OH
Ginkgolide M:	H	OH	OH

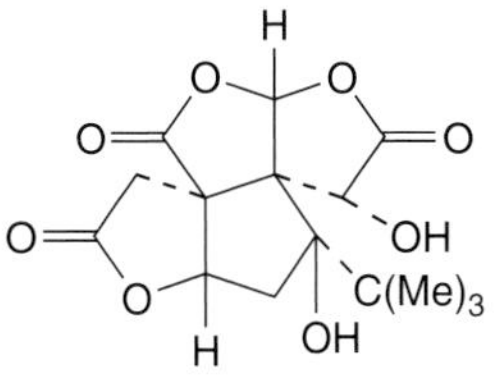

Bilobalide

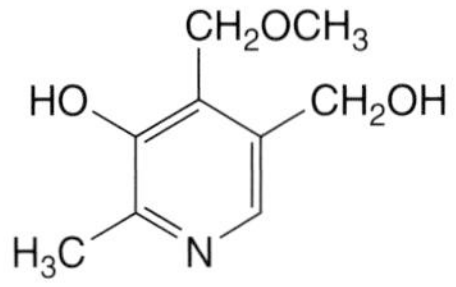

Ginkgotoxin

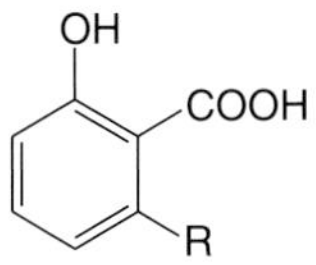

R = C_{13}, C_{15} or C_{17} aliphatic
side-chain with 0, 1 or 2
double bonds
Ginkgolic acids

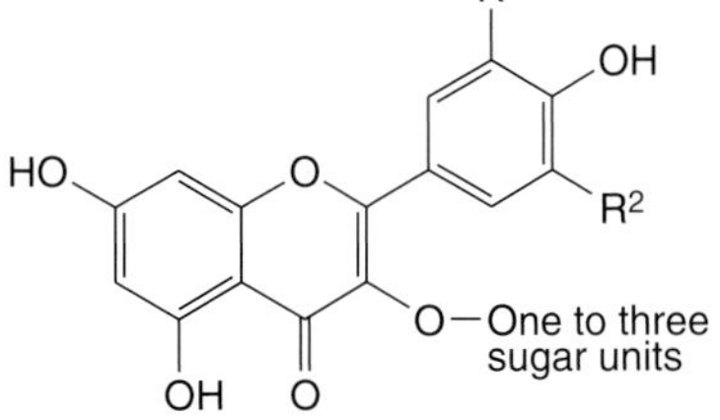

Flavonol structures

Kaempferol derivatives: R^1= OH; R^2= H
Quercetin derivatives: R^1= OH; R^2= H
Myricetin derivatives: R^1= OH; R^2= OH
Isorhamnetin derivatives: R^1= OMe; R^2= H

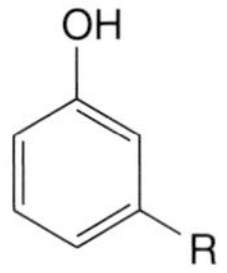

R = C_{13}, C_{15} or C_{17} aliphatic
side-chain with 0 or 1
double bonds
Cardanols

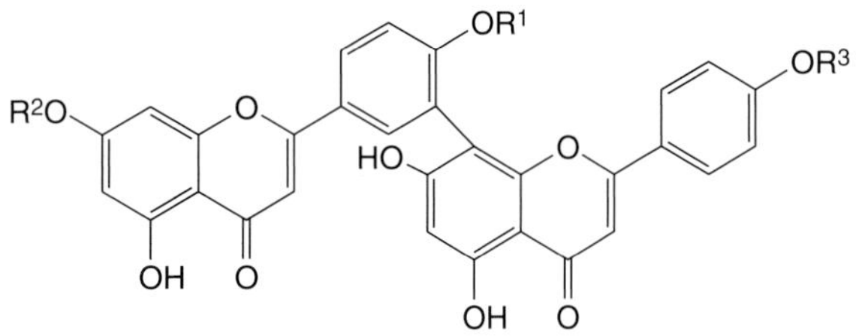

Biflavonoid structures

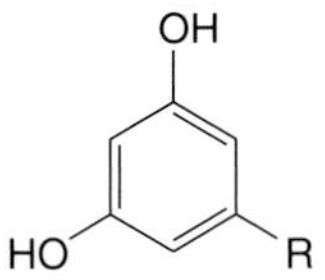

R = C_{15} aliphatic
saturated side-chain
a Cardol

	R^1	R^2	R^3
Amentoflavone:	H	H	H
Bilobetin:	Me	H	H
Sequojaflavone:	H	Me	H
Ginkgetin:	Me	Me	H
Isoginkgetin:	Me	H	Me
Sciadopitysin:	Me	Me	Me

Fig. 24.5
Some constituents of *Ginkgo biloba* leaves.

Further reading

Ghisalberti EL 1997 The biological activity of naturally occurring kaurane diterpenes. Fitoterapia 68(4): 303–325. *Review with 180 references*

Singh B, Kaur P, Gopichand, Singh RD, Ahuja PS 2008 Biology and chemistry of *Ginkgo biloba*. Fitoterapia 79(6): 401–418. *Review with 113 references*

Van Beek TA (ed), Hardman R (series ed) 2000 Medicinal and aromatic plants—industrial profiles, Vol 12. *Ginkgo biloba*. Harwood Academic, Amsterdam

SESTERTERPENES

This relatively recently recognized family of C_{25} compounds, formed by the addition of a C_5 isopentenyl unit to geranylgeranyl diphosphate, is at the moment of limited medicinal interest. Examples are confined principally to the fungi, some marine organisms (e.g. sponges of the genus *Ircinia*) and insect waxes (e.g. gascardic acid).

TRITERPENOIDS

These C_{30} constituents are abundant in nature, particularly in resins, and may occur as either esters or glycosides. They may be aliphatic (e.g. the squalene found in animals and in the unsaponifiable matter of many oils such as arachis and olive), tetracyclic or pentacyclic. Tetracyclic ones include the limonoids, the sterols found in wool fat and yeast and the cardioactive glycosides. The triterpenoid saponins, most of which are pentacyclic, are discussed elsewhere.

This is again a very active area of research and is regularly reviewed in *Natural Product Reports*.

One group of compounds showing a range of interesting biological activity is the quassinoids. These are degradation and rearrangement products of triterpenes and are described under 'Quassia' below and in Chapter 27.

Quassia Wood

Quassia (*Jamaica Quassia*) is the stem wood of *Picrasma excelsa* (*Picroena excelsa* or *Aeschrion excelsa*) (Simaroubaceae), which is known in commerce as Jamaica quassia. The tree, 15–20 m high, grows in the West Indies (Jamaica, Guadeloupe, Martinique, Barbados and St Vincent).

Characters. Quassia occurs in logs, chips or raspings. The logs are of variable length and up to 30 cm diameter (those of Surinam quassia never exceed 10 cm diameter). The logs are covered with a dark grey cork which readily separates from the phloem. The wood is at first whitish but becomes yellow on exposure. It frequently shows blackish markings owing to the presence of a fungus. The logs split readily and the commercial chips, which are cut across the grain, break very readily into smaller fragments. The drug has no odour but an intensely bitter taste.

A small piece of quassia wood should be smoothed and the transverse, radial and tangential surfaces examined with a lens.

A transverse section of quassia shows medullary rays, which are mostly two to five cells wide. The xylem is composed of vessels, wood fibres, and wood parenchyma. The vessels are large (up to 200 μm diameter) and occur singly or in groups of 2–11 which often extend from one medullary ray to the next. Single prisms of calcium oxalate, each 6–30 μm long and enclosed in a delicate membrane, occur scattered in the medullary ray cells and wood parenchyma cells. Starch grains are few; mostly simple, spherical and about 5–15 μm, occasionally two-compound.

Constituents. Quassia contains the amaroid (terpenoid) compound quassin, an intensely bitter lactone; also neoquassin, 18-hydroxyquassin, and scopoletin.

The quassins have been traditionally estimated by sensory means (*BP*, 1973) but Wagner and colleagues (*Planta Med.*, 1980, **38**, 204) described three equally effective methods for the quantitative determination of the individual quassinoids. These involve separation by TLC, HPLC and circular chromatography, followed by absorption measurements.

Quassia wood also contains alkaloids, as illustrated by cathine-6-one.

Quassin   Neoquassin

Allied drugs. Surinam quassia is derived from *Quassia amara* (Simaroubaceae), a shrub growing in the Guianas, northern Brazil and Venezuela. It occurs in smaller billets than those of Jamaica quassia. The medullary rays are only 1 or 2 cells wide but up to 30 cells deep. Calcium oxalate is absent. Cathine-6-one type alkaloids and quassinoids have been isolated from the wood. For a recent phytochemical study see J. A. Dou *et al.*, *Int. J. Pharmacognosy*, 1996, **34**, 349.

A number of *Picrasma* species produce similar constituents to the above. Three novel C_{18} quassinoids have been isolated from the leaves of *Samadera madagascariensis* leaves (P. H. Coombes *et al.*, *Phytochemistry*, 2005, **66**, 2734).

Uses. Quassia is used as a bitter tonic, as an insecticide, and as an enema for the expulsion of thread worms.

Q. amara wood is used in S. American traditional medicine for its stomachic, antiamoebic, antimalarial and antianaemic activity. The commercial 'quassin' prepared from *Q. amara* contains principally quassin and neoquassin and is widely used to give a bitter taste to beverages. It is also used as an insecticide because of its antifeedant properties.

Other quassinoids. Various parts of a number of plants of the family Simaroubaceae have been used in traditional medicine for the treatment of a variety of diseases including cancer, amoebic dysentery and malaria, and research has established that it is the quassinoid (simaroubolide) content of these plants that is responsible for this activity. Such compounds, and in some instances their glycosides, have also been shown to have antileukaemic, antiviral, anti-inflammatory, and (for insects) antifeedant properties. Recent studies are discussed in Chapter 28.

BLACK HOREHOUND

The dried aerial parts of *Ballota nigra* L. family Labiatae collected during the flowering period are included in the *BP/EP* and *BHP* 1996. Dispersed throughout Europe, N. Africa, western Asia, the USA and Australia, the plant is common to roadsides, hedges, etc. and is often regarded as a weed.

Characters of this species, many common to other Labiatae, are the erect square stems, often reddish-brown in the lower parts and up to 100 cm in height; leaves arranged oppositely, 2–5 cm in length, petiolate, rounded to ovate in outline, margin coarsely toothed, surfaces rugose and covered with whitish hairs, venation particularly prominent on the lower surface, depressed on the upper; flowers numerous in whorls in the axils of bracts, calyx about 1 cm in length ten-nerved with five teeth; corollas purple or more rarely white and two-lipped; fruits consist of four small, three-sided achenes. The plant has an unpleasant odour.

Features of the powdered drug include numerous jointed uniseriate trichomes, various glandular trichomes, predominantly anisocytic but some anomocytic stomata on the lower leaf surface, portions of corolla with a papillose epidermis, pollen grains 25–30 μm in diameter with a smooth exine.

Constituents. The constituents of black horehound have been extensively studied during the last 35 years, commencing principally with the work of G. Savona and colleagues in 1976, who characterized the diterpenoid content. Marrubiin, recognized for many years as a constituent of white horehound, is present in very small amounts, its derivates ballotinone, ballonigrine, 7α-acetoxymarrubiin, ballotenol and 13-hydroxyballonigrinolide form the major representatives of the group.

Flavonoids include derivatives of luteolin and apigenin.

The *BP/EP* states a minimum requirement of 1.5% of total *ortho*-dihydroxycinnamic derivatives for the dried drug expressed as acteoside (verbascoside) (for formula see 'Mullein'); this also includes apiosyl, xylosyl and arabinosyl derivatives of verbascoside.

WHITE HOREHOUND

White horehound consists of the dried leaves and flowering tops of *Marrubium vulgare* L., family Labiatae. It is described in the *BP/EP*, *BHP* and the *Complete German Commission E* monographs. The plant is common throughout Europe, including the UK, having become naturalized in many places. Small amounts are obtained commercially for medicinal purposes from S.E. Europe, Morocco, Italy and France. Its principal use is as an expectorant and antispasmodic in the treatment of bronchitis and whooping cough; it also possesses choleretic properties.

The active principals appear to be diterpenes. Marrubiin is one such, which, on the opening of its lactone ring, gives marrubinic acid, to

which is ascribed the choleretic property of the drug. Related compounds present to a lesser extent are the diterpene alcohols marrubenol and vulgarol. Other constituents are: ubiquitous flavonoids including vitexin, apigenin and luteolin together with their glycosides; the alkaloids betonicine and stachydrine; and a small amount of volatile oil (0.06%) giving the drug its pleasant smell.

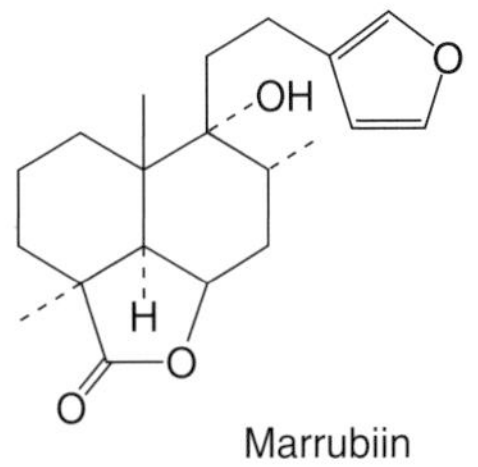

Marrubiin

The *BP/EP* gives a TLC test for the drug and requires a minimum content of 0.7% marrubiin determined by liquid chromatography using a solution of marrubiin in methanol as a reference solution with absorption measurements at 217 nm.

TETRATERPENES—CAROTENOIDS

Important among these compounds are the C_{40} yellow or orange-red carotenoid pigments of which about 500 have been reported. As indicated in Chapter 18 they are formed by the tail to tail union of two molecules of the C_{20} geranylgeranyl diphosphate to give an acyclic intermediate with a *cis*-configuration of the central double bond. By a change of configuration of the latter to *trans* and further desaturation of the isoprenoid chain, lycopene, the all-*trans* pigment of the ripe tomato fruit is formed. The various carotenes and derivatives can be envisaged by cyclization of one or both ends of the lycopene molecule (Fig. 24.6); all are all-*trans*. *Cis*-isomers, usually present in extracted carotenoid preparations, are probably artefacts.

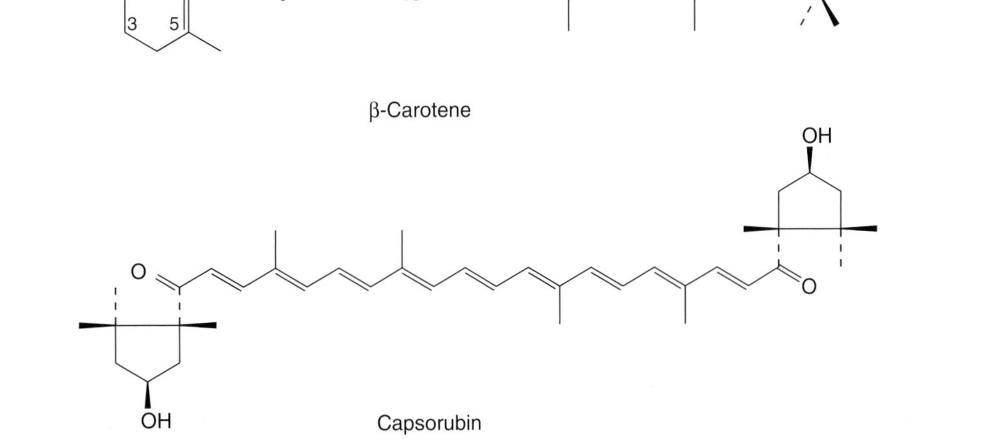

Lycopene

β-Carotene

Capsorubin

Fig. 24.6
Structures of carotenoids.

Table 24.1 Examples of oxygenated carotenoids.

Carotenoid	Formula	Occurrence
Bixin	$C_{25}H_{30}O_4$	Annatto
Capsanthin	$C_{40}H_{56}O_3$	*Capsicum* spp.
Capsorubin	$C_{40}H_{60}O_4$	*Capsicum* spp.
Crocetin	$C_{20}H_{24}O_4$	Saffron
Crocin	$C_{44}H_{64}O_{24}$	Saffron
Fucoxanthin	$C_{40}H_{60}O_6$	Brown algae
Lutein	$C_{40}H_{56}O_2$	*Tagetes erecta*

In association with chlorophyll, carotenes participate in photosynthesis, but also occur in other non-photosynthetic plant organs such as the carrot and in fungi and bacteria. 'Carotene', a mixture of all the carotenes but with β-carotene predominating, was isolated from carrots as early as 1831. Between 1913 and 1915 a fat-soluble growth factor, vitamin A, was recognized to be present in materials such as butter and cod-liver oil and was subsequently shown to be a diterpenoid produced in the livers of animals by enzymic hydrolysis from β-carotene. There are many derivatives of the carotene molecule; some are oxygenated (Table 24.1), some have allenic and acetylenic bonds while others are formed by the loss of a portion of one end of the molecule as with β-citraurin, the characteristic apocarotenoid of citrus fruits. The striking pigments of the red peppers, capsanthin and capsorubin illustrate a contraction of either one (capsanthin) or two (capsorubin) of the usual cyclohexene end groups to a cyclopentane ring.

In addition to the pro-vitamin A activity of β-carotene, the carotenoids have more recently come to be recognized as essential for human health not only as antioxidants but also for specific functions such as normal vision and actions favouring the immune system. Thus, in 1997 J. T. Landrum and colleagues (*Exper. Eye Res.*, **65**, 57) established that the lutein of the 'macula lutea' of the retina of the eye is chemically identical to that giving the colour of marigold flowers (*Tagetes erecta*, Compositae). This accords with the use of lutein in nutritional supplements as preventatives of age-related macular degeneration and for other health benefits. Importantly, it has been demonstrated (P. Molnar *et al.*, *Carotenoid Sci.*, 2006, **10**, 1) that the natural lutein ester, as extracted from marigold, remains virtually stable at gastric pH and body temperature, in contrast to lutein (unesterified), which is degraded by over 60% with the concurrent formation of anhydroluteins and 3′-epilutein. This implies that, for a given dose, relatively more of the ester will reach the intestinal absorption sites than will free lutein.

In 1835 Marquart observed that certain yellow flowers (e.g. buttercup), when treated with strong sulphuric acid, gave dark blue, green or violet colours. This reaction is characteristic of carotenoids and serves as a means of distinguishing them from other natural pigments such as the anthocyanins. The test is best carried out by stratifying an ether or chloroform solution of the carotenoid with 85% sulphuric acid, when a blue colour is formed at the junction of the two layers. Most carotenoids give a blue colour with antimony trichloride in chloroform (Carr–Price test), or a dark-blue colour with concentrated hydrochloric acid containing a little phenol. These tests have been adapted for use as TLC reagents for the identification of relevant crude drugs.

The considerable commercial demand for carotenes has encouraged the development of biotechnological methods for their production. These include mass-culture production from algae, yeast, fungi and recombinant DNA systems. Immobilized enzyme systems for carotenoid production have been studied.

For a concise and informative article (75 refs) on the biological properties of carotenoids, see N. L. Krinsky *Pure Appl. Chem.*, 1994, **66**, 1003. See also this book, Chapter 32: The plant nutraceuticals.

POLYTERPENOIDS

Polyterpenes are composed of many isoprene units. Common examples, both having macromolecules of molecular weight over 100 000, are found in indiarubber and gutta-percha. Doubtless the rubber-like substances of many other plants have a similar composition. Chemically pure rubber is *cis*-1,4-polyisoprene $(C_5H_8)_n$, although in the natural state other materials are present; its occurrence is confined to the dicotyledons, and the one important commercial source is *Hevea brasiliensis*. Gutta-percha (see below) is *trans*-1,4-polyisoprene, and chicle, obtained from *Manilkara sapota*, contains a mixture of low molecular weight *cis*- and *trans*-polyisoprenes. No biological function for polyisoprenes has yet been discovered.

Rubber
A number of species of the families Euphorbiaceae, Apocynaceae, Moraceae, Asclepiadaceae and others produce a latex either in specialized cells or in anastomosing canals (Chapter 42), from which rubber can be prepared.

In Malaysia, *Hevea brasiliensis* (Euphorbiaceae) is cultivated for commercial use. Tapping is carried out mainly by women in the early morning when the internal latex pressure is highest. Trees are tapped by making an overlapping spiral groove, initially 1.5 m above the ground, with a knife called a *jebong*. The exuded latex is collected in cups placed at the lower end of the groove. After about 11 years the spiral has reached ground level. Following an initial cleaning of the latex in vats it is coagulated and bleached by treatment with formic acid and a bleaching agent. The latex emerges as blocks which are then passed through a mill 30 times to give thin layers ready for further processing.

Rubber consists of linear chains of about 1500 to 60 000 C_5-isoprenoid units linked by *cis* double bonds (Fig. 18.20C). Compounds initiating the biosynthesis of rubber in *H. brasiliensis* have been characterized (Y. Tanaka *et al.*, *Phytochemistry*, 1996, **41**, 1501) and possible mechanisms controlling the molecular weights of rubber produced investigated (J. Tangpakdee *et al.*, *Phytochemistry*, 1996, **42**, 353).

Gutta-percha
Gutta-percha is purified, coagulated latex obtained from trees of the genera *Palaquium* and *Payena* (Sapotaceae), which are found both wild and cultivated in Malaysia and Indonesia. The method of collection resembles that used for rubber but the latex flows less readily. Depletion of these natural sources has led to the use of *Parthenium argentatum* (Compositae) for limited production. Gutta-percha differs from rubber in being almost incapable of vulcanization, and in that it becomes plastic when heated to about 45–60°C. Gutta-percha contains a white, polymerized hydrocarbon gutta, composed of C_5-units linked by *trans* double bonds (Fig. 18.20B); it has fewer units than rubber.

Gutta-percha was used in the form of chloroformic solution as a means of applying drugs to the skin, as gutta-percha tissue for covering moist dressings, and in the manufacture of surgical instruments. The *USP/NF* (1995) directs that it should be preserved under water in well-closed containers protected from light.

Chicle
Chicle is a polyisoprenoid consisting of a mixture of *cis*- and *trans*-C_5 isoprenoids obtained from *Manilkara zapota* (Sapotaceae), the sapodilla plum. It was the base used for the original chewing-gum.

25

Cyanogenetic glycosides, glucosinolate compounds, cysteine derivatives and miscellaneous glycosides

In addition to the important groups of glycosides discussed in previous chapters, there are a number of other groups of some medicinal interest. Two of these, the cyanogenetic glycosides and the glucosinolate compounds, are characteristic of certain groups of plants and have similarities in their biosynthetic origins.

CYANOGENETIC GLYCOSIDES

The poisonous properties of the roots of *Manihot utilissima* (cassava) have long been known to primitive tribes; they use it as an important foodstuff, having first found methods to remove its poison. In 1830 the cyanogenetic glycoside manihotoxin was isolated from it, and in the same year amygdalin was obtained from bitter almonds, linamarin from linseed and phaseolunatin from a bean, *Phaseolus lunatus*. These yield prussic acid on hydrolysis and were the first discovered cyanogenetic or cyanophoric glycosides. Over 2000 plant species involving about 110 families are estimated to be cyanogenetic. Professor Lindley, a teacher of pharmaceutical students in London, realized as early as 1830 that the presence or absence of HCN was of taxonomic importance and used it as a character for separating the subfamilies of the Rosaceae. At the species level the presence or absence of prussic acid may denote varieties or different chemical races of the same species (e.g. *Prunus amygdalus* yields both bitter and sweet almonds). Interest in cyanogenetic principles as chemotaxonomic characters continues to receive much attention, as does the general biochemistry of cyanide in plants and microorganisms.

Many of these glucosides, but not all, are derived from the nitrile of mandelic acid. Although they contain nitrogen their structure is that of *O*-and not *N*-glycosides. The sugar portion of the molecule may be a monosaccharide or a disaccharide such as gentiobiose or vicianose. If a disaccharide, enzymes present in the plant may bring about hydrolysis in two stages, as in the case of amygdalin (amygdaloside), Fig. 25.1.

Table 25.1 gives some well-known cyanogenetic glycosides isolated from various sources between 1830 and 1907.

Tests

To test for a cyanogenetic glycoside qualitatively the material is well broken and placed in a small flask with sufficient water to moisten. In the neck of the flask a suitably impregnated strip of filter-paper is suspended by means of a cork. The paper may be treated in either of the following ways to give a colour reaction with free hydrocyanic acid. Either sodium picrate (yellow), which is converted to sodium isopurpurate (brick-red), or a freshly prepared solution of guaiacum resin in absolute alcohol which is allowed to dry on the paper and treated with very dilute copper sulphate solution. The latter test-paper turns blue with prussic acid. If the enzymes usually present in the material have not been destroyed or inactivated, the hydrolysis takes place within about an hour when the flask is kept in a warm place. More rapid hydrolysis will result if a little dilute sulphuric acid is added and the flask gently heated. The depth of colour produced with sodium picrate paper can be used for semiquantitative evaluations.

For materials containing a fairly high percentage of cyanogenetic glycosides (e.g. bitter almonds) the amount may be determined quantitatively by placing the plant in a flask with water and tartaric acid and passing steam through until all the hydrocyanic acid has distilled into a receiver. The distillate is then adjusted to a definite volume and aliquots titrated with standard silver nitrate solution. More sensitive methods including the direct determination of individual glycosides by GLC of their TMS derivatives are now available.

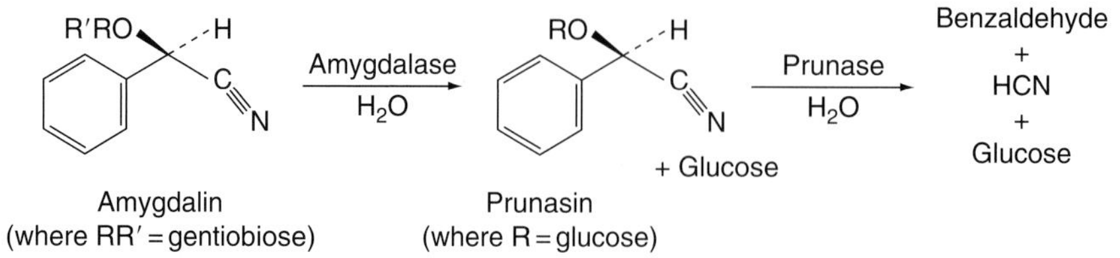

Fig. 25.1
Hydrolysis of amygdalin.

Amygdalin
(where RR′ = gentiobiose)

Prunasin
(where R = glucose)

Benzaldehyde
+
HCN
+
Glucose

Table 25.1 Some cyanogenetic glycosides and their sources.

Glycoside	Source	Family	Constitution
Amygdalin	*Prunus amygdalus*	Rosaceae	D(−)-Mandelonitrile-gentiobioside
Linamarin	*Linum usitatissimum*	Linaceae	Acetone-cyanohydrin-glucoside
Prulaurasin	*Prunus laurocerasus*	Rosaceae	DL-Mandelonitrile-D-glucoside
Manihotoxin	*Manihot utilissima*	Euphorbiaceae	Identical with linamarin (q.v.)
Dhurrin	*Sorghum vulgare*	Gramineae	β-Glucoside of *p*-hydroxymandelonitrile
Sambunigrin	*Sambucus nigra*	Caprifoliaceae	L(+)-Mandelonitrile-D-glucoside
Vicianin	*Vicia angustifolia*	Leguminosae	Mandelonitrile-vicianoside
Phaseolunatin	*Phaseolus lunatus*	Leguminosae	Identical with linamarin (q.v.)
Prunasin	*Prunus serotina*	Rosaceae	D(−)-Mandelonitrile-D-glucoside

Biogenesis

The aglycones of cyanogenetic glycosides are derived solely from nitrogen intermediates. The biosynthesis of prulaurasin (DL-mandelonitrile glucoside) has been studied in the leaves of *Prunus laurocerasus*. Phenyl[3-^{14}C]alanine, phenyl[2-^{14}C]alanine and phenyl[1-^{14}C] alanine were fed to the leaves and the hydrolytic products of the isolated glycosides were examined. The three labelled precursors gave, respectively, active benzaldehyde and inactive hydrocyanic acid; inactive benzaldehyde and active hydrocyanic acid; and inactive benzaldehyde and active hydrocyanic acid; and inactive hydrolytic products consistent with the following incorporation:

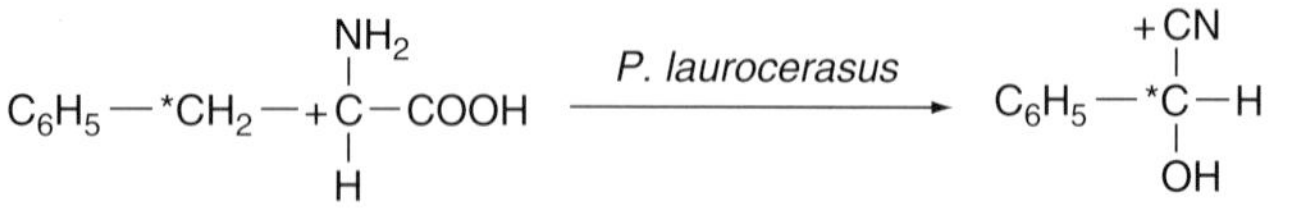

Similarly, phenyl[2-^{14}C]alanine fed to *P. amygdalus* gives amygdalin with most activity in the carbon atom of the nitrile. Experiments with doubly labelled amino acids have shown that the nitrile nitrogen of the cyanogen is derived from the nitrogen atom of the amino acid. Similar results have been obtained with dhurrin isolated from sorghum seedlings fed with labelled tyrosine. More recent work has sought to

determine the nature of the intermediates involved in the above conversions and, for prunasin and linamarin, the participation of oximes and nitriles has been demonstrated (Fig. 25.2).

For a report of a lecture on the biosynthesis, compartmentation and catabolism of cyanogenetic glycosides including amygdalin, linamarin and lotaustralin see E. E. Conn, *Planta Med.*, 1991, **57** (Suppl. Issue No 1), SI. Nahrstedt (*Proc. Phytochem. Soc. Europe*, 1992, **33**, 249) reviewed (84 refs) progress concerning the biology of cyanogenetic glycosides.

A review (107 refs) asking 'Why are so many plants cyanogenetic?' (D. A. Jones, *Phytochemistry*, 1998, **47**, 155) illustrates the continuing interest in these plants, an interest which is, however, largely non-pharmaceutical.

Wild cherry bark

Wild cherry bark (*Wild Black Cherry* or *Virginia Prune Bark; Prunus Serotina*) is the dried bark of *Prunus serotina* (Rosaceae). The plant is a shrub or tree widely distributed in Canada and the USA, extending from Ontario to Florida and westward to Dakota and Texas. Commercial supplies are obtained from Virginia, North Carolina and Tennessee. The most esteemed bark is collected in the autumn, at which time it is most active. After careful drying it should be kept in airtight containers.

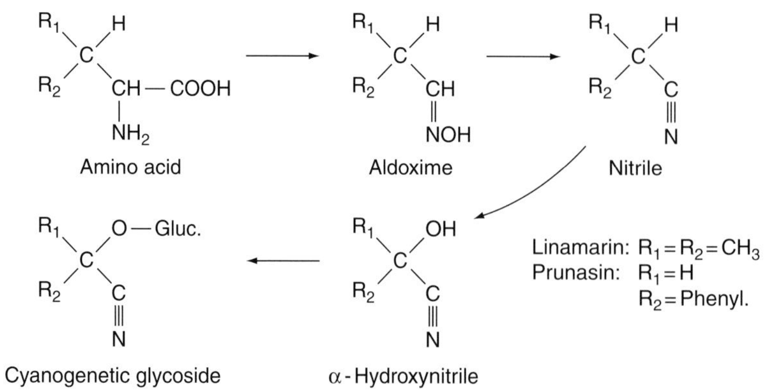

Fig. 25.2
Biosynthetic pathway for cyanogenetic glycosides.

Amino acid

Aldoxime

Nitrile

Cyanogenetic glycoside

α-Hydroxynitrile

Linamarin: R$_1$ = R$_2$ = CH$_3$
Prunasin: R$_1$ = H
R$_2$ = Phenyl.

History. The drug was introduced into American medicine about 1787 and appeared in the *USP* in 1820. It first attracted notice in Britain about 1863.

Macroscopical characters. The drug usually occurs in curved or channelled pieces up to 10 cm long, 5 cm wide and 0.3–4.0 mm thick (Fig. 25.3). Much larger pieces of trunk bark, up to 8 mm thick, may be found but the *BP* (1980) maximum thickness is 4.0 mm and is known commercially as 'Thin Natural Wild Cherry Bark'. The branch bark, if unrossed, is covered with a thin, glossy, easily exfoliating, reddish-brown to brownish-black cork, which bears very conspicuous whitish lenticels. In the rossed bark pale buff-coloured lenticel scars are seen and the outer surface is somewhat rough, some of the cortex having been removed and the phloem exposed. The inner surface is reddish-brown and has a striated and reticulately furrowed appearance, which is caused by the distribution of the phloem and medullary rays. Patches of wood sometimes adhere to the inner surface. The drug breaks with a short, granular fracture. When slightly moist it has an odour of benzaldehyde. Taste is astringent and bitter.

Features of the microscopy (Fig. 25.3) are numerous groups of sclereids, prismatic and cluster crystals of calcium oxalate, cork cells with brown contents, and starch granules.

Constituents. The bark contains prunasin (see above) and the enzyme prunase. Samples on hydrolysis yield glucose, benzaldehyde and about 0.07–0.16% of hydrocyanic acid, Also present are benzoic acid, trimethylgallic acid, *p*-coumaric acid, some tannin and a resin which gives scopoletin on hydrolysis. Modern methods of analysis have allowed detection, for the first time, of amygdalin in the leaves of several *Prunus* spp. including *P. serotina* and a cultivar of *P. virginiana* (F. S. Santamour, *Phytochemistry*, 1998, **47**, 1537).

Uses. Wild cherry bark in the form of a syrup or tincture is mainly used in cough preparations, to which it gives mild sedative properties and a pleasant taste. It was regarded as particularly useful for irritable and persistent coughs.

Cherry-laurel leaves

Cherry-laurel leaves are obtained from *Prunus laurocerasus* (Rosaceae), an evergreen shrub common in Europe. They were formerly official in the fresh state.

The leaves have little odour when entire, but when crushed an odour of benzaldehyde is soon apparent and a positive test for cyanogenetic glycoside is obtained. The cyanide content of small young leaves is reported as 5%, rapidly dropping to about 0.4–1.0% as leaf-size increases. For the structure and hydrolysis of the glucoside prulaurasin, see Table 25.1.

GLUCOSINOLATE COMPOUNDS

Over a century ago sinigrin and sinalbin were isolated in crystalline form from black and white mustards. These and similar glycosides have since been isolated from many plants, particularly those used as condiments (e.g. horseradish) or in folk medicine; they have the general structure:

$$R-C\begin{array}{c}N-O.SO_2.O.X\\\\S.C_6H_{11}O_5\end{array}$$

In the above formulae, R represents $CH_2=CHCH_2$ in sinigrin and $p\text{-}HOC_6H_4CH_2$ in sinalbin; in sinigrin the X represents an atom of

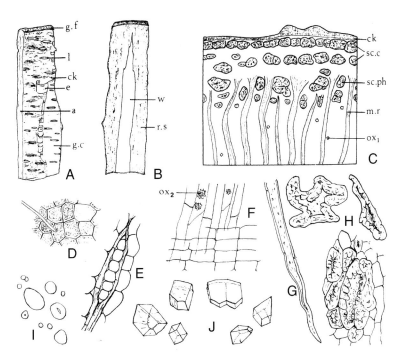

Fig. 25.3
Wild cherry bark. A, Outer surface of bark; B, inner surface (both × 0.5); C, distribution of tissues in TS (× 25). D–J, fragments of powder (all × 200): D, cork cells in surface view with associated fungal hypha; E, medullary ray in TLS; F, medullary ray in RLS with associated parenchyma; G, portion of fibre of the pericycle; H, sclereids; I, starch; J, prismatic crystals of calcium oxalate. a, Obliquely cut edge of bark; ck, cork; e, exfoliating cork; g.c, greenish cortex; g.f, granular fracture; l, lenticel; m.r, medullary ray; ox₁, ox₂, prismatic and cluster crystals respectively of calcium oxalate; r.s, reticulately marked inner surface; sc.c, sclereid groups of cortex; sc.ph, sclereid groups of secondary phloem; w, adhering wood.

potassium but can take the form of a more complex cation—for example, sinapine ($C_{16}H_{25}O_6N$), in sinalbin. A suggestion made in 1961 to rationalize the nomenclature of this enlarging group appears to have found acceptance. This is that the anion of the formula be designated a glucosinolate; thus, sinalbin becomes sinapine, 4-hydroxybenzyl-glucosinolate. Many such glycosides, with a variety of side-chains, including indolyl, are now known; all contain the β-D-1-glucopyranosyl residue. They have been found only in dicotyledonous plants and are particularly abundant in the families Cruciferae, Capparidaceae and Resedaceae with sporadic occurrences in the Euphorbiaceae, Tovariaceae, Moringaceae, Tropaeolaceae and Caricaceae. The enzyme myrosinase has a similar wide distribution. With the Cruciferae it has been shown that the mustard oil glycosides significantly increase the non-specific resistance of the plants to microorganisms which disrupt plant cells; they do not appear to affect the resistance of cruciferous plants to club root infections. Many glucosinolates have an antithyroid and goitre-inducing effect in man.

Biosynthesis

Biosynthesis of the glucosinolates of the relevant Cruciferae takes place principally in the fruit wall with subsequent translocation to the seed. However it has been shown for oilseed rape (*Sinapis alba*) that the necessary enzymes for the biosynthesis of *p*-hydroxybenzylglucosinolate (derived from tryosine) are present in the seed where a limited synthesis does occur (L. Du and B. A. Halkier, *Phytochemistry*, 1998, **48**, 1145).

The earlier feeding experiments with those members of the Cruciferae which produce mustard oil glucosides showed that suitable amino acids are converted to thioglucosides by the plant. Doubly labelled (^{14}C, ^{15}N) amino acids afforded glucosides with $^{14}C:^{15}N$ ratios consistent with direct incorporation (Fig. 25.4).

This means that all intermediates in this conversion are nitrogenous compounds giving a similar situation to that found in the biosynthesis of cyanogenetic glycosides (see above). Following the work on cyanogenetic compounds, it was then demonstrated (1967) by different groups of workers that appropriate aldoximes were effective precursors of these compounds in flax (linamarin), *Cochlearia officinalis* (glucoputranjivan), *Lepidium sativum* (benzylglucosinolate) and *Tropaeolum majus* (benzylglucosinolate).

With sinigrin, the thioglucoside found in horseradish leaves and in black mustard seeds, the most effective precursor of the carbon chain appears to be homomethionine rather than allylglycine which inspection of the sinigrin structure might suggest. Homomethionine arises by chain lengthening of methionine with acetate by a mechanism analogous to the formation of leucine from valine (see Fig. 18.16). Although the sulphur atom on the thioglucoside moiety may be introduced by feeding with methionine, Matsuo (1968) showed the sulphur of DL-[^{35}S]cysteine to be a more efficient precursor. The sulphur of the bisulphite portion of the molecule is more readily introduced from

inorganic sources. Some incorporations consistent with the envisaged pathway for sinigrin are illustrated in Fig. 25.4.

Mustard seed

Black or brown mustard (*Sinapis*) is the dried ripe seed of *Brassica nigra* or of *B. juncea* (Cruciferae) and their varieties. The former species is cultivated in Europe and the USA, while *B. juncea* is grown in India and the former USSR.

Characters. The seeds are globular and 1–1.6 mm diameter. The testa is dark reddish-brown to yellow and minutely pitted. The cells of the outer epidermis of the testa contain mucilage. The embryo is oily and greenish-yellow or yellow in colour; it consists of two cotyledons folded along their midribs to enclose the radicle. Powdered mustard acquires a much brighter yellow colour on treatment with alkali.

Constituents. Black mustard seeds contain sinigrin and myrosin and yield after maceration with water 0.7–1.3% of volatile oil. The latter contains over 90% of allylisothiocyanate. The seeds also contain about 27% of fixed oil, 30% of proteins, mucilage and traces of sinapine hydrogen sulphate (cf. white mustard).

Allied drug. White mustard, the seeds of *Sinapsis alba*, are globular and 1.5–2.5 mm diameter. The testa is yellowish and almost smooth, and contains mucilage in its outer epidermal cells. The kernel is oily and the cotyledons are folded as in black mustard. On treatment with water the powder develops a pungent taste but the pungent odour of the black variety is absent. With alkali the powder acquires a bright yellow colour.

White mustard seeds contain the glucoside sinalbin and myrosin. In the presence of moisture decomposition takes place with the formation of isothiocyanate, sinapine hydrogen sulphate and glucose. The isothiocyanate is an oily liquid with a pungent taste and rubefacient properties but, owing to its slight volatility, it lacks the pungent odour of allylisothiocyanate. Sinapine hydrogen sulphate, which is also found in black mustard, is the salt of an unstable alkaloid. The seeds also contain about 30% of fixed oil, 25% of proteins and mucilage.

Uses. The mustards have been traditionally used, particularly in the form of plasters, as rubefacients and counterirritants. In large doses they have an emetic action. Both varieties are used as condiments.

CYSTEINE DERIVATIVES

Derivatives of the amino acid cysteine occur as sulphoxides in the genus *Allium* and are responsible for the lachrymatory factor of onions, garlic etc. Variations in the structure of these compounds are found in different species, thus S-(trans-propen-1-yl)-cysteine

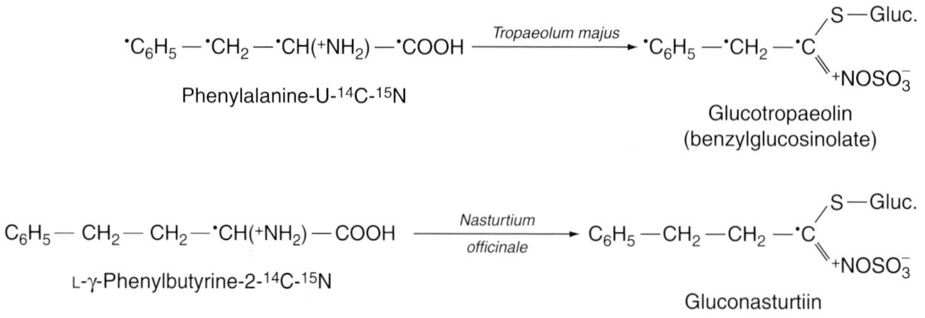

$$\cdot C_6H_5 - \cdot CH_2 - \cdot CH(+NH_2) - \cdot COOH \xrightarrow{\textit{Tropaeolum majus}} \cdot C_6H_5 - \cdot CH_2 - \cdot C \begin{matrix} S-Gluc. \\ \\ +NOSO_3^- \end{matrix}$$

Phenylalanine-U-^{14}C-^{15}N

Glucotropaeolin
(benzylglucosinolate)

Fig. 25.4
Incorporation of doubly labelled amino acids by cruciferous species.

$$C_6H_5 - CH_2 - CH_2 - \cdot CH(+NH_2) - COOH \xrightarrow{\textit{Nasturtium officinale}} C_6H_5 - CH_2 - CH_2 - \cdot C \begin{matrix} S-Gluc. \\ \\ +NOSO_3^- \end{matrix}$$

L-γ-Phenylbutyrine-2-^{14}C-^{15}N

Gluconasturtiin

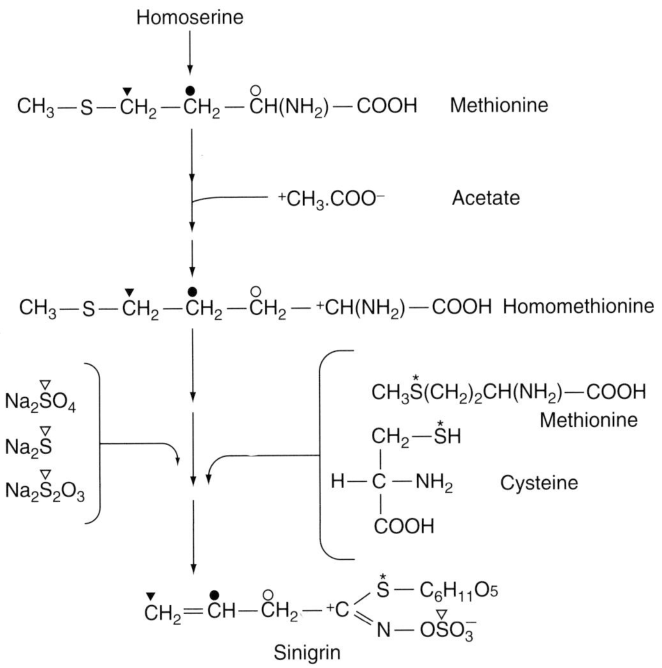

Fig. 25.5
Biosynthesis of sinigrin.

sulphoxide is the active component of the onion and the S-allyl derivative of garlic. As well as its considerable culinary interest, the latter also has medicinal usage.

GARLIC

Garlic bulbs (*Allium sativum* L., family Liliaceae) and the separated cloves need little description, being universally available for culinary purposes. Powdered garlic is prepared from bulbs, cut, freeze-dried or dried at a temperature no greater than 65°C. Conditions are important in order to maintain a uniform product but, even so, powders from different commercial sources may vary in their constituents and the *BHP* cites different standards for two major producers, Egypt and China.

A microscopical examination of the powder shows much parenchymatous tissue accompanied by groups of spiral or annular vessels.

In the plant itself the principal constituent of interest is the sulphur compound alliin. When the bulb is chopped or crushed alliin is brought into contact with the enzyme allinase, normally stored in separate cells, and under moist conditions alliin is rapidly transformed via allylsulphenic acid to allicin the main component of the commercial powder. Under dry conditions both alliin and allicin are relatively stable but the latter when formed is readily converted during processing of the powder to other sulphur compounds (Fig. 25.6) including

diallyldisulphide, diallyltrisulphide and other linear and cyclic sulphur compounds. These reactions produce the characteristic garlic odour.

The *BP/EP* requires a minimum allicin content of 0.45% calculated with reference to the dried drug. Liquid chromatography is used for the assay employing butyl parahydroxybenzoate as an internal standard.

Votalile oil distilled from the drug contains the above sulphur compounds (no alliin or allicin), and various terpenes.

The pharmacological activities and reputed beneficial effects of garlic are numerous and for details and references (138) the reader is referred to J. Barnes *et al.*, *Herbal Medicines*, 3rd edn. 2007, Pharmaceutical Press, London.

MISCELLANEOUS GLYCOSIDES

Attention is drawn to the following types of glycoside, some of which have been mentioned under other headings.

Steroidal alkaloidal glycosides

These are particularly abundant in the families Solanaceae and Liliaceae. Like saponins, they have haemolytic properties. Examples are α-solanin (potato, *Solanum tuberosum*), soladulcin (bitter-sweet, *S. dulcamara*), *tomatin* (tomato, *Lycopersicon esculentum*) and rubijervine (*Veratrum* spp.). The sugar components, one to four in number, are attached in the 3-position and may be glucose, galactose, rhamnose or xylose. The formulae (as shown below), in which part of the steroidal structure is omitted, illustrate three variations in the E and F ring systems of the aglycones. Solasodine and 5-dehydrotomatidine are stereoisomeric spirosolanes and the configuration of the nitrogen atom is apparently always linked to that at C-25.

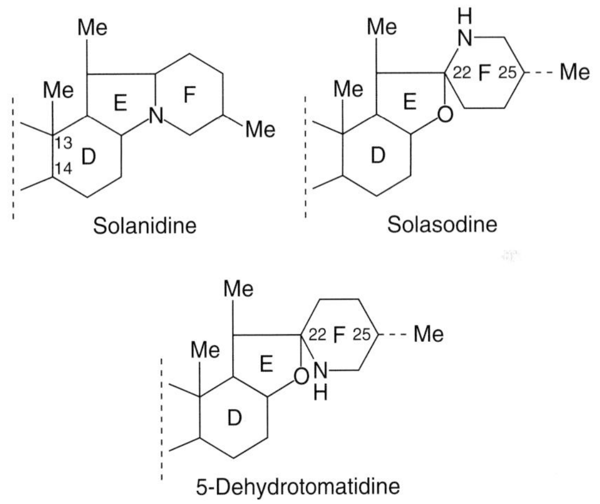

Solanidine

Solasodine

5-Dehydrotomatidine

Thus, solasodine, the nitrogen analogue of diosgenin (q.v.), is Δ⁵,22β,25α-spirosolen-3β-ol and 5-dehydrotomatidine is $\Delta^5,22\alpha,25\beta$-spirosolen-3β-ol (see also 'Chemical Races', Chapter 14 and 'Saponins', Chapter 23).

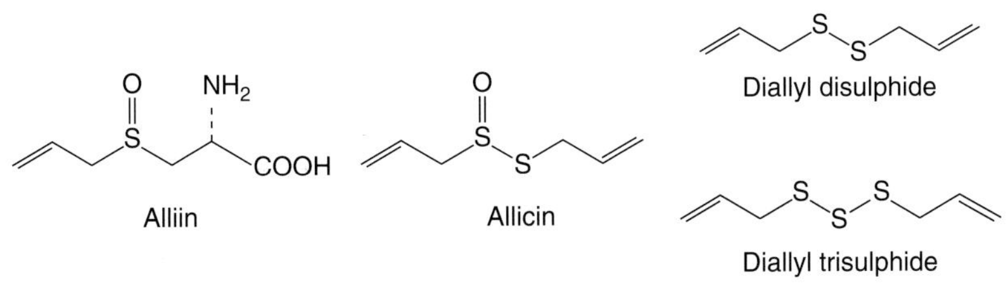

Alliin

Allicin

Diallyl disulphide

Diallyl trisulphide

Fig. 25.6
Constituents of garlic.

Glycosidal resins

The complex resins of the Convolvulaceae such as those found in jalap and scammony (q.v.) are glycosidal; they yield on hydrolysis sugars such as glucose, rhamnose and fucose together with normal fatty acids and the hydroxyl derivatives.

Glycosidal bitter principles

While many glycosides have a bitter taste, certain of them were described as 'bitter principles' long before their chemical nature was elucidated. These compounds include gentiopicrin or gentiopicroside of gentian root (q.v.); picrocrocin or picrocroside of saffron (q.v.); and cucurbitacins of the Cucurbitaceae (e.g. colocynth, q.v.).

Betalains

For many years a group of plant pigments, associated with the order Centrospermae and containing nitrogen, had been known. These compounds were termed 'nitrogenous anthocyanins'. Following the initial isolation in crystalline form of one such compound in 1957, the structures of two groups of pigments have now been determined; these are the betacyanins and betaxanthins, the former being red-violet in colour and the latter yellow. These names were derived from a combination of *Beta vulgaris* (the red beet) and the anthocyanin and anthoxanthin pigments to which they were thought to be related. That these new compounds contained nitrogen was confirmed, but they are not flavonoid derivatives (see structures below). Betanin, on hydrolysis, gives the aglycone betanidin; indicaxanthin, although not a glycoside, is included here for completeness. Betalains are also responsible for the bright colorations of the flowers and fruits of the Cactaceae. In this case the sugar moiety of betanin may be substituted at C-2 and C-6 by malonyl, apiosyl and feruloyl groups. For a report on betalains from Christmas cactus see N. Kobayashi *et al.*, *Phytochemistry*, 2000, **54**, 419. Muscaaurin and muscapurpurin are betalain pigments of the fly agaric, *Amanita muscaria*. *Opuntia dillenii* fruits have been suggested as an industrial source of betanins. Chemotaxonomically these compounds are of considerable interest and are of importance as food colourants (Chapter 33).

R = β-D- Glucosyl (Betanin)   Indicaxanthin

Further reading

Strach D, Vigt T, Schlieman W 2003 Recent advances in betalain research. Phytochemistry 62(3): 247–269

Antibiotic glycosides

Certain antibiotics are of glycosidal nature. Streptomycin, for example (see Table 30.1) is formed from the genin streptidin (a nitrogen-containing cyclohexane derivative) to which is attached the disaccharide streptobiosamine. The latter is constituted from one molecule of the rare methylpentose streptose and one molecule of *N*-methylglucosamine.

Nucleosides or nucleic acids

These substances, which are of the highest biological importance, have three components: a sugar unit (either ribose or 2-desoxyribose), a purine or pyrimidine base or bases (e.g. adenine, guanine and cytosine) and phosphoric acid. These are *N*-glycosides. When conjugated with proteins (q.v.) they form nucleoproteins.

26

Alkaloids

Alkaloid-containing plants constitute an extremely varied group both taxonomically and chemically, a basic nitrogen being the only unifying factor for the various classes. For this reason, questions of the physiological role of alkaloids in the plant, their importance in taxonomy, and biogenesis are often most satisfactorily discussed at the level of a particular class of alkaloid. A similar situation pertains with the therapeutic and pharmacological activities of alkaloids. As most alkaloids are extremely toxic, plants containing them do not feature strongly in herbal medicine but they have always been important in the allopathic system where dosage is strictly controlled and in homoeopathy where the dose-rate is so low as to be harmless.

INTRODUCTION

A precise definition of the term 'alkaloid' (alkali-like) is somewhat difficult because there is no clear-cut boundary between alkaloids and naturally occurring complex amines. Typical alkaloids are derived from plant sources, they are basic, they contain one or more nitrogen atoms (usually in a heterocyclic ring) and they usually have a marked physiological action on man or other animals. The name 'proto-alkaloid' or 'amino-alkaloid' is sometimes applied to compounds such as hordenine, ephedrine and colchicine which lack one or more of the properties of typical alkaloids. Other alkaloids, not conforming with the general definition, are those synthetic compounds not found in plants but very closely related to the natural alkaloids (e.g. homatropine). In practice, those substances present in plants and giving the standard qualitative tests outlined below are termed alkaloids, and frequently in plant surveys this evidence alone is used to classify a particular plant as 'alkaloid-containing'.

HISTORY

The first isolations of alkaloids in the nineteenth century followed the reintroduction into medicine of a number of alkaloid-containing drugs and were coincidental with the advent of the percolation process for the extraction of drugs. The French apothecary Derosne probably isolated the alkaloid afterwards known as narcotine in 1803 and the Hanoverian apothecary Sertürner further investigated opium and isolated morphine (1806, 1816). Isolation of other alkaloids, particularly by Pelletier and Caventou, rapidly followed; strychnine (1817), emetine (1817), brucine (1819), piperine (1819), caffeine (1819), quinine (1820), colchicine (1820) and coniine (1826). Coniine was the first alkaloid to have its structure established (Schiff, 1870) and to be synthesized (Ladenburg, 1889), but for others, such as colchicine, it was well over a century before the structures were finally elucidated. Modern methods and instrumentation have greatly facilitated these investigations, and it is interesting to note that the yields of 'minor' alkaloids, too small for further investigation, isolated by chemists during the first quarter of the last century would now be sufficient, several thousand times over, for a complete structure analysis. In the second half of the twentieth century alkaloids featured strongly in the search for plant drugs with anticancer activity. A notable success was the introduction of *Catharanthus* alkaloids and paclitaxel into medicine and there is much current interest in other alkaloids having anticancer properties as well as those exhibiting antiaging and antiviral possibilities.

DISTRIBUTION

Some 150 years of alkaloid chemistry had resulted by the mid-1940s in the isolation of about 800 alkaloids; the new technology of the next 50 years increased this figure to the order of 10 000.

True alkaloids are of rare occurrence in lower plants. In the fungi the lysergic acid derivatives and the sulphur-containing alkaloids, e.g. the gliotoxins, are the best known. Among the pteridophytes and gymnosperms the lycopodium, ephedra and *Taxus* alkaloids have medicinal interest. Alkaloid distribution in the angiosperms is uneven. The dicotyledon orders Salicales, Fagales, Cucurbitales and Oleales at present appear to be alkaloid-free. Alkaloids are commonly found in the orders Centrospermae (Chenopodiaceae), Magnoliales (Lauraceae, Magnoliaceae), Ranunculales (Berberidaceae, Menispermaceae, Ranunculaceae), Papaverales (Papaveraceae, Fumariaceae), Rosales (Leguminosae, subfamily Papilionaceae), Rutales (Rutaceae), Gentiales (Apocynaceae, Loganiaceae, Rubiaceae), Tubiflorae (Boraginaceae, Convolvulaceae, Solanaceae) and Campanulales (Campanulaceae, sub-family Lobelioideae; Compositae, subfamily Senecioneae).

Hegnauer, who has made an intensive study of alkaloid distribution, while recognizing the undoubted potential chemotaxonomic significance of this group, is cautious about its use without due regard to all the other characters of the plant. Nevertheless it continues to be a popular area of research.

Nearly 300 alkaloids belonging to more than 24 classes are known to occur in the skins of amphibians along with other toxins. They include the potent neurotoxic alkaloids of frogs of the genus *Phyllobates*, which are among some of the most poisonous substances known. Other reptilian alkaloids are strongly antimicrobial. Alkaloids derived from mammals include ones of indole and isoquinoline classes a few are found in both plants and animals.

PROPERTIES

Most alkaloids are well-defined crystalline substances which unite with acids to form salts. In the plant they may exist in the free state, as salts or as *N*-oxides (see below). In addition to the elements carbon, hydrogen and nitrogen, most alkaloids contain oxygen. A few, such as coniine from hemlock and nicotine from tobacco, are oxygen-free and are liquids. Although coloured alkaloids are relatively rare, they are not unknown; berberine, for example, is yellow and the salts of sanguinarine are copper-red.

A knowledge of the solubility of alkaloids and their salts is of considerable pharmaceutical importance. Not only are alkaloidal substances often administered in solution, but also the differences in solubility between alkaloids and their salts provide methods for the isolation of alkaloids from the plant and their separation from the non-alkaloidal substances also present. While the solubilities of different alkaloids and salts show considerable variation, as might be expected from their extremely varied structure, it is true to say that the free bases are frequently sparingly soluble in water but soluble in water but soluble in organic solvents; with salts the reverse is often the case, these being usually soluble in water but sparingly soluble in organic solvents. For example, strychnine hydrochloride is much more soluble in water than is strychnine base. It will soon be realized that there are many exceptions to the above generalizations, caffeine (base) being readily extracted from tea with water and colchicine being soluble in either acid, neutral or alkaline water. Again, some alkaloidal salts are sparingly soluble—for example, quinine sulphate is only soluble to the extent of 1 part in 1000 parts of water, although 1 part quinine hydrochloride is soluble in less than 1 part of water.

STRUCTURE AND CLASSIFICATION

Alkaloids show great variety in their botanical and biochemical origin, in chemical structure and in pharmacological action. Consequently, many different systems of classification are possible. In the arrangement

of the well-known drugs which follow later in the chapter, the phytochemical arrangement introduced in the eleventh edition of this book and based on the origin of the alkaloids in relation to the common amino acids has been used. For practical purposes it is useful, therefore, to maintain the well-established classifications based on chemical structures, Fig. 26.1, and Table 26.1 closely follows that used by a number of authors. There are two broad divisions:

I. Non-heterocyclic or atypical alkaloids, sometimes called 'protoalkaloids' or biological amines.
II. Heterocyclic or typical alkaloids, divided into 14 groups according to their ring structure.

The nitrogen of alkaloids

Alkaloids, taken in their broadest sense, may have a nitrogen atom which is primary (mescaline), secondary (ephedrine), tertiary (atropine) or quaternary (one of the N atoms of tubocurarine), and this factor affects the derivatives of the alkaloid which can be prepared and the isolation

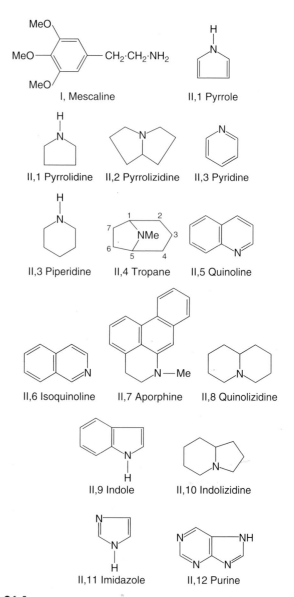

Fig. 26.1
Skeletal structures of alkaloids found in medicinal plants. (Numbers refer to location in Table 26.1).

Table 26.1   Types of alkaloid and their occurrence.

I. Non-heterocyclic alkaloids

Hordenine or N-methyltyramine	In germinating barley, *Hordeum distochon*
Mescaline, related to tryptamine (see formula)	*Lophophora williamsii* (Cactaceae)
Ephedrine	*Ephedra* spp. (Ephedraceae)
Colchicine (tropolone nucleus with nitrogen in side-chain)	*Colchicum* spp. and related genera (Liliaceae)
Erythromycin (an antibiotic)	*Streptomyces erythreus* (Bacteriophyta, Actinomycetales)
Jurubin (steroid with 3-amino group)	*Solanum paniculatum* (Solanaceae)
Pachysandrine A (steroid with N-containing C-17 side-chain)	*Pachysandra terminalis* (Buxaceae)
Taxol (a modified diterpene pseudo alkaloid)	*Taxus brevifolia* (Taxaceae)

II. Heterocyclic alkaloids

1. *Pyrrole and pyrrolidine*

Hygrines	*Coca* spp. (Erythroxylaceae); often associated with tropane alkaloids of the Solanaceae
Stachydrine	*Stachys tuberifera* (Labiatae), soya bean and other Leguminosae

2. *Pyrrolizidine*

Symphitine, echimidine	*Symphytum* spp.
Senecionine, seneciphylline, etc.	*Senecio* spp.

3. *Pyridine and piperidine*

Trigonelline	Fenugreek (Leguminosae), strophanthus (Apocynaceae), coffee (Rubiaceae)
Coniine	*Conium maculatum* (Umbelliferae)
Arecoline	*Areca catechu* (Palmae)
Lobeline	*Lobelia* spp. (Lobeliaceae)
Pelletierine	*Punica granatum*, the pomegranate (Punicaceae)
Nicotine (pyridine + pyrrolidine)	*Nicotiana tabacum* and other spp. (Solanaceae)
Anabasine	*Nicotiana glauca*; *Anabasis aphylla* (Chenopodiaceae)
Piperine	*Piper* spp. (Piperaceae)
Ricinine	*Ricinus communis* (Euphorbiaceae)

4. *Tropane* (piperidine/N-methyl-pyrrolidine)

Hyoscyamine, atropine, hyoscine, meteloidine, etc.	Species of *Atropa, Datura, Hyoscyamus, Duboisia, Mandragora* and *Scopolia* (Solanaceae)
Calystegines	*Convolvulus* spp., *Ipomoea polpha* (Convolvulaceae), some solanaceous spp., *Morus* spp. (Moraceae)
Cocaine	*Coca* spp. (Erythroxylaceae)
Pesudo-pelletierine	*Punica granatum* (Punicaceae)

5. *Quinoline*

Quinine, quinidine, cinchonine, cinchonidine	*Cinchona* spp. (Rubiaceae), *Remijia* spp. (Rubiaceae)
Cusparine	*Angostura* or *cusparia* bark, *Galipea officinalis* (Rutaceae)

6. *Isoquinoline*

Papaverine, narceine, narcotine	*Papaver somniferum* (Papaveraceae)
Corydaline	*Corydalis* and *Dicentra* spp. (Fumariaceae)
Hydrastine, berberine	Numerous genera of the Berberidaceae, Ranunculaceae and Papaveraceae
Emetine, cephaeline	*Cephaelis* spp. (Rubiaceae)
Tubocurarine	Curare obtained from plants of Menispermaceae
Morphine, codeine	*Papaver somniferum* (Papaveraceae)
Erythraline	*Erythrina* spp. (Leguminosae)
Galanthamine	*Leucojum aestivum* (Amaryllidaceae)

7. *Aporphine* (reduced isoquinoline/naphthalene)

Boldine	*Peumus boldus* (Monimiaceae)

8. *Quinolizidine*

Sparteine, cytisine, lupanine, laburnine	Sometimes called 'the lupin alkaloids'. Occur particularly in the Leguminosae, subfamily Papilionaceae, e.g. broom. *Cytisus scoparius*; dyer's broom, *Genista tinctoria*; *Laburnum* and *Lupinus* spp.

9. *Indole or benzopyrrole*

Ergometrine, ergotamine	*Claviceps* spp. (Hypocreaceae)
Lysergic acid amide, clavine alkaloids	*Rivea corymbosa, Ipomoea violacea* (Convolvulaceae)
Physostigmine	*Physostigma venenosum* (Leguminosae)
Ajmaline, serpentine, reserpine	*Rauwolfia* spp. (Apocynaceae)
Yohimbine, aspidospermine	*Aspidosperma* spp. (Apocynaceae)
Vinblastine, vincristine	*Catharanthus roseus* (Apocynaceae)
Calabash curare alkaloids	*Strychnos* spp. (Loganiaceae)
Strychnine, brucine	*Strychnos* spp. (Loganiaceae)

26

(Continued)

Table 26.1 Types of alkaloid and their occurrence. (Cont'd)

10. *Indolizidine*	
Castanospermine	*Castanospermum australe* (Leguminosae), *Alexa* spp. (Leguminosae)
Swainsonine	*Swainsona* spp. (Leguminosae), Loco plants (Leguminosae)
11. *Imidazole or glyoxaline*	
Pilocarpine	*Pilocarpus* spp. (Rutaceae)
12. *Purine* (pyrimidine/imidazole)	
Caffeine	Tea (Ternstroemiaceae), coffee (Rubiaceae), maté (Aquifoliaceae), guarana (Sapindaceae), cola nuts (Sterculiaceae)
Theobromine	Cocoa (Sterculiaceae)
13. *Steroidal* (some combined as glycosides)	
Solanidine (glycoside = solanine)	Shoots of potato (Solanaceae), etc.
Veratrum alkamine esters and their glycosides	*Veratrum* spp. and *Schoenocaulon* spp. (Liliaceae)
Conessine	*Holarrhena antidysenterica* (Apocynaceae)
Funtumine	*Funtumia elastica* (Apocynaceae)
14. *Terpenoid*	
Aconitine, atisine, lyctonine, etc.	*Aconitum* and *Delphinium* spp. (Ranunculaceae)

procedures. In the plant, alkaloids may exist in the free state, as salts or as amine or alkaloid *N*-oxides.

Alkaloid *N*-oxides. *N*-oxidation products of alkaloids, particularly the *N*-oxides of tertiary alkaloids, are well-known laboratory products, easily prepared from the original base. As early as the 1920s quite extensive pharmacological and toxicological comparisons had been made of common alkaloids such as morphine, strychnine and hyoscyamine and their corresponding *N*-oxides. Some enthusiasm for the clinical use of *N*-oxides was engendered by their purported delayed-release properties, low toxicities and low addictive properties compared with the corresponding tertiary alkaloids.

Although the formation of *N*-oxides and other *N*-oxidation products of alkaloids in animal systems is well-known, forming part of the wider scheme for the metabolism of amines, the occurrence of such compounds in plants has, until relatively recently, received little attention. This was possibly due to a belief that such compounds represented artefacts arising during the extraction and work-up of tertiary alkaloids. Secondly, because of the high polarity, and water-solubility of alkaloid *N*-oxides, they were discarded by the normal alkaloid extraction procedures.

One group of alkaloids known to occur extensively as the natural *N*-oxides comprises the quinolizidines of the Boraginaceae, Compositae and Papilionaceae; these are alkaloids, including those of *Senecio* spp., which cause extensive liver damage in animals using plants containing them as fodder. A number of *N*-oxide alkaloids of the indole series have been isolated from plant materials, and among those of pharmaceutical significance are the simple hallucinogenic indole derivatives of *Amanita* spp., reserpine, strychnine, and some *Mitragyna* alkaloids. Fresh *Atropa, Datura, Hyoscyamus, Scopolia* and *Mandragora* each contain the two isomeric *N*-oxides of hyoscyamine.

One of the two possible *N*-oxides of hyoscine has been isolated from species of the first four genera above. Morphine and codeine *N*-oxides are natural constituents of the opium poppy latex, and *Nicotiana* spp. contain two isomeric nicotine *N*-oxides based on the pyrrolidine nitrogen. Some *N*-oxides—for example, aspergillic acid and iodinin (1,6-dihydroxyphenazine dioxide)—isolated from microorganisms, possess antibacterial activity.

As with the tertiary alkaloids themselves, there is little evidence to suggest what role the *N*-oxides may play in the plant's metabolism. Ontogenetic studies of hyoscyamine *N*-oxide production in belladonna indicate a dynamic role for the *N*-oxide with a maximum build-up in the developing fruits. Oxidation–reduction involving *N*-oxides and tertiary bases is a probability. It has been suggested that *N*-oxides may be involved in demethylations and their participation in the biosynthesis of benzylisoquinoline alkaloids has also been proposed. The solubility properties of *N*-oxides could influence the transport of alkaloids both throughout the plant and also within the cell itself.

Tests for alkaloids

Most alkaloids are precipitated from neutral or slightly acid solution by Mayer's reagent (potassiomercuric iodide solution), by Wagner's reagent (solution of iodine in potassium iodide), by solution of tannic acid, by Hager's reagent (a saturated solution of picric acid), or by Dragendorff's reagent (solution of potassium bismuth iodide). These precipitates may be amorphous or crystalline and are of various colours: cream (Mayer's), yellow (Hager's), reddish-brown (Wagner's and Dragendorff's). Caffeine and some other alkaloids do not give these precipitates (see below). Care must be taken in the application of these alkaloidal tests, as the reagents also give precipitates with proteins. During the extraction of alkaloids from the plant and subsequent evaporation, some proteins will not be extracted and others will be made insoluble (denatured) by the evaporation process and may be filtered out. If the original extract has been concentrated to low bulk and the alkaloids extracted from an alkaline solution by means of an organic solvent, and then transferred into dilute acid (e.g. tartaric), the latter solution should be protein-free and ready to test for alkaloids.

As mentioned above, caffeine, a purine derivative, does not precipitate like most alkaloids. It is usually detected by mixing with a very small amount of potassium chlorate and a drop of hydrochloric acid, evaporating to dryness and exposing the residue to ammonia vapour. A purple colour is produced with caffeine and other purine derivatives. This is known as the murexide test. Caffeine easily sublimes and may be extracted from tea by heating the broken leaves in a crucible covered with a piece of glass. Colour tests are sometimes useful—for example, the yellow colour given by colchicine with mineral acids or the bluish-violet to red colour given by indole alkaloids when treated with sulphuric acid and *p*-dimethylaminobenzaldehyde. Other examples will be given under individual drugs.

For the identification of drugs containing known alkaloids, pharmacopoeias commonly employ TLC separations using reference compounds to establish the presence of individual alkaloids. In this respect, some of the alkaloid reagents quoted above are useful for detection of the separated bases.

EXTRACTION OF ALKALOIDS

Extraction methods vary with the scale and purpose of the operation, and with the raw material. For many research purposes chromatography gives both speedy and accurate results. However, if an appreciable quantity of alkaloid is required, one of the following general methods will usually serve.

Process A. The powdered material is moistened with water and mixed with lime which combines with acids, tannins and other phenolic substances and sets free the alkaloids (if they exist in the plant as salts). Extraction is then carried out with organic solvents such as ether or petroleum spirit. The concentrated organic liquid is then shaken with aqueous acid and allowed to separate. Alkaloid salts are now in the aqueous liquid, while many impurities remain behind in the organic liquid.

Process B. The powdered material is extracted with water or aqueous alcohol containing dilute acid. Pigments and other unwanted materials are removed by shaking with chloroform or other organic solvents. The free alkaloids are then precipitated by the addition of excess sodium bicarbonate or ammonia and separated by filtration or by extraction with organic solvents.

Large-scale extractions based on the above principles are sometimes done in the field and the crude mixtures of alkaloids afterwards sent to a factory for separation and purification. This has been done for both cinchona and coca alkaloids in South America and Indonesia, the crude alkaloids then being sent to Europe, USA or Japan for purification. The separation and final purification of a mixture of alkaloids may sometimes be done by fractional precipitation or by fractional crystallization of salts such as oxalates, tartrates or picrates. Chromatographic methods are particularly suitable if the mixture is a complex one and if small quantities of alkaloids will suffice. Supercritical fluid extraction (Chapter 17), although not yet applied to many alkaloids, will probably become of increasing importance for these compounds.

Volatile liquid alkaloids such as nicotine and coniine are most conveniently isolated by distillation. An aqueous extract is made alkaline with caustic soda or sodium carbonate and the alkaloid distilled off in steam. Nicotine is an important insecticide, and large quantities of it are prepared from those parts of the tobacco plant which cannot be used for tobacco manufacture.

Cell, tissue and organ culture

The production of alkaloids using cell, tissue and organ cultures has now been extensively investigated for its commercial potential, as a means of obtaining new alkaloids and for elucidating biosynthetic pathways. These aspects are considered in Chapter 13 and under individual drugs.

FUNCTIONS OF ALKALOIDS IN PLANTS

The characteristic nature of alkaloids and their often very marked pharmacological effects when administered to animals naturally led scientists to speculate on their biological role in the plants in which they occurred. In spite of many suggestions over the years, however, little convincing evidence for their function has been forthcoming. The following points are noteworthy.

1. Being of such diverse nature, alkaloids as a group could not be expected to have a common role (if any) in the plant, except possibly in situations requiring a non-specific basic compound. In this respect the increase in putrescine in barley seedlings when grown in a medium deficient in potassium is of interest.
2. Alkaloids often occur in plants in association with characteristic acids—for example, the tropane alkaloids of the Solanaceae and Erythroxylaceae are esters, the cinchona alkaloids occur with quinic and cinchotannic acids, opium alkaloids are associated with meconic acid. In some cases the alkaloids could provide either a means of storing or transporting in soluble form the particular acids. In the case of solanaceous plants it has been shown that tropane esters formed in the roots are translocated to the aerial parts, where hydrolysis of the alkaloid and breakdown of the liberated acid occurs.
3. As the majority of alkaloids are biosynthesized from readily available units by a series of ubiquitous reactions, their presence in the plant may be purely chance, depending on the enzymes present and the availability of precursors. Being apparently harmless to the plant, they are not eliminated through necessity by natural selection.
4. By the use of suitable grafts, plants which normally accumulate alkaloids in the aerial parts (e.g. *Nicotiana*, *Datura*) are produced free of alkaloids. The lack of alkaloid in the scion appears in no way to impair its development, which suggests the non-essential nature of the alkaloid.
5. Plants which do not normally contain alkaloids appear usually to suffer no adverse reaction when administered alkaloids (colchicine is an exception). Some 'foreign' alkaloids may be metabolized.
6. Current research constantly demonstrates not only that alkaloids participate in plant metabolism over the long term, but also that daily variation in alkaloid content (qualitative and quantitative) is very common in some species. This implies that even if the presence of alkaloids is not vital to the plant, they do participate in metabolic sequences and are not solely the waste, endproducts of metabolism.
7. Pertinent to the above, it has been suggested (R. A. Larson and K. M. Marley, *Phytochemistry*, 1984, **23**, 2351; R. A. Larson, *Phytochemistry*, 1988, **27**, 969) that alkaloids may have a role in the defence of the plant against singlet oxygen ($^1O_2$), which is damaging to all living organisms and is produced in plant tissues in the presence of light. Of 15 alkaloids tested, most showed a good ability to quench singlet oxygen, with brucine and strychnine being especially efficient. Circumstantial evidence quoted is the turnover of poppy alkaloids on a diurnal basis and the formation of oxidized serpentine at the expense of the reduced ajmaline when *Catharanthus roseus* tissue cultures are exposed to light. Further, to concur with the above hypothesis, one would expect plants inhabiting regions with a high ultraviolet light intensity to accumulate more alkaloids, and confirmatory examples quoted are berberine in *Berberis* and tomatidine in *Lycopersicum*. To these could be added quinine in *Cinchona*.

Further reading

Cordell GA (ed) 1991 The alkaloids. Chemistry and pharmacology, Vols 41–. Academic Press, London. *Vol. 53 appeared in 2000. This is a continuation of the original Manske and Holmes series started in 1950; followed by A Brossi as editor, Vols 23–41*
Roberts MR, Wink M (eds) 1998 Alkaloids. Biochemistry, ecology and medical applications. Plenum, New York
Southon IW, Buckingham J 1989 Dictionary of alkaloids. Chapman and Hall, London

ORNITHINE-DERIVED ALKALOIDS

As indicated in Fig. 26.2, the amino acid ornithine, its decarboxylation product, putrescine, and proline constitute the basic unit of the tropane, ecgonine, nicotine (pyrrolidine ring), necine and stachydrine groups of alkaloids. Biogenetically ornithine is linked to arginine (Fig. 18.13); putrescine can also be formed from arginine without the involvement of ornithine and this has led to problems in the understanding of the

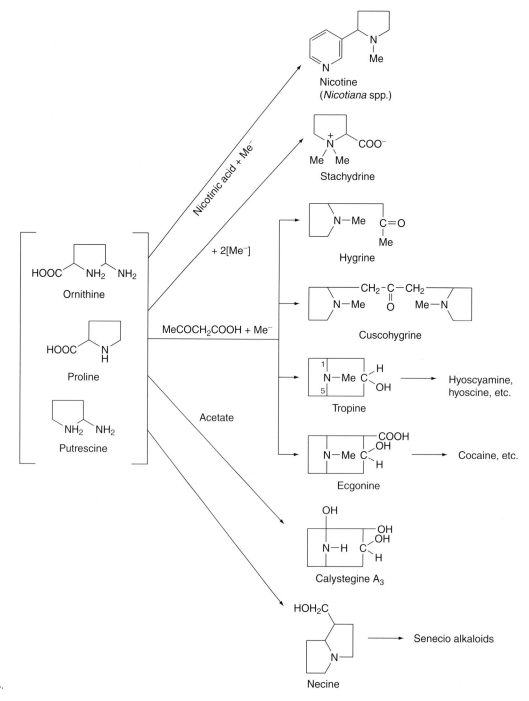

Fig. 26.2
Some ornithine-derived alkaloids.

stereospecific incorporation, or otherwise, of precursors into particular alkaloids, see below. Pharmaceutically, the tropane group is important.

TROPANE ALKALOIDS

The principal alkaloids of medicinal interest in this group are (−)-hyoscyamine; its more stable racemate atropine, and hyoscine (scopolamine). The compounds are esters and are hydrolysed by heating at 60°C with baryta water; atropine yields tropic acid and tropine; hyoscine gives tropic acid and oscine (scopine is actually formed by enzymatic hydrolysis but the chemical treatment converts it to the more stable geometric isomer, oscine).

Hyoscyamine, Atropine   Hyoscine (Scopolamine)

These three specific alkaloids are confined to the Solanaceae, in which some 40 different ester bases of the tropane type have now been discovered; they constitute an interesting chemotaxonomic study within the family. Examples of tropanol esters are given in Table 26.2. Dimeric and trimeric tropanol ester alkaloids involving the dicarboxylic acids mesaconic and itaconic acids are found in *Schizanthus*. For isolations from *S. porrigens* see O. Muñoz and S. Cortés, *Pharm. Biol.*, 1998, **36**, 162, and from *S. hookeri* see M. Jordan *et al.*, *Phytochemistry*, 2006, **67**, 570. Other tropane bases occur in the Erythroxylaceae (see cocaine in coca leaves), Convolvulaceae, Dioscoreaceae, Rhizophoraceae, Cruciferae and Euphorbiaceae.

Schizanthine Z—a tropandiol mesaconic acid diester

Altogether over 200 tropane alkaloids have now been recorded. Semisynthetic derivatives, e.g. hyoscine butylbromide (Buscopan), are of medicinal importance.

BIOGENESIS OF TROPANE ALKALOIDS

As the characteristic alkaloids of the group are esters of hydroxytropanes and various acids (tropic, tiglic, etc.) there are, for each alkaloid, two distinct biogenetic moieties which warrant consideration. Most studies in this connection have utilized various species of *Datura* because, for a number of reasons, they are one of the most convenient of the Solanaceae with which to work. However, with the advent of isolated root culture techniques the study of alkaloid formation in other genera has become more evident and Japanese workers in particular have employed species of *Hyoscyamus* and *Duboisia* with considerable success.

Tropane moiety.   The available evidence suggests that the formation of the tropane ring system is generally similar for all Solanaceae studied but there are still apparent variations between species, particularly in the stereospecific incorporation of some precursors.

Early work with isotopes indicated that ornithine and acetate were precursors of the tropane nucleus; later, the incorporation of ornithine was shown to be stereospecific. Hygrine can also serve as a precursor of the tropane ring but is not now considered to lie on the principal pathway. The *N*-methyl group of the tropane system can be supplied by methionine and can be incorporated at a very early stage of biosynthesis, as demonstrated by the intact incorporation of *N*-methylornithine into hyoscine and hyoscyamine of *Datura metel* and *D. stramonium*. Early involvement of the *N*-methyl group was reinforced by the isolation in 1981 of naturally occurring δ-*N*-methylornithine from belladonna plants. Also supporting the stereospecificity of the ornithine incorporation was the work of McGaw and Woolley (*Phytochemistry*, 1982, **21**, 2653) which showed that for *D. meteloides* the C-2 of hygrine was specifically incorporated into the C-3 of the tropine moiety of the isolated alkaloid. Putrescine (the symmetrical diamine formed by the decarboxylation of ornithine) and its *N*-methyl derivative also serve as precursors, which, taken in conjunction with the stereospecific incorporation of ornithine, makes it difficult to construct a single pathway for tropane ring formation. A scheme for the biogenesis of the tropane moiety, consistent with the above findings, is shown in Fig. 26.3.

Studies on the enzyme putrescine *N*-methyltransferase in cultured roots of *Hyoscyamus albus* support the role of this enzyme as the first committed enzyme specific to the biosynthesis of tropane alkaloids. (N. Hibi *et al.*, *Plant Physiol.*, 1992, **100**, 826.)

It will be observed from Fig. 26.3 that the reduction of tropinone yields both tropine (3α-hydroxytropane) and pseudotropine (3β-hydroxytropane). These reductions are brought about by two independent tropinone reductases (EC 1.1.1.236), often referred to as TR-I and TR-II, which accept NADPH as coenzyme. After considerable research involving principally *D. stramonium* root cultures both enzymes were separately purified and characterized. Furthermore, cDNA clones coding for the two separate enzymes TR-I and TR-II have been isolated and shown to involve polypeptides containing 272

Table 26.2   Examples of ester components of tropane alkaloids of the Solanaceae.

Genera of pharmaceutical interest	*Atropa, Acnistus, Scopolia, Physochlaina, Przewalskia, Hyoscyamus, Physalis, Mandragora, Datura, Solandra, Duboisia, Anthocercis*

Tropanol components of esters

R¹ = H or CH₃
R² = H or OH
R³ = H or OH
(Tropine: R¹ = CH₃, R² = R³ = H)

Scopine: R¹ = CH₃
Norscopine: R¹ = H
(Esterified with tropic or atropic acid only)

φ-Tropine
(Esterified with tiglic acid only)

Esterifying acids	Acetic, propionic, isobutyric, isovaleric, 2-methylbutyric, tiglic, nonanoic, tropic, atropic, 2-hydroxy- 3-phenylpropionic, 2,3-dihydroxy-2-phenylpropanoic, *p*-methoxyphenylacetic, anisic

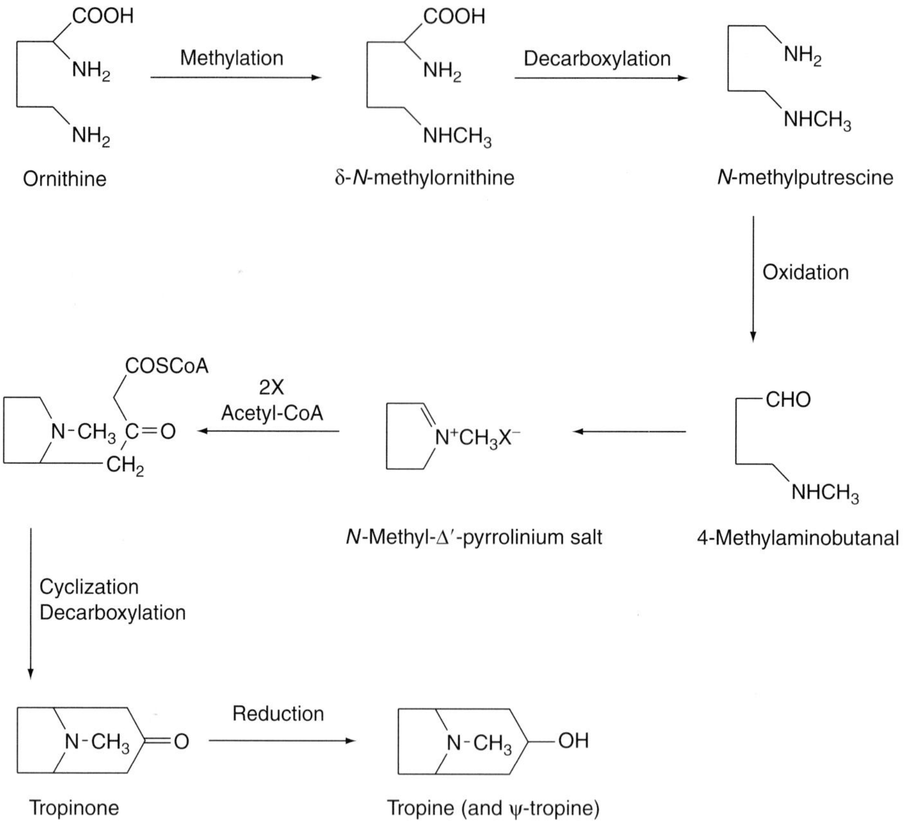

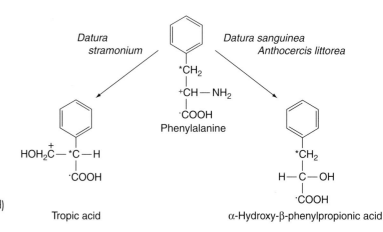

Fig. 26.3
Possible biogenetic routes for tropine and pseudotropine (see text for additional comments).

and 260 amino acids respectively: These clones were expressed in *Escherichia coli* and the same reductive specificity demonstrated as for the natural TRs isolated from plant material.

As indicated in Table 26.2 for solanaceous alkaloids, hydroxyls and ester groups are also common at C-6 and C-7 (R² and R³) of the tropane ring system. Current evidence suggests that hydroxylation of these carbons probably occurs after the C-3 hydroxyl has been esterified.

Esterification. The next stage in the biosynthesis of hyoscyamine, the esterification of tropine and tropic acid, has been demonstrated by feeding experiments and isolated enzymes. It was some 40 years ago that Kaçzkowski first recorded the presence of a hyoscyamine esterase in *D. stramonium*; later, Robins *et al.* (*FEBS Lett.*, 1991, **292**, 293) demonstrated the involvement of two acetyl-CoA-dependent

acyltransferases in the respective formation of 3α- and 3β-acetoxytropanes in *D. stramonium*-transformed root cultures.

Acid moiety. The tropic acid fragment of hyoscine and hyoscyamine is derived from phenylalanine, as is the α-hydroxy-β-phenylpropionic acid (phenyllactic acid) of the tropane alkaloid littorine. The specific incorporations obtained with phenylalanine are given in Fig. 26.4. The sequence involved in the rearrangement of the side-chain in the conversion of phenylalanine to tropic acid has been the subject of longstanding debate. Ansarin and Woolley (*Phytochemistry*, 1994, **35**, 935), by feeding phenyl [1,3¹³C₂]lactic acid to *D. stramonium* and examining the ¹³C-NMR spectra of the subsequently isolated hyoscine and hyoscyamine, have substantiated the hypothesis that tropic acid is formed by an intramolecular rearrangement of phenyllactate. Furthermore, it has been demonstrated that hyoscyamine is biosynthesized from littorine by a

Fig. 26.4
Demonstrated incorporations of phenylalanine into the tropic acid and α-hydroxy-β-phenylpropionic acid (phenyllactic acid) moieties of hyoscyamine and littorine, respectively.

process involving the intramolecular rearrangement of the phenyllactate moiety of the alkaloid. In concordance with this, transformed roots of *Datura stramonium* will convert exogenously added littorine to hyoscyamine (35% metabolism recorded) but, in contrast, exogenously added hyoscyamine is not metabolized to littorine.

Isoleucine serves as a precursor of the tigloyl and 2-methylbutanoyl moieties of various mono- and di-esters of the hydroxytropanes.

Biogenesis of hyoscine (scopolamine). Work initiated by Romeike in 1962 showed that hyoscine appeared to be formed in the leaves of *D. ferox* from hyoscyamine via 6-hydroxyhyoscyamine and 6,7-dehydrohyoscyamine. The former intermediate has been well substantiated, as indicated below, and occurs in quantity in some other genera (*Scopolia*, *Physochlaina*, *Przewalskia*) but the latter, although incorporated into hyoscine when fed as a precursor to *D. ferox*, has never been isolated from normal plants. Some 25 years later Hashimoto's group, using *Hyoscyamus niger* cultured roots, isolated and partially purified the enzyme responsible for the conversion of hyoscyamine to 6-hydroxyhyoscyamine. They used this enzyme to prepare [6-^{18}O]-hydroxyhyoscyamine from hyoscyamine and showed that when the labelled compound, fed to *Duboisia myoporoides*, was converted to hyoscine the ^{18}O was retained, thus eliminating 6,7-dehydrohyoscyamine from the pathway (Fig. 26.5). For this reaction to proceed the epoxidase enzyme requires 2-oxo-glutarate, ferrous ions and ascorbate as cofactors, together with molecular oxygen.

The elucidation of the above pathway, which has spanned many years, aptly illustrates the value of biotechnology and enzymology in contributing to the resolution of some uncertainties resulting from traditional labelled-precursor experiments.

Ontogenesis. In some plants of the Solanaceae (e.g. belladonna and scopolia) hyoscyamine is the dominant alkaloid throughout the life cycle of the plant. In *D. stramonium* hyoscyamine is the principal alkaloid at the time of flowering and after, whereas young plants contain principally hyoscine; in many other species of *Datura* (e.g. *D. ferox*) hyoscine is the principal alkaloid of the leaves at all times. The relative proportions of hyoscine and hyoscyamine in a particular species not only vary with age of the plant, but also are susceptible to other factors, including day length, light intensity, general climatic conditions, chemical sprays, hormones, debudding and chemical races. Isolated organ cultures of belladonna, stramonium and hyoscyamus indicate that the root is the principal site of alkaloid synthesis; however, secondary modifications of the alkaloids may occur in the aerial parts, for example, the epoxidation of hyoscyamine to give hyoscine, and the formation of meteloidine from the corresponding 3,6-ditigloyl ester.

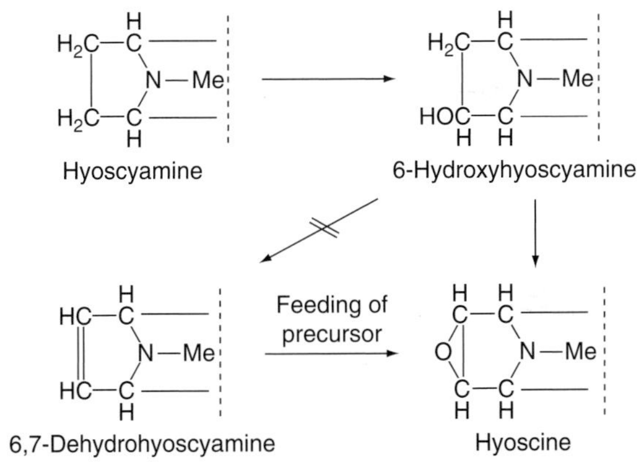

Fig. 26.5
Route for the formation of hyoscine from hyoscyamine (partial formulae).

Further reading

Griffin WJ, Lin GD 2000 Chemotaxonomy and geographical distribution of tropane alkaloids. Phytochemistry 53: 623–637

Lounasmaa M, Tamminen T 1993 Tropane alkaloids. In: Cordell GA (ed) The alkaloids. Chemistry and pharmacology, Vol 44. Academic Press, London. *A review with 484 references listing all known tropane alkaloids*

Robins RJ, Walton NJ 1993 The biosynthesis of tropane alkaloids. In: The alkaloids. Chemistry and pharmacology. *A review with 191 references*

STRAMONIUM LEAF

Stramonium Leaf *BP/EP* (*Thornapple Leaves; Jimson* or *Jamestown Weed*) consists of the dried leaves or dried leaves and flowering tops of *Datura stramonium* L. and its varieties (Solanaceae). The drug is required to contain not less than 0.25% of alkaloids calculated as hyoscyamine. The plant is widespread in both the Old and New Worlds. British supplies are derived mainly from the Continent (Germany, France, Hungary, etc.).

Plant. *D. Stramonium* is a bushy annual attaining a height of about 1.5 m and having a whitish root and numerous rootlets. The erect aerial stem shows dichasial branching with leaf adnation. The stem and branches are round, smooth and green. The flowers are solitary, axillary and short-stalked. They have a sweet scent. Each has a tubular, five-toothed calyx about 4.5 cm long, a white, funnel-shaped corolla about 8 cm long, five stamens and a bicarpellary ovary. The plant flowers in the summer and early autumn. The fruit is originally bilocular but as it matures a false septum arises, except near the apex, so that the mature fruit is almost completely four-celled. The ripe fruit is a thorny capsule about 3–4 cm long. Stramonium seeds (see Fig. 41.6) are dark brown or blackish in colour, reniform in outline and about 3 mm long. The testa is reticulated and finely pitted. A coiled embryo is embedded in an oily endosperm.

D. stramonium var. *tatula* closely resembles the above; its stems are reddish and the leaves have purplish veins, as also have the lavender-coloured corollas. Varieties of both the above forms occur with spineless capsules.

History. Stramonium was grown in England by Gerarde towards the end of the sixteenth century from seeds obtained from Constantinople. The generic name, *Datura*, is derived from the name of the poison, *dhât*, which is prepared from Indian species and was used by the Thugs.

Macroscopical characters. Fresh stramonium leaves or herbarium specimens should first be examined, since the commercial leaves are much shrunken and twisted, and their shape can only be ascertained by careful manipulation after soaking them in water.

The dried leaves are greyish-green in colour, thin, brittle, twisted and often broken. Whole leaves are 8–25 cm long and 7–15 cm wide; they are shortly petiolate, ovate or triangular-ovate in shape, are acuminate at the apex and have a sinuate-dentate margin. They are distinguished from the leaves of the Indian species, *D. innoxia*, *D. metel* and *D. fastuosa*, by the margin, which possesses teeth dividing the sinuses, and by the lateral veins which run into the marginal teeth.

The commercial drug contains occasional flowers and young capsules, which have been described above. The stems are often flattened, longitudinally wrinkled, somewhat hairy and vary in colour from light olive brown (*D. stramonium*) to purplish-brown (var. *tatula*). Stramonium has a slight but unpleasant odour, and a bitter taste.

Microscopical characters. A transverse section of a leaf (Fig. 26.6) shows that it has a bifacial structure. Both surfaces are covered with a

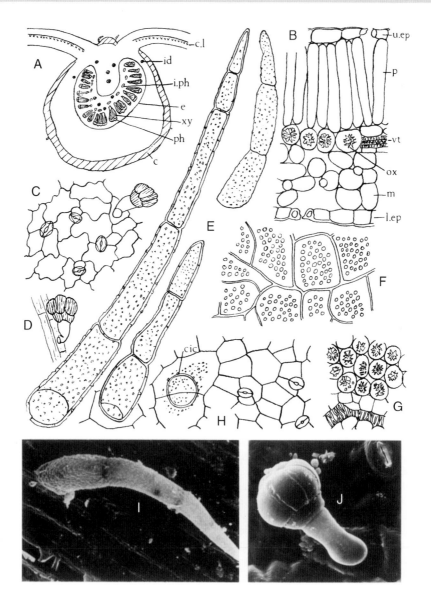

Fig. 26.6

Datura stramonium leaf. A, Transverse sections of midrib (×15); B, transverse section portion of lamina; C, lower epidermis with stomata and glandular trichome; D, glandular trichome over vein; E, clothing trichomes (all ×200); F, arrangement of calcium oxalate crystals in crystal layer, surface view (×50); G, calcium oxalate crystals in cells; H, upper epidermis showing cicatrix and stomata (G and H, ×200). I, J, Scanning electron micrographs of (I) clothing trichome and (J) glandular trichome. c, Collenchyma; cic, cicatrix; c.l, crystal layer; e, endodermis; id, idioblast containing micro-crystals; i.ph, intraxylary phloem; l.ep, lower epidermis with stoma; m, mesophyll; ox, calcium oxalate crystal; p, palisade layer; ph, phloem; u.ep, upper epidermis with stoma; vt, veinlet; xy, xylem. (Photographs: L. Seed and R. Worsley.)

smooth cuticle and possess both stomata and hairs. Cluster crystals of calcium oxalate are abundant in the mesophyll (Fig. 26.6F, G), and microsphenoidal and prismatic crystals are also found. The stomata are of the anisocytic and anomocytic types. The epidermal cells have wavy walls, particularly those of the lower epidermis. The uniseriate clothing hairs are three- to five-celled, slightly curved, and have thin, warty walls (Fig. 26.6E). The basal cell is usually more than 50 μm long (distinction from *D. metel*). Small glandular hairs with a one- or two-celled pedicel and others with a two-celled pedicel and an oval head of two to seven cells are also found. If portions of the leaf are cleared with chloral hydrate solution, the abundance of the cluster crystals of calcium oxalate and their distribution with regard to the veins may be noted.

The midrib shows a bicollateral structure and characteristic subepidermal masses of collenchyma on both surfaces. The xylem forms a strongly curved arc. Sclerenchyma is absent.

Stems are present, but few of these should exceed 5 mm diameter. They possess epidermal hairs up to 800 μm long and have perimedullary phloem. The stem parenchyma contains calcium oxalate similar to that found in the leaf.

Constituents. Stramonium usually contains 0.2–0.45% of alkaloids, the chief of which are hyoscyamine and hyoscine, but a little atropine may be formed from the hyoscyamine by racemization. At the time of collection these alkaloids are usually present in the proportion of about two parts of hyoscyamine to one part of hyoscine, but in young plants hyoscine is the predominant alkaloid. The TLC test for identity given in the *BP/EP* enables other *Datura* species containing different proportions of alkaloids to be detected. The larger stems contain little alkaloid and the official drug should contain not more than 3% stem with a diameter exceeding 5 mm. Stramonium seeds contain about 0.2% of mydriatic alkaloids and about 15–30% of fixed oil. The roots contain, in addition to hyoscine and hyoscyamine, ditigloyl esters of 3,6-dihydroxytropane and 3,6,7-trihydroxytropane, respectively, and a higher proportion of alkamines than the aerial portions. For a recent report on the distribution of alkaloids in different organs and in three varieties of *D. stramonium*, see S. Berkov *et al.*, *Fitoterapia*, 2006, **77**, 179. *D. stramonium* cell and root cultures have been considerably utilized in biogenetic studies.

Prepared Stramonium BP/EP is the finely powdered drug adjusted to an alkaloid content of 0.23–0.27%.

Allied species. All *Datura* species examined to date contain those alkaloids found in stramonium, but frequently hyoscine, rather than hyoscyamine, is the principal alkaloid.

Commercial 'datura leaf' consists of the dried leaves and flowering tops of *D. innoxia* and *D. metel*; it is obtained principally from India. Like those of stramonium, the dried leaves are curled and twisted, but are usually somewhat browner in colour, with entire margins and with differences in venation and trichomes. The leaves contain about 0.5% of alkaloids. Variations in hyoscine and atropine contents in different organs of *D. metel* during development have been studied (S. Afsharypuor *et al.*, *Planta Med.*, 1995, **61**, 383). Over 30 alkaloids have been characterized from *D. innoxia* by capillary GLC–mass spectrometry. For studies on the anatomy of the leaf of *D. metel*, see V. C. Anozie, *Int. J. Crude Drug Res.*, 1986, **24**, 206; and for the isolation of 3α-anisoyloxytropane see S. Siddiqui *et al.*, *J. Nat. Prod.*, 1986, **49**, 511. 'Datura seeds' are derived from *D. metel* and possibly other species. Each seed is light brown in colour and ear-shaped. They are larger and more flattened than stramonium seeds but resemble the latter in internal structure. The alkaloid content, hyoscine with traces of hyoscyamine and atropine, is about 0.2%. *D. ferox*, a species having very large spines on its capsules, contains as its major alkaloids hyoscine and meteloidine.

The 'tree-daturas' constitute Section Brugmansia of the genus; these arboraceous, perennial species are indigenous to South America and are widely cultivated as ornamentals. They produce large, white or coloured trumpet-shaped flowers and pendant unarmed fruits. Some species constitute a potential source of hyoscine (W. C. Evans, *Pharm. J.*, 1990, **244**, 651) and *D. sanguinea*, in particular, has proved a most interesting plant with respect to its wide range of tropane alkaloids and has been cultivated commercially in Ecuador. It yields about 0.8% hyoscine. Plantations have an economically useful life of about 10 years. Chemical races of *D. sanguinea* are evident, particularly one producing relatively large amounts of 6β-acetoxy-3α-tigloyloxytropane. Various tree datura hybrids developed at Nottingham University, UK, have been used by a number of workers for alkaloid studies involving hairy root and root cultures; as an example see P. Nussbaumer *et al.*, *Plant Cell Rep.*, 1998, **17**, 405.

The South American Indians have long cultivated various races of these plants for medicinal and psychotropic use (for a comparison of

native assessment of their potency with alkaloid content, see Bristol *et al.*, *Lloydia*, 1969, **32**, 123).

Withanolides (q.v.) have also been recorded in a number of species of the genus; these include various hydroxywithanolides.

Adulteration. Adulterants cited are the leaves of species of *Xanthium* (Compositae), *Carthamus* (Compositae) and *Chenopodium* (Chenopodiaceae), which are, however, easily distinguished from the genuine drug.

Uses. Atropine has a stimulant action on the central nervous system and depresses the nerve endings to the secretory glands and plain muscle. Hyoscine lacks the central stimulant action of atropine; its sedative properties enable it to be used in the control of motion sickness. Hyoscine hydrobromide is employed in preoperative medication, usually with papaveretum, some 30–60 min before the induction of anaesthesia. Atropine and hyoscine are used to a large extent in ophthalmic practice to dilate the pupil of the eye.

HYOSCYAMUS LEAF

Hyoscyamus Leaf (*Henbane*) *BP/EP* 2001 consists of the dried leaves or the dried leaves and flowering tops of *Hyoscyamus niger* (Solanaceae). It is required to contain not less than 0.05% of total alkaloids calculated as hyoscyamine. The pharmacopoeial description refers to petiolate as well as sessile leaves, the first-year biennial leaves being thus admitted. Henbane is no longer cultivated commercially in Britain and supplies are imported from central Europe. The plant is also cultivated in the USA.

Plant. Henbane is a biennial (var. α-*biennis*) or annual (var. β-*annua*) plant. It is found wild, chiefly near old buildings, both in the UK and in the rest of Europe, and is widely cultivated. Before examining commercial henbane leaves it is advisable to study growing plants or herbarium specimens. The differences tabulated in Table 26.3 should be noted.

Henbane flowers have the formula K(5), C(5), A5, G(2). The hairy, five-lobed calyx is persistent. The fruit is a small, two-celled pyxis (see Fig. 41.6B), which contains numerous seeds.

Henbane seeds are dark grey in colour, somewhat reniform in shape and about 1.5 mm long. They have a minutely reticulated testa and an internal structure closely resembling that of stramonium seeds. Henbane seeds contain about 0.06–0.10% of alkaloids (hyoscyamine with a little hyoscine and atropine) together with calystegines (nortropane alkaloids). A number of non-alkaloidal components include various lignanamides (C.-Y. Ma *et al.*, *J. Nat. Prod.*, 2002, **65**, 206).

History. Henbane, probably the Continental *H. albus*, was known to Dioskurides and was used by the ancients. Henbane was used in

Table 26.3 Comparison of commercial varieties of hyoscyamus.

First-year biennial	Second-year biennial	Annual
Stem very short	Stem branched and up to 1.5 m high	Stem simple and about 0.5 m high
Leaves in a rosette near the ground. Ovate-lanceolate and petiolate, up to 30 cm long, the lamina being up to 25 cm long. Hairy	Leaves sessile, ovate-oblong to triangular-ovate. 10–20 cm long. Margin deeply dentate or pinnatifid. Very hairy, especially in the neighbourhood of the midrib and veins	Leaves sessile. Smaller than those of the biennial plant, with a less incised margin and fewer hairs
Does not normally flower in the first year	Flowers May or June. Corolla yellowish with deep purple veins	Flowers July or August. Corolla paler in colour and less deeply veined

England during the Middle Ages. After a period of disuse in the eighteenth century the drug was restored to the *London Pharmacopoeia* of 1809, largely owing to the work of Störck.

Collection and preparation. Biennial henbane was the variety traditionally grown in England, but much of the current drug is now of the annual variety or is derived from the allied species *H. albus*. The germination of henbane seeds is slow and often erratic and may often be assisted by special treatments (e.g. concentrated sulphuric acid, gibberellic acid or splitting of the testa). The plant may be attacked by the potato beetle, and spraying with derris or pyrethrum may be necessary.

The annual plant usually flowers in July or August and the biennial in May or June. The leaves should be dried rapidly, preferably by artificial heat at a temperature of about 40–50°C.

Macroscopical characters. Commercial henbane consists of the leaves and flowering tops described above. The leaves are more or less broken but are characterized by their greyish-green colour, very broad midrib and great hairiness. If not perfectly dry, they are clammy to the touch, owing to the secretion produced by the glandular hairs. The stems are mostly less than 5 mm diameter and are also very hairy. The flowers are compressed or broken but their yellowish corollas with purple veins are often seen in the drug. Henbane has a characteristic, heavy odour and a bitter, slightly acrid taste.

Microscopical characters. A transverse section of a henbane leaf shows a bifacial structure (Fig. 26.7A). Both surfaces have a smooth cuticle, epidermal cells with wavy walls, stomata of both anisocytic and anomocytic types, and a large number of hairs, which are particularly abundant on the midrib and veins. The hairs are up to 500 μm long; some are uniseriate and two to six cells long, while others have a uniseriate stalk and a large, ovoid, glandular head, the cuticle of which is often raised by the secretion (Fig. 26.7E). Similar hairs are found on the stems. The spongy mesophyll contains calcium oxalate, mainly in the form of single and twin prisms, but clusters and microsphenoidal crystals are also present (Fig. 26.7B,D). The broad midrib contains a vascular bundle, distinctly broader than that of stramonium, showing the usual bicollateral arrangement, which is also to be seen in the stems. The mesophyll of the midrib is made up of two thin zones of collenchyma immediately within the epidermi and a ground mass of colourless parenchyma showing large, intercellular air spaces and containing prisms or, occasionally, microsphenoidal crystals of calcium oxalate.

The calyx possesses trichomes and stomata, as in the leaf. The corolla is glabrous on the inner surface but exhibits trichomes on the outer surface, particularly over the veins (Fig. 26.7G). Those cells of the corolla which contain bluish anthocyanins turn red with chloral hydrate solution. Numerous pollen grains are present, about 50 μm diameter, tricolpate with three wide pores and an irregularly, finely pitted exine (Fig. 26.7F). The testa of the seeds has an epidermis with lignified and wavy anticlinal walls, and sclereids are present in the pericarp.

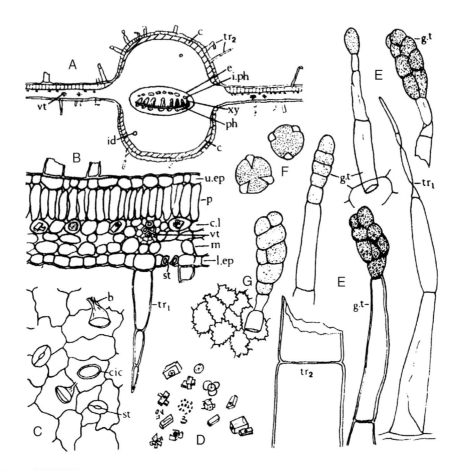

Fig. 26.7

Hyoscyamus niger. A, Transverse section of midrib of leaf (×40); B, transverse section of portion of leaf lamina; C, portion of leaf upper epidermis, surface view; D, calcium oxalate crystals; E, trichomes; F, pollen grains; G, portion of epidermis of corolla with attached glandular trichome (all ×200). b, Base of trichome; c, collenchyma; cic, cicatrix; c.l, crystal layer; e, endodermis; g.t, glandular trichome or portion of; id, idioblast; i.ph, intraxylary phloem; l.ep, lower epidermis; m, mesophyll; p, palisade layer; ph, phloem; st, stoma; tr_1, tr_2, whole and broken clothing trichomes, respectively; u.ep, upper epidermis; vt, veinlet; xy, xylem.

Constituents. Henbane leaves contain about 0.045–0.14% of alkaloids and yield about 8–12% of acid-insoluble ash (*BP/EP* 2001 not more than 12%). Hyoscyamine and hyoscine are the principal alkaloids. The petiole appears to contain more alkaloid than the lamina or stem.

Prepared Hyoscyamus BP/EP 2001 is the drug in fine powder adjusted to contain 0.05–0.07% of total alkaloids. It has a 'loss on drying' requirement of not more than 5.0%.

Allied drugs. *Hyoscyamus albus* is grown on the Continent, particularly in France, and in the Indian subcontinent. It has petiolate stem-leaves and the flowers have pale yellow, non-veined corollas. Unlike *H. niger*, the fruits are barely swollen at the base. Quantitatively and qualitatively its alkaloids appear similar to those of *H. niger*. It has been used in biogenetic studies (q.v.) and the hairy roots (transformed with *Agrobacterium rhizogenes*) have been analysed for 7β- and 6β-hydroxyhyoscyamine, littorine, hyoscine and hyoscyamine (M. Sauerwein and K. Shimomura, *Phytochemistry*, 1991, **30**, 3277). In traditional medicine of the Tuscan archipelago the seeds are pressed into the cavities of decayed teeth to obtain pain relief (R. E. Uncini Manganelli and P. E. Tomei, *J. Ethnopharmacology*, 1999, **65**, 181).

Hyoscyamus muticus is indigenous to India and Upper Egypt; it has been introduced into Algiers. For further details, see below.

Indian henbane. Under this name considerable quantities of drug were imported into Britain during World War II. Although *H. niger* is grown in India and Pakistan, much of the drug came from a closely related plant, *H. reticulatus*. This contains hyoscine and hyoscyamine and microscopically it is almost identical to *H. niger*.

Hyoscyamus aureus and *H. pusillus* are two species which produced hyoscine as the principal alkaloid.

Uses. Henbane resembles belladonna and stramonium in action but is somewhat weaker. The higher relative proportion of hyoscine in the alkaloid mixture makes it less likely to give rise to cerebral excitement than does belladonna. It is often used to relieve spasm of the urinary tract and with strong purgatives to prevent griping.

Hyoscyamus for Homoeopathic Preparations. This is described in the *BP/EP* Vol. III and consists of the whole, fresh, flowering plant of *Hyoscyamus niger* L. There is a limit for foreign matter (max. 5%) and a *minimal* loss on drying at 100–105°C for 2 h of 50%. An assay is described for the Mother Tincture.

Egyptian henbane

Egyptian henbane consists of the dried leaves and flowering tops of *Hyoscyamus muticus* (Solanaceae). The plant is a perennial about 30–60 cm in height. It is indigenous to desert regions in Egypt, Arabia, Iran, Baluchistan, Sind, western Punjab, and has been introduced into Algiers and is cultivated in southern California. In Egypt it is collected from wild plants by Arab shepherds.

Macroscopical characters. The drug consists of leaves, stems, flowers and fruits. The leaves are usually matted and form a lower proportion of the drug than in the case of European henbane. The leaves are pubescent, pale green to yellowish, rhomboidal or broadly elliptical and up to about 15 cm long. Midrib broad, venation pinnate, margin entire or with about five large teeth on each side. Petiole almost absent or up to 9 cm long. The stems are greyish-yellow, striated, slightly hairy and hollow. The flowers are shortly stalked, with large hairy bracts, a tubular five-toothed calyx and a yellowish-brown corolla which in the dry drug may show deep purple patches. The fruit is a cylindrical pyxidium surrounded by a persistent calyx and containing numerous yellowish-grey to brown seeds. Odour, slightly foetid; taste, bitter and acrid.

Microscopical characters. Egyptian henbane is easily distinguished from *H. niger* by the numerous branched and unbranched glandular trichomes, which have a one- to four-celled stalk and unicellular heads. Additional characters are the striated cuticle, the prisms of oxalate 45–110 μm, twin prisms and occasional clusters and microsphenoids.

Constituents. Ahmed and Fahmy found about 1.7% of alkaloids in the leaves, 0.5% in the stems and 2.0% in the flowers. The chief alkaloid is hyoscyamine for the isolation of which (as atropine) the plant is principally used. The alkaloidal mixture of plants grown in Afghanistan had the following composition: hyoscyamine 75%, apoatropine 15%, hyoscine 5%, with smaller quantities of noratropine and norhyoscine. A number of non-alkaloidal ketones, an acid and sitosterol have been characterized from plants raised in Lucknow, India. The formation of alkaloids in suspension cell cultures has been widely investigated with variable results; with callus cultures the addition of phenylalanine to the medium produced maximum alkaloid production (3.97%) whereas isoleucine gave the greatest growth (M. K. El-Bahr *et al.*, *Fitoterapia*, 1997, **68**, 423).

BELLADONNA LEAF

Belladonna Leaf *BP/EP* (*Belladonna Herb*) consists of the dried leaves and, occasionally fruit-bearing flowering tops of *Atropa belladonna* L. (Solanaceae); it contains not less than 0.30% of total alkaloids calculated as hyoscyamine. Traditionally the *BP* drug consisted of all the aerial parts (Belladonna Herb) but under the European requirements there is a limit (3%) of stem with a diameter exceeding 5 mm. The *USP*, which requires 0.35% alkaloid, also admits *A. acuminata* (see below) in the Belladonna Leaf monograph.

A. belladonna is cultivated in Europe and the USA.

Plant. The deadly nightshade, *A. belladonna*, is a perennial herb which attains a height of about 1.5 m. Owing to adnation, the leaves on the upper branches are in pairs, a large leaf and a smaller one.

The flowers appear about the beginning of June. They are solitary, shortly stalked, drooping and about 2.5 cm long. The corolla is campanulate, five-lobed and of a dull purplish colour. The five-lobed calyx is persistent, remaining attached to the purplish-black berry. The latter is bilocular, contains numerous seeds and is about the size of a cherry (see Fig. 41.6C). In the USA the plant is often known as the 'Poison Black Cherry', while the German name is 'Tollkirschen' (i.e. Mad Cherry). A yellow variety of the plant lacks the anthocyanin pigmentation; the leaves and stems are a yellowish-green and the flowers and berries yellow.

History. Belladonna was probably known to the ancients but it is not clearly recorded until the beginning of the sixteenth century. The leaves were introduced into the *London Pharmacopoeia* of 1809, but the root was not used in Britain until a liniment prepared from it was introduced by Squire in 1860.

Cultivation, collection and preparation. Belladonna is grown from seed. The leaves are said to be richest in alkaloid at the end of June or in July, and a sunny position is said to give more active leaves than a shady one. Plants about 3 years old are sufficiently large to give a good yield of leaves and, if the roots are being collected, it would seem to be best to replant about every third year (see also 'Belladonna Root'). Two or more crops of leaves may be collected annually. Leaves left in an imperfectly dry state deteriorate and give off ammonia. They should therefore be dried immediately after collection and be carefully stored. Leaves of a good colour may be obtained by drying in thin layers starting with a moderate heat which is gradually increased to about 60°C and then gradually decreased. Sometimes the leaves are badly attacked by insects and the roots by a fungus.

Macroscopical characters. The drug consists of leaves and the smaller stems, the latter seldom exceeding 5 mm diameter, together with flowers and fruits as described above. If the drug is little broken, the arrangement of the leaves in unequal pairs may be seen. The leaves are dull green or yellowish-green in colour, the upper side being somewhat darker than the lower. Each has a petiole about 0.5–4 cm long and a broadly ovate, slightly decurrent lamina about 5–25 cm long and 2.5–12 cm wide. The margin is entire and the apex acuminate. A few

flowers and fruits may be found. If the leaves are broken, the most useful diagnostic characters are the venation and roughness of the surface. The latter is due to the presence of calcium oxalate in certain of the mesophyll cells which causes minute points on the surface of the leaf as the other cells contract more on drying.

Microscopical characters. A transverse section of the leaf of *A. belladonna* is shown in Fig. 26.8A. It has a bifacial structure. The epidermal cells have wavy walls and a striated cuticle (Fig. 26.8E). Stomata of the characteristic anisocytic type and also some of the anomocytic type are present on both surfaces but are most common on the lower. Hairs are most numerous on young leaves. Some of the hairs are uniseriate, two- to four-celled clothing hairs; others resemble these but have a unicellular glandular head; while a third kind has a short pedicel

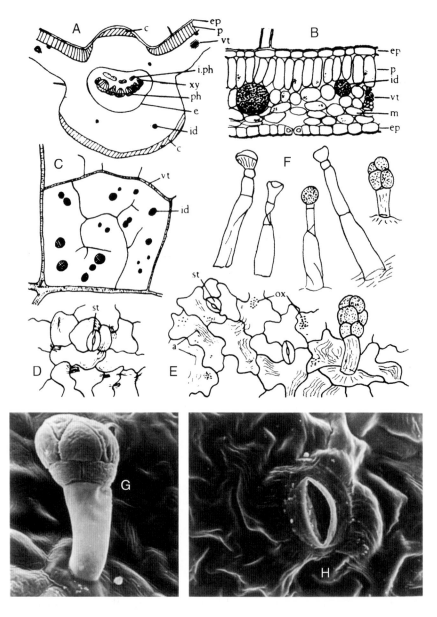

Fig. 26.8
Atropa belladonna leaf. A, Transverse section of midrib (×40); B, transverse section of portion of lamina (×200); C, distribution of idioblasts, surface view of leaf cleared in chloral (×50); D, upper epidermis; E, lower epidermis; F, trichomes (all ×200); G and H, Scanning electron micrographs (G) of glandular trichome and epidermal cells with striated cuticle and (H) stoma and striated cuticle. a, Striations of cuticle; c, collenchyma; e, endodermis; ep, epidermis; id, idioblast containing crystals of calcium oxalate; i.ph, intraxylary phloem; m, mesophyll; ox, calcium oxalate crystals; p, palisade layer; ph, phloem; st, stoma; vt, veinlet; xy, xylem. (Photographs, L. Seed and R. Worsley.)

and a multicellular glandular head (Fig. 26.8F). Certain of the cells of the spongy mesophyll are filled with microsphenoidal ('sandy') crystals of calcium oxalate (Fig. 26.8B, C). The midrib is convex above and shows the usual bicollateral vascular bundle. A zone of collenchyma underlies both epidermi in the region of the midrib.

Constituents. The drug from *A. belladonna* contains 0.3–0.60% of alkaloids, the chief of which is hyoscyamine. Small quantities of volatile bases, such as pyridine and *N*-methylpyrroline, are present, and if not removed during the assay of the drug by heating, increase the titration and appear in the result as hyoscyamine. The leaves also contain a fluorescent substance, β-methylaesculetin (scopoletin), and calcium oxalate. They yield about 14% of ash and not more than 4% of acid-insoluble ash.

Prepared Belladonna Herb is the finely powdered drug adjusted to contain 0.28–0.32% of total alkaloids. Note the 'loss on drying' requirement.

Allied drugs. *Indian belladonna* from *A. acuminata* Royle ex Lindley differs from that derived from *A. belladonna* in that its flowers are yellowish-brown and its leaves brownish-green, oblong-elliptical and tapering towards both base and apex. It grows wild in the Himalayan regions of northern India (1800–3400 m) and is cultivated in the Kashmir valley.

Atropa baetica Willk. is a species native to southern Spain and northern Morocco; it produces yellow flowers and black berries and is regarded as an endangered species. R. Zárate *et al.* have described a rapid *in vitro* propagation method for the plant, and from hairy root cultures have isolated tigloylpseudotropine—alkaloid not found in the mature plant (*Plant Cell Rep.*, 1999, **18**, 418).

Adulterants. Of the numerous recorded adulterants of belladonna leaves, those of *Phytolacca decandra* (Phytolaccaceae) and *Ailanthus glandulosa* (Simaroubaceae) are perhaps the most important. In *Phytolacca* the lamina is denser and less decurrent than in belladonna; the epidermal cells have straight walls, the stomata are of the anomocytic type and some of the mesophyll cells contain bundles of needle-shaped crystals of calcium oxalate. *Ailanthus* leaves are triangular-ovate, have straight-walled epidermal cells showing a strongly striated cuticle, cluster crystals of calcium oxalate, and on both surfaces white, unicellular clothing hairs which are lignified (Fig. 42.3F).

Uses. Belladonna leaves are mainly used for internal preparations which are used as sedatives and to check secretion. Preparations of the root are mainly used externally.

Belladonna root

Belladonna root consists of the dried roots or rootstock and roots of *Atropa belladonna* (Solanaceae).

Collection and preparation. Much of the *A. belladonna* drug is of small size and poor quality. The first-year roots are not profitable to collect from the commercial point of view, although they contain a high proportion of alkaloids. The autumn of the third year would seem to be a suitable time for collection. The roots are dug up, washed, sliced and dried.

Macroscopical characters. *Atropa belladonna* rapidly develops a large branching root. The aerial stems die back each year and new ones arise independently from the large crown. Dried roots of 3-year-old plants are about 3 cm diameter and roots over 4 cm diameter are exceptional. Most commercial drug is about half this thickness.

The drug is usually cut into short lengths, which are sometimes split longitudinally. The outer surface is a pale greyish-brown. The root breaks with a short fracture and then shows a whitish or, if overheated during drying, brownish interior. A yellowish-green colour in the region of the cambium is often seen.

A transverse section of the bark is non-fibrous and the wood does not show a radiate appearance. The wood consists of scattered groups of vessels, tracheids and fibres which are most abundant near the cambium; there is a central mass of primary xylem (Fig. 41.8G). The extensive parenchyma of bark and wood contains sandy crystals of calcium oxalate and abundant simple and compound starch grains.

The structure gradually changes as the roots pass into rhizome, the wood becoming denser and exhibiting a distinctly radiate structure; the rhizome also shows a distinct pith and internal phloem. The aerial stems found on the upper surface of the crown are hollow.

Constituents. *Atropa belladonna* root contains about 0.4–0.8% of alkaloids calculated as hyoscyamine.

Samples of belladonna root examined by Kuhn and Schäfer showed 0.3–1.0% of alkaloids, of which 82.8–97.3% was hyoscyamine, 2.7–15.2% atropine, and 0.0–2.6% scopolamine. Capillary GLC–mass spectrometry data revealed the presence of hygrine, hygroline, cuscohygrine, tropinone, tropine, pseudotropine and nine tropanol esters (F. Oprach *et al.*, *Planta Med.*, 1986, 513). Other constituents previously reported include belladonnine together with β-methylaesculetin, calcium oxalate and starch.

A pseudotropine-forming, tropinone reductase (see biogenesis of tropane alkaloids), not entirely similar in chemical and catalytic properties to other samples of the enzyme previously described, has been isolated from transformed belladonna root cultures. The pseudotropine could have implications for the formation of calystegines (q.v). Littorine has been detected in both non-transformed and hairy root-cultures (F. Nakanishi *et al.*, *Plant Cell Rep.*, 1998, **18**, 249).

Allied drug. *Indian belladonna root* from *Atropa acuminata* (see under 'Belladonna Leaf') consists of brownish-grey roots, stolons, rootstock and stem bases. It has been described in detail by Melville. The roots are cylindrical, longitudinally wrinkled, occasionally branched, and 0.5–3 cm diameter. Young roots resemble those of *A. belladonna* but older ones show concentric zonation of the secondary xylem. The rootstock is 3–9 cm diameter at the top and bears the bases of 4–12 aerial stems. The rootstock, stem bases and stolons all possess a pith which becomes hollow in the stem bases. The constituents are similar to those of European belladonna.

Adulterant. The root of *Phytolacca decandra* (Phytolaccaceae) is sometimes sliced and mixed with samples of belladonna. It bears little resemblance to belladonna root, but a casual and inexperienced observer might perhaps mistake it for pieces of an old belladonna crown. The transverse section shows a number of concentric cambia, each producing a ring of wood bundles. The parenchyma contains abundant acicular crystals of calcium oxalate.

DUBOISIA LEAVES

Three species of *Duboisia* are indigenous to Australia and two of these, *D. myoporoides* and *D. leichhardtii*, have for over 55 years been a major world source of tropane alkaloids, particularly hyoscine. The third species, *D. hopwoodii*, contains principally nicotine and related alkaloids and was used by the Australian aborigines for the preparation of 'pituri' by mixing powdered leaves with an alkaline wood ash to form a quid which was held in the cheek pouch.

26

D. myoporoides, discovered by Robert Brown, naturalist to the Flinders expedition of 1802, occurs along the east coast of Australia, where the rainfall exceeds a monthly mean of 5 cm for 11 months of the year and where frosts rarely occur. *D. leichhardtii* was described by Mueller in 1877 and is named after the explorer Ludwig Leichhardt, who originally collected the plant; it occurs naturally in a limited area of south-east Queensland known locally as the South West Burnett. *D. hopwoodii* is of wide distribution in Western and Central Australia.

Of the two tropane alkaloid-containing species *D. myoporoides* is the larger and more densely leaved; both, however, are bushy trees and have the advantage that in one year repeated harvests can often be taken from the same plants. For collection, the small branches are removed, tied in bundles and stood in sheds to dry; the leaves are then easily removed by beating.

In addition to hyoscine and hyoscyamine, minor alkaloids occur in variable amounts and include norhyoscyamine, 6β- hydroxyhyoscyamine, valeroidine, tigloidine, poroidine, isoporoidine, valtropine, 3α-tigloyloxytropane, 3α-acetoxytropane, 3α-nonanoyloxytropane, butropine and apohyoscine. Two discopine esters were identified in 1980 in *D. leichhardtii* and the greenhouse leaves have yielded calystegines B$_1$, B$_2$, B$_4$, C$_1$, and C$_2$ (A. Kato *et al.*, *Phytochemistry*, 1997, **45**, 425). Other constituents include the triterpenoids ursolic acid and betulonic acid and a number of recently reported aliphatic constituents.

A number of chemical races occur, particularly in *D. myoporoides*, and include the well-established 'northern' and 'southern' races which differ in their relative contents of hyoscine and hyoscyamine, and a race which contains nicotine and anabasine as principal bases.

For a number of years, growers have also been cultivating a hybrid of the two species, the origin of which is doubtful, but which Griffin considers may derive from the experimental work of the CSIRO carried out in the early 1950s. Established plantations of the hybrid exhibit no morphological differences and propagation is carried out vegetatively. In a series of experiments on the hybrid, Griffin and Luanratana (*J. Nat. Prod.*, 1980, **43**, 552; 1982, **45**, 270) have shown that the total alkaloid content of the leaves does not vary throughout the year but there is a decrease in hyoscine content from January to June (summer to autumn) and a gradual increase from June to September; the reverse is true for hyoscyamine. Repeated sprayings of plants with cytokinin solution (which also has a beneficial effect on plant growth), in the form of a sea-weed extract, prevented the hyoscine decline. Such treatment of plants could possibly enhance the hyoscine yield from all-year harvesting. There is evidence (Y. Kitamura *et al.*, *Phytochemistry*, 1996, **42**, 1331) that in the plant the tropic acid moiety of atropine may be recycled.

Addition of putrescine and spermidine to the culture medium of *D. myoporoides* root cultures has been shown to increase the hyoscine content.

Most of the Australian crop (some 1200 tonnes) is exported to West Germany, Switzerland and Japan for processing. Plantations have also been established in Ecuador.

Scopolia

All species of *Scopolia* investigated appear to contain tropane alkaloids similar to those found in belladonna (q.v.). Although little used in western Europe, these plants constitute a useful source of hyoscyamine and galenicals in regions where the plant is available locally. *Scopolia carniolica* is a central and eastern European species somewhat smaller than belladonna. In shape the leaves resemble those of belladonna, although they are more lanceolate and translucent. The cuticle is striated but less markedly so than in belladonna, sandy crystals are less numerous, hairs are rare or absent, and stomata are present on the lower surface only. The fruit, a pyxis, may often be found in the drug.

The rhizomes (*BPC* 1934), which are nearly black in colour and bear numerous depressed stem scars, are used similarly to belladonna root. In addition to hyoscyamine and hyoscine, other alkaloids reported in this species are cuscohygrine, 3α-tigloyloxytropane, pseudotropine and tropine. *S. caucasia*, *S. lurida* and *S. tangutica* all appear to be suitable as sources of hyoscyamine; the last two also contain 6-hydroxy-hyoscyamine and an alkaloid named daturamine (anisodine) which is a 'hydroxyhyoscine'. Both these alkaloids are produced commercially in China. The dried rhizomes of *S. japonica* ('Japanese Belladonna Root') were official in the *Japanese Pharmacopoeia* 1961; the isolation of steroidal glycosides (scopolosides) has been reported from this species (S. Okamura *et al.*, *Chem. Pharm. Bull.*, 1992, **40**, 2981).

Przewalskia tangutica is a related tropane alkaloid-containing plant and is used in Tibetan traditional medicine. The roots have a high content of hyoscyamine with total alkaloids amounting to 1.7–3.8%; 6β-hydroxyhyoscyamine and small amounts of hyoscine are also present.

Mandrake

The true mandrake, *Mandragora officinarum*, is one of several Mediterranean species. It was well known to Dioskurides (see R. T. Gunther's English edition of *The Greek Herbal of Dioscorides*, 1934, Oxford, UK: OUP). B. P. Jackson, in an investigation of the botanical source of the drug, found that the species *M. autumnalis* is also involved. The leaves and roots were official in France (1818–1883) and in Spain. The roots occur in fusiform or two-branched pieces and their microscopical structure and distinction from belladonna root has been described by Berry and Jackson (*Planta Med.*, 1976, **30**, 281). The plant is surrounded with much folklore and superstition and even the collection of the root was formerly accompanied by special rites. The drug, like belladonna, has long been known to contain atropine and the fluorescent substance scopoletin. Recent investigations have established the presence of several other solanaceous alkaloids.

For a review of the isolated constituents of *Mandragora* spp., including alkaloids, volatile compounds, lipids and related compounds, coumarins and pigments (78 refs), see L. O. Hanus *et al.*, *Phytochemistry*, 2005, **66**, 2408.

COCA LEAF AND COCAINE

Coca leaves are derived from two cultivated shrubs of the Erythroxylaceae, namely *Erythroxylum coca* Lam. and *E. novogranatense* (Morris) Hieron. Each comprises two subspecies, as indicated below.

History. Coca leaves have been used in South America as a masticatory from very early times. They were formerly reserved for the sole use of the native chiefs and Incas. Coca was introduced into Europe about 1688 and cocaine was isolated in 1860. By employing the alkaloid in ophthalmic surgery in 1884 Carl Koller was the first to introduce it into clinical practice so heralding the era of modern anaesthetics. For reviews covering both the historical and other aspects of coca see the special issue of *The Journal of Ethnopharmacology* (1981), Vol. 3: *Coca and Cocaine*.

Cultivation and collection. These differ depending on geographical source. For Andean coca, plants are raised from seed and cultivated at an altitude of 500–2000 m. Pruning limits the height to about 2 m and traditionally three harvests are collected annually, the first from the pruned twigs, the second in June and the third in November. The leaves are artificially or sun dried and packed into bags. On the other hand, in the Amazon, plants are raised from cuttings, often in jungle clearings and interplanted between other staple crops.

Varieties and characters:

1. *Huanco* or *Bolivian coca* consists of the leaves of *E. coca* var. Lam; it is produced as described above on the eastern slopes of the Andes in Bolivia and Peru. The leaves are shortly petiolate, oval, 2.5–7.5 cm long and 1.5–4 cm wide. The lamina is greenish brown to brown and glabrous; margin entire. The midrib is prominent on the lower surface, bears a ridge on its upper surface, and projects slightly beyond the lamina as an apiculus. The latter is often broken in the commercial drug but the leaves are otherwise fairly entire. The lower surface shows two, very characteristic, curved lines, one on either side of the midrib. Odour, characteristic; taste, at first bitter and slightly aromatic, the alkaloids afterwards causing numbness of the tongue and lips.

2. The subspecies *E. coca* var. *ipadu* Plowman is an Amazonian coca cultivated sparingly in the western area of the Amazon basin. The leaves are broadly elliptic and rounded at the base; on the lower surface the characteristic 'parallel lines' of *E. coca* var. *coca* are often indistinct or lacking and the cocaine content is consistently lower.

3. *Columbian coca* comprises the leaves of *E. novogranatense* var. *novogranatense*; it has been cultivated throughout the mountains of present Columbia and Venezuela since pre-Columbian times. It thrives at lower altitudes and in hotter drier climates than does *E. coca*; this variety was widely planted in the Old World tropics, especially in the former British colonies, as an ornamental plant and minor source of cocaine.

4. *Truxillo, Trujillo* or *Peruvian coca*, derived from *E. novogranatense* var. *truxillense*, is the well-known commercial variety of the drug. It is well adapted to the desert conditions of N. Peru and was cultivated for 'coca chewing' and the manufacture of coca-based soft drinks (originally containing cocaine but now legally devoid of the alkaloid). Leaves of a Truxillo-type coca were formerly exported from Indonesia for the manufacture of cocaine (*Javanese coca* leaves). The leaves are pale green in colour, are more papery in texture than the Huanuco and are usually broken. Lamina about 1.6–5 cm long; lines on the lower surface usually indistinct. Flowers of a species of *Inga* (Leguminosae, subfamily Mimosoideae) are sometimes added to the leaves.

Microscopical characters. A transverse section of a coca leaf shows upper epidermis, palisade parenchyma containing prisms of calcium oxalate, spongy parenchyma and a very characteristic lower papillose epidermis with numerous stomata. The midrib is partly surrounded by an arc of pericyclic fibres, above and below which is a considerable amount of collenchyma. A surface preparation of the lower epidermis shows the papillae as well-marked circles, and numerous stomata (see Fig. 42.2J), each with four subsidiary cells, two of which have their long axes parallel to the pore.

DNA analysis. For a report on the differentiation of the cocaine-producing species and varieties of *Erythroxylum* using AFLP DNA analysis, see E. L. Johnson *et al.*, *Phytochemistry*, 2003, **64**, 187; 132 *Erythroxylum* samples were examined.

Constituents. Coca leaves contain about 0.7–1.5% of total alkaloids, of which cocaine, cinnamylcocaine and α-truxilline are the most important (Fig. 26.9). They occur in different proportions in different commercial varieties. Javanese leaves are usually richest in total alkaloids, of which the chief is cinnamylcocaine, while the Bolivian and Peruvian leaves contain less total alkaloid but a higher proportion of cocaine. Other substances isolated from various varieties of the leaves are hygrine, hygroline, cuscohygrine, dihydrocuscohygrine, tropacocaine (3β-benzoyloxytropane), crystalline glycosides and cocatannic acid. 1-Hydroxytropacocaine (free hydroxyl situated at a bridgehead carbon) has been isolated as a major alkaloid of greenhouse-cultivated *E. novogranatense* var. *novogranatense*; much lower amounts were detected in var. *truxillense* and in field cultivated coca from Colombia and Bolivia (J. M. Moore *et al.*, *Phytochemistry*, 1994, **36**, 357).

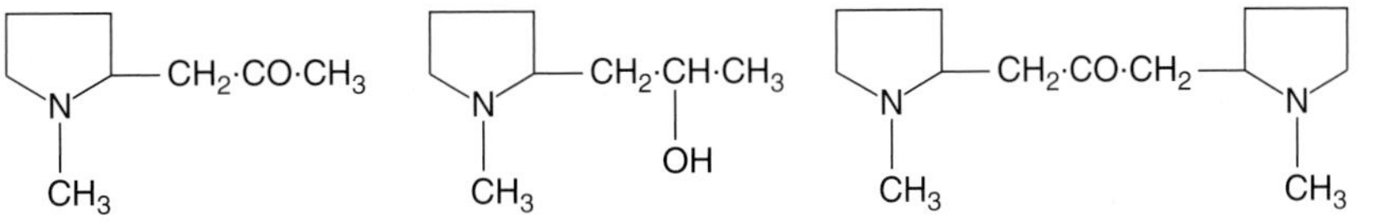

The leaves also contain essential oil and as early as 1894 Van Romburgh identified methyl salicylate as a component; this was confirmed (13.6%) in a recent study, together with *N*-methylpyrrole (3.7%) and possibly *N,N*-dimethylbenzylamine (0.5%) and two dihydrobenzaldehydes (38.9%). The grassy odour of the leaves is explained to a large extent by the presence in the oil of *trans*-2-hexenal (10.4%) and *cis*-3-hexen-1-ol (16.1%); no mono- or sesquiterpenes were detected (M. Novák *et al.*, *Planta Med.*, 1987, **53**, 113).

Although it had been generally assumed that ecgonine, the basic moiety of the cocaines, was ornithine-derived (Fig. 26.2), the practical demonstration of the incorporation of the usual precursors proved difficult. Then Leete (*J. Am. Chem. Soc.*, 1982, **104**, 1403) obtained a significant level of radioactivity in cocaine isolated from *Erythroxylum coca*, the leaves of which were painted with an aqueous solution of DL-[5-¹⁴C]ornithine HCl. The pathway to ecgonine appears to be similar to that for tropine except that the carboxyl is retained and the different stereospecificities need to be accommodated. The benzoyl moiety of cocaine is derived from phenylalanine. For work on the incorporation of labelled 1-methyl-Δ¹-pyrrolinium chloride into cuscohygrine, indicating the alkaloid to be a mixture of its *meso* and optically active diastereomers, see E. Leete *et al.*, *Phytochemistry*, 1988, **27**, 401.

Manufacture of cocaine. The crude alkaloids may be extracted with dilute sulphuric acid or by treatment with lime and petroleum or other organic solvents. Non-alkaloidal matter is roughly separated by

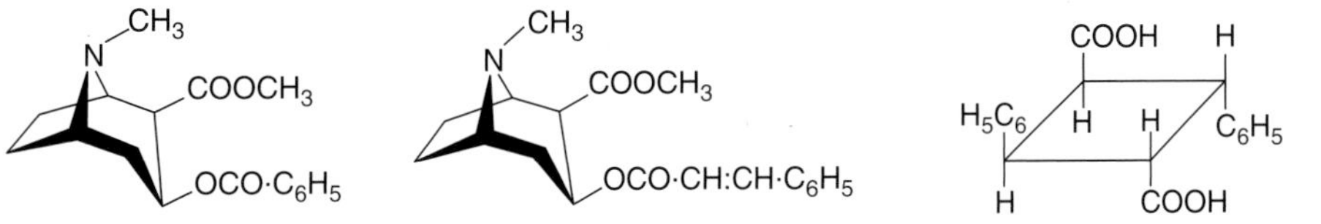

Fig. 26.9
Constituents of coca.

transferring the alkaloids from one solvent to another. The crude alkaloids are obtained in solid form either as free bases by precipitation with alkali, or as hydrochlorides by concentrating an acidified solution.

Pure cocaine is prepared from the leaves, the crude bases or the crude hydrochlorides. The process depends on the fact that cocaine, cinnamylcocaine and α-truxilline are closely related derivatives of ecgonine (Fig. 26.2), which is produced by hydrolysing them with boiling dilute hydrochloric acid.

Cocaine → ecgonine + methyl alcohol + benzoic acid
Cinnamylcocaine → ecgonine + methyl alcohol + cinnamic acid
α-Truxilline (1 mol) → ecgonine (2 mols) + methyl alcohol (2 mols) + α-truxillic acid (1 mol)

The ecgonine hydrochloride is purified and converted into the free base. This is benzoylated by interaction with benzoic anhydride and the benzoylecgonine purified. The benzoylecgonine is methylated with methyl iodide and sodium methoxide in methyl alcohol solution, to give methylbenzoylecgonine or cocaine. The latter is converted into the hydrochloride and purified by recrystallization.

Much illicit cocaine is extracted locally in South America and despite the unsophisticated methods employed a high degree of purity can be attained.

In view of the importance of quantitatively determining cocaine and its metabolite, benzoylecgonine, in body fluids, etc., many assays are available for these alkaloids.

Allied species. There are over 200 species of *Erythroxylum* found throughout the tropical and pantropical regions of the world. Few of the non-cocaine-producing species have been systematically examined but the majority of those that have contain a range of tropane alkaloids (W. C. Evans, *J. Ethnopharmacol.*, 1981, **3**, 265 and for Pt. 12 of a further series of papers see P. Christen *et al.*, *Phytochemistry*, 1995, **38**, 1053). Subsequently, other workers have isolated a number of the same alkaloids from other species, together with the characterization of new tropane alkaloids, some named pervilleines and others catuabines. Nortropanols (calystegins, see below) are present in some species. Trimethoxybenzoic acid and trimethoxycinnamic acid commonly occur as esterifying acids. D. Bieri *et al.* (*J. Ethnopharmacology*, 2006, **103**, 439) have studied the cocaine distribution in 51 species of *Erythroxylum* from S. America, 28 of which had received no previous phytochemical examination; cocaine was reported for the first time in 14 species, with *E. laetevirens* having the highest cocaine content of the wild species. It is of interest to note that in this study, the time between collection and analysis of the samples varied from 20 to 25 years.

Uses. Cocaine and its salts were the earliest of the modern local anaesthetics but, because of their toxic and addictive properties, their use is now almost entirely confined to ophthalmic, ear, nose and throat surgery.

Calystegines

These relatively new alkaloids are trihydroxy-, tetrahydroxy- or penta-hydroxy derivatives of nortropane. They were originally isolated from the roots of the bindweed *Calystegia sepium* and given the names calystegine A₃ (a 1,2,3-trihydroxynortropane) (Fig. 26.2) and calystegine B₂ (a 1,2,3,4-tetrahydroxynortropane). By 1998 the structures of nine such alkaloids had been elucidated including the 3-*O*-β-D-glucopyranoside of calystegine B₁. In chemotaxonomic studies of the Convolvulaceae involving GC-MS analyses, T. Schimming *et al.* (*Phytochemistry*, 1998, **49**, 1989; 2005, **66**, 469) record the occurrence of 11 calystegines and the calystegine patterns in 135 species.

Calystegines have also been reported in the Solanaceae including belladonna and hyoscyamus root cultures. R. J. Nash *et al.*,

(*Phytochemistry*, 1993, **34**, 1281) found these compounds to be present in the tubers and leaves of potato plants and that these alkaloids can be isolated from certain moths and butterflies, the larvae of which feed on the plant. Other sources are the Brassicaceae, Erythroxylaceae (see 'Coca' above) and the Moraceae.

The formation of calystegines in root cultures of *Calystegium sepium* involves tropinone and pseudotropine as metabolic intermediates (Y. Scholl *et al.*, *Phytochemistry*, 2003, **62**, 325).

Pharmaceutically, interest lies in the calystegines because they are potent inhibitors of glycosidases (R. J. Molyneux *et al.*, *Arch. Biochem. Biophysics*, 1993, **304**, 81) making them possible candidates for the development of antiviral, anticancer and antidiabetic drugs (cf. the trihydroxyindolizidine alkaloids castanospermine and swainsonine and the tetrahydroxypyrrolizidine alkaloid australine).

Further reading
Biastoff S, Dräger B 2007 Calystegines. The Alkaloids 64: 49–102.
A review with 347 refs covering structures, chemical properties, occurrence, biosynthesis, chemical syntheses, activities

Tobacco alkaloids
The principal alkaloids of the genus *Nicotiana* have a pyridine moiety associated with either a pyrrolidine ring (ornithine-derived) or a piperidine ring (lysine-derived). The former group is represented by nicotine (Fig. 26.2) and the latter by anabasine (Fig 26.11).

Although, with the exception indicated below, no drugs are derived from these alkaloids, they have been extensively studied in relation to tobacco manufacture and smoking, and as insecticides (see Chapter 40). Consequently, much is known of their plant biochemistry and genetics of formation.

A pharmaceutical introduction is that of nicotine chewing-gum, nasal spray or patch, intended to help smokers who want to give up smoking but who experience great difficulty in so doing because of their nicotine dependence.

PYRROLIZIDINE ALKALOIDS

Although these alkaloids have at present no great medicinal significance they are important in that they constitute the poisonous hepatotoxic constituents of plants of the genus *Senecio* (Compositae), well-known for their toxicity to livestock. Some of the alkaloids also show carcinogenic and mutagenic properties and have caused concern in that they occur in small quantities in some herbal products such as comfrey (Boraginaceae) and coltsfoot (Compositae). These alkaloids are known to have an ecological role in some species of butterfly affording protection to some and converting to female flight arrestants in others. In the first demonstration of its kind, the presence of alkaloids on leaf surfaces has been indicated in eight different samples of *Senecio jacoboea* (K. Vrieling and S. Derridj, *Phytochemistry*, 2003, **64**, 1223). Indicine *N*-oxide has antitumour properties (q.v.). Australine, recently characterized from the seeds of the leguminous tree *Castanospermum australe*, is a tetrahydroxypyrrolizidine alkaloid. It was obtained by use of repeated preparative centrifugal TLC. Like the polyhydroxyindolizidine alkaloids it exhibits glycosidase inhibitory activity (for further details see R. J. Molyneux *et al.*, *J. Nat. Prod.*, 1988, **51**, 1198). The alkaloids frequently occur as esters, being linked with characteristic mono- or dibasic acids called the necic acids. They are biosynthesized from ornithine via a symmetrical intermediate and labelling experiments have shown the involvement of putrescine and homospermidine. Two molecules of putrescine are required to form one of homospermidine. This pathway

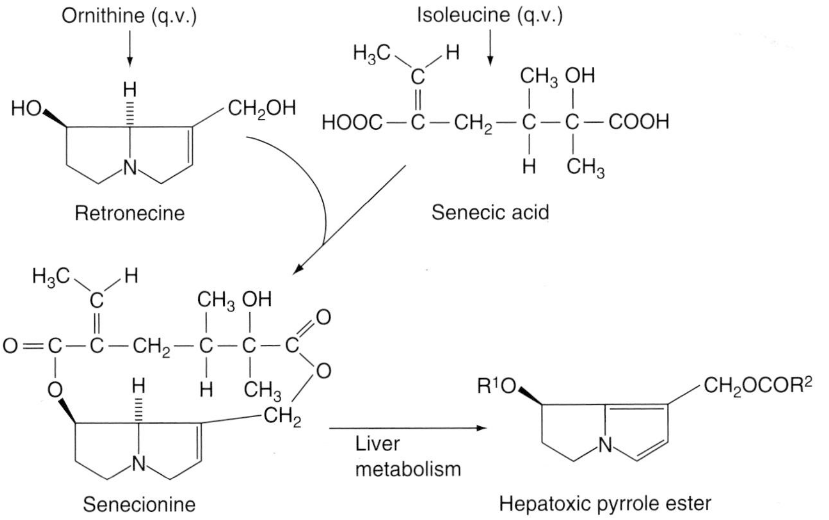

Fig. 26.10
Formation and liver metabolism of pyrrolizidine-ester alkaloids.

has been supported by the isolation, partial purification and characterization of the NAD⁺-dependent enzyme homospermidine synthase, the first pathway-specific enzyme in pyrrolizidine alkaloid biosynthesis (F. Böttcher *et al.*, *Phytochemistry*, 1993, **32**, 679). The components of senecionine are illustrated in Fig. 26.10. The hepatotoxic properties are believed to arise by breakdown of the alkaloids in the liver to strongly alkylating pyrrole esters.

For reports on pyrrolizidine alkaloids see: T. Hartmann and L. Witte (1995), *Alkaloids, Chemical and Biological Perspectives* (ed. S. W. Pelletier), Vol. 9, New York: Wiley, p. 155. A general review: K. Ndjoko *et al.*, *Planta Med.*, 1999, **65**, 562. Determination in *Senecio* species.

LYSINE-DERIVED ALKALOIDS

As the next homologue to ornithine, lysine and its associated compounds give rise to a number of alkaloids, some of which are analogous to the ornithine group (see Fig. 26.11). The lycopodium alkaloids are also derived from lysine. Although in some cases, such as the quinolizidine lupin alkaloids, lysine is incorporated via a symmetrical precursor, e.g. cadaverine, in the majority of examples (anabasine, sedamine, *N*-methylpelletierine) the incorporation is asymmetric. In general, for the simple α-substituted piperidines, the C-2 of lysine becomes the point of attachment of the α side-chain.

The wide distribution of these bases throughout the plant kingdom is illustrated by the drugs which follow.

LOBELIA

Lobelia *BHP, BP* 1988 (*Lobelia Herb, Indian Tobacco*) consists of the dried aerial parts of *Lobelia inflata* (Campanulaceae), an annual herb indigenous to the eastern USA and Canada. It is cultivated in the USA and Holland.

History. Lobelia has long been used by the North American Indians. It was recommended for use in asthma by Cutler in 1813 and was introduced to the English medical profession by Reece in 1829.

Cultivation and collection. Lobelia is grown from seed which is sown either in the autumn or in March and April. The plant produces an aerial stem about 50 cm high. It bears alternate leaves 3–8 cm long and pale blue, bilabiate flowers. The inferior ovary develops into an inflated capsule. The plants are cut in August or September, when they bear numerous capsules. After drying, the drug is exported in bales or compressed packets. The seeds are sometimes separated by thrashing.

Macroscopical characters. Up to about 60% (*BP*, 1988, upper limit) of the drug consists of stems. These are green or purplish, winged and very hairy in the upper part but becoming more rounded and channelled and less hairy below. The pale green leaves are usually more or less broken and are covered with bristly hair. Entire leaves are ovate to ovate-lanceolate in shape. The margin is irregularly serrate-dentate and the teeth bear water-pores. The flowers are rarely seen in the drug. The fruits are 5–8 mm long, ribbed and crowned by the calyx teeth. Each is bilocular and contains numerous oval-oblong, brown reticulated seeds about 0.5–0.7 mm long. The drug has a slightly irritating odour and an acrid taste.

Microscopical characters. The epidermis of the stem is composed of rectangular cells, covered with a striated cuticle and with anticlinal walls clearly pitted, giving a characteristic beaded appearance. The epidermis bears stomata with the pore parallel to the stem axis and large, conical, warty-walled, unicellular hairs up to 600 μm long (Fig. 42.3). The cortex is composed of rounded, thin-walled, chlorophyll-containing parenchyma except in the wings, where the cells are collenchymatous. The endodermis is well-differentiated, the cells clearly showing the Casparian strip. A pericycle composed of small groups of fibres is distinguishable in the lower part of the stem. The phloem is composed of small groups of delicate sieve-tube tissue enclosing the anastomosing latex vessels, readily seen after staining with iodine. The xylem is composed of elongated, thick-walled xylem fibres and spiral and scalariform vessels. The pith is composed of pitted lignified parenchyma.

With the leaf the upper epidermis is composed of straightwalled, papillose cells with the anticlinal walls showing the beaded appearance (Fig. 42.2). The lower epidermal cells have wavy walls, and numerous stomata, without special subsidiary cells, are present. Unicellular covering hairs, like those present on the stem, are borne on both epidermal surfaces. The mesophyll is differentiated into a single-layered palisade tissue and a spongy mesophyll. The mesophyll cells contain small fat crystals. The palisade tissue is interrupted in the midrib and groups of collenchyma occur above and below the midrib bundle. The phloem contains the characteristic latex vessels. Numerous water-pores occur on the upper surface of the marginal teeth.

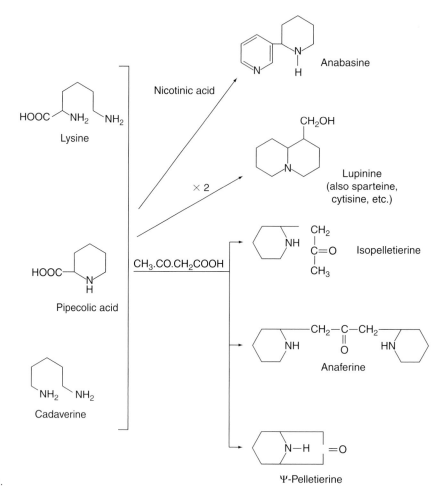

Fig. 26.11
Lysine as a precursor of alkaloids.

The surface of the seed is characteristically reticulate. The pollen grains are roughly spherical, 20–30 μm diameter, and show three pores.

Constituents. Lobelia contains about 0.24–0.4% of alkaloids (*BP* 1988, not less than 0.25% as determined by a standard Stas-Otto procedure) the most important of which is lobeline. This and many related alkaloids including lobelidine, lobelanine, lobelanidine and isolobelanine, have a piperidine nucleus (Fig. 26.12). Others are piperideines (i.e. the ring system is unsaturated).

By analogy with the biosynthesis of coniine (Fig. 26.38), the above alkaloids could be formed from a polyketo acid involving two benzoyl units and acetate. However, the demonstration that phenylalanine can be incorporated by the plant into the lobelia alkaloid lobinaline and into the related sedamine (*Sedum acre*, Crassulaceae), and the incorporation of lysine into the piperidine ring of lobeline, does not support this hypothesis. A number of Brazilian species contain similar constituents.

Root cultures of *L. inflata* transformed by *Agrobacterium rhizogenes* have been shown to produce lobeline at the same concentration as normal pot-grown plants (H. Yonemitsu *et al.*, *Plant Cell Rep.* 1990, **9**, 307).

Uses. Lobelia is used in spasmodic asthma and chronic bronchitis; it is included in some antismoking preparations. In its pharmacological action, lobeline resembles nicotine in having both central and peripheral effects. In toxic doses the drug has a paralytic effect and its continuous use should be avoided.

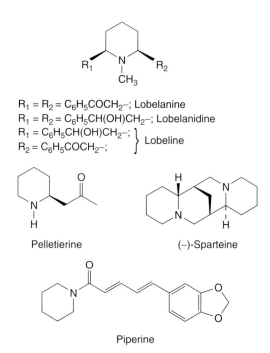

$R_1 = R_2 = C_6H_5COCH_2-$; Lobelanine
$R_1 = R_2 = C_6H_5CH(OH)CH_2-$; Lobelanidine
$R_1 = C_6H_5CH(OH)CH_2-$;
$R_2 = C_6H_5COCH_2-$; } Lobeline

Pelletierine   (–)-Sparteine

Piperine

Fig. 26.12
Alkaloids of lobelia, pomegranate, broom and pepper.

Indian lobelia

This drug, which is official in India, consists of the dried aerial parts of *L. nicotianaefolia*, a biennial or perennial herb found in many parts of India at altitudes of 700–2200 m. The leaves and stems are larger than those of the American lobelia and in the form of powder the drug may be distinguished by the trichomes and palisade ratio. Indian lobelia contains not less than 0.8% alkaloids calculated as lobeline.

Pomegranate

The pomegranate, *Punica granatum* L. Punicaceae, is cultivated throughout subtropical and tropical regions of the world; some 800 000 metric tons are produced annually, principally for dietary purposes. However, the barks, fruit-rind, flowers and seeds all find medicinal use.

Both stem and root barks are used and occur in curved or channelled pieces about 5–10 cm long and 1–3 cm wide. The outer surface of the stem bark shows longitudinal corky furrows, a few shallow depressions and the bark apothecia of lichens, while that of the root bark shows depressions where the outer layers have exfoliated. The barks are smooth and yellowish on their inner surfaces and break with a short granular fracture. They contain about 0.5–0.9% of volatile liquid alkaloids, the chief of which are pelletierine and pseudopelletierine, together with about 22% of tannin.

Pelletierine tannate, a mixture of the tannates of the alkaloids, was included in the *BP* 1948 and was used as an anthelminthic with a specific action on tapeworms.

The dried pericarp of the fruit occurs in thin, curved pieces about 1.5 mm thick, some of which bear the remains of the woody calyx or a scar left by the stalk. The outer surface is brownish-yellow or reddish and the inner surfaces bear impressions left by the seeds. A high tannin content (28%) affords its use as an astringent in the treatment of diarrhoea.

The seeds have been studied for their bioactive constituents with new compounds recently reported. Major components are monoacyl-glycerols, glycerides, sterols, proteins, pectins and sugars (M. Yusuph and J. Mann, *Phytochemistry*, 1997, **44**, 1391; R.-F. Wang *et al.*, *J. Nat. Prod.*, 2004, **67**, 2096). The validity of a seed extract for use in the treatment of diarrhoea, as practised in traditional Indian and Bangladesh medicine, has been experimentally verified (A. K. Das *et al.*, *J. Ethnopharm.*, 1999, **68**, 205).

The flowers are used in Chinese medicine; a new polyphenol and six known compounds including maslinic acid (see 'Olive Leaf') have been reported (R. Wang *et al.*, *Fitoterapia*, 2006, **77**, 534).

For a study on the antioxidant, antimalarial and antimicrobial tannin-rich fractions, ellagitannins and phenolic acids of pomegranate, see M. K. Reddy *et al.*, *Planta Medica*, 2007, **73**, 461.

N. P. Seeram *et al.* (see 'Further reading') have listed 122 compounds isolated from various organs of the pomegranate; they are classed as ellagitannins and gallotannins, ellagic acid derivatives, catechin and procyanidins, anthocyanins and anthocyanidins, flavonols, organic acids, simple galloyl derivatives, fatty acids and triglycerides, sterols and terpenoids, alkaloids and other compounds.

For studies on the biosynthesis of *N*-methylpelletierine involving the feeding of ^{13}C-labelled acetoacetate and acetate see Hemscheidt and Spenser (*J. Am. Chem. Soc.*, 1990, **112**, 6360). Their results constitute evidence in support of the classical biogenetic concepts regarding the incorporation of acetate into the alkaloid (compare findings for the incorporation of acetate into the tropane skeleton).

The role of pomegranate juices and extracts as nutraceuticals is discussed in Chapter 32: The plant nutraceuticals.

Further reading

Seeram NP *et al* (eds), Hardman R (series ed) 2006 Medicinal and aromatic plants industrial profiles, Vol 43. Pomegranates – ancient roots to modern medicine. CRC, Taylor and Francis Group, Boca Raton, FL

Broom

The broom, *Cytisus scoparius* (Leguminosae), is a perennial shrub about 1–2 m high. The lower part is woody but the long, straight branches are green and glabrous. The upper parts of the stem bear five prominent, longitudinal ridges. The lower leaves are stalked and consist of three obovate leaflets, but the upper leaves are sessile and usually reduced to a single leaflet.

The flowers are typical of the subfamily Papilionaceae. The fruit is a black, hairy pod about 3–5 cm long.

Broom tops are described in the *BHP* 1988 and *BPC* 1949. An aqueous decoction or other extract was used as a mild diuretic. Their chief constituents are quinolizidine alkaloids, including the volatile liquid alkaloid sparteine (Fig. 26.12), a yellow isoflavone scoparin, and flavonoids. The drug has diuretic and cathartic actions but is now little used.

Pepper

Black pepper (*Piper nigrum*) consists of the dried, unripe fruits of *Piper nigrum* (Piperaceae), a perennial climbing plant cultivated in the Malay Archipelago, southern India, South America and the West Indies. Large quantities are obtained from Indonesia, Sarawak and Brazil. The structure of the pepper market is extremely complex and highly speculative, with dealers often selling one shipment of pepper several times over on behalf of various principals.

Pepper was known to Theophrastus and other ancient writers. It was the most important spice used in the Middle Ages and was imported into England about AD 1000. The high cost of pepper and other Eastern spices was a big inducement to the Portuguese to find a sea route to India; competition for the spice trade has played a large part in the colonial expansion of European nations.

Pepper is essentially a crop of the wet tropics and is propagated from cuttings (Sarawak) or runners (India). However, it is subject to various diseases which are transmitted by vegetative propagation so that shoot-culture techniques designed for the mass culture of selected disease-free vines have been investigated (V. J. Philip *et al.*, *Plant Cell Reps.*, 1992, **12**, 41).

Production. The vines are grown on poles or trees. The inflorescence is a spike of about 20–30 sessile flowers, which develop into sessile fruits (see earlier editions for diagrams). The latter are picked when the lower fruits of the spike turn red. They are then removed from the axis and dried, either in the open air or by artificial heat. The fire-dried spice is most esteemed but the ground spice is usually a blend of different varieties.

White pepper, which is largely used in the East, is also obtained from *P. nigrum*, but the fruits are allowed to become more completely ripe. After storing them for some days or soaking them in water, the outer part of the pericarp is removed by rubbing and washing and the fruits are dried.

Black pepper fruits are almost globular and 3.5–6 mm diameter. The surface is dark brown or greyish-black and strongly reticulated. The apex shows the remains of the sessile stigmas and a basal scar indicates the point of attachment to the axis. Pepper has an aromatic odour and pungent taste.

Bacterial and fungal contamination of the stored peppers can be reduced by washing and redrying with subsequent maintenance of the moisture content at less than 11%.

In white pepper, owing to the removal of the outer part of the pericarp, the vascular bundles, about 16 in number, run on the outside of the fruit from base to apex.

Constituents. Pepper contains 1–2.5% of volatile oil, 5–9% of the crystalline alkaloids piperine and piperettine, and a resin. The aroma of the spice is due to the volatile oil, which consists largely of terpenes, while the pungency is ascribed to piperine and the resin. Piperine, first isolated in 1819, is also found in the long pepper (1–2%) and in Ashanti pepper, the fruits of *Piper guineense*. Analyses for the volatile oil are given as β-caryophyllene (21.59–27.70%), limonene (21.06–22.17%), sabinene (8.5–17.6%), β-pinene (9.16–11.08%), α-pinene (5.07–6.18%), myrcene (2.2–2.3%), *p*-cymeme (0.0–0.18%) and oxygenated constituents (3.39–5.68%); 40 compounds were identified in oil from Sao Tome e Principe (A. P. Martíns *et al.*, *Phytochemistry*, 1998, **49**, 2019).

Pepper was once employed in the treatment of gonorrhoea and chronic bronchitis. Large quantities are used as a condiment.

Long pepper is the dried unripe fruit of *Piper retrofractum* (*P. officinarum*) and *P. longum*, grown in Indonesia, India and the Philippines. The spice consists of whole spikes of small fruits forming a structure about 4 cm long and 6 mm in diameter. Individual fruits show a similar structure to black pepper. For a report on the component alkamides and other constituents see B. Das *et al.*, *Planta Med.*, 1996, **62**, 582. Guineesine, a recently isolated alkaloid, is an acyl-CoA:cholesterol acyltransferase inhibitor and has been proposed as an attractive target for the prevention and treatment of hypercholesterolemia and atherosclerosis (S. W. Lee *et al.*, *Planta Medica*, 2004, **70**, 678).

Cubebs or tailed pepper are the dried, full-grown fruits of *Piper cubeba*, a native of Indonesia, Borneo and Sumatra. The fruits are collected while green and dried in the sun. They were used in Europe as a spice as early as the eleventh century. The spikes of cubebs bear more fruits than those of pepper and become falsely stalked as they mature, owing to an abnormal development of the base of the pericarp. The upper part of the cubeb fruit is globular, 3–6 mm diameter and covered with a greyish-brown, reticulated pericarp, which is prolonged at the base into a straight stalk. Cubebs yield 10–18% of volatile oil containing terpenes and sesquiterpenes, a crystalline inodorous substance (−)-cubebin (formula Table 21.7) and a number of other lignans, a white amorphous substance cubebic acid (1%), and amorphous resin (3%).

The above gives only a token appreciation of the genus as a whole—there are some 700 species of *Piper* globally of which only about 12% have been studied phytochemically. Nevertheless the literature is extensive and in a review (341 refs) covering the secondary metabolites (V. S. Parmar *et al.*, see 'Further reading') nearly 600 constituents are listed. Classes of metabolites considered are alkaloids/amides, propenylphenols, lignans, neolignans, terpenes, steroids, kawa pyrones, piperolides, chalcones, dihydrochalcones, flavones, flavanones and miscellaneous compounds.

Further reading

Parmar VS, Jain SC, Bisht KS *et al* 1997 Phytochemistry of the genus *Piper*. Phytochemistry 46(4): 597–673

Ravindran PA (ed), Hardman R (series ed) 2000 Medicinal and aromatic plants—industrial profiles, Vol 13. Black pepper, *Piper nigrum*. Harwood Academic, Amsterdam

Lycopodium

Lycopodium consists of the spores of the clubmoss, *Lycopodium clavatum* (Lycopodiaceae, Phylum Pteridophyta). Most of the commercial drug is collected in Poland and E. Europe, but Indian and Pakistani supplies are obtained from the Himalayas. The sporangial spikes are cut and dried, and the spores are separated by shaking and then freed from vegetable debris by sieving through four sieves. The drug is exported in sacks, which are usually enclosed in matting.

Lycopodium is a light, yellow, extremely mobile powder without odour or taste. It floats on water without being wetted. The spores are 25–40 µm diameter and have the shape of a three-sided pyramid with a convex base. The surface is covered with polygonal-shaped reticulations which form a projecting ridge at the edge of the spore. Viewed from the apex of the pyramid, the edges of the flat sides form a distinct, triradiate marking. On crushing, yellowish drops of oil exude.

Lycopodium consists about 50% of fixed oil, which consists mainly of the glycerides of lycopodiumoleic acid. The drug also contains about 3% of sugars, phytosterin and alkaloids of the annotine type, which are characteristic of the genus, together with traces of nicotine. The lycopodium alkaloid lycopodine, first reported in 1881, is, like pelleterine, derived from lysine and acetate (for the role of the latter in its biosynthesis in the intact plant see T. Hemscheidt and I. D. Spenser, *J. Amer. Chem. Soc.*, 1993, **115**, 2052). For a review of the lycopodium alkaloids see Ayer (*Nat. Prod. Rep.*, 1991, **8**, 455).

Adulteration with the pollen of *Pinus* species, *Corylus avellana*, *Typha latifolia*, etc., or with roasted and coloured starches, dextrin, sulphur or inorganic salts, can readily be detected by means of the microscope.

Lycopodium was once used to a limited extent in dusting powders and medicated snuffs, and as a dusting powder for pills. It is employed in quantitative microscopy (see Chapter 43).

Further reading

Kobayashi J, Morita H 2005 The lycopodium alkaloids (*a review with 154 refs*). The Alkaloids 61: 1–57

PHENYLALANINE-, TYROSINE- AND DIHYDROXYPHENYLALANINE-DERIVED ALKALOIDS

The title compounds and their corresponding decarboxylation products are the precursors of a large number of alkaloids which include simple protoalkaloids, the benzylisoquinolines, phthalideisoquinolines, aporphines and proaporphines, protoberberines, protopines, naphthaphenanthridines, the *Erythrina*, Amaryllidaceae and ipecacuanha alkaloids and the morphine and rhoeadine-type alkaloids. A group of compounds, first recognized in 1965, is that comprising the phenethylisoquinoline alkaloids; it is from these that colchicine arises. Some of the pharmaceutically more important groups are illustrated in Fig. 26.13.

In addition to the reading matter quoted at the end of the first section of this chapter, see also the following reviews: Isoquinoline alkaloids, H. Guinaudeau and J. Brunetonin *Methods in Plant Biochemistry* (ed. P. G. Waterman) 1993, Vol 8. London: Academic, p. 373; bisbenzylisoquinoline alkaloids, P. L. Schiff, *J. Nat. Prod.*, 1983, **46**, 1; 1987, **50**, 529; 1991, **54**, 645; dimeric aporphinoid alkaloids, H. Guinaudeau *et al.*, *J. Nat. Prod.*, 1988, **51**, 1025; 1994, **57**, 1025.

PROTOALKALOIDS

Those alkaloid-like amines which do not have the nitrogen as part of a heterocyclic ring system are often termed protoalkaloids. They are not restricted to any particular class of alkaloids and are often classified according to the amino acids from which they are derived. Some are quaternary bases as, for example, the protoberberine alkaloids which constitute a large group with diverse structures and a wide distribution

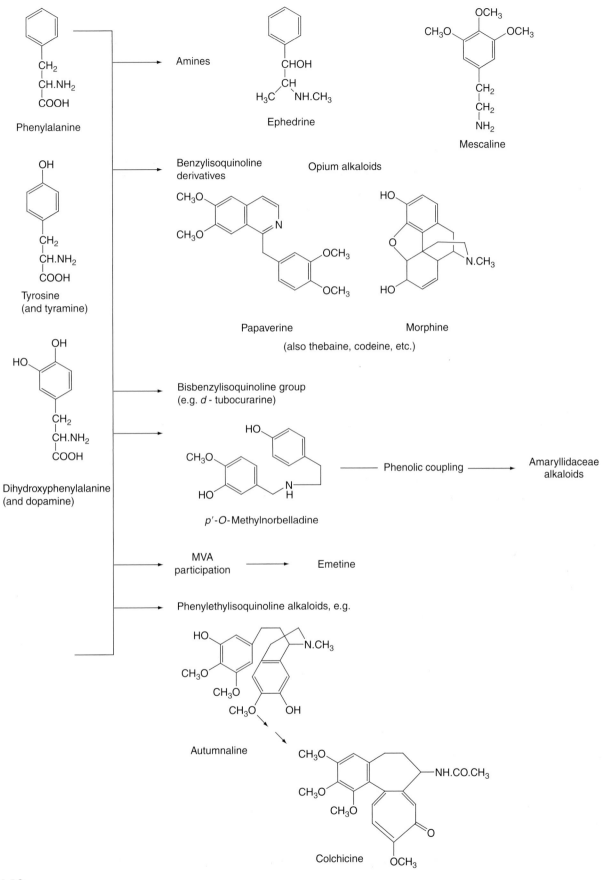

Fig. 26.13
Some bases derived from phenylalanine, tyrosine and dihydroxyphenylalanine.

in nature. Although not prominent in common herbal drugs the alkaloids are being studied for their antibacterial, antimalarial (Chapter 28) and potential genotoxic properties. For reviews with many references see E. V. L. Da-Cunha *et al.*, *The Alkaloids*, 2005, **62**, 1–75; L. Grycova *et al.*, *Phytochemistry*, 2007, **68**, 150.

Ephedra

Various species of *Ephedra* (*Ma-huang*) (Ephedraceae) are used as a source of the alkaloids ephedrine and pseudoephedrine, which may also be prepared by synthesis. Among these are the Chinese species *Ephedra sinica* and *E. equisetina* and the Indian and Pakistani *E. gerardiana*, *E. intermedia* and *E. major*.

Although ma-huang was known to the Chinese over 5000 years ago and ephedrine was isolated in 1887, it only came into extensive use during the last century.

Collection.   The drug is collected in the autumn, this being important, as the amount of alkaloid present shows considerable variation at different seasons. The drug is imported in bales. It consists of slender, more or less broken aerial stems which are woody and usually branch only at the base.

Characters.   The stems of the ephedras bear numerous, fine, longitudinal ridges. The leaves are small, connate at the base, and usually in whorls of two (less commonly, whorls of three or four) and decussate.

1. *Ephedra sinica* Stapf. The stems are about 30 cm long, ashy greyish-green in colour, and slightly rough. The diameter at the lowest green node is about 1 or 2 mm, while the internodes are about 3–6 cm long. The leaves, which are about 4 mm long, have a subulate, recurved apex; the lamina is whitish and the base reddish-brown. In the transverse section the young stem 9 shows 6–10 bundles. The pith is largely unlignified.
2. *E. equisetina* Bunge. The stems are very woody and much branched, 25–200 cm in length and ashy yellow-green in colour. The internodes are shorter than *E. sinica*, being about 1–2.5 cm long. The apex of the leaves is shorter than the cup and not recurved. The leaves are of a brownish-purple colour, the lower ones tending to go black. Transverse sections show that the number of bundles in the stem is not constant (usually about 10). The pith is lignified.

3. *E. distachya*. The stems are slightly woody and branching takes place from the upper and lower parts of the main stem. Stems about 37 cm long, rough and greenish-yellow in colour. Internodes 2.5–6 cm long. Leaf apex short but acute and often fissured at the base. There are no cortical or perimedullary fibres, but the pith is lignified. *Ephedra*, when dry, has little odour. The taste is slightly bitter.

Constituents.   The ephedras contain about 0.5–2.0% of alkaloids. Of the total, ephedrine (and its isomers) forms from 30 to 90%, according to the species. Pseudoephedrine is also present (see Fig. 26.14). The roots also contain a number of macrocyclic alkaloids (ephedradines) and feruloylhistamine which have hypotensive properties.

Biosynthesis of ephedrine and related alkaloids.   These alkaloids are formed by a union of a C_6–C_1 unit and a C_2 unit. For many years it has been known that phenylalanine is the originator of the C_6–C_1 moiety, being converted first to benzaldehyde or benzoic acid. GrueSørensen and Spenser (*J. Am. Chem. Soc.*, 1993, **115**, 2052 and references quoted therein) using ^{13}C- and ^{2}H-labelled precursors in feeding experiments with *E. gerardiana* have shown that benzoic acid combines with the intact CH_3CO group of pyruvic acid to form ephedrine and related alkaloids with 1-phenylpropan-1,2-dione and (*S*)-(−)-2-amino-1-phenylpropan-1-one (cathinone) serving as intermediates. The route is illustrated in Fig. 26.14. 1-Phenylpropan-1,2-dione and cathinone are known constituents of *Catha edulis* (see below) but the previous non-isolation of cathinone from ephedra is attributed to its high efficiency of incorporation into the nor-alkaloids.

Uses.   Ephedrine is used for the relief of asthma and hay fever. Its action is more prolonged than that of adrenaline, and it has the further advantage that it need not be given by injection but may be administered by mouth. In oriental medicine the ephedras are also used as anti-inflammatory drugs and this action is ascribed to an oxazolidone related to ephedrine. In contrast to the herb, which has a sudorific action, the root has been used clinically in China for its antisudorific effect.

Khat or Abyssinian tea

This consists of the fresh leaves of *Catha edulis* Forsk. (Celastraceae). The plant is cultivated in Abyssinia, in parts of east and southern Africa,

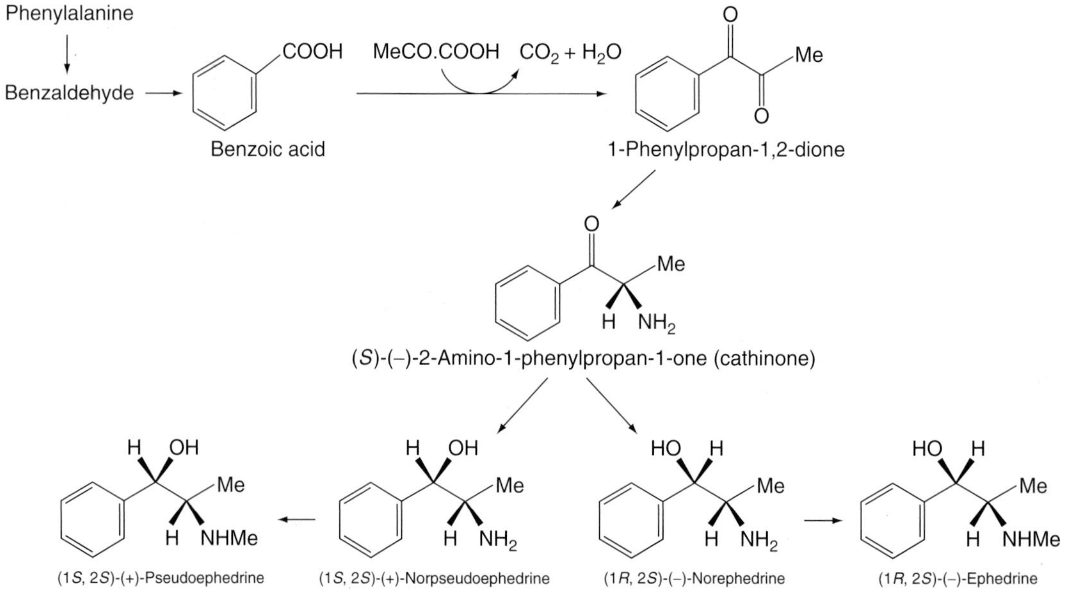

Fig. 26.14
Biogenesis of ephedrine and related alkaloids.

and in southern Arabia. There appear to be a number of different varieties of the plant varying in 'khatamine' content between 0.1% (Yemen, Madagascar) and 0.5% (Kenya). It is widely employed in African and Arab countries, particularly in the Yemen, for chewing, and its misuse has been surveyed by the WHO. Its traditional use is similar to that of coca in that the fresh leaves, when chewed, have a stimulatory effect with the alleviation of depression and of the sensations of hunger and fatigue. The drug constitutes a problem in the West.

On a dry weight basis the leaves contain about 1.0% of (+)-norpseudoephedrine, and for many years this was thought to be the principle responsible for the stimulant effect of the drug. In 1975 another phenylpropane, (−)-α-aminopropiophenone (cathinone), was isolated at UN laboratories and is considered the principal CNS stimulant of the fresh plant. (−)-Cathinone has pharmacological properties analogous to those of (+)-amphetamine, possessing a similar potency and the same mechanism of action. Many other components (alkaloids, sesquiterpenes, triterpenes, flavonoids, numerous acids as esters), including an essential oil containing about 40 components, have been characterized. Tissue cultures of the plant have been shown to produce quinone-methide triterpenes; these compounds do not appear to be present in the normal plant although they have been reported in several other members of the Celestraceae. Crombie and Whiting have reviewed (64 refs) the alkaloids of khat (*Alkaloids*, 1990, **39**, 139).

BENZYLISOQUINOLINE DERIVATIVES

A number of important drugs come within this heading. Phytochemically the group is often subdivided.

Opium poppy

The opium poppy, *Papaver somniferum* L., is an annual herb about 50–150 cm in height. The stem and leaves are glaucous. The latter are about 10 cm in length, entire, sessile and amplexicaul. The margin is dentate but varies somewhat in the different varieties. The flowers, which are borne on a slightly hairy peduncle, are solitary, nodding in the bud, and have caducous sepals. They have the floral formula K2, C2 + 2, A$_\infty$, G(∞). The unilocular ovary contains numerous ovules attached to parietal placentas. It bears at its apex a flat disc formed by the union of the radiating stigmas. The capsule opens by means of small valves, which are equal in number to the carpels and situated immediately below the stellate stigma.

In addition to numerous garden hybrids, the following varieties are recognized:

P. somniferum var. *glabrum* Boiss., cultivated in Turkey; flowers purplish but sometimes white; capsule subglobular; stigmata, 10–12; seeds, white to dark violet.

P. somniferum var. *album* D.C., cultivated in India; flowers and seeds white; capsules more or less egg-shaped, 4–8 cm diameter, no pores under the stigma.

P. somniferum var. *nigrum* D.C., cultivated in Europe for the seeds, which are slate-coloured and are known as 'maw seeds' (probably a corruption of *Mohnsamen*). The leaves and calyx are glabrous, the flowers violet and the capsules somewhat smaller and more globular than those of the var. *album*.

P. somniferum var. *setigerum* D.C., a truly wild form found in southern Europe. The peduncles and leaves are covered with bristly hairs. The leaf lobes are sharply pointed and each terminates in a bristle.

Poppy capsules contain, when ripe, 0.18–0.28% of morphine. Poppy seeds contain only very small quantities of narcotine, papaverine and thebaine in addition to morphine and codeine, all detectable by GC/MS. It has been pointed out that the detection of the former three bases

in urine samples may be used to differentiate between poppy seed consumption and the illegal use of morphine or heroin (B. D. Paul *et al.*, *Planta Med.*, 1996, **62**, 544). Importantly the seeds also contain 50–60% of a drying oil which is used by artists and also for cooking.

Papaver breeding has received some attention; a morphine-rich strain suitable for mechanical harvesting and a low-morphine variety for seed production have been described. Other strains with little alkaloid, and ones with a higher proportion of codeine, have also been produced.

The red or corn poppy, *Papaver rhoeas*, was formerly used in pharmacy. The fresh scarlet petals were particularly used as a colouring matter in the form of a syrup and are described in more detail in Chapter 33. They contain the anthocyanidin glucoside mecocyanin, an isomer of the cyanin found in red rose petals. A number of alkaloids are produced (e.g. rhoeadine of the benzyltetrahydroisoquinoline type); they have no morphine-like activity.

OPIUM

Opium (*Raw Opium*) is the latex obtained by incision from the unripe capsules of *Papaver somniferum* (Papaveraceae) and dried partly by spontaneous evaporation and partly by artificial heat. It is worked into irregularly shaped masses and is known in commerce as Indian opium. Indian opium is specifically stated because this is a legally available source of the drug. However, a number of countries e.g. Turkey, former USSR and Yugoslavia and Australia (Tasmania) grow considerable quantities of the opium poppy for alkaloid extraction and seed production. For strategic purposes, a relatively small crop is raised in southern England. Much illegal opium is produced in S.E. Asia.

The *BP/EP* monograph for Raw Opium states that it is intended only as a starting material for the manufacture of galenical preparations (e.g. Tincture of Opium) and is not dispensed as such. It should contain not less than 10% of morphine and not less than 2.0% of codeine. The thebaine content is limited to 3%. The alkaloidal assays are performed by liquid chromatography on the drug dried at 100–105°C.

Prepared Opium BP/EP is raw opium powdered and dried at a temperature not exceeding 70°C. It contains 9.8–10.2% morphine and a minimum 1.0% of codeine; thebaine is limited to 3.0%. The powder may be adjusted to strength by the addition of raw opium or a suitable excipient, which must be recorded on the label.

History. Opium was well known to the ancients. Dioskurides, about AD 77, distinguishes between the latex of the capsules, *opos*, and an extract of the whole plant, *mekonion*. The use of opium spread from Asia Minor to Persia, where opium eating became popular, and from there to India and China. However, it was not until the second half of the eighteenth century that opium smoking began to be extensively practised in China and the Far East.

Asia Minor has from very early times been an important source of opium production. In Macedonia cultivation was started as recently as 1865. Persian opium was imported into England from about 1870 to 1955. Opium was cultivated in India during the Middle Ages, and the monopoly of the Mogul Government was taken over first by the East India Company and then by the British Government. Formerly, Indian opiums, being prepared mainly for smoking, were little esteemed for pharmaceutical purposes. However, that now imported is of good quality and constitutes the principal British source for the manufacture of alkaloids.

Production. The plant cultivated in India under licence is *P. somniferum* var. *album*. Sowing takes place in November and collection from April to June. The incisions are made in the afternoon with an instrument known as a 'nushtur'. This bears narrow iron spikes which are drawn down the capsule to produce several longitudinal cuts. The incision must not penetrate into the interior of the capsule or latex will be lost. The latex, which is at first white, rapidly coagulates and turns brown. Early in the morning of the day following the making of the incisions the partly dried latex is scraped off with a trowel-like 'see-tooar'. Each capsule is cut several times at intervals of 2 or 3 days. After collection the latex is placed in a tilted vessel so that the dark fluid (pussewah) which is not required may drain off. By exposure to air the opium acquires a suitable consistency for packing.

Indian opium is exported in 5 kg blocks, packed 12 to a lightweight wooden case to facilitate air transport. Each block is wrapped in grease-proof paper, tied with tape and placed in a polythene bag. The drug has a soft consistency and so arrives as rounded, somewhat flattened, cakes. It contains about 9–12% of morphine. Being difficult to dry and powder because of its plastic nature, Indian opium is less suitable than some other types for the preparation of powdered opium.

Former varieties of legal opium were obtained from Turkey (Turkish Government Monoply Opium) and the former Yugoslavia, and opium is also produced in former Kirghiz SSR and China under government control for national use. Iran and Egypt, former producers, no longer cultivate the plant. Such opiums were very characteristic in appearance and packaging, and illustrations of some different varieties together with tools for production will be found in the 10th edition (1972) of this book. Turkish government opium was until relatively recently much used and consisted of cubical stamped blocks each weighing 2 kg; it was much easier to powder than the Indian drug.

In addition to the above countries, opium has been produced, often only on an experimental scale, in most European countries, the USA, the East Indies and parts of Africa. Experiments have shown that a hot climate is not essential—opium of excellent quality has been produced in Scotland and Norway.

Microscopy. Opium examined under the microscope shows agglomerated latex granules in irregular masses. Other smaller amounts of characteristic material which arise as a result of the preparation process are best seen by examining the residue left after water-extraction of the opium. These particles include occasional spherical pollen grains, fragments of vessels and portions of the epicarp of the capsule the latter showing in surface view polygonal thick-walled cells with a stellate lumen. Pointed trichomes and a few starch grains may be present.

Constituents. Opium contains some 30 alkaloids, which are largely combined with the organic acid meconic acid; the drug also contains sugars, salts (e.g. sulphates), albuminous substances, colouring matters and water. Six principal alkaloids are listed in Table 26.4.

The first group (e.g. morphine) consists of alkaloids which have a phenanthrene nucleus whereas those of the papaverine group have a benzylisoquinoline structure. Some of the less important opium alkaloids (e.g. protopine and hydrocotarnine) are of different structural

types. The morphine molecule has both a phenolic and an alcoholic hydroxyl group, and when acetylated forms diacetyl morphine or heroin. Codeine is an ether of morphine (methylmorphine), and other morphine ethers which are used medicinally are ethylmorphine and pholcodine.

New alkaloids continue to be isolated from *P. somniferum*—a number were recognized during investigations on the biogenesis of morphine and Repasi *et al.* (*Planta Med.*, 1993, **59**, 477) obtained 5′-*O*-demethylnarcotine during the purification of narcotine from poppy straw; it was also detected in a sample of Indian opium.

Meconic acid, a dibasic acid, is easily detected either in the free state or as a meconate by the formation of a deep red colour on the addition of a solution of ferric chloride. As it is invariably found in opium, its presence has long been used to indicate opium. However, research has shown that some species of *Papaver* which produce no morphine but other morphinanes may also contain this acid; it may serve as a chemotaxonomic marker for the Papaveraceae. It is notable that the related acid, chelidonic acid, is found in some other members of the Papaveraceae such as in the root of Greater Celandine (q.v.).

Meconic acid   Chelidonic acid

Papaveretum *BP*

Papaveretum *BP* is a mixture of the hydrochlorides of opium alkaloids containing 80.0–88.4% anhydrous morphine HCl, 8.3–9.2% papaverine HCl and 6.6–7.4% codeine HCl. It is assayed by liquid chromatography. Well-known preparations of papaveretum are the trade products Omnopon and Nepenthe which are used mainly for premedication and as analgesics during and after operations. Formerly, Papaveretum (*BPC*, 1973) also contained the opium alkaloid noscapine but this has now been removed from the preparation on account of its genotoxicity. Noscapine has also been a constituent of many cough mixtures and these have now been withdrawn by the manufacturers.

BIOGENESIS OF THE OPIUM AND RELATED ALKALOIDS

The step-by-step elucidation of the biogenetic pathway of the opium alkaloids constitutes a brilliant chapter in the history of phytochemical research. The principal features of the biosynthesis of thebaine, codeine and morphine as now envisaged are given in Fig. 26.15; a further consideration of the initial stages of this scheme follows later.

In 1910 Winterstein and Trier suggested that there was a structural relationship between the benzylisoquinoline alkaloids and dihydroxyphenylalanine. This was extended by Robinson's observation that morphine could be derived from these alkaloids by rotation of the

Table 26.4 Historic isolations of principal opium alkaloids.

Alkaloid	Formula	Discoverer	Date	Properties
Morphine	$C_{17}H_{19}O_3N$	Sertürner	1816	Strong bases, which are alkaline to litmus and highly toxic
Codeine	$C_{18}H_{21}O_3N$	Robiquet	1832	
Thebaine	$C_{19}H_{21}O_3N$	Thiboumèry	1835	
Noscapine	$C_{22}H_{23}O_7N$	Derosne	1803	Feeble bases, which are slightly toxic
Narceine	$C_{23}H_{22}O_8N$	Pelletier	1832	
Papaverine	$C_{22}H_{21}O_4N$	Merck	1848	

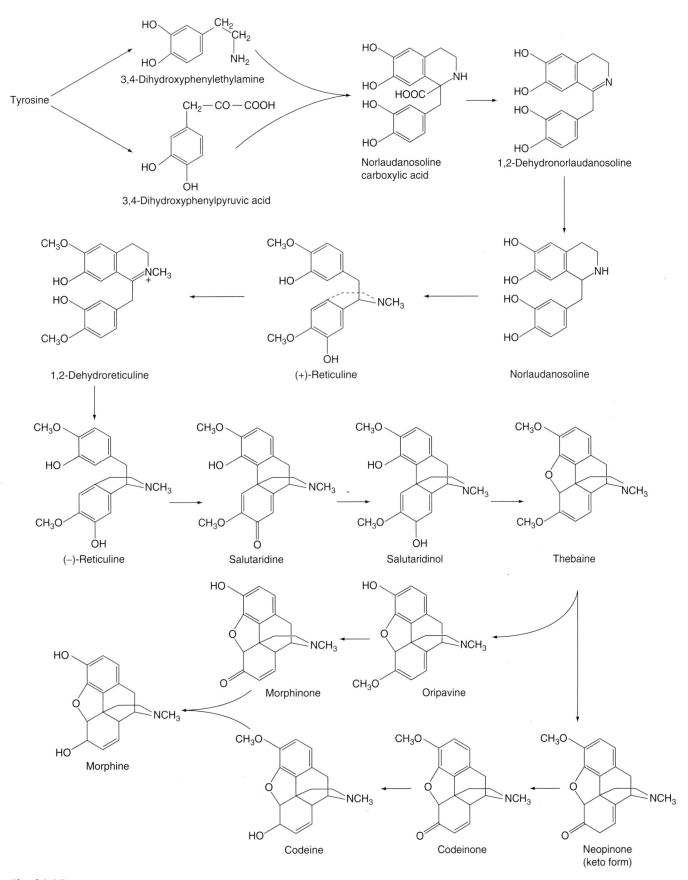

Fig. 26.15
Biogenesis of thebaine, codeine and morphine; see also Fig. 26.16.

tetrahydroisoquinoline residue followed by oxidative ring closure. The validity of such schemes remained untested until the advent of radiochemical techniques, when in 1958–60 experiments with labelled tyrosine, administered to poppy capsules, demonstrated that two molecules of precursor were incorporated into the morphine molecule, in full accord with Robinson's theory. Further, the intermediate stage was confirmed by the demonstration that norlaudanosoline acted as a more efficient precursor for morphine than did tyrosine and yielded a product labelled as required by the theory. By the cultivation of poppy plants in $^{14}CO_2$, and by injection of labelled alkaloids into the plant, it was shown that the first major alkaloid formed is thebaine; this is irreversibly converted to codeine and then to morphine.

Many details of the above outline pathway have now been filled in. Theory required that in the oxidative coupling of norlaudanosoline, the hydroxyl groups not involved in the reaction be protected. A base of the type required, in which two of the hydroxyls were methylated, had previously been isolated from another plant (*Annona reticulata*, Annonaceae, order Magnoliales); this was reticuline. Labelled reticuline and norreticuline both proved to be very efficient precursors of morphine in the poppy, surpassing norlaudanosoline in this respect. Subsequently in 1964 reticuline was found to be a normal, minor component of *P. somniferum*; this is another instance of the isolation of a natural product from a plant after its presence has been suggested on phytochemical grounds. It also illustrates the point that what may be a principal alkaloid in one plant (reticuline in *Annona*) is, in another, a transient metabolite, which is essential to some metabolic pathway but which does not accumulate. In support of the theory, when tetrahydropapaverine (all hydroxyl groups methylated) was fed to the opium poppy, negligible incorporation into the alkaloids was obtained. The stages in the conversion of reticuline to thebaine and of thebaine to codeine were demonstrated by the feeding of appropriate labelled intermediates, alkaloids which have since been isolated as minor components of the opium alkaloid mixture.

One sequence of the pathway shown in Fig. 26.15, which has been difficult to establish unequivocally involves the initial stages leading to the formation of (+)-reticuline. Now norcoclaurine (also called higenamine, and a constituent of *Annona squamosa*, q.v.) is a favoured tri-

hydroxylated precursor. In 1987 the (*R*)-isomer was shown to be specifically incorporated into thebaine when applied as a labelled precursor to *P. somniferum* seedlings. Also with cell cultures and plants of *Berberis*, *Peumus*, *Eschscholtzia* and *Argemone* spp. it was specifically incorporated into protoberberine, aporphine and benzophenanthridine alkaloids (see R. Stadler *et al.*, *Phytochemistry*, 1989, **28**, 1083). The experiments indicated that dopamine and *p*-hydroxyphenylacetaldehyde (both derived from tyrosine) condense to give norcoclaurine, thus explaining the observed lack of incorporation of DOPA and dopamine into the benzylic portion of reticuline-derived alkaloids. The origin of (+)-reticuline by this route is shown in Fig. 26.16.

A second pathway for the terminal steps in the biosynthesis of morphine has been demonstrated (E. Brochmann-Hanssen, *Planta Med.*, 1984, **50**, 343) by using two strains of the opium poppy—a Tasmanian strain known to contain the alkaloid oripavine and the Indra strain. Both species converted labelled oripavine to morphine, and morphinone was also isolated with good incorporation of radioactivity, albeit in small quantity owing to its unstable nature. Codeine and thebaine were not radioactive, demonstrating that the demethylation of the phenolic ether of thebaine is not reversible. This alternative final stage would therefore appear to be thebaine → oripavine → morphinone → morphine (Fig. 26.15).

Two alkaloids which arise as branches of the principal biogenetic pathway are neopine, the presence of which in opium is explained as a reduction product of neopinone, and papaverine, which arises by methylation of norreticuline (Fig. 26.17) followed by dehydrogenation. The presence of some of the other minor alkaloids of opium can be explained by various methylations and dehydrogenations of laudanosoline, reticuline and their nor-derivatives. Various oxidative couplings of reticuline account for other minor alkaloids (e.g. corytuberine and isoboldine).

Role of reticuline in alkaloid biosynthesis. The alkaloids involved in Fig. 26.15 are derived from (−)-reticuline, and the enzymic racemization of reticuline, which is essential for the biosynthesis of the principal opium alkaloids, is very substrate specific. Thus the *N*-ethyl, 6-ethoxy and 4′-ethoxy analogues of reticuline are completely resistant to racemization. (+)-Reticuline also gives rise to a

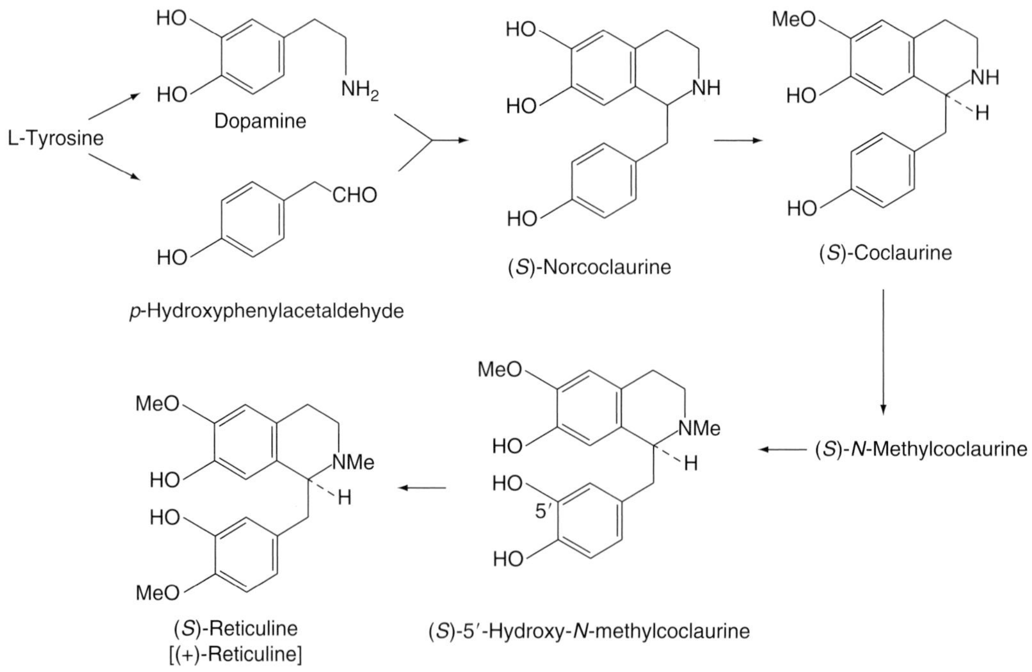

Fig. 26.16
A revised biogenetic route from L-tyrosine to (*S*)-reticuline.

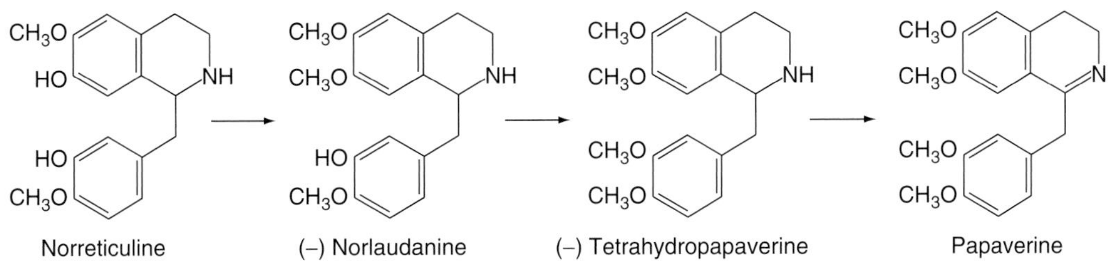

Fig. 26.17
A major pathway in the biogenesis of papaverine.

Norreticuline   (−) Norlaudanine   (−) Tetrahydropapaverine   Papaverine

number of bases: narcotine (noscopine) and narceine of opium; canadine, berberine and hydrastine of *Hydrastis* (Berberidaceae); and sinomenine (the enantiomer of the opium alkaloid salutaridine, Fig. 26.15, of *Sinomenium acutum*, Menispermaceae). With the exception of sinomenine, these alkaloids are termed 'berberine bridged' alkaloids and they arise from norlaudanosoline and a one-carbon unit, which is derived from the *N*-methyl group of (+)-reticuline. The methylenedioxy group of these alkaloids is formed by oxidative cyclization of an *o*-methoxyphenol function. A scheme indicating the origin of some of these alkaloids is given in Fig. 26.18. For berberine, 13 enzymes are involved in its biosynthesis from two molecules of tyrosine. The enzyme associated with the final reaction, the formation of the methylenedioxy bridge, has now been detected in microsomal preparations from different Ranunculaceae and Berberidaceae cell cultures (M. Rueffer and M. H. Zenk, *Phytochemistry*, 1994, **36**, 1219).

Enzyme studies.   As indicated in Chapter 13 cell cultures of *P. somniferum* do not produce morphine-type alkaloids but accumulate large amounts of sanguinarine and other alkaloids. However, some of the enzymes of the morphinan pathway are present in such cell cultures as shown by the reduction of codeinone to codeine by immobilized cells of *P. somniferum* and by the isolation from cell cultures of the enzyme

which reduces salutaridine to (7*S*)-salutaridinol. This enzyme has been fully characterized (R. Gerardy and M. H. Zenk, *Phytochemistry*, 1993, **34**, 125) as has 1,2-dehydroreticuline reductase isolated from poppy seedlings. The same group has shown (R. Wilhelm and M. H. Zenk, *Phytochemistry*, 1997, **46**, 701) that the enzyme necessary for the enol cleavage in the conversion of thebaine to neopinone (Fig. 26.15) is present in cell cultures, as evidenced by the formation of a new alkaloid, thebainone, as a result of feeding labelled thebaine to low-thebaine producing *P. somniferum* cultures. For work on genes encoding (*S*)-*N*-methylcoclaurine-5′-hydroxylase and codeinone reductase see F.-C. Huang and T. M. Kutchan, *Phytochemistry*, 2000, **53**, 555.

Tests for opium alkaloids.   Tests for morphine and other alkaloids are given in the pharmacopoeias. The solubility of morphine in sodium hydroxide solution is explained by its phenolic nature. Conversely, codeine is precipitated by sodium hydroxide.

Storage.   Opium requires careful storage if the morphine content is to be maintained. In the past, Indian opium appears to have suffered more morphine loss during preparation and storage than the other varieties, but when it is dried at 100°C and stored out of contact with air, the loss of morphine is small. Abraham and Rae (1926) ascribe the loss

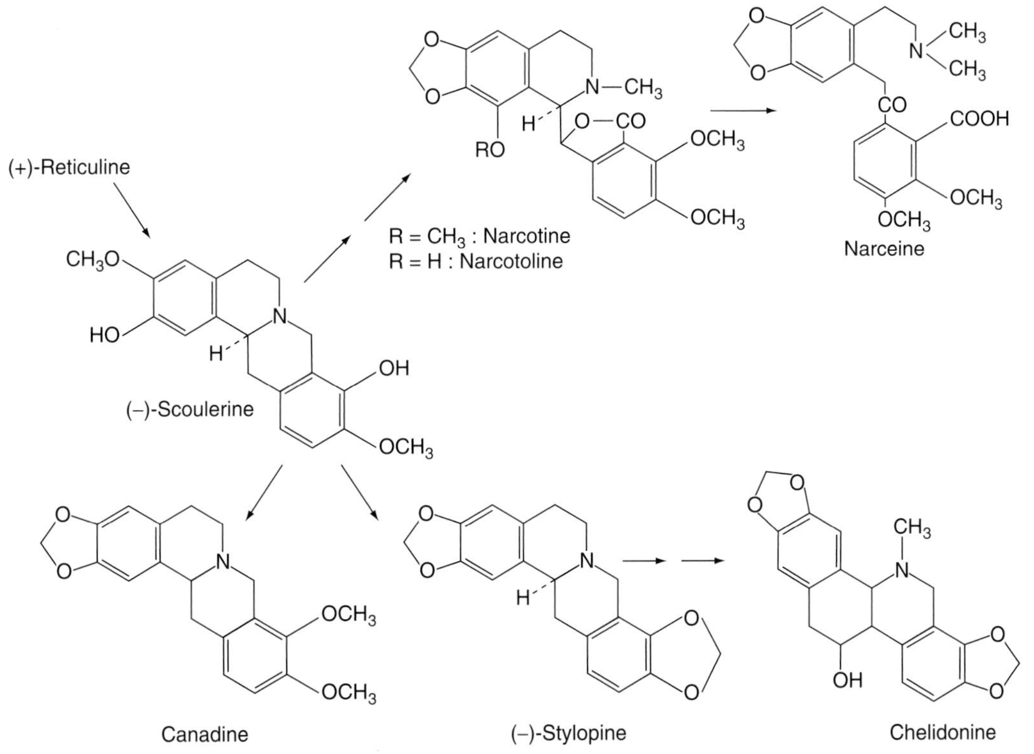

(+)-Reticuline

(−)-Scoulerine

R = CH₃ : Narcotine
R = H : Narcotoline

Narceine

Canadine

(−)-Stylopine

Chelidonine

Fig. 26.18
Some alkaloids derived from (+)-reticuline.

of morphine to a peroxidase which they called opiase. More recently a phenoloxidase which acts on morphine has been isolated from poppy capsules.

Adulteration. Opium has been adulterated with sugary fruits, gum, powdered poppy capsules and other substances too numerous to mention. As far as legitimate commerce is concerned, such adulteration is now pointless because the product is analysed and the price paid is governed by the content of morphine and other alkaloids.

Uses. The alkaloids present in opium in greatest proportion decrease in narcotic properties in the order morphine, codeine, noscapine. Opium and morphine are widely used to relieve pain and are particularly valuable as hypnotics, as, unlike many other hypnotics, they act mainly on the sensory nerve cells of the cerebrum. Codeine is a milder sedative than morphine and is useful for allaying coughing. Both morphine and codeine decrease metabolism, and the latter, particularly before the introduction of insulin, was used for the treatment of diabetes. Opium, while closely resembling morphine, exerts its action more slowly and is therefore preferable in many cases (e.g. in the treatment of diarrhoea). Opium is also used as a diaphoretic. The habitual use of codeine may, in some individuals, produce constipation.

Manufacture of opium alkaloids. The majority of legal opium is used for the isolation of its constituent alkaloids, and in Britain some 90% of the morphine produced is converted into other bases such as codeine, ethylmorphine and pholcodine. In recent years attempts have been made to reduce the illicit traffic in opium either by banning the cultivation of the opium poppy or by cultivation under strict licences. However, two methods by which the opium stage is eliminated are by extraction of the whole poppy capsule and by the use of other species (e.g. *P. bracteatum*) which do not contain morphine.

Extraction of poppy capsules and straw. The feasibility of extracting poppy straw has long been known and utilized in Europe and recently there has been a world-wide trend towards the extraction of the dried poppy capsules (e.g. in Hungary, former USSR, Tasmania). In a study of poppy capsule drying and storage under commercial conditions in Tasmania it has been shown that kiln-drying of immature capsules (42 days old) at various temperatures (40–100°C) resulted in a loss of morphine content of up to about 11% without effect on codeine and thebaine. However, this morphine loss was significantly less than with the field-dried material. To avoid deterioration of the dried product the moisture content should not exceed 16%. Processes have also been developed in France and in the UK for the harvesting and processing of the green capsule, one technical difficulty being the separation of the seed from the fruit at this stage of development.

Use of morphine-free species of *Papaver*. The increasing abuse of opiates has stimulated the search for raw materials other than *Papaver somniferum* which would meet the requirements of the pharmaceutical industry. Thus, plants containing non-addictive thebaine as principal alkaloid could be used for the manufacture of codeine, naloxone (a narcotic antagonist prescribed for babies of heroin addicts) and etorphine (a 'Bentley' compound used for sedating large wild animals).

In this respect attention focused on three closely related perennial species of *Papaver* of the section *Oxytona* Bernh. of the family, namely, *P. bracteatum*, *P. orientale* and *P. pseudo-orientale*. These are indigenous to the mountainous districts of Iran, eastern Turkey and the Transcaucasian former USSR. Confusion concerning the identity of the characteristic alkaloids for each species had arisen from various factors, including incorrect identification, variations of chromosome number within a species, the existence of chemical races and geographical influences.

Papaver bracteatum

Thebaine is the predominant alkaloid of this species and in a UN-backed programme of large-scale cultivation trials were organized in various countries. High yielding strains were introduced, for example, Ayra II, a race obtained from west Iran in 1974 which gives 3.5% thebaine in the dried capsules. Problems associated with the development were the insufficiency of seed of high-yielding strains and the poorer crops obtained when the plants were removed from their normal environment. However, political decisions also jeopardized the continuation of the programme.

P. bracteatum produces some 27 alkaloids belonging to 10 of the 14 alkaloid groups described for *Papaver*. The biogenesis of thebaine follows the same pathway as in *P. somniferum*. Feeding experiments with labelled intermediates have shown that the plant is capable of converting codeinone to codeine but cannot perform either of the demethylations leading to codeine or directly to morphine. Thebaine does not appear to be entirely an end-product and undergoes further metabolism to unknown products (for a report, see H. G. Theuns *et al.*, *Phytochemistry*, 1985, **24**, 581). A more recently described new alkaloid is salutaridine-*N*-oxide (G. Sariyar *et al.*, *Planta Med.*, 1992, **58**, 368).

Papaver orientale

This species is commonly cultivated as the ornamental poppy and a number of alkaloid chemotypes have been described. Generally, oripavine (formed by demethylation of the aromatic ring of thebaine, Fig. 26.15) is the principal alkaloid, but Phillipson *et al.* (*Planta Med.*, 1981, **43**, 261) described one chemotype with mecambridine (a berberine type alkaloid) as principal constituent.

Papaver pseudo-orientale

The plant ($2n = 42$) is intermediate in many of its characters between those of the above two species and may have arisen as an allohexaploid from them. Phillipson (above reference) divided 16 Turkish samples in three cytological and alkaloid groups. Thirteen samples contained isothebaine, mecambridine and orientalidine as major alkaloids, two contained principally salutaridine and thebaine, and one sample possessed salutaridine as the major component. (For other alkaloids and biogenetic transformations see G. Sźariya *et al.*, *Phytochemistry*, 1986, **25**, 2403.)

(For a comprehensive review of the morphine alkaloids covering general chemistry, biogenesis, occurrence and structure elucidation (391 refs) see C. Sźantay *et al.*, *The Alkaloids*, 1994, **45**, 128.)

BOLDO LEAVES

Boldo leaves *BP/EP* are derived from *Peumus boldus* (Monimiaceae); they contain aporphine-type alkaloids, chiefly boldine. The drug has antihepatoxic activity and is described in Chapter 29.

GOLDENSEAL ROOT

Goldenseal root *BP/EP*, *BHP* 1990 consists of the dried rhizome and roots of *Hydrastis canadensis* (Berberidaceae), a small perennial plant indigenous to the woods of eastern Canada and the eastern USA.

The wild plants have been exterminated in many districts and the species now has CITES listing (q.v.) for the USA and Canada. Most of the commercial drug is now obtained from cultivated plants grown in America and in Europe. The use of hydrastis, both as a drug and as a dye, was learned by the early European settlers from the Cherokee Indians.

Characters. The drug consists of almost cylindrical rhizomes about 1–5 cm long and 2–10 mm diameter. The rhizomes grow more or less obliquely and bear numerous, short branches, which terminate in cup-shaped scars and bear encircling cataphyllary leaves. Similar scale leaves are found on the rhizome, the outer surface of which is yellowish-brown or greyish-brown. The roots, which originate on the ventral and lateral surfaces, are long and wiry, and in the commercial drug are often broken at a distance of a centimetre or so from the rhizome. The drug breaks with a short, waxy fracture. It has a slight but distinctive odour and bitter taste.

A transverse section of the rhizome shows a fairly thick, yellow or yellowish-brown bark; 12–20 radially elongated, bright yellow wood bundles, separated by wide medullary rays; a large pith.

Constituents. Hydrastis contains the alkaloids hydrastine, berberine, canadine and other minor ones. Commercial samples yield 1.5–4% of hydrastine and 0.5–6.0% of berberine. The latter, as a constituent of an extract of the root, is responsible for activity against multiple drug resistant *Mycobacterium tuberculosis* (see E. J. Gentry *et al.*, *J. Nat. Prod.*, 1998, **61**, 1187)

The *BP/EP* requires a minimum content of 2–5% (dried drug) for hydrastine and a minimum of 3.0% for berberine. These are determined by liquid chromatography with absorbance measurements at 235 nm using a reference solution of the above alkaloids for comparison. These alkaloids are also identified in the TLC test for the drug using visualization with UV light at 365 nm.

Uses. The use of hydrastis to check uterine haemorrhage, as a bitter stomachic and locally in the treatment of catarrhal conditions of the genito-urinary tract is largely based on empirical observations. Hydrastine hydrochloride and hydrastinine hydrochloride have been used in various forms to control uterine haemorrhage.

FUMITORY

Fumitory *BP/EP*, *BHP* consists of the dried aerial parts of *Fumaria officinalis* L., family Fumariaceae, collected when in flower. It is an annual herb common as a weed and on roadsides throughout most of Europe; it has spread world-wide. The leaves are greyish-green, stalked, each pinnately divided several times giving flattened lanceolate, often toothed segments. The flowers are arranged in racemes with pink, red-tipped petals forming a tubular corolla. Fruits are somewhat flattened achenes, 2.0–2.5 mm, with rough surfaces. Microscopical features of the olive-green powder include leaf epidermi with anomocytic stomata and spherical pollen grains, about 35–40 μm in diameter, with pitted exine and six large pores; also in abundance are features of the stems, flowers and fruits.

Constituents. A range of isoquinoline-type alkaloids includes protoberberines, spirobenzylisoquinolines, benzophenanthridines and indenobenzazepines. Protopine (Fig. 26.19) is the principal alkaloid, the *BP/EP* requiring a minimum total alkaloid content of 0.40% calculated as this alkaloid. A titrimetric assay is employed, sonication being used for dissolving the plant extract produced in the alkaloid purification procedure.

Other constituents include flavonoids, principally glycosides of quercetin, and acids, including chlorogenic and caffeic acids.

Uses. Fumitory is employed for its choleretic action, see Chapter 29.

GREATER CELANDINE

Greater celandine *BP/EP* consists of the dried whole or cut aerial parts of *Chelidonium majus* L. family Papaveraceae, collected parts of *Chelidonium majus* L. family Papaveraceae, collected during the flowering period. There is a minimum requirement of 0.6% for total alkaloids expressed as chelidonine.

This perennial herb is widespread throughout Europe, northern Asia and the north-eastern USA, growing along banks, in hedgerows, against walls and in waste areas. The hollow, ribbed stems are up to about 90 cm in height, branched and leafy. When fresh, the stems and leaves exude a milky sap, which turns to orange–red

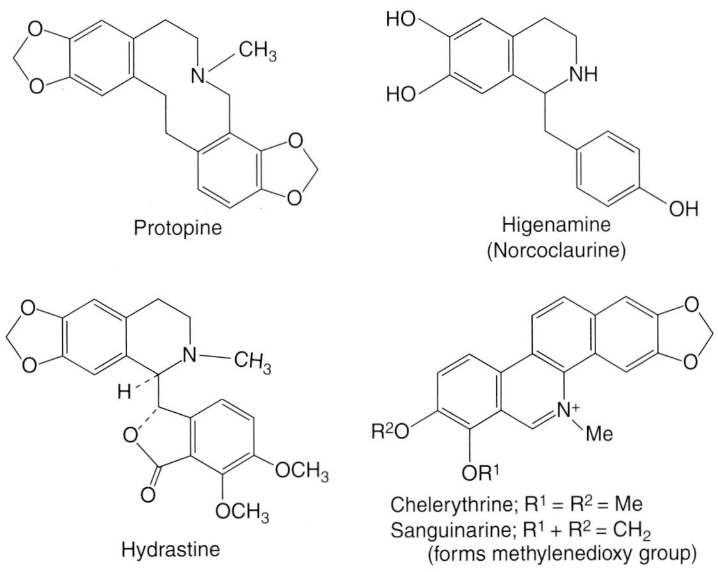

Fig. 26.19
Selected alkaloids of drugs described in the accompanying text.

when exposed to the air and is a skin irritant. The leaves are almost pinnate and divided into five to seven ovate to oblong leaflets, the terminal ones often three-lobed; margins are crenately toothed, the upper surfaces glabrous and dark green and the lower somewhat glaucous. The bright yellow flowers, 2–2.5 cm in diameter each have two greenish-yellow sepals and four petals. Stamens are yellow and numerous. Fruit is a capsule 3–5 cm in length, containing black seeds having a white appendage; mature fruits are rarely to be found in the drug.

Microscopic features include: anomocytic stomata on the lower leaflet surfaces, uniseriate possibly fragmented covering trichomes, vascular tissues, associated latex canals with brown contents, corolla fragments with oil droplets, spherical three-pored pollen grains up to 40 μm in diameter.

Constituents. Greater celandine contains up to 4% of alkaloids including α- and β-allocryptopine, berberine (Fig. 28.1), chelerythrine (Fig. 26.19), chelidonine (Fig. 26.18), chelirubine, choline, coptisine, hydroxychelidonine, hydroxysanguinarine, protopine (Fig. 26.19), sanguinarine (Fig. 26.19), sparteine (Fig. 26.12), and others.

The *BP/EP* TLC test for identity produces a number of unidentified separated components; the assay for total alkaloids is performed on an extract of the drug treated in acid solution with the *BP* chromotropic, sodium salt reagent and absorbance measurements at 570 nm.

Uses. The drug has many traditional uses based on its reputed anodyne, antispasmodic, caustic, diaphoretic, diuretic, hydragogue, narcotic and purgative properties, Some of these activities have support from pharmacological tests involving particular alkaloids. *C. majus* is also used in homoeopathic practice and in Chinese medicine.

Annona squamosa (Annonaceae)

Various parts of this plant have featured in the folk medicine of Africa, India and the Far East for the treatment of a number of conditions including heart disorders. The cardioactive effect has been attributed to the alkaloid higenamine (Fig. 26.19) an important precursor of a number of other isoquinolines.

Bloodroot

Bloodroot consists of the dried rhizomes and roots of *Sanguinaria canadensis* (Papaveraceae), a perennial herb widely distributed in the woods of North America. The drug consists of dark brown, more or less cylindrical pieces of rhizome, 2–7 cm long and 5–15 mm diameter. Some of the pieces are branched and some show numerous wiry roots. The latter, however, are usually broken off in the commercial drug. The rhizome breaks with a short fracture and, if not overheated during drying, shows numerous red dots (secretion cells) distributed throughout the starch-containing parenchyma of the bark and large pith. If dried at too high a temperature, the secretion escapes from its containing cells and the whole section assumes a deep red or brownish-red colour. A ring of small, yellow, fibrovascular bundles lies about 1 mm from the outside. Odour, slight; taste, acrid and bitter. Bloodroot contains the benzophenanthridine alkaloids sanguinarine, chelerythrine (Fig. 26.19), allocryptopine, protopine and dihydrosanguilutine. Sanguinarine and chelerythrine, although themselves colourless, form red and yellow salts, respectively. The drug also contains red resin and starch.

In a report by Rho *et al.* (*Appl. Microbiol. Biotechnol.*, 1992, **36**, 611) *S. canadensis* cultured cells produced sanguinarine (about 80%

of the total alkaloid) together with chelirubine and chelerythrine. In contrast, in the normal rhizome sanguinarine and sanguirubine together account for some 70% of the total alkaloids. (For elicitor studies see G. B. Mahady and C. W. W. Beecher, *Phytochemistry*, 1994, **37**, 415.)

Bloodroot is used mainly in the USA, where it is an ingredient of Compound White Pine Syrup. Sanguinarine, like colchicine, causes the doubling of the chromosomes in cells.

Calumba root

Calumba is the dried, sliced root of *Jateorhiza palmata* (*J. columba*) (Menispermaceae), a dioecious climbing plant indigenous to the forests of Mozambique and Madagascar (Malagasy Republic) and other east African countries. It is exported to Europe from Tanzania and the name derives from the fact that it was at one time exported from Colombo (Sri Lanka).

Collection. Attempts to cultivate the drug in various areas do not appear to have been successful and collection is from the wild. The plant possesses a somewhat slender rhizome from which numerous large fusiform roots arise. The older reports state that these are dug up during dry weather (March), the rhizomes are rejected and the roots cut into transverse or oblique slices and dried in the shade. The imported 'natural calumba' is frequently washed, brushed and graded, the product being known as 'washed calumba'.

Macroscopical characters. Calumba occurs in circular or oblique slices. These are usually 2–8 cm diameter and 3–12 mm thick.

The cork is thin, greyish-brown or reddish-brown in colour and longitudinally wrinkled. Within it lies a broad, greenish-yellow zone which extends to the cambium and contains in its outer part isolated sclerenchymatous cells within which are dark-grey, sinuous strands of sieve tissue. The greyish wood, which is separated from the bark by a dark cambium line, shows numerous narrow, radiating lines of yellow vessels separated by abundant parenchyma. The vessels are close together in the region near the cambium and again in the extreme centre of the root, but they are less numerous in the intermediate zone, which therefore shrinks considerably and becomes depressed on drying. Some pieces show two or more concentric zones of wood. The fracture is short and starchy; odour, slight and somewhat musty; taste, bitter.

Calumba frequently contains occasional slices of *calumba rhizome*. These average about 2–3 cm diameter. The structure is markedly radiate and, owing to its greater woodiness in that region, is not depressed in the centre.

Microscopical characters. The drug is characterized by the sclereids which have unevenly thickened, yellow walls and contain a number of prisms of calcium oxalate, by abundant parenchymatous cells containing starch grains, each grain measuring about 20–85 μm long and having an eccentric, very distinct radiate or cleft hilum, and by the yellow reticulate vessels. The walls of both the sclerenchymatous cells and vessels on treatment with 66% v/v sulphuric acid change colour from yellow to green.

Constituents. Calumba contains about 2–3% of isoquinoline alkaloids, palmatine, jatrorrhizine and columbamine. Bisjatrorrhizine is a quaternary dimeric alkaloid formed by *ortho*-oxidative coupling of the phenolic group of jatrorrhizine. Other constituents are the non-alkaloidal furanoditerpenes columbin, isocolumbin, palmarin, chasmanthin, jateorin and isojateorin. Some of these occur as glucosides and have been named palmatosides A to G.

Palmatine: R¹ = R² = CH₃
Jatrorrhizine: R¹ = H, R² = CH₃
Columbamine: R¹ = CH₃, R² = H

Columbin: R¹ = ◄ H, R² = H
Isocolumbin: R¹ = — H, R² = H
Columbinyl glucoside: R¹ = ◄ H, R² = glycosyl

Other diterpenes are similar isomers differing in the positions of the epoxide ring and in the stereochemistry of the C-12–C-13 bond.

Uses. Calumba is used as a bitter tonic and, as it contains no tannin, may be prescribed with iron salts. In the *BHP* it is specifically indicated for anorexia and flatulent dyspepsia.

Serpentary

Serpentary consists of the dried rhizome and roots of *Aristolochia reticulata* (Aristolochiaceae). This is known in commerce as Texan or Red River snake-root and is collected in the woods of Texas, Louisiana, Arkansas and Oklahoma.

Macroscopical characters. The drug has a yellowish colour when fresh, becoming brown on keeping. It consists of small rhizomes bearing the remains of subaerial stems and numerous wiry roots. The rhizomes are about 1–2 cm long and 2–3 mm diameter, while the roots are about 10 cm long and 0.2–1.2 mm diameter. The drug contains up to 10% of subaerial stems. Odour, camphoraceous; taste, camphoraceous and bitter.

A transverse section of the rhizomes shows a starchy, eccentric pith (nearer the upper surface of the rhizome than the lower), wedge-shaped, yellowish vascular bundles separated by wide medullary rays, and a narrow bark.

Allied drugs. *Virginian snake-root*, from *Aristolochia serpentaria*, was formerly official but its regular importation has now ceased. It closely resembles the Texan drug, but has smaller rhizome and more wiry roots. *Indian aristolochia* or Indian birthwort consists of the roots and rhizome of *Aristolochia indica*; it contains aristolochic acid together with other phenanthrene derivatives, an *N*-glycoside and steroids. *A. heterophylla* is used in China, and *A. constricta*, recently investigated (L. Pastrelli *et al.*, *J. Nat. Prod.*, 1997, **60**, 1065), is widely employed in folk medicine in S. America. *A. clematis* (birthwort) is European and has been used both internally and externally. It contains similar constituents to other species.

Constituents. Many species of *Aristolochia* including *A. reticulata* contain aristolochic acid and the tumour-inhibiting properties of this compound are of interest. However, in experimental animals it can cause tumour formation and has been associated with cases of renal failure. Aristolochic acid is not alkaloidal, belonging to a small group of naturally occurring nitro-compounds, but is included here because of its direct derivation from isothebaine derivatives in the plant.

Isothebaine isomer   Aristolochic acid

(For a review on the structure of the aristolochic acids and their corresponding lactams (aristolactams) see D. B. Mix *et al.*, *J. Nat. Prod.*, 1982, **45**, 657 and for the isolation of aristolochic acids I–IV and aristolactams I–III from *A. auricularis* see P. J. Houghton and M. Ogutveren, *Phytochemistry* 1991, **30**, 253.)

Uses and dangers. Snakeroot has been traditionally employed as an aromatic bitter but other *Aristolochia* spp. have also been employed in Chinese herbal medicines for various treatments. As from 28 July 1999 an emergency ban on the import, sale and supply of medicinal products containing *Aristolochia* spp. came into force for the UK. This arose in part from two UK cases of end-stage renal failure in patients using Chinese medicines containing *Aristolochia* and from many cases of renal failure in Belgium when *Aristolochia* was substituted for *Stephania* in a herbal preparation. Apparently in Chinese herbal preparations it is liable to be substituted for other innocuous components such as *Stephania*, *Akebia* or *Clematis* (MCA/CSM, UK, *Current Problems in Pharmacovigilance*, 1996, **22**, 10; see also the report, *Pharm. J.*, 2000, **265**, 10).

CURARE

The term 'curare' is a generic one applied to various South American arrow poisons. These extracts are made from a number of different plants, particularly members of the Menispermaceae (e.g. *Chondrodendron*) and the Loganiaceae. From the former, tubocurarine is obtained and the (+)-hydrochloride of this is included in the *BP/EP* as a muscle relaxant.

Curares from the upper Amazon (Brazil and Peru) seem to be mainly menispermaceous in origin. The original genus *Chondrodendron* has been divided into two by Barneby and Krukoff (*Mem. N. Y. Bot. Gdn*, 1971, **22**, 1); *Chondrodendron* itself with three species (*Ch. tomentosum*, *Ch. platyphyllum*, *Ch. microphyllum*) and *Curarea* with four species (*Cu. toxicofera*, *Cu. candicans*, *Cu. tecunarum* and *Cu. cuartecasasii*).

The principal ones used in curare are *Ch. tomentosum* (the only plant known to contain tubocurarine), and the first three of the *Curarea* species. Several other genera of Menispermaceae are known to have been, or to be, ingredients of curares including species of *Sciadotenia*, *Abuta*, *Telitoxicum* and *Cissampelos*, but little is known about the muscle-relaxant activity, if any, of their alkaloids.

The curares from Guyana, Venezuela and Colombia owe much of their activity to species of *Strychnos* (Loganiaceae); around 20 species are known to have been incorporated into curares and these include *S. toxifera*, *S. jobertiana*, *S. peckii* and *S. guianensis*.

(For reviews covering the history, uses, botany and chemistry of curare see N. G. Bisset, *J. Ethnopharmacology*, 1992, **36**, 1; *Alkaloids*, *Chem. Biol. Perspect.*, 1992, **8**, 1.)

History. There is a close botanical relationship between Pareira Brava Radix of the seventeenth- and eighteenth-century pharmacopoeias and the menispermaceous plants yielding curare. In both cases the botanical source of the drugs has long been in doubt. It is now known that Pereira Brava is obtained from two species of *Chondrodendron*, namely, *C. microphyllum*, which contains (+)-bebeerine, and *C. platyphyllum*, which contains (−)-bebeerine. A similar case is the so-called *C. tomentosum*, which sometimes yields

(+)-Tubocurarine

(+)-tubocurarine and sometimes the less active (−)-tubocurarine. This led King (1948) to write: 'It seems very probable therefore that two species are involved under the name *C. tomentosum*'.

Boehm (1895) distinguished three kinds of curare differentiated first by their containers, and second by their different chemical characteristics.

1. *Tube-curare*, packed in bamboo tubes. This came from Brazil and Peru, was mainly menispermaceous in origin and contained the alkaloid which Boehm (1895) isolated as amorphous 'tubocurarine' and which King (1935) first prepared crystalline as tubocurarine chloride.
2. *Calabash-curare* is packed in gourds and comes mainly from Guiana, Venezuela and Columbia. It was formerly the type of curare most commonly found in commerce. Chemical investigations of Wieland *et al.* (1937–41), King (1949) and Karrer (1946–54) show that *Strychnos* species furnish important constituents.
3. *Pot-curare*, which is no longer a commercial article, was packed in earthenware pots. These varied in size and were glazed, unglazed or ornamented with paint. King's examination of one small pot led him to the conclusion that it was menispermaceous in origin and contained no *Strychnos* spp. However, Bauer (1969, 1981) showed in an extensive investigation of museum samples of curare that pot curares were usually of mixed Loganiaceae/Menispermaceae origin.

Curare in tins. Much curare has been imported in tins containing about 1 kg of a viscous dark-brown or blackish extract. It has little odour but a very bitter taste.

This drug is similar to the specimen examined by King (1948), who received it from Asher Kates y Cia S.A. of Lima, Peru, together with

the leaves of the plant from which it was prepared. These leaves were indistinguishable from those of *C. tomentosum* and its menispermaceous nature, and similarity to the old tube-curare, was confirmed by the isolation of (+)-tubocurarine chloride and four other alkaloids.

Constituents. (1) *Menispermaceous* tube-curare and the form now imported in tins contain tubocurarine. From the tin-curare King (1948) isolated (+)-tubocurarine chloride and four non-quaternary bases (isochondrodendrine dimethyl ether, (−)-curine (bebeerine), (+)-chondrocurine and (+)-isochondrodendrine). (2) *Loganiaceous* calabash-curare derives its activity largely from *Strychnos* species, particularly *S. toxifera*. King (1949) has shown that the bark of this species contains 12 crystalline quaternary alkaloids, the toxiferines I–XII, of which two had previously been isolated by Wieland *et al.* (1937–41). These latter authors examined calabash-curare, probably from Venezuela, and isolated several alkaloids known as C-curarines (C signifies calabash). Toxiferines I and II have been found in calabash-curare.

More recently calabash-curares and *Strychnos* spp. have been examined by Karrer and his colleagues with the isolation of a large number of new alkaloids. (+)-Tubocurarine is a bisbenzylisoquinoline alkaloid and as such is derived from dopamine, whereas the Loganiaceous curares are indolic and contain C_{40} compounds of the dimeric strychnine type.

Uses. Curare is now little used except as a source of alkaloids. Tubocurarine chloride, official in the *BP/EP*, is used to secure muscular relaxation in surgical operations and in certain neurological conditions.

TETRAHYDROISOQUINOLINE MONOTERPENOID ALKALOIDS AND GLYCOSIDES

These alkaloids and alkaloid-glycosides derive from the condensation of dopamine with secologanin (a C_{10} monoterpene) to give two series of compounds. The best-known examples of their limited occurrence are in species of *Cephaëlis* (Rubiaceae) and *Alangium* (Alangiaceae). The former gives ipecacuanha root, and the root, bark, fruits and leaves of *A. lamarckii* are used in Ayurvedic medicine for the treatment of a number of conditions.

IPECACUANHA

Ipecacuanha (*Ipecacuanha Root*) of the *BP* is the dried root or rhizome and root of *Cephaëlis ipecacuanha* (Brotero) A. Richard (Rubiaceae), known in commerce as Matto Grosso Ipecac. or of *Cephaëlis acuminata* Karsten, known in commerce as Costa Rica Ipecac. A mixture of both species is also permissible. It should contain a minimum of 2% of ether-soluble alkaloids.

C. ipecacuanha is a shrub 20–40 cm high found over a large area in Brazil, particularly in the moist and shady forests of Matto Grosso and Minãs Geraes; plantations have been established in the Matto Grosso area. It is cultivated to some extent in Malaya, Burma and the Darjeeling Hills of West Bengal. *C. acuminata* is exported from Colombia, Nicaragua and Costa Rica; Costa Rica is at present the principal source of the drug. However India is now in full production of Costa Rican type root which is of high quality (in excess of 3.5% total alkaloid) and extremely competitive in price; extracts of the Indian root are now being produced and exported.

History. What appears to have been ipecacuanha was mentioned, under the name of *Igpecaya*, by a Portuguese friar around 1600. It was introduced into Europe in 1672.

Collection and preparation. In the Matto Grosso district of Brazil the drug is collected from wild plants. The collector, using a pointed stick, levers the plant from the ground and, having removed most of the roots, replaces it in the ground, where it usually lives to produce further crops. The roots are dried in the sun or by fires and transported down river to ports such as Rio de Janeiro, Bahia and Pernambuco from which they are exported in bales. Other South American ipecacuanhas are collected in a similar way. The supply of S. American ipecacuanha has been erratic for many years as a result of habitat destruction, overcollection and the uprooting of plants. The high price of the drug has stimulated both cultivation in other areas (see above) and the promotion of cell and root cultures for alkaloid production (see below).

Macroscopical characters. The underground portion consists of thin, horizontal rhizomes from the lower surface of which roots are given off. Some of the latter remain thin, while others develop an abnormally thick bark and become annulated.

The Matto Grosso drug occurs in tortuous pieces up to 15 cm long and 6 mm diameter, but it is usually smaller. The colour of the outer surface varies from a deep brick-red to a very dark brown, the colour being very largely dependent on the type of soil in which the plant has been grown. Most of the roots are more or less annulated externally, and some have a portion of the rhizome attached (Fig. 26.20A), while separate portions of rhizome and non-annulated roots are also found. Generally, the drug of present-day commerce is less markedly annulated than was formerly the case, a fact that points to earlier collection. The ridges are rounded and completely encircle the root; here and there the bark has completely separated from the wood.

The root breaks with a short fracture and shows a thick greyish bark and a small, dense wood, but no pith. The rhizomes, on the other hand, have a much thinner bark and a definite pith (Fig. 26.20C, D). The drug has little odour, but is irritating and sternutatory when in fine powder, and has a bitter taste.

The Costa Rica drug (Fig. 26.20B) is exported from Cartagena and Savanilla. The main differences between the Rio and Cartagena drugs are listed in Table 26.5.

Ipecacuanha stems, although containing the same alkaloids as the roots, usually contain them in smaller proportion. An excessive amount of stem must, therefore, be regarded as an adulteration.

Microscopical characters. A transverse section of the root (Fig. 26.20C) shows a thin, brown cork, the cells of which contain brown, granular material. Within this is a wide secondary cortex (phelloderm), the cells of which are parenchymatous and contain starch, usually in compound grains with from two to eight components, or raphides of calcium oxalate. The individual starch grains are muller-shaped and up to 15 or 20 μm diameter. The phloem is entirely parenchymatous, containing no sclerenchymatous cells or fibres. The compact central mass of xylem is composed of small tracheidal vessels, tracheids, substitute

Table 26.5 Comparison of ipecacuanha (*Cephaëlis*) roots.

	C. ipecacuanha	*C. acuminata*
Usual diameter	1–4 mm	4–6.5 mm
Colour	Brick-red to brown	Greyish-brown
Annulations	Very crowded	Less crowded and less projecting
Starch	Individual grains up to 15 μm	Individual grains up to 20 μm

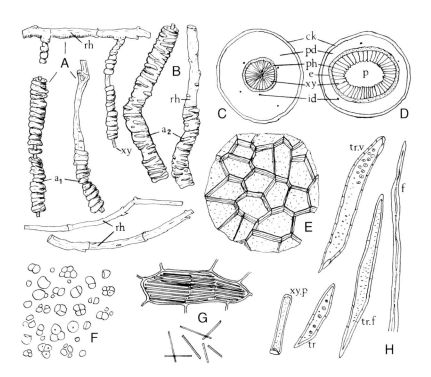

Fig. 26.20
Ipecacuanha. A, *Cephaëlis ipecacuanha* roots with rhizome; B, *C. acuminata* roots with rhizome (both ×1); C, transverse section of root; D, transverse section of rhizome (both ×4); E, cork cells in surface view; F, starch granules (mounted in cold lactophenol); G, idioblast containing calcium oxalate crystals; H, elements from Schultze maceration of wood (all ×200). a₁, Complete annulation of *C. ipecacuanha*; a₂, incomplete annulation of *C. acuminata*; ck, cork; e, endodermis; f, fibrous cell; id, idioblast containing calcium oxalate; p, pith; pd, phelloderm; ph, phloem; rh, rhizome; tr.v, tracheid vessel; xy, xylem; xy.p, xylem parenchyma.

fibres, xylem fibres and xylem parenchyma. Starch is present in the xylem parenchyma and substitute fibres contain starch (Fig. 26.20E–H).

The transverse section of ipecacuanha rhizome (Fig. 26.20D) shows the presence of a ring of xylem and a large pith. The pericycle contains characteristic sclerenchymatous cells. Spiral vessels occur in the protoxylem. The pith is composed of pitted parenchyma which shows some lignification.

Adulterants. At one time other 'ipecacuanhas' were regularly imported, the name being applied in South America to a number of different roots which were reputed to have emetic properties. Most of these, briefly described in the 10th edition, are very easily distinguished from the genuine drug and are now rarely imported.

Constituents. Ipecacuanha contains the alkaloids emetine (Pelletier and Magendie, 1817), cephaëline (Paul and Cownley, 1894), psychotrine, psychotrine methylether and emetamine. These are isoquinoline derivatives of a group only known with certainty to occur in the families Alangiaceae, Icacinaceae and Rubiaceae. However, emetine-type alkaloids are not necessarily a characteristic of the genus *Cephaëlis* as a whole as Solis *et al.* (*Phytochemistry*, 1993, **33**, 1117) recorded a new *indole* alkaloid and four other known indole alkaloids from the aerial parts of *C. dichroa* from Western Panama.

In a review (411 refs) of the ipecacuanha and related bases (T. Fujii and M. Ohba, *The Alkaloids*, 1998, **51**, 271) 39 new alkaloids from ipecacuanha and *Alangium* are recorded for the 14 years to 1997. For further new alkaloids of *A. longiflorum*, see for example N. Sakurai *et al.*, *Phytochemistry*, 2006, **67**, 894.

Other constituents of the official drug are monoterpenoid isoquinoline glucosides including ipecoside (Fig. 26.22), alangiside and, reported in a series of papers (1989–), a number of other novel glycosides closely related to the known ipecacuanha alkaloids (A. Itoh *et al.*, *Phytochemistry*, 2002, **59**, 91 and the refs cited therein). The iridoid glucosides sweroside and 7-dehydrologanin together with starch and calcium oxalate are also found in the root. Ipecacuanhin and ipecacuanhic acid, originally designated glycosidal tannins, are now thought to have been impure mixtures of ipecoside and sucrose.

As may be seen from Fig. 26.21, the principal alkaloids are closely related to one another; emetine and psychotrine methylether are non-phenolic, whereas cephaëline and psychotrine are phenolic.

Thus, emetine, which is the alkaloid usually required in medicine, may be prepared by methylating the cephaëline originally present in the drug. These alkaloids may be regarded as being formed in the plant from two phenylethylamine units and a C_9 terpenoid precursor. The latter is provided in the plant by secologanin and is incorporated via desacetylisoipecoside into the emetine alkaloids (Fig. 26.22). The glucosidic compound ipecoside is formed from the epimer desacetylipecoside (cf. Fig. 26.22, which illustrates the involvement of secologanin in the formation of some indole alkaloids; in this case, however, only the α-epimer, strictosodine, is formed, but it can serve as a precursor for alkaloids with β-configuration). The isolation by Itoh *et al.*, (*Chem. Pharm. Bull.*, 1994, **17**, 1460) of tetrahydroisoquinoline-monoterpenoid glucosides, from *Alangium lamarckii* fruits, with the same stereo-configuration as desacetylisoipecosides supported the role of the latter as an intermediate in the formation of emetine-type alkaloids. Furthermore cell-free extracts of *A. lamarckii* have been shown to contain two enzyme activities promoting the condensation of dopamine and secologanin to give the (*S*)- and (*R*)-products respectively (W. De-Eknamkul *et al.*, *Phytochemistry*, 1997, **45**, 477).

Various varieties of ipecacuanha contain different proportions of the principal alkaloids. Thus, the Rio drug, which is now difficult to obtain commercially and is the most esteemed, contains 2–2.4% alkaloids, of which 60–75% is emetine. Those varieties derived from *C. acuminata* yield 2–3.5% alkaloids, of which emetine may constitute 30–50%.

Cell and root cultures. Production of the ipecacuanha alkaloids by artificial culture would be commercially highly desirable and some research in this area has been reported. The composition of the culture medium and the nature of the added hormones greatly influences alkaloid production but generally root cultures appear to be more satisfactory than callus or suspension cultures. Increased growth of roots is obtained by the induction of hairy roots. In contrast to whole roots, cell cultures produce more cephaëline than emetine, and immobilized cell systems give higher amounts of cephaëline compared with static cell cultures. (For original research papers see K. Yoshimatsu *et al.*, *Phytochemistry*, 1991, **30**, 507; S. Jha *et al.*, *ibid.*, **30**, 3999; C. Veeresham *et al.*, *ibid.*, 1994, **35**, 947.) The roots of *C. ipecacuanha* transformed with *Agrobacterium rhizogenes* grow well in a gamboge medium yielding 112 mg/l of cephaeline and 14 mg/l of emetine after eight weeks of culture (K. Yoshimatsu *et al.*, *Planta Med.*, 2003, **69**, 1018).

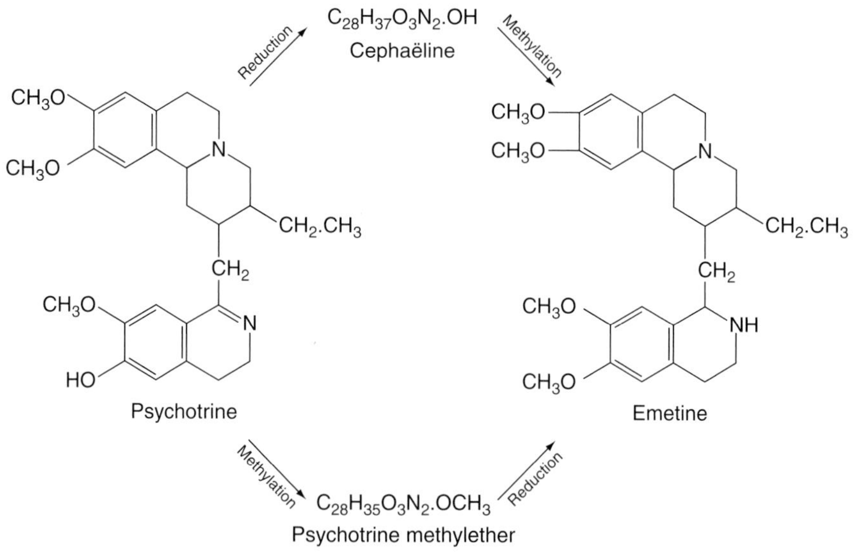

Fig. 26.21
Relationship between the principal alkaloids of ipecacuanha.

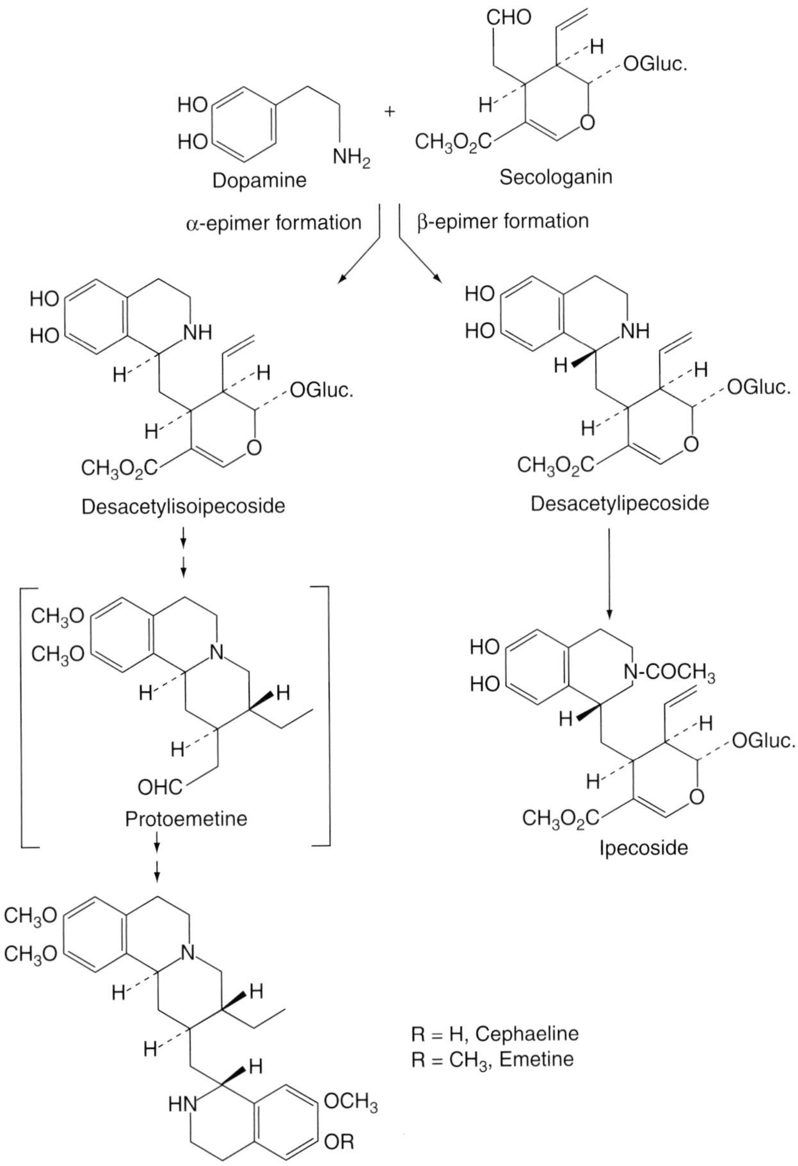

Fig. 26.22
Biosynthetic sequence for the biosynthesis of cephaeline, emetine and the alkaloidal glucoside ipecoside.

A simple one-step method for the production of ipecacuanha plants from root cultures has been described (K. Yoshimatsu and K. Shimomura, *Plant Cell Rep.*, 1994, **14**, 98).

Test for emetine. Mix 0.5 g of the powdered drug with 20 ml of hydrochloric acid and 5 ml of water; filter, and to 2 ml of the filtrate add 0.01 g of potassium chlorate; if emetine is present, a yellow colour appears, which, on standing for about 1 h, gradually changes to red.

Prepared Ipecacuanha is the drug reduced to a fine powder and adjusted to contain 1.90–2.10% of total alkaloids. It is assayed (*BP/ EP*) by extraction of the alkaloids followed by back-titration of the standarized acid solution with sodium hydroxide.

Uses. Ipecacuanha is used as an expectorant and emetic and in the treatment of amoebic dysentery (Chapter 28). Emetine has a more expectorant and less emetic action than cephaëline, a fact that accounts for the preference shown for the Brazilian drug. In the treatment of amoebic dysentery emetine hydrochloride is frequently given by injection, and emetine and bismuth iodide by mouth. Psychotrine and its *O*-methyl ether are selective inhibitors of human immunodeficiency virus and their study could lead to the development of therapeutically useful agents (G. J. Tan *et al.*, *J. Biol. Chem.*, 1991, **266**, 23529).

Cocillana

Cocillana *BP* 2001 (Grape Bark, Guapi Bark) is the dried bark of *Guarea rusbyi* (Meliaceae) and other closely related species. The trees are native to the South American Andes and the bark is collected in Bolivia and Haiti.

Macroscopical characters. The commercial bark which has a slight aromatic odour, occurs in fairly large flattish or curved pieces, up to 60 cm long and 5–20 mm thick. Externally, the cork may be quite extensive and fissured, but the outer layers are missing in some areas and covered by lichen patches in others. The inner surface shows longitudinal striations and is lighter in colour than the grey-brown or orange brown outer tissues.

Microscopical characters. The lignified cork cells occur in bands alternating with layers of lignified parenchyma and sclereids. In the phloem the narrow medullary rays, some cells of which are sclerenchymatous, run between numerous fibre groups, each containing a prism sheath. Many cells contain pigmented contents and a little starch is present. For illustrations showing the macroscopical and microscopical features of the drug, see previous editions.

Constituents.   There appears to be no recent work which delineates the active constituents of the drug and it is placed in this position because of its association with ipecacuanha. Arising from work carried out at the end of the nineteenth century, the bark is described as containing 2.3% resins, 2.5% fixed oil, tannin, a small quantity of alkaloid and possibly a glycoside. A study carried out in 1966, which duplicated the earlier methods of extraction and fractionation, gave different results and added credence to the widespread belief that present commercial supplies may not be identical with the earlier ones.

Uses.   A liquid extract, with other ingredients, is used in the form of a linctus as an expectorant giving an alternative to ipecacuanha in the treatment of coughs.

AMARYLLIDACEAE ALKALOIDS

The bulbs of this family are well-known for their toxic properties, at least one fatality in the UK being recorded in 1999 as a result of mistaken consumption of daffodil bulbs for onions.

The alkaloids are derived from one molecule of phenylalanine and one of tyramine and biochemically fall into three series depending on the type of oxidative phenolic coupling undergone by the precursor p'-O-methylnorbelladine (formula Fig. 26.13). These series are represented by the alkaloids haemanthamine (p,p'coupling, lycorine (o,p' coupling) and galanthamine (o',p coupling) (Fig. 26.23), all three types often co-occurring in one species. Some 20 genera of the family produce these alkaloids but in the past they have been of minor significance in Western medicine. However *Narcissus tazetta* var. *chinensis*,

Haemanthamine

Lycorine

Galanthamine

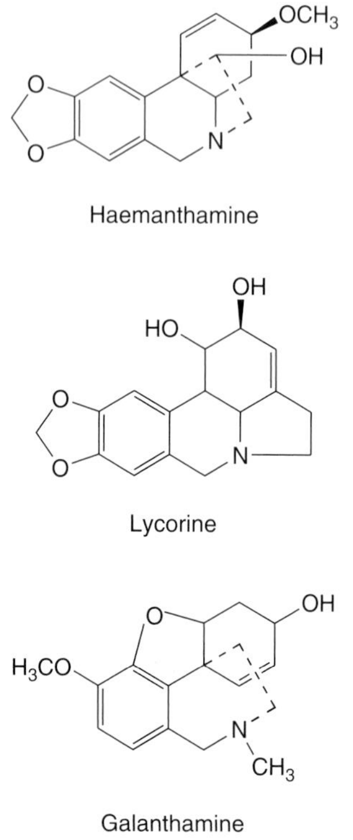

Fig. 26.23
Structural types of Amaryllidaceae alkaloids.

the bulbs of which contain lycorine, pseudolycorine and tazettine, is described in Chinese traditional and herbal remedy texts.

O. Hoshino has reviewed (203 refs) the Amaryllidaceae alkaloids considering ten types plus miscellaneous alkaloids (*The Alkaloids*, 1998, **51**, 323).

Currently there is much interest in galanthamine which has emerged as a useful drug for the treatment of Alzheimer's disease.

Galanthamine (Galantamine)

This base was first isolated from the Caucasian snowdrop *Galanthus woronowi* by Russian workers in 1952 and subsequently by other scientists from the common snowdrop *G. nivalis*. It was rapidly shown to be a metabolite of many species of the family (J. J. Willaman and H.-L. Li, *J. Nat. Prod.*, 1970, **33**, 17) from which *Leucojum aestivum* has emerged as a commercial source with the consequence that wild plants are, like many other medicinal plants, becoming an endangered species.

A. Poulev *et al.* (*Planta Medica*, 1993, **59**, 442) have used ELISA techniques (Ch. 16) for the quantitative determination of galanthamine in plant materials and obtained yields of from 0.1 to 2.0% for the dried bulbs of *L. aestivum* with *Phaedranassa negistrophylla* from Peru giving 7.4%. Various *Narcissus* cultivars have been examined for the alkaloid and it has been shown that planting depth, planting density, bulb size and flower bud removal did not affect the galanthamine content (R. M. Moraes-Cerdeira *et al.*, *Planta Medica*, 1997, **63**, 472). *N. confusus*, endemic to Spain, is reported to have the highest galanthamine content of the genus reaching in the emerging bulb a maximum concentration of up to 2.5%, dry weight (S. Lopez *et al.*, *Planta Medica*, 2003, **69**, 1166).

There is a considerable body of literature on the pharmacology of galanthamine (see review by A. L. Harvey, *Pharmac. Ther.*, 1995, **68**, 113) and readers will note a possible confusion in nomenclature in a number of the more recent publications by use of the designation 'galantamine', a name also employed by the manufacturer to describe the new product mentioned below.

Galanthamine is an acetylcholinesterase inhibitor and as such has been used extensively since the late 1950s in Eastern Europe and the former Soviet Union in anaesthesia as a curare reversal agent. Secondly, the alkaloid also acts centrally by penetrating the blood–brain barrier to serve as a modulator of nicotinic cholinergic receptors, thus augmenting central cholinergic neurotransmission. It is the latter which has invoked investigation into its use in the palliative treatment of Alzheimer's disease.

Clinical trials with the isolated alkaloid involving patients presenting with mild to moderate symptoms of Alzheimer's disease have given positive findings for the improvement of memory and intellectual functioning. The drug, as Reminyl®, was granted European marketing approval in July 2000.

Further reading

Hanks GR (ed), Hardman R (series ed) 2002 Medicinal and aromatic plants – industrial profiles, Vol 21. Narcissus and daffodil – the genus *Narcissus*. CRC Press, Taylor and Francis Group, Boca Raton, FL
Heinrich M, Teoh HL 2004 Galanthamine from snowdrop – the development of a modern drug against Alzheimer's disease from local Caucasian knowledge. J Ethnopharmacology 92: 147–162. *Review with about 80 references*

PHENETHYLISOQUINOLINE ALKALOIDS

This group of alkaloids was first recognized in 1966 during investigations on the biosynthetic origin of colchicine, the principal alkaloid of the autumn crocus. They represent analogues of the benzyltetrahydroisoquinoline alkaloids and are found in a number of genera of the Liliaceae.

Colchicine-type alkaloids are present in many species of *Colchicum* (e.g. *C. luteum* and *C. speciosum*). Also, the genera *Androcymbium*, *Bulbocodium*, *Camptorrhiza*, *Dipidax*, *Gloriosa*, *Iphigenia*, *Littonia*, *Merendera*, *Ornithoglossum* and *Sandersonia* possess similar constituents.

Colchicum seed and corm; Colchicine

Colchicum seed and corm are derived from the autumn crocus or meadow saffron, *Colchicum autumnale* (Liliaceae). The plant, whose life cycle is described below, is found in Britain and in many other parts of Europe. Commercial supplies come from Poland, Czechoslovakia, former Yugoslavia and The Netherlands. *Colchicum luteum* is used in Indian medicine.

History. Drugs believed to have been derived from species of *Colchicum* have long been known under the names of 'colchicum', 'hermodactyl', 'surinjan' and 'ephemeron', and some have been identified as *C. autumnale*. Dioskurides was aware of the poisonous nature of a *Colchicum* which may or may not have been the species now used in medicine. The genus derives its name from Colchis on the Black Sea, one of the places where this plant is found. The drug was recommended in Arabian writings for use in gout, but it was little employed in either classical or mediaeval times, owing to the wholesome fear inspired by its poisonous properties. Colchicum corm appeared in the *London Pharmacopoeias* of 1618, 1627, 1632 and 1639. It was then deleted but reappeared in the edition of 1788. The uncertain action of the corm led Dr W. H. Williams, of Ipswich, to introduce the use of the seeds about 1820, and these were admitted to the *Pharmacopoeia* of 1824. Colchicine was isolated by Pelletier and Caventou in 1820.

Life cycle. The corm consists of an enlarged underground stem bearing foliage leaves, sheathing leaves and fibrous roots. If the plants are examined in the latter part of the summer, it will be found that a new corm is developing in the axil of a scale leaf near the base of the old corm, the new plant occupying an infolding in the side of the parent corm. In September the parent corm bears the remains of recently withered leaves and is very much larger than the daughter corm. For medicinal purposes the corm would have been collected shortly after the withering of the leaves ('early summer') and before the enlargement of its axial bud. The corms are surrounded by a dark, membranous coat. The young corm develops fibrous roots at its base, and in August or September two to six flowers emerge from it, but its foliage leaves do not appear above ground until the following spring. The flowers are 10–12 cm long. Each has six stamens and a perianth consisting of six lilac or pale-purple segments which fuse into an exceptionally long perianth tube, at the base of which lies the superior ovary. More than half the length of the flower is below ground, and the fruit lies protected throughout the winter by the surrounding corm and earth. The fruit is a three-lobed, three-celled, septicidal capsule, which is carried above ground in the spring by the expanding leaves. The fully grown leaves are radical, linear-lanceolate and about 12 cm long. During these changes the daughter corm grows at the expense of the parent, which now gradually perishes. Before doing so, however, it may produce in its second spring one or more small corms by means of which the number of plants may be increased.

Characters of seed. The seeds are collected when ripe, usually in July or August, and dried. They are ovoid or globular in shape and 2–3 mm in diameter. They are extremely hard and have a reddish-brown, minutely pitted testa. During drying the seeds darken in colour and become covered with a sugary exudation. The seed, as in most Liliaceae, develops from an amphitropous ovule. From a slight projection at the hilum there extends for about one-quarter of the circumference a well-marked strophiole. The small embryo lies embedded in horny endosperm.

Microscopical examination shows that the testa consists of somewhat thick-walled reddish-brown parenchyma; that the endosperm cells have pitted walls and contain fixed oil and aleurone grains up to 5 mm in diameter; and that the strophiole contains starch.

Colchicum seeds contain 0.6–1.2% of colchicine, a number of other colchicine-type alkaloids, a resin, fixed oil and reducing sugars.

Characters of corm. The corms are collected about July, cut into transverse slices and dried at a temperature not exceeding 65°C. The outer membranes are rejected. The whole corms are 2–3 cm diameter, but the dried drug consists of somewhat reniform, transverse slices and occasional more ovate longitudinal slices, about 2–5 mm thick. The epidermal surface is cinnamon-brown and slightly wrinkled. The interior is white and starchy and, if carefully smoothed, shows scattered fibrovascular bundles. The drug breaks with a short mealy fracture. The odour is much less marked than in the fresh drug. Taste, bitter.

Microscopical examination shows numerous starch grains contained in parenchyma, some simple but the majority consisting of two to seven components. Individual grains are from 6 to 30 μm diameter, and show a triangular or star-shaped hilum. Their shape varies from spherical or ovoid to polygonal. Vessels with a spiral or annular thickening and portions of brownish epidermis with very occasional circular stomata may also be seen.

On treating the drug with 60–70% sulphuric acid or with concentrated hydrochloric acid, a yellow colour, due to colchicine, is produced. The corms contain up to about 0.6% colchicine, other related alkaloids and starch.

Colchicine

This is an amorphous, yellowish-white alkaloid, which darkens on exposure to light and gives a yellow coloration with strong mineral acids. Colchicine readily dissolves in water, alcohol or chloroform but is only slightly soluble in ether or petroleum spirit. It is a weak base and may be extracted from either acid or alkaline solution by means of chloroform. Colchicine *BP/EP* is assayed by non-aqueous titration.

The rather unusual chemical structure of colchicine meant that its probable biogenetic origin from simpler molecules could not be easily predicted. Examples of the occurrence of the tropolone ring (ring C) are rare in higher plants, although it features in mould metabolism; also, the position of the nitrogen atom is unusual. Owing mainly to the work of Battersby, Leete and their coworkers involving tracer studies on *C. autumnale* and *C. byzantium*, the principal pathway for the biogenesis of colchicine has now been established.

Ring A and carbons 5, 6 and 7 are derived from phenylalanine; the tropolone moiety arises from tyrosine by ring cleavage followed by closure to give a seven-membered ring. In contrast to mould metabolism, acetate does not contribute directly to the tropolone ring but is merely effective in supplying the *N*-acetyl group. An intermediate formed early in the pathway as the result of union of the two amino acids is a 1-phenylethylisoquinoline derivative. This is a member of a class of alkaloids first reported in 1966, the first two representatives being androcymbine and the dimer melanthioidine, alkaloids of *Androcymbium melanthioides*, a close relative of colchicum. Demecolcine, also a constituent of *Colchicum* spp., is a more immediate precursor of colchicine. The sequential formation of these compounds is indicated in Fig. 26.24. (For a study on the early stages of colchicine biosynthesis leading to the formation of phenethylisoquinoline intermediates see R. B. Herbert *et al.*, *Tetrahedron*, 1990, **46**, 7119 and for more recent refinements to the biosynthetic sequence see A. Nasreen *et al.*, *Phytochemistry*, 1997, **46**, 107).

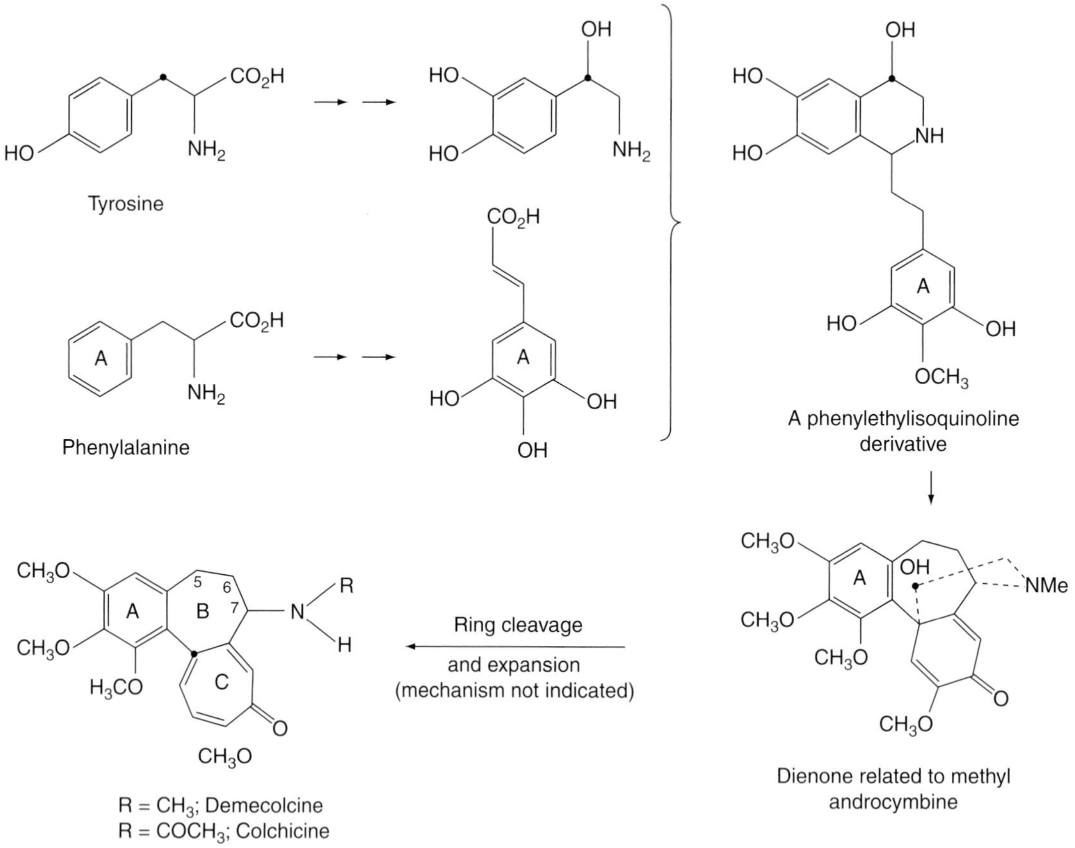

Fig. 26.24
Steps in the biogenesis of colchicine.

The richest sources of colchicine are the corms and seeds, but the difficulty of obtaining adequate supplies of these has led Šantavý and coworkers (*Planta Med.*, 1979, **36**, 119; 1981, **43**, 153) to investigate the possibility of using leaves and flowers for extraction purposes. In colchicine content the flowers compare with the seeds. The leaves contain only one-fifteenth the alkaloid content of the seeds but, compared with the corms, they contain half the amount of 2-demethyl-demecolcine. The latter alkaloid can be chemically converted to demecolcine. On slow drying of the leaves, the proportion of 2- and 3-demethylated derivatives of colchicine increases; these are not glycosidic breakdown products but arise from unknown compounds as a result of enzymatic liberation. Suspension and callus cultures of *C. autumnale* have been shown to produce colchicine.

Uses. Colchicum preparations are used to relieve gout, but must be employed with caution. Colchicine is frequently prescribed in tablet form and transdermal preparations containing colchicine are the subject of a Japanese patent (1991). The alkaloid is also used in biological experiments to produce polyploidy or multiplication of the chromosomes in a cell nucleus (see Chapter 14).

Further reading

Lettello C 2000 The pharmacology and therapeutic aspects of colchicine. Alkaloids 53: 287–352

TRYPTOPHAN-DERIVED ALKALOIDS

With a few minor exceptions, tryptophan and its decarboxylation product, tryptamine, give rise to the large class of indole alkaloids. These bases usually contain two nitrogen atoms; one is the indolic nitrogen and the second is generally two carbons removed from the β-position of the indole ring. Of the several alkaloid groups within the indole class, two may be produced, depending on the type of condensation occurring between tryptamine and an aldehyde or ketoacid. A Mannich reaction involving the α-carbon atom of the indole nucleus affords a β-carboline derivative; reaction involving the β-position gives rise to an indolenine (Fig. 26.25).

A number of simple tryptamine derivatives and β-carbolines have psychomimetic properties; for a review of their phytochemistry, chemotaxonomy and pharmacology, see Allen and Holmstedt (*Phytochemistry*, 1980, **19**, 1573).

Some examples of alkaloids of pharmaceutical interest, derived from tryptamine, are given in Fig. 26.26. It will be noted that the more complex indole alkaloids contain a non-tryptophan-derived portion of the molecule and this is supplied by mevalonic acid, which in the case of the ergot alkaloids is a C_5-isopentenyl unit and with the alkaloids of the Apocynaceae, Loganiaceae, Rubiaceae etc., a C_{10}-geraniol (monoterpenoid) contribution. Some 2000 monoterpenoid alkaloids are known and Fig. 26.27 illustrates how a number of alkaloid types within this group can arise.

A key intermediate in the biogenesis of the monoterpene indole alkaloids is $3\alpha(S)$-strictosidine; it was first isolated in 1968 by G. N. Smith from *Rhazya stricta* and until 1997 its structure was based on compounds of known stereochemistry, then, direct instrumental measurements furnished its first detailed stereochemical analysis (Á. Patthy Lukats, *J. Nat. Prod.*, 1997, **60**, 69). It is formed by the enzymatic condensation of tryptamine and secologanin (Fig. 26.28). The enzyme responsible for this important reaction, strictosidine synthase, has been isolated and characterized from

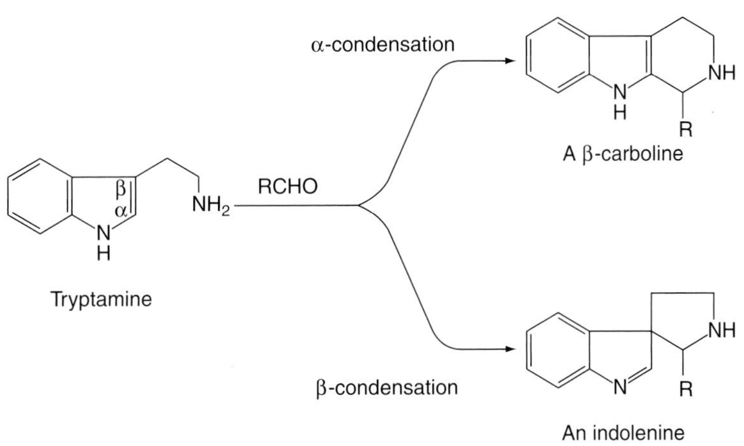

Fig. 26.25
Formation of the indole alkaloids.

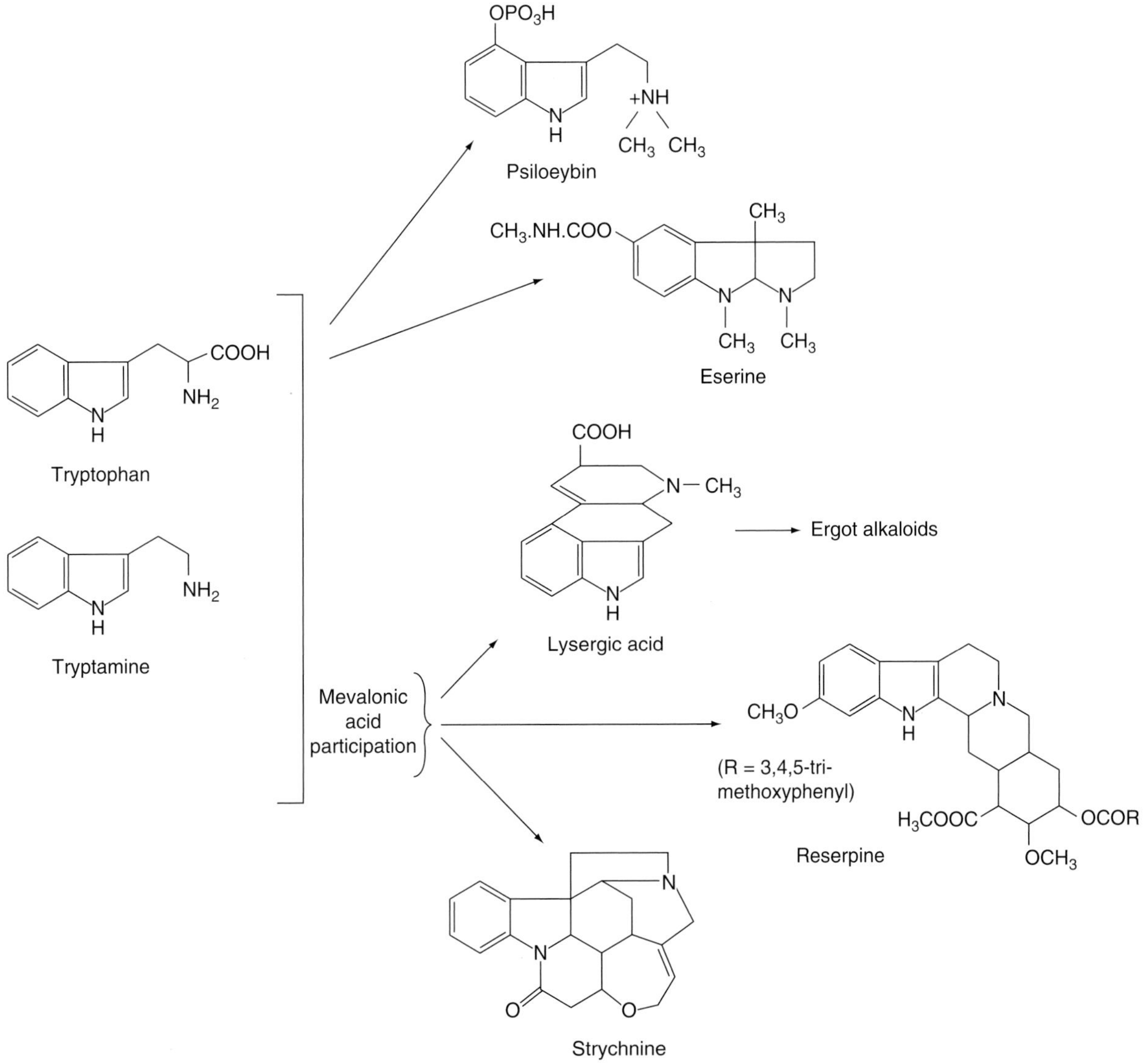

Fig. 26.26
Tryptophan and tryptamine as precursors of indole alkaloids.

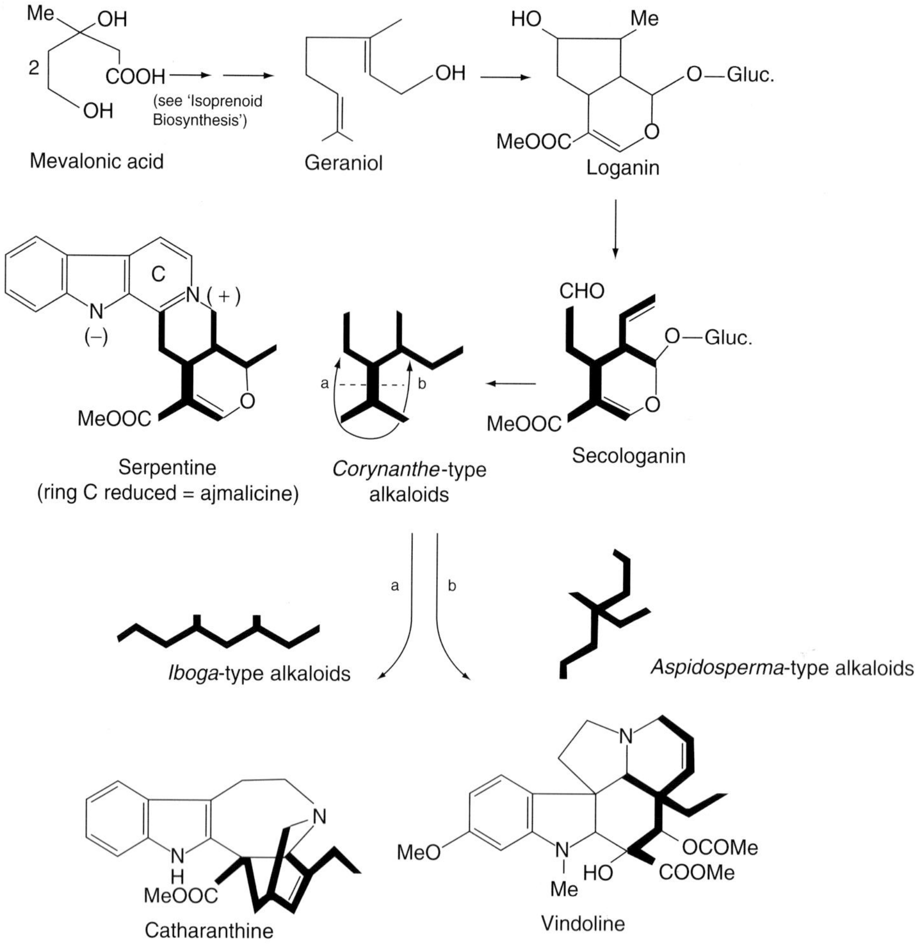

26

Fig. 26.27
Incorporation of mevalonic acid into some
indole alkaloids.

cell cultures of a number of species including *Rauwolfia serpentina*, *Cinchona robusta* and *Catharanthus roseus* and a number of isoforms have been described. The *R. serpentina* gene relating to this enzyme has been cloned and heterologously expressed in microorganisms including *Escherichia coli* and *Saccharomyces cerevisiae* (baker's yeast). This example represented the first cloning of cDNA for an enzyme of alkaloid biosynthesis. The gene is a single polypeptide M_r about 34 000, possessing a 5.3% carbohydrate content. An investigation of 10 spp. of *Rauwolfia* using a polymerase chain reaction comparison showed the gene to be highly conserved, which was unexpected considering the geographical range of the species and the fact that it would be conventionally considered as an unimportant gene of secondary metabolism.

Strictosidine glucosidase was reported in 1996 from a suspension cell culture of *Tabernaemontana divaricata* (T. J. C. Luijendijk *et al.*, *Phytochemistry*, 1996, **41**, 1451).

Prior to 1977, 3β(*R*)-vincoside (Fig. 26.28), the epimer of 3α(*S*)-strictosidine was accepted as the naturally occurring precursor of the monoterpenoid indole alkaloids and elaborate biomimetric models had to be conceived to accommodate the necessary inversion of configuration at C-3 to give the natural alkaloids. Quinine is also derived from tryptophan but this is not immediately obvious by inspection of its formula; its biogenesis is outlined under 'Cinchona'. The antileukaemic alkaloids of *Catharanthus roseus*, vinblastine and vincristine are dimeric alkaloids of this group (see Chapter 27) and their biogenesis, production in artificial culture and enzymic aspects remain a most active area of research.

ERGOT AND ERGOT ALKALOIDS

Ergot (*Ergot of Rye*) is the dried sclerotium of a fungus, *Claviceps purpurea* Tulasne (Clavicipitaceae), arising in the ovary of the rye, *Secale cereale*. Controlled field cultivation on rye is the main source of the crude drug. The most important producers are Czechoslovakia, Hungary, Switzerland and former Yugoslavia. With modern farming the supply of 'natural' ergot is decreasing and fields of rye are devoted to its cultivation. Different selected strains of *C. purpurea* are used for the production of the alkaloids ergotamine, ergocristine, or ergocornine and ergokryptine. Commercially, ergot of rye is becoming less important and by 1994 UK dealers were trading mainly in ergot of wheat.

History. There is considerable doubt as to whether ergot and ergotism were known to the ancients, and it is impossible to say whether the 'ignis sacer' of the Romans referred to ergotism. The outbreaks of 'ignis St Antonii', or St Antony's fire, which occurred during the Middle Ages, do, however, appear to have been of ergot origin. Outbreaks of ergotism occurred in Germany in 1581, 1587 and 1596 and at intervals in Europe until recent years. Ergotism was never common in England, probably owing to the fact that rye is little grown, and the only serious outbreak recorded, which took place in 1762, was caused by wheat.

World-wide, sporadic reports of ergot poisoning still appear in the literature and in 1992 an analysis of rye flour sold in Canada showed that low-level contamination by the fungus still exists; of 128 samples tested 118 proved positive for ergot alkaloids at concentrations of 70–414 ng g^{-1} whereas with wheat flour the incidence and levels were much lower.

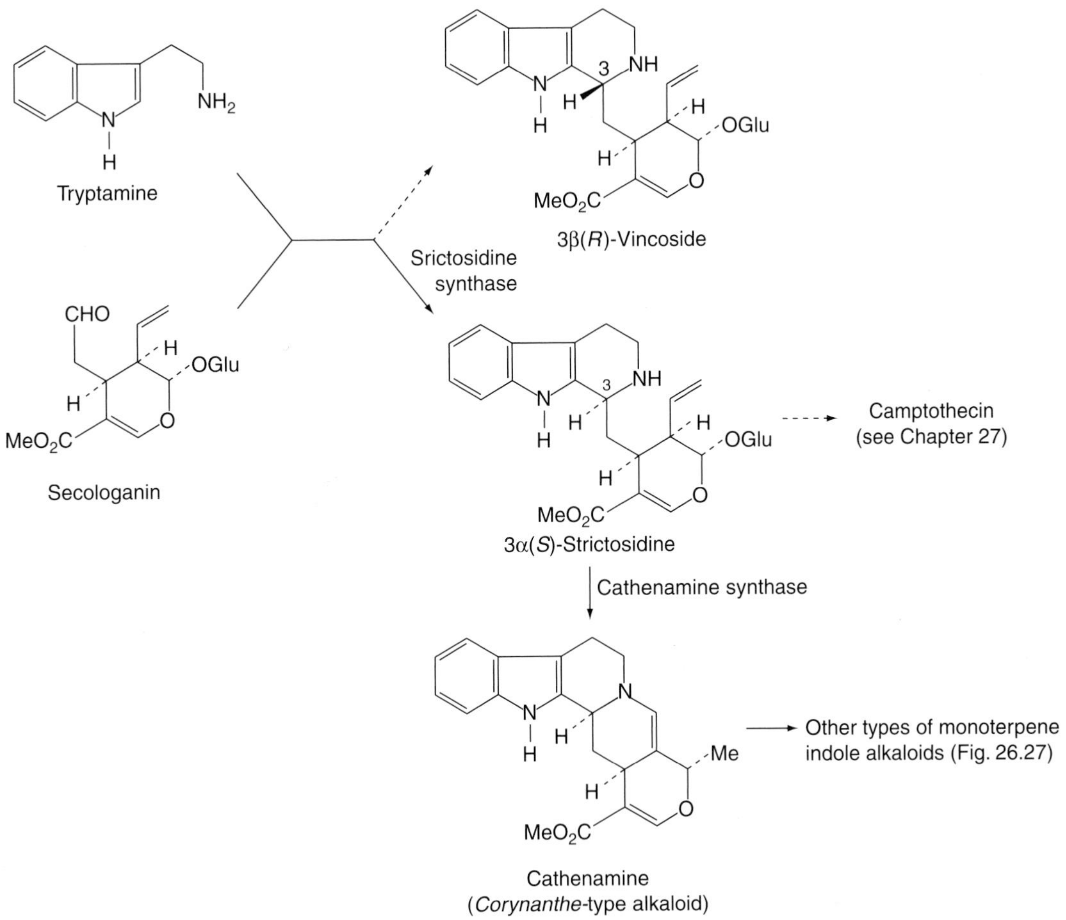

Fig. 26.28
Formation and metabolism of strictosidine.

The obstetric use of ergot was known in the sixteenth century, but the drug was not widely employed until the nineteenth century. It was first introduced into the *London Pharmacopoeia* of 1836. The fungoid origin of ergot was recognized by Münchausen in 1764, while the life history of the fungus was worked out and the name *Claviceps purpurea* given to it by Tulasne in 1853.

Life history and collection. The fungus *C. purpurea* and other species such as *C. microcephala* Wallr., *C. nigricans* Tul. and *C. paspali* produce ergots on many members of the Gramineae (including the genera *Triticum, Avena, Festuca, Poa, Lolium, Molinia* and *Nardus*) and Cyperaceae (including the genera *Scirpus* and *Ampelodesma*). Many of these ergots appear to be extremely toxic and to produce typical ergotism.

For the life-cycle and illustrations of the fungus, see earlier editions.

Macroscopical characters. The drug consists almost entirely of sclerotia, the amount of other organic matter being generally limited to not more than 1%. Each sclerotium is about 1.0–4 cm long and 2–7 mm broad; fusiform in shape and usually slightly curved. The outer surface, which is of a dark, violet-black colour, is often longitudinally furrowed and may bear small transverse cracks. Ergot breaks with a short fracture and shows within the thin, dark outer layer a whitish or pinkish-white central zone of pseudoparenchyma in which darker lines radiating from the centre may be visible. Ergot has a characteristic odour and an unpleasant taste.

Powdered ergot when treated with sodium hydroxide solution develops a strong odour of trimethylamine. In filtered ultraviolet light it has a strong reddish colour by means of which its presence in flour may be detected.

Microscopical characters. Ergot shows an outer zone of purplish-brown, rectangular cells, which are often more or less obliterated. The pseudoparenchyma consists of oval or rounded cells containing fixed oil and protein, and possessing highly refractive walls which give a reaction for chitin. Cellulose and lignin are absent.

Constituents. The ergot alkaloids (ergolines) can be divided into two classes: (1) the clavine-type alkaloids, which are derivatives of 6,8-dimethylergoline and have been extensively studied in cultures of the mycelium of the ergot fungus; and (2) the lysergic acid derivatives, which are peptide alkaloids. It is the latter class that contains the pharmacologically active alkaloids that characterize the ergot sclerotium (ergot). Each active alkaloid occurs with an inactive isomer involving isolysergic acid; the inactive isomers are not formed initially in the sclerotium but tend to accumulate as a result of unsuitable processing and poor or long storage. These alkaloids have been studied over many years and were not easy to characterize. Thus 'ergotoxine', which since its isolation in 1906 (by Barger and Carr and independently by Kraft) had been accepted as a pure substance, and in the form of ergotoxine ethanosulphonate was formerly used as a standard, was shown to be a mixture of the three alkaloids ergocristine, ergocornine and ergocryptine.

Six pairs of alkaloids predominate in the sclerotium and fall into either the water-soluble ergometrine (or ergonovine) group or the water-insoluble ergotamine and 'ergotoxine' groups. Table 26.6 gives the more

Table 26.6 Alkaloids of ergot.

	Alkaloid	Formula	Discovered
I. Ergometrine group	Ergometrine Ergometrinine	$C_{19}H_{22}O_2N_3$	Dudley and Moir (1935)
II. Ergotamine group	Ergotamine Ergotaminine	$C_{33}H_{35}O_5N_5$	Spiro and Stoll (1920)
	Ergosine Ergosinine	$C_{30}H_{37}O_5N_5$	Smith and Timmis (1937)
III. Ergotoxine group	Ergocristine Ergocristinine	$C_{35}H_{39}O_5N_5$	Stoll and Burckhardt (1937)
	Ergocryptine Ergocryptinine	$C_{32}H_{41}O_5N_5$	
	Ergocornine Ergocorninine	$C_{31}H_{39}O_5N_5$	Stoll and Hoffmann (1938, 1943)

physiologically active member of each pair first. Alkaloids of groups II and III are polypeptides in which lysergic acid or isolysergic acid is linked to other amino acids. In the ergometrine alkaloids lysergic acid or its isomer is linked to an amino alcohol. Ergometrine was synthesized by Stoll and Hofmann in 1943. Other, new, peptide alkaloids have been isolated from submerged cultures of *C. purpurea* and from the field-growing fungus (L. Cvak *et al.*, *Phytochemistry*, 1996, **42**, 231; 1997, **44**, 365).

Among the less important constituents of ergot may be mentioned histamine, tyramine and other amines and amino acids; acetylcholine; colouring matters; sterols (ergosterol and fungisterol); and about 30% fat. The cell walls are chitinous.

Variation in alkaloid constituents. Not only are chemical races very evident in *C. purpurea* with respect to alkaloid production but also the host plant is not without influence. Thus a new commercial strain of ergot adapted from a wild grass (*Anthraxon lancifolius*) to rye gave sclerotia containing 0.5% total alkaloids involving ergometrine (33%), ergotamine (17.6%), ergocornine (18.7%) and ergocryptine (22.7%). However, sclerotia produced on the grass as a result of natural infection did not contain ergometrine (K. K. Janardhanan *et al.*, *Planta Med.*, 1982, **44**, 166). The application of specific amino acids to maturing sclerotia can also be used to influence the type of alkaloids produced (a technique also used with saprophytic cultures).

For recent studies and references on the investigation of the alkaloid gene cluster in *C. purpurea* see T. Haarmann *et al.*, *Phytochemistry*, 2005, **66**, 1312.

Alkaloid production in artificial cultures. The artificial culture of the ergot fungus has received considerable attention, and, obviously, large-scale submerged fermentation with selected strains to give alkaloids of choice has commercial possibilities. Abe's initial work in Japan showed that submerged cultures did not produce the typical alkaloids associated with the sclerotium but, rather, a series of new non-peptide bases (clavines) which unfortunately possessed no significant pharmacological action. Attempts were made by many workers to influence alkaloid production by modification of the culture medium and the fungus strain. As a result of successful experiments in 1960, the commercial manufacture of simple lysergic acid derivatives by fermentative growth of a strain of *Claviceps paspali* became feasible. The alkaloids produced are converted to lysergic acid which is used for the part-synthesis of ergometrine and related alkaloids. Other strains are now available which produce the peptide alkaloids in culture; not only can different chemical races of the fungus be used to produce specific groups of alkaloids but synthesis can also be directed by the addition of certain amino acids or their analogues to the fermentation liquid. In this way new unnatural alkaloids can be produced.

Flieger *et al.* (*J. Nat. Prod.*, 1989, **52**, 1003) found that with submerged cultures in the postproduction stage both the alkaloid concentration and the composition of the alkaloid mixtures underwent dramatic changes including the production of two new alkaloids, 8-hydroxyergine and 8-hydroxyerginine. (For papers pertaining to the isolation of new and unnatural alkaloids from submerged cultures of *C. purpurea* see N. C. Perellino *et al.*, *J. Nat. Prod.*, 1992, **55**, 424; 1993, **56**, 489.)

Biosynthesis. The majority of biosynthetic studies were at first directed to the clavine alkaloids, which could be easily produced in cultures but, until recently, their biological relationship to the lysergic acid derivatives remained obscure. The ergoline nucleus is derived from tryptophan and mevalonate, and current work has involved elucidating the biosynthetic relationship between the various clavine alkaloids, determining which of these intermediates is the true natural precursor of lysergic acid, and studying the initial hydrogen elimination from the C-4 of mevalonate to yield the stereo-configuration of chanoclavine-I. Possible biosynthetic routes for lysergic acid involving two isomeric intermediates are given in Fig. 26.29. A major problem has been not so much in discovering which reactions the fungus can effect when supplied with a given substrate as which route is actually involved in its normal metabolism. As a result of work with cell-free systems, Abe assigned a primary role to 4-isopentenyltryptophan and lysergene rather than to the dimethylallyl compound, agroclavine or chanoclavine. Later work by Gröger *et al.* (*Planta Med.*, 1980, **40**, 109) appeared to favour a scheme involving the latter compounds and this has now been generally substantiated with the intermediates involved with the ring closure between dimethylallyltryptophan and chanoclavine having been investigated (A. P. Kozikowski *et al.*, *J. Amer. Chem. Soc.*, 1993, **115**, 2482).

Work on the origin of the nitrogen of the peptide portions of the ergot alkaloids indicates that appropriate amino acids are specifically incorporated. Abe's scheme is shown in Fig. 26.30 and he obtained intact incorporation of the units shown, in certain strains, but workers in Germany were unable to confirm these results. As has been mentioned earlier, unnatural amino acids can also be incorporated into the alkaloids.

Varieties. Commercial ergot varies considerably in activity from batch to batch, and the differences cannot be fully explained by differences in storage; further, it is often found that inferior-looking ergot is highly active. Such variations are apparently due to the fact that there are a number of different chemical races of *C. purpurea* and in cultivating ergot by modern methods it is obviously important to prepare the spore-cultures used for infecting the rye from a race of the fungus known to develop ergots having a high content of the required

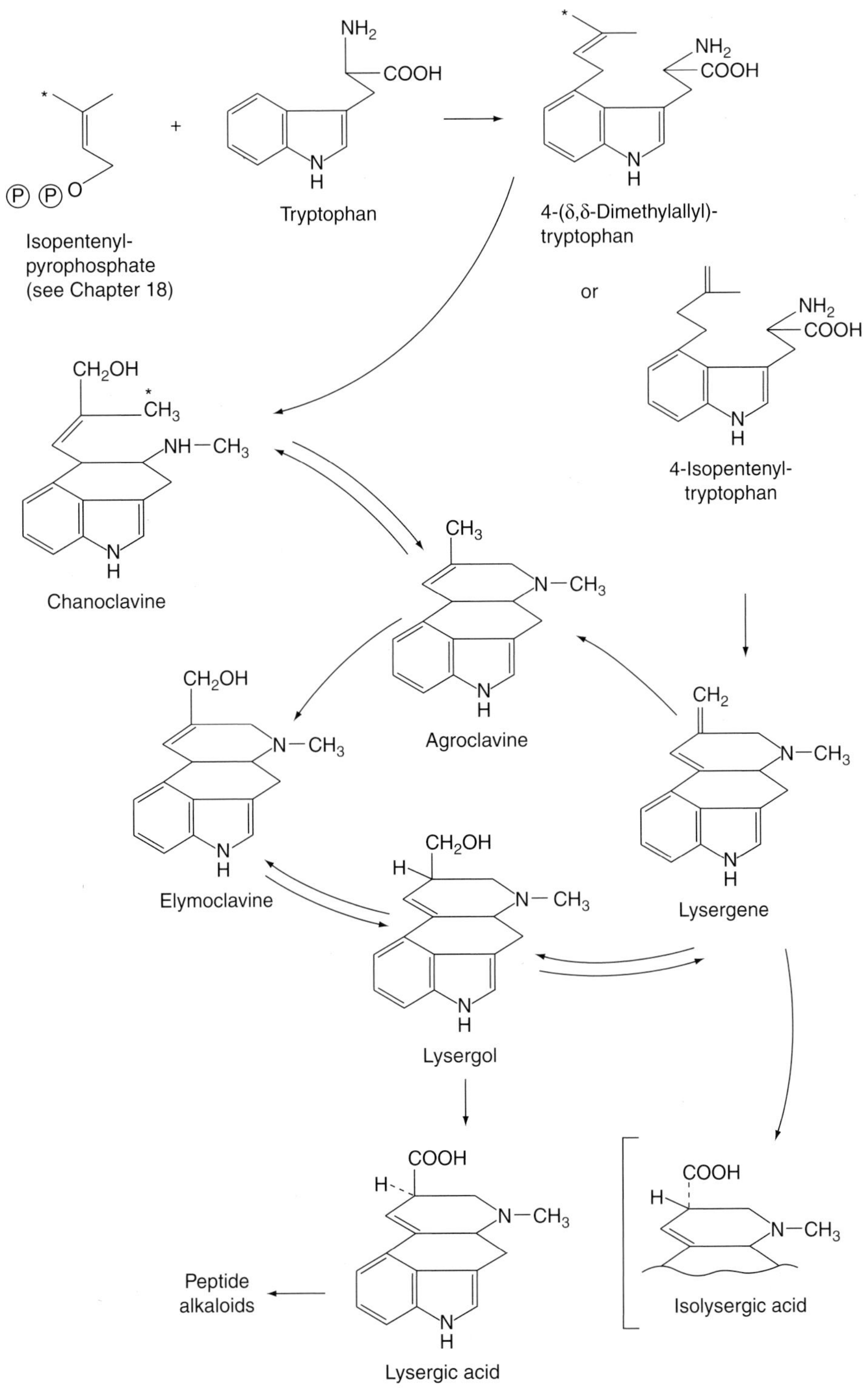

Fig. 26.29
Possible biogenesis of lysergic acid.

alkaloids. Cultivated ergot may contain up to 0.5% of total alkaloids, and 0.15% is a minimum commercial value. In addition, there may be a minimal requirement for water-soluble alkaloids. The alkaloids can be determined by colorimetry, as they give a blue colour with a solution of p-dimethylaminobenzaldehyde.

Substitutes. *Ergot of wheat* is now imported into Britain and has been used medicinally in France. The sclerotia are shorter and thicker than those of rye. Instances of ergot on barley and rye in Britain, and on wheat and rye in the USA and Canada have been reported.

Ergot of oats has been used medicinally in Algiers. The sclerotia are black in colour, 10–12 mm long and 3–4 mm diameter.

Ergot of diss, which is produced on the Algerian reed *Ampelodesma tenax*, has appeared in commerce and is said to be highly active. The sclerotia may attain as much as 9 cm in length and are spirally twisted.

Storage. Ergot is particularly liable to attack by insects, moulds and bacteria. After collection it should be thoroughly dried, kept entire, and stored in a cool, dry place. If powdered and not immediately defatted, the activity decreases, but if defatted and carefully stored in an air-tight

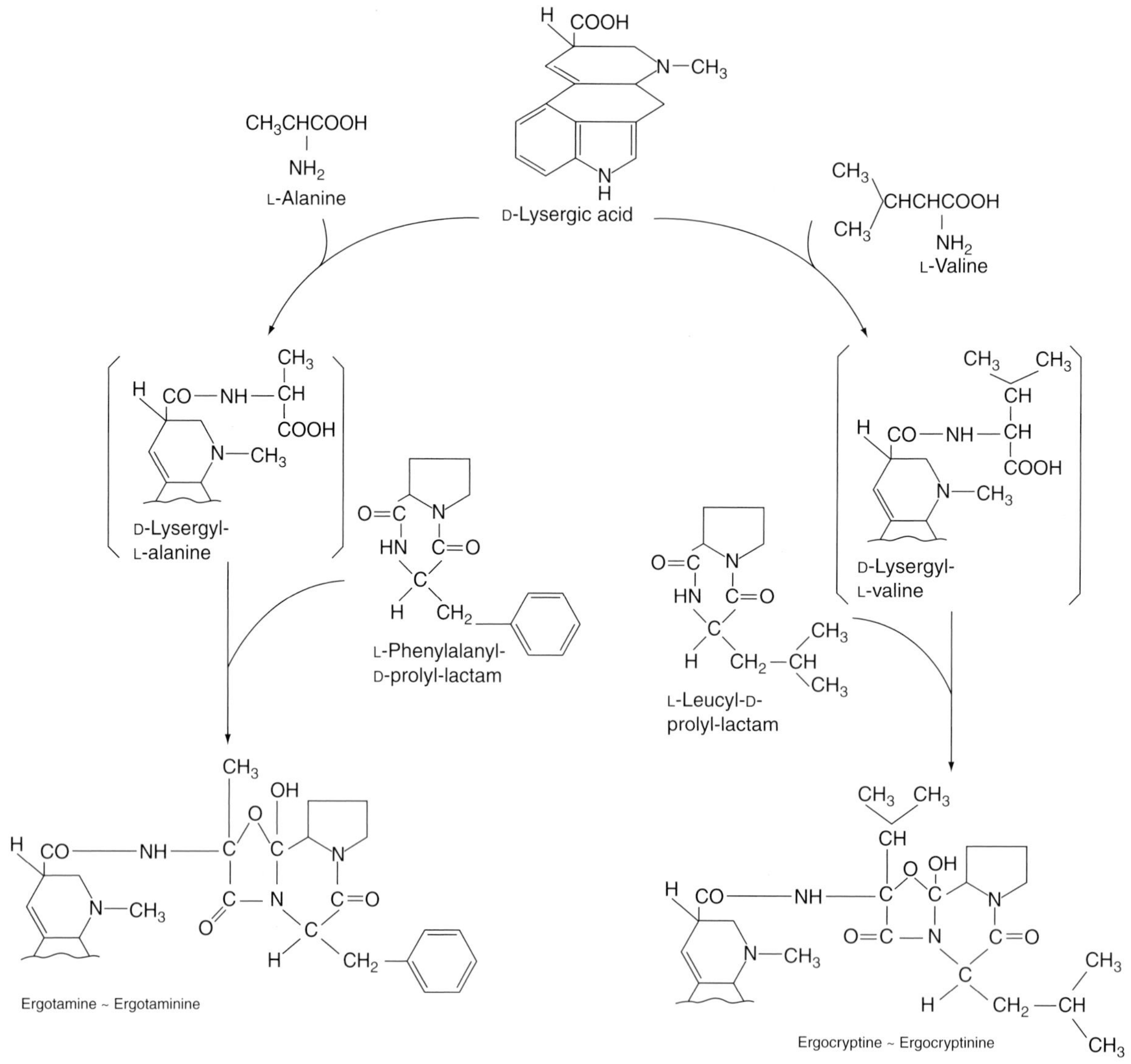

Fig. 26.30
Biogenesis of ergot peptide alkaloids (after Abe).

container, it will remain active for a long period. However, as indicated above, under certain conditions, loss of activity arises by the conversion of the pharmacologically important alkaloids to inactive isomers. Any sample of ergot which shows worm holes or a considerable amount of insect debris will almost certainly deteriorate further on storage.

Uses. Although whole ergot preparations were traditionally used in labour to assist delivery and to reduce post-partum haemorrhage, ergot itself has been largely replaced in the pharmacopoeias by the isolated alkaloids. Only ergometrine produces an oxytocic (literally 'quick delivery') effect, ergotoxine and ergotamine having quite a different action. Ergometrine is soluble in water or in dilute alcohol. It is often known, particularly in the USA, as ergonovine. Ergotamine and the semisynthetic dihydroergotamine salts are employed as specific analgesics for the treatment of migraine. Lysergic acid diethylamide (LSD-25), prepared by partial synthesis from lysergic acid, is a potent specific psychotomimetic.

Calabar bean and physostigmine

Calabar beans (*Ordeal beans*) are the dried ripe seeds of *Physostigma venenosum* (Leguminosae), a perennial woody climber found on the banks

of streams in West Africa. The plant bears typical papilionaceous flowers, and legumes about 15 cm long, each containing two or three seeds.

History. The seeds were formerly used by the west African tribes as an 'ordeal poison'. They were first known in England in 1840. The myotic effect of the drug was noted in 1862 by Fraser, and physostigmine was isolated in 1864 by Jobst and Hesse.

Characters. Calabar beans have a somewhat flattened, reniform shape. They are 15–30 mm long, 10–15 mm wide and up to 15 mm thick. The seeds are extremely hard. The dark brown testa is smooth, except in the neighbourhood of the grooved hilum, which runs the whole length of the convex side and round one end, where it is somewhat wrinkled. On either side of the groove is a well-marked ridge and in the groove itself are the greyish, papery remains of the funiculus. A transverse section shows a large central cavity and two, very hard, concavo-convex cotyledons.

Constituents. The seeds contain the alkaloids physostigmine or eserine, eseramine, isophysostigmine, physovenine, geneserine, *N*-8-norphysostigmine, calabatine and calabacine. The structure of geneserine, long regarded as an *N*-oxide, has been revised to include the oxygen in a ring system. The chief alkaloid, physostigmine, is present to the extent of about 0.15%. It is derived from tryptophan (see Fig. 26.26). On exposure to air it oxidizes into a red compound, rubreserine, and should therefore be protected from air and light. Both physostigmine salicylate and sulphate are included in the *BP/EP*. The former of the two is more stable and non-deliquescent. For both salts there is a colorimetic test for the elimination of eseridine and a non-aqueous titration assay.

Uses.   Physostigmine salicylate is used for contracting the pupil of the eye, often to combat the effect of mydriatics. It has also been investigated as an intravenous injection for reversing the effects of a number of sedatives. With Alzheimer's disease it has shown some evidence of inducing a slight improvement in intellectual and cognitive performance (*Pharm. J.*, 1992, **249**, 376) but galanthamine (q.v.) may prove superior. Physovenine has the same order of activity but that of eseramine is much lower.

Nux vomica

Nux vomica consists of the dried, ripe seeds of *Strychnos nux-vomica* (Loganiaceae), a tree 10–13 m high with a distribution including Ceylon, India, East Bengal, Burma, Thailand, Laos, Cambodia and S. Vietnam. The drug is mainly collected in India and exported from Mumbai (Bombay), Madras, Cochin, Cocanada and Calcutta.

History.   Nux vomica was known in Europe in the sixteenth century and was sold in England in the time of Parkinson (1640), mainly for poisoning animals. Strychnine was isolated in 1817 and brucine in 1819.

Collection and preparation.   The fruit is a berry about the size of a small orange. When ripe it has a rather hard orange-yellow epicarp and a white, pulpy, interior in which 1–5 seeds are embedded. The seeds are washed free from pulp and dried. They are exported in small sacks, known as 'pockets', holding about 18–25 kg.

Macroscopical characters.   Nux vomica seeds are extremely hard and should be boiled in water for at least an hour in order to soften them sufficiently for dissection. The seeds are greenish-grey, disc-shaped, 10–30 mm diameter and 4–6 mm thick. Most of the seeds are nearly flat and regular in shape, but a few are irregularly bent and somewhat oval in outline. The edge is rounded or acute. The testa is covered with silky, closely appressed, radiating hairs. In the centre of one of the flattened sides is a distinct hilum, and a small prominence on the circumference marks the position of the micropyle, which is joined to the hilum by a radial ridge. To examine further, a boiled seed should be cut transversely and another one opened like an oyster by inserting the blade of a small knife or scalpel at a point on the circumference opposite the micropyle. The small embryo with two cordate cotyledons and a cylindrical radicle, the latter directed towards the micropyle, will be seen embedded in a grey, horny endosperm (Fig. 26.31). In the centre of the seed is a slit-like cavity. The seeds are odourless when dry; but if soaked in water and left for a day or two, they develop a very unpleasant odour. They have a very bitter taste.

Microscopical characters.   A radial section shows a very thin testa consisting of collapsed parenchyma and an epidermal layer of very characteristic lignified hairs (Fig. 41.7M). The latter have a very large, thick-walled base with slit-like pits. Surface irregularities in the bases of the hairs cause them to interlock with one another. The upper portions of the hairs are set at almost a right angle to the bases and all radiate out towards the margin of the seed, giving the testa its characteristic silky appearance. On the ridge connecting hilum and micropyle, however, the hairs are irregularly arranged. The upper part of the wall

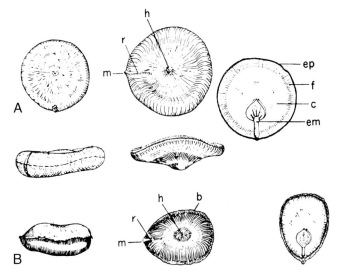

Fig. 26.31
A, *Strychnos nux-vomica* seed; B, *S. nux-blanda* seed. Surface and lateral views of entire seed and inner surface of horizontally split seeds. All ×0.8. m, Micropyle; r, ridge; h, hilum; b, lateral ridge; ep, epidermis; f, area of fusion of two endosperm halves; c, area of central cavity; em, embryo. (Drawn by Dr. T. D. Turner. For further details, see *J. Pharm. Pharmacol.*, 1963, **15**, 594.)

of the hair is composed of about 10 longitudinal ridge-like thickenings united by a thin wall so that the lignified ribs readily separate from one another on powdering. The lumen is circular in the upper part, but in the base has branches corresponding with the oblique pits in the wall. Fragments of testa, removed from a soaked seed, may be disintegrated by treatment with 50% nitric acid and a little potassium chlorate; the hairs can then be separated.

The endosperm consists of large, thick-walled cells, which are non-lignified and yield galactose and mannose on hydrolysis. When mounted in solution of iodine, they show well-marked protoplasmic threads (plasmodesma) passing through the walls (see Fig. 42.1G) and an oily plasma containing a few aleurone grains and the alkaloids strychnine and brucine. Strychnine is most abundant in the inner part of the endosperm and brucine in the outer layers. The presence of strychnine is shown by mounting a section in a solution of ammonium vanadate in sulphuric acid, when a violet colour is produced; of brucine, by mounting in nitric acid, when a crimson colour is observed.

The length of lignified ribs of the hairs per milligram of nux vomica seed has been used for the determination of the content of seeds in veterinary medicines, see 'Quantitative Microscopy'.

Constituents.   Nux vomica usually contains about 1.8–5.3% of the indole alkaloids strychnine and brucine. Strychnine (formula Fig. 26.26) is physiologically much more active than brucine and the seeds are therefore assayed for strychnine and not for total alkaloids. They usually contain about 1.23% of strychnine and about 1.55% of brucine. Minor related alkaloids include α-colubrine, β-colubrine, icajine, 3-methoxyicajine, protostrychnine, vomicine, novacine, *N*-oxystrychnine, pseudo-strychnine and isostrychnine.

For a review (188 refs) of recent studies concerning the synthesis of strychnine, see M. Shibasaki and T. Ohshima, *The Alkaloids*, 2006, **64**, 103.

Iridoids of the seeds include the glycoside loganin (Fig. 26.27), loganic acid and 7-*O*-acetyl loganic acid together with three new iridoids, 6'-*O*-acetyl loganic acid, 4'-*O*-acetyl loganic acid and 3'-*O*-acetyl loganic acid (X. Zhang *et al.*, *Phytochemistry*, 2003, **64**, 1341).

The seeds also contain chlorogenic acid (see Fig. 19.5) and about 3% of fixed oil.

Loganic acid: $R_1 = R_2 = R_3 = R_4 = H$
Acetyl loganic acids: acetyl groups occur singly on R_1, R_2, R_3, or R_4 (see text)

Loganin, although present only in small amounts in the seed, occurs to the extent of about 5% in the fruit pulp together with secologanin; these compounds are intermediates in the biogenesis of the strychnine-type alkaloids (Fig. 26.27).

Seasonal variations in alkaloid content of *S. nux-vomica* have been studied (K. H. C. Baser and N. G. Bisset, *Phytochemistry*, 1982, **21**, 1423).

Uses. The action of the whole drug closely resembles that of strychnine. The alkaloid was formerly used as a circulatory stimulant in such cases as surgical shock, but its use is now more limited to that of a respiratory stimulant in certain cases of poisoning. Like other bitters, strychnine improves the appetite and digestion, but it has been considerably misused as a 'general tonic'. Nux vomica is used in Chinese medicine for much the same purposes as in Western medicine and the seeds are usually processed to reduce their toxicity. Heat-treatment of the seeds reduces the normal levels of the principal alkaloids and the amounts of isostrychnine, isobrucine, strychnine *N*-oxide and brucine *N*-oxide are increased (B.-C. Cai *et al.*, *Chem. Pharm. Bull.*, 1990, **38**, 1295).

Allied drugs. The genus *Strychnos* continues to attract considerable attention. (For extensive reviews on the taxonomy, chemistry and ethnobotany of the American, African and Asian species see N. G. Bisset *et al.*, *Lloydia*, **33**, 201; **34**, 1; **35**, 95, 193; **36**, 179; **37**, 62; **39**, 263; also Bisset's review on alkaloids of the Loganiaceae in *Indole and Biogenetically Related Alkaloids*, 1980 (eds J. D. Phillipson and M. K. Zenk) p. 27, London: Academic Press; and J. Quetin-Leclercq *et al.*, *J. Ethnopharm.*, 1990, **28**, 1, review with *c.* 150 refs.)

Ignatius beans are the seeds of *Strychnos ignatii*, a plant occurring in the Philippines, Vietnam and elsewhere. The fruits are larger than those of nux vomica and may contain as many as 30 seeds. These are about 25 mm long, dark grey in colour and irregularly ovoid in shape. The structure closely resembles that of nux vomica, but the testa, which bears irregularly arranged greyish hairs, is easily rubbed off and is almost entirely absent in the commercial drug. The seeds contain about 2.5–3.0% of total alkaloids, of which about 46–62% is strychnine. They are mainly used for the preparation of strychnine and brucine. The seeds of *S. ignatii* from Java (*S. tieute*) contain 1.5% strychnine and no brucine and from Hainen (*S. hainanensis*) mainly brucine with little strychnine.

In addition to the seeds, other parts of the plants of *Strychnos* spp. may contain alkaloids including strychnine (B. De Datta and N. G. Bisset, *Planta Med.*, 1990, **56**, 133; G. Massiot *et al.*, *Phytochemistry*, 1992, **31**, 2873).

S. potatorum, from India, and *S. nux-blanda*, from Burma, have been substituted for nux vomica; although they contain no strychnine or brucine, seeds of the former have been reported to contain the alkaloid diaboline and its acetyl derivative, triterpenes and sterols. They are best distinguished by means of the ammonium vanadate reagent. The seeds of *S. potatorum* are used in India for clearing water, whence the specific name. They will also flocculate heavy metal contaminants in water and are capable of mopping up radioactive isotopes from nuclear waste. The protein responsible for this property has now been isolated (*Pharm. J.*, 1994, **252**, 238). The tannins present in the seeds are suggested as the possible active constituents associated with the folklore treatment of chronic diarrhoea (S. Biswas *et al.*, *Fitoterapia*, 2002, **73**, 43).

Gelsemium

Gelsemium consists of the dried rhizomes and roots of the American yellow jasmine, *Gelsemium sempervirens* (*G. nitidum*) family Loganiaceae, indigenous to southern USA. It is a climbing plant and produces scented yellow flowers; it should not be confused with the yellow-flowering jasmine (*Jasminum nudiflorum*, family Oleaceae) cultivated as an ornamental in Europe.

The drug occurs in cylindrical pieces 3–20 cm long and 3–30 mm diameter. The outer cork cells of the rhizome are reddish-brown and the inner ones yellowish. As growth takes place, the outer cork cells crack and the inner cork shows itself as a yellowish-brown reticulation. The roots are somewhat smaller than the rhizome and have a uniform yellowish-brown cork. Gelsemium breaks with an irregular splintery fracture. It has a slightly aromatic odour and a bitter taste. A transverse section of the rhizome shows a thick cork, a cortex containing groups of sclerenchyma, a dense wood, internal as well as external phloem and a small pith. The roots, on the other hand, have no sclerenchyma in the cortex and no pith.

Gelsemine

Gelsedine: R = H
Gelsemicine: R = OCH$_3$

Gelsemium contains extremely toxic alkaloids of unique skeletal type. Gelsemine is the principal alkaloid and is the one most studied although it is not as toxic as gelsemicine. Other oxindole bases characterized are sempervirine, 1-methoxy- and 21-oxo-gelsemine, 14-hydroxygelsemicine, gelsedine and 14-hydroxy-gelsedine. Three new alkaloids of the gelsidine type, together with an iridoid, have been reported by M. Kitajima *et al.*, *Chem. Pharm. Bull.*, 2003, **51**, 1211.

In a review (129 refs) H. Takayama and S. Sakai list 45 alkaloids derived from *G. elegans*, *G. sempervirens* and *G. rankinii*; they are classified into five groups according to structure (*The Alkaloids*, 1997, **49**, 1).

Scopoletin is responsible for the blue fluorescence of the broken drug in ultraviolet light. Iridoids and glucoiridoids have been isolated from the aerial parts.

Gelsemium is used (*BHP*, 1983) in the treatment of trigeminal neuralgia and migraine, but its use requires great care, as dangerous side-effects may develop. It has been studied for its anticancer properties.

G. elegans is used in Oriental folk medicine for much the same purposes as *G. nitidum*. For information on new and known alkaloids of the leaves and stems of this species see Y.-K. Xu *et al.*, *J. Nat. Prod.*, 2006, **69**, 1347.

Rauwolfia (Rauvolfia)

Rauwolfia consists of the dried rhizome and roots of *Rauwolfia serpentina* (*Rauvolfia serpentina*), Apocynaceae, a small shrub found in India, Pakistan, Burma, Thailand and Java. The geographical source appears to influence the alkaloidal content, and manufacturers tend to prefer drug obtained from India or Pakistan. Reserpine, the most important constituent, is contained in many other species of *Rauwolfia* (see 'African Rauwolfia' below); it is included in the *BP/EP*.

History.   Although used in India from time immemorial, it was not until 1942 that favourable reports were published of the use of the drug in powdered form. Since then research workers have studied the pharmacognosy, chemistry, pharmacology and clinical uses of many species of *Rauwolfia* and of the alkaloids obtained from them.

Collection and preparation.   The drug is collected mainly from wild plants, but cultivation of the drug will probably increase as wild plants become more scarce; in parts of India collectors are required to leave some root from each plant in the ground for future growth. Nevertheless, and coupled with the low seed viability, the plant is regarded as an endangered species in India. Consequently, the potential for the regeneration of plants from cell cultures and the possible utilization of nodal culture has received some attention (see C. M. Ruyter *et al.*, *Planta Med.*, 1991, **57**, 328; N. Sharma and K. P. S. Chandel, *Plant Cell Rep.*, 1992, **11**, 200).

As other species of *Rauwolfia* are found in India, care is needed to identify the correct plant. When first imported, many commercial samples were found to be adulterated; this was due in many cases to lack of knowledge, and substitution of, or adulteration with, other species has become much rarer in recent years. After collection the drug is cut transversely into convenient-sized pieces and dried.

Macroscopical characters.   The first detailed description of the drug was made by Wallis and Rohatgi in 1949. It usually occurs in cylindrical or slightly tapering, tortuous pieces about 2–10 cm long and 5–22 mm in diameter (Fig. 26.32A). The roots are rarely branched and rootlets, 0.5–1 mm in diameter, are rare. Pieces of rhizome closely resemble the root but may be identified by a small central pith; they occasionally have attached to them small pieces of aerial stem.

The outer surface is greyish-yellow, light brown or brown with slight wrinkles (young pieces) or longitudinal ridges (older pieces); occasional circular scars of rootlets. In this species the bark exfoliates readily, particularly in the older pieces, and may leave patches of exposed wood. The drug breaks readily with a short fracture. The smoothed transverse surface shows a narrow, yellowish-brown bark and a dense pale yellow wood, which occupies about three-quarters of the diameter. Both bark and wood contain abundant starch. Some commercial samples show mould. The recently dried drug has a slight odour which seems to decrease with age. Taste, bitter.

Microscopical characters.   The cork is stratified into about two to eight zones (Fig. 26.32E), which consist of smaller and radially narrower suberized but unlignified cells alternating with larger radially broader cells which are lignified. In many pieces much of the cork is exfoliated, and for section cutting it may be best to select pieces with little exfoliation, separate these from the wood and cut sections of the bark and wood separately. Most of the cells of the secondary cortex are parenchymatous and contain starch; isolated latex cells may occur in this region, particularly in the Dehra Dun variety. The phloem is narrow and consists mainly of parenchyma with scattered sieve tissue. Sclerenchyma is absent (distinction from many other species such as *R. tetraphylla* (*R. canescens*), *R. micrantha*, *R. densiflora*, *R. perakensis* and *R. vomitoria*; see Fig. 26.32 C, D). Most of the parenchymatous cells of the bark contain starch grains, and others prisms or conglomerate crystals of calcium oxalate.

The xylem is entirely lignified and usually shows three to six annual rings. The medullary rays, which are one to five cells wide, contain starch and alternate with the rays of the secondary xylem, which consist of vessels, fibres and xylem parenchyma. Compared with many other species of *Rauwolfia*, the vessels of *R. serpentina* are small (up to 57 μm) and are less numerous than in most of the likely adulterants. The starch grains are larger in the wood than in the bark and measure from 5–8 to 12–20 μm.

Constituents.   Rauwolfia contains at least 40 alkaloids, which total some 0.7–2.4%. Other substances present include phytosterols, fatty acids, unsaturated alcohols and sugars.

In 1931 Siddiqui and Siddiqui isolated ajmaline (rauwolfine), ajmalinine, ajmalicine, serpentine and serpentinine. The chief therapeutically important alkaloids are reserpine (isolated in 1952; formula Fig. 26.26) and rescinnamine (isolated in 1954). These are esters derived from methyl reserpate and trimethoxybenzoic acid in the case of reserpine and trimethoxycinnamic acid in the case of rescinnamine. New alkaloids continue to be isolated; recently, five anhydronium bases (e.g. 3,4,5,6-tetradehydroyohimbine) for the first time (O. Wachsmuth and R. Matusch, *Phytochemistry*, 2002, **61**, 705) and five new indole alkaloids together with a new iridoid glycoside, 7-epiloganin, a new sucrose derivative and 20 known compounds (A. Itoh *et al.*, *J. Nat. Prod.*, 2005, **68**, 848).

Cell and root cultures.   *R. serpentina* cell suspension cultures have proved an important tool in the elucidation of monoterpenoid indole alkaloid biogenesis and in this connection the significance, and isolation, of strictosidine synthase has been considered. By the use of cell cultures Stöckigt in 1988 was able to clarify a 10-step biosynthetic pathway from strictosidine to the typical rauwolfia alkaloid, ajmaline. His group has also shown that the principal alkaloid of cell suspension cultures of *R. serpentina* is raucaffricine occurring in amounts of up to 1–6 g l^{-1} in the nutrient medium, representing 2.3% of the dried cells, a value some 67 times higher than found for the roots. Ajmalicine, an antiarrhythmic drug, is also produced to the extent of 0.6% (cell dry wt.) together with over 30 different monoterpenoid alkaloids in trace amounts including five glucoalkaloids. Addition of high levels of ajmaline to the cell culture medium promoted the formation of a new group of alkaloids, the raumaclines, not found in the roots (for further details see S. Endress *et al.*, *Phytochemistry*, 1993, **32**, 725 and references cited therein).

Hairy root cultures of *R. serpentina*, produced by *Agrobacterium rhizogenes* transformation, synthesized ajmaline (0.045% dry wt.) and serpentine (0.007% dry wt.) (B. D. Benjamin *et al.*, *Phytochemistry*, 1994, **35**, 381); minor alkaloids have also been recorded (H. Falkenhagen *et al.*, *Can. J. Chem.*, 1993, **71**, 2201). *R. verticillata* hairy roots have been shown to produce reserpine and aimaline. Working on hairy root cultures, Stockigt's group has reported on the isolation of three new monoterpenoid indole alkaloids of the sarpagine group along with 16 known compounds together with the first *natural* occurrence (cf. cell cultures above), of the rare raumacline type alkaloids (Y. Sheludko *et al.*, *J. Nat. Prod.*, 2002, **65**, 1006; *Planta Medica* 2002, **68**, 435).

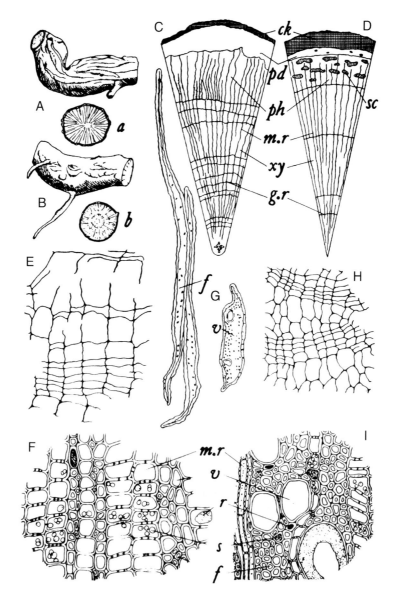

Fig. 26.32

Rauwolfia serpentina and *R. vomitoria* roots. A, Root of *R. serpentina* (×1); a, transverse section (TS) of same (×1); B, root of *R. vomitoria*, ×1; b, TS of same (×1); C, diagrammatic TS of *R. serpentina* root (×15); D, diagrammatic TS of *R. vomitoria* root (×15); E, TS of cork of *R. serpentina*; F, TS of the secondary wood of *R. serpentina*; G, fibres and vessel of *R. serpentina*, isolated by maceration; H, TS of cork of *R. vomitoria*; I, TS of the secondary wood of *R. vomitoria*; E, F, G, H and I, (all ×150). ck, cork; f, fibre; g.r, growth ring; m.r, medullary ray; pd, phelloderm; ph, phloem; r, resinous material; s, starch; sc, group of sclereids; v, wood vessel; xy, xylem (J. D. Kulkarni, partly after T. E. Wallis and S. Rohatgi (*R. serpentina*) and W. C. Evans (*R. vomitoria*))

Two monoterpenoid indole alkaloids and four β-carbolines have been isolated from cultured hybrid cells of *Rauwolfia serpentina* and *Rhazya stricta*, not all of the compounds being found in the parent plants (N. Aimi *et al.*, *Chem. Pharm. Bull.*, 1996, **44**, 1637).

Standardization. An assay for total alkaloids is not a true measure of therapeutic activity, since only some of the alkaloids have the desired pharmacological action. The *BPC* 1988 and *USP/NF* 1995 determine the reserpine-like alkaloids by utilizing the colour reaction between an acid solution of reserpine (and rescinnamine) and sodium nitrite solution.

Allied drugs. The 110 *Rauwolfia* species classified by Pichon in 1947 were reduced by Woodson in 1957 to 86. Some of these occur in

more than one geographic area but their approximate geographic areas are as follows: Central and South America 34, Africa 20, Far East 24, India and Burma 7, Hawaii, New Guinea and New Caledonia 6. A large number of these species have been examined for reserpine and related alkaloids.

In the identification of the roots of species of *Rauwolfia* useful characters to be seen in transverse sections are: cork (whether stratified or lignified); cortex and phloem (presence or absence of sclereids or fibres); wood (relative number, distribution and size of vessels). As the species vary from herbs to large trees, the roots vary considerably in size. Some samples of drug contain aerial stems, which usually contain less reserpine than the roots and have unlignified pericyclic fibres.

R. tetraphylla (*R. canescens*, *R. hirsuta*) is a species of wide distribution—tropical South America, the Caribbean, India, Australia

(Queensland). The root was at one time occasionally substituted for *R. serpentina* and could be recognized by its non-stratified cork, and sclereid groups in the phloem. It has served as a commercial source of reserpine and the alkaloid deserpidine, possibly particularly important as *R. serpentina* is now classed as an endangered species. Micropropagation protocols have been described for *in vitro* mass multiplication of the plant (D. Sarma *et al.*, *Planta Medica*, 1999, **65**, 277).

R. nitida is a West Indian species from the root-bark of which 33 indole alkaloids have been isolated.

Uses.

Rauwolfia preparations and reserpine are used in the management of essential hypertension and in certain neuropsychiatric disorders. Ajmaline, which has pharmacological properties similar to those of quinidine, is marketed in Japan for the treatment of cardiac arrhythmias.

An estimated 3500 kg of ajmalicine is isolated annually from either *Rauwolfia* or *Catharanthus* spp. by pharmaceutical industries for the treatment of circulatory diseases.

Conflicting reports on the possible involvement of the rauwolfia alkaloids in breast cancer engendered a natural hesitation in their use. A report in *the Lancet* (1976) suggested that the alkaloids do not initiate the carcinogenic process but that they promote breast cancer from previously initiated cells.

African Rauwolfia (African Rauvolfia)

African rauwolfia consists of the dried roots of *Rauwolfia vomitoria* Afz. The plant is a bush or tree widely distributed in tropical Africa from the west coast to Mozambique. It is the most important African rauwolfia for the commercial preparation of reserpine.

Collection and preparation.   As the tree may attain a height of 10 m, the roots are larger than those of *R. serpentina*. Before drying they are cut transversely, but are rarely sliced longitudinally. Roots up to 5 cm or more in diameter are sometimes found but the commercial drug usually consists of much smaller pieces. Occasional shipments have been made consisting of the bark only.

Macroscopical characters.   The first detailed description of the drug was published by Evans in 1956. It occurs in cylindrical or flattened pieces, usually 0.15–1.5 cm diameter and up to 30 cm long. The roots taper slightly and are occasionally branched. The outer surface is greyish-brown, longitudinally furrowed or rubbed smooth, since the outer cork easily flakes off. Pieces do not break easily, but the fracture is short in the bark and splintery in the wood. The smoothed transverse surface shows a narrow brown bark and a buff or yellowish, finely radiate wood. Odourless; taste, bitter. Pieces of rootstock with attached stem-bases are sometimes found in the drug.

Microscopical characters.   The drug is easily distinguished from *R. serpentina* by the groups of sclereids in the bark arranged in up to five discontinuous bands and by the large vessels of the wood which are up to 180 μm in diameter (Fig. 26.32 D and I).

Constituents.   African rauwolfia contains reserpine and rescinnamine and alkaloids of the same type such as reserpoxidine and seredine. Many other alkaloids such as ajmaline, alstonine and yohimbine are also present. Court's group (see *Planta Med.*, 1982, **45**, 105) isolated 42 indole alkaloids from the stem-bark and identified 39. The major alkaloids were heteroyohimbines (especially reserpiline) and N_a-demethyldihydroindoles. The interrelationship of these alkaloids with those in the root of the plant is discussed in the same paper. New indole alkaloids from *R. vomitoria* extracts have continued to be reported.

Allied drugs.   Other African rauwolfias containing reserpine are *R. caffra* (*R. natalensis*), *R. mombasiana*, *R. oreogiton*, *R. obscura*, *R. cumminsii*, *R. volkensii* and *R. rosea*. Court and coworkers have made a systematic study of the microscopy and chemistry of African species (for a report see W. E. Court, *Planta Med.*, 1983, **48**, 228). The roots of *R. caffra* closely resemble those of *R. vomitoria* but the cork has not the same tendency to flake off. In sections the main difference is that in *R. vomitoria* there are alternating lignified and unlignified cork cells, while in *R. caffra* all the cork cells are lignified. *R. caffra* contains the alkaloid raucaffricine—one of relatively few examples of monoterpenoid indole glucoalkaloids within the group. *R. mombasiana* differs from *R. vomitoria* in the structure of the wood of the root; *R. rosea*, *R. volkensii* and *R. obscura* lack sclereid development.

Alstonia barks

Several *Alstonia* species (Apocynaceae) have been used in the past as antimalarials, and the barks of the Indian *Alstonia scholaris* and the Australian *A. constricta* were included in the 1914 edition of the *British Pharmacopoeia*. At least 11 species are known to contain alkaloids, such as alstonine, alstoniline, cillastonine and echitamine. Interest in them was again awakened by the isolation in 1955 of reserpine in moderate yield from the root-bark of *A. constricta*; reserpine has since been isolated from *A. venenata*. For a report on the isolation of a new indole alkaloid and a new glycosidic indole alkaloid from the trunk bark of Indonesian *Alstonia scholaris*, see A. A. Salim *et al.*, *J. Nat. Prod.*, 2004, **67**, 1591. Descriptions of *Alstonia* barks will be found in the older editions of reference books (e.g. the 22nd edition of the *USD*, p. 1227).

Yohimbe bark

Yohimbe bark is derived from *Pausinystalia yohimbe* (Rubiaceae), a tree growing in the Cameroon Republic. It occurs in flat or slightly quilled pieces up to 75 cm long and 2 cm thick. The grey-brown cork has furrows and cracks and patches of lichen. The inner surface is reddish-brown and striated. Taste, bitter. It contains the indole alkaloid yohimbine, which is structurally related to reserpine.

The bark is well-recognized for its aphrodisiac property and yohimbine is effective in the symptomatic treatment of erectile dysfunction, producing fewer side-effects than invasive treatments (M. H. Pittler, *Fortschritte der Medizin*, 1998, **116**, 32).

Aspidosperma barks

The large genus *Aspidosperma* (Apocynaceae) contains many alkaloid-containing South American trees. The alkaloids are of various indole types formed by a number of different biogenetic pathways. Among the many investigated are yohimbine, which is structurally related to reserpine, and aspidospermine, which has the same general structure as vindoline (see Fig. 26.27). The *Aspidosperma* barks are therefore potential sources of alkaloids, because the trees are large and the barks would be commercially available cheaply and in almost unlimited quantities.

Catharanthus roseus.

For an account of this important plant, see Chapter 27.

Mitragyna leaves

The genus *Mitragyna* (Rubiaceae) occurs in West and East Africa, India and S.E. Asia. More than 30 different alkaloids have been characterized, and the majority of these are indole or oxindole structures with an open or closed ring E; they exist in various isomeric forms. One alkaloid, mitragynine, isolated from *Mitragyna speciosa* has analgesic and antitussive properties similar to those of codeine.

Shellard and coworkers published extensively on the genus during the 1960s and 1970s (for more recent work on *M. speciosa* from the same Department see P. J. Houghton *et al.*, *Phytochemistry*, 1991, **30**, 347). The mis-use of mitragyna as an hallucinogen is considered in Chapter 39.

Uncaria species

In addition to *Uncaria gambir*, the source of catechu (q.v.), the genus is notable for its alkaloids, which resemble those of *Mitragyna*. Uncaria hooks, the dried climbing hooks and stems of *U. sinensis*, have sedative and antispasmodic properties. They are used in Chinese medicine for the relief of headaches and dizziness caused by hypertension and for the treatment of convulsions in children. The drug contains indole alkaloids, e.g. rhyncophylline and indole alkaloid glycosides which exhibit a long-lasting hypotensive effect (K. Endo *et al.*, *Planta Med.*, 1983, **49**, 188; S. Kawazoe *et al.*, *ibid.*, 1991, **57**, 47).

Uncaria rhynchophylla, a species also used in Chinese medicine, is reported to contain various alkaloids including rhynchophylline, corynoxeine, corynantheine and among others, hirsutine which exhibit antihypertensive, neuroprotective and vasodilator effects; (+)-catechin and (−)-epicatechin have been isolated for the first time from this species (W.-C. Hou *et al.*, *J. Ethnopharmacology* 2005, **100**, 216). Other research suggests this species to be an effective anxiolytic agent acting via the serotonergic nervous system (K. W. Jung *et al.*, *J. Ethnopharmacology*, 2006, **108**, 193).

U. tomentosa, one of two species found in S. America, features in the traditional medicine of Peru. It produces similar hooks to *U. sinensis* being known locally by the Spanish as 'una degato' (tomcat's claw).

In a number of reports on this species, M. Kitajima *et al.*, have recorded a new glucoindole akaloid, 3,4-dehydro-5-carboxystrictosodine, various triterpenes including nor-triterpene glycosides and cincholic acid glycosides (see *Chem. Pharm. Bull.*, 2004, **52**, 1258 and references cited therein). The plant has a potential immunostimulant action and has been examined for its pharmacological and toxicological properties (K. Keplinger *et al.*, *J. Ethnopharmacology*, 1999, **64**, 23; I. Lemaire *et al.*, *J. Ethnopharmacology*, **64**, 109). It is being used traditionally to treat a large number of conditions, including cancer (R. Pilarski *et al.*, *J. Ethnopharmacology*, 2006, **104**, 18; L. De Martino *et al.*, *J. Ethnopharmacology*, 2006, **107**, 91; G. Gonçalves *et al.*, *Phytochemistry*, 2005, **66**, 89).

Further reading

Heitzman ME, Neto CC, Winiarz E *et al* 2005 Ethnobotany, phytochemistry pharmacology of *Uncaria* (Rubiaceae). Phytochemistry 66(1): 5–29

Vinca major and *V. minor*

The greater periwinkle (*Vinca major*) together with the lesser periwinkle (*V. minor*) are the only members of the essentially tropical and subtropical family Apocynaceae found wild in the British Isles. The former is listed in the *BHP* (1983) for the treatment of menorrhagia and topically as an application for haemorrhoids but is now seldom used. The following indole alkaloids have been characterized: reserpine, majdine, akuammicine, strictosidine (Fig. 26.34), pseudo-akuammigine, akuammine and possibly 10-hydroxycathofoline. New alkaloids continue to be reported e.g. Atta-ur-Rahman *et al.*, *Phytochemistry*, 1995, **38**, 1057. More than 50 alkaloids have been isolated from the leaves of *V. minor*, a few of them quaternary (for a recent report see D. Uhrin *et al.*, *J. Nat. Prod.*, 1989, **52**, 637). Vincamine, first isolated from *V. minor* in 1953, is available as a vasodilatory drug.

CINCHONA

Cinchona bark consists of various species, races and hybrids of *Cinchona* (Rubiaceae), large trees indigenous to Colombia, Ecuador, Peru and Bolivia. The *BP/EP* recognizes the whole or cut, dried bark of *Cinchona pubescens* Vahl (*C. succirubra* Pavon), *C. calisaya* (Weddell), of *C. ledgeriana* (Moens ex Trimen) or its varieties or hybrids, containing not less than 6.5% of total alkaloids, 30–60% of which consists of quinine-type alkaloids. The former importance of cinchona bark and its alkaloids in the treatment of malaria has been lessened by the introduction of synthetic drugs, but it remains of great economic importance, and salts of quinine and quinidine are included in most pharmacopoeias.

Collection from wild trees was soon replaced by cultivation, and most research was undertaken by the Dutch in Java and the British in India to obtain hybrids which are rich in alkaloids. While Indonesia and India remain important producers of cinchona, a high percentage of the total crop is now grown on plantations in Tanzania, Kenya, Guatemala and Bolivia.

History. The natives of South America do not appear to have been acquainted with the medicinal properties of cinchona bark, the bitter taste of which inspired them with fear. Although Peru was discovered in 1513, the bark was first used for the cure of fevers about 1630. The name 'Cinchona' is said to be derived from a Countess of Chinchon, wife of a viceroy of Peru who it was long believed was cured in 1638 from a fever by the use of the bark. According to recent study of the Count's diary, it appears that the Countess never suffered from malaria or other fever during her stay in Peru, and although the Count himself did so, there is no record of his having been treated with cinchona bark. The remedy, which became known as 'Pulvo de la Condesa', acquired a considerable reputation and was known in Spain in 1639. The further distribution of the bark was largely due to the Jesuit priests, and the drug became known as Jesuit's Powder or Peruvian Powder. It first appeared in the *London Pharmacopoeia* in 1677 under the name of 'Cortex Peruanus'.

The bark was originally obtained by felling the wild trees, which were exterminated in many districts. Ruiz (1792) and Royle (1839) suggested the cultivation of cinchonas in other parts of the world. Weddell germinated seeds in Paris in 1848, and the plants were introduced into Algiers in the following year but without much success. A further attempt by the Dutch was made in 1854, seeds and plants being obtained from Peru by Hasskarl and introduced into Java. An English expedition under Markham in 1860 led to the introduction of *C. succirubra* (the most hardy species), *C. calisaya*, and *C. micrantha* into India. Seeds of *C. ledgeriana* were obtained in Bolivia by Charles Ledger in 1865 and were bought by the Dutch for their Javanese plantations. A fascinating book covering Ledger's exploits is *The Life of Charles Ledger (1818–1905)* by G. Grammicia, Macmillan Press, London, 1988. World War II and subsequent fighting in Malaya and Vietnam increased the demand for cinchona and stimulated cultivation in Africa and Central and South America.

Cultivation, collection and preparation. The production of cinchona bark is a highly specialized section of tropical agriculture. An acid soil, rainfall and altitude are all important factors in cinchona production. Selection of high-yielding strains is of paramount importance, and grafting techniques with *C. succirubra* as stock may be employed. Seedlings need careful treatment and propagation to avoid disease attack, etc. Since the mid-1970s a disease of the cinchona tree, known as stripe canker, has posed a threat to the plantations of Central Africa. The disease, also known in Central America, is caused by the phytopathogenic fungus *Phytophthora cinnamomi*, which causes sunken necrotic stripes in the bark and kills thousands of trees a year.

26

General characters

1. *Stem-bark*. The commercial 'druggist's' quills are up to 30 cm long and usually 2–6 mm thick. Bark for manufacturing purposes is frequently in small curved pieces. The outer surface frequently bears moss or lichen. The cork may or may not be longitudinally wrinkled, and usually bears longitudinal and transverse cracks, which vary in frequency and distinctness in the different varieties. The inner surface is striated and varies in colour from yellowish-brown to deep reddish-brown. The fracture is short in the outer part but somewhat fibrous in the inner part. Odour, slight; taste, bitter and astringent.

2. *Root-bark*. Root-bark occurs in channelled, often twisted pieces about 2–7 cm long. Both surfaces are of similar colour, the outer, however, being somewhat scaly, while the inner surface is striated.

Special characters.   In view of the number of hybrids which are cultivated, the distinction of the various commercial cinchona barks is a matter of some difficulty. In Table 26.7 the notes on four important

species have been made as concise as possible to facilitate comparison.

Microscopical characters.   Cinchona barks have the general microscopical structure shown in Fig. 26.33. The cork is composed of several layers of thin-walled cork cells, arranged in regular radial rows and appearing polygonal in surface view. Their cell contents are dark reddish in colour. Within the cork cambium is a phelloderm of several layers of regular cells with dark walls. The cortex is composed of tangentially elongated, thin-walled cells containing amorphous reddish-brown matter or small starch grains 6–10 μm diameter. Scattered in the cortex are idioblasts containing microcrystals of calcium oxalate and secretion cells. The phloem consists of narrow sieve-tubes showing transverse sieve plates, phloem parenchyma resembling that of the cortex and large characteristic spindle-shaped phloem fibres with thick conspicuously striated walls traversed by funnel-shaped pits. The phloem fibres occur isolated or in irregular radial rows. The distribution and size of the phloem fibres differ in the various species

Table 26.7   Comparison of *Cinchona* species.

C. succirubra (Fig. 26.33)	*C. calisaya*	*C. ledgeriana*	*C. officinalis*
Frequently 20–40 mm diameter, and 2–6 mm thick	Diameter 12–25 mm and 2–5 mm thick	Similar to *C. calisaya*	Up to 12 mm diameter, and 1 mm thick
Well-marked longitudinal wrinkles, relatively few transverse cracks. Some pieces, but by no means all, show reddish warts	Broad longitudinal fissures; transverse cracks about 6–12 mm apart	Similar to *C. calisaya*, but cracks more numerous and less deep. Some pieces show longitudinal wrinkles and reddish warts	Transverse cracks, very numerous, often less than 6 mm apart
Powder reddish-brown	Powder cinnamon-brown	Powder cinnamon-brown	Powder yellowish

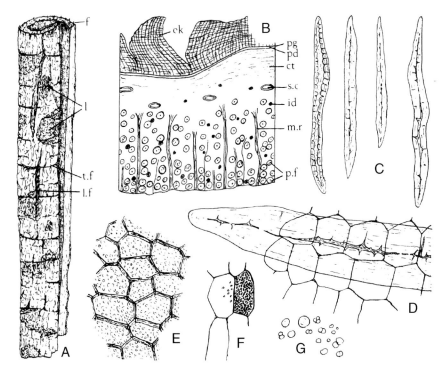

Fig. 26.33
Cinchona bark. A, specimen of *Cinchona succirubra* (× 0.5); B, transverse section of bark (×25); C, isolated phloem fibres (×50); D, portion of phloem fibre with surrounding parenchyma; E, cork cells in surface view; F, idioblast with calcium oxalate; G, starch (all × 200). ck, Cork; ct, cortex; f, fibres protruding from fracture; id, idioblast; l, lichen patches; l.f, longitudinal fissure; m.r, medullary ray; pd, phelloderm; pg, phellogen; p.f, phloem fibres; s.c, secretory cell; t.f, transverse fissure.

(those of *C. succirubra* are 350–**600**–**700**–1400 μm long and 30–**40**–70–100 μm in diameter; for other species see 10th edition). The medullary rays are two or three cells wide, the cells being thin-walled and somewhat radially elongated.

Constituents. Cinchona bark contains quinoline alkaloids (see Fig. 26.34). The principal alkaloids are the stereoisomers quinine and quinidine and their respective 6′-demethoxy derivatives, cinchonidine and cinchonine. The quinine series has the configuration 8S, 9R and the quinidine 8R, 9S (Fig. 26.34); other alkaloids of lesser importance have been isolated. Some of these (e.g. quinicine and cinchonicine) are amorphous. The amount of alkaloids present and the ratios between them vary considerably in the different species and hybrids, also according to the environment of the tree and the age and method of collection of the bark.

The alkaloids appear to be present in the parenchymatous tissues of the bark in combination with quinic acid and cinchotannic acid. Quinic

acid (see Fig. 19.5) is present to the extent of 5–8%. Cinchotannic acid is a phlobatannin and a considerable amount of its decomposition product, 'cinchona red', is also found in the bark. Other constituents are quinovin (up to 2%), which is a glycoside yielding on hydrolysis quinovaic acid and quinovose (isorhodeose).

Anthraquinones, which as a group of compounds are associated with the family Rubiaceae (see Table 21.3), are not normally found in quantity in the bark of cinchona as indicated by the isolation of norsolorinic acid, a tetrahydroxyanthraquinone, in 0.0008% yield from the bark of *C. ledgeriana*. However, they are produced in cell cultures of the plant and by infection of the bark with *Phytophthora cinnamomi*. The latter case may be associated with a phytoalexin defence mechanism; in infected material, alkaloid production is lowered. In connection with the production of anthraquinones in cell cultures, enzymes associated with the later stages of glycoside formation have been isolated. This work involved glucosidases in *C. succirubra* cell cultures and the

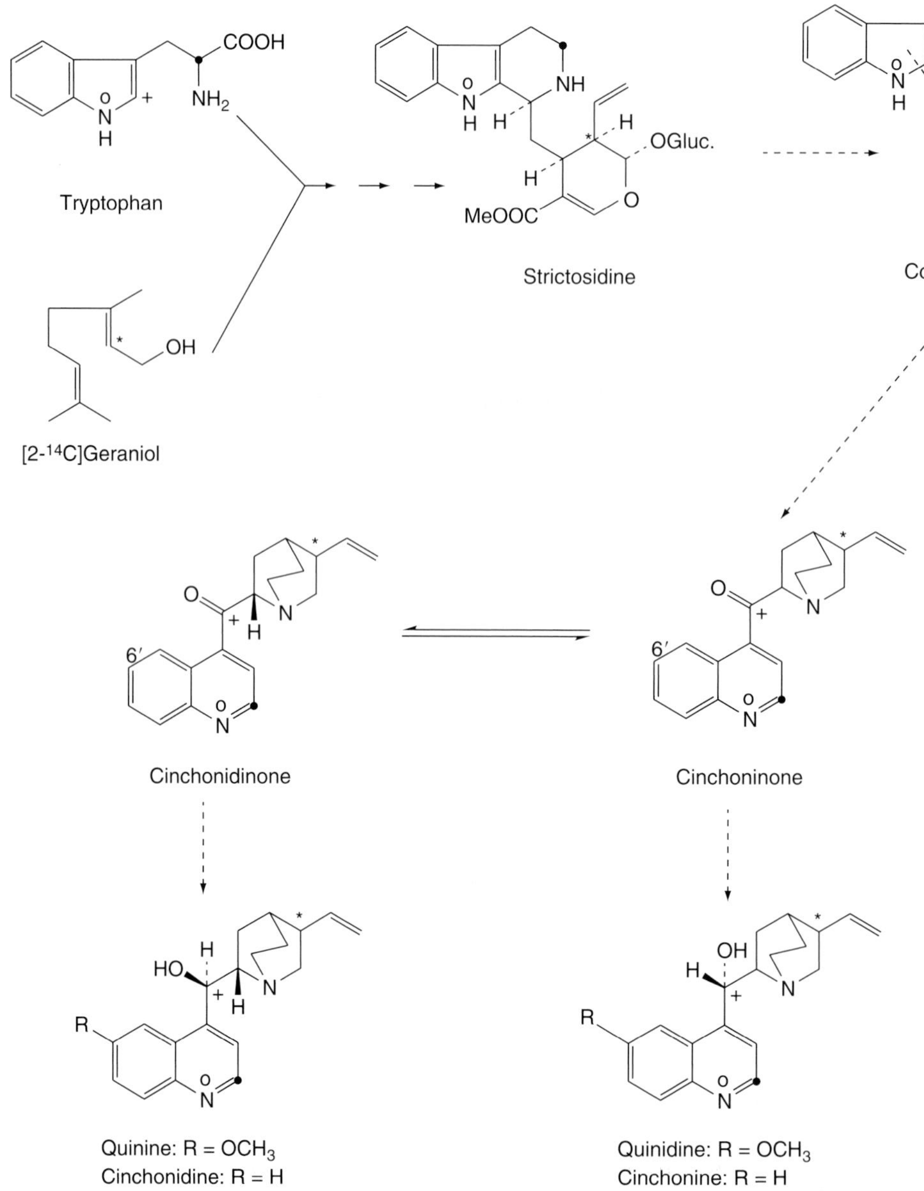

Fig. 26.34
Outline of possible biogenetic pathway for *Cinchona* alkaloids. Marked atoms illustrate the structural changes.

isolation of five distinct glucosyltransferases (EC 2,4,1,-) which catalyse the transfer of the glucosyl moiety from UDP-glucose to the hydroxyl groups of those anthraquinones found in cinchona cultures (e.g. emodin, anthrapurpurin, quinizarin, etc.).

Biosynthesis of alkaloids. Grafting experiments and organ culture suggest that the alkaloids are formed principally in the aerial parts of the plant. Although the quinoline alkaloids have structures which by inspection might suggest anthranilic acid as a biological precursor, they are, in fact, as originally suggested by Janot *et al.* in 1950, derived from indolic precursors. This has been demonstrated by the specific incorporation of tryptophan (indole moiety), loganin and geraniol (terpenoid moiety) into the quinine of *Cinchona* spp. The pathway, largely established by Battersby's and Leete's groups, involves alkaloids of the serpentine type as illustrated in Fig. 26.34.

The proposed biosynthetic route has been supported and elaborated by enzyme studies. The important role of strictosidine synthase in the initial stages of the biogenesis of some tryptophan-derived alkaloids and its isolation from *C. robusta* was mentioned at the beginning of this section. The enzyme tryptophan decarboxylase (EC 4.1.1.28), which provides tryptamine, is also involved in these early reactions. An enzyme (cinchoninone: NADPH oxidoreductase) associated with the pathway has been isolated from cells of a suspension culture of *Cinchona ledgeriana*; it catalyses the reduction of cinchoninone to an unequal mixture of cinchonine and cinchonidine. The enzyme can be resolved (by ion exchange) into two isoenzymic forms both of which have an absolute requirement for NADPH and catalysed reversible reactions. Isoenzyme I acts specifically on cinchoninone in the forward direction of the pathway and on cinchonidine and cinchonine in the reverse direction. Isoenzyme II has a broad specificity acting on all the quinoline alkaloids of cinchona tested.

Allied drugs. The barks of certain species of *Remijia* (Rubiaceae) contain alkaloids. That of *R. pedunculata* is quoted (*USP*) as a source of quinidine. It also contains cupreine, an alkaloid which responds to the thalleioquin test and by methylation forms quinine. False cuprea bark (*R. purdiena*) contains no quinine but an alkaloid cusconidine and small proportions of cinchonine and cinchonamine.

Cinchona leaf alkaloids. Alkaloids of the indole type (e.g. cinchophylline) are generally considered to typify the leaves, so that it is of interest that Phillipson *et al.* (*J. Pharm. Pharmacol.*, 1981, **33**, 15P) isolated quinine from leaves of *C. succirubra* grown in Thailand. Thirteen alkaloids have been separated by HPLC.

Uses. Galenicals of cinchona have long been used as bitter tonics and stomachics. On account of the astringent action, a decoction and acid infusion are sometimes used as gargles. Before World War II, quinine was the drug of choice for the treatment of malaria but became largely superseded by the advent of synthetic antimalarials developed during that period. It has, however, remained of importance in Third World countries and has re-emerged as suitable for the treatment of *Plasmodium falciparum* infections (falciparum malaria) in the many areas where the organism is now resistant to chloroquine and other antimalarials.

Quinidine is employed for the prophylaxis of cardiac arrhythmias and for the treatment of atrial fibrillation; it also has antimalarial properties and like quinine is effective against chloroquine-resistant organisms.

MISCELLANEOUS ALKALOIDS

There are a number of relatively small groups of alkaloids, some of whose biosynthetic relationships to particular amino acids have not been firmly established or whose formation does not involve direct amino acid participation.

INDOLIZIDINE ALKALOIDS

Only a small number of indolizidine alkaloids are currently known but they have recently become of pharmaceutical interest through the discovery of the tetrahydroxy alkaloids castanospermine and 6-epicastanospermine, which are possible lead compounds in the search for anti-AIDS drugs (see Chapter 30). Also, like the above, swainsonine, the toxic constituent of locoweeds and Australian *Swainsona* spp., is a powerful glycosidase inhibitor; this alkaloid is a trihydroxy-indolizidine. Both alkaloids are biosynthesized from lysine via pipecolic acid.

(For a review of the simple indolizidine alkaloids (154 refs) see J. Takahata and T. Momose, *Alkaloids*, 1993, **44**, 189.)

IMIDAZOLE ALKALOIDS

The most important pharmaceutical examples of this group are the *Pilocarpus* alkaloids, pilocarpine finding use as an ophthalmic cholinergic drug. Possible biosynthetic routes to pilocarpine (see formula under 'Jaborandi Leaf and Pilocarpine', below) could involve either of the amino acids histidine or threonine.

JABORANDI LEAF AND PILOCARPINE

The name 'jaborandi' is now applied to the leaflets of various species of *Pilocarpus* (Rutaceae), a genus of trees and shrubs well represented in South America and found to a lesser extent in the West Indies and Central America. The principal jaborandi now imported, Maranham jaborandi, is that derived from the Brazilian plant *Pilocarpus microphyllus*.

The state of Maranhão accounts for about 90% of the Brazilian leaf. Traditionally the crop is collected from wild plants but over the years production has fallen due to non-sustainability of the supply and attempts to cultivate the plant commercially have been undertaken. As with a number of medicinal plants, transforming a wild species into a cultivable crop is not necessarily easy and a balanced collection between wild and cultivated plants may be desirable.

A comprehensive account relating to jaborandi production is given by C. U. B. Pinheiro (*Economic Botany*, 1997, **51**, 49).

Jaborandi was formerly official but is now used mainly as a source of the medicinally important alkaloid pilocarpine.

Characters of principal sources

1. *Maranham jaborandi.* The plant *P. microphyllus*, which produces the Maranham drug, bears imparipinnate compound leaves with about seven leaflets (Fig. 26.35). The leaflets are attached to a somewhat winged rachis which is almost glabrous (*Swartzia* is hairy). The drug consists of separated leaflets, a certain amount of rachis and an occasional fruit. The leaflets are 2–5 cm long, 1–3 cm broad, and emarginate at the apex. The terminal leaflets are oval, symmetrical and have a petiolule 5–15 mm long, with a winged margin which passes imperceptibly into the lamina. The remaining leaflets are

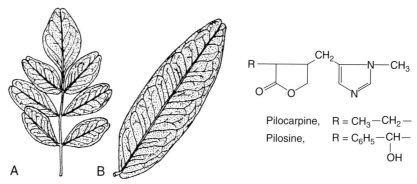

Fig. 26.35
Jaborandi. A, Leaf of *Pilocarpus microphyllus*; B, leaflet of *P. jaborandi* (×0.5).

obovate, asymmetrical and sessile. Leaflets of the left and right sides of the leaf may be distinguished from one another by the fact that the broader side of each leaflet lies away from the rachis. The veins are pinnate and anastomose near the margin. The drug is greyish-green to greenish-brown and brittle in texture. Numerous small oil cells may be seen by transmitted light. Odour, when crushed, slightly aromatic; taste, bitterish and aromatic with induction of salivation.

2. *Pernambuco jaborandi*. Pernambuco jaborandi consists of the leaflets of *Pilocarpus jaborandi* Holmes, which are obtained from a compound imparipinnate leaf with 1–9 leaflets. Leaflets 4–12 cm long and 2–4 cm broad (Fig. 26.35), petiolules short; apex emarginate; base usually asymmetric; margin entire and slightly revolute. Upper surface glabrous and greyish to brownish-green; lower surface yellowish- or greenish-brown and slightly pubescent. Midvein not prominent on the upper surface but very prominent on the lower surface (in the midveins of the Maranham leaflets the reverse is the case). A transverse section of the midveins is often useful for distinguishing between the various species of *Pilocarpus*—for example, the Pernambuco variety shows a complete ring of pericyclic sclerenchyma, the Maranham a broken ring.

A compound, 1-phenyl-5-vinyl-5,9-dimethyl decane has been obtained from the foliar epicuticular wax of *P. jaborandi* and by TLC it can be used to distinguish this species from others of *Pilocarpus* (G. Negri *et al.*, *Phytochemistry*, 1998, **49**, 127).

3. *Paraguay jaborandi*. Paraguay jaborandi, derived from *P. pennatifolius* Lemaire. Greyish-green; papery in texture; usually equal at base; veins not prominent on the upper surface and the anastomoses not marked. Pericyclic sclerenchyma more broken than in Maranham or Pernambuco. The above three varieties have a single palisade layer, a point which distinguishes them from the Guadeloupe and Aracati varieties.

4. *Ceara jaborandi*. Ceara jaborandi is derived from *P. trachylophus* Holmes and is exported from the Brazilian provinces of Ceara and Maranhão. Leaflets are smaller than those of *P. jaborandi*; oblong or elliptical; coriaceous; both surfaces bearing short curved hairs, which are particularly abundant on the lower surface.

Constituents. Maranham leaves contain about 0.7–0.8% of the alkaloids, pilocarpine, isopilocarpine, pilosine and isopilosine and about 0.5% of volatile oil. An examination of the volatile oil composition of a number of species indicated a total of 22 components occurring throughout the samples. These included monoterpenes (e.g. limonene, sabiene, α-pinene) sesquiterpenes (e.g. caryophyllene) but not in *P. jaborandi*, and 2-undecanone or 2-tridecanone.

Pilocarpine, the lactone of pilocarpic acid, contains a glyoxaline nucleus and with heat or alkalis is converted into its isomer isopilocarpine. Isopilocarpine occurs in small quantity in the leaf but more is formed during the extraction process. The dried leaves soon lose their activity on storage.

Uses. Salts of pilocarpine (e.g. Pilocarpine Hydrochloride *BP/EP* and Nitrate *BP/EP*) are used in ophthalmic practice, as they cause contraction of the pupil of the eye, their action being antagonistic to that of atropine. In early glaucoma treatment they serve to increase the irrigation of the eye and relieve pressure. A study in the USA involving 207 patients suffering from dry mouth resulting from radiation treatment for head or neck cancer indicated that oral pilocarpine can possibly offer relief (*Pharm. J.*, 1993, **251**, 215). In 1994 its use was approved for this purpose by the US Food and Drug Administration.

PURINE ALKALOIDS

The purine nucleotides, together with the pyrimidine nucleotides, constitute vital structural units of the nucleic acids; they also function as coenzymes (Chapter 18) and as portions of complex substrate molecules. Adenine and guanine are the purines most commonly involved in these roles, but xanthine and hypoxanthine feature in their biosynthesis.

'Purine alkaloids' constitute secondary metabolites and are derivatives of xanthine; three well-known examples are caffeine (1,3,7-trimethylxanthine), theophylline (1,3-dimethylxanthine) and theobromine (3,7-dimethylxanthine).

Beverages such as tea and coffee owe their stimulant properties to these substances. Caffeine stimulates the central nervous system and has a weak diuretic action, whereas theobromine acts in the reverse way. Theophylline has generally similar properties to the above, with a shorter, though more powerful diuretic action than caffeine; it relaxes involuntary muscles more effectively than either caffeine or theobromine. The three alkaloids are official in the *EP* and *BP*.

Adenine

Guanine

Xanthine

Biogenesis. The ring formation of the purine alkaloids appears to follow the classical scheme for the biosynthesis of purine nucleotides with C_1-moieties arising from such compounds as formates and formaldehyde. Methylamine is also effectively incorporated into the ring system; studies by Suzuki *et al.* indicated that methylamine is oxidized to formaldehyde and then metabolized as a C_1 compound. For caffeine, the purine bases such as hypoxanthine, adenine and guanine, and the nucleosides can also be incorporated by the plant into the molecule.

In both tea and coffee plants and in suspension cultures of *Coffea arabica* it has been clearly demonstrated that theobromine is methylated to caffeine. In 1979, as a result of work involving *N*-methyltransferases, Roberts and Waller suggested the pathway 7-methylxanthosine → 7-methylxanthine (heteroxanthin) → 3,7-dimethylxanthine (theobromine) → 1,3,7-trimethylxanthine (caffeine) which has been substantiated by later work. *S*-Adenosylmethionine is utilized as a donor of the methyl groups. Attempts to isolate the individual *N*-methyltransferase enzymes do not yet appear to have been successful due partly to their extreme lability. However progress has been made on their biochemical characterization and their time course during leaf development of *Coffea arabica* (S. S. Mösli Waldhauser *et al.*, *Phytochemistry*, 1997, **44**, 853). The origin of the caffeine molecule is shown in Fig. 26.36.

(For a review on this aspect see T. Suzuki *et al.*, *Phytochemistry*, 1992, **31**, 2575.)

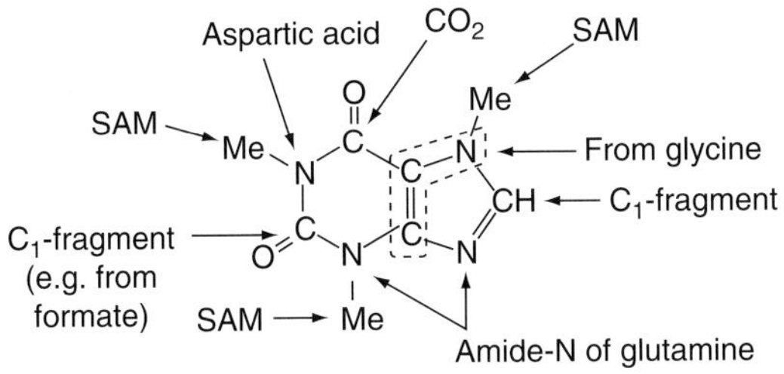

Fig. 26.36
Biogenetic origin of the caffeine molecule (SAM = S-adenosylmethionine).

COLA

Commercial cola (*Kola seeds*, *bissy* or *gooroo* nuts) consists of the dried cotyledons of the seeds of various species of *Cola* (Sterculiaceae), trees found in West Africa, the West Indies, Brazil and Java. The colour of the fresh seeds varies, those of *C. acuminata* being white or crimson, *C. astrophora* red, *C. alba* white and *C. vera* (*C. nitida*) (which is possibly a hybrid of the two latter species) either red or white. The *BP/EP* specifies *C. nitida* and its varieties as well as *C. acuminata*, containing not less than 1.5% caffeine. The dried cotyledons are usually of a dull, reddish-brown colour and more or less broken. They are usually graded as 'halves' and 'quarters'. The whole seeds are 2–5 cm long, and in the seeds usually imported there are two cotyledons. A microscopical examination of the powder shows portions of thick-walled, reddish polygonal cells of the cotyledons containing concentrially striated starch granules, reniform to ovoid in shape and 5–25 μm in size. Odourless; taste, slightly astringent.

Kola seeds contain caffeine (1–2.5%) and a little theobromine, which appear to be partly in the free state and partly combined. Cola also contains about 5–10% of tannoids (the 'kolatin' of earlier workers),

particularly catechol and epicatechol. During preparation, oxidation and polymerization of these produces the insoluble phlobaphene 'kola-red'. It has been suggested (C. Maillard *et al.*, *Planta Med.*, 1985, 515) that the differences in the stimulatory action between fresh and dried seeds may be due to the formation of a caffeine–catechin complex in the latter.

The pharmacopoeia uses a TLC test for identity using caffeine and theobromine as reference compounds. Liquid chromatography is used for the official assay with absorption measurements at 272 nm.

COCOA SEED

Cocoa seeds (*Cocoa Beans*) are obtained from *Theobroma cacao* (Sterculiaceae), a tree usually 4–6 m high. Cocoa is produced in South America (Ecuador, Colombia, Brazil, Venezuela and Guiana), Central America, the West Indies, West Africa (Ivory Coast, Nigeria and Ghana), Ceylon and Java.

History. Cocoa has long been used in Mexico and was known to Columbus and Cortez. Cocoa butter was prepared as early as 1695.

Collection and preparation. Cocoa fruits are 15–25 cm long and are borne on the trunk as well as on the branches. Cocoa plantations are very vulnerable to pest attack and recently modern pheromone technology has been used to control the cocoa pod borer, also known as the cocoa moth (*Conopomorpha cramerella*), the most serious pest of the crop in S.E. Asia. Collection continues throughout the year, but the largest quantities are obtained in the spring and autumn. The fruits have a thick, coriaceous rind and whitish pulp in which 40–50 seeds are embedded. In different countries the seeds are prepared in different ways, but the following may be taken as typical: the fruits are opened and the seeds, embedded in the whole pulp or roughly separated from it, are allowed to ferment. Fermentation occurs in tubs, boxes or cavities in the earth; the process lasts 3–9 days, and the temperature is not allowed to rise above 60°C. In Jamaica fermentation is allowed to proceed for 3 days at a temperature of 30–43°C. During this process a liquid drains from the seeds, which change in colour from white or red to purple, and also acquire a different odour and taste. After fermentation the seeds may or may not be washed. They are then roasted at 100–140°C, when they lose water and acetic acid and acquire their characteristic odour and taste. Roasting facilitates removal of the testa. The seeds are cooled as rapidly as possible and the testa removed by a 'nibbling' machine. The nibs or kernels are separated from the husk by winnowing. Sometimes the seeds are simply dried in the sun but these are not as highly regarded owing to their astringent and bitter taste.

Plain or *bitter chocolate* is a mixture of ground cocoa nibs with sucrose, cocoa butter and flavouring. Milk chocolate contains in addition milk powder.

Macroscopical characters. Cocoa seeds are flattened ovoid in shape, 2–3 cm long and 1.5 cm wide. The thin testa is easily removed from prepared cocoa beans, but is difficult to remove from those that have not been fermented and roasted. The embryo is surrounded by a thin membrane of endosperm. The cotyledons form the greater part of the kernel and are planoconvex and irregularly folded. Each shows on its plane face three large furrows, which account for the readiness with which the kernel breaks into angular fragments. Both testa and kernel are of a reddish-brown colour, which varies, however, in different commercial varieties and depends on the formation of 'cacao-red' during processing.

Constituents. Cocoa kernels contain 0.9–3.0% of theobromine and the husks contain 0.19–2.98% of this alkaloid. The seeds also contain 0.05–0.36% caffeine, cocoa fat or butter (nibs 45–53%, husk 4–8%). During the fermentation and roasting, much of the theobromine originally present in the kernel passes into the husk. The constituents other than fat and theobromine are extremely complex and have been intensely studied in recent years. The fresh seeds contain about 5–10% of water-soluble polyphenols (epicatechol, leucoanthocyanins and anthocyanins) which are largely decomposed during processing, forming the coloured complex formerly known as 'cocoa-red'. Condensed tannins are also present, and some 84 different volatile compounds, including glucosinolates, are responsible for the aroma (see M. S. Gill et al., Phytochemistry, 1984, **23**, 1937).

Theobromine is produced on the commercial scale from cocoa husks. The process consists of decocting the husks with water, filtering, precipitating 'tannin' with lead acetate, filtering, removing excess of lead and evaporating to dryness. Theobromine is extracted from the residue by means of alcohol and purified by recrystallization from water.

Theobromine is 3,7-dimethylxanthine (see p. 409), the lower homologue of caffeine (trimethylxanthine). It is isomeric with theophylline (1,3-dimethylxanthine), which occurs in small quantities in tea. Theobromine crystallizes in white rhombic needles. It gives the murexide reaction (see p. 356), and may be distinguished from caffeine by the fact that it is precipitated from a dilute nitric acid solution by silver nitrate. Theobromine sublimes at 220°C, caffeine at 178–180°C.

Callus and suspension cultures of cocoa both produce caffeine, theobromine and theophylline and are considered useful for studying secondary metabolism *in vitro*.

Uses. Cocoa has nutritive, stimulant and diuretic properties. Theobromine is used as a diuretic. It has less action on the central nervous system than caffeine but is more diuretic. With its isomer, theophylline, the diuretic effect is even more marked. Oil of theobroma (q.v.) is used in pharmacy chiefly as a suppository base.

Allied products. *Guarana* (*Pasta Guarana* or *Brazilian cocoa*) is a dried paste prepared mainly from the seeds of *Paullinia cupana* (Sapindaceae). The seeds are collected from wild or cultivated plants in the upper Amazon basin by members of the Guaranis tribe. The kernels are roughly separated from the shell, broken and made into a paste with water, starch and other substances being frequently added. The paste is then made into suitable shapes and dried in the sun or over fires.

The drug usually occurs in cylindrical rolls 10–30 cm long and 2.5–4 cm diameter. Portions of broken seed project from the dark chocolate-brown outer surface. When broken, similar fragments project from the fractured surface. The drug has no marked odour but an astringent bitter taste.

Guarana contains 2.5–7.0% of caffeine, other xanthine derivatives, tannins about 12% ('guarana red') and other constituents resembling, as far as is known, those of cola and cocoa. Guarana resembles tea and coffee in its action and the powder grated from the masses is used in South America with water to make a drink. In the West it is now a popular remedy for combating fatigue, for slimming, and for the treatment of diarrhoea. The fat content of the drug is stated to effect a slow but steady release of the alkaloids (for a short article on guarana see P. Houghton, Pharm. J., 1995, **254**, 435).

Coffee consists of the seeds of *Coffea arabica* and other species of *Coffea* (Rubiaceae). It contains caffeine (1–2%), tannin and chlorogenic (caffeotannic) acid (see Fig. 19.5), fat, sugars and pentosans.

Prepared coffee is the kernel of the dried ripe seeds of various species, including *C. arabica* (Arabica coffee), *C. liberica* and *C. canephora* (Robusta coffee) (Rubiaceae), deprived of most of the seed coat and roasted. The kernels are dark brown, hard and brittle, elliptical or planoconvex and about 1.0 cm long. Coffee has a characteristic odour and taste. A decoction is used as a flavouring agent in Caffeine Iodide Elixir BPC (1979). Prepared coffee contains about 1–2% of caffeine, probably combined with chlorogenic acid and potassium. Other constituents include nicotinic acid, fixed oil and carbohydrates caramelized during roasting.

C. arabica, both as whole plants and as cell suspension cultures, has been considerably employed to study purine alkaloid variations and biosynthesis (q.v.).

Tea consists of the prepared leaves of *Camellia sinensis* (*Thea sinensis*) (Theaceae), a shrub cultivated in India, Sri Lanka, East Africa, Mauritius, China and Japan. The leaves contain thease, an enzymic mixture containing an oxidase, which partly converts the phlobatannin into phlobaphene. This oxidase may be destroyed by steaming for 30 s. Tea contains 1–5% of caffeine and 10–24% of tannin; also small quantities of theobromine, theophylline and volatile oil. The alkaloid content of the leaves is very much dependent on age and season.

C. sinensis is known locally as the Chinese tea plant, the flower buds and seeds of which contain acylated oleane-type triterpenes (theasaponins) with antiallergic activities (M. Yashikawa et al., Chem. Pharm. Bull., 2007, **55**, 57; **55**, 598). The flower buds of *C. japonica* yield noroleane and oleane-type triterpenoids having gastroprotective and platelet aggregation activities (M. Yashikawa et al., Chem. Pharm. Bull., 2007, **55**, 606).

Callus and root suspension cultures of *C. sinensis* have been shown to accumulate caffeine and theobromine (A. Shervington et al., Phytochemistry, 1998, **47**, 1535).

The possible beneficial effects of drinking black or green tea have received considerable coverage in the medical and national press. An infusion of tea contains in addition to caffeine a mixture of polyphenols including epigallocatechin-3-gallate possessing strong antioxidant and free-radical scavenging properties. Possible beneficial effects are: inhibition of angiogenesis, a process involving the growth of blood vessels necessary for tumour growth and metastasis; the treatment of genetic haemochromatosis by the inhibition of absorption of iron by tannates and other ligands; treatment of blindness caused by diabetes (an angiogenic related condition); and a lowering of the risk of ischemic heart disease in older men (a finding not substantiated with tea with milk added) see M. G. L. Hertog et al., Amer. J. Clin. Nutr., 1997, **65**, 1489; J. P. Kaltwasser, E. Werner, K. Schalk et al., Gut, 1998, **43**, 649; Y. Cao and R. Cao, Nature, 1999, **398**, 381.

Maté leaf

Maté (*Yerba maté; Paraguay tea*) consists of the dried and cured leaves of *Ilex paraguensis* (Aquifoliaceae) and other species of *Ilex*, small trees or shrubs indigenous to the region where Argentina, Paraguay and Brazil meet. The drug is obtained partly from wild plants (e.g. in Brazil) and partly from cultivated ones (in Argentina).

The branches are cut when the fruits are ripe and 'toasted' for a moment over a fire until they show blisters. The leaves are then separated and spread on a platform over a small wood fire for about 24–36 h. They are then reduced to a coarse powder and put into sacks (formerly into hide serons), in which the leaf should be allowed to mature for at least a year. Rapid drying in ovens gives an inferior product.

The whole leaves, seldom seen in commerce, are shortly petiolate, ovate or oblong-lanceolate, 5–15 cm long, and dark green to yellowish-green. They have a crenate-serrate margin and a coriaceous texture. The commercial drug consists of fragments of leaf with a variable amount of 'stalk'. It has a characteristic odour and a somewhat bitter-ish taste.

Maté contains about 0.2–2% of caffeine, about 10–16% of chloro-genic acid (caffeotannic acid) and a little volatile oil. It is said to be very rich in vitamins. Maté tea is very widely used in South America with some consumption in Europe and America. (For studies on maté drinking in S. America, see A. Vázquez and P. Moyna, *J. Ethnopharm.*, 1986, **18**, 267.)

Comfrey

The roots and aerial parts of *Symphytum officinale* (comfrey), family Boraginaceae, have long been important drugs in herbal medicine for the treatment of pulmonary and gastric conditions and various rheu-matic complaints. In addition to mucilage and tannin these contain allantoin (0.6–0.8% in the roots) which can be regarded as a break-down product of uric acid. Allantoin stimulates tissue regeneration and therefore the drug has been used for external injuries and gastric ulcers. A new saponin involving oleanic acid glycosylated at C-3 with arabi-nose-glucose-glucose has been reported (V. U. Ahmad *et al.*, *J. Nat. Prod.*, 1993, **56**, 329). (For a report on the isolation of other bidesmo-sidic triterpenoidal saponins see F. V. Mohammed *et al.*, *Planta Med.*, 1995, **61**, 94.) The relatively recent discovery of a range of pyrroliz-idine alkaloids in comfrey and in Russian comfrey (*S. × uplandicum*) has cast doubt on the desirability of using the drug for internal medica-tion (see p. 370). N.-C. Kim et al. (*J. Nat. Prod.*, 2001, **64**, 251) have described the separation of three such alkaloids by counter-current chromatography, each having 1,2-unsaturation of the pyrrolizidine nucleus and ester functions on two side-chains (variously angelic, tiglic, viridifloric or echimidinic acids), e.g. symphytine q.v. Only the root is included in the *BHP* 1996 and is listed as a vulnerary.

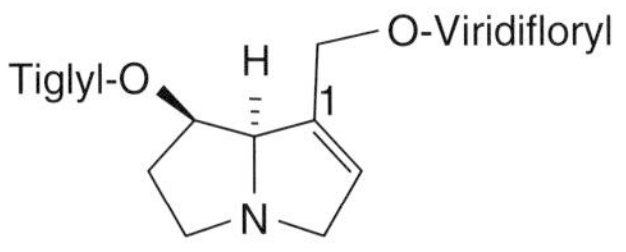

Symphytine

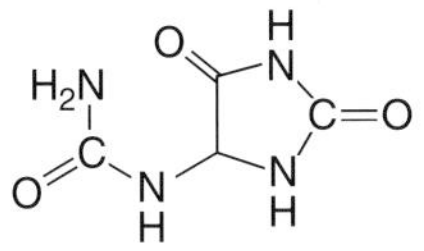

Allantoin

REDUCED PYRIDINE ALKALOIDS

In addition to the lysine-derived alkaloids (see Fig. 26.11), there are a number of other alkaloids having a reduced pyridine moiety. They include coniine (from hemlock), arecoline (see 'Areca Nut') and rici-nine, the alkaloid of the castor seed (q.v.). Ricinine has been shown to be derived from nicotinic acid or other participants of the pyridine nucleotide cycle; hence, glycerol and succinic acid proved to be good precursors but quinolinic acid was not detected as an intermediate, as originally expected in the pathway shown in Fig. 26.37.

Hemlock fruit

(*Conii Fructus*). The drug consists of the dried unripe fruits of *Conium maculatum* (Umbelliferae), the spotted hemlock, a poisonous biennial plant indigenous to Europe.

Hemlock was the plant used by the Greeks for preparing a draught by means of which criminals were put to death. It was employed in

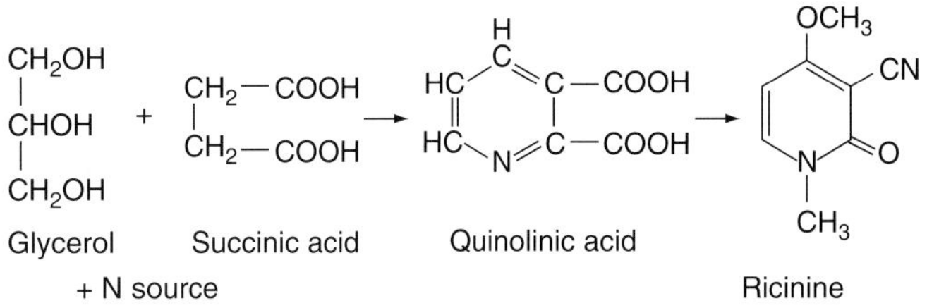

Fig. 26.37
Biosynthesis of ricinine.

Anglo-Saxon medicine and was in considerable use until about 80 years ago. Although now rarely employed, it merits attention as one of the commonest of our indigenous poisonous plants and on account of the fact that coniine was the first alkaloid to be synthesized (Ladenburg, 1886).

The fruit is a broadly ovate, somewhat laterally compressed cremo-carp about 3 mm long. It bears a small stylopod and the remains of the stigmas. Each mericarp has five prominent, primary ridges, the width of which is constantly altering so as to give them a beaded appearance. The transverse section differs from that of most umbelliferous fruits in not showing conspicuous vittae, although numerous very small ones are actually present. The endosperm is deeply grooved and is surrounded by well-marked, alkaloid-containing layers.

When hemlock is treated with solution of potassium hydroxide, it develops a strong, mouse-like odour owing to liberation of the alkaloid coniine. The latter is volatile and may be steam-distilled. It is present to the extent of 1–2.5% together with *N*-methyl coniine, conhydrine, pseudoconhydrine, conhydrinone and γ-coniceine. Roberts reported (*Phytochemistry*, 1981, **20**, 447) South African *Conium* to contain a high volatile oil composition, the main component being myrcene. The alkaloids were similar to those of European plants but consisted, in addition, of *N*-methyl pseudoconhydrine.

Daily fluctuations in the proportions of these alkaloids in the living plant have been reported. Unlike a large number of alkaloids, coniine does not appear to be biosynthesized in the plant directly from an amino acid, but from four molecules of acetic acid with the participa-tion of ammonia or some other nitrogen source. Leete's experiments (*J. Am. Chem. Soc.*, 1972, **94**, 5472) involving the isolation of [1′-^{14}C]-coniine and γ-[1′-^{14}C]-coniceine after feeding hemlock plants with 5-oxo[6-^{14}C]octanol and 5-oxo[6-^{14}C] octanoic acid are consis-tent with Fig. 26.38 for the biogenesis of coniine and related alkaloids from acetate.

The origin of the nitrogen may be indicated by Roberts' work, in which an enzyme, mol. wt 56 200, catalysing a transamination between 5-ketooctanal and L-alanine to give γ-coniceine and pyruvic acid, has been isolated.

Further reading
Reynolds T 2005 Hemlock alkaloids from Socrates to poison aloes.
  Phytochemistry 66(12): 1399–1406

Areca nut
Areca nuts (*betel nut*) are the seeds of *Areca catechu* (Palmae), a feather-palm 15–17 m high, which is cultivated in tropical India, Sri Lanka, Malaysia, south China, the East Indies, the Philippine Islands and part of East Africa (including Zanzibar and Tanzania). Large quantities are exported from Madras, Singapore, Penang and Sri Lanka.

History. Areca was known in China under the name *pinlang* (prob-ably a corruption of the Malay name for the tree *pinang*) from at least

26

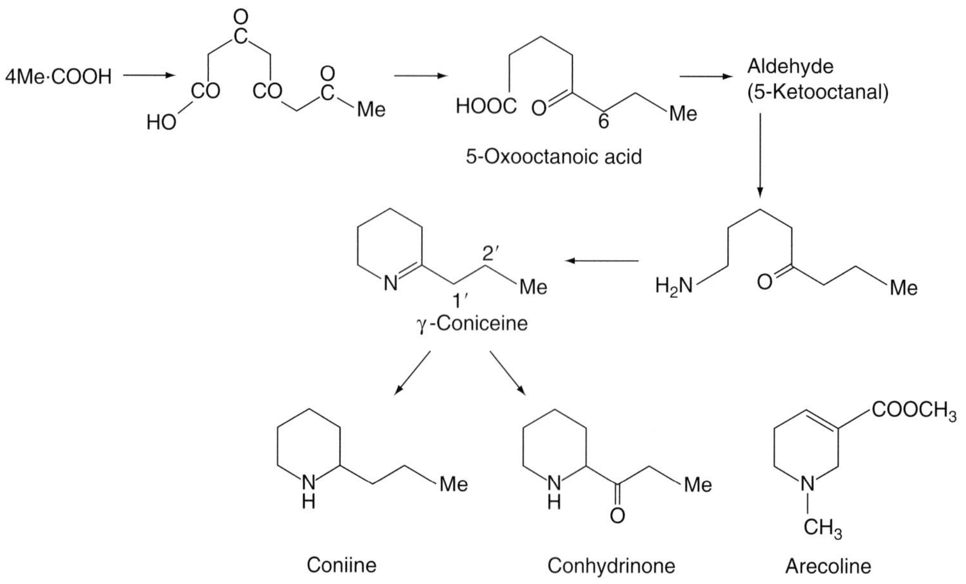

Fig. 26.38
Biogenesis of hemlock alkaloids.
Formula of arecoline.

100 BC. Immense quantities have been consumed in the East from very early times in the form of a masticatory known as betel, which consists of a mixture of areca nuts, the leaves of *Piper betle*, and lime. The value of areca as a taenicide was also known in the East.

Collection and preparation. The fruits, of which about 100 are annually borne on each tree, are detached by means of bamboo poles and the seeds extracted. The latter, before exportation, are usually boiled in water containing lime, and dried.

Characters. The areca nut is about 2.5 cm long and rounded conical in shape. Patches of a silvery coat, the inner layer of the pericarp, occasionally adhere to the testa. The deep brown testa is marked with a network of depressed, fawn-coloured lines. The seed is very hard, has a faint odour when broken and an astringent, somewhat acrid taste. Sections of the seed show dark-brown, wavy lines (folds of testa and perisperm) extending into the lighter-coloured interior (ruminate endosperm). At the flattened end of the seed is a small embryo.

Constituents. Areca contains alkaloids which are reduced pyridine derivatives. Of these, arecoline (methyl ester of arecaine) (Fig. 26.38), arecaine (*N*-methylguvacine) and guvacine (tetrahydronicotinic acid) may be mentioned. Only arecoline, which is present to the extent of 0.1–0.5%, is medicinally important. Ether extraction yields about 14% of fat, consisting mainly of the glycerides of lauric, myristic and oleic acids; subsequent extraction with alcohol yields about 15% of amorphous red tannin matter (areca red) of phlobaphene nature.

TERPENOID ALKALOIDS

Included in the terpenoid alkaloids are monoterpenes (e.g. skytanthine), sesquiterpenes (e.g. patchoulipyridine) and diterpenes (e.g. the alkaloids of *Aconitum*, *Delphinium* and *Taxus* spp.). Various *Taxus* spp. are considered elsewhere and aconite, which has some medicinal interest, is described below. Valerian root, which contains monoterpene alkaloids of the skytanthine type, is grouped

with the iridoids in Chapter 24. (For reviews of the literature covering diterpenoid alkaloids for the period 1985–92 (308 refs in all) see N. S. Yunusov, *Nat. Prod. Rep.*, 1991, **8**, 499; 1993, **10**, 471; also F. P. Wang and X. T. Liang, *Alkaloids*, 1992, **42**, 151 (196 refs) and Atta-ur-Rahman and M. I. Choudhary, *Nat. Prod. Rep.*, 1995, **12**, 361).

Aconite root

Aconite (*Wolfsbane Root*) consists of the dried roots of *Aconitum napellus* (Ranunculaceae), collected from wild or cultivated plants. *A. napellus* is a polymorphic aggregate extending from Western Europe to the Himalayas. Cultivated forms have deeper coloured flowers, and darker green and less narrowly divided leaves than the wild plants; the former are in considerable demand in Europe as cut flowers and to meet this demand a rapid micropropagation method using floating membrane rafts and shoot tips has been developed (A. A. Watad *et al.*, *Plant Cell Rep.*, 1995, **14**, 345). The greater part of the commercial drug is derived from wild plants grown in central and southern Europe, particularly Spain.

Macroscopical characters. Aconite differs in appearance according to the season of collection. The aconite formerly cultivated in England was harvested in the autumn and consisted of both parent and daughter roots. Both are obconical in shape, dark-brown in colour, 4–10 cm long and 1–3 cm diameter at the crown. Most Continental aconite is collected from plants at the flowering stage and therefore consists mainly of parent roots. The parent roots bear the remains of aerial stems and are more shrivelled than the daughter roots, which bear large, apical buds. Rootlets may be present but these are usually broken off. The odour is usually slight but samples vary in this respect. Taste at first slightly sweet, followed by tingling and numbness (taste with care; long chewing may be painful).

Transverse sections cut about one-third of the length from the crown show a stellate cambium with five to eight angles. The amount of lignified tissues is small, the greater part of the root consisting of starch-containing parenchyma of the pith and secondary phloem.

Constituents. Aconite contains terpene ester alkaloids, of which the most important is aconitine.

	R¹	R²
Aconine	H	H
Benzoylaconine	$CO \cdot C_6H_5$	H
Aconitine	$CO \cdot C_6H_5$	$CO \cdot CH_3$

Aconite also contains other alkaloids such as mesaconitine, hypaconitine, neopelline, napelline and neoline. Hikino *et al.* (*J. Nat. Prod.*, 1984, **47**, 190) isolated eight alkaloids from roots of Swiss origin, five being new to the species.

From ssp. *vulgare* Arlandini *et al.*, (*J. Nat. Prod.*, 1987, **50**, 937) isolated *N*-deethylaconitine, and Chen *et al.*, (*J. Nat. Prod.*, 1999, **62**, 701) obtained twelve diterpenoid alkaloids, characterized by NMR and MS, from the herb and flowers.

The percentage of total alkaloid in the drug is about 0.3–1.2%. About 30% of the total is ether-soluble aconitine. In view of the different groups of alkaloids reported by workers over the years, and the large variation in aconitine contents of roots, it seems that in all probability there is considerable chemical variation between varieties of *A. napellus*. Aconite also contains aconitic acid (see p. 177) and abundant starch.

Other *Aconitum* species may contain aconitine or similar alkaloids of very varied toxicity and the hydrolysis products of those given in Table 26.8 may be compared with aconitine. According to Zhu *et al.* (*Phytochemistry*, 1993, **32**, 767) more than 96 spp. of *Aconitum* have been studied chemically, resulting in reports regarding over 250 C_{19}-diterpene alkaloids and a number of C_{20}-diterpene alkaloids. For a recent report on the alkaloids of the aerial parts of *A. variegatum* from the Carpathians and Pyrenees, see J. G. Diaz *et al.*, *Phytochemistry*, 2005, **66**, 837.

The employment of *Aconitum* spp. as arrow poisons in China, India and other parts of Asia has been reviewed by Bisset in a series of publications (*J. Ethnopharmacology*, 1981, **4**, 247; 1984, **12**, 1; 1989, **25**, 1; 1991, **32**, 71).

Japanese aconite

Japanese aconite was formerly an article of European commerce. The roots are shorter and plumper than the European drug, and dark grey or brownish in colour. *Aconitum japonicum* possesses cardiotonic properties and the principal alkaloid associated with this activity is higenamine [(±)- demethylcoclaurine], formula Fig. 26.19, which is active

at about the same dosage levels as the *Digitalis* glycosides. The only other cardioactive alkaloid obtained is coryneine chloride (dopamine methochloride) from *A. carmichaelii*. The reported yield of both alkaloids was small. These species are important in Oriental medicine and have clinical usage.

Chinese aconites

A. carmichaelii, *A. kusnezofii* and *A. brachypodum* are three species employed in Chinese medicine. Traditionally, as with other very poisonous drugs, such as nux vomica, the toxicity is reduced by processing—in this case by soaking or boiling in water which causes some hydrolysis of the alkaloids. However this treatment may not always be properly controlled and as reported in the *Lancet* (1992), in Hong Kong 17 Chinese were poisoned, two fatally, as a result of consuming a herbal preparation involving the above species.

For the characterization of trans-2,2',4,4'-tetramethyl-6,6'-dinitroazobenzene from the traditional Chinese medicinal plant, *A. sungpanense* see X. Wang *et al.*, *Fitoterapia*, 2004, **75**, 789.

Indian aconites

The *Indian Pharmacopoeia* includes the dried root of *A. chasmanthum*. This it describes as being 2.5–4.5 cm long. It contains indaconitine. Several other aconites have been imported from India and Pakistan, including roots from *A. deinorrhizum* and *A. balfourii*, with smaller quantities of *A. spicatum* and *A. laciniatum*. In 1970 Mehra and Purie considered that some six species were being collectively exported under the commercial name of *A. ferox*. Samples often consist of daughter roots about 15 cm long and 4 cm diameter at the crown. The surface is dark brown and coarsely wrinkled. The drug is very hard and horny, the starch being usually gelantinized by excessive heating. (For the isolation of alkaloids from *A. ferox* see J. B. Hanuman and A. Katz, *J. Nat. Prod.*, 1993, **56**, 801.)

Uses. Aconite is a very potent and quick-acting poison which is now rarely used internally in the UK, except in homeopathic doses. The drug was included in the *BPC* (1973) and was formerly used for the preparation of an antineuralgic liniment.

STEROIDAL ALKALOIDS

Steroidal alkaloids arise by the inclusion of a basic nitrogen at some point in the steroid molecule. Those of the C_{27} group include the *Solanum* alkaloids mentioned in Chapter 23 in relation to their potential as steroid precursors, and the *Veratrum* alkaloids, considered in more detail below, which have a similar structure. A second, C_{21} group, of which many examples are found in the Apocynaceae (*Holarrhena* and *Funtumia*) and in the Buxaceae, probably arise from pregnenolone by amination at either C-3 or C-20 (see formulae of examples overleaf). Conessine is a common alkamine of the group and represents a desirable starting material for the synthesis of some hormones (e.g. aldosterone). Whereas

Table 26.8 Hydrolysis products of *Aconitum* alkaloids.

Alkaloid	Base	Acids
Hypaconitine	Hypaconine	Acetic and benzoic acids
Jesaconitine	Aconine	Acetic acid and anisic acid (*p*-methoxybenzoic acid)
Pseudaconitine	Pseudaconine	Acetic acid and veratric acid (Fig. 19.5)
Lycaconitine	Lycoctonine	Lycoctoninic acid (*N*-succinyl anthranilic acid)

Holaphylline

Conessine

holaphylline has little toxicity, the quaternary diamine malouetine, which is found in the same family, is a potent curare-type poison.

For reviews of steroidal alkaloids see R. Shakirov *et al.*, *Nat. Prod. Rep.*, 1990, **7**, 557; Atta-ur-Rahman and M. I. Choudhary, *ibid.*, 1995, **12**, 361. References pertaining to the investigation and traditional uses of neotropical S. American steroidal akaloids may be found in J. Nino *et al.*, *Pharm. Biol.*, 2006, **44**, 14.

Veratrums

American veratrum (Green Hellebore), *Veratrum viride* (Liliaceae), and European veratrum (White Hellebore), *V. album*, are very similar perennial herbs, whose rhizomes and roots are almost indistinguishable either macroscopically or microscopically. Some alkaloidal constituents are common to both species. The American drug is collected in the eastern parts of Canada and the USA and white hellebore in central and southern Europe.

History. The North American Indians were aware of the therapeutic activity of American hellebore and it was employed by the early European settlers. Its use spread to England about 1862. In Europe the closely allied drug obtained from *V. album* had long been used. Until about 1950 veratrums, except as insecticides, were being little used. Since then they have been the subject of much research and are now employed in the treatment of hypertension.

Collection and preparation. The rhizome is dug up in the autumn, often sliced longitudinally into halves or quarters to facilitate drying, and sometimes deprived of many of the roots.

Macroscopical characters. The rhizome, if entire, is more or less conical and 3–8 cm long and 2–3.5 cm wide; externally brownish-grey. The roots, if present, are numerous and almost completely cover the rhizome. Entire roots are up to 8 cm long and 4 mm diameter, light brown to light orange, and usually much wrinkled (for transverse section, see Fig. 41.8H). Commercial American veratrum is more frequently sliced than is the drug from *V. album*, and more of the roots remain attached to the rhizome. Odourless, but sternutatory; taste, bitter and acrid.

Microscopical characters. The various species of *Veratrum* resemble one another very closely in microscopical structure. The rhizomes of *V. viride* and *V. album* are virtually identical microscopically but minor differences occur in the roots. Microscopical distinction of the powders is nevertheless difficult.

Allied drugs. Youngken (1952) reported on the following substitutes for *V. viride*, which have been offered commercially: *V. album*, *V. eschscholtzii*, *V. woodii*, *V. californicum* and what is believed to be a variety of *V. viride* from Montana. In addition to these, *V. fimbriatum* has been the subject of chemical investigation.

Constituents. Numerous steroidal alkaloids are present in both *V. album* and *V. viride*; over 100 have been recorded in the former and new alkaloids of both groups (see below) continue to be isolated (Atta-ur-Rahman *et al.*, *J. Nat. Prod.*, 1992, **55**, 565; K. A. El Sayed *et al.*, *Int. J. Pharmacognosy*, 1996, **34**, 111). *V. nigrum* L. var. *ussuriense* is used for the preparation of the Chinese drug 'Li-lu', together with other species (W. Zhao *et al.*, *Chem. Pharm. Bull.*, 1991, **39**, 549). Both drugs have long been used as insecticides, but their more recent importance results from those alkaloids that have hypotensive properties. Alkaloids present in some other species, e.g. *V. californicum*, can cause serious damage to livestock grazing in locations where the plant occurs as they have teratogenic properties (see 'Teratogens of Higher Plants', Chapter 39).

There are two distinct chemical groups of veratrum steroidal alkaloids and these are now referred to as the jerveratrum and ceveratrum groups.

Jerveratrum alkaloids contain only 1–3 oxygen atoms and occur in the plant as free alkamines and also combined, as glucosides, with one molecule of D-glucose. Examples are pseudojervine derived from jervine and veratrosine derived from veratramine.

Ceveratrum alkaloids are highly hyroxylated compounds with 7–9 oxygen atoms. They usually occur in the plant esterified with two or more various acids (acetic, α-methylbutyric, α-methyl-α-hydroxybutyric, α-methyl-α,β-dihydroxybutyric), but are also found unconjugated. It is these ester alkaloids that are responsible for the hypotensive activity of veratrum; examples are the esters of germine, protoverine and veracevine.

Uses. American veratrum is used for the preparation of Veriloid, a mixture of the hypotensive alkaloids. European veratrum is used for the preparation of the protoveratrines. Both drugs, and the closely related cevadilla seeds (*Schoenocaulon officinale*), are used as insecticides.

Cevadilla seeds

Cevadilla seeds, which contain alkaloids similar to those of veratrum, are considered under 'Pesticides', Chapter 40.

Kurchi or holarrhena bark

The stem-bark of *Holarrhena pubescens* (*H. antidysenterica*) (Apocynaceae), has long been valued for its antidysenteric properties. The plant is a small tree found in many parts of India and up to about 1250 m in the Himalayas; Than reports that the Burmese material is also satisfactory. The drug should be obtained from trees about 8–12 years old, which yield a stem bark about 6–12 mm in thickness.

The pieces are recurved. The outer surface shows deep cracks and is buff to brownish in colour. Fracture, brittle and splintery. Odour, none; taste, bitter.

Kurchi contains numerous steroidal-type alkaloids (1.8–4.5%) including conessine, norconessine, isoconessine and kurchine. Bhutani *et al. (Phytochemistry*, 1988, **27**, 925; 1990, **29**, 969) isolated six new steroidal alkaloids named regholarrhenines A–F, and P. J. Houghton and M. L. Dias Diogo (*Int. J. Pharmacognosy*, 1996, **34**, 305) have reported on two bark samples from Malawi showing levels of conessine comparable with those of Nepalese material.

The bark, official in India, is required to contain not less than 2% of alkaloids and Kurchin Bismuth Iodide, a preparation much used for amoebic dysentery, 23–27% of total alkaloids. Conessine hydrobromide is manufactured from the seeds of *H. antidysenterica* and the polymorphous W. African species *H. floribunda* has been cultivated for the same purpose. For the isolation of a new steroidal alkaloid from the seeds of holarrhena and for other references associated with the drug see A. Kumar and M. Ali, *Fitoterapia*, 2000, **71**, 101.

The root-bark also contains conessine and other steroidal alkaloids.

New isolated flavonoids of the leaves are recorded by P. Tuntiwachwuttikul *et al.*, *Fitoterapia*, 2007, **78**, 271.

Callus and cell suspension cultures of *H. antidysenterica* produce principally conessine and the addition of cholesterol to the nutrient medium has been shown to enhance alkaloid production.

26

27

The search for naturally derived anticancer agents*

In the endeavour to discover effective drugs for the treatment of various cancerous diseases, the natural kingdoms, especially the plant kingdom, have been extensively researched. The research involved has been enormous and although the number of successful outcomes appears very modest, the effective drugs produced rank among the most common chemotherapeutic agents employed. Also, the wide diversity and complexity of the compounds isolated have afforded valuable material for the manufacture of semi-synthetic derivatives, often less toxic and clinically superior to the original isolate.

It has been estimated (2005) that over 60% of the anticancer drugs in current use are in some way derived from plants and micro-organisms; marine products are in the process of evaluation. A successful anticancer drug should kill or incapacitate cancer cells without causing excessive damage to normal dividing cells. This ideal is difficult, or perhaps impossible, to attain and is why cancer patients frequently suffer unpleasant side-effects when undergoing treatment.

PLANTS IN CANCER TREATMENT

Plant materials have been used in the treatment of malignant diseases for centuries; a comprehensive survey of the literature describing plants used against cancer listed over 1400 genera (Hartwell, 1967–71, see *Lloydia*, 1971, **34**, 427 for index). Recent phytochemical examination of plants which have a suitable history of use in folklore for the treatment of cancer has indeed often resulted in the isolation of principles with antitumour activity. Podophyllum was used over 2000 years ago by the ancient Chinese as an antitumour drug, and resins from the root of the plant *Podophyllum hexandrum* (syn. *P. emodi*) and the related American species, the May-apple (*P. peltatum*) have yielded a number of lignans and their glycosides having antitumour activity. Although the major constituents from these two species, podophyllotoxin and the peltatins, are unsuitable for systemic drug use, two semi-synthetic derivatives of podophyllotoxin, etoposide and teniposide, gave particularly good results in clinical trials. Etoposide is currently available for the treatment of small-cell lung cancer and testicular cancer, and teniposide is used in paediatric cancers, though both compounds have a similar anticancer spectrum. Other podophyllotoxin-related analogues have been developed and tested. Podophyllotoxin itself may be used topically, and is most effective in the treatment of venereal warts. From the time of Galen (about AD 180), the juice expressed from woody nightshade (*Solanum dulcamara*) has been used to treat cancers, tumours and warts, and references to its use have appeared in the literature of many countries. The active tumour-inhibitory principle has been identified as the steroidal alkaloid glycoside β-solamarine. Various lichens, e.g. species of *Cladonia, Cetraria* and *Usnea*, also have a history of use in folk medicine against cancer since about AD 970. These are all rich sources of usnic acid, a compound which has been recognized for many years as an antibacterial and antifungal agent, but only more recently as an antitumour compound. Similarly, many centuries ago, the druids claimed that mistletoe (*Viscum album*) could be used to cure cancer; protein fractions with marked antitumour activity have been isolated from mistletoe extract. Mezereon (*Daphne mezereum*), despite its toxic properties, has also been used in many countries for the treatment of cancer. The active antitumour constituent of this plant has been identified as a diterpene derivative mezerein, which is structurally very similar to the toxic principle daphnetoxin.

Very successful higher plant materials used in cancer chemotherapy are the alkaloids of *Catharanthus roseus*. Research on this plant, the Madagascan periwinkle, was stimulated by its mention in folklore,

*Based on an original chapter 'Tumour inhibitors from plants', by P. M. Dewick.

not as a cure for cancer, but in the treatment of diabetes. No hypoglycaemic activity was detected, but treated test animals became susceptible to bacterial infection, and this led the researchers to undertake extensive examination for possible immunosuppressive principles causing these effects. A number of bisindole alkaloids showing antileukaemic activity have subsequently been isolated and two of these, vincaleukoblastine (vinblastine) and leurocristine (vincristine), are now extracted commercially from *Catharanthus roseus* and used, either alone, or in combination with other forms of therapy for cancer treatment. Another important, more recent, addition to the list of anticancer drugs is paclitaxel (Taxol), a diterpene derivative isolated initially from the bark of the Pacific Yew, *Taxus brevifolia*. Although reportedly used by Native North Americans for various conditions, it does not appear to have had any traditional cancer usage and was obtained as part of the random collection programme of the US National Cancer Institute (NCI). Taxol and related taxanes are treated below.

METHODS OF INVESTIGATION

An intensive survey of plants, microorganisms and marine animals (starfish, corals, etc.) for antitumour activity began in the late 1950s, mainly because the United States National Cancer Institute (NCI) instigated and funded a major screening programme. A random-selection screening programme was adopted, since novel compounds may be found anywhere in the plant or animal kingdom, and it is known that some natural products are restricted to a single genus, or even species. Random mass-screening is naturally an expensive operation, and probably only justified in certain areas, where our present range of drugs is seriously inadequate or inefficient. Cancer was considered to be in this category.

Since the beginning of the programme, which continued until 1983, a vast number of extracts from various sources has been tested for antitumour activity. About 4% of the extracts tested have shown reproducible activity. Over about 25 years, some 114 000 plant samples representing 40 000 species were tested. Different parts of a plant—seeds, leaves, roots, etc.—were separately examined wherever possible. It is estimated that between a quarter and half a million plant species exist worldwide, and thus the plant kingdom still represented a vast untapped source of material.

The isolation of biologically active constituents, probably minor constituents, from a crude plant extract involves techniques differing from those of conventional phytochemical evaluation. With these, it was customary to study those chemicals which were most easily separated from a plant extract; these were usually those present in the largest quantities and which crystallized readily, or those which represented the researcher's field of interest, e.g. alkaloids, terpenoids, phenols, etc. Only after characterization of their structures were such compounds subjected to biological testing, e.g. for hypotensive, antibacterial, anticancer activities, etc., and this would depend on sufficient material being available. Countless medicinally useful compounds have been missed in this type of approach.

In the more recent systematic studies for useful plant constituents, every portion of the plant and every fraction of the extract is tested biologically before any constituent is isolated and characterized. Usually only those fractions showing biological activity are studied further. Thus, one may isolate almost any class of compound as an active constituent, and it may not be one traditionally associated with a particular plant family. Even procedures involving continuous monitoring of fractions for biological activity are not free from anomalies. It is quite well known that isolated constituents of a plant drug may not give the same clinical response as a crude preparation of that plant drug. Very often, the total therapeutic activity is greater than, or different from the therapeutic activities of the individuals. Synergism or antagonism (see Chapter 7) due to the complex nature of the extract are probably the causes of such observations. It is thus possible that a fraction from a plant extract, although showing significant biological activity, possesses no single constituent with this activity. Conversely, a fraction showing no activity may still contain an active constituent. A further complication is that crude fractions may contain additional substances with delayed toxicity, causing test animals to die at about the same time as control animals.

An effective screening procedure in which a large number of crude plant extracts are to be assayed for biological activity should fulfil several criteria. It should be sufficiently selective to limit the number of leads for follow-up evaluation yet it should be highly sensitive in order to detect low concentrations of active compounds, and it should be specific so that the assay is not affected by a wide variety of inactive compounds. The preliminary screens employed in the NCI studies changed during the lifetime of the programme to avoid detecting weakly active common plant products such as polyphenols, tannins, saponins and sterols not capable of being developed into useful drugs; such dereplication (Chapters 8, 9) is now commonly employed. The routine testing of extract fractions for antitumour activity is frequently done via an *in vitro* cytotoxity assay, although *in vitro* cytotoxicity is not always an effective or reliable means of predicting *in vivo* antitumour activity. However, since the *in vitro* cytotoxicity bioassay is rapid and inexpensive, and only small amounts of extract are necessary, it is the popular method for initial tests.

Promising chemicals are subsequently tested against a range of standard experimental neoplasms, and then considered for preclinical toxicological studies if these results are sufficiently encouraging. At this stage, relatively large amounts of material will be required, and larger-scale extractions and fractionation may be necessary. Very few compounds will reach clinical trials. A low or very narrow therapeutic index (the ratio of maximum tolerated dose to minimum effective dose), undesirable side-effects or high toxicity can outweigh beneficial tumour-inhibitory activity. From some 25 000 screens conducted annually by the NCI (including both synthetic and natural materials), only eight to twelve compounds are likely to be selected for preclinical testing, and perhaps only six to eight go on to clinical trials. Slightly less than half of these may be plant-derived.

Should a plant-derived natural product or derivative be considered worthy of development as a drug, the availability of future supplies of the plant becomes critical. Collections from the wild may be exploited if the plant is common, but mass cultivation should be considered. With slow-growing crops, e.g. trees, this could mean a considerable delay before significant supplies are available. Alternative plants might be richer sources of the compound, or be more accessible; other species of the same genus or closely related genera from the same family should also be analysed. Thus, wild sources could not supply the huge amount of *Taxus brevifolia* bark needed to satisfy demand for the manufacture of taxol but the discovery of baccatin III and deacetylbaccatin III (readily convertible to taxol) in the leaves of the common yew (*T. baccata*) has ensured the future supply of the drug. For commercial exploitation, agreements giving some slice of any profit arising from the sale of a product derived from wild plant material must be arranged with the country of origin.

Plant tissue cultures might provide a reliable source. If total synthesis of the active chemical is feasible, this will always be the preferred option.

However, the extremely complex structures of most bioactive natural products frequently preclude satisfactory commercial syntheses.

Although the random-selection screening programme for natural products was terminated by the NCI in 1983, the number of cytotoxic and antitumour agents identified was enormous, and these have increased our understanding of the cancer process, and the mechanisms of action of the agents. Synthetic work has enabled structure–activity studies to be undertaken, and there is every hope that synthetic or semi-synthetic analogues may, in time, be developed and become useful drugs.

Over the years, separation techniques (TLC, HPLC, chiral chromatography, etc.) and chemical structure determination (MS, NMR, UV, X-ray crystallography) have reached high levels of sophistication. For the examination of large numbers of samples, high-throughput screening is now employed (Chapter 9).

Following on from the above, partly as a result of new screening techniques, the NCI in 1986 revived its collection of plants, focusing on tropical and subtropical species which had local medicinal use.

Considerable recent research has been, and still is, carried out by National Cooperative Drug Discovery Groups (NCDDGs); these groups result from cooperative agreement awards funded essentially by the NCI, which supports all aspects of preclinical anticancer drug discovery and treatment strategies. In 2003, there were 13 funded groups of which five were natural-product based. Such groups may involve the participation world-wide, of universities, research centres and industry, together with the resource countries of plant or marine materials. The complex nature of such groups is evident from the number of authors involved in ensuing publications. For updated reports from a number of such groups, see 'Further reading'. For an article giving explanatory details of the NCDDGs project, see Y. F. Hallock and G. M. Cragg, *Pharm. Biol.*, 2003, **41**(supplement), 78.

Another multinational group involving collaboration of seven S. American countries and supported by the Organization of American States has prioritized 314 Latin American plant species for screening for cytotoxic properties. Results for some 70 species from 40 families tested against breast, lung and central nervous system human cancer cell lines have been reported (A. I. Calderon *et al.* (11 authors), *Pharm. Biol.*, 2006, **44**, 130).

For cytotoxicity testing, human cancer cell lines obtained from the NCI are frequently employed. Plant selection for screening can be assisted by initially choosing those from an ethnomedical database and submitting them to a search for biological and chemical information in the libraries held by NAPRALERT (see Chapter 2), industry or other research centres.

Research groups in which there is a commercial interest should establish agreements with the countries of origin of the plant material giving the latter a fair share of any profits that might arise from the marketing of any successful products. This follows from the 1992 UN Convention on Biological Diversity, which calls for recognition of the sovereign rights of countries to control the utilization of their natural resources and genetic materials. Further, some countries, e.g. the Philippines, have instituted their own regulations concerning bioprospecting.

ESTABLISHED NATURAL PRODUCTS AS TUMOUR INHIBITORS

The tumour-inhibitory principles isolated in screening tests are usually new natural products, spanning a wide range of structural types.

Examples of these, subdivided into phytochemical groups, are listed in Table 27.1, and structures of the more promising chemicals which were subsequently evaluated in clinical tests are shown in Fig. 27.1. However, a number of the compounds isolated were, in fact, previously known natural products. These were presumably compounds which had not been subjected to rigorous testing for biological, particularly antitumour, activity. Amongst these are usnic acid, ellagic acid, the anthraquinone aloe-emodin, the quinones juglone and lapachol, pyrrolizidine alkaloids retronecine and monocrotaline, the nitrophenanthrene aristolochic acid (see 'Serpentary'), the bufadienolide hellebrigenin acetate, the *Colchicum* alkaloids colchicine, demecolcine and 3-demethylcolchicine (see 'Colchicum'). Other known compounds that proved active but were rejected on terms of toxicity, low therapeutic index, etc. were the alkaloids of *Senecio*, indicine N-oxide from *Heliotropium indicum* and the cucurbitacins. Further examples established as tumour inhibitors at much later dates than the above were the alkaloids acronycine, ellipticine, emetine and nitidine. Acronycine, from *Acronychia baueri*, failed in phase 1 clinical trials. The pyridocarbazole alkaloids ellipticine and 9-methoxyellipticine from *Ochrosia elliptica* and other related plants, together with a number of synthetic analogues appeared useful but exhibited unacceptable side-effects. However, the quaternization of 9-hydroxyellipticine to give the water-soluble 9-hydroxy-2-N-methylellipticinium acetate (elliptinium acetate) (Fig. 27.2) has produced a highly active material, of value in some forms of breast cancer, and perhaps also in renal cell cancer. A variety of such quaternized derivatives is being tested, and some water-soluble N-glycosides also show high activity. *Cephaelis ipecacuanha* has been used for many years as an emetic and expectorant and the principal alkaloid, emetine, was shown to have antitumour properties. Clinical usefulness was marginal, however, and some toxic effects were noted. Nitidine is a benzophenanthridine alkaloid isolated from *Zanthoxylum nitidum*, and has more recently been obtained from screens of *Fagara* species (Rutaceae). Nitidine was selected for development based on its exceptional antileukaemic activity, but was dropped owing to erratic toxicity. The closely related alkaloid fagaronine is less toxic than nitidine. Similar benzophenanthridine derivatives are present in *Chelidonium majus* (Papaveraceae), a plant with substantial folklore history of use in the treatment of cancers. More recently, NK 109 (Fig. 27.2), a synthetic isomer of fagaridine found in *Fagara xanthoxyloides*, has been found to have greater antitumour activity than any of the natural benzophenanthridine structures, coupled with excellent stability, and was entered for clinical trials in Japan.

NEW NATURAL PRODUCTS WITH ANTITUMOUR ACTIVITY

The systematic studies have also resulted in the isolation of many new natural products exhibiting antitumour activity, and a number of these were considered sufficiently active for clinical studies to be commenced (Fig. 27.1 and Table 27.1). Tylocrebine, a phenanthroindolizidine alkaloid from *Tylophora crebiflora* was sufficiently active for further development, but in a clinical trial unmanageable CNS effects precluded continuation of the studies. Two bis-benzylisoquinoline alkaloids, thalicarpine from *Thalictrum dasycarpum* and tetrandrine from *Cyclea peltata* appeared particularly promising and were selected for development. Clinical trials showed no antitumour activity, and these compounds were dropped from further study. Camptothecin and derivatives, alkaloids from the Chinese tree *Camptotheca acuminata*, showed broad-spectrum activity and produced a fair response in

Table 27.1 Some antitumour compounds from plants.

Class	Compound	Plant Source	Family
Monoterpene	Allamandin	*Allamanda cathartica*	Apocynaceae
	4-Ipomeanol	*Ipomoea batatas*	Convolvulaceae
	Penstimide	*Penstemon deutus*	Scrophulariaceae
Sesquiterpene	Baccharin	*Baccharis megapotamica*	Compositae
	Elephantopin	*Elephantopus elatus*	Compositae
	Helenalin	*Helenium autumnale*	Compositae
	Liatrin	*Liatris chapmanii*	Compositae
	Phyllanthoside	*Phyllanthus acuminatus*	Euphorbiaceae
	Phyllanthostatin 1	*P. acuminatus*	Euphorbiaceae
	Vernolepin	*Vernonia hymenolepis*	Compositae
Diterpene	Gnidin	*Gnidia lamprantha*	Thymelaeaceae
	Jatrophone	*Jatropha gossypiifolia*	Euphorbiaceae
	Mezerein	*Daphne mezereum*	Thymelaeaceae
	Taxodione	*Taxodium distichum*	Taxodiaceae
	Taxol	*Taxus brevifolia*	Taxaceae
	Tripdiolide	*Tripterygium wilfordii*	Celastraceae
	Triptolide	*T. wilfordii*	Celastraceae
Quassinoid/Simaroubolide	Bruceantin	*Brucea antidysenterica*	Simaroubaceae
	Glaucarubinone	*Simarouba glauca*	Simaroubaceae
	Holacanthone	*Holacantha emoryi*	Simaroubaceae
Triterpenoid, Steroid, etc.			
Cucurbitacin	Cucurbitacin E	*Marah oreganus*	Cucurbitaceae
Saponin	Acer saponin P	*Acer negundo*	Aceraceae
Cardenolide	Strophanthidin	*Parquetina nigrescens*	Asclepiadaceae
Bufadienolide	Hellebrigenin acetate	*Bersama abyssinica*	Melianthaceae
Withanolide	Withaferin A	*Acnistus arborescens*	Solanaceae
Stilbene	Combretastin A-4	*Combretum caffrum*	Combretaceae
Lignan	α- and β-Peltatin	*Podophyllum peltatum*	Berberidaceae
	Podophyllotoxin	*P. hexandrum, P. peltatum*	Berberidaceae
		Juniperus chinensis	Cupressaceae
	Steganacin	*Steganotaenia araliacea*	Umbelliferae
Quinone	Jacaranone	*Jacaranda caucana*	Bignoniaceae
	Lapachol	*Stereospermum suaveolens*	Bignoniaceae
Alkaloid			
Pyrrolizidine	Monocrotaline	*Crotalaria spectabilis*	Leguminosae
	Indicine-*N*-oxide	*Heliotropium indicum*	Boraginaceae
Isoquinoline	Emetine	*Cephaelis acuminata*	Rubiaceae
Bis-isoquinoline	Tetrandrine	*Cyclea peltata*	Menispermaceae
	Thalicarpine	*Thalictrum dasycarpum*	Ranunculaceae
Benzophenanthridine	Fagaronine	*Fagara zanthoxyloides*	Rutaceae
	Nitidine	*F. macrophylla*	Rutaceae
Phenanthroindolizidine	Tylocrebine	*Tylophora crebiflora*	Asclepiadaceae
Acridone	Acronycine	*Acronychia baueri*	Rutaceae
Pyridocarbazole	Ellipticine	*Ochrosia elliptica, O. moorei*	Apocynaceae
	9-Methoxyellipticine	*O. maculata*	Apocynaceae
Pyrroloquinoline	Camptothecin	*Camptotheca acuminata*	Nyssaceae
		Nothapodytes foetida (formerly *Mappia foetida*)	Icacinaceae
Cephalotaxine	Harringtonine	*Cephalotaxus harringtonia*	Cephalotaxaceae
	Homoharringtonine	*C. harringtonia*	Cephalotaxaceae
Bis-indole	Leurosine	*Catharanthus lanceus, C. roseus*	Apocynaceae
	Vinblastine	*C. roseus*	Apocynaceae
	Vincristine	*C. roseus*	Apocynaceae
Maytansinoid/Ansa macrolide	Maytanacine	*Maytenus buchananii*	Celastraceae
	Maytansine	*M. buchananii, M. serrata*	Celastraceae
		Putterlickia verrucosa	Celastraceae
	Maytanvaline	*Maytenus buchananii*	Celastraceae
Non-heterocyclic	Colchicine	*Colchicum speciosum*	Liliaceae
Peptide	Bouvardin	*Bouvardia ternifolia*	Rubiaceae
	Deoxybouvardin	*B. ternifolia*	Rubiaceae

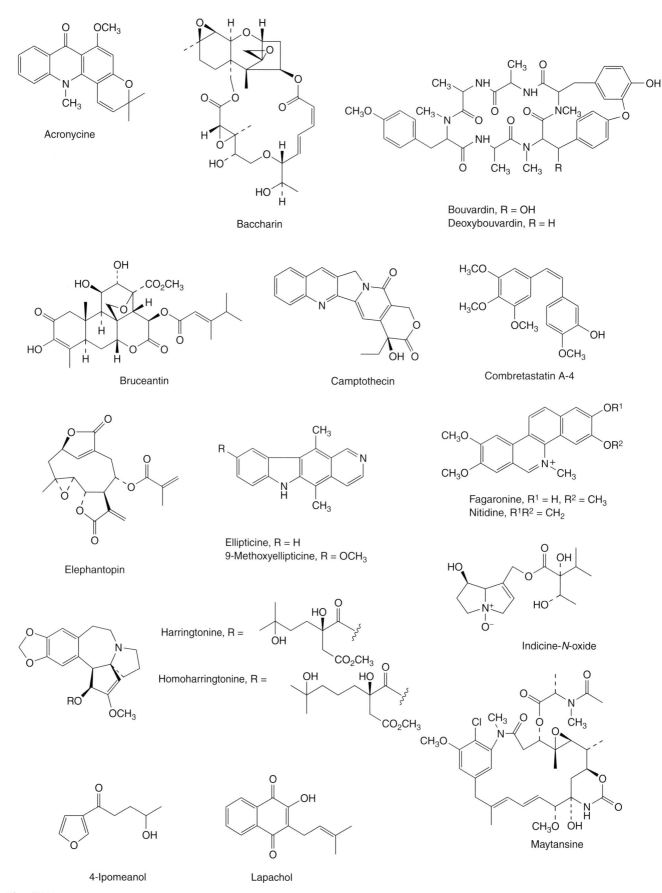

Fig. 27.1
Structures of some antitumour compounds of plant origin.

(Continued)

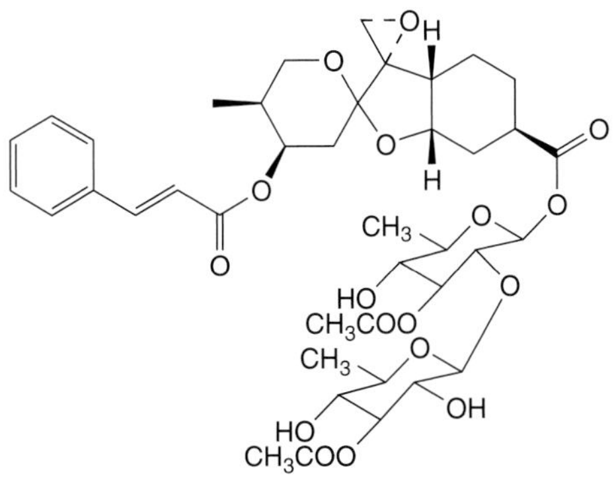

Phyllanthoside

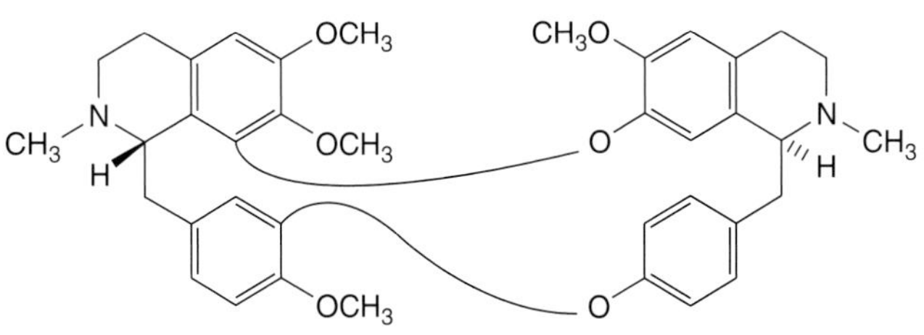

Tetrandrine

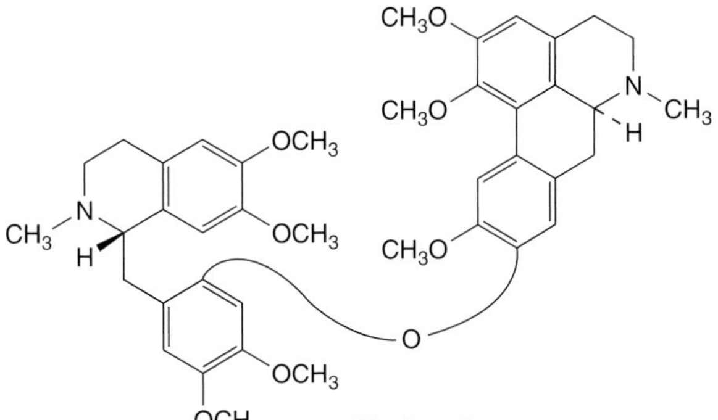

Thalicarpine

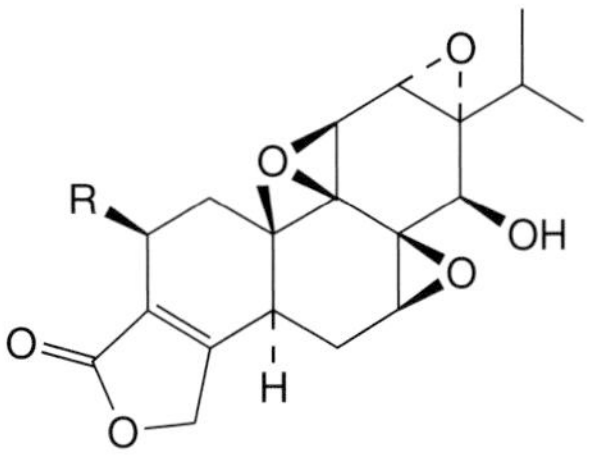

Triptolide, R = H
Tripdiolide, R = OH

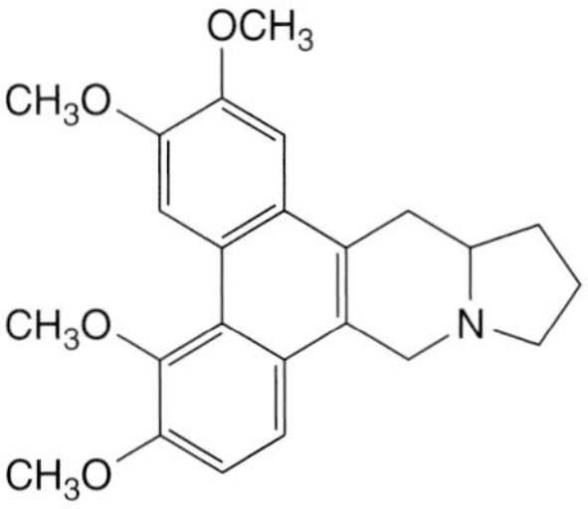

Tylocrebine

Fig. 27.1—Cont'd

limited clinical trials, but toxicity and poor solubility were problems. The natural 10-hydroxycamptothecin is more active than camptothecin, and is used in China against cancers of the neck and head. Synthetic analogues 9-aminocamptothecin and particularly the water-soluble derivatives topotecan and irinotecan (Fig. 27.2) showed good responses in a number of cancers; topotecan and irinotecan were made available for the treatment of ovarian cancer and colorectal cancer, respectively. Irinotecan is a carbamate pro-drug of 10-hydroxy-7-ethylcamptothecin, and is converted into the active drug by liver enzymes.

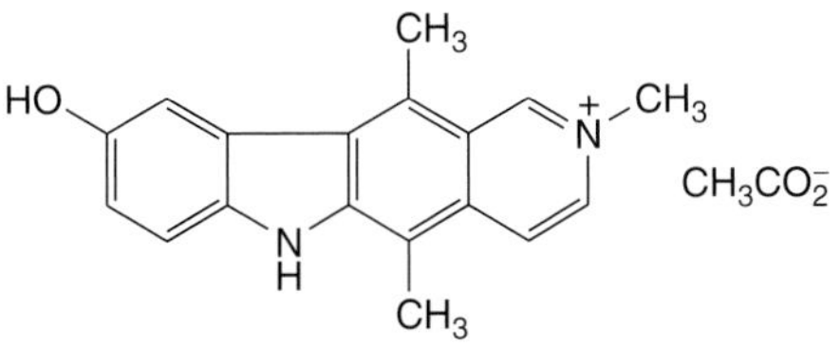

Elliptinium acetate

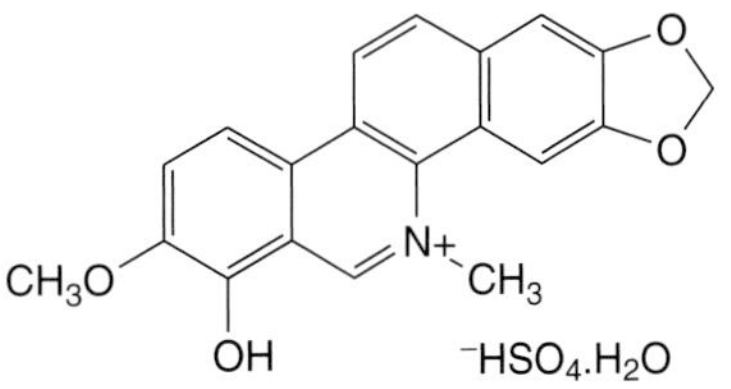

NK 109

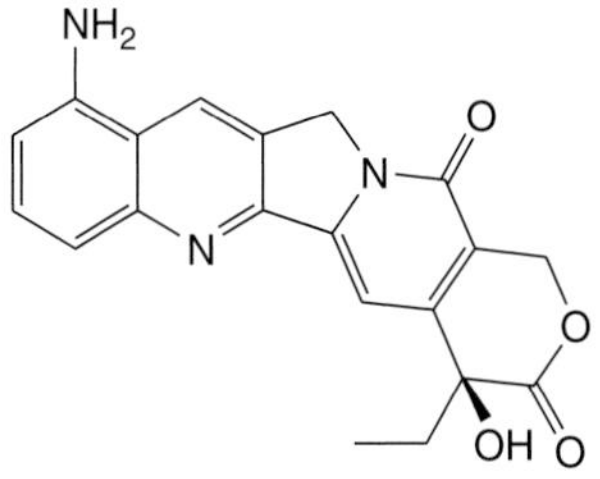

9-Aminocamptothecin

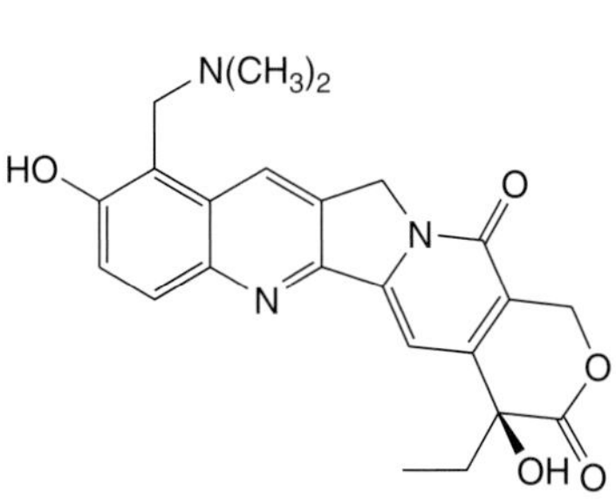

Topotecan

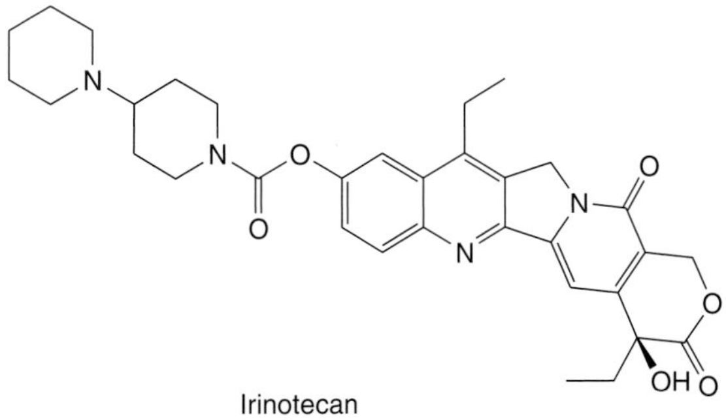

Irinotecan

Fig. 27.2
Some drugs based on plant natural products.

The quassinoids or simaroubolides are a group of terpenoid-related compounds isolated from a variety of plants in the Simaroubaceae (q.v.). Many of these plants have folk-medicine history, particularly for antiamoebic activity, and a number of the isolated quassinoids are currently of interest for their antitumour properties. Thus, *Brucea antidysenterica* is used in Ethiopia in the treatment of cancer, and systematic fractionation of this plant has led to the isolation of bruceantin, which shows high antileukaemic activity at low dosages, and over a wide dose range. Bruceantin acts through inhibition of protein synthesis, and has undergone clinical trials in man. No significant therapeutic activity has been noted in these early studies, but research on a whole range of quassinoids related to bruceantin continues. *Maytenus serrata* (Celastraceae) and other species of *Maytenus* contain maytansine, an ansa macrolide, which was regarded as an antitumour agent of exceptional promise. It is active against several of the experimental neoplasms at very low dosage and shows a favourable therapeutic index. It acts through inhibition of mitosis. In clinical trials, maytansine was a big disappointment, and showed few beneficial effects. Synthetic or semi-synthetic derivatives may offer more hope. Other maytansinoids isolated from *Maytenus* are also highly active; maytansine was originally chosen for study simply because of its relatively higher concentration in the plants. There is now the opportunity of producing maytansinoids via microorganisms. A species of *Nocardia* has been shown to produce ansamitocin, which is a mixture of esters of maytansinol, the parent alcohol of maytansine. This compound could then serve as starting material for semi-synthesis of a whole range of derivatives, and there is still potential for developing these compounds.

Several other natural products have also proved sufficiently interesting to justify clinical trials, or toxicological testing prior to further study. The diterpenes triptolide and tripdiolide isolated from *Tripterygium wilfordii* are potent antileukaemic agents that contain a reactive triepoxide system. The plant is not readily accessible and contains only small amounts of these compounds; large-scale isolation thus delayed their evaluation, and no further development occurred. Nevertheless, in China crude extracts of *T. wilfordii* are used in inflammatory and immune disorders, and triptolide underwent extensive evaluation in the treatment of these conditions. Of many sesquiterpene lactones tested, few show useful *in vivo* antitumour activity, but several of the best *in vivo* active compounds, e.g. the germanacrolide elephantopin from *Elephantopus elatus*, have been evaluated. Baccharin is a trichothecene sesquiterpene isolated from the Brazilian plant *Baccharis megapotamica* and is closely related to the fungal trichothecene toxins (q.v.). This and some of the fungal-derived compounds have undergone thorough evaluation. A series of novel alkaloidal esters from *Cephalotaxus* species are currently being isolated on a large scale for toxicological studies preliminary to clinical trials. The parent alkaloid cephalotaxine is inactive, but the esters harringtonine and homoharringtonine from *C. harringtonia* show good activity in a number of systems. Chinese researchers have reported favourable results in clinical studies using alkaloidal fractions of *C. harringtonia*, and homoharringtonine in particular is active in patients with leukaemia resistant to existing chemotherapies. Homoharringtonine is only a minor constituent in *Cephalotaxus*, but can be obtained by semi-synthesis from the more abundant cephalotaxine. Tissue cultures of *Cephalotaxus* also synthesize cephalotaxine and the active esters and may offer potential access to these alkaloids in useful quantities. The Central American tree *Phyllanthus acuminatus* contains in its roots a complex mixture of glycosides, two of which, phyllanthostatin 1 and phyllanthoside, have demonstrated marked antitumour properties. Phyllanthoside has undergone early clinical trials. The *cis*-stilbene combretastatin A-4 is one of the most potent antimitotic agents from about 20 active substances isolated from the African tree *Combretum caffrum*. A water-soluble phosphate pro-drug (CA4) has shown promise in early clinical trials and a number of other CA4 mimics are now under investigation.

The milk-thistle (*Silybum marianum*), established as a hepatoprotective remedy, contains a mixture of flavonolignans termed silymarin (Chapter 29). Recent research has shown this mixture and its individual components to possess anticancer activity; a phase I clinical study involving prostate cancer patients was recently reported (T. W. Flaig *et al.*, *Invest. New Drugs*, 2007, **25**, 139). The antitumour-promoting effects of seven silymarin flavonolignans on Epstein–Barr virus activation has been studied and in this research silychristin B proved to be the most active compound (A.-S. Lin *et al.*, *Pharm. Biol.*, 2007, **45**, 735).

The fractionation schemes employed in the NCI programme are based on the rationale that a balance between hydrophilicity and lipophilicity is important for substances to reach biological receptors. Thus, extremely polar plant extracts (aqueous) or extremely non-polar extracts (petrol) are unlikely to show as much activity as extracts of intermediate polarity (ethanol, chloroform, etc.) which are normally screened. Recently, many peptides and proteins from microorganisms have shown high antitumour activity, as have some water-soluble polysaccharides, and consideration is thus being given to the testing of aqueous extracts from plants. Already, screening of the Mexican plant *Bouvardia ternifolia* has yielded the bicyclic hexapeptides bouvardin and deoxybouvardin as active principles. Bouvardin was selected for further development, but was subsequently dropped because of its narrow spectrum of activity. The mistletoe proteins mentioned earlier offer a further example. Future work on plant peptides could thus prove most valuable.

Numerous research papers regularly appear in the literature citing cytotoxicity tests for extracts and constituents of plants. As an example, N. R. Monks *et al.* (*Pharm. Biol.*, 2002, **40**, 603) scanned 145 Brazilian plants (538 extracts) from 34 families for antitumour activity against two human cell lines. Families containing a high proportion of active species were the Anacardiaceae, Annonaceae, Asteraceae, Celestraceae, Leguminosae (Fabaceae), Meliaceae and Myrtaceae.

An NCDD Group have reported on novel strategies for the discovery of plant-derived anticancer drugs; examples of plants containing alkaloids, diterpenoids, naphthoquinones, polyacetylenes, phenols, flavones, stilbenes and xanthones add to the list previously cited in Table 27.1 (A. D. Kinghorn *et al.* (16 authors), *Pharm. Biol.*, 2003, **41**(supplement), 53). For a review of a project devoted to the investigation of anticancer agents from unique natural product sources (includes fungi), see C. M. Ireland *et al.* (23 authors), *Pharm. Biol.*, 2003, **41**(supplement), 15.

The search for new antitumour compounds in nature is by no means confined to plants. Microorganisms, widely employed as sources of antibiotics (see Chapter 30), produce a considerable number of metabolites having antitumour activity. Many of these also have antibiotic properties. Amongst materials in general use against cancers are dactinomycin (actinomycin D), bleomycin, doxorubicin (adriamycin), daunorubicin, mithramycin and mitomycin C. Microorganisms have particular advantages over plants as far as ease of culture and the opportunity for genetic manipulation are concerned. The recent identification of epothilones from the bacterium *Sorangium cellulosum* has thus generated considerable interest, since these agents mimic the effects of taxol, and some analogues are much more potent than taxol, especially towards multidrug-resistant cell lines.

Marine animals, e.g. corals and starfish, may also be a fruitful source of potentially useful anticancer agents and this area of research is also producing a number of natural products with antitumour activity.

Compounds of particular note are the depsipeptide didemnin B, isolated from the Caribbean sea-squirt *Trididemnum solidum*, the bryostatins, a group of macrocyclic lactones from the marine bryozoan *Bugula neritina*, and dolastatin 10, a linear peptide from the sea hare, *Dolabella auricularia*. Didemnin B shows activity against several human cancers (including prostate, lung and brain cancers and lymphomas) and bryostatin I has been found to bind to and activate protein kinase C which mediates growth of cancer cells. Dolastatin 10 is a very potent inhibitor of microtubule assembly, and synthetic material is now available for testing. All three compounds are in clinical trials. An NCDD Group has reported on new anticancer compounds derived from cultured and collected marine organisms; these include cancer cell growth inhibitors from marine invertebrates (sponges), selected marine microalgae (dinoflagellates), marine fungi and bacteria (W. Fenical *et al.* (21 authors), *Pharm. Biol.*, 2003, **41**(supplement), 6).

PLANTS CONTAINING ANTICANCER AGENTS IN CURRENT USE

CATHARANTHUS ROSEUS

The Madagascan periwinkle, *Catharanthus roseus*, has been variously designated *Vinca rosea* and *Lochnera rosea* (Apocynaceae). It is indigenous to Madagascar but is now widely distributed throughout warm regions and is much cultivated as an ornamental; it grows profusely in southern Florida. Commercial supplies of the drug are obtained from both wild and cultivated plants produced in various locations, including Africa, India, Thailand, Taiwan, eastern Europe, Spain, USA and Australia.

Characters.   *C. roseus* is a herbaceous subshrub, 40–80 cm high, becoming woody at the base. The leaves are oppositely arranged,

oblong with a petiolate acute base, a rounded or mucronate apex and an entire margin. In form the flowers resemble those of the common periwinkle *Vinca major* and are coloured violet, rose, white (var. *albus*) or white with a red eye (var. *ocellatus*). The fruit is a divergent follicle. Tetraploid plants are reported to have a more vigorous growth habit and larger flowers than diploid ones.

History.   Although the plant has a certain reputation in folk medicine for the treatment of diabetes, modern investigators have been unable to confirm this property. Instead Canadian workers, during 1955–1960, discovered that extracts of the leaves produced leukopenic actions in rats. These observations led researchers at Eli Lilly to undertake an intensive phytochemical investigation of the plant with a view to the isolation of constituents of value in cancer chemotherapy. Six alkaloids proved active in this respect and two are now available commercially (see R. L. Noble, *Biochem. Cell Biol.*, 1990, **68**, 1344–1351).

Catharanthus is an example of a drug plant which has been introduced into medicine during recent years, and it is used for the isolation of pure substances rather than for galenical preparation. Indeed, simple galenicals, prepared from the dried plant material and containing a wide spectrum of alkaloids, would be quite useless therapeutically. Hence, in normal circumstances, the raw material is handled by the manufacturer and does not reach the pharmacist as such.

Constituents.   About 150 alkaloids have now been isolated from *C. roseus*; some, for example, ajmalicine, lochnerine, serpentine and tetrahydroalstonine, occur in other genera of the family. Of particular interest is a group of about 20 bisindole alkaloids which contains those having antineoplastic activity, including leurocristine (vincristine) and vincaleukoblastine (vinblastine). Vinblastine is produced by coupling

Vinblastine, R = CH₃

Vincristine, R = CHO

Vindesine

Vinorelbine

27

of the indole alkaloids catharanthine and vindoline, both of which occur free in the plant. Formation of 3′,4′-anhydrovinblastine from these monomers has been effected with peroxidase isozymes isolated from *C. roseus* suspension cultures and with commercial horseradish peroxidase (see J. P. Kutney, *Nat. Prod. Rep.*, 1990, **7**, 85–103). Vincristine is structurally similar to vinblastine, but has a formyl group rather than a methyl on the indole nitrogen in the vindoline-derived portion. Because these alkaloids are only minor constituents of the plant (vincristine is obtained in about 0.0002% yield from the crude drug), large quantities of raw material are required and chromatographic fractionations are extensively employed in the isolation procedures. In addition, there is a growing demand for vincristine rather than vinblastine, but the plant produces a much higher proportion of vinblastine. Fortunately, it is now possible to convert vinblastine into vincristine either chemically, or via a microbiological *N*-demethylation using *Streptomyces albogriseolus*.

Cell cultures. In efforts to improve the production of alkaloids, cell cultures of *C. roseus* have received considerable attention (Chapter 13). Success has been achieved in obtaining total alkaloid yields corresponding to 0.1–1.5% dry weight cultured cells, but cultures produced catharanthine and tabersonine, and not vindoline, so lacked one of the essential precursors for formation of the bisindole alkaloids. A similar problem arises with transformed root cultures although the feeding of loganin alone at the early stationary phase has been shown to increase the ajmalicine production 2.3-fold and the serpentine 1.8-fold when compared with control cultures; catharanthine levels are unaffected by a single feed of the precursor. Research is still necessary to find means of inducing the production of the useful alkaloids.

Uses. Vinblastine is used mainly for the treatment of generalized Hodgkin's disease, and non-Hodgkin's lymphomas. Vincristine is used principally in the treatment of acute lymphocytic leukaemia in children. It has other applications for lymphomas, small-cell lung cancer, cervical and breast cancers. The semi-synthetic vindesine is also used in the treatment of acute lymphoid leukaemia in children. Vincristine has a superior antitumour activity compared to vinblastine, but is more neurotoxic. Vinorelbine is a newer, orally active, semi-synthetic anhydro derivative of 8′-norvinblastine with a broader anticancer activity and lower neurotoxic side-effects than the other *Catharanthus* alkaloids.

Other species. A number of other *Catharanthus* species have been investigated and found to contain vindoline-type alkaloids; some (e.g. *C. longifolius*, *C. trichophyllus* and *C. lanceus*) contain dimeric alkaloids similar to vincristine and vinblastine.

PODOPHYLLUM AND PODOPHYLLUM RESIN

Podophyllum (Podophyllum Rhizome, May-apple Root, Wild Mandrake) consists of the dried rhizome and roots of *Podophyllum peltatum* (Berberidaceae, sometimes Podophyllaceae), a perennial herb common in moist shady situations in the eastern parts of Canada and the USA. The drug is collected in Virginia, Kentucky, North Carolina, Tennessee and Indiana.

Collection. The rhizome, which is about a metre in length, is dug up, cut into pieces about 10 cm in length, and dried.

History. The drug has long been used by the North American Indians as a vermifuge and emetic, and was introduced into the 1864 *Pharmacopoeia*. Podophyllin, a crude resin obtained from the rhizomes and roots, was subsequently employed as a purgative, but usage declined, until in 1942 podophyllin was recommended for the treatment of venereal warts. Since then, extensive research has led to an appreciation of podophyllum's antitumour properties, and the development of successful anticancer agents.

Macroscopical characters. Podophyllum occurs in subcylindrical reddish-brown pieces about 5–20 cm long and 5–6 mm thick. The outer surface is smooth (autumn rhizome) or wrinkled (summer rhizome). The nodes are enlarged to from two to three times the diameter of the internodes. On these swellings the remains of the aerial stems are visible on the upper surface as large cup-shaped scars surrounded by the remains of the cataphyllary leaves, some of which have buds in their axils. On the lower side of each node are about 5–12 root scars or portions of roots. The latter, if entire, are 2–7 cm in length and about 1.5 mm in diameter. The drug breaks with a short fracture and shows a starchy or horny interior. The transverse section of the internode shows a starchy bark and pith and a ring of 20–30 small fibrovascular bundles. The latter are not radially elongated (cf. Indian podophyllum). A section of the node is similar but shows branches from the ring of bundles running upwards to the cup-shaped scar of the aerial stem or downwards to the roots. Odour, slight; taste, disagreeably bitter and acid.

Microscopical characters. A transverse section of the rhizome shows a dark-coloured epidermis, one or two layers of cork cells, a large collenchymatous and parenchymatous cortex and pith, and a ring of small vascular bundles. The small vessels of the latter have simple pores or reticulate thickening. Many of the cells of the ground tissue contain reddish-brown masses of resin, cluster crystals of calcium oxalate, and starch. The cluster crystals are 30–**60**–100 μm in diameter, many exceeding 60 μm (cf. Indian podophyllum). The starch occurs in simple grains 3–**15**–25 μm in diameter and in compound grains with 2–15 components. In those rhizomes breaking with a horny fracture the starch shows gelatinization. The roots have a central wood occupying about one-sixth of the total diameter.

Constituents. The active principles of podophyllum are contained in the resin, podophyllum resin or 'podophyllin', which is prepared by pouring an alcoholic extract of the drug into water and collecting and drying the precipitate. American podophyllum yields about 2–8% and Indian podophyllum (see below) about 6–12% of resin. Podophyllum Resin of the *USP* was obtained solely from the American drug but that of the *BP* may be either American or Indian, although the resins from these two sources are not identical.

The chief constituents of the root belong to the group of lignans, which are C_{18} compounds derived biosynthetically by dimerization of two C_6–C_3 units (e.g. coniferyl alcohol) at the β-carbon of the side-chains. The most important ones present are podophyllotoxin (about 0.25%), β-peltatin (about 0.33%) and α-peltatin (about 0.25%) (see D. E. Jackson and P. M. Dewick, *Phytochemistry*, 1984, **23**, 1147–1152). In the root, all of these occur both free and as glucosides. Preparation of the resin results in considerable losses of the glucosides. The root also contains smaller amounts of the closely related 4′-demethylpodophyllotoxin and its glucoside, desoxypodophyllotoxin and podophyllotoxone. These compounds all possess cytotoxic or antitumour activity, but activity is lost on mild base treatment. Epimerization, α to the carbonyl, results in the formation of the thermodynamically more stable *cis*-fused lactone ring, rather than the severely strained *trans* arrangement of the natural compounds.

C. Canel *et al.* (*Planta Medica*, 2001, **67**, 97) have suggested that to avoid destruction of the natural population of *P. pelatum* by root collection the harvested leaves of cultivated plants be utilized. The authors found that rehydration of the powdered dried leaves and subsequent

Podophyllotoxin, R = CH₃

Demethylpodophyllotoxin, R = H

β-Peltatin, R = CH₃

α-Peltatin, R = H

Etoposide

organic solvent extraction, gave yields of 5.2% podophyllotoxin exceeding levels previously reported from any source. This increase in yield resulted from hydrolysis of lignan 4-O-β-O-glucosides *in situ* during the rehydration period.

Uses. Podophyllum resin has long been used as a purgative but has largely been replaced by less drastic drugs. It has a cytotoxic action and is used as a paint in the treatment of soft venereal and other warts. Podophyllotoxin is also used for this purpose. Etoposide (4′-demethyl-epipodophyllotoxin ethylideneglucoside) is a lignan derivative obtained semi-synthetically from podophyllotoxin and used in the treatment of small-cell lung cancer and testicular cancer as well as lymphomas and leukaemias. The water-soluble pro-drug etopophos (etoposide 4′-phosphate) is also available. The related thenylidene derivative teniposide has similar anticancer properties and though not as widely used as etoposide has value in paediatric neuroblastoma, lymphocytic leukaemia, and brain tumours in children (see H. Stähelin and A. von Wartburg, *Cancer Res.*, 1991, **51**, 5–15).

INDIAN PODOPHYLLUM

Indian podophyllum consists of the dried rhizome and roots of *Podophyllum hexandrum*, syn. *P. emodi* (Berberidaceae), a perennial herb found in Tibet, Afghanistan and the Himalayan areas of Pakistan and India. The drug is collected in India, Pakistan and China.

Macroscopical characters. The drug, at first glance, shows little resemblance to American podophyllum. The roots frequently break off and some samples consist almost entirely of rhizomes, while others consist largely of roots.

The rhizomes occur in much contorted pieces of an earthy brown colour, about 2–4 cm long and 1–2 cm in diameter. The internodes are much shorter than in the American drug, with the result that each piece bears the remains of about 3–6 branches ending in cup-shaped scars and about 20–40 roots or root scars. The rhizome is hard and somewhat difficult to break. Internally it is pale brown in colour and horny (usually) or starchy. The general arrangement of the tissues resembles that found in American podophyllum, but the vascular bundles are more elongated radially. The odour and taste resemble those of the American drug.

Microscopical characters. The calcium oxalate cluster crystals are fewer and smaller, 20–**30**–60 μm. The starch grains are simple or 2–20 compound; individual grains 2–**7**–34 μm (cf. American podophyllum).

Constituents. Indian podophyllum contains more resin (about 6–12%) than the American drug and the percentage of podophyllotoxin in the

resin (up to 40%) is much higher. The root contains about 4% podophyllotoxin, 0.45% 4′-demethylpodophyllotoxin and smaller amounts of related lignans (see D. E. Jackson and P. M. Dewick, *Phytochemistry*, 1984, **23**, 1147–1152). Only traces of the peltatins are present, but the range of constituents is much the same as in the American resin.

Root cultures of *P. hexandrum* have been shown to contain higher proportions of podophyllotoxin than normal roots (B. P. S. Sagar and R. Zafar, *Pharm. Biol.*, 2005, **43**, 404).

Uses. Indian podophyllum is used for the preparation of the resin and isolation of podophyllotoxin for drug use and semi-synthesis of etoposide. Other less common species of *Podophyllum* (e.g. *P. pleianthum*) and related genera (e.g. *Diphylleia*) also contain podophyllotoxin and structurally related lignans (see A. J. Broomhead and P. M. Dewick, *Phytochemistry*, 1990, **29**, 3831–3837).

TAXUS BREVIFOLIA AND TAXOL

A note on nomenclature: the name taxol was given to a diterpene ester with anticancer properties when it was first isolated in 1971 from *Taxus brevifolia*. When this compound was subsequently exploited commercially as a drug, Taxol was registered as a trademark. Accordingly, the generic name paclitaxel has been assigned to the compound. The literature now contains an unhappy mixture of the two names, though the original name taxol is most often employed.

The Pacific yew, *Taxus brevifolia* (Taxaceae) is a slow-growing shrub/tree found in the forests of North-West Canada (British Columbia) and the USA (Washington, Oregon, Montana, Idaho and N. California). Although the plant is not rare, it does not form thick populations, and needs to be mature (about 100 years old) to be large enough for exploitation of its bark. At this age, the tree will be some 6–9 m high, and have a trunk of about 25 cm in diameter. The bark is removed from mature trees during the period May–August. The wood of *T. brevifolia* is not suitable for timber, and in some areas, plants have been systematically destroyed to allow cultivation of faster-growing commercially exploitable conifers. Harvesting is now strictly regulated. Although taxol is currently extracted from the dried bark, it is realized that this cannot be expected to provide a satisfactory long-term supply of the drug. It requires the bark from about three mature 100-year-old trees to provide one gram of taxol, and a course of treatment may need 2 grams of taxol. Current demand for taxol is in the region of 100–200 kg per annum.

Constituents. All parts of *Taxus brevifolia* contain a wide range of diterpenoid derivatives termed taxanes, which are structurally related to the toxic constituents found in other *Taxus* species, e.g. the common yew, *Taxus baccata*. Over a hundred taxanes have been characterized

27

Taxol
(Paclitaxel)

10-Deacetylbaccatin III

Taxotere
(Docetaxel)

from various *Taxus* species, and taxol is a member of a small group of compounds possessing a four-membered oxetane ring and a complex ester side-chain in their structures, both of which are essential for antitumour activity. Taxol is found predominantly in the bark of *T. brevifolia*, but in relatively low amounts (0.01–0.02%). Up to 0.033% of taxol has been recorded in some samples of leaves and twigs (see N. C. Wheeler *et al.*, *J. Nat. Prod.*, 1992, **55**, 432–440), but generally the taxol content is much lower than in the bark. Significant variation in taxol content depending on season, geographical location, and environmental factors as well as individual populations of trees have been noted. The content of some other taxane derivatives in the bark is considerably higher, e.g. up to 0.2% baccatin III. Other taxane derivatives characterized include 10-deacetyltaxol, 10-deacetylbaccatin III, cephalomannine and 10-deacetylcephalomannine.

TAXUS BACCATA AND OTHER TAXUS SPP.

A more satisfactory solution now employed for the long-term supply of taxol and derivatives for drug use is to produce these compounds by semi-synthesis from more accessible structurally related materials. Both baccatin III and 10-deacetylbaccatin III may be efficiently transformed into taxol. 10-Deacetylbaccatin III is readily extracted from the leaves and twigs of *Taxus baccata*, and although the content is variable, it is generally present at much higher levels (up to 0.2%) than taxol can be found in *T. brevifolia*. *Taxus baccata*, the common yew, is widely planted as an ornamental tree in Europe and the USA and is much faster growing than the Pacific yew; it therefore provides a sustainable source of raw material. Five new taxanes and forty known ones have been reported from *T. baccata* grown in Israel (Q.-W. Shi *et al.*, *J. Nat. Prod.*, 2004, **67**, 168). *T. baccata* pollen contains taxine alkaloids (yield 0.08%) and the taxoids taxol, baccatin III and 10-deacetylbaccatin III (overall yield 0.004%). It is suggested that exposure to yew pollen could be the origin of the atopic manifestations attributed to the tree (M. Vanhaelen *et al.*, *Planta Medica*, 2002, **68**, 36).

New taxane analogues have been reported from the needles of *T. canadensis* (J. Zhang *et al.*, *J. Nat. Prod.*, 2001, **64**, 450; Q.-W. Shi *et al.*, *Nat. Prod.*, 2003, **66**, 470). This species (Canada yew), occurring wild in the north-eastern United States and eastern Canada, is harvested

commercially for its content of paclitaxel and 10-deacetylbaccatin III. S. L. Cameron and R. F. Smith (*Pharm. Biol.*, 2008, **46**, 35) have reported on taxane levels in both older and younger components of twigs throughout a season and find that the lowest levels occur during periods of active growth (April–July), with peak levels following; overall, the preferable harvesting time is August and September. For a review of the chemistry and biological activity of the taxoids (120) of *T. cuspidata* (Japanese yew), see H. Shigemori *et al.*, *J. Nat. Prod.*, 2004, **67**, 245. Three new oxetane-ring-containing taxoids have been isolated from *T. chinensis*; the availability of such C-14 oxygenated taxoids with an oxetane functionality has great potential, allowing the synthesis of additional oxygenated derivatives of taxol (F.-S. Wang *et al.*, *J. Nat. Prod.*, 2004, **67**, 905).

Advances in the identification of the genes involved in the biosynthesis of taxol have been reported. By 2001 five cDNA encoding pathway enzymes had been isolated from a *Taxus* cDNA library and functionally expressed from an appropriate vector or in bacteria or yeast as host (K. Walker and R. Croteau, *Phytochemistry*, 2001, **58**, 1).

Cell cultures of *Taxus* species also offer excellent potential for production of taxol of 10-deacetylbaccatin III; taxol yields of up to 0.2% dry weight cultured cells have been reported. *Taxus cuspidata* (Japanese yew): large-scale cell cultures have produced approximately 3 mg/1 of taxol and 74 mg/1 total taxanes after 27 days of growth (S. H. Son *et al.*, *Plant Cell Rep.*, 2000, **19**, 628).

A number of reports deal with the effect of various added precursors on taxol production; species so studied include *T. baccata*, *T. brevifolia*, *T. chinensis*, *T. cuspidata* and *T. wallichiana*, see C. Veersham *et al.*, *Pharm. Biol.*, 2003, **41**, 426. Abietane diterpenoids have been isolated from callus cultures of *T. baccata* (B. Monacelli *et al.*, *Planta Medica* 2002, **68**, 764).

Uses. Taxol® (paclitaxel) is being used clinically in the treatment of ovarian cancers, breast cancers and non-small-cell lung cancer. It may also have potential value against other cancers. Taxotere® (docetaxel) is a side-chain analogue of taxol, which has also been produced by semi-synthesis from 10-deacetylbaccatin III. It has improved water-solubility and is used in treatment of breast cancers.

Further reading

Banerjee S, Wang Z, Mohammad M, Sarkar FH 2008 Efficacy of selected natural products as therapeutic agents against cancer. J. Nat. Prod. 71: 492–496

Canel C, Moraes RM, Dayan FE, Ferreira D 2000 Molecules of interest— 'Podophyllotoxin', Phytochemistry 54(2): 115–130

Cassady JM et al 2004 Recent developments in the maytansinoid antitumour agents. Chemical and Pharmaceutical Bulletin 52(1): 1–26. *A review listing 27 compounds*

Cragg GM, Newman DJ 2005 Plants as a source of anti-cancer agents. J Ethnopharmacology 100: 72–79

Ge G-B et al 2008 Chemotaxonomic study of medicinal *Taxus* species with fingerprint and multivariate analysis. Planta Medica 74: 773–779

Itokawa H, Lee KH (eds), Hardman R (series ed) 2003 Medicinal and aromatic plants, Vol 32. *Taxus*–the genus *Taxus*. CRC Press, Taylor and Francis Group, Boca Raton, FL. *A comprehensive coverage, 1584 refs*

Kinghorn AD and 15 other authors 2003 Novel strategies for the discovery of plant-derived anticancer agents. Pharmaceutical Biology 41 (supplement): 53–67

28

Antiprotozoal natural products

C. W. Wright

Diseases caused by protozoa are responsible for considerable mortality and morbidity, especially in the developing world. Many plant species are used in the preparation of traditional medicines for the treatment of protozoal diseases and plants are the source of the clinically used antimalarial drugs quinine (Fig. 28.1 (**1**)) (from *Cinchona* spp.) and artemisinin (Fig. 28.3 (**8**)) (from *Artemisia annua*). Other examples of natural-product-derived antiprotozoal agents are the nitroimidazoles, which are based on the antibiotic azomycin (Fig. 28.1 (**2**)) produced by a species of *Streptomyces* that was collected on the Island of Réunion. Azomycin was found to be active against the protozoan *Trichomonas vaginalis*, the causative agent of trichomoniasis, and the synthetic analogue metronidazole was the first effective treatment for this disease. Later, it was found that the latter was also highly effective in the treatment of infections caused by anaerobic bacteria. A more recent example of a natural-product-derived antiprotozoal drug is the antimalarial atovaquone, which was derived from lapachol (Fig. 28.4 (**14**)), a naphthoquinone found in S. American species of the *Bignoniaceae*. Natural products have made a significant contribution to the chemotherapy of protozoal diseases and it is possible that the continued investigation of natural-product-derived compounds will provide new antiprotozoal drugs in the future. As shown in the following sections, many of the available antiprotozoal agents have serious limitations due to their toxicity and/or the development of drug-resistant parasites, so that new drugs are urgently needed.

DISEASES CAUSED BY PROTOZOA

Malaria

In the mid-1950s it was confidently anticipated that malaria would be eradicated, but by the 1990s the disease had reached epidemic proportions throughout the tropical world. The failure to eradicate malaria was due to a number of factors, including the emergence of malaria parasites resistant to the antimalarial chloroquine, resistance of the vector female Anopheline mosquitoes to insecticides such as DDT and the avoidance of insecticide use because of toxiciological and ecological considerations. It is estimated that between 1 and 2 million people, mostly children under the age of 5 years, die from the disease each year, and that some 300–800 million people contract malaria annually. Malaria caused by *Plasmodium falciparum* is the most serious type because it often proves fatal due to the complication of cerebral malaria unless prompt treatment is given. There is now widespread resistance of *P. falciparum* to chloroquine and to some other antimalarial drugs. *P. vivax* is also a common cause of malaria but it is usually sensitive to treatment with chloroquine (followed by a course of primaquine to eradicate parasites, which lie dormant in the liver and may later cause relapses—these do not occur with *P. falciparum* malaria). Recently, chloroquine-resistant strains of *P. vivax* have been reported. The other species of malaria parasite which (less commonly) infect man are *P. malariae* and *P. ovale*.

Trypanosomiasis

African sleeping sickness (African trypanosomiasis) is caused either by *Trypanosoma brucei gambiense* (W. African form) or by *T. brucei rhodesiense* (E. African form). The disease is transmitted by the tsetse flies (*Glossina* species) and initially causes a feverish illness. Later stages of the disease are characterized by effects on the central nervous system, including movement disorders and convulsions, excessive sleepiness and finally coma. About 50 million people live in areas where the disease is endemic and, in addition to the threat to humans, it is also a major

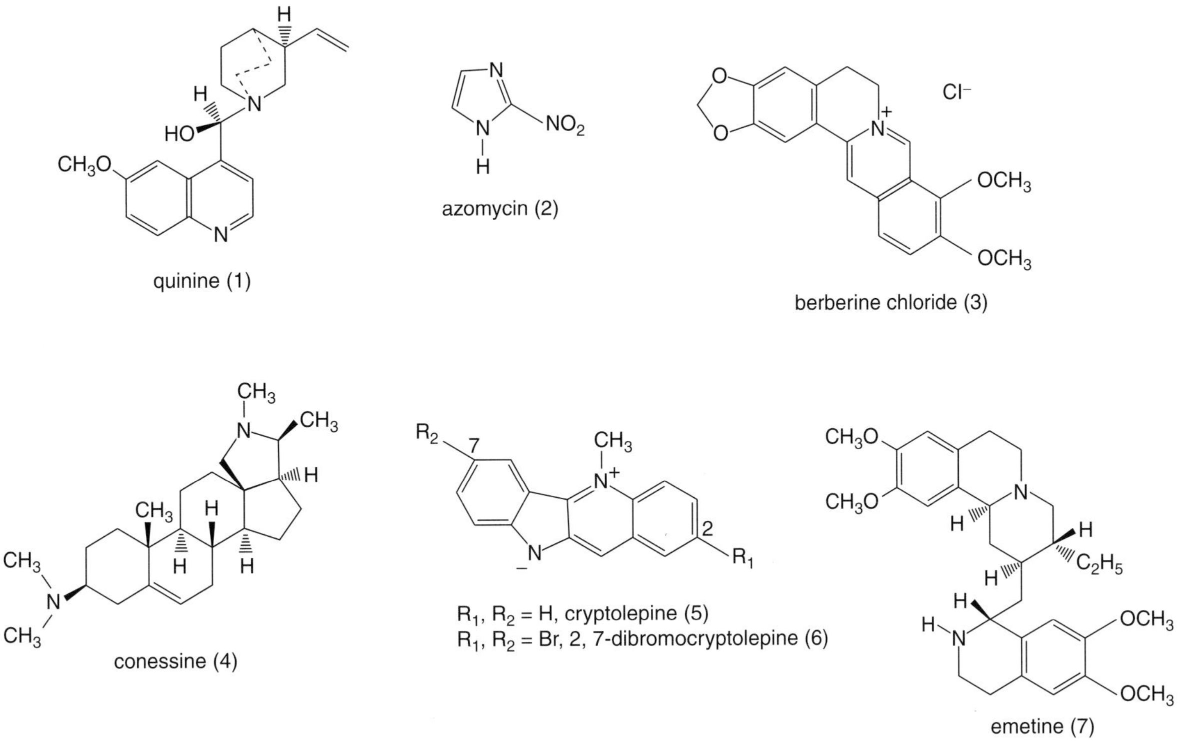

Fig. 28.1
Examples of some alkaloids with antiprotozoal properties.

problem for livestock. Current drug treatment is limited as suramin and pentamidine are only effective in the early stages of the disease while the arsenical drug melarsoprol, which is used in the late stages, is toxic. Treatment has improved with the development of eflornithine (α-difluoromethylornithine), an inhibitor of polyamine synthesis but this drug is not effective against the E. African form of the disease.

In S. America, Chagas' disease results from infection with *T. cruzi*, which is transmitted by house bugs living in the cracks of mud-walled houses. Chagas' disease causes heart failure and other complications; it is estimated that some 20 million people are infected with *T. cruzi*. Only the acute stages of the disease are amenable to treatment but the available drugs, nifurtimox and benznidazole, are poorly tolerated.

Leishmaniasis

Leishmaniasis affects more than 20 million people worldwide and is caused by various species of *Leishmania*, which are transmitted by female sand-flies of the genus *Phlebotomus*. In S. America, cutaneous leishmaniasis (infections of the skin and mucous membranes) is caused by *L. mexicana* and *L. braziliensis*; in the Old World it is caused by *L. tropica* and *L. major*. Another form of the disease, known as visceral leishmaniasis (kala azar), occurs in northern India and is caused by *L. donovani*, which infects the reticuloendothelial system; unless treated, this condition is rapidly fatal. Immunocompromised patients, such as those with AIDS, are susceptible to infection with *L. infantum* in Mediterranean countries. The antimonial drugs diamidines and amphotericin B are used in the treatment of severe forms of leishmaniasis but toxic effects are common and it is hoped that treatment will improve with the introduction of a new drug, miltefosine, which has given encouraging results in clinical trials.

Gastrointestinal diseases

Diarrhoeal disease is often the result of protozoal infections in the gastrointestinal tract. Giardiasis, caused by *Giardia intestinalis* (also known as *G. duodenalis* and *G. lamblia*) is thought to infect 200 million people each year and is responsible for an estimated 10,000 deaths. Amoebic dysentery is caused by *Entameoba histolytica*, which, if untreated, may give rise to serious complications including liver abscesses. There are some 42 million cases annually and an estimated 75,000 deaths. Both diseases are treatable with metronidazole, although this drug is poorly tolerated by some patients. As a result of the AIDS pandemic, the importance of *Cryptosporidium parvum* as a common cause of diarrhoea in both normal and immunocompromised patients has been recognized; currently there is no effective treatment for cryptosporidiosis.

METHODS OF INVESTIGATION

The study of antiprotozoal compounds from plants has required the development of bioassay techniques, especially *in vitro* methods that allow large numbers of plant extracts to be screened for activity against pathogenic species of protozoa. *In vitro* assays are particularly useful for bioassay-guided fractionation of plant extracts. It is not always possible to test against the species or stages of the lifecycle that actually infect man because they cannot be cultured or will not infect animal models; for example, *in vitro* tests against *Trypanosoma* spp. are often carried out using epimastigotes, which are found in the insect vector. An *in vitro* assay for activity against *Plasmodium falciparum* was developed in 1979 following the development of *in vitro* methods for the cultivation of this parasite, and it is not possible to infect animal models so that the most common *in vivo* antimalarial assays utilize the rodent malaria parasite *P. berghei* in mice. Brief descriptions of the antimalarial and antiamoebic tests are given here to illustrate some of the techniques that are employed.

28

Antimalarial assays

In vitro **(antiplasmodial) assays.** *Plasmodium falciparum* is cultured in human red blood cells in 96-well microtitre plates. The inhibition of parasite growth in the presence of drugs may be assessed by measuring the incorporation of [³H]-hypoxanthine into the parasite. More recently, a new method has been developed that does not require the use of radiolabelled compounds. Instead, parasite growth is assessed by measuring parasite lactate dehydrogenase (LDH) activity by adding a reagent containing an analogue of NAD, acetylpyridine adenine dinucleotide (APAD) and a tetrazolium compound. APAD is reduced by parasite LDH (but not by red cell LDH) and then the reduced APAD in turn reduces tetrazolium to give a blue colour, which is measured spectrophotometrically; the intensity of the colour is proportional to parasite growth.

In vivo **assays.** Two different tests are commonly employed utilizing *P. berghei* in mice. In the 4-day suppressive test (Peters' test), mice are inoculated with red blood cells infected with *P. berghei*. The plant extract or compound under test is administered daily for 4 days, starting on the day of infection, and may be given orally or by subcutaneous or intraperitoneal injection. Different dose levels are administered to groups of five mice and, on the fifth day, a blood sample is taken from each mouse. Blood films are prepared and stained (e.g. using Giemsa's stain) so that malaria parasites may be observed and counted microscopically. The percentage of parasitized red blood cells in the test groups and control group of mice are determined and the ED_{50} value (i.e. the dose of extract/compound that causes a 50% reduction in parasitaemia) is calculated. If any test animals die before the end of the assay, death is considered to be due to the toxicity of the substance under test.

The Rane test utilizes an alternative procedure in which mice are given a standard inoculation of *P. berghei*, which would normally be expected to kill the animals within 6 days. On day 4, a single dose of the extract/compound under test is given at a series of different dose levels. The test material is considered to be active if the mice survive for 12 days or more. The minimum effective dose is compared with the maximum tolerated dose (i.e. the dose that produces no more than one in five toxic deaths). In this way, a measure of the difference between the effective dose and the toxic dose is obtained.

Antiamoebic assays

In vitro **assays.** The development of axenic cultures of *E. histolytica* has enabled the development of *in vitro* assays. Before the development of axenic media it was only possible to grow amoebae in the presence of bacteria (polyxenic culture), which made interpretation of test results extremely difficult. *E. histolytica* is grown in 96-well microtitre plates in the presence of serial dilutions of extracts/compounds. Following a suitable incubation time, the growth of amoebae may be assessed by visual observation with a microscope. Alternatively, a colorimetric method may be used, in which the culture medium is removed leaving healthy amoebae attached to the bottom of the wells while dead amoebae are washed away. A measure of the number of amoebae remaining in the wells is obtained by fixing and staining the parasites. The quantity of stain taken up is proportional to the number of amoebae and is determined spectrophotometrically.

In vivo **assays.** Rats are used for the determination of activity against intestinal infections and hamsters are used for assessing activity against hepatic infections. *E. histolytica* is introduced into the caecum via the rectum and the intestine is examined for the presence of amoebae and ulceration. Liver infections are inititiated by injection of amoebae into the lobes. In practice, such *in vivo* tests are difficult to perform, are time consuming and are unpleasant for the animals.

MODES OF ACTION OF NATURAL ANTIPROTOZOAL AGENTS

The effectiveness of any chemotherapeutic agent is dependent upon a favourable therapeutic ratio, i.e. the drug must kill or inhibit the parasite but have little or no toxicity to the host. Although a large number of natural products have been shown to be able to inhibit the growth of one or more species of protozoa, very few have been shown to be selectively toxic to the parasite. Selectivity depends on differences in biochemistry between the parasite and the host, such that a drug can act on a biochemical target in the parasite that is either absent in, or significantly different from, that in the host. Marked differences in metabolism from that in mammalian cells have been found in some species of pathogenic protozoa. For example, *Trypanosoma* spp. are unique in that glycolysis takes place in an organelle known as the glycosome, rather than in the cytosol as in all other organisms. The unusual pathways found in the glycosome may provide viable biochemical targets. The following sections describe some of the biochemical differences between parasites and host cells that are exploited by antiprotozoal drugs. However, the modes of action of many natural products with antiprotozoal activities are, at present, unknown and it is possible that some of these may act on biochemical targets unique to protozoa.

EXAMPLES OF ANTIPROTOZOAL NATURAL PRODUCTS

ALKALOIDS

Berberine

This benzylisoquinoline alkaloid, common in members of the Menispermaceae, has been used clinically in the treatment of cutaneous leishmaniasis and has been shown to eliminate *L. major* amastigotes from macrophages, although it was less effective in animal models of cutaneous leishmaniasis. Berberine (Fig. 28.1 (**3**)) and a number of related alkaloids, including palmatine and jattrorhizine, have potent *in vitro* activities against *P. falciparum* but they have little activity against *P. berghei* in mice; by contrast, berberine has been reported to be effective against intestinal amoebiasis in mice but it is only weakly active against *E. histolytica in vitro*. These findings illustrate the limitations of *in vitro* tests for the prediction of activity *in vivo*, as compounds may need to be metabolically activated *in vivo* and thus may be inactive in *in vitro* tests. Conversely, drugs that are active *in vitro* might also be metabolized to inactive metabolites *in vivo* and lack of activity *in vivo* may also be due to problems related to the absorption and distribution of the drug.

Conessine

In India, the bark of *Holarrhena pubescens* (Apocynaceae) known as kurchi bark has been used traditionally for the treatment of amoebic dysentery. A number of steroidal alkaloids have been isolated from the bark and a few of these, including the major alkaloid conessine (Fig. 28.1 (**4**)) have been shown to have *in vitro* activity against *E. histolytica*.

Cryptolepine

A decoction of the roots of *Cryptolepis sanguinolenta* (Asclepiadaceae), a climbing plant, is used in West Africa for the treatment of malaria and various other infectious diseases. The indoloquinoline alkaloid cryptolepine (Fig. 28.1 (**5**)) is the main alkaloid present and this has potent *in vitro* activity against *P. falciparum* but it is also cytotoxic as a result of intercalation into DNA as well as inhibition of DNA synthesis and of topisomerase II. Cryptolepine is toxic to mice when given by intraperitoneal injection, but not toxic when given orally, and has little *in vivo* antimalarial activity when given by this latter route. The reasons for this appear to be related to poor absorption and/or metabolism to inactive metabolites. It has been shown that cryptolepine is oxidized by the liver enzyme aldehyde oxidase to form cryptolepine-11-one, a metabolite that is inactive against *P. falciparum in vitro*. A number of synthetic derivatives of cryptolepine have been made that have more potent activities against malaria parasites *in vitro* but that do not have the DNA-interacting properties of cryptolepine. One of these, 2,7-dibromocryptolepine (Fig. 28.1 (**6**)), has been shown to have promising *in vivo* activity against *P. berghei* in mice when given by intraperitoneal injection without causing toxic effects to the mice. The antiplasmodial mode of action of cryptolepine and its derivatives appears to involve the inhibition of β-haematin formation (see under quinine, below), but it appears that 2,7-dibromocryptolepine has another mode of action that explains its higher potency compared to cryptolepine. Recently, 2,7-dibromocryptolepine has been shown to have potent activity against *T. brucei in vitro* as well as activity *in vivo*.

Emetine

This alkaloid was discovered as a result of investigating *Cephaelis ipecacuanha* (Rubiaceae), a plant used by S. American Indians as a treatment for dysentery. Emetine (Fig. 28.1 (**7**)) is highly active against *E. histolytica in vitro* and is effective in the treatment of both hepatic and intestinal amoebiasis but has toxic effects, especially on the heart. It inhibits protein synthesis, which is probably responsible for its antiamoebic action and the toxic effects seen in man. The related (synthetic) compound dehydroemetine is less toxic, probably because it is eliminated from the body more rapidly than emetine.

Quinine

The barks of various species of *Cinchona* originating from S. America were used for the treatment of fevers including malaria from about 1630 until they were superseded by quinine (Fig. 28.1 (**1**)) (isolated from *Cinchona* bark in 1820). For more than a century, quinine was the only effective antimalarial available until the development of chloroquine and other synthetic antimalarials, following which the use of quinine declined. (*Note:* chloroquine was not, as is sometimes stated, derived from quinine but derived from products of the synthetic dyestuffs industry.) With the development of *P. falciparum* strains resistant to chloroquine and other antimalarials, there has been a resurgence in the use of quinine for the treatment of chloroquine-resistant malaria, although this may decline with the increasing use of the safer artemisinin derivatives. Although quinine is a relatively toxic drug, it has a selective action against *Plasmodia* due to differences between the host and the parasite; two distinct mechanisms are involved. First, the drug is able to accumulate in the parasite to concentrations higher than those in the host cells. Malaria parasites growing in red blood cells digest haemoglobin in an acid food vacuole; quinine, being a basic drug is concentrated in the acidic vacuole by an 'ion trapping' mechanism. Second, in the food vacuole haemoglobin is broken down into amino acids (which may be utilized by the parasite) leaving the haem ring as an unwanted residue. Haem is toxic and in mammalian cells it is broken down by the enzyme haem oxidase, but this enzyme is not present in malaria parasites. To detoxify haem, the parasite converts it into a polymeric substance, haemozoin, also known as malaria pigment. Quinine and some other antimalarials such as chloroquine and mefloquine, as

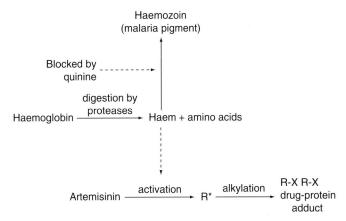

Fig. 28.2
Scheme illustrating the antimalarial modes of action of quinine and artemisinin.

well as cryptolepine (see above), bind to haem, thus preventing the formation of haemozoin; the haem–drug complex is toxic and causes parasite death (Fig. 28.2).

Other alkaloids

In addition to the above, many other alkaloids have been investigated for their antiprotozoal properties. Bisbenzylisoquinoline alkaloids have been isolated from a number of Menispermaceous plant species used traditionally for malaria treatment and some of them, e.g. tetrandrine and phaeanthine, have *in vitro* antiplasmodial activities; interestingly, these compounds were found to be more active against chloroquine-resistant than against chloroquine-sensitive strains. The above alkaloids have also been shown to reverse chloroquine-resistance in *P. falciparum*, an action that might be related to their calcium-channel-blocking activity, whereas others, such as gyrocarpine, daphnandrine and obaberine, have activities against promastigotes of *Leishmania* sp. The African medicinal plants *Ancistrocladus abbreviatus* (Ancistrocladaceae) and *Triphyophyllum peltatum* (Dionchophyllaceae) contain naphthylisoquinoline alkaloids that have *in vitro* and *in vivo* antimalarial activity; dionchophylline C appears to be a promising lead for further investigations.

A number of alkaloids related to emetine have been shown to have antiprotozoal activities; two alkaloids isolated from *Pogonopus tubulosus* (Rubiaceae), cephaeline and tubulosine, showed potent *in vitro* antiplasmodial activities and tubulosine was active against malaria in mice. Several alkaloids isolated from *Strychnos usambarensis* were found to be active against *E. histolytica*, *P. falciparum* and *Giardia intestinalis in vitro* but in contrast to emetine they were less toxic to cells. An interesting series of 2-substituted quindoline alkaloids isolated from *Galipea longifolia* (Rutaceae), a species used in Bolivia to treat cutaneous leishmaniasis and fever, have been assessed for *in vitro* and *in vivo* antileishmanial activities. Chimanine D, (2-[1′,2′-transepoxypropyl]quinoline) was more potent than meglumine antimonate (Glucantime) against cutaneous disease caused by *L. amazonensis* and was effective in suppressing parasitaemia in mice with visceral leishmaniasis due to *L. donovani*. Another constituent, 2-n-pentylquinoline was not active against *Leishmania* spp., but has *in vitro* and *in vivo* antimalarial activity. The β-carboline alkaloid harmaline, a constituent of *Peganum harmala* and some related tryptamine derivatives, have been tested against *L. amazonensis*; harmaline has potent *in vitro* activity but α-ethyltryptamine was orally active in mice infected with the same organism. The related compound harmine was found to have activity against *T. cruzi* epimastigotes. Ellipticine, a constituent of *Ochrosia elliptica*, and a number of derivatives have been investigated for their effects against *T. cruzi*. These compounds interact with DNA but it appears that in trypanosomes the kinetoplast DNA is more susceptible than the nuclear DNA to these compounds and may therefore be a potential biochemical target. Several alkaloids of the acridone type have been shown to have *in vitro* antiplasmodial activity; atalaphillinine isolated from *Atalantia monophylla* (Rutaceae) was also active in mice infected with *P. berghei*. The aporphine alkaloid (−)-roemrefidine from *Sparattanthelium amazonum* (Hernandiaceae) also has *in vitro* antiplasmodial activity (against chloroquine-sensitive and chloroquine-resistant strains) and is active *in vivo* against *P. berghei* in mice.

Species of *Alstonia* (Apocynaceae) are widely used in traditional medicine for the treatment of malaria but the monoterpenoid indole alkaloids they contain have, with few exceptions been found to have little or no activity against malaria parasites. Those that have been shown to have *in vitro* antiplasmodial activity, such as villastonine and macralstonine (present in *A. angustifolia*), are dimeric alkaloids, whereas monomeric *Alstonia* alkaloids such as alstonerine, echitamine and pleiocarpamine are only weakly active. It is possible that the major alkaloids present in *Alstonia* species have other effects, e.g. antipyretic properties which may explain the widespread use of these species in malaria treatment. In this context it is interesting to note that the 4-quinazole derivative, febrifugine, found in the Chinese antimalarial plant *Dichroa febrifuga* (Saxifragaceae) is effective against malaria in mice and also enhances nitric oxide production in activated macrophages. It is suggested that the antimalarial activity of febrifugine is due to enhanced host defence mechanisms.

TERPENES

Artemisinin

For hundreds of years the Chinese have used the herb known as Qing Hao (*Artemisia annua*, Asteraceae) for the treatment of fevers including malaria but it was not until 1971 that Chinese scientists isolated the sesquiterpene lactone artemisinin (Fig. 28.3 (**8**)) and showed that it was highly active against *P. falciparum*. Clinical trials showed that the drug was effective in treating malaria including chloroquine-resistant malaria as well as the often fatal complication of cerebral malaria. However, after 1 month many patients had a recurrence of malaria (known as recrudescence), because not all of the parasites in the red cells had been killed by the drug. In an attempt to overcome this problem and to develop drugs with improved formulation characteristics, a number of derivatives have been prepared by reduction of the lactone carbonyl to give dihydroartemisinin (Fig. 28.3 (**9**)) followed by the preparation of ether (Fig. 28.3 (**10**)) or ester (Fig. 28.3 (**11**)) derivatives. The methyl ether, artemether, is soluble in oil and is given by intramuscular injection, whereas esters such as sodium artesunate and sodium artelinate are water soluble and can be given orally or by intravenous injection. Recrudescence is still a problem with these derivatives and, more importantly, malaria parasites with reduced sensitivity to artemisinin derivatives have recently been isolated from malaria patients. To prevent the possibility of artemisinin-resistant malaria parasites developing the WHO has directed that artemisinin and its derivatives should never be used alone for malaria treatment and that a second drug (e.g. mefloquine) should be given in addition. This also has the advantage of reducing the risk of recrudescence. In the body, all of the artemisinin derivatives are metabolized to dihydroartemisinin, which is more active against malaria parasites than artemisinin. Some derivatives such as sodium artesunate are so rapidly hydrolysed that the latter may be considered to be a 'pro-drug', whereas artemether is metabolized more slowly so that both the parent and the metabolite contribute to the antimalarial action.

Artemisinin and its derivatives are the most rapidly acting antimalarials known and are highly selective against malaria parasites. As with quinine, haem is involved in their mode of action but the mechanism is quite different (Fig. 28.2). Artemisinin is unusual in that the molecule contains an endoperoxide group and this reacts with the iron in haem, giving rise to highly reactive free radicals. Parasite death is believed to result from the reaction of these free radicals with parasite molecules, such as proteins and nucleic acids. Artemisinin does not react with the iron in haemoglobin so that uninfected red cells are unaffected. In the clinic, artemisinin derivatives are remarkably non-toxic and although animal experiments raised fears that neurotoxicity might be a problem, this has not yet been shown in malaria patients. Artemisinin may, however, be embryotoxic so that the use of these drugs is not recommended in early pregnancy. One interesting feature of the artemisinin derivatives is that they are active against the gametocyte form of the malaria parasites, which is responsible for the transmission of the disease from man to mosquito during feeding; thus these drugs not only cure the patient but may help to reduce transmission of the disease.

Although artemisinin has been synthesized, the process is complex and not economically viable, so that artemisinin is extracted from *A. annua* herb and then derivatized as required. The amount of artemisinin present in the plant is about 0.5% of the dry weight of the herb but some strains of *A. annua* have higher amounts and plant breeding programmes are being carried out to increase the yield further. In addition, plants contain larger amounts of the compound artemisinic acid, which may be converted chemically into artemisinin, thus increasing the yield. Currently there is interest in Africa in growing *A. annua* for local use as a herbal antimalarial but at the present time there is little clinical evidence to support this practise. In China, a clinical trial in which malaria patients received capsules containing crude alcoholic extracts of *A. annua* found that while patients did respond to treatment initially, recrudescence rates were very high. As it is imperative to prevent the emergence of parasites resistant to artemisinin, it would seem unwise to use herbal preparations that could result in parasites being exposed to sub-lethal concentrations of drug, thus encouraging the development of resistance.

As artemisinin is a complex molecule, much effort has been put into synthesizing compounds based on the 1,2,4-trioxane ring of artemisinin. Many compounds have been made, some of which have promising *in vivo* activities in animal models. Endoperoxide-containing sesquiterpenes have also been found in another Chinese species, *Artrobotrys unciatus* (Annonaceae), also known as Ying Zhao. Yingzhaosu A (Fig. 28.4 (**12**)) and C were active against *P. berghei* in mice, although they were less potent than artemisinin. A synthetic derivative known as arteflene was evaluated in clinical trials but was abandoned due to high rates of recrudescence.

Quassinoids

The quassinoids are derived biosynthetically from triterpenoid precursors and are bitter principles present in species of the *Simaroubaceae*, which were found to be active against avian malaria in a screening programme in the 1940s. Quassin itself is not active but a number of quassinoids possessing an unsaturated A-ring, a lactone ring and a methylene oxygen bridge in the C-ring, such as in brusatol (Fig. 28.4 (**13**)) (a constituent of *Brucea javanica*), have very potent antiprotozoal properties against several species, including *P. falciparum*, *E. histolytica* and *G. intestinalis*. Unfortunately, these compounds are also very toxic to mammalian cells and attempts to improve their selectivity by making structural changes have not so far been very successful. Both the antiprotozoal and cytotoxic activities are due to the inhibition of protein synthesis and, as these processes appear to be similar in protozoa and mammalian cells, it is likely to be difficult to improve selectivity.

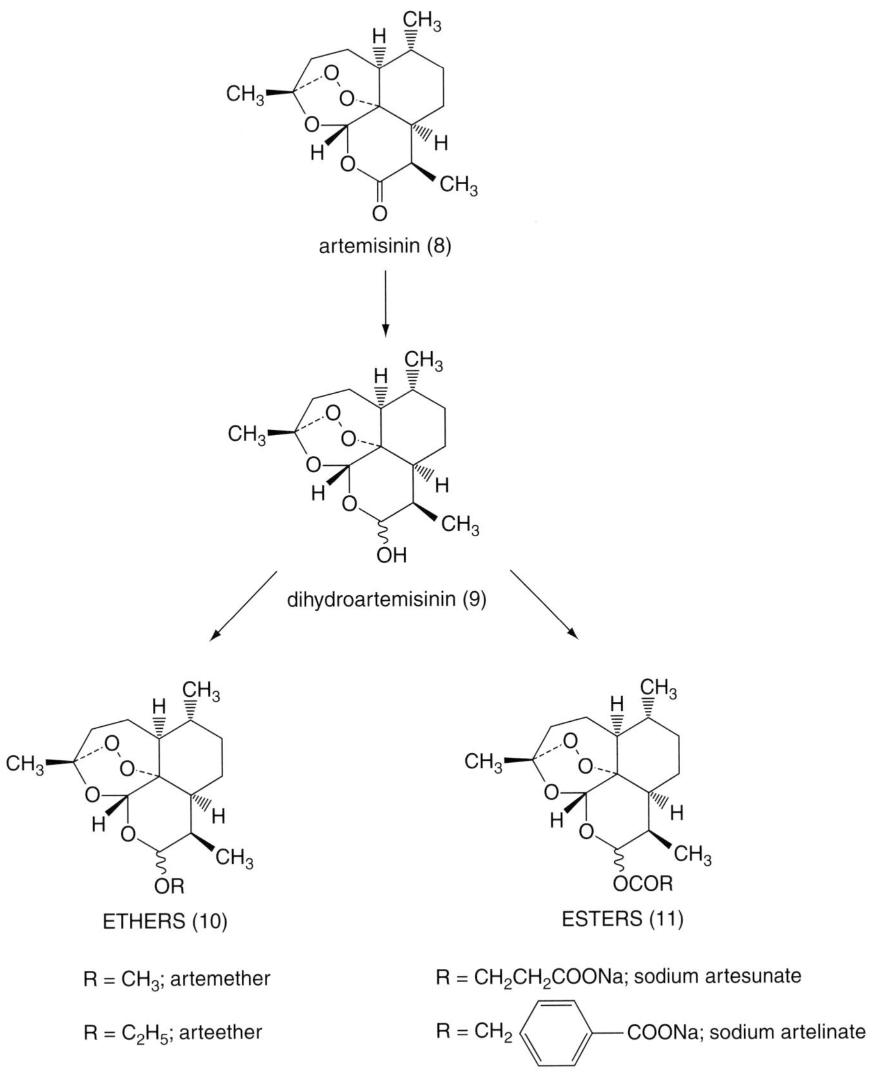

artemisinin (8)

dihydroartemisinin (9)

ETHERS (10)

ESTERS (11)

R = CH$_3$; artemether

R = C$_2$H$_5$; arteether

R = CH$_2$CH$_2$COONa; sodium artesunate

R = CH$_2$ —⟨benzene ring⟩— COONa; sodium artelinate

Fig. 28.3
Artemisinin and some clinically used derivatives.

However, it is of interest to note that one quassinoid, glaucarubinone, found in *Simarouba glauca*, was formerly used in France for the treatment of amoebic dysentery. The Meliaceae is a plant family related to the Simaroubaceae that produces bitter terpenoids chemically related to the quassinoids, known as limonoids. The neem tree, *Azadirachta indica*, is widely used in Asia for malaria treatment and contains a number of limonoids, such as gedunin, which have *in vitro* antiplasmodial activities but they are less potent than the quassinoids.

Other terpenoids that have reported antiprotozoal activities include the triterpene tingenone, a red–orange pigment present in some species of the Celastraceae and Hypocrataceae. It is highly active against *T. cruzi* epimastigotes *in vitro* and it appears to interact with DNA but is also an inhibitor of mitochondrial electron transport and has antineoplastic properties. Jatrophone is a diterpene found in *Jatropha isabelli* (Euphorbicaceae), which has activity against *Leishmania* promastigotes and *T. cruzi* epimastigotes and was effective in treating mice infected with *L. amazonensis*. The polyoxygenated monoterpene iridoid, arbortristoside A, from *Nycanthes arbortristis* (Oleaceae) was as effective against *L. donovani* infection in mice as a standard drug, although it was only weakly active against *L. donovani* amastigotes *in vitro*. Interest in natural products isolated from marine sources is growing and a number of diterpenes (isocyanoisocylcoamphilectanes) have

been reported from the sponge *Cymbastella hooperi*, which possesses potent *in vitro* activities against chloroquine-sensitive and chloroquine-resistant *P. falciparum* with relatively low cytotoxicity.

QUINONES

Lapachol derivatives

Lapachol (Fig. 28.4 (**14**)) is a naphthoquinone found in the heartwood of S. American species of *Bignoniaceae*, for example *Tabebuia rosea*. Although lapachol itself has only weak antiprotozoal properties, a number of synthetic derivatives are more potent. β-Lapachone and allyl-β-lapachone were found to be active against *T. cruzi* epimastigotes and the latter was shown to reduce the infectivity of trypomastigotes inoculated into mice. β-Lapachone was not effective *in vivo* as it reacts with haemoglobin with the formation of methaemoglobin. The action of these compounds appears to depend on their intracellular reduction to free radical species that stimulate the production of hydrogen peroxide by acting as electron carriers between NADH or NADPH and oxygen. Hydrogen peroxide is especially toxic to trypanosomes as they have unsusual antioxidant pathways; *T. cruzi* is particularly vulnerable as it lacks the enzyme superoxide dismutase. Research on lapachol derivatives has led to the development of atovaquone, a synthetic naphthoquinone now licensed for use (in combination with proguanil) for the treatment of falciparum malaria.

Plumbagin

The S. American species *Plumbago benensis* (Euphorbiaceae) is used traditionally for the treatment of leishmainiasis and contains the naphthoquinones plumbagin (Fig. 28.4 (**15**)) as well as the dimers 3,3′-plumbagin and 8,8′-plumbagin. These compounds are active against *Leishmania* species *in vitro*, and some activity *in vivo* has also been shown. Plumbagin has also been reported to have *in vitro* activities against *P. falciparum* and epimastigotes of *T. cruzi*. Diospyrin, a constituent of *Diospyros montana* (Ebenaceae), is another naphthoquinone dimer and has been shown to inhibit the growth of *L. donovani* promastigotes *in vitro*. However, the tetraacetoxy and tetrahydroxy derivatives of diospyrin were much more active than the parent compound against *P. falciparum* (multi-drug-resistant strain K1) and were generally more active against *L. donovani* amastigotes, *T. b. brucei* trypomastigotes and *T. cruzi* amastigotes. It is likely that the above compounds have a similar mode of action to that of the lapachol derivatives.

Other quinones with antiprotozoal properties include the prenylated preanthraquinones, vismiones H and D, constituents of *Visnia guineenis* (Guttiferaceae) which have potent *in vitro* antiplasmodial activities. The quinones, 2-(1-hydroxyethyl)naphtha[2,3*b*]furan-4,9-quinone and isopinnatal isolated from *Kigelia pinnata* (Bignoniaceae) were found to possess potent *in vitro* activities against *T. b. brucei* and *T. b. rhodesiense* trypomastigotes.

PHENOLIC COMPOUNDS

Lichochalcone A

The Chinese liquorice species (*Glycyrrhiza uralensis glabra* and *G. inflata*) are the source of an oxygenated chalcone, licochalcone A (Fig. 28.4 (**16**)), which has *in vitro* activities against *P. falciparum*

as well as against amastigotes and promastigotes of *L. major* and *L. donovani*. Activity has also been shown in animal models of both the cutaneous and visceral forms of leishmaniasis, as well as in mice infected with *P. yoellii*. Studies have shown that this compound alters the ultrastructure and function of mitochondria in *Leishmania* parasites. Licochalcone A is considered to be a promising lead compound for the development of new antileishmanial agents but to date no clinical studies in man have been carried out.

Phloridzin

This naturally occurring flavonoid glycoside is of interest as it was once used as a treatment for malaria, as, like quinine, it has a bitter taste. It inhibits the growth of malaria parasites *in vitro* by inhibiting the increase in permeability of the red cell membrane which occurs in infected cells, thus depriving the parasite of glucose and other nutrients. Unfortunately, phloridzin (Fig. 28.4 (**17**)) also blocks the reabsorption of glucose by the kidney tubules so that it is not suitable for clinical use.

Examples of some other phenolic compounds active against protozoa include the polyphenol gossypol, a constituent of cottonseed oil which is well known for its use as a male contraceptive in China, but is also active against *P. falciparum*, *T. cruzi* and *E. histolytica in vitro*. In *T. cruzi* gossypol inhibits the oxidoreductase enzymes α-hydroxyacid dehydrogenase and malate dehydrogenase. In the body, gossypol is concentrated in the liver and colon as a result of being excreted in the bile and therefore may be worth investigating for the treatment of amoebiasis where amoebae may be present both in the liver and in the gut lumen. A few flavonoids have *in vitro* activity against *P. falciparum* including the exiguaflavones isolated from *Artemisia indica* (Asteraceae). The methoxylated flavones artemetin and casticin have been shown to act synergistically with artemisinin *in vitro* and it has been suggested that flavonoids present in *A. annua* might contribute to the antimalarial action of extracts or herbal teas prepared from this species but there is no evidence to support this.

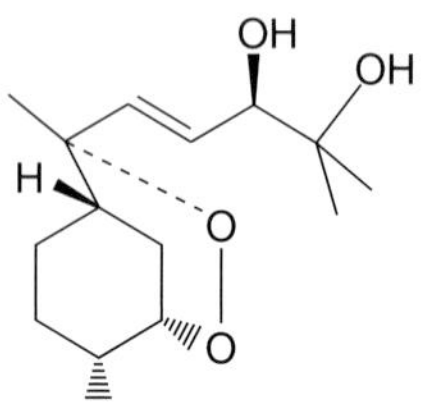

yingzhaosu A (12)

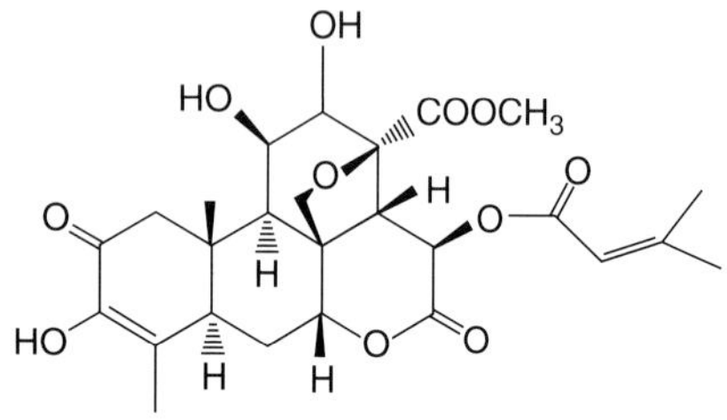

brusatol (13)

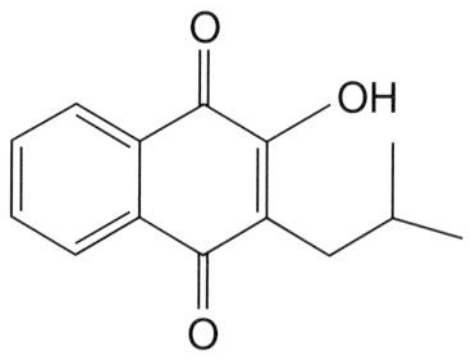

lapachol (14)

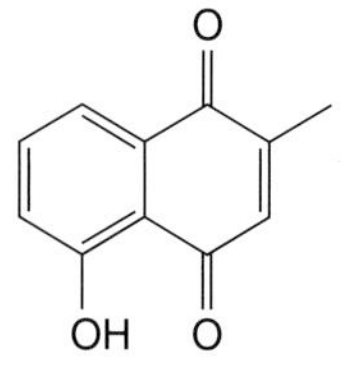

plumbagin (15)

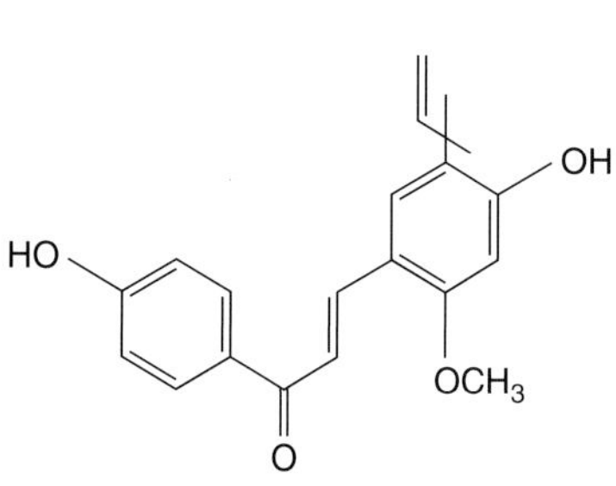

licochalcone A (16)

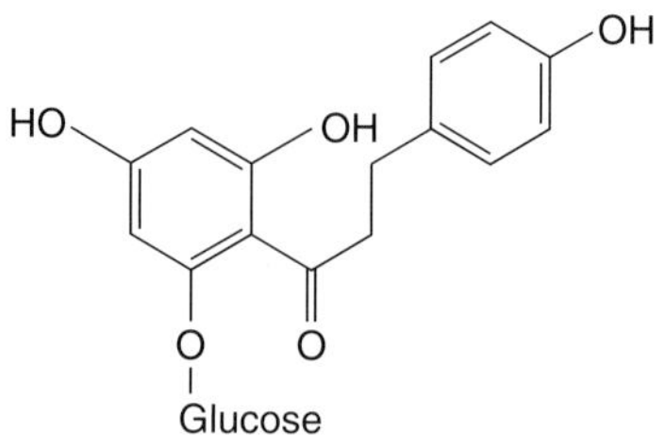

phloridzin (17)

Fig. 28.4
Examples of some non-alkaloidal antiprotozoal compounds.

CONCLUSIONS

In recent years, the artemisinin derivatives have become important antimalarial drugs and this illustrates very well the potential of natural products to provide highly effective antiprotozoal agents. This chapter illustrates the wide range of compounds found in plant species that possess antiprotozoal activities and it is likely that natural products will continue to provide novel compounds, which may lead to new antiprotozoal drugs. However, many of the people who are afflicted with protozoal diseases do not have the resources to afford pharmaceuticals and it is important to assess locally used traditional remedies to determine their efficacy and safety. One initiative that has been set up to encourage this is the Research Initiative on Traditional Antimalarial Methods (RITAM) which is a network of researchers and others interested in the study and use of traditional, plant-based antimalarials.

Further reading

Salem MM, Werbovetz KA 2006 Natural products from plants as drug candidates and lead compounds against leishmaniasis and trypanosomiasis. Current Medicinal Chemistry 13: 2571–2598

Willcox M, Bodeker G, Rasoanaivo P (eds) 2004 Traditional medicinal plants and malaria. CRC Press, London

28

29

An overview of drugs with antihepatotoxic and oral hypoglycaemic activities

The botanicals considered in this chapter are ones which, although not normally encountered in orthodox medicine, have important roles in traditional medicine for the treatment of two widespread and life-threatening conditions. In recent years new technologies have led to rapid advances in the biological testing and chemical elucidation of the active constituents of many of these plants. Much, but not all, of the research is attributable to workers in Asian institutions. In the space available here it is possible to provide a few examples only to illustrate the wide variety of chemical structures involved. For further information readers are referred to the various reviews and references quoted.

PLANTS IN THE TREATMENT OF LIVER AND BILIARY TRACT DISEASES

The liver, the principal organ of metabolism and excretion is subject to a number of diseases which may be classed as liver cirrhosis (cell destruction and increase in fibrous tissue), acute chronic hepatitis (inflammatory disease) and hepatitis (non-inflammatory condition). Jaundice, a yellow discoloration of the skin and eyes caused by bile in the blood is a symptom of blockage of the bile duct, or disease within the tissue of the liver itself.

The predominant type of liver disease varies according to country and may be influenced by local factors. In 1989 it was estimated that there were some 200 million chronic carriers of the hepatitis B virus of which 40% were expected eventually to die of hepatocellular carcinoma and 15% of cirrhosis. Causative factors of liver disorders include: virus infection; exposure to, or consumption of, certain chemicals, e.g. the excessive inhalation of chlorinated hydrocarbons or overindulgence in alcohol; medication with antibiotics, chemotherapeutic agents and possibly plant materials such as those containing pyrrolizidine alkaloids (q.v.); contaminated food containing toxins such as aflatoxins (q.v.) or peroxides in oxidized edible oils; ingestion of industrial pollutants, including radioactive material. Drug abuse in Western society and poor sanitary conditions in Third World countries are contributing factors to the above.

Except for the use of the appropriate vaccine for the treatment of hepatitis caused by viral infection, there are few effective cures for liver diseases. It is not surprising therefore that there has developed a considerable interest in the examination of those numerous worldwide traditional plant remedies which are used for such treatment and that in recent years *in vivo* and *in vitro* test models have been developed for the evaluation of plants for their antihepatotoxic activities. These systems measure the ability of the test plant extract to prevent or cure in rats or mice liver toxicity induced by various hepatotoxins. The latter include carbon tetrachloride (the most commonly used), D-galactosamine (this produces liver lesions comparable to those found in viral hepatitis) and peroxides. In such liver damage the serum level of the liver enzymes, particularly serum glutamic-pyruvic transaminase, is raised and the extent of its control by the antihepatotoxic drug under test is used as a basis for estimation. Other effects of induced liver damage which can also be used in the evaluation of plant extracts are: the prolonged lengthening of the time of lost reflex induced by short-acting barbiturates; reduction of prothrombin synthesis giving an extended prothrombin time; reduction in clearance of certain substances such as bromosulphalein.

In order to reduce the number of animal experiments involved in these surveys H. Hikino and colleagues developed (1983–85) assay methods for antihepatotoxic activity using hepatotoxin-induced cytotoxicity in primary cultured hepatocytes. The fractionated plant extract under test and the hepatotoxin (e.g. CCl_4) are added to the hepatocyte medium and incubated; the activity of the transaminases released into the medium are then determined. The results obtained by this method were comparable with the *in vivo* assays. (For further details and references readers should consult H. Hikino in *Biologically Active Natural Products*, eds K. Hostettman; P. J. Lea, *Proc. Phytochemical Soc. Europe*, 1987, No. 27, p. 143; R. Gebhardt, *Planta Med.*, 2000, **66**, 99).

Handa and his group (*Fitoterapia*, 1991, **62**, 229) reported that about 170 phytoconstituents isolated from 110 plants belonging to 55 families were stated to possess liver-protective activity; about 600 commercial herbal formulations with claimed hepatoprotective activity are being marketed world-wide. The active constituents elucidated to date involve a wide range of components including terpenoids, curcuminoids, lignoids, flavonoids, cyanogenetic glycosides etc., and some examples are given in Fig. 29.1. The terminal events in the attack on the liver by carbon tetrachloride involve the production of a highly reactive radical leading to lipid oxidation and the inhibition of the calcium pump of the microsome giving rise to liver lesions. Glycyrrhizin, glycyrrhetinic acid (Table 23.5) and wuweizisu C (Table 21.7) and gomisin A (lignoid constituents of *Schizandra chinensis* fruits) exert their activity as antioxidants. Similarly, the patented flavonoid extract (Kolaviron) of *Garcinia kola* seeds for the treatment of hepatic disorder has been shown to have antioxidant and scavenging properties E. O. Farombie *et al.*, *Pharm. Biol.*, 2002, **40**, 107. Based on lignan content, high pressure liquid chromatography has proved useful for the identification and differentiation of samples of *Schisandra chinensis* and *S. sphenanthera* collected from different regions of China (Zhu Min *et al.*, *Chromatographia*, 2007, **66**, 125).

A number of plant drugs used for treating biliary disorders are cholagogues (they promote the flow of bile). Herbalists prescribe such drugs either singly or more commonly as mixtures; a cholagogue tea, for example, may consist of a mixture of Peppermint leaves 50.0% (principal cholagogue), Melissa leaves 20.0% (sedative adjuvant), Fennel fruits 20.0% (complementary carminative), Frangula bark 10.0% (gentle laxative).

In Europe the most widely used plant hepatoprotective agent is silymarin, a purified extract from *Silybum marianum*. Silymarin is also used as a standard against which to test other drugs. This and other antihepatotoxic and cholagogue drugs are listed below.

Silybum marianum. This plant, syn. *Carduus marianus* (Compositae) is one of the milk-thistles. Indigenous to the Mediterranean region, it has been introduced to most areas of Europe, North and South America and Southern Australia. In addition to cultivation as a medicinal crop the plant is grown as an annual or biennial for its attractive foliage. The glabrous leaves are dark green, oblong sinuate-lobed or pinnatifid, with spiny margins. White veins give the leaves, which initially form a flat rosette, a diffusely mottled appearance. The terminal heads which appear from July to September are also spiny with deep violet and slightly fragrant flowers. The achenes, 6–7 mm in length and transversely wrinkled, are dark in colour, grey-flecked with a yellow ring near the apex. Attached to the achene is a long white pappus.

G. Ram *et al.* (*Fitoterapia*, 2005, **76**, 143) studied 15 accessions of the plant and suggest that an improved crop (seed yield/plant, number of capsules/plant) could be obtained by direct selection.

As a bitter the milk-thistle has a long history but more recently it has become recognized in Germany and continental Europe as a most effective liver remedy, particularly in those forms of hepatitis affecting the liver parenchyma.

Milk-thistle fruit *BP/EP, BHP* 1996 consists of the mature fruit, devoid of pappus, of *Silybum marianum* L. Gaertner. Several so-called flavanolignans with marked hepatoprotective properties have been isolated from the fruits. A mixture of these, termed silymarin, is available commercially as a dried, purified and standarized extract. Principal components of the extract are three pairs of diastereoisomers: silybin (silibinin) A and silybin (silibinin) B, isosilybin (isosilibinin) A and isosilybin (isosilibinin) B and, silychristin (silicristin) and silychristin (silicristin) B; see Fig. 29.2 for formulae. Other related constituents are silandrin, 3-deoxysilychristin, silymonin and silydianin. A new compound, silyamandin, has recently been isolated from incubated tincture of milk thistle; it may arise from the degradation of silydianin (Fig. 29.2) (S. L. Mackinnon *et al.*, *Planta Medica*, 2007, **73**, 1214). The literature nomenclature for these compounds can be confusing as recommended international proprietary names (in brackets above) may also be used and both nomenclatures still appear to be used by authors. For isolation and structural reports on the above see DY-W. Lee and Y. Liu, *J. Nat. Prod.*, 2003, **66**, 1171, 1632; W. A. Smith *et al.*, *Planta Med.*, 2005, **71**, 877. The levels of these flavonolignans vary markedly in samples of *S. marianum* from different sources; they are formed by various couplings of the flavonoid taxifolin and the lignan precursor coniferyl alcohol. Silymarin, in addition to the above flavonolignans, contains 20–30% of polyphenolic compounds. The scavenging (antioxidant) properties of the silymarin components have been tested against phenylglyoxylic ketyl radicals (F. Sersen *et al.*, *Fitoterapia*, 2006, **77**, 525).

Other non-specific constituents reported for the fruits involve flavonoids including taxifolin, sterols, dehydrodiconiferyl alcohol and fixed oil based principally on linoleic and oleic acids.

Silybin-like metabolites have been isolated from cell suspension cultures and although, to date, no glycosides of silybin have been reported in the plant, silybin-7-*O*-β-D-glucopyranoside can be produced by cell cultures of *Papaver somniferum* var. *setigerum* with added silybin (V. Kren *et al.*, *Phytochemistry*, 1998, **47**, 217.

The *BP/EP* test for milk-thistle fruit identifies silybin, silychristin and taxifolin and the liquid chromatography assay involves separation of the flavonolignans, summation of their peak areas and calculation of their total content in the drug by use of a reference solution of the same constituents; absorbance measurements are made at 282 nm.

Apart from the established use of silymarin as an antihepatotoxic agent, recent research together with clinical studies, have shown the flavonolignans to have anticancer properties (see Chapter 27).

For a 1995 extensive review of the drug (211 refs) see P. Morazzoni and E. Bombardelli, *Fitoterapia*, 1995, **66**, 3.

Cynaria scolymus (Asteraceae/Compositae). The leaves of the globe artichoke have been described in Chapter 19, the drug being used principally as a cholagogue (stimulation of bile production in the liver and promotion of emptying of the gall bladder and bile ducts). There has been more recent interest in the hepatoprotective properties of the plant and significant antioxidative activity has been demonstrated involving chlorogenic acid and cynarin; other constituents are, however, also implicated. For further details and references, see J. Barnes *et al.*, *Herbal Medicines*, 3rd ed., 2007, p. 67. Pharmaceutical Press, London.

Peumus boldus. Boldo leaves (*BP/EP; BHP* 1996) are collected from the small tree *Peumus boldus* Molina (Monimiaceae) indigenous to Chile. The leaves are up to about 8 cm long, of coriaceous texture with a strong camphoraceous lemony odour owing to the presence of volatile oil (2%) containing ascaridole, linalool, *p*-cymene and cineole. E. Miraldi *et al.* (*Fitoterapia*, 1996, **67**, 227) identified 46 components of the oil, 22 of which were recorded for the first time in *P. boldus*. The active constituents have been shown by laboratory testing to be alkaloids of the aporphine type (1–3%) the chief of which is boldine (Fig. 29.1).

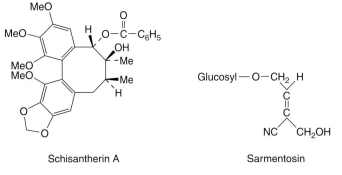

Curcumin R¹ = R² = OMe
Bis-(4-hydroxycinnamoyl)methane R¹ = R² = H
Feruloyl-(4-hydroxycinnamoyl)methane R = H; R² = OMe

Androgapholide

Kutkoside

Boldine

Silybin

Saikosaponin a, R¹ = < OH / H

Saikosaponin d, R¹ = < OH / H

Saikosaponin b₂, R¹ = < OH / H

Saikosaponin b₁, R¹ = < OH / H

Sugars = glucose and fructose

Schisantherin A

Sarmentosin

Sarmentol F
(Type of structure giving rise
to megastigmane glycosides)

Fig. 29.1
Plant constituents possessing antihepatotoxic activity.

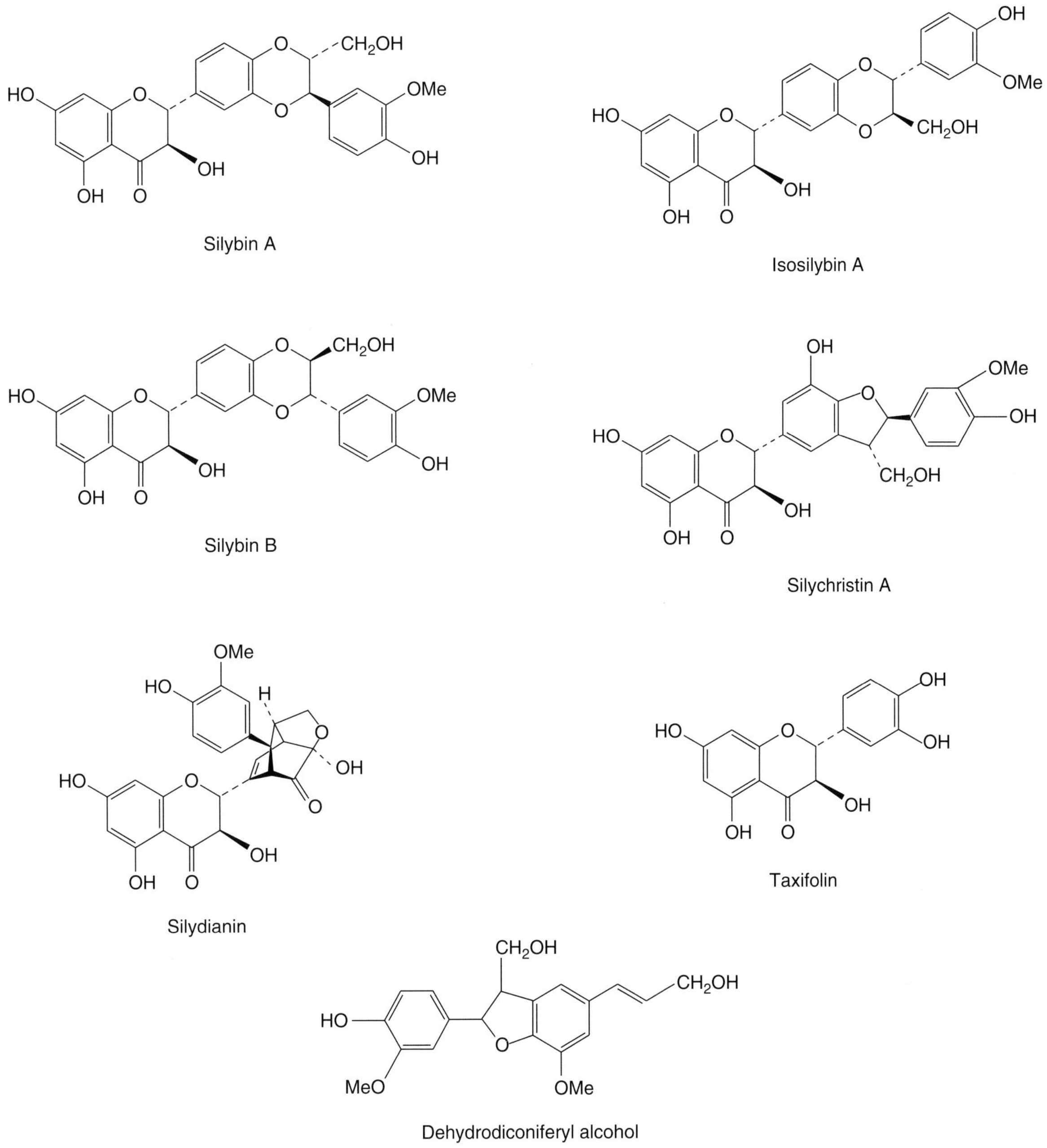

Silybin A

Isosilybin A

Silybin B

Silychristin A

Silydianin

Taxifolin

Dehydrodiconiferyl alcohol

Fig. 29.2
Constituents of milk-thistle fruit.

Boldine is reported to be a potent scavenger of hydroxyl, lipid and alkyl peroxyl radicals and experimental evidence supports its cytoprotective and anti-inflammatory properties (M. Gotteland *et al.*, *Planta Medica*, 1997, **63**, 311).

Studies on the genetic variation of the essential oil and alkaloid composition of the drug (H. Vogel *et al.*, *Planta Medica*, 1999, **65**, 90) indicated no significant differences in boldine concentration in samples from North, Central and South Chile; highest values for ascaridole were in northern collections and for *p*-cymene in the southern ones. There appeared to be considerable potential for the selection of superior strains. The *BP* requirement for volatile oil is not more than 2.0% (whole drug) and 1.5% (fragmented drug), and for alkaloid content (as boldine), not less than 0.1%. Reticuline and flavonoid glycosides have also been recorded. The bark, which contains a higher content of alkaloids (6–10%), is exported from Chile for the commercial production of boldine.

The leaves have a stimulant action on the liver and diuretic properties. An extract of the total alkaloids has a greater activity than boldine itself. The drug is also used in proprietary slimming preparations.

***Taraxacum officinale* root (Compositae). Syn: Dandelion root.**
Although now obsolete as a drug in the allopathic system of medicine dandelion root has maintained its importance in herbal medicine in which it is used as a hepatic stimulant, diuretic, tonic and antirheumatic. Commercial supplies of the cultivated drug come principally from Eastern Europe.

The drug consists of the dried vertical rhizome and tap-root which pass imperceptibly into one another. Up to 30 cm long when fresh and

2.5 cm diameter, it is frequently branched with an apical crown bearing brownish hairs. The rhizome has a ring of vascular bundles and a pith; the root has a central yellow wood. Concentric zones of latex vessels occur in the thick bark. Dandelion root contains up to 25% of inulin and other polysaccharides, sesquiterpene lactones including taraxacoside, triterpenes including taraxerol, taraxol and B-amyrin, various acids including caffeic and *p*-hydroxyphenylacetic acids, and carotenoid yellow colouring matter.

In addition to its use in medicine the dandelion root is useful botanically for the demonstration of latex vessels (Fig. 42.7) and inulin (Fig. 42.1). The leaf has similar medicinal uses. Flavonoids, cinnamic acids and coumarins from different plant tissues and medicinal preparations have been recorded (C. A. Williams *et al.*, *Phytochemistry*, 1996, **42**, 121). For a review of the phytochemistry and pharmacology of the drug (over 90 refs + formulae), see K. Schultz *et al.*, *J. Ethnopharmacol.* 2006, **107**, 313.

Other drugs used to treat liver ailments as exemplified by the *BHP* (1983, 1991) and R. F. Weiss (1988, *Herbal Medicine* Ab Arcanum, Gothenberg, Sweden; Beaconsfield Publishers Ltd, Beaconsfield, UK), are listed below:

***Chionanthus virginicus* (Oleaceae).** Bark a cholagogue and hepatic stimulant.

***Euonymus atropurpureus* (Celastraceae).** Bark is used in combination with other drugs for the treatment of gall bladder and liver disorders; it is essentially a cholagogue.

***Fumaria officinalis* (Fumariaceae), syn. Common fumitory.** The whole herb, which also features in a number of commercial Indian preparations, is used for liver disorders; it contains isoquinoline alkaloids including canadine, dicentrine, fumaricine and sanguinarine.

***Hydrastis canadensis* (Ranunculaceae).** The root is employed in atonic dyspepsia with hepatic symptoms. A fuller description of the drug is given in Chapter 26.

***Iris versicolor* and *Iris caroliniana* (Iridaceae), syn. Blue flag.** The rhizome is used for biliousness with liver dysfunction.

***Juglans cinerea* (Juglandaceae), syn. White walnut, Butternut.** The inner bark contains naphthoquinones including juglone together with fixed oil, volatile oil and tannins. Extracts are used for various conditions including use as a cholagogue.

***Veronicastrum virginicum* (Scrophulariaceae), syn. Black root.** Used as a cholagogue.

The bulk of modern research into the testing of plant antihepatotoxic drugs has focused on those that are used in the Asian and Oriental systems of medicine in which these medicines have an important role. On the Indian market there are available many patent polyherbal preparations involving a variety of combinations of Indian herbs (for details of the components of these preparations see A. Sharma *et al.*, *Fitoterapia*, 1991, **62**, 229). In many instances the liver protective properties ascribed to these long-established drugs have been corroborated by clinical and animal testing. For this group of drugs more modern work appears to have been reported on the Asian and Oriental drugs than on the corresponding plants used in the traditional European system. Research from other geographical areas is now appearing in the literature. A few notes on those which have received considerable attention are given below.

***Andrographis paniculata* (Acanthaceae).** This plant is found throughout the plains of India and all parts have been extensively used in Unani and Ayurvedic medicine; it is also utilized in Chinese medicine. The leaf juice is a household remedy for many ailments of the alimentary tract. Sharma *et al.* (*loc. cit.*) find this plant to be one of the most active ingredients of the Indian polyherbal preparations used to treat liver ailments. A number of researchers have described the isolation of flavonoids, xanthones, sesquiterpenes, lactones and other groups of compound from the plant. (M. K. Reddy *et al.*, *Phytochemistry*, 2003, **62**, 1271; V. K. Dua *et al.*, *J. Ethnopharmacol.*, 2004, **95**, 247; W. Li *et al.*, *Chem. Pharm. Bull.*, 2007, **55**, 455). More than 20 diterpenoids and not less than 10 flavonoids are known). The active antihepatotoxic principle is probably the diterpene lactone andrographolide (Fig. 29.1), which has been shown to protect against alcohol- and carbon tetrachloride-induced hepatic microsomal lipid peroxidation. For a report on the antiallergic activity of andrographolide and neoandrographolide see P. P. Gupta *et al.*, *Pharm. Biol.*, 1998, **36**, 72. In a systematic review of the safety and efficacy of the drug for the treatment of uncomplicated upper respiratory tract infections, J. T. Coon and E. Ernst record adverse effects as mild and infrequent with preliminary evidence for a protective effect for the above condition (*Planta Medica*, 2004, **70**, 293).

***Aralia elata* (Araliaceae).** A Japanese patent (*Chem. Abs.*, 1991, **115**, 132150) exists for the isolation from this plant of pentacyclic triterpenoid saponins for the treatment of liver disorders.

***Boerhavia diffusa* (Nyctaginaceae).** A plant with uses in the Ayurvedic system, including the treatment of jaundice; recently, it has also been shown to be a source of phytoecdysones. A number of pharmacological actions have been demonstrated for plant extracts including inhibition of increased serum aminotransferase activity in arthritic animals and an increase in liver ATP phosphohydrolase activity. A study on the whole-plant extract indicated hepatoprotective activity in CCl_4-induced hepatotoxicity in rats; the extract is considered to be a safe and potent antihepatotoxic. A number of compounds have been isolated from the roots and hepatoprotective properties demonstrated; the most active roots were those collected in May (Lucknow) (A. K. S. Rawat *et al.*, *J. Ethnopharm.*, 1997, **56**, 61).

***Bupleurum falcatum* roots (Umbelliferae).** This is one of the most important drugs in kampo, the traditional medicine of Japan, and in Chinese medicine. It is used for the treatment of chronic hepatitis, nephrosis syndrome and auto-immune diseases. A kampo formula which has shown promise in clinical trials for the treatment of chronic hepatitis B infection consists of a mixture of *Bupleurum falcatum*, licorice roots, *Panax ginseng*, *Scutellaria baicalensis*, *Zizyphus jujuba*, ginger root and *Pinellia ternata* (R. Reichert, *Quart. Rev. Nat. Med.*, 1997 (Summer), 103; thro' *HerbalGram*, 1998, No 43, 20).

The roots contain a group of oleanene saponins called saikosaponins a, b_{1-4}, c, d and f (Fig. 29.1) and in addition a coumarin, several flavonoid derivatives, polyacetylenes, and other common constituents. Minor components include three saikogenins, two polyhydroxy sterols, a trihydroxy fatty acid, a lignan and a simple chromone designated saikochromone. The total pharmacological activity of the roots is not entirely accounted for by the saikosaponin content and H. Yamanda *et al.* (*Planta Med.*, 1991, **57**, 555) have pointed out that the root polysaccharides have a potent antiulcer effect against HCl/ethanol-induced ulcerogenesis in mice.

Saikosaponins a and d are more active on the liver enzymes than b_1, b_2 and c. The former pair also have the stronger haemolytic and anti-inflammatory properties. Hashimoto *et al.* (*Planta Med.*, 1985,

29

51, 401) have shown that the saikosaponins enhance the activity of low doses of corticosterone with respect to the induction of liver tyrosine aminotransferase. (For summaries of the pharmacological effects, see the above paper and K. Ohuchi *et al.*, *Planta Med.*, 1985, **51**, 208.)

Saikosaponins have been produced by cell culture and by root culture; in the former, the dried cells are recorded as containing 0.26% saikosaponin d, similar to that found in the normal roots and in the latter this saponin occurred in high concentrations in 3-month-old adventitious roots derived from callus.

In experiments in which plants were cultivated from seven collections of seeds from different habitats in Japan it was shown that the species was polymorphic with respect to the saikosaponin contents of the roots.

It appears that a number of drugs are sold on the Far East markets under the name Bupleurum Root. For Taiwanese material *Bupleurum falcatum* contains the highest saikosaponin content followed by the indigenous *B. kaoi*.

For further information on the botany, cultivation, chemistry, pharmacology, clinical applications and patents for plants of the genus see S.-L. Pan (ed.), R. Hardman (series ed.) 2006 Traditional Herbal medicines for Modern Times (Vol 7): *Bupleurium* Species. CRC Press/ Taylor and Francis Group, Boca Raton, Fl.

Eclipta alba (**Compositae**). This species is a common annual weed found throughout India and elsewhere at altitudes up to 2000 m. In India it is a common component of polyherbal mixtures used for the treatment of liver disorders. The juice of the leaves is used as a hepatic tonic and deobstruent. The herb is reported to contain an alkaloid principle (ecliptine), lactones (e.g. wedelolactone) and resin. DNA-damaging steroidal alkaloids have been reported in material obtained from the Surinam rain forest (M. S. Abdel-Kader *et al.*, *J. Nat. Prod.*, 1998, **61**, 1202).

Opuntia fuliginosa, **prickly pear cactus** (**Cactaceae**). This cactus is used traditionally in Mexico for the treatment of oral diabetes mellitus. Research has demonstrated its value for human subjects and a purified extract, precluding a dominant role for dietary fibre, can achieve control of experimentally induced diabetes in rats. The active constituent(s) have not been identified. (A. Trejo-González *et al.*, *J. Ethnopharm.*, 1996, **55**, 27).

Picrorrhiza kurroa (**Scrophulariaceae**). There are two species only of this genus, both perennial herbs and found in the North-western Himalayan region at 3000–4000 m. *P. kurroa* rhizome (*kutaki* in Hindi) is used for liver ailments and as a cholagogue in Indian remedies. In 1965 clinical studies on the drug by Chaturvedi and colleagues indicated that, in patients with infective hepatitis and jaundice, there was a rapid fall in serum bilirubin levels towards the normal range and a quicker recovery with no untoward effects. In 1969 extracts of *P. kurroa* were shown to exert hepatoprotective activity in rats against CCl$_4$-induced toxicity and in 1971 a hydrocholagogue activity was demonstrated. As indicated by the references given below the drug is still under intensive investigation.

The rhizome contains iridoid glycosides which have been named picroside I, picroside II, kutkoside (Fig. 29.1) and pikoroside. Various mixtures of these glycosides have been shown to possess hepatoprotective properties. For references to the above and reports on the protective action of 'Picroliv' (a product containing about 60% picroside I and kutkoside, 1:1.5) against hepatotoxic agents see R. A. Asari *et al.*, *J. Ethnopharm.*, 1991, **34**, 61; P. K. S. Visen *et al.*, *Phytotherapy Res.*, 1991, **5**, 224; S. Srivastava *et al.*, *Fitoterapia*, 1996, **67**, 252; Qi Jia *et al.*, *J. Nat. Prod.*, 1999, **62**, 901; R. Ananden and T. Devaki, *Fitoterapia*, 1999, **70**, 54; K. L. Joy and R. Kuttan, *J. Ethnopharm.*, 1999, **67**, 143; B. Saraswat *et al.*, *J. Ethnopharm.*, 1999, **66**, 263.

A US patent exists for the extraction of these pharmacologically active compounds (*Chem. Abs.*, 1992, **117**, 220069).

Sedum sarmentosum (**Crassulaceae**). A number of *Sedum* species have found use in Chinese medicine. In 1982 Chinese scientists reported the isolation of a new cyanogenetic glycoside, sarmentosin (Fig. 29.1), from plants of the genus; this compound significantly lowered the serum glutamic-pyruvic transaminase (SGPT) level of patients with chronic viral hepatitis. A considerable number of various megastigmanes and their glycosides based on the type of structure illustrated by sarmentol F (Fig. 29.1) have recently been reported in the whole plant (T. Morikawa *et al.*, *Chem. Pharm. Bull.*, 2007, **55**, 435; M. Yoshikawa *et al.*, *J. Nat. Prod.*, 2007, **74**, 575).

Schisandra chinensis (**Magnoliaceae**). The fruits and seeds of this East Asian liana and other species of the genus are used in Chinese medicine to treat a chronic persistent type of hepatitis. In addition to its antihepatotoxic activity, the drug has been shown to have anticancer, antioxidant and physical performance improvement properties; clinical effectiveness has yet to be established. The active constituents are various biphenyl octenoid lignans; compounds isolated and characterized include wuweizisu C (Table 21.7), wuweizichun B, schisantherin A (Fig. 29.1), B, C and D which all produce a lowering of the level of SGPT. The structure–activity relationships of these lignans as PAF antagonists has been studied (I. S. Lee *et al.*, *Biol. Pharm. Bull.*, 1999, **22**, 265). The herb Wu Wei Zi is becoming familiar in Western health food stores as a general tonic, being sold either singly or as a component of a mixture.

For a review of the botany, chemistry and pharmacology of *Schisandra chinensis* see J. L. Hancke *et al.*, *Fitoterapia*, 1999, **70**, 451; for an overview of Russian research and medicinal uses see A. Panossian and G. Wikman, *J. Ethnopharm.*, 2008, **118**, 183.

Other species of *Schisandra* recently investigated for their biologically active constituents, chiefly lignans and triterpenoids, include *S. sphaerandra* and *S. propinqua*; for a report on the Thai species *S. verruculosa*, and further references, see R. Wilairat *et al.*, *Pharm. Biol.*, 2006, **44**, 411. The composition and biological activity of different extracts from *S. chinensis* and *S. spheranthera* have been studied (C. Huyke *et al.*, *Planta Medica*, 2007, **73**, 1116).

Turmeric. Turmeric (Curcuma) is the dried rhizome of *Curcuma longa* (Zingiberaceae), cultivated in India, West Pakistan, China and Malaya. The primary and secondary rhizomes are dug up, steamed or boiled, and dried.

The primary rhizomes are ovate or pear-shaped and are known as 'bulb' or 'round' turmeric, while the more cylindrical secondary, lateral rhizomes are about 4–7 cm long and 1–1.5 cm wide. The latter are known as 'fingers' and contain more yellow colouring matter than the bulb variety. Turmeric has an aromatic odour and a warm somewhat bitter taste.

Turmeric contains about 5% of diaryl heptanoid colouring materials known as curcuminoids, the chief of which is curcumin (diferuloylmethane), together with smaller quantities of dicaffeoylmethane and caffeoylferuloylmethane (Fig. 29.1). Dihydrocurcumin was reported in 1980. The volatile oil (about 5%) contains sesquiterpenes (e.g. zingiberene, 25%), sesquiterpene alcohols and ketones, and monoterpenes. A detailed study of the distribution of components of the oil in various organs of the plant has been reported (R. P. Bansal *et al.*, *Pharm. Biol.*, 2002, **40**, 384). Enzymes associated with the biosynthesis of curcuminoids in turmeric and ginerols in ginger have been identified (M. del C. Ramirez-Ahumada *et al.*, *Phytochemistry*, 2006, **67**, 2017).

29

In a series of papers Japanese workers reported on the characterization of the constituents of a polysaccharide fraction of the drug, which has a marked immunological activity. The acid glycans designated ukonan A, B and C show remarkable reticuloendothelial system (RES) potentiating properties. Ukonan A, for example, is composed of L-arabinose, D-xylose, D-galactose, D-glucose, L-rhamnose and D-galacturonic acid in addition to small amounts of peptide moieties. Ukonan D, a neutral polysaccharide, also shows RES-potentiating activity as indicated in a carbon clearance test; it has an estimated molecular mass of 28 000 and is composed of L-arabinose, D-galactose, D-glucose and D-mannose in the molar ratio 1:1:12:0.2, plus a small peptide fraction. (For further details and references concerning these polysaccharides see R. Gonda *et al.*, *Chem. Pharm. Bull.*, 1992, **40**, 185.)

The rhizomes also contain free arabinose (about 1.0%), fructose (12%) and glucose (2%). Abundant zingiberaceous starch grains, about 30–60 μm long and often gelatinized, are present.

Turmeric is used in Indian and Oriental medicine as an aromatic stomachic and diuretic as well as a treatment for jaundice and hepatitis. The choleretic activity of curcumin was described in 1956–7 and *in vitro* experiments have now demonstrated the strong antihepatotoxic action of the curcuminoids. For a review of the pharmacology of the drug see H. P. T. Ammom and M. A. Wahl, *Planta Med.*, 1991, **57**, 1.

Large quantities of turmeric are used in the preparation of curries and sauces. Paper impregnated with an alcoholic extract of turmeric is used as a test for boric acid and borates.

Javanese turmeric. The rhizome of this plant, *Curcuma xanthorrhiza*, is described in the *BP/EP*. As the name implies it is obtained from Indonesia with smaller quantities coming from India. Its constituents are similar in chemical nature and pharmacological properties to those of *C. longa*.

The official requirement for volatile oil content is not less than 5%, one sesquiterpene component (xanthorrhizol) being characteristic for the species. Dicinnamoyl methane derivatives (≮0.1%), expressed as curcumin, are assayed by absorbance measurement at 530 nm.

Curcuma zedoaria rhizome (zedoary) finds medicinal use in the East as a carminative and digestive stimulant and in the treatment of colds and infections. It occurs as circular slices of rhizome resembling bulb turmeric and contains many types of sesquiterpenoids. An active curcuminoid, demethoxycurcumin, has been isolated by bioassay-directed fractionation (W.-J. Syn *et al.*, *J. Nat. Prod.*, 1998, **61**, 1531). The antimicrobial properties of both *C. zedoaria* and *C. malanarica* have been demonstrated (B. Wilson *et al.*, *J. Ethnopharmacol.*, 2005, **99**, 147).

C. wenyujin is a Chinese medicinal plant, the constituents of which exhibit antitumour activity. Among other constituents the essential oil contains a novel superoxidized sesquiterpene named wenjine.

Wendelia calendulaceae (Compositae). This herb is ascribed medicinal properties similar to those of *Eclipta* spp, and may be used as a single plant remedy in Asian medicine. An alcoholic extract of the plant has been shown to possess hepatoprotective activity.

Other plants for which positive antihepatotoxic properties have been recorded include: *Aeginetia indica* (Orobanchaceae); *Artemesia capillaris* buds, *A. maritima* (Compositae); *Atractylodes* sp., rhizome (Compositae); *Berberis* spp. (Berberidaceae); *Citrus limon* fruits (Rutaceae); *Glycyrrhiza* spp. (Leguminosae), principally glycyrrhetinic acid and glycyrrhizin (q.v.); *Mallotus japonicus* (Euphorbiaceae); *Panax ginseng* roots (Araliaceae) (q.v.); *Phyllanthus niruri* (Euphorbiaceae); *Plumbago zeylanica* (Plumbaginaceae); *Salvia plebeia* (Labiatae); *Swertia japonica* (Gentianaceae); *Tephrosia purpurea* (Leguminosae); *Tetrapanax papyriferum* leaves (Araliaceae); *Uncaria gambir* (Rubiaceae); *Withania somnifera* (Solanaceae).

There is obviously much further scope for the clinical testing of these drugs to ascertain whether toxicity levels and side-effects of the constituents would permit them to be recognized in Western medicine.

PLANTS WITH ORAL HYPOGLYCAEMIC ACTIVITY

Diabetes arises from a deficient production of insulin by the β-cells of the pancreatic islets. The endocrine hormone operates at various sites throughout the body regulating carbohydrate, triglyceride and protein metabolism and controlling entry of glucose into the blood. Insufficient insulin results in hyperglycaemia and the symptoms of diabetes, namely, an excess of sugar in the blood and urine, hunger, thirst and a gradual loss of weight. The disease is estimated to affect 4–5% of the population and patients are generally classified as either insulin-dependent diabetics (type 1) or non-insulin-dependent diabetics (type 2). A third type, malnutrition-related diabetes mellitus, affects young people in poor tropical countries and is associated with a history of nutritional deficiency. The type 1 group includes all diabetic children, the majority of those under 40 years of age and a few over 40 years. These individuals lack the functional β-cells necessary to synthesize the hormone and insulin therapy is the only satisfactory treatment. Type 2 diabetics, constituting some 75% of the diabetic population, have functional pancreatic β-cells but there is, nevertheless, a deficiency in insulin production; patients are those in which the disease has usually manifested after the age of 40.

In many cases the type 2 condition can be controlled by a suitable diet and exercise but if this is not successful treatment with oral hypoglycaemics in conjunction with a suitable dietary regimen may prove satisfactory. These drugs act in a variety of ways: (1) by stimulating the β-cells to produce insulin; (2) by decreasing gluconeogenesis and increasing peripheral utilization of glucose—success is still dependent on some limited production of insulin by the pancreas; (3) retardation of carbohydrate absorption from the gut resulting in a reduction of excessive postprandial plasma-glucose concentration. In Western medicine these three aspects are effectively accommodated by the respective use of (1) sulphonylureas, (2) biguanides and (3) Guar gum.

It is important however to appreciate that there are also many plants and plant extracts which possess marked hypoglycaemic activity. From ancient times such materials have been used for the treatment of diabetes mellitus and still find extensive use in traditional medicine world-wide. Apart from their importance *per se* these plants represent possible sources of new drugs which may act in ways additional to those indicated above; as long-established traditional remedies they may be less toxic than some previously untried medicaments. As emphasized in Chapter 36, traditional cures are much used by immigrants who seek advice from their own healers and it is important that medical staff at hospitals recognize that such patients may be taking drugs about which little is known in orthodox medicine. Diabetic patients taking such traditional oral hypoglycaemics present a particular problem.

There have been several comprehensive reviews covering plant hypoglycaemics. Oliver-Bever and Zahnd (*Quart. J. Crude Drug Res.*, 1979, **17**, 139) reviewed the literature up to 1978 and Ivorra *et al.* (*J. Ethnopharm.*, 1989, **27**, 243, *c.* 165 refs) covered the subsequent 10 years and have tabulated both constituents and plant species. Atta-ur-Rahman and Zaman's review (*J. Ethnopharm.*, 1989, **26**, 1, 383 refs) of the published literature on the antidiabetic activity of some 343 plants covers the period 1907–88 and their Table illustrates well the world-wide usage of these plants; the chemical structures of over 40 hypoglycaemic phytochemicals are given. Handa *et al.* (*Fitoterapia*, 1989, **60**, 195) reviewed (260 refs) about 150 plants reported to have hypoglycaemic activity and, where available, have incorporated information on active principles. A. Andrade-Cetto and M. Heinrich have recorded 306 species of Mexican plants traditionally used for their hypoglycaemic effect in the treatment of diabetes; seven of these spp. are discussed in some detail highlighting current knowledge and the enormous gaps regarding toxicity, pharmacokinetics and metabolism of the active constituents (*J. Ethnopharmacol.*, 2005, **99**, 325). See also 'Further reading' for more recent reviews.

Methods of studying oral hypoglycaemics include: clinical trials involving both normal human volunteers and type 2 diabetics; effect on glucose levels of normal animals (rabbits, rats, mice and dogs have been used); measurement of the reduction of blood sugar levels of animals having glucose-induced hyperglycaemia, and also with alloxan- and streptozotocin-induced diabetic animals. Such tests do not evaluate toxicity, and specifically, a number of drugs which are hepatotoxic and affect liver enzymes involved in gluconeogenesis will lower the blood sugar level, thus giving false-positive results. An example of this concerns the unripe fruits of the akee tree, *Blighia sapida* (Sapindaceae), which contain the toxic principles hypoglycin A and B. These cyclopropanoid amino acids (formula Table 39.1) have marked hypoglycaemic properties and act on the liver by blocking the oxidation of fatty acids. The resulting depletion of liver glycogen leads to a lowering of the blood sugar level. In the West Indies green akee fruits are eaten parboiled, the cooking water being discarded, but over the years many fatalities appear to have occurred in Jamaica as a result of the consumption of uncooked fruits.

The wide range of structures of those plant constituents which appear to be the active hypoglycaemic principles suggests different sites of action within the body. *Polysaccharides* feature prominently in antidiabetic plants and they include the glycans of *Aconitum carmichaelii* roots (a traditional oriental drug), *Ephedra distachya* (the oriental crude drug Mao), *Gymnema sylvestre* leaves (an Ayurvedic drug used to control blood sugar levels in diabetics), *Lithospermum erythrorhizin* (q.v.), *Panax ginseng* and *P. quinquefolium* (q.v.) and the non-sucrose portion of the juice of stems of *Saccharum officinarum*. The traditional use of various *Dioscorea* species in oriental medicine appears justified by demonstration of the hypoglycaemic activity of their polysaccharides in animal tests. In Mexican traditional medicine one of the most important antidiabetic remedies is a root decoction of *Psacalium decompositum* (syn. *Cacalia decomposita*), Compositae. F. J. Alarcon-Aguilar *et al.* (*J. Ethnopharm.*, 2000, **69**, 207) have found the hypoglycaemic effect on healthy mice to lie, not in the known sesquiterpenes (cacalol, cacalone, maturin), but in two polysaccharide fractions of the freeze-dried water decoction of the roots. Some polysaccharide seaweed extracts have been shown to be active. Plant mucilages with similar pharmacological properties include those from some members of the Malvaceae (*Abelmoschus* spp., *Althaea* spp.) and *Plantago* (Plantaginaceae). Generally, deacetylation of mucilages enhances activity.

Some *flavonoids, phenols* and related compounds have been shown to have hypoglycaemic activity. One such compound is (−)-epicatechin (formula, Fig. 21.7), which is contained in the bark of the tree *Pterocarpus marsupium* (Leguminosae). As a drug it is popular with Ayurvedic physicians for the treatment of diabetes mellitus and has been the subject of a number of clinical trials in India. The heartwood is similarly used and beakers turned from the wood are filled with water and allowed to stand overnight to give 'Beeja wood water'. This cold infusion is stated to maintain the blood sugar of diabetics at normal concentrations until treatment is withdrawn. The wood contains pterostilbene (Fig. 29.3) the positive activity of which has been confirmed. The dried juice of this tree is the source of Malabar kino.

Steroid-containing plants known to exhibit antidiabetic activity include the barks of various species of *Ficus*, the roots of ginseng [the ginsenosides (steroids) as well as the pannaxosides (glycans, above) have been shown to be active in many animal tests], fenugreek, and the fruits and seeds of various Cucurbitaceae. The last includes *Momordica charantia* or karela fruit, extracts of which are commonly used on the Indian subcontinent for the treatment of diabetes. The seeds of the related *M. cochinchinensis* (Sprengel seeds) contain two active glycosides as tested on streptozotocin-induced diabetic rats. Both glycosides have oleanolic acid as aglycone; one involves glucose and the other glucose and arabinose. *Balanites aegyptica* (Zygophyllaceae) finds a variety of uses as a folk medicine in many countries of Africa. In Egypt the fruits, after removal of the epicarp, are used as an oral antidiabetic. Aqueous extracts have been shown to exhibit a pronounced effect by oral administration to streptozotocin-induced diabetic mice. The fruits contain steroidal saponins which are active as a recombinant mixture but not singly. The saponins of *B. aegyptica* are also molluscicidal (q.v.). The genus *Ajuga* contains steroidal withanolides (q.v.) and *A. bracteosa* and *A. iva* are used in Pakistan and N. Africa respectively for the treatment of diabetes. The active constituents are stated to potentiate the effects of insulin.

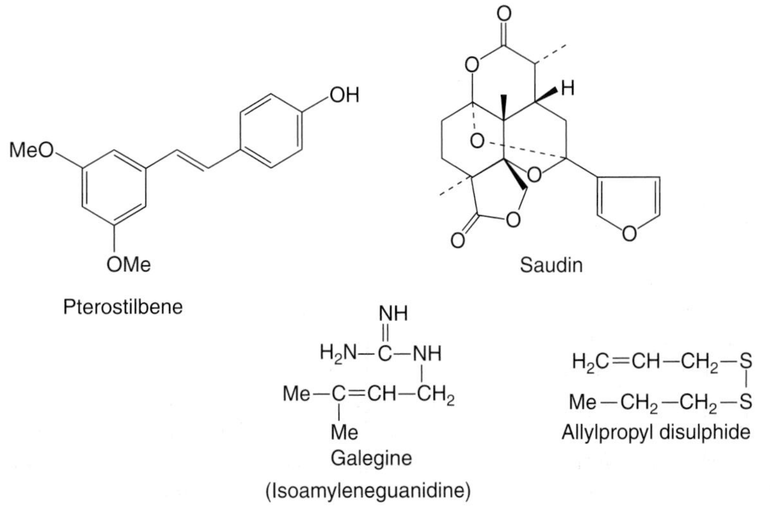

Fig. 29.3
Phytochemicals having oral hypoglycaemic activity illustrated by a phenol, a diterpene, a guanidine derivative and a disulphide. For other groups of active compounds see text.

29

In a series of papers Mossa and associates reported on a *diterpenoid* compound named saudin (Fig. 29.3) with a novel 6,7-secolabdane skeleton (*Int. J. Crude Drug Res.*, 1990, **28**, 163 and references cited therein). Saudin was isolated from the euphorbiaceous plant *Cluytia richardiana* which grows in the mountainous regions of western and southern Saudi Arabia. It has marked hypoglycaemic effects and its use in the treatment of diabetes mellitus has been patented (US).

Comparatively speaking, the number of *alkaloid-containing plants* reported to have antidiabetic properties appears to be small. *Coptis chinensis* (Ranunculaceae), a Chinese medicinal herb, contains berberine, and active simpler nitrogen compounds are found in *Capsicum, Allium, Lathyrus, Lepidium* and *Galega. Galega officinalis* (Leguminosae), syn. Goat's Rue, is a herb native to S.E. Europe but introduced elsewhere including Britain. An erect glabrous perennial up to 150 cm high, it has leaves composed of 13 or 15 oblong or oblong-ovate, mucronate or marginate leaflets with white, lilac or pinkish papilionate flowers. It is included in the *BHP* (1983) and the active principle is galegine (isoamyleneguanidine) (Fig. 29.3), which shows hypoglycaemic activity when tested on alloxan-diabetic rats. Other constituents are 4-hydroxygalegine, peganine, saponins and flavonoids. Peganine and related alkaloids are well-known as constituents of *Peganum harmala* (Zygophyllaceae) seeds which are themselves used in some areas for treating diabetes. However, these seeds have other marked pharmacological actions and on the basis of their toxicity to rats M. M. Al-Zaid *et al.* (*Int. J. Pharmacognosy*, 1991, **29**, 81) have suggested that their use should be discouraged.

A plant, the various parts of which have been used in antidiabetic preparations in Europe and India, is *Syzygium cumini* (Myrtaceae) syn. *Eugenia jambolana*. The dried fruits are described in the *BHP* (1983) and may be prescribed with Galega (see above). Constituents of the seed include phenols, tannins, essential oil in small quantity, an alkaloid and glycoside, and triterpenes. The hypoglycaemic action of the fruit extract seeds (M. R. M. Rafiullah *et al.*, *Pharm. Biol.*, 2006, **44**, 95), and seed kernels (K. Ravi *et al.*, *Pharm. Biol.*, 2003, **41**, 578) have been experimentally verified. Likewise for the seed kernels of the fever nut, *Caesalpinia bonducella*, (S. Parameshwar *et al.*, *Pharm. Biol.*, 2002, **40**, 590).

A number of complex indole alkaloids of the Apocynaceae have been shown to exhibit hypoglycaemic activity with animal models and include those of *Rauwolfia, Vinca* and *Catharanthus*. It is of interest that Handa records (*loc. cit.*) that the Madagascan periwinkle *C. roseus*, now used as a source of anticancer alkaloids was, during World War II, used as a tea by diabetic natives of the Philippine Islands and apparently served as a successful substitute for the then unavailable insulin.

The onion (*Allium cepa*) and garlic (*A. sativum*) (Liliaceae) have long been used in traditional medicine but have recently been a source of much interest because of their antithrombitic, hypolipidaemic, hypoglycaemic, hypotensive, diaphoretic, expectorant and antibiotic medicinal properties. Their hypoglycaemic action derives from *disulphides* such as allicin (diallyldisulphide oxide) and allylpropyldisulphide (Fig. 29.3) both of which have been shown to be active in animals and humans. It has been envisaged that, by virtue of their thiol groups, these disulphides act as sparing agents for insulin by competing with it for inactivating compounds.

The inorganic materials such as potassium, zinc, calcium, manganese and small amounts of chromium found in plants are believed to have a beneficial effect in the treatment of diabetes mellitus. In preliminary studies using the oral glucose tolerance test, A. Kar *et al.* (*J. Ethnopharmacol.*, 1999, **64**, 179) investigated the inorganic constituents of 30 medicinal plants which are used in the traditional treatment of hyperglycaemia in the form of their ash. The results included: *Syzygium cumini* (*Eugenia jambolana*) seed and *Momordica chirantia* afforded ashes having a superior action to the organic plant extract; *Ficus glomeratus* and *Gymnema sylvestre* showed activity for both the organic and inorganic samples; *Vinca rosea* and *Zingiber officinale* had greater activity in the organic state than as ashes.

There are also numerous plants that by traditional experience and pharmacological tests have proven hypoglycaemic activity but for which the chemical constitution is lacking. One such example concerns the leaves of *Globularia alypum* (Globulariaceae) used in Morocco for the treatment of diabetes and shown to have hypoglycaemic activity in rats. Enhanced peripheral metabolism of glucose and increased insulin release has been advanced to explain its pharmacological activity (F. Skim *et al.*, *Fitoterapia*, 1999, **70**, 382). A similar situation exists for the flowers of *Punica granatum* which are also recommended in Unani medicine for the treatment of diabetes, see N. A. Jafri *et al.*, *J. Ethnopharmacol.*, 2000, **70**, 309. *Viscum album* (mistletoe) leaves are widely used in Nigerian folkloric medicine for the treatment of diabetes and positive hypoglycaemic properties have been reported using alloxan-induced diabetic animals (F. C. Ohiri *et al.*, *Pharm. Biol.*, 2003, **41**, 184). In similar experiments, positive results have been obtained with an ethanolic leaf extract of *Nymphaea stellata*, a plant used traditionally in Indian medicine to treat a variety of conditions including diabetes (S. P. Dhanabal *et al.*, *Fitoterapia*, 2007, **78**, 288). The traditional use in Indian medicine of *Curculigo orchioides* tubers (family Hypoxidaceae) for the treatment of diabetes has also been supported by experiment (V. Makhavan *et al.*, *Pharm. Biol.*, 2007, **45**, 18).

The above examples serve to show that there is potential scope for the use of oral plant antidiabetics in medicine. However it must be remembered that with experimental models the most pronounced hypoglycaemic dose is not necessarily achieved with the normal recommended therapeutic dose of starting plant material. In most cases further toxicity studies must be undertaken and clinical trials and stability of the plant extract generally require further study. Meanwhile, diabetic patients hoping to find a 'natural' cure for their condition should be dissuaded from embarking on unsuperivsed herbal treatment to the neglect of their diet and insulin therapy. High acetone levels or diabetic polyneuritis which may arise by inadequate therapy then require much skill and time to remedy.

Further reading

Li WL, Zhen HC, Bukuru J, De Kimpe N 2004 Natural medicines used in the traditional Chinese medical system for therapy of diabetes mellitus. Journal of Ethnopharmacology 92(1): 1–21. *Over 80 plants considered, chemical formulae, over 200 references*

Mukherjee PK, Maiti K, Mukherjee K, Houghton PJ 2006 Leads from Indian medicinal plants with hypoglycemic potentials. Journal of Ethnopharmacology 106(1): 1–28. *Over 60 spp. listed, alkaloids, imidazoline compounds, polysaccharides, flavonoids, dietary fibres, saponins, ferulic acid*

Soumyanath A (ed), Hardman R (series ed) 2006 Traditional herbal medicine for modern times: antidiabetic plants. CRC/Taylor and Francis Group, Boca Raton, FL, 527 pp. *42-page table of plants, chapters covering polysaccharides, saponins and polyphenols*

30

Antibacterial and antiviral drugs

Antibacterial and antiviral compounds constitute two of the groups of antimicrobial substances; other representatives are antiprotozoal drugs (Chapter 28) and antifungal drugs. Antimicrobial agents can also be categorized according to whether they are antibiotics (derived from the growth of microorganisms), chemotherapeutic agents (synthetic compounds not found in nature) or derivatives from non-microbial natural sources (lichens, higher plants, animals).

ANTIBACTERIAL DRUGS

For the student of pharmacy, these compounds are of utmost importance and in the UK are usually studied outside the field of pharmacognosy. For this reason, and because space precludes the in-depth treatment afforded by other works available to readers, an introduction only is given below.

Sources

Waksman's 1951 definition of antibiotics was limited to substances produced by microorganisms. The term 'antibacterial' is consequently used to include those active compounds prepared synthetically or isolated from higher plants. Most of the clinically used antibiotics are produced by soil microorganisms or fungi but many examples of antibacterial agents from the other groups have been recorded and are mentioned below.

History. The first scientific recording of antibiotic activity was made by Louis Pasteur, who in 1877 reported that animals injected with an inoculation containing *Bacillus anthracis* and certain other common bacilli failed to develop anthrax.

In 1881, Tyndal in his *Essays on the Floating Matter of the Air in Relation to Putrefaction and Infection* reported that in some tubes containing a nutritive infusion and bacteria which had become contaminated also with *Penicillium glaucum*, the bacteria lost their 'transilatory power and fell to the bottom of the tube'. Tyndal attributed this phenomenon to the cutting off of the oxygen supply to the bacteria by the pellicles formed by the mould. Ten years after Pasteur's discovery, Emmerich (1887) accidentally discovered that a guinea-pig which had previously been injected with *Streptococcus erysipelatis* failed to develop cholera when injected with virulent cultures of *Vibrio cholerae*. He immediately recognized the significance of the discovery and was able to prevent anthrax in experimental animals by administering *S. erysipelatis* prior to the injection of *B. anthracis*.

Bouchard (1889) noticed that *Pseudomonas aeruginosa* prevented the development of anthrax in the rabbit; this observation was extended in scope by Woodhead and Wood (1889), who found that sterilized cultures of *P. aeruginosa* exerted the same protective effect against anthrax. The lytic action of certain Actinomycetes on various microorganisms was observed by Brunel. Emmerich with his colleague Low further studied the protective action of culture filtrates of *P. aeruginosa*; they concentrated these cell-free filtrates to 1/10th of their original volume and demonstrated that they destroyed *Corynebacterium diphtheriae*, staphylococci, streptococci, the pneumococcus, the gonococcus, *Vibrio cholerae* and *Shigella paradysenteria in vitro*. The active principle present in this preparation has now been isolated and purified and its structure determined. The recognition of the phenomenon of antibiosis had now been established but in 1928 Fleming noted the inhibition of bacteria by a colony of *Penicillium notatum* that had developed as a contaminant on a Petri dish. He advocated in his paper (Fleming, 1929) the possible clinical use of the substance formed by the *Penicillium* culture.

The advent of World War II launched a large-scale programme for the production and testing of the substance now known as penicillin, and the resources of industry and academic institutions were devoted to the study of this substance and the search for other antibiotics. This led to the discovery of streptomycin, aureomycin, chloromycetin and many other antibiotics involving notably various species of *Streptomyces*. High-yielding strains of *Penicillium chrysogenum* which produce little pigment have now replaced *P. notatum* for penicillin manufacture. Preferential synthesis of benzylpenicillin is achieved by the addition of phenylacetic acid to the fermentation medium.

Clinical use. Of the antibiotics in clinical use, most are of bacterial or fungal origin (Table 30.1). Among the bacteria, the genus *Streptomyces*

is particularly noteworthy, as it produces antibiotics such as streptomycin, chloramphenicol, chlortetracycline, tetracycline, erythromycin and neomycin. The penicillins, griseofulvin (an antifungal agent) and cephalosporins are of fungal origin.

The cephalosporins (cefalosporins) are broad-spectrum antibiotics related both structurally and clinically to the penicillins. Being stable in acid solutions, some can be administered orally. Cephalosporin C arises by fermentation utilizing *Cephalosporium acrimonium*. As shown in Fig. 30.1, cephalosporin possesses two side-chains and substitution of these with a variety of groups has given rise to a considerable number of clinically effective drugs; some twelve, with their

Table 30.1 Some clinically important antibiotics.

Types and examples	Sources	Notes
Penicillins	Various *Penicillium* spp.	Based on β-lactam structure with various side-chains mainly at position 6
Benzylpenicillin (Penicillin G)	Suitable strains of *P. notatum*	Acts by interfering with the synthesis of bacterial cell membranes. Inactivated by bacterially produced penicillinases
Phenoxymethyl penicillin (Penicillin V)	As above, with phenoxyacetic acid added to the culture medium	Unlike benzyl penicillin it is resistant to acid gastric juice
Semisynthetic penicillins	By enzymatic removal of side-chain of penicillin and re-esterification with other acids	Have modified properties of penicillin G such as acid resistance, penicillinase resistance (flucloxacillin), broad-spectrum activity (ampicillin) and antpseudomonal activity (ureidopenicillins)
Cephalosporins		Core structure similar to that of the penicillins and based on 7-aminocephalosporic acid
Cephalosporin C	*Cephalosporium acremonium*	Has only moderate antibacterial activity
Modified cephalosporins	Side-chain substitution — see text	They have a higher degree of resistance to staphylococcal penicillinase compared with the penicillins. Wide spectrum of activity against Gram-negative bacteria
Tetracyclines		
Tetracycline, chlortetracycline, oxytetracycline and others	*Streptomyces* spp., *S. aureofaciens, S. rimosus*	Broad-spectrum antibiotics to which bacterial resistance has greatly increased. Bacteriostatic rather than bactericidal. Most commonly prescribed for chronic bronchitis
Chloramphenicol	*S. venezuelae*: now by synthesis	Because of its toxicity chloramphenicol should be reserved for life-threatening diseases such as typhoid fever, meningitis, infections of *Haemophilus influenzae* and other conditions where no other antibiotic is effective. Widely used as eye drops
Aminoglycosides	Various soil organisms	All are bactericidal and active against many Gram-negative and some Gram-positive organisms
Streptomycin	Strains of *Streptomyces griseus* and other spp.	Discovered shortly after penicillin, streptomycin was used for the treatment of tuberculosis. Resistance was rapidly developed by the tubercle bacilli and it is now little used
Gentamicin	*Micromonospora purpurea*	The most widely used of the aminoglycosides; *BP* drug is a mixture of various gentamicin sulphates. Used in a variety of preparations
Neomycin	Selected strains of *Streptomyces fradiae*	Not used systemically. Administered prior to colonic surgery to suppress bowel flora. Topical applications. Eye preparations
Macrolides		
Erythromycin	Certain strains of *Streptomyces erythreus* which produce principally erythromycin A	An alternative therapy for penicillin-hypersensitive patients
Nystatin	*Streptomyces* spp.	A polyene macrolide used for local treatment of the fungus *Candida albicans*
Peptides	Principally *Bacillus* spp.	Composed of a polypeptide chain linked to another group such as a long-chain fatty acid
Bacitracin	*B. subtilis, B. licheniformis*	In combination with other antibiotics it is used principally to treat skin infections
Polymyxin B	*B. polymyxa*	Effective against Gram-negative organisms particularly *Pseudomonas aeruginosa*. Included in bladder instillations, eye and ear drops and as other topical preparations
Colistan (Polymyxin E)	*B. colistinus*	Uses include bowel sterilization regimens
Cytotoxic antibiotics		
Actinomycin D, daunorubicin and others	Various *Streptomyces* spp.	Anticancer therapy

preparations, are listed in the current *British National Formulary*. They are usually graded, somewhat arbitrarily into first-, second- and third-generation cephalosporins, which roughly conform to the dates they were introduced and the particular type of derivative. Drugs from all generations are currently in use.

Other antibiotics of bacterial origin are the actinomycin, bacitracin, tyrothrycin and polymixin groups. These are all polypeptides and although their strong antibacterial properties were recognized early in the development of antibiotics their cytotoxicity prevented clinical use as internal medicines. However, the subsequent quest for anticancer agents led to a renewed interest in their antitumour action and now some of them (e.g. doxorubicin, daunorubicin, actinomycin D) are used to treat a variety of cancers. Such cytotoxic antibiotics can completely block RNA replication and are among the most potent antitumour compounds discovered but, like others of

this group, cause unwanted side-effects owing to their non-selective action.

Unfortunately, due in part to the widespread and often indiscriminate use of antibiotics, together with poor hygiene, many pathogenic organisms have acquired a resistance to specific antibiotic treatments and these strains are particularly evident in the hospital environment. The problem is further compounded by the fact that resistance to a particular antibiotic can be transferred from one organism to another (jumping genes). Thus, the clinician's antibiotic armamentarum is being steadily eroded and research directed towards the isolation or synthesis of new drugs is still a matter of considerable urgency.

Antibiotics are employed topically, orally or as injections but in order to reduce the development of antibiotic-resistant strains of microorganisms, they are now being prescribed in a more restrictive manner than was originally the case. For this reason the use of topical

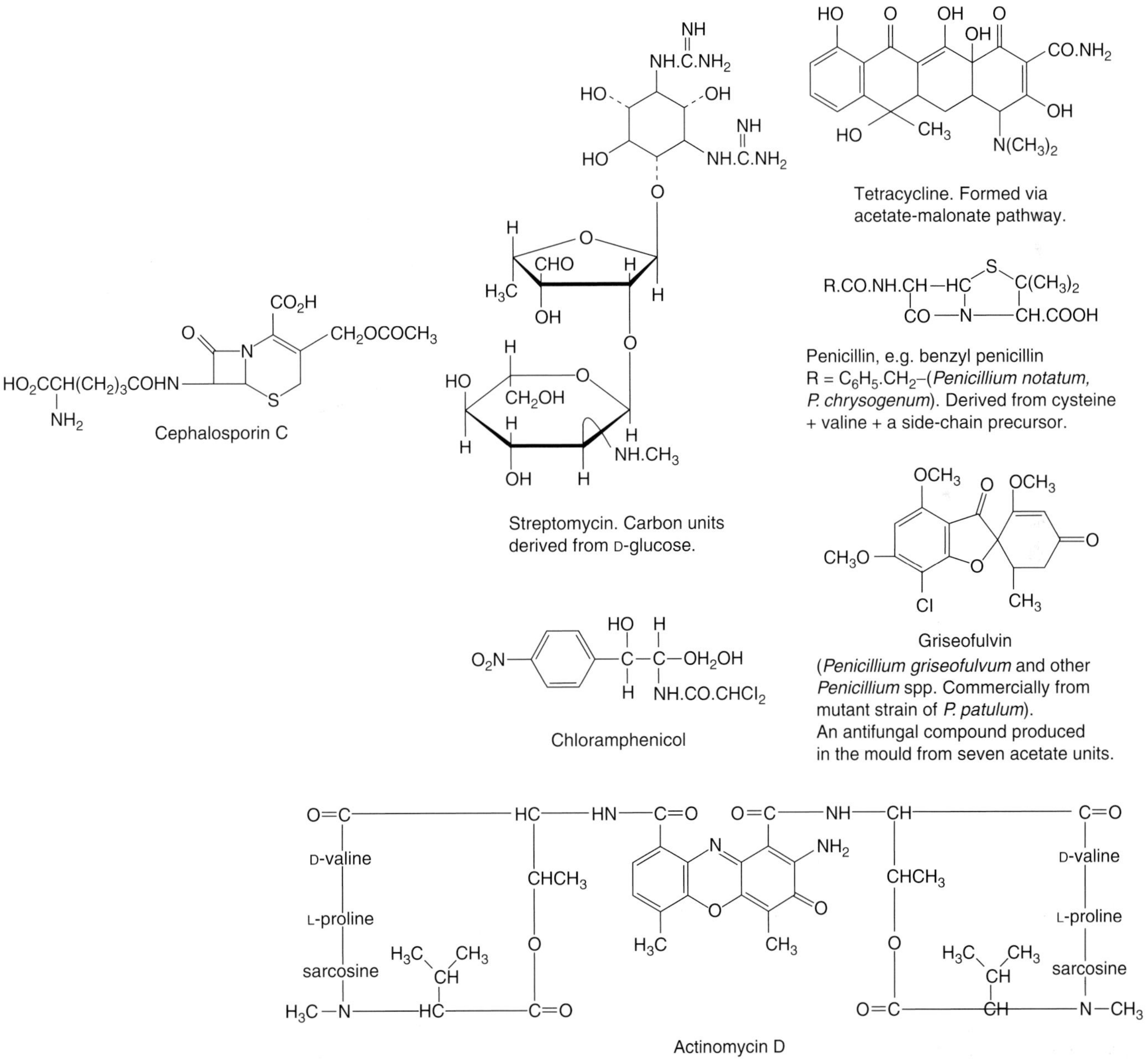

Fig. 30.1
Structures of some antibiotics.

creams and ointments has declined although topical ocular preparations remain important.

The varied chemical nature of a number of antibiotics is illustrated in Fig. 30.1.

Non-microbial sources of antibacterials

Lichens. Many of these appear to owe their bacteriostatic and antifungal properties to usnic acid or vulpinic acid.

Order Coniferae. Various essential oils from *Juniperus* and *Pinus* spp. have antibacterial activity.

Monocotyledons. Fresh garlic owes its antibiotic action to alliine, a sulphur-containing amino acid; ginger has antibacterial properties, so too aloe vera gel.

Dicotyledons. Examples from this group are: the sesquiterpene ketones of hops (humulene and lupulene) and those of myrrh (furanodiene-6-one and methoxyfuranoguaia-9-ene-8-one); protoanemonine, a lactone present in *Anemone pulsatilla* and many other Ranunculaceae; various sulphur-containing compounds found in the Cruciferae; plumbagin (2-methyl-5-hydroxyl-1,4-napthaquinone), found in *Drosera*; and compounds found in compositous plants such as burdock, thistle and *Hieracium pilosella*. The last plant, mouse-ear hawkweed, has been used clinically for the treatment of Malta fever. Mastic gum is effective in the treatment of gastric ulcers and has been shown to be active in low doses against *Helicobacter pylori*, an organism associated with this condition, (F. U. Huwez *et al.*, *New Engl. J. Med.*, 1998, **339**, 1946). Cinnamon extracts have been shown to inhibit the growth and urease activity of the same organism (M. Tabek *et al.*, *J. Ethnopharm*, 1999, **67**, 269). Many other plants have been screened for antimicrobial activity and new reports continually appear in the literature.

Marine organisms. *Cephalosporium acremonium*—see above. The marine streptomycete, *Streptomyces tenjimariensis* produces istamycin A and B, active against Gram-negative and Gram-positive bacteria.

Plants/insects. Propolis (bee glue) prepared by bees from the pollen of various species of tree (q.v.) has bacteriostatic activity irrespective of geographical source.

ANTIVIRAL AGENTS

The success achieved in tackling bacterial infection by the use of natural antibiotics derived from microorganisms was not paralleled in the quest for antiviral agents. Virus diseases still remain an area of medicine for which specific treatments are lacking. Apart from the paucity of drugs which can prevent replication of the virus within the living cell there is also the problem that the peak rate of growth of the virus is usually over before the clinical symptoms appear. Treatment is often, of necessity, symptomatic. In some instances, e.g. for various types of influenza, vaccines are available.

Added impetus was given to the search for antiviral drugs by the recognition that the retrovirus termed human immunodeficiency virus (HIV) was the causative agent of acquired immunodeficiency syndrome (AIDS) [a retrovirus is one which utilizes the enzyme reverse transcriptase (RT) for the conversion of its RNA into DNA, in this way enabling it to become incorporated into the DNA of the host]. This prompted the large-scale screening of natural products and synthetic compounds for anti-HIV activity by pharmaceutical companies and organizations such as the US National Cancer Institute.

It is considered that there are some ten stages in the replication of the HIV virus which could be targeted in the search for effective drugs. One such stage of critical importance is the reverse transcription step mediated by the enzyme RT and many compounds have now been shown to have HIV-RT inhibitory properties.

Few of the compounds showing activity in the initial screens reach the stage of clinical testing, most being of low potency, too cytotoxic or, as with the tannins and flavonoids, being non-specific in their action. The removal of the latter such 'nuisance compounds' in the testing of crude plant extracts has already been discussed in Chapter 9. Successful compounds may well serve as lead compounds for the semisynthetic preparation of less toxic derivatives.

As is often the case in science, a significant discovery came from an unrelated area of research. Bell and colleagues at London University, working on possible pesticidal non-protein amino acids, discovered in the seeds of *Castanospermum australe* (Leguminosae), a new alkaloid of the tetrahydroxyindolizidine group which was named castanospermine. This alkaloid had unusual solubility properties and was isolated in experiments designed to separate amino acids rather than alkaloids. Castanospermine was found to exert its biological effect on insect larvae by inhibiting the carbohydrase enzymes which are essential for the elaboration of the oligosaccharide side-chains on glycoproteins. This led to the testing of the alkaloid against HIV on the basis that as the compound inhibits α-glucosidase I and II, which control the formation of glycoproteins in the viral coat, then, without the essential envelope structure the virus would be unable to infect healthy white blood cells. The antiviral tests proved positive and various *O*-acyl derivatives have since been shown to be up to 20 times more active than castanospermine itself. The enzyme inhibitory properties of the alkaloid have now been considerably studied. Although the toxicity levels are unsatisfactory for clinical use it constitutes a prime lead compound for the development of other glucosidase inhibitors. Castanospermine is isolated in yields of up to 0.3% from the seeds and has also been isolated from the closely related genus *Alexa*. Two other inhibitors of α-glucosidase isolated from the seeds of *C. australe* are 6-*epi*-castanospermine and the tetrahydroxypyrrolizidine alkaloid australine.

One significant discovery in this field to date relates to a series of coumarins—the calanolides. In 1991 calanolide A and calanolide B were isolated in small yield from the leaves and twigs of the tropical rainforest tree *Calophyllum lanigerum* (Guttiferae) and shown to possess anti-HIV activity. Botanists returned to Sarawak in 1992 to discover the trees had been destroyed; other collections from the same locality proved to be inactive, demonstrating once again the problems of securing sustainable sources of raw material. However the structures of the active (+)-calanolide A (Fig. 30.2) and (−)-calanolide B were established together with some structure–activity correlations; synthesis gave a less active racemate. Although (+)-calanolide A is now unavailable as a natural product (−)-calanolide B (also known as costatolide) and the related soulattrolide are apparently available in high yield from the latex of *C. teysmannii* which can be collected without destruction of the tree. Other HIV-inhibitors named inophyllums, and related to the calanolides, have been isolated from *C. inophyllum*; in these compounds a phenyl ring replaces the propyl side-chain at C-4. By 1998 preclinical trials of calanolide A racemate were in progress.

Sumbul root (*Ferula sumbul*, Umbelliferae), a drug formerly used for its stimulant and antispasmodic properties, contains at least 27 coumarins and possesses anti-HIV activity (P. Zhou *et al.*, *Phytochemistry*, 2000, **53**, 689).

Sometimes anti-AIDS agents of more than one chemical class occur in the same plant, e.g. coumarins, flavonoids and pentacyclic triterpenoids in liquorice (Table 30.2). Also salaspermic acid, a pentacyclic triterpene, from the roots of *Tripterygium wilfordii* (Celastraceae)

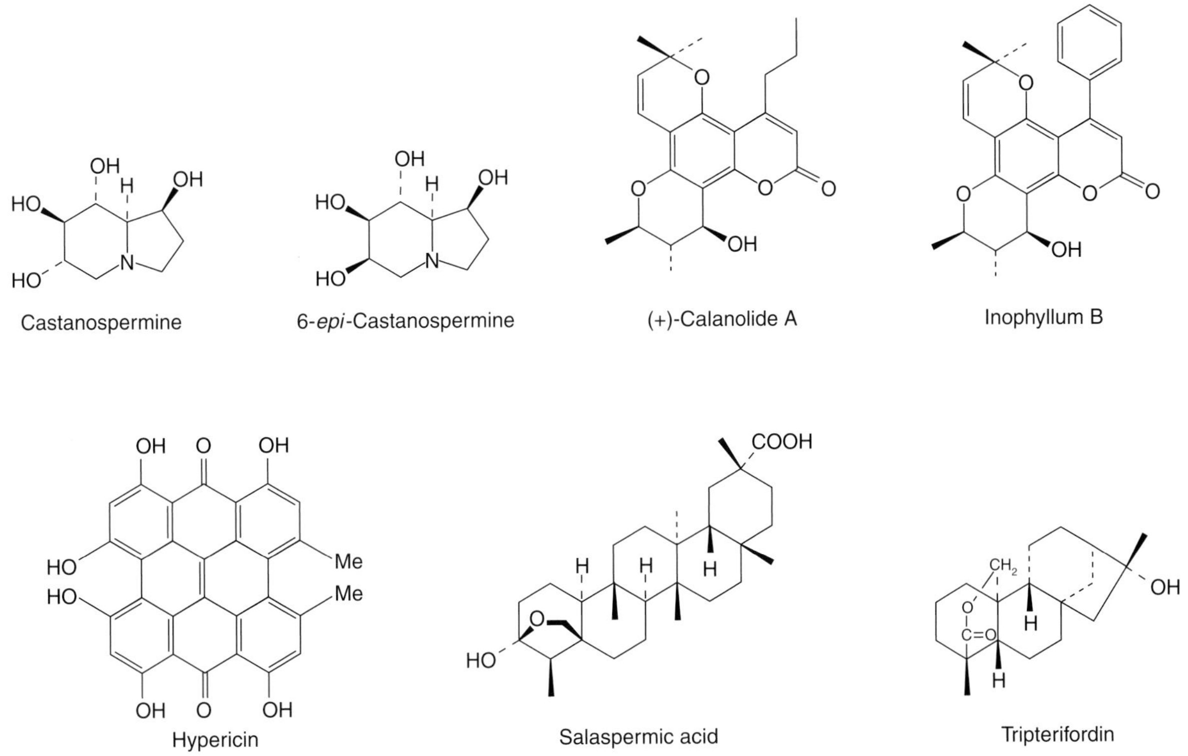

Fig. 30.2
Structures of potentially useful natural products for the treatment of AIDS. For other compounds see Table 30.2.

Table 30.2   Plant constituents with anti-HIV activity.

Constituent	Plant source	Observations
Alkaloids		
Castanospermine (Fig. 30.2)	See text	
Michellamines A–C (Naphthylisoquinoline dimers)	Ancistrocladus korupensis (Ancistrocladaceae)	Michellamine B has broad range of anti-HIV activity. Submitted for pre-clinical trials (see Chapter 38)
Anthraquinones		
Hypericin (Fig. 30.2)	Hypericum spp. (Guttiferae)	Antiretroviral activity; clinical trials (1991)
Coumarins		
Calanolides A and B (Fig. 30.2)	See text	Inhibition of giant cell formation in HIV-infected cell cultures
Lycopyranocoumarin	Glycyrrhiza glabra	
Glycycoumarin		
Dimeric sesquiterpenes		
Gossypol (Fig. 24.3)	Seeds of Gossypium spp.	Inhibitory effect on HIV replication
Diterpene lactones		
Tripterifordin (Fig. 30.2)	See text	
Flavonoids		
Glycyrrhizoflavone Isolicoflavonol Licochalcone	Glycyrrhiza glabra	Similar action to liquorice coumarins
Lignans		
(–)-Trachelogenin	Ipomoea cairica (Convolvulaceae)	Suppresses the integration of proviral DNA into cellular genome
Pentacyclic triterpenoids		
Glycyrrhizin (Fig. 23.12)	Glycyrrhiza glabra and other spp.	Asymptomatic HIV carriers experienced delayed development of AIDS symptoms
Salaspermic acid (Fig. 30.2)	See text	
Polysaccharides		
Sulphated polysaccharides	Various Chinese herbal medicines including Viola yedoensis (Violaceae); Prunella vulgaris (Labiatae); Alternanthera philoxeroides (Amaranthaceae)	In vitro inhibitory activity against HIV
Tannins		
Tetragalloylquinic acids	Commercial tannic acid	HIV reverse transcriptase inhibitors

shows inhibition of HIV reverse transcriptase and HIV replication in HG lymphocyte cells. Also active, from the same plant, is tripterifordin, a kaurene-type diterpene lactone. The plant is a toxic liane known for its pesticidal properties and since 1960 has been shown to possess a number of other biological actions.

Several species of a genus of gourds (*Trichosanthes*, Cucurbitaceae) widespread in Asia, contain a toxic protein trichosanthin. Preparations based on this compound appear to have ribosome-inactivating properties and selectively kill cells infected with HIV. Although the roots of *T. kirilowii* have traditional medicinal uses in China, Taiwan and Korea a number of AIDS sufferers in the US who took this preparation on their own initiative suffered severe side effects, including death, illustrating the necessity for adequate testing of such materials.

Most of the major chemical groups of natural products have yielded compounds with anti-HIV activity and more continue to appear in the literature. As an illustration, a few plants and their active consituents are given in Table 30.2 and formulae in Fig. 30.2.

Plant constituents showing activity against *Herpes simplex* are the podophyllotoxin lignan deoxypodophyllotoxin (from *Thuja occidentalis*), saponins of the oleane type which inhibit viral DNA synthesis, and ursane-type saponins which interfere with the formation of capsidal proteins. Of the numerous 3-methoxyflavones some are active against polio and rhino-viruses. A standardized extract of elderberry (*Sambucus nigra*) proved effective in the treatment of individuals during an outbreak of influenza B Panama; it also inhibited, *in vitro*, several other strains of the virus.

The use of shikimic acid as a starting material for the synthesis of oseltamivir (Tamiflu®) has been discussed elsewhere (q.v.).

31

Vitamins and hormones

Both vitamins and hormones constitute a range of many different types of organic molecule which are essential to the proper functioning of the human organism. Their absence or depletion gives rise to deficiency diseases, and, particularly with hormones, an excess can also be harmful. Vitamins are obtained largely from the diet, whereas hormones are manufactured in the body.

VITAMINS

Vitamins, formerly known as 'accessory food factors', are present in many animal and vegetable foods. Their absence from the diet causes deficiency diseases such as scurvy, beri-beri, rickets and night blindness. The value of citrus juices in the treatment of scurvy was realized in the eighteenth century. Systematic feeding experiments began about 1873 and much work on the subject was done by Gowland Hopkins from 1906 to 1912. Fraser and Stanton established that beri-beri was produced in people living mainly on polished rice, who could be cured if 'rice-polishings', the outer part of the grain removed in making polished rice, were added to the diet. In 1911 Funk coined the name 'vitamine' now usually spelt vitamin, for the active fraction of rice-polishings.

The existence of vitamin A was proved in 1915 and other letters were applied to later vitamins discovered. Many vitamins have since been proved to be extremely complex mixtures, and one now speaks, for example, of the vitamin B complex, components of which can be referred to as B_1, B_2, etc., or by their chemical or other names. As the chemical nature of the vitamins has been discovered and vitamin complexes have been resolved into their constituents, there is an increasing tendency in the scientific and medical literature to discard the term 'vitamin' with its associated letter (and number) in favour of the chemical name for the material under consideration (see, for example, the *BP* monographs on Hydroxocobalamin, Riboflavine and Thiamine Hydrochloride). However, in the lay literature the original vitamin terminology persists and pharmacists need to be familiar with this. Some vitamins have as yet no proved role in the treatment of human diseases but others are valuable items of the materia medica. A large number of different pharmacopoeial and proprietary vitamin preparations are available but with a well-balanced diet the normal individual should require no vitamin supplementation (Table 31.1). However, people on a strict vegetarian diet who eat no eggs or dairy produce need a supplement of vitamin B_{12}; and alcoholics need vitamin B_1, which is required for the complete metabolism of ethanol. Other groups, such as narcotic drug users, whose diet is generally inadequate are also prone to vitamin deficiency. Need for vitamins is still great in many underdeveloped countries. Notwithstanding the above, the consumption by the general public of vitamin preparations is enormous and this is one of the larger areas of the pharmaceutical industry. Numerous publications on healthy foods and promotional leaflets ensure that these substances are universally recognized.

It will be noted in Table 31.1 that a number of gaps appear in the naming of the vitamins and this is because some substances once regarded as vitamins (e.g. vitamin F and a number of the B group) are of indefinite character or have been reclassified as essential nutritional factors.

Chemically, vitamins vary from very simple compounds to very complex ones. They belong to no one chemical type. Vitamin A has already been mentioned under 'Diterpene compounds'; vitamin C has affinity with the sugars, being the enolic form of 3-oxo-L-gulofuranolactone; B_{12}, which first became official in 1963, has a very complex molecule. Several forms of vitamin D occur. Vitamin K_1 is 2-methyl-3-phytyl-1,4-naphthoquinone. As might be expected from

Table 31.1 Sources of vitamins.

Vitamin	Alternative names	Distribution
A (A$_1$, A$_2$)	Anti-infective or antixerophthalmic vitamin, retinol	Fish livers (cod, halibut, shark, etc.) and other animal fats. Plants contain proto-vitamin A, the vitamin precursors (e.g. α-, β- and γ-carotene) and cryptoxanthine; these are converted to vitamin A in liver
B$_1$	Aneurine, thiamine	Rice polishings, cereal germ, animal organs, yeast or prepared synthetically
B$_2$	Riboflavine	Widely distributed in both plants and animals; bacteria, yeasts and other fungi, cereal grains and many fruits
B$_3$	Niacin, nicotinic acid, nicotinamide, niacinamide, pellagra-preventing or PP vitamin	Milk, eggs, liver, yeast, malted barley, or may be prepared by fermentation
B$_5$	Pantothenic acid	Yeast, liver, red meat, chicken, milk, mushrooms, beans, bananas, nuts, avocados, potatoes
B$_6$	Pyridoxine, pyridoxine hydrochloride	Prepared synthetically but present in many foodstuffs, including yeast, liver, red meat, fish, yoghurt, bananas, cabbage, wholegrains
B$_9$	Folic acid, folacin, vitamin M	Yeast, liver, green plants, wholemeal bread, oranges, nuts
B$_{12}$	Cyanocobalamin, megaloblastic anaemia vitamin	From livers or from the metabolic products of microorganisms such as *Streptomyces griseus*
C	Ascorbic acid	Fruits, particularly citrus fruits, tomatoes, potatoes, capsicums; raw vegetables; or made synthetically
D$_2$	Antirachitic vitamin; calciferol, ergocalciferol	Calciferol is produced by irradiation of ergosterol
D$_3$	Cholecalciferol	Formed by irradiation of cholesterol. It is found in fish-liver oils (e.g. cod, halibut) and in human skin following exposure to sunlight
E	Tocopherols, alpha tocopheryl acetate	Embryos of cereals (wheat and maize germ oils); other vegetable oils (palm, olive, etc.); fresh vegetables, nuts, eggs, butter
H	Biotin (two forms), coenzyme R	Yeast, peanuts, chocolate, carrots, liver, kidney, eggs
K$_1$	Phytomenadione, coagulation factor, antihaemorrhagic vitamin	From plants (e.g. alfalfa, lucerne, tomatoes, etc.); or by synthesis. Abundant in the human intestine, where it is synthesized by intestinal bacteria
P	Permeability factor (significance now doubtful)	Flavonoids derived especially from *Citrus, Ruta, Sophora* and other genera
Ubiquinone 10	Ubidecanenone; coenzyme Q$_{10}$. Has been referred to as Vitamin Q$_{10}$	A coenzyme found in liver; also in other metabolic tissues of plants and animals

these wide variations in structure, vitamins differ from one another in physical properties such as solubility. They have been traditionally classified according to their water-solubility and fat-solubility properties and this division is still useful. In the main, the water-soluble vitamins are non-toxic and can be consumed in large doses without harm; they also remain in the body for a relatively short time. Conversely, the fat-soluble vitamins are more toxic in large doses and are stored in the fatty reserves of organs of the body for long periods of time. The solubilities also determine the type of food products in which the two groups occur, e.g. fatty dairy products as opposed to plant juices.

FAT-SOLUBLE VITAMINS

Vitamin A (A$_1$; A$_2$)

Vitamin A is found as such only in the animal kingdom and is particularly abundant in fish-liver oils. The preparation of cod-liver oil is described below. Vitamin A occurs in three or more forms termed vitamers. Vitamin A$_1$, retinol (see Fig. 31.1), is an alcohol and retinal is its corresponding aldehyde. Vitamin A$_2$, dehydroretinal, has a second unsaturated bond in the ring system and also occurs as the aldehyde dehydroretinol. The carotenes (see Chapter 24) are C$_{40}$ compounds found in the plant kingdom and are converted to vitamin A in the small intestine and other organs. Although the formulae of the carotenes might suggest that each molecule would give rise to two molecules of vitamin A, the successive oxidations of the molecule in fact give rise

to only one molecule of the vitamin. Infants and young children have only a limited capacity to effect this conversion and true carnivores (e.g. cats) and invertebrate animals are unable to utilize carotene in this respect.

Vitamin A is decomposed by exposure to light and may be assayed in fish-liver oils and other preparations by ultraviolet absorption and spectrophotometry.

Vitamin A is essential for the normal functioning of the body epithelia and the retina. Deficiency is indicated by night blindness and by a drying and crusting of the mucous membranes.

Vitamin D

The compounds comprising this group have antirachitic activity and are individually designated D$_2$–D$_6$; they are formed by the opening of ring B of a steroidal provitamin. Vitamin D$_3$ (cholecalciferol, see Fig. 31.1) is the only member to occur naturally in higher animals and is formed photochemically from 7-dehydro-cholesterol by the sun's irradiation of the skin. Vitamin D$_2$ (calciferol, ergocalciferol) differs from D$_3$ in having an unsaturated side-chain. D$_4$, D$_5$ and D$_6$ are produced artificially by the irradiation of 22-dihydroergosterol, 7-dehydrositosterol and 2-dehydrostigmasterol respectively. These vitamins are relatively stable and preparations containing them are assayed (*BP/EP*) by liquid chromatography using, as a standard, a preparation of crystalline vitamin D$_3$.

Vitamin D regulates the calcium and phosphorus balance in the body by direct action on phosphorus metabolism. It promotes calcium

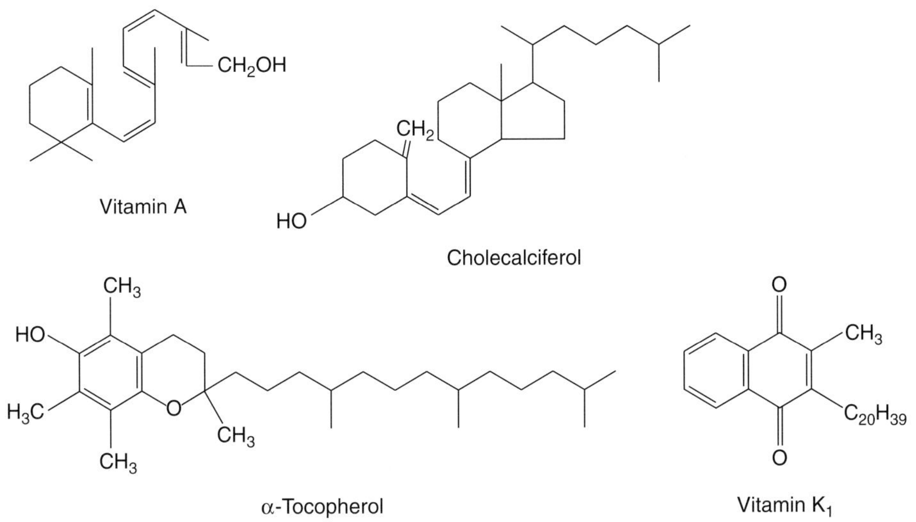

Fig. 31.1
Structures of some fat-soluble vitamins.

absorption and is an essential factor in bone formation (a deficiency causes rickets). Excessive doses of the vitamin should be avoided.

Vitamin E

Contained in this group are a number of tocopherols, prefixed α-, β-, γ-, etc, which are of wide occurrence in plants, being particularly abundant in the germ oil of cereals. For the preparation of vitamin products the cereal embryos are conveniently separated during the manufacture of the appropriate starches; α- (see Fig. 31.1), β- and γ-tocopherols are among those found in the germ of wheat, barley and rye, whereas others are found in soya beans, ground nuts and maize. Oats contains some five different tocopherols. The various tocopherols differ in the methylation patterns of the ring system. Virgin Wheat-germ Oil and Refined Wheat-germ Oil are included in the *BP/EP*; also seven monographs based on derivatives of the racemic and RRR-α-tocopherols. These are evaluated by gas chromatography.

Discovered in 1922, vitamin E is a powerful antioxidant and has an important role in the preservation of the well-being of cells, for slowing their ageing effects and in counteracting the harmful aspects of toxins in the blood and lungs. It may assist protection of the cardiovascular system by preventing blood–lipid peroxidation with the subsequent formation of sticky deposits. Traditionally the vitamin has been associated with the improvement of fertility.

A normal diet supplies adequate amounts of the vitamin; deficiency leads to the destruction of red blood cells with resultant anaemia. It may be added to cod-liver oil (q.v.).

Vitamin K (phytomenadione, phylloquinone)

This vitamin occurs in several natural forms. Vitamin K_1 (Fig. 31.1) is found in many plant sources and has a C_{20} side-chain with one unsaturated linkage. K_2, originally prepared from decaying fish, has a polyunsaturated isoprenoid side-chain which is of variable length. These compounds, termed menaquinones (MK), are produced by bacteria and, as an example, MK-8 refers to a menaquinone produced by *Escherichia coli* with 8 isoprene units and 40 carbon atoms in the side chain. (For the biogenesis of these compounds, see R. Bentley and R. Meganathan, *J. Nat. Prod.*, 1983, **46**, 44.) The formation of phylloquinone in green plants has received less attention; chorismic acid (q.v.) and 2-succinylbenzoic acid are probable intermediates. Similar compounds with vitamin K activity have been synthesized.

Vitamin K is a necessary factor in the blood-clotting process; it acts indirectly by activating those substances which are necessary for the conversion of prothrombin to thrombin. In healthy individuals it is possible that the intestinal flora provides an adequate supply of the vitamin. Deficiency symptoms are prolonged bleeding and excessive bruising.

COD-LIVER OIL

Medicinal cod-liver oil is a fixed triglyceride oil prepared from the fresh liver of the cod, *Gadus morhua* L. and other species of *Gadus* (family Gadidae) under conditions which give a palatable oil containing a due proportion of vitamins. To comply with European requirements, two oils (Type A and Type B) are described in the *BP*. Both have identical standards for vitamin contents but the former has a limit test governing secondary oxidation of the oil (see standardization). The Type B oil is the principal commercial product. In Western Europe the principal producers and suppliers of the raw material are now Norway and Iceland with much of the crude oil coming to the UK for subsequent refining and processing. (*Note*: the production of fish-liver oils should not be confused with that of fish-body oils; some tonnage of the latter is produced in the UK but more of the requirement is satisfied by imported material).

History.   Cod-liver oil was exported from Norway during the Middle Ages but it appears to have been used solely for non-medical purposes. Its introduction into medicine was largely due to Dr Samuel Kay, a physician at Manchester Infirmary from 1752 to 1784. The original method of preparation was the 'rotting process', in which the livers were allowed to rot in barrels and the oil rising to the surface was skimmed off. The more modern 'steaming process' was introduced about 1850.

Collection and extraction.   The following account is based largely on information supplied by Seven Seas Health Care Ltd., leading refiners and processors of cod-liver oil worldwide.

The cod livers, which contain about 50% oil, are removed immediately the fish are boarded and transferred to steamers in which the oil is released from the tissue, or stored in chilled conditions for later processing at a shore station. All this takes place mainly on Norwegian and Icelandic vessels. On arrival in port the oil is stored in land-based tanks prior to bulk shipment to the UK for refining and processing, although some preliminary refining of oils is now conducted at the extraction plants in Norway and Iceland.

Preparation. The principal stages in the preparation of the medicinal oil are (1) refining of the crude oil, (2) drying, (3) winterization, (4) deodorization, (5) standardization for vitamin content.

Refining. Quality and flavour of cod-liver oil are improved by refining under air-free conditions to avoid oxidation; at Marfleet, UK, this is carried out in a continuous, automatic, hermetic refining plant consisting of a battery of mixers linked to centrifuges. The crude oil is rapidly heated to 77°C in a heat exchanger and passed to disc-type mixers, where controlled addition of an aqueous reagent takes place which removes impurities and causes further dissolution of the small amount of liver tissue present. Oil and water phases are separated in a hermetic separator (centrifuge: 7000 r.p.m.) without contact with air. The refined oil is then mixed with water, reheated and the separation process is repeated in a second and third set of centrifuges.

Drying. Drying is effected in a vacuum drying tower which continuously evaporates any small amount of residual water and discharges a clear, bright, highly refined oil. The plant can refine 50–60 tonnes of oil per day.

Winterization. All medicinal oil and veterinary oils are cooled to about 0°C, which causes stearin (triglycerides with a higher saturated fatty acid content) to separate. The solid is removed by cold filtration and a polyunsaturated (enriched) product is left. Photographs illustrating the above processes can be found in the 14th edition of this book.

Deodorization. Final deodorization is achieved by steaming under vacuum which removes about 0.02% of aldehydic and ketonic impurities, and once again protects the oil from oxidation. This process establishes the palatable flavour of the finished oil.

Standardization. The medicinal oil is finally standardized for vitamin content by blending. The *BP/EP* oil is required to contain in 1 g, 600 to 2500 Units of vitamin A and 60 to 250 International Units of vitamin D_3. The former is assessed by the HPLC method of the *Pharmacopoeia*, the Unit being equivalent to 0.344 mg of *all-trans*-vitamin A acetate or 0.3 mg of the corresponding alcohol. The determination of the vitamin D content requires two chromatographic procedures—the first for purification of the solution under test and the second for the separation of ergocalciferol and cholecalciferol. Ergocalciferol EPCRS is used as an internal standard and peak heights or areas are measured.

The fatty acid composition of the oil is determined by gas chromatography and limits are given for 15 individual acids classified as saturated, mono-unsaturated and poly-unsaturated fatty acids.

As mentioned above, the *BP/EP* includes Type A and Type B oils; both have identical vitamin-content requirements but Type A has, in addition, an anisidine value of $\not> 30.0$. The latter represents a limit of aldehydes and ketones produced by secondary oxidation of the oil. For determination, the oil is reacted with anisidine in glacial acetic acid and the yellow–brown colour produced measured at 350 nm (anisidines are methyl ethers of *o-* and *p*-aminophenol).

It is now common practice to add some vitamin E to cod-liver oil (often as dl-α-tocopheryl acetate) to assist in the *in vivo* protection against reduction of the user's vitamin E status, owing to higher intake of polyunsaturates.

Storage. The oil should be kept in well-filled airtight containers, protected from light and in a cool place. The addition of small amounts (0.01%) of certain antioxidants (e.g. dodecyl gallate, octyl gallate) is permitted.

Characters. Medicinal cod-liver oil is a very pale yellow liquid with only a slightly fishy odour and taste. The acid value should not exceed 2.0 but varies with age. The iodine value, as may be inferred from the constituents, is high (150–180). In contrast to halibut-liver oil, the unsaponifiable matter is low (1.5%).

Constituents. The medicinal properties of cod-liver oil are mainly due to vitamin A and vitamins of the D group. The main antirachitic activity appears to be due to D_3 (cholecalciferol). The oil consists of glycerides of unsaturated (about 85%) and saturated (about 15%) acids. In the unsaturated group the acids possess 14, 16, 18, 20 or 22 carbon atoms, and up to 6 ethylenic linkings; in the ω-3 series eicosapentaenoic acid (C20:5) and decosahexaenoic acid (C22:6) are preeminent with smaller amounts of docosapentaenoic acid (C22:5) (see Fatty acids, Chapter 19 for explanation of nomenclature). Evidence is increasing that these polyunsaturated acids are significant for human health. The saturated acids include myristic acid (C14:0), palmitic acid (C16:0) and traces of stearic acid (C18:0).

Uses. Cod-liver oil is still widely used in underdeveloped countries for the prevention and cure of rickets. In Europe and the USA its use has changed somewhat as in addition to its traditional use as a vitamin supplement it now finds application in the relief of rheumatic pains and joint and muscle stiffness. Cod-liver oil has the established activity of reducing blood cholesterol levels and affording protection against cardiovascular disease (see also Chapter 6). It has extensive veterinary use.

Allied drugs. Halibut-liver Oil *BP* is a fixed oil obtained from the livers of the halibut, *Hippoglossus vulgaris* (Pleuronectidae). It is a pale golden-yellow liquid containing relatively large amounts of vitamins A and D, assayed spectrophotometrically. The standard for unsaponifiable matter is not less than 7.0%. It is used for the same purposes as cod-liver oil but in proportionately smaller doses, often in capsule form diluted with a vegetable oil to achieve specific vitamin potencies. Many other fish-liver oils resemble cod-liver oil, and shark-liver oil, Oleum Selachoidei, is included in the *Indian Pharmacopoeia*.

WATER-SOLUBLE VITAMINS

Vitamin B₁ (thiamine, aneurine)

The vitamin B_1 molecule is comprised of a pyrimidine and a thiazole unit connected by a methylene bridge (Fig. 31.2). It is official (*BP/EP*) as the hydrochloride and nitrate and is widely available from plant and animal sources (Table 31.1). In plants it is biosynthesized in the leaves and transported to the roots where it acts as a growth factor. Animals accumulate either the pyrophosphate (cocarboxylase) or a protein-magnesium complex.

Vitamin B_1 in food is destroyed by boiling and its preparations should be protected from light. The *BP/EP* assay for the hydrochloride and nitrate is by non-aqueous titration.

In the body, carbohydrate metabolism and the normal functioning of the nervous system are dependent on adequate supplies of the vitamin. Severe deficiency causes beri-beri and was classically observed when people whose staple diet was whole ground rice were converted to polished rice. Initially symptoms of deficiency include loss of appetite, muscular atrophy and mental disturbances.

Vitamin B₂ (riboflavine, lactoflavine)

Vitamin B_2 is built up from a ribose and an isoalloxazine residue, the name riboflavin(e) being derived from the sugar component and the intense yellow fluorescence of its aqueous solution. It is of wide occurrence in nature and constitutes a component of the flavin coenzyme systems. Synthesis by microorganisms of the intestinal flora of humans can result in a higher excretion in the faeces of vitamin B_2 than is actually present in the diet. The vitamin is unstable to light and strong alkalis and should be stored in a well-closed container.

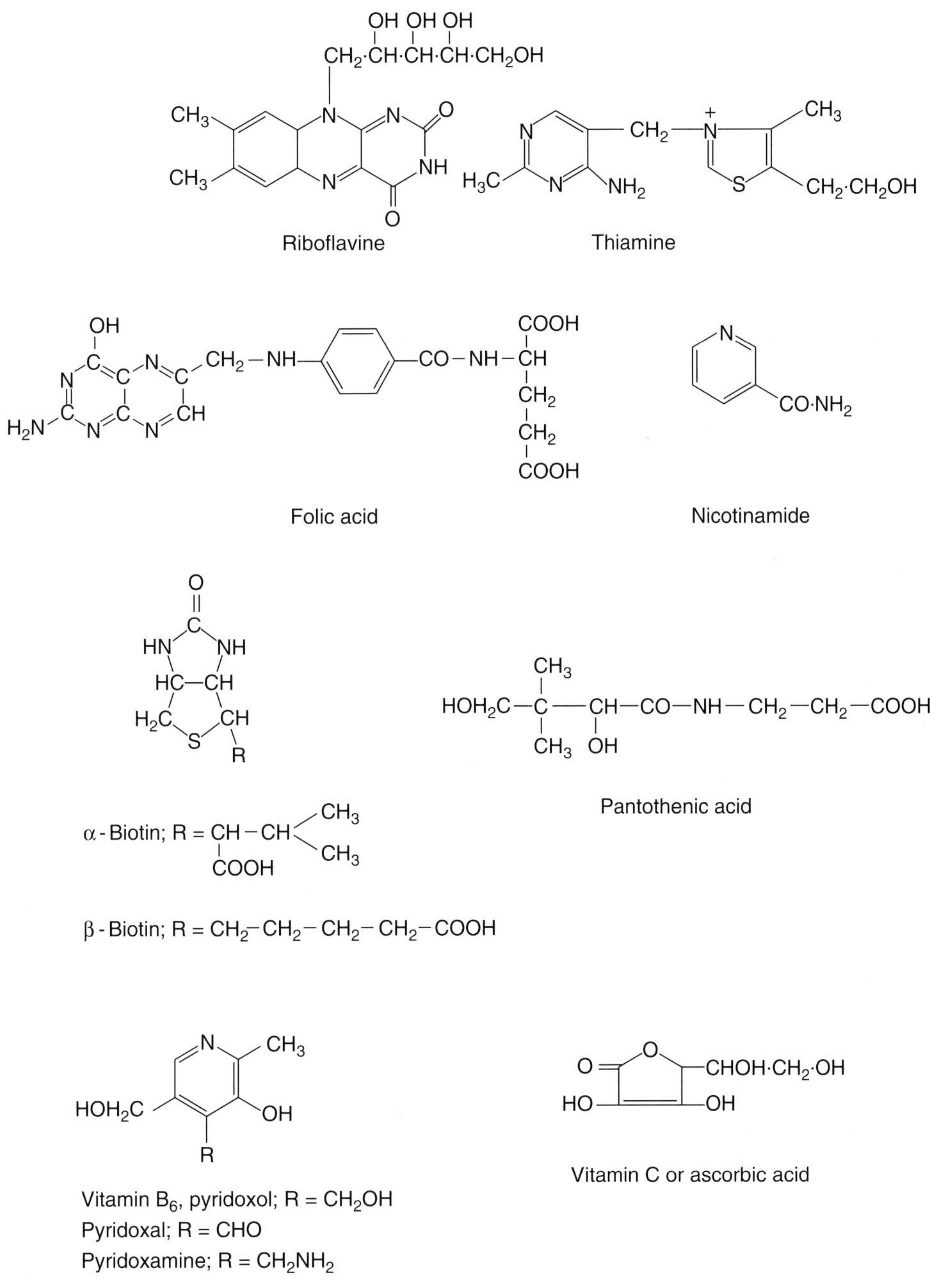

Fig. 31.2
Structures of some water-soluble vitamins.

It is assayed (*BP/EP*) by measurement of the absorbance of a solution of the acetate at 444 nm.

Deficiency in humans is rarely encountered; symptoms include a cracking of the corners of the mouth, dermatitis and conjunctivitis.

Pantothenic acid (vitamin B₃ or B₅)

This compound (Fig. 31.2) is a component of coenzyme A (q.v.). Deficiency symptoms are not well-defined and differ appreciably with different species of animal.

Vitamin B₆ (pyridoxine)

Pyridoxol (Fig. 31.2), pyridoxal and pyridoxamine are three forms of the vitamin. The first is found in large quantity in plant sources and the other two in animal tissues. In man, B₆ is synthesized by microorganisms of the large gut, but how much of this is utilized appears uncertain.

The vitamin participates in an important coenzyme system in protein synthesis and is involved in fat metabolism. It has been tested for various disorders of the body and is indicated by the *BP/EP* for the treatment of sideroblastic anaemias. Although not medically proven, many women appear to derive beneficial effects from large doses of the vitamin taken to combat premenstrual tension. Deficiency symptoms, which are rare in humans, resemble those for other B vitamins and include convulsions, polyneuritis and skin disease.

Pyridoxine Hydrochloride of the *BP/EP* is assayed by non-aqueous titration; it should be stored protected from light.

Nicotinamide (vitamin B₇, vitamin PP) and nicotinic acid (niacin)

These compounds (Fig. 31.2) are found, principally as the amide, in a variety of foods and are manufactured in the body, with the aid of other B vitamins, from tryptophan. Nicotinamide is a component of a

31

number of coenzymes (Chapter 18) which play an important role in the primary metabolism of the cell.

The classical deficiency disease associated with the vitamin is pellagra but other supplementary factors involving a lack of other B vitamins, an unbalanced diet, and exposure to the sun are also involved. Symptoms of deficiency are skin inflammation, diarrhoea and delirium. Nicotinic acid has a vasodilatory effect.

The vitamin is stable in foodstuffs; nicotinic acid should be protected from light and nicotinamide should be stored in well-closed containers. The *BP/EP* assay utilizes non-aqueous titration (nicotinamide) and acid–base titration (nicotinic acid).

Vitamin B₁₂ (cyanocobalamin)

This vitamin is not found in plants or yeasts but occurs in meat, in particularly large quantities in livers and kidneys. In the serum it is largely combined with serum globulins. B₁₂ is also produced by a number of microorganisms (e.g. species of *Streptomyces* and *Bacillus*) and these are used for the commercial production of the vitamin. The molecule is a porphyrin derivative complexed with cobalt and linked to a nucleotide. As a natural complexed porphyrin derivative it may be compared with chlorophyll (Mg^{2+}) and haemoglobin (Fe^{2+}), which together have been described as 'pigments of life'. The vitamin complex exists in a number of forms designated B₁₂ (cyanocobalamin), B₁₂ₐ (hydroxocobalamin), B₁₂ᵦ etc., the term cobalamin being restricted to those members having 5,6-dimethylbenzimidazole as the basic portion of the nucleotide. Hydroxocobalamin (B₁₂ₐ) has, in alkaline solution, a hydroxy group instead of the cyanide ion of B₁₂. Cyanocobalamin *BP/EP* is assayed by absorbance measurements at 361 nm and hydroxocobalamine, official as the acetate, chloride and sulphate by measurements at 351 nm.

Cyanocobalamin
(vitamin B₁₂); R = CN.
Hydroxocobalamin
(vitamin B₁₂ₐ); R = OH.

Nearly 40 years after the structure elucidation of vitamin B₁₂ by the late Dorothy Hodgkin in 1956, the biosynthetic pathway for this compound was finally established in what Battersby has described as the Everest of biosynthetic problems [for an account (19 refs) see L. R. Milgrom, *Chemistry in Britain*, 1994, **31**, 923].

In the body, vitamin B₁₂ is involved with the metabolism of amino acids particularly the methylation of homocysteine to give methionine (see Fig. 18.15) and the breakdown of other amino acids.

Vitamins B₁₂ and B₁₂ₐ are used for the treatment of pernicious anaemia; they are best given by injection and replace the former treatment with raw liver and liver extracts. Hydroxocobalamin binds more strongly with the serum proteins than does B₁₂ and so has a longer period of action.

Cyanocobalamin (⁵⁷Co) and (⁵⁸Co) are radioactive forms of the vitamin used in diagnostic tests for pernicious anaemia; they have radioactive half-lives of 271.7 days and 70.8 days respectively, and are prepared by cultivating suitable microorganisms on a medium containing the radioactive cobaltous ions. Owing to its long radioactive half-life (5.27 years), cyanocobalamin (⁶⁰Co) should not be used in this test.

Folic acid (folacin, vitamin B_c, vitamin M, factor V)

Folic acid refers to pteroylmonoglutamic acid (Fig. 31.2), as distinct from the tri- and heptaglutamic acids also found in this group of substances. The structure of the original vitamin-like material isolated from spinach leaves in 1941 and named 'folic acid' is not known. In the body, folic acid is necessary for cell division and for the normal production of red blood cells. With normal diets, deficiency is rare, but supplementation may be required during pregnancy and as a result of taking oral contraceptives. Lack of the vitamin produces diarrhoea, loss of weight and megaloblastic anaemia. The last two symptoms resemble those of vitamin B₁₂ deficiency and correct diagnosis and avoidance of self-medication is essential.

Vitamin C (ascorbic acid)

Ascorbic acid (Fig. 31.2) is prepared synthetically or by extraction from plant materials such as rose hips, blackcurrants and the juice of citrus fruits (q.v.). One of the richest sources appears to be the fruit of an edible Combretaceous tree, *Terminalia ferdinandiana*, found along the north-west coast of Australia. The edible fruits contain some 2300–3150 mg ascorbic acid per 100 g of edible fruit, a figure two to three times higher than that for rose hips. In the plant ascorbic acid is biosynthesized from D-glucose and a pathway involving fructose, mannose and galactose derivatives has also been proposed (G. L. Wheeler *et al.*, *Nature*, 1998, **393**, 365; see also F. A. Loewus, *Phytochemistry*, 1999, **52**, 193).

Vitamin C is essential for the normal functioning of living cells and is involved in many enzymic reactions. It is required for the development of cartilage, teeth and bones, for wound healing and for aiding the absorption of iron from the intestine. Gross deficiency causes scurvy; early signs of a lack of the vitamin in individuals are muscular weakness, tiredness, reduced resistance to infection and easy bruising. Large doses of vitamin C have been tested for the prevention of the common cold, but without significant success.

The pharmacopoeial assay involves titration with 0.05 M iodine solution with starch as indicator.

The reducing and associated antioxidant properties of vitamin C are utilized in the food industry and in the formulation of some pharmaceutical preparations.

Biotin (vitamin H)

Biotin occurs in so-called α- and β-forms, which differ in their side-chain structure (Fig. 31.2). In the body, these substances, in some instances, operate with other water-soluble vitamins and enzymes and are required for digestion and carbohydrate metabolism. Large quantities are produced by the intestinal microorganisms and deficiency conditions such as dermatitis are rare.

The pharmacopoeia illustrates the β form, which is assayed by potentiometric titration with 0.1 M tetrabutylammonium hydroxide. Various possible impurities, largely involving the structure of the side-chain, are listed. Tests include TLC and IR spectrometry.

Ubiquinone (ubidecarenone, coenzyme Q10)

In the mitochondria of plants and animals this coenzyme is involved in electron transport. It may act as a free radical scavenger and function as an antioxidant and membrane stabilizer. For patients with cardiovascular disorders it is regarded as a useful addition to orthodox treatment but a double-blind study involving 46 patients failed to give a positive result; for a brief report see *Pharm. J.*, 1999, **263**, 848. It is sold to the general public as a popular food supplement for protection against heart and gum disease and for maintaining general well-being.

DOG ROSE (ROSE HIPS)

Dog rose consists of the incompletely dried, almost ripe hips, with the achenes removed, of various species of *Rosa* (Rosaceae) including the common dog roses (*R. canina* L.), downy-leaved roses (*R. villosa* L.) and 'alpine rose' (*R. pendulina* L.). The hips should be collected between the period when they just begin to change colour and when they are fully red, and used for the preparation of galenicals as soon as possible.

The hip is an aggregate fruit formed from the apocarpous gynacecium of a single flower. Fruits of different species of *Rosa* naturally vary in size and shape. That of *R. canina* is urn-shaped, almost 2 cm long, bright red and glossy when ripe. As the commercial drug, it occurs as broken fragments of the fleshy, hollow receptacle, strongly wrinkled on the convex surface and bristly on the inner. The upper end of the receptacle bears the scars of the five fallen sepals. A characteristic feature of the powder is the large unicellular trichomes up to 2 mm in length which arise from lignified cells of the inner epidermis.

Rose hips are used for their vitamin content containing 0.1–1.0% ascorbic acid (Vitamin C) (Fig. 31.2) and smaller amounts of vitamin A, aneurine, riboflavine and nicotinic acid. The *BP/EP* requires a minimum 0.3% ascorbic acid for the dried drug, which is determined spectrophotometrically.

The syrup, prepared from the fresh fruit, is unstable and loses up to 50% of its ascorbic acid within 6 months.

BLACKCURRANT

The *BP* material requires little description and consists of the fresh ripe fruits of *Ribes nigrum* L. (Grossulariaceae, but often included in the Saxifragaceae) together with their pedicels and rachides. The plants are commonly cultivated in most temperate regions. The fruits contain various acids (e.g. citric and malic), pectin, colouring matter and ascorbic acid. The ascorbic acid content varies from 100 to 300 mg 100 g^{-1}. They are used for the preparation of Black Currant Syrup and in some lozenges. The leaves are used in Europe as a traditional treatment for rheumatic diseases; the active constituents may be prodelphinidin oligomers. Other species of *Ribes*, for example, the gooseberry (*R. grossularia*) and red currant (*R. rubrum*), have also been used in medicine.

Citrus juices

Lemon juice is produced on a large scale in many lemon-growing countries. The fruits yield about 30% of juice, which may be packed at natural strength or after concentration. Large quantities are used for citric acid manufacture. Lemon juice is used for its vitamin C content, but orange juice is richer in this vitamin and is more suited to infant feeding. Decitrated orange and lemon juices are used for making vitamin C concentrates. Vitamin C, or ascorbic acid, may be prepared from other vegetable sources (e.g. the ripe fruits of *Capsicum annuum*) or made synthetically.

Dried yeast

Dried yeast consists of the cells of a suitable strain of *Saccharomyces cerevisiae* (Order Protoascales, Saccharomycetaceae) dried so as to preserve the vitamins present.

Collection and preparation.   Yeast is produced by growing the parent cells in a liquid containing sugars and nitrogenous compounds. Distillers' or bakers' compressed yeast is separated from the medium by the use of filter presses and is a by-product in the manufacture of alcoholic liquors. However, yeast may be the sole product of a yeast factory. Compressed yeast contains about 70% of moisture and is converted into dried yeast by heating at a temperature not exceeding 30°C until the moisture content is reduced to below 9%.

Characters.   Dried yeast occurs as a pale buff powder. Under the microscope it shows spherical, elliptical or ovate cells up to 8 μm long, some showing budding. They are transparent and have a cell wall enclosing a granular protoplasm in which are one or two glycogen vacuoles. The nucleus exists as a small mass near the centre of the cell and cannot usually be seen without the use of a special staining procedure. Yeast should contain no starchy material.

Constituents.   Important constituents of yeast are the vitamins of the B group (aneurine, nicotinic acid, riboflavine, folic acid and B$_{12}$). It also contains about 46% of protein, 36% of carbohydrates (particularly glycogen), fats, sterols and enzymes (the zymase complex, glycogenase, invertase, maltase and emulsin).

Uses.   Yeast is used in the treatment of furunculosis and as a source of the B vitamins. It is a rich source of biologically complete protein and is used in the manufacture of nucleic acid. In addition to the yeast described above, Torula yeast, derived from *Candida utilis* (Cryptococcaceae), is used. It contains about 45% of protein and is rich in vitamins.

In molecular genetics *S. cerevisiae* has been utilized as a suitable organism for the overexpression of active enzymes of other plants and of animals (e.g. hirudin of the medicinal leech).

HORMONES

Some textbooks of pharmacognosy include endocrine organs and hormones; others do not. The pharmacy student usually acquires knowledge of these partly in pharmacology, pharmaceutical chemistry and pharmaceutics. The brief account which follows may form a useful starting point.

Hormones, or 'chemical messengers', are substances secreted by the endocrine or ductless glands of animals. Until recently it was fashionable to deride the therapeutic use of animal products; for example, livers from various animals by the ancient Egyptians and toad-skins by the ancient Chinese. Research has since shown that such materials often contain therapeutically valuable substances. This is especially true of the ductless glands, whose function was a mystery to men such as Galen. An early example of the rational use of endocrine organs was the employment of hog testis by Magnus in the thirteenth century for male impotence. For a long period it was known that abnormalities of the thyroid produced myxoedema and cretinism, and when in 1891 Horsley showed that such patients benefited from the administration by mouth of animal thyroid glands, the modern period of organotherapy started. Suprarenal extracts were introduced about 1894 and two thyroid preparations (a dry powder and a solution) were included in the *BP* 1898. The practice of using the glands or more or less crude preparations of them (organotherapy) has gradually been displaced by

Table 31.2 Distribution of hormones.

Hormones	Nature and occurrence
Gonadotropins	Water-soluble glycoproteins. Pituitary glands of man, horse, sheep and pig
Corticotropins	Polypeptides of pituitary glands
Thyrotropin	Protein combined with carbohydrate. Pituitary gland
Oxytocin and vasopressin	Octapeptides. Pituitary gland
Thyroxin	An iodine-containing compound. Thyroid gland
Adrenalin	(−)-α-3,4-Dihydroxy-phenyl-β-methyl aminoethanol. Suprarenal gland or prepared synthetically
Insulin	Molecule contains two unbranched polypeptide chains linked by two disulphide bridges. Islets of Langerhans of pancreas
Corticosteroids	From adrenal cortex from which over 40 steroids, many having hormonal activity, have been isolated. Examples: cortisone, aldosterone. Many others have been prepared synthetically
Oestrogens	Steroidal female sex hormones. From pregnant mares or human urine, hog ovaries, etc.
Androgens	Steroidal male sex hormones (e.g. testosterone and androsterone). From urine or by partial synthesis

the use of their active principles (hormone therapy). With a knowledge of their chemical structure some hormones can now be best made synthetically. Adrenaline was first used in 1901 and became official in 1914. Thyroxin was isolated in 1915, was synthesized in 1928 and has gradually replaced the use of thyroid glands. In Britain, on grounds of safety and in the light of the more reliable alternatives available, the licensing authority removed all thyroid extract products from the market from October 1982. One of the most notable advances was the discovery of insulin by Banting and Best in 1921, which revolutionized the treatment of diabetes; the hormone became official in the *BP* 1932. In another big step forward, insulin has continued in the forefront of pharmaceutical development in that human insulin is now produced by microorganisms which have been engineered to contain the necessary human genetic material for hormone production. The first sex

hormones were isolated from urine in 1931; testosterone became official in 1948 and testosterone implants in 1963. Oral contraception greatly increased the demand for substances of this class (see Chapter 24).

Hormones, like vitamins, are chemically a diverse class (Table 31.2). Some are related to the polypeptides and proteins, while others are steroidal. The preparation and purification of hormones such as insulin from natural sources at first presented difficult technical problems. Chemists also had formidable tasks in determining structures and evolving methods for synthesis.

Phyto-oestrogens   are non-steroidal plant substances of flavonoid constitution exhibiting oestrogenic properties. They have recently received considerable press and scientific attention and are described in Chapter 21, p. 252.

32

The plant nutraceuticals

G. B. Lockwood

A number of plant nutraceuticals are common food constituents, and extracts of many others are used as nutraceuticals.

There are a number of definitions of nutraceuticals, but the first and most straightforward is that coined by De Felice, of the Foundation of Innovation in Medicine, who defined a 'nutraceutical' as a 'food, or parts of a food, that provide medical or health benefits, including the prevention and treatment of disease'.

Nutraceuticals are rarely legally classed as medicines, but instances exist in certain countries for particular entities, for example coenzyme Q10 in Japan and melatonin in the UK. This consequent lack of regulation for most nutraceuticals has resulted in a number of poor quality products being available on the market.

There are a number of sources of nutraceuticals, including basic human and mammalian metabolites, dietary components of plant and animal origin, synthetic constituents and plant secondary metabolites; increasingly, they are also produced by microbial fermentation. Arguably the greatest number are derived from plants and are used either as single purified components, such as resveratrol, purified multi-component products, such as pycnogenol, or whole plant foods, such as flaxseed. The most researched nutraceuticals of plant origin are those derived from soy and tea, but large numbers of scientific and medical publications relate to the constituents of grapes and wine, and also the many plants rich in polyphenolic components. Table 32.1 lists plant sources and therapeutic activities of a number of commercially available single-component nutraceuticals, which often occur in a number of plants. Various purified multi-component nutraceuticals are also obtained from specific plants (Table 32.2). Those from grape, soy and tea could realistically be obtained from the diet. Increasingly, a number of foods are being promoted as sources of nutraceuticals specifically for consumers who prefer eating a healthy diet instead of taking supplements; Table 32.3 depicts a wide variety of such products. The last group of nutraceuticals occurs in the plant kingdom either widely, such as coenzyme Q10 and S-adenosylmethionine (SAMe), or only in a few specific plants but at insubstantial levels, and are therefore not suitable for realistic incorporation in the diet. These latter nutraceuticals are often produced by chemical or biotechnological synthesis (Table 32.4).

The range of therapeutic applications is wide, encompassing many areas in which conventional pharmaceuticals treat only the symptoms of the disease state. A number of these nutraceuticals have been shown to treat the underlying cause of the illness, e.g. α-linolenic acid. As a consequence of this, many nutraceutical manufacturers and pharmaceutical companies are increasingly investigating the possibility of formulating and marketing plant based nutraceuticals.

Many of the nutraceuticals owe their activities to antioxidant activity (activity is highlighted in Tables 32.1–32.4), but this may not be the full story. It has been claimed that many also have other activities, including enhancement or inhibition of Phase I and II metabolizing enzymes, and modulation of DNA repair.

In addition to the increasing number of clinical trials being published to support the use of plant nutraceuticals, evidence is accumulating regarding synergistic interactions, adverse effects, and quality of commercially available single and multicomponent nutraceuticals.

Carotenoids

A number of plant-derived carotenoids such as lycopene, lutein and zeaxanthin are currently commercially available as single entities and have wide-ranging activities; their structures are shown in Fig. 32.1. Lycopene is present in red fruits and vegetables, particularly tomatoes, and lutein is present in spinach, peas and watercress. Foods that are yellow—maize, orange juice, honeydew melon and orange pepper—are also good sources of lutein.

Table 32.1   Single-component nutraceuticals.

Nutraceutical	Antioxidant	Plant sources	Major application(s)
Lycopene	√	Tomato (*Lycopersicon esculentum*), spinach (*Spinacea oleracea*)	Cardiovascular health and cancer prevention
Lutein	√	Tomato (*Lycopersicon esculentum*), butternut squash (*Cucurbita moschata*)	Cardiovascular and eye health
Zeaxanthin	√	Tomato (*Lycopersicon esculentum*), butternut squash (*Cucurbita moschata*)	Eye health
γ-Linolenic acid	√	Evening primrose (*Oenothera biennis*), borage seed (*Borago officinalis*)	Skin, joint and women's health
Policosanol/octacosanol	√	Sugar cane (*Saccharum officinarum*)	Cardiovascular health
Resveratrol	√	Grapes (*Vitis vinifera*), wine, cranberry juice	Cardiovascular health and cancer prevention
Sterols/stanols	×	Seed oils, e.g. tall oil	Cardiovascular health
Theanine	×	Tea (*Camellia sinensis*)	Cardiovascular health, relaxant and memory enhancement

Table 32.2   Multi-component products.

Nutraceutical	Antioxidant	Source	Typical constituents	Major applications
GSPE	√	Grape	Catechins and derivatives	Cardiovascular health
Pycnogenol	√	Maritime pine (*Pinus pinaster*)	Procyanidins	Cardiovascular and respiratory health
Soy isoflavones	√	Soy (*Glycine max*)	Isoflavones	Cardiovascular, mental, women's health, cancer prevention
Tea catechins	√	Tea (*Camellia sinensis*)	Catechins	Cardiovascular health and cancer prevention

Table 32.3   Dietary sources of nutraceuticals.

Dietary source	Antioxidant	Plant source	Constituent(s)	Major application(s)
Cocoa/chocolate	√	*Theobroma cacao*	Flavonoids	Cardiovascular health
Cranberry	√	*Vaccinium macrocarpon*	Polymers of epicatechin, epigallocatechin and gallic acid	Reduction of urinary tract infections
Flaxseed	√	*Linum usitatissimum*	α-Linolenic acid, lignans	Cancer prevention, cardiovascular and women's health
Olives	√	*Olea europoea*	Oleuropein, hydroxytyrosol, lignans	Cardiovascular health, cancer prevention
Pomegranate	√	*Punica granatum*	Ellagitannins and other polyphenols	Cardiovascular health
Soy	√	*Glycine max*	Isoflavonoids, protein	Cancer prevention, cardiovascular health
Tea	√	*Camellia sinensis*	Catechins, theaflavins	Cardiovascular health, cancer prevention

The recommended daily intake of lycopene is 35 mg, but a number of Western societies consume from 5–25 mg, with processed products accounting for at least 50% of the total intake, therefore supplementation is often advised. A wide range of lycopene levels has been reported in tomatoes (1–15 mg/100 g), and lutein has been found to occur at 0.08 mg/100 g in tomatoes and 2.38 mg/100 g in butter squash. The mixture of lutein and zeaxanthin stereoisomers have also been reported at levels of 40 mg/100 g in kale and 12 mg/100 g in spinach. Zeaxanthin also co-occurs with lutein at 0.28 mg/100 g in butter squash.

Lycopene.   Lycopene has antioxidant and free-radical scavenging activity, and serum levels have been shown to be protective against myocardial infarction (MI). Many researchers believe that these mechanisms are most likely to account for its beneficial effects in cancers. Reactive oxygen species (ROS) are the main source of oxidative damage that can generate structural alterations in DNA and decrease DNA repair by damaging essential proteins, and ultimately cause cancer. A number of trials have shown levels of cancer of the oral cavity, pharynx, oesophagus and colorectum, decreased with increasing levels of lycopene intake. An association with lycopene intake is less likely in ovarian and breast cancers.

Epidemiological literature has shown that diets rich in tomatoes are associated with lower lung cancer rates. The presence of lycopene in the human lung following lycopene supplementation has been demonstrated, and it is believed that an increased intake of lycopene might

Table 32.4 Nutraceuticals present in plants but commercially obtained from other sources.

Nutraceutical	Antioxidant	Typical sources	Major application(s)
Co Q10	√	Mitochondria of plants	Cardiovascular health and cancer prevention
Melatonin	√	Banana (*Musa sapientum*), grape (*Vitis vinifera*)	Sleep improvement, jet lag, bone formation and cancer prevention
MSM	×	Capers (*Capparis spinosa*)	Joint health
SAMe	√	Banana (*Musa sapientum*)	Joint and mental health

provide an additional level of protection against oxidative damage. A high intake of tomato products is associated with a 35% lower risk of total prostate cancer, and a 53% lowered risk of advanced prostate cancer. A decline in protective effect of a range of tomato products have been shown to correspond to a decline in plasma lycopene levels.

Overall, preliminary evidence suggests that lycopene intake, and serum lycopene levels are associated with a reduced risk of developing cancer, most notably prostate and lung cancer.

Lutein. Plasma lutein concentration is believed to be inversely related to heart disease, and an inverse relationship has been reported between serum lutein levels and progression of intima-media thickness in carotid arteries.

Lutein and zeaxanthin have been implicated in maintenance of eye health and they selectively accumulate in the retina of mammals, which gives the macula lutea its yellow colour, and makes up a screen-

ing pigment known as the macular pigment. This pigment may have both acute and chronic effects on visual performance. Lutein and zeaxanthin are carried in human serum, mainly by high-density lipoproteins (HDL). Lutein and zeaxanthin are both antioxidant and are able to filter blue light. There is evidence that a diet high in carotenoids is associated with a lower risk of age-related macular degeneration (AMD). One case control study found a 43% lower risk of AMD in individuals consuming the highest levels of carotenoids (especially lutein and zeaxanthin) compared with those consuming the least. A strong inverse association was found for consumption of spinach containing high levels.

γ-Linolenic acid

γ-Linolenic acid occurs in *Oenothera* spp., notably *O. biennis*, at levels of 7–9 % in the fixed oil. Borage oil yields 25%, but it is not widely found elsewhere in substantial amounts, although it is also present in starflower oil and blackcurrant seed oil. γ-Linolenic acid is not usually purified and the complete oil is used for oral supplementation.

It is an essential intermediate between linoleic acid and dihomogammalinolenic acid (DGLA), and thereafter prostaglandins, thromboxanes and leukotrienes. Disruption of its production by the action of delta-6-desaturase on linoleic acid is thought to be responsible for a number of human disease states. Atopic eczema and premenstrual syndrome are two of the most popular applications. Metabolism of γ-linolenic acid to DGLA in healthy individuals may reduce inflammation via competitive inhibition of leukotrienes and 2-series prostaglandins. Trials using 1.4 or 2.8 g/daily of γ-linolenic acid for up to 12 months have shown progressive improvements in symptoms of rheumatoid arthritis.

Policosanol/octacosanol

Policosanol is found in sugar cane waste and the leaves of alfalfa and wheat, and is also present in wheat germ. The major component, octacosanol is present at levels of 67% in material obtained from sugar cane waste and wheat germ.

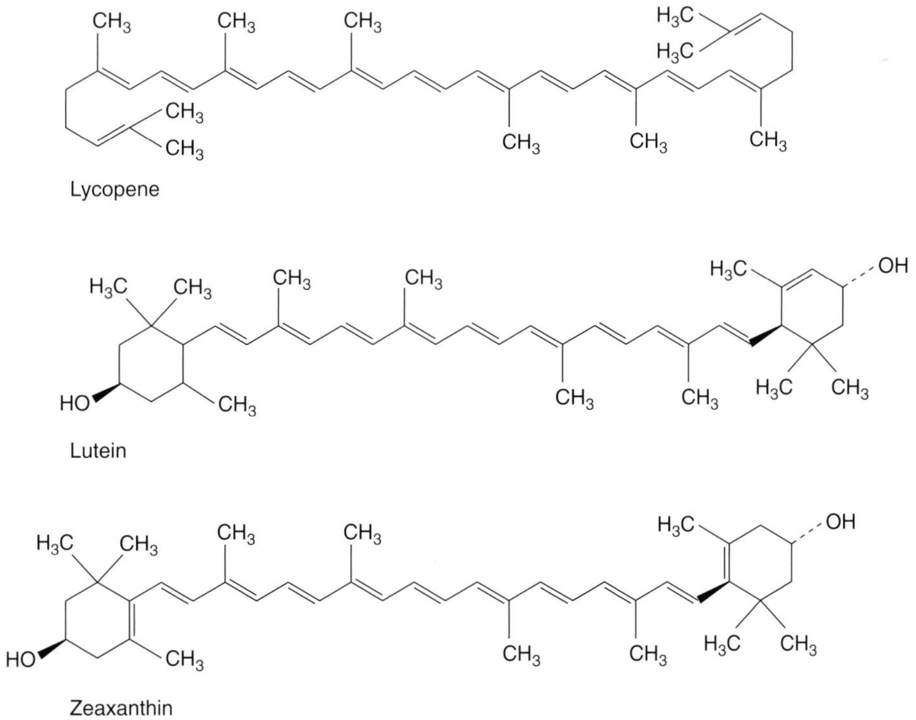

Fig. 32.1
Structures of plant-derived carotenoids.

Policosanol was developed in Cuba, and the majority of the reseach (over 60 clinical trials) was carried out there. Most studies confirm effective lipid-lowering effects at doses of 10–20 mg/day. Typical improvements include a lowering of low-density lipoprotein-cholesterol (LDL-C) by 18–26%, total cholesterol by 13–17%, and an increase in HDL-C by 15–28%. Comparison of policosanol (10 mg) with lovastatin (20 mg) showed similar effects on lipid levels, but none of the statin side effects were observed with policosanol. Policosanol is also thought to act by inhibition of cholesterol biosynthesis, but direct inhibition of HMG-CoA reductase as seen with the statins is not the mode of action.

Antiplatelet activity also occurs, at 20% of the dose as with aspirin.

Resveratrol

Resveratrol is found in the leaves, skins and petals of *Vitis vinifera*, and also wines and grape juice, and levels are elevated when the vine is infected with the fungus, *Botrytis cinerea*. Red wines contain increased levels due to extended time in contact with the skins. A number of other stilbene derivatives are also found in grape products. Resveratrol is also present in other plant products, such as peanut butter. Wide-ranging levels of resveratrol have been found in wines from different varieties of grapes and different geographical sources; 0.3–4.7 mg/l (French Barolo, French Chateauneuf). Concommitant levels of catechin, 23–136 mg/l (French Barolo, French Burgundy) and epicatechin, 17–64 mg/l (French Barolo, French Beaujolais) are also present.

Research in animals and humans has demonstrated a range of biological activities, including antioxidant activity, inhibition of platelet aggregation and modulation of hepatic apolipoprotein and lipid synthesis. Red wine is the major dietary source of resveratrol, and it is implicated in risk reduction for a number of cancers, including upper digestive tract, lung and colon cancers. Resveratrol inhibits metabolic activation of carcinogens, induces apoptosis and is anti-inflammatory.

Sterols/stanols

These both exist in all plants, and the major sources are the vegetable oils. Cholesterol absorption ranges from 35 to 70%, but sitosterol and camposterol, which are the major plant sterols, are both poorly absorbed in the intestine (0.4–4%), and the stanols even less so (0.02–0.3%). They are thought to act by inhibition of cholesterol absorption. Plant sterols and stanols are being actively used for reduction in blood cholesterol levels, and the majority of these investigations have involved sterol and stanol enrichment of the subjects' diet, and a positive association has been found for cholesterol reduction. The effects of a plant-sterol-enriched reduced-fat spread have been monitored over 5 weeks, with patients receiving either 1.1 and 2.2 g daily of sterol and a 40% reduced-fat spread. Total cholesterol and LDL-C values were reduced by 5.2% and 6.6%, and 7.6% and 8.1%, respectively, at these two levels of supplementation. A later comparison of trials using a number of sterols and stanols in fortified diets, revealed that effective doses ranged from 1.5 to 3.0 g daily, and total cholesterol reduction was of the order of 10%, while LDL-C reductions were between 8% and 15%. The mode of action was thought to be due to interference with the solubilization of cholesterol in intestinal micelles, consequently reducing cholesterol absorption. However, other mechanisms have also been postulated. Tablets and capsules containing sterols and stanols are commercially available, but there is no evidence that these have the same beneficial effects as sterol- and stanol-enriched spreads.

Theanine

Theanine is a non-protein amino acid present in tea, and other species of the genus *Camellia*. It is the major amino acid in tea, and constitutes 1–2% of the dry weight of tea. Theanine has been shown to possess three potentially useful properties: namely, relaxant, hypotensive activity and memory enhancement.

Oral supplementation with 50–200 mg theanine once weekly, has been reported to increase production of α-brain waves, which causes a state of relaxed alertness. In addition, theanine shows the ability to modulate moods, which is possibly linked to its effects on serotonin, dopamine and other neurotransmitters.

It has been postulated that the reduction in blood pressure may be responsible for mental calming. A reduction in serotonin, and also dopamine, may have an effect on memory and learning ability. It has been reported that doses of theanine up to 2000 mg/kg produced significant reduction in blood pressure in spontaneously hypertensive rats.

Theanine is increasingly being incorporated into a range of convenience foods, as well as pharmaceutical formulations. Confectionary containing 72 mg has been reported to cause relaxation, as indicated by increased generation of α-waves. Whole tea obviously contains both theanine and the catechins (see later), therefore is responsible for a range of activities, often not assigned to specific components.

Long-term social tea drinking appears to have no side effects apart from the effects of the caffeine content, therefore it may be assumed that realistic levels of theanine consumption comparable to those obtained from tea drinking should be safe. The structures of a number of single component nutraceuticals are shown in Fig. 32.2.

GSPE

Grapeseed proanthocyanidin extract (GSPE) constituents are based on either catechin or epicatechin, and monomers, dimers, trimers and other oligomers. The procyanidins are polymers of catechin or epicatechin monomers, composed of 2–12 monomers. Dimeric procyanidins named procyanidin B1 (PCB1), B2, B3 and B4, depending on the configuration of catechin and epicatechin subunits, are present. A number of these catechin derivatives are present as their gallates in addition to the free form. The structures of epicatechin and procyanidin B2 are shown in Fig. 32.3.

Levels of proanthocyanidins have been estimated in a number of wines, Greek red seed extracts have been quantified, PCB1 17 mg/100 g, PCB2 16 mg/100 g, catechin 191 mg/100 g, and epicatechin 100 mg/100 g, and white seed extracts found to contain marginally less. Japanese grape extracts have been found to contain much lower levels.

GSPE is a powerful antioxidant, with higher activity than vitamins C and E, and it is believed that this is responsible for its cardioprotective activity against cardiovascular disease and circulation defects. Most research has shown that GSPE causes a 60–90% reduction in oxidation of LDL-C, and consequently a reduction in atherosclerosis. GSPE is widely used for treatment of vascular disorders such as varicose veins, venous insufficiency and microvascular problems in Europe.

Pycnogenol

Pycnogenol is the registered name of a standardized extract of the bark of the French maritime pine, *Pinus pinaster* Aiton, subspecies Atlantica des Villar, containing mainly phenolic acids and procyanidins. A number of phenolic acids that are derivatives of benzoic acid, vanillic acid or gallic acid, or cinnamic acid derivatives, exist both free and in combination with glucose. The major procyanidin dimers include B1, consisting of catechin and epicatechin, and B3, consisting of two catechin monomers and lower concentrations of the equivalent dimers. Monomeric catechin, free taxifolin and its glucoside, as well

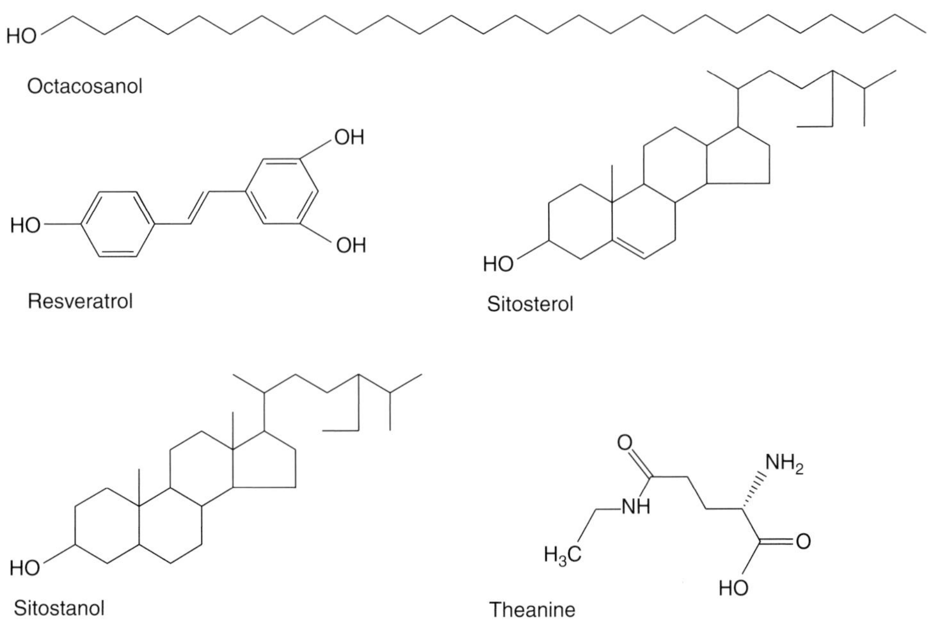

Fig. 32.2
Structures of a number of single-component nutraceuticals.

as vanillin are also present. The structures of procyanidin B3 and B6 are shown in Fig. 32.3.

Historically, pine bark has been used for treating inflammatory diseases, which gives some credence to the use of pycnogenol. A range of cardiovascular effects has also been reported, including vaso-relaxant effects, ability to inhibit angiotensin-converting enzyme (ACE) and increase in the microcirculation by increasing capillary resistance.

Pycnogenol, is a highly potent antioxidant with a high affinity for collagen. Larger procyanidins bind to proteins of damaged blood vessels to lower capillary permeability and reduce basement membrane leakage. Pycnogenol increases production of nitric oxide, which may be impaired in certain disease states, such as diabetes, by stimulating endothelial nitric oxide synthetase, and the nitric oxide produced relaxes constricted blood vessels. Pycnogenol reduces leukocyte-mediated degeneration of retinal capillaries, and has also been shown to prevent increased platelet activity without increasing bleeding time.

Adults taking pycnogenol have been reported to have significantly reduced serum leukotrienes. A study conducted in children with mild-to-moderate asthma using the supplement for 3 months showed significantly more improvement in pulmonary functions and asthma symptoms and found that they could reduce their use of prescription medication.

Soy isoflavones

The major soy consumers live in East Asia, and their foods include a wide variety of different forms, some examples being whole soybeans, soy sauce, tofu (soybean curd), tempeh, soymilk, miso (fermented soybean paste) and natto (fermented soybeans).

The major isoflavones present in soybeans in order of concentration are genistein, daidzein, and glycitein, and they occur as β-glycosides. The isoflavone content varies between 0.4 and 2.4 mg/g, depending on growing conditions and crop variety. Processed products contain a much lower isoflavone content due to manufacturing methods, such as alcohol washing of soy concentrates. Genistein occurs in the range of 1–150 mg/100 g in the raw soybean, and is converted to its β-glycoside genistin in biological fluids. Daidzein and its β-glycoside daidzin occur in lower concentrations, at levels of 0.5–91 mg/100 g.

Glycitin and its aglycone glycitein, are also present and only found in relatively small amounts.

Daidzein is metabolized by human intestinal flora to give equol in 30–50% of the population. Babies are unable to produce equol, and the ability is developed in susceptible individuals. Equol is powerfully oestrogenic, more so than estradiol, and is therefore probably the major active component in hormone-dependent conditions. Fig. 32.4 shows the structures of the major soy isoflavones and equol.

In 1999, the FDA approved manufacturers of soy foods to state the health claim that 'consumption of at least 25g of soy protein per day may be beneficial to a reduced risk of developing CHD'. It has been claimed that much of the support for this decision was obtained from a meta-analysis published in 1999. The results of this analysis showed that consumption of soy protein instead of animal protein reduced LDL-C levels by 7–24%, depending on initial cholesterol levels. However, it was not clear whether the benefits reported were due to the soy protein or to the constituent isoflavones. A more recent meta-analysis in 2005 reported that soy protein containing isoflavones significantly reduced total cholesterol, LDL-C and triglycerides, while increasing HDL-C. Soy has been reported to improve vascular function and to have beneficial effects in preventing onset and development of atherosclerosis.

Low levels of isoflavones (60–100 mg) taken for up to 12 weeks have been reported to increase memory, pattern recognition and mental flexibility. Improvements in both young males and females, in both short- and long-term memory, and also in mental flexibility, have been reported.

Epidemiological data suggest that consumption of soy isoflavones at typical Chinese or Japanese dietary levels should potentially reduce the risk of developing cancer. Japanese adults are thought to consume around 30–40 mg daily, but the quantity of soy products that need to be consumed to reach these levels of intake varies considerably depending on the dietary form of the soy. The mortality from clinically diagnosed prostate cancer has been shown to be lower in countries with high soy consumption. The death rate of men dying from prostate cancer in Japan is about 25% the level found in the US, and in Japanese men with prostate cancer, many tumours are much

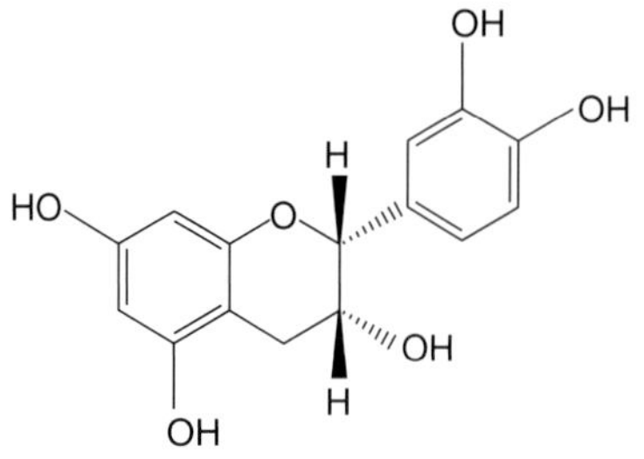

Epicatechin

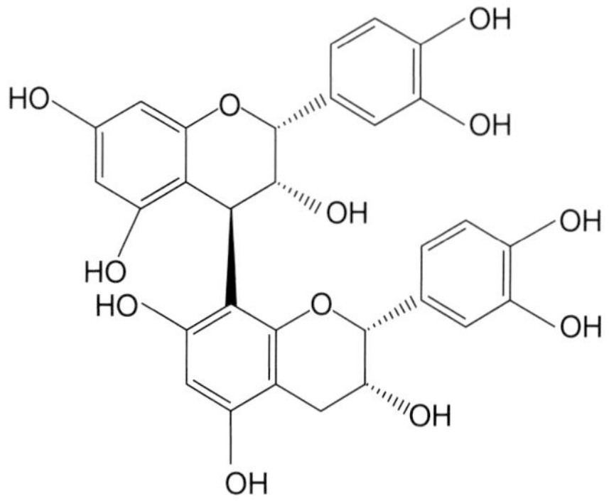

Procyanidin B2

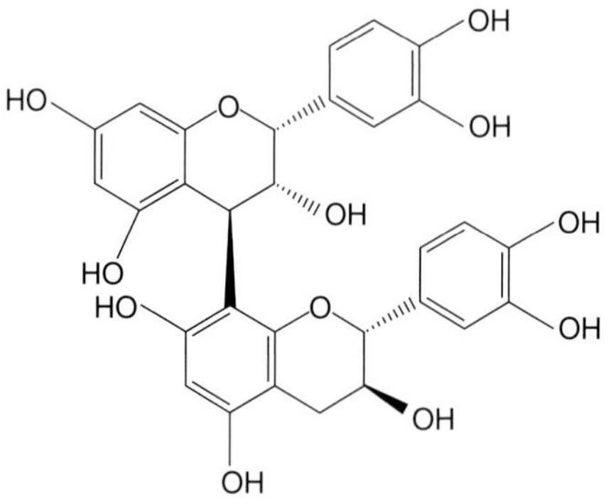

Procyanidin B3

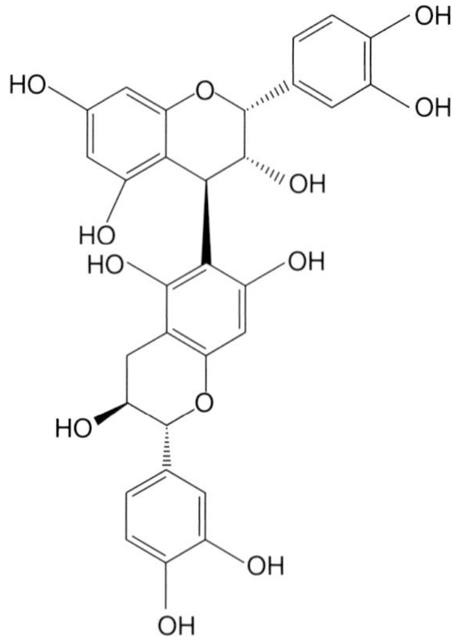

Procyanidin B6

Fig. 32.3
Structures of typical phenolic constituents
of GSPE and pycnogenol.

smaller on average. However, Asian emigrants who move to the US and change their dietary habits show a marked increase in the risk of developing prostate or breast cancer, reaching levels comparable to those found in indigenous inhabitants. This is likely to be a result of higher fat and much lower soy isoflavone content of the diet, suggesting that the protective effect found in inhabitants of Asia is diet related. Also, women who had consumed tofu during adolescence were less likely to develop both premenopausal and postmenopoausal breast cancer as adults.

Recent research has identified a further two bioactive constituents, the Bowman–Birk protease inhibitor, and lunasin, a unique 43-amino-acid peptide. Both of these have anticancer activity and may be partially responsible for the beneficial effects of soy consumption.

Soy isoflavones, up to 100 mg per day, may be a safe and effective alternative therapy for many menopausal symptoms. They are thought to be promising as supplements in preventing and treating postmenopausal osteoporosis, due to their oestrogenic activity, and consequently as potential replacements for estrogen deficiency. Most studies with soy isoflavones in osteoporosis have therefore restricted themselves to female subjects during or after the menopause.

Epidemiological studies have shown strong evidence that soy isoflavones have a positive effect on bone mineral density (BMD). Far lower rates of osteoporosis and fractures have been observed in oriental women than in their Western counterparts. Over 4.5 years, the level of consumption of soy protein and isoflavones by Chinese women was found to be possibly associated with a reduction in bone fracture, particularly in the early years following menopause. Data from intervention studies are limited, and have shown contradicting results. Clinical trials in postmenopausal and perimenopausal women that have analysed bone mineral content and BMD have demonstrated that isoflavones can significantly increase BMD at the lumbar spine.

Whole soybean contains many constituents, as well as protein and isoflavonoids, so there is the possibility that unknown synergistic effects may be seen.

Studies with isoflavones in humans, suggest that doses ranging from 1 to 16 mg/kg body weight are reasonably safe, although higher doses are being recommended for prevention of bone loss in postmenopausal women. Genistein at high doses, such as 600 mg per day, has been shown *in vitro* to inhibit cell growth and induce apoptosis. In addition, some reproductive disturbances, such as uterotropic effects,

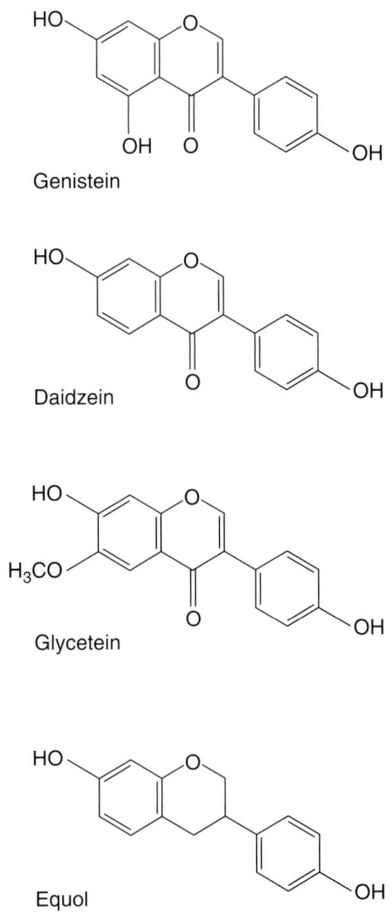

Fig. 32.4
Structures of soy-derived isoflavones.

have been reported in animals fed a diet rich in isoflavones or other phytoestrogens.

Tea catechins

Tea has been discussed previously (see section Alkaloids, Purine alkaloids), and is known to contain caffeine and a number of polyphenols. Black tea accounts for approximately 78% of the total tea consumed world wide, with green tea representing 20% and oolong tea accounting for less than 2%.

The polyphenols include catechins, quercetin, myricetin and kaempferol; these account for 30–42% of the dry weight of tea. Catechins are the main components and the four principal ones found in tea are (−)-epicatechin (EC), (−)-epicatechin gallate (ECG), (−)-epigallocatechin (EGC) and (−)-epigallocatechin gallate (EGCG). EGCG is the most abundant, accounting for 50–80% of the catechins. A typical brewed cup of green tea, approximately 240 ml, can contain up to 200 mg of EGCG. Fig. 32.5 shows the structures of typical tea constituents.

A number of epidemiological surveys have been carried out on the effects of tea consumption, initially with green tea but later with black and oolong teas. The major findings are decreased serum total-cholesterol and triglyceride, with an increase in HDL-C and reduction in the proportion of lipoprotein cholesterol and very-low-density lipoprotein cholesterol (VLDL-C). In particular, black tea consumption has positive effects on endothelial function, atherosclerosis of coronary arteries and hypertension. Subjects consuming 120 ml

tea/day for a year have been shown to have a 46% lower risk than non-tea-drinkers.

Tea polyphenols are also thought to have antiplatelet, antithrombotic and anti-inflammatory activity, and thereby reduce the risk of congestive heart disease. Meta-analysis of 17 studies has shown that an increase in tea consumption of three cups/day is associated with an 11% reduction in incidence of myocardial infarction.

EGCG has been claimed to be the most important active constituent, although it is known to have low bioavailability. Studies in human lung cancer cell lines found ECG to be most active in inhibiting growth, followed by EGCG, then EGC, but EC was inactive. Theaflavin-3-3′-digallate appears to have similar activity to that of EGCG and therefore the inhibitory activity of black tea (containing theaflavin-3-3′-digallate) against the development of cancer may be due to the combination of catechins and theaflavins. Tea polyphenols have been proposed to act via a number of different mechanisms to exert their cancer chemopreventive effects.

Studies have shown that EGCG acts specifically on certain cancer cells by mechanisms such as induction of apoptosis, cell-cycle arrest and inhibition of cell growth, but that it does not cause these effects in normal cells. The inhibition of cell growth is thought to be caused by the involvement of tea polyphenols in the activation of genes, via signalling mechanisms.

Laboratory animals with lung cancer treated with black tea had a 19% incidence of tumours, compared with 47% in the control. Apparently contradictory results in Japanese patients have been published. The age of cancer onset in females was increased from 65.7 years, in those who drank less than three cups of green tea a day, to 74.4 years in those consuming over ten cups a day. The age of cancer onset in males was shown to increase from 63.3 years to 68.3 years. The smaller delay in age seen in males was thought to be attributable to the higher number of male smokers. However, the incidence of cancer increased in individuals consuming over ten cups of tea a day, over the age of 80 years. The increase in incidence was higher than in those who drank fewer cups of green tea.

Lung, oral and oesophageal cancers are particularly caused by cigarette smoking. The incidence of lung cancer in males in the US is twice that in Japan, even though the prevalence of smokers in Japan is nearly twice that of the US. This could be due to a number of other factors, including genetic and environmental factors. Green tea is consumed far more in Japan than in the US, a fact that has suggested the possible chemopreventive effects of tea against smoking-induced cancers.

Consumption of ten cups of green tea a day, providing approximately 3000–4000 mg of EGCG, has been shown to produce a chemopreventive effect, and it is possible that there is a dose–response relationship between consumption of tea and cancer prevention.

Cocoa/chocolate

The fresh seed of the cocoa plant, *Theobroma cacao*, contains epicatechol, leucoanthocyanins and anthocyanins, which are decomposed during processing (see Cocoa seed, Alkaloids). Chocolate, which is derived from the fermented seeds, contains 0.8 mg/g of catechin monomers and 4.6 mg/g procyanidins, the latter occurring at levels five to ten times greater than in cranberry juice. The content of catechin and epicatechin represents 10 mg/g. The structure of epicatechin is shown in Fig. 32.5. *In vitro* experiments have shown chocolate to inhibit LDL oxidation. Concentrations used are consistent with plasma epicatechin levels observed following consumption of realistic amounts of dark chocolate. The activity of chocolate in atherosclerosis might be due to its effects on improving endothelial function, which has been demonstrated in both healthy and impaired individuals. This could be caused

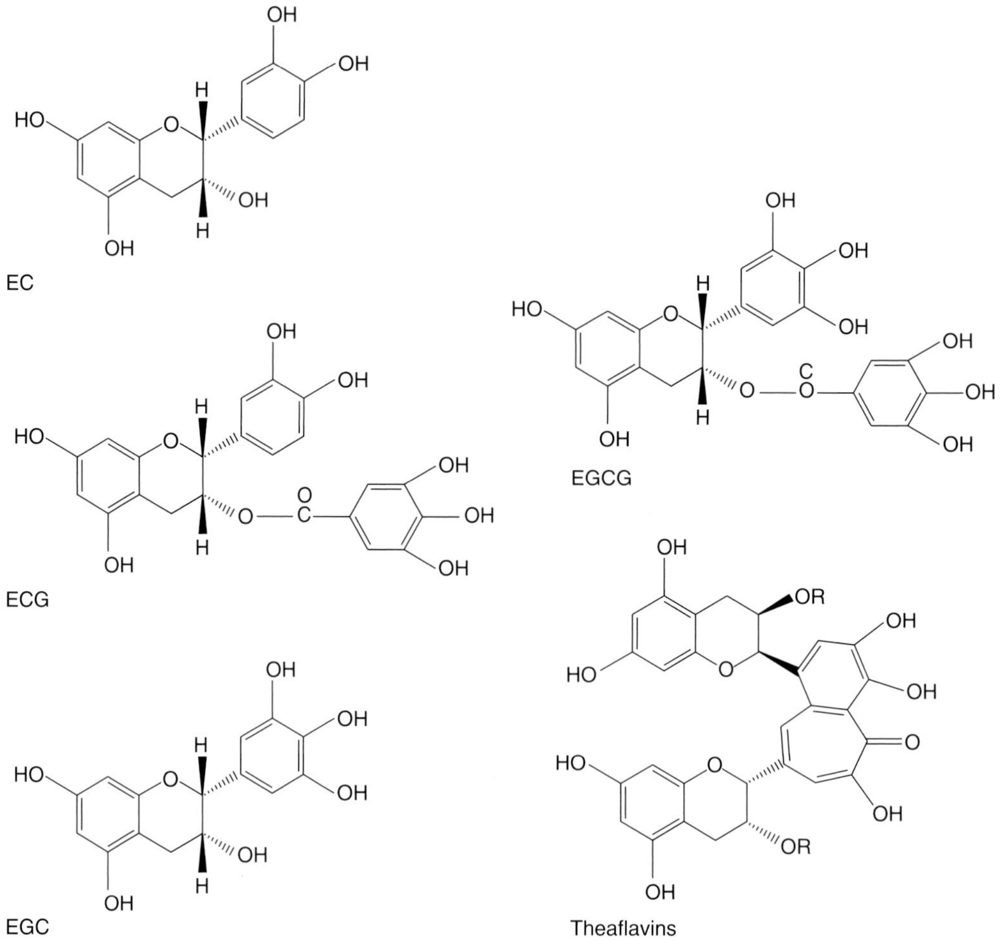

Fig. 32.5
Structures of representative
catechins and theaflavins of tea.

by its antioxidant activity, but it is also able to modulate platelet activity, inhibiting platelet activation and reducing platelet function, and hence inflammation.

Cranberry

A number of polyphenols have been identified, including ursolic acid, benzoic acid and derivatives, quercitin and hydroxyl flavonol glycosides, such as quercitin glucoside and galactoside. Typical constituents are shown in Fig. 32.6. Cranberry also contains polymeric proanthocyanidins that are thought to be responsible for beneficial health effects, especially those relating to interference with microbial adhesion. Evidence is seen, particularly in the urinary tract, of *Esherichia coli*, and in the gastrointestinal tract of *Helicobacter pylori*. A large body of epidemiological and clinical evidence, and evidence of the mechanism of action of cranberry and its components, exists in the area of urinary tract infections (UTIs). Initial research suggested that the anti-adhesive effect on *E. coli*, with consumption of 300 ml/day of cranberry juice, reduced the risk of UTIs. The action of a large-molecular-weight, non-dialysable polymer of cranberry (NDM) on the pathogenicity of *H. pylori* has only been examined *in vitro*, but it may be possible that it could be inhibited from adhering *in vivo* and prevent the development of stomach ulcers. A number of Gram negative anaerobic bacteria are particularly prone to form dental biofilms. NDM can inhibit the co-aggregation of various oral bacteria in the gingival cavity and produce a 90% inhibitory effect on the enzymes responsible for synthesis of biofilm polysaccharides. Manipulation of the ecology of bacteria in the gingival cavity using cranberry could be an effective approach in controlling periodontal diseases.

Flaxseed

Lignans.   Flax contains two major lignans—secoisolariciresinol diglucoside and matairesinol—the major mammalian metabolites of which are enterolactone and enterodiol. Six other lignans have been identified, and these are variably converted to enterolactone and enterodiol, and also to enterofuran. Levels of 370 mg secoisolariciresinol diglucoside per 100 g flax have been reported, but there are other sources, and a low level of 273 μg per 100 g is present in soy. Fig. 32.7 outlines the human metabolism of the major flax lignans.

α-Linoleic acid.   There are many sources of α-linoleic acid, flaxseed being the richest, but candlenut, hemp seed, pumpkin seed, canola, walnut and soy contain lesser amounts. Flaxseed oil contains more than 50% α-linoleic acid, which is an essential fatty acid. A high consumption of dietary α-linoleic acid has been shown to result in a reduced prevalence of carotid artery plaques and reduced intima-media thickness of the arteries. However, epidemiological studies have shown that a high intake or blood level of α-linoleic acid can increase the incidence of prostate cancer. Flax lignans have been shown to produce a 73% reduction in the development of hypercholesterolaemic atherosclerosis.

Flaxseed has reported anticancer properties, which are thought to be caused by the lignans, but flaxseed oil (containing α-linoleic acid as the major fatty acid) has also been shown to have activity against metastasis. A significant inverse relationship between the metabolite serum enterolactone level and breast cancer incidence has been reported.

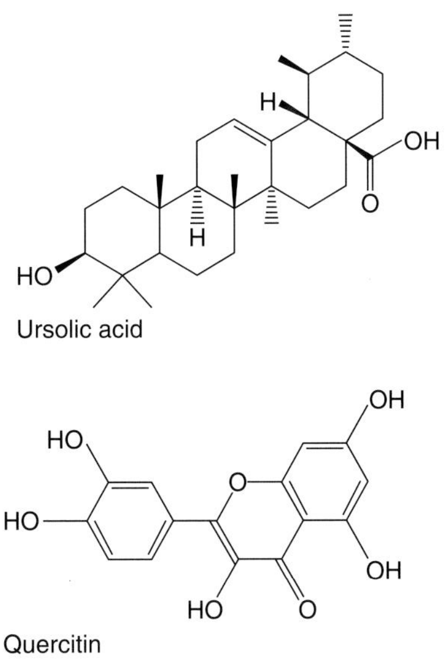

Ursolic acid

Quercitin

Fig. 32.6
Structures of typical cranberry polyphenols.

The lignan metabolites, enterodiol and enterolactone, are thought to be weakly oestrogenic and/or antioestrogenic, and may be of use against hormone-dependent cancers.

In one study into menopausal symptoms, supplementation of women's diets with 40 g/day of flaxseed was shown to produce a decrease in the number of hot flushes, and attenuated menopausal symptoms. A number of studies have confirmed the positive benefits of flax on hot flushes and vaginal dryness, and it is likely that consumption of 40 g or more of flaxseed is required to elicit beneficial effects, whereas 25 g is insufficient.

Olives

The oil extracted from the flesh contains at least 30 phenolic constituents, the major ones being oleuropein, hydroxytyrosol and tyrosol, and these are all powerful antioxidant and radical scavengers. Hydroxytyrosol is a hydrolysis product of oleuopein, and increases in concentration during ripening of the fruit. Both of these have antimicrobial activity. In addition, a hydroxycinnamic derivative, verbascocide, and pinoresinol lignans have been identified. Fig. 32.8 shows a number of major olive phenolics.

There is a large amount of epidemiological data concerning the 'Mediterranean diet', and olive oil in particular. Studies have shown that populations with high olive oil consumption (c. 50 g/day) have a low incidence of associated coronary heart disease, and this is thought to be due to the 25 mg of olive phenolics ingested daily. Animal studies have shown oleuropein to lower blood pressure, relieve arrhythmias and prevent internal muscle spasms. Oleuropein and verbascoside have been found to inhibit platelet aggregation. Bactericidal and bacteriostatic activity of oleuropein and its metabolites have been demonstrated against many organisms, and also inhibit growth and enterotoxin B production by *Staphylococcus aureus*. Oleuropein and other olive phenolics have been found to inhibit growth of *E. coli* and other organisms, and verbascoside also has similar activity.

The antioxidant ability of most of these constituents is thought to be responsible for protective activity against a number of cancers, notably breast, prostate and colon cancers, coronary heart disease and the effects of ageing.

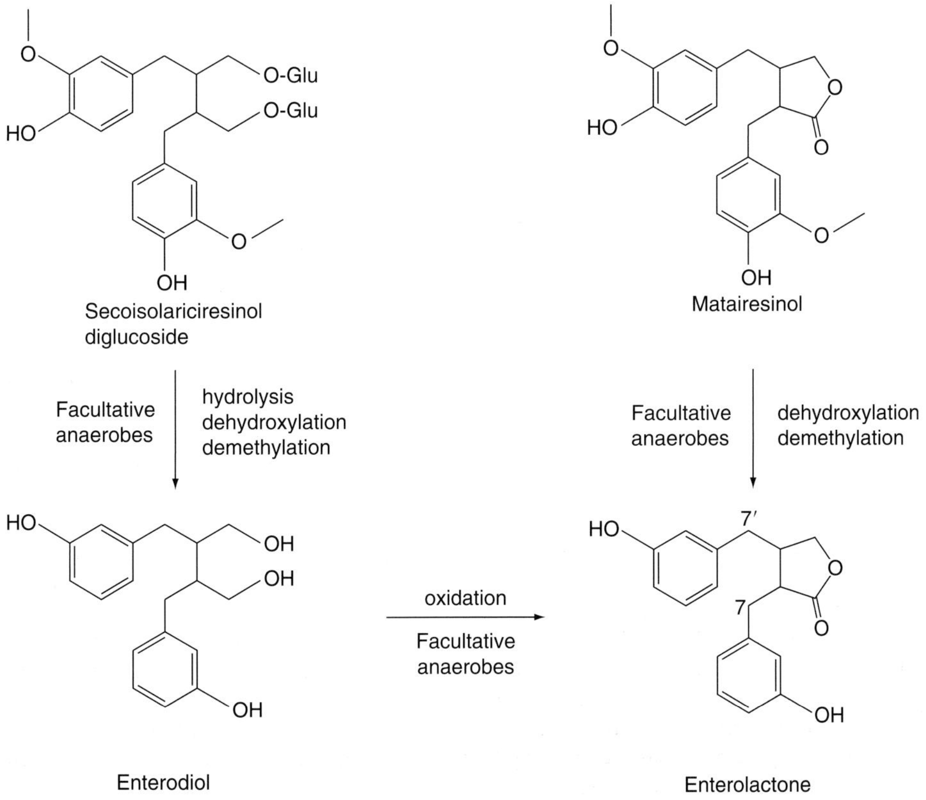

Secoisolariciresinol diglucoside

Matairesinol

Facultative anaerobes | hydrolysis dehydroxylation demethylation

Facultative anaerobes | dehydroxylation demethylation

Enterodiol

oxidation

Facultative anaerobes

Enterolactone

Fig. 32.7
Structures of secoisolariciresinol diglucoside and matairesinol, showing their major human metabolites. Reproduced from Rowland I, Faughnan M, Hoey L, *et al.* Bioavailability of phyto-oestrogens. *Brit J Nutr* 2003; 89: S45–S58, with permission granted by the authors and *British Journal of Nutrition*.

Pomegranate

The constituent present in the highest concentration is punicalagin, which is the major fruit ellagitannin. It also contains ellagic acid in free and bound forms, gallotannins and anthocyanins (cyanidin, delphinidin and pelargonidin glycosides), and other flavonoids (quercitin, kaempferol and luteolin glycosides). The structure of ellagic acid is shown in Fig. 32.8. There is great variability in levels of these constituents between the juice and pericarp, and a range of extracts and individual components has been investigated for biological activity. Comparison of activities of these extracts and individual entities with the popular commercially available pomegranate juice can lead to difficulties.

The antibacterial activity of four different extracts from pomegranate fruit rind on a number of organisms have been reported, and the methanolic extract has also been shown to act synergistically with five different antibiotics against isolated strains of methicillin-resistant *Staphylococcus aureus* (MRSA) and methicillin-sensitive *Staphylococcus aureus* (MSSA) have been reported. The antiviral activity of pomegranate has been investigated, and it was found that a mixture of ferrous salt and pomegranate rind extract reduced the infectivity of the poliovirus, herpes simplex virus type 1 (HSV-1) and human immunodeficiency virus type 1 (HIV-1) in cell culture assays, indicating a possible use in halting the spread of these diseases. A link between the antioxidant activity of juice polyphenols and antiatherogenic effects has been reported, using both humans and mice. This activity was attributed to the antioxidant capacity of the juice to reduce lipid peroxidation in lipoproteins, macrophages and platelets, with tannins being implicated in some of these effects. Evidence indicates a possible therapeutic use of pomegranate juice in realistic daily doses (50 ml/day, and for 240 ml/day in CHD).

A methanolic extract of pomegranate flower has been investigated for activity in diabetes, and was found to inhibit the increase in plasma glucose in rats loaded with glucose after 6 weeks of treatment.

The effects on a range of cancers have been researched. Pomegranate constituents may interfere with colon cancer cell formation and progression at multiple points. A significant effect of pomegranate fermented juice on breast cancer *in vitro*, has been reported, however, few *in vivo* data are available.

Possibly due to its antioxidant effects, pomegranate is an inhibitor of the markers of skin tumour promotion, along with other markers that could signify further anticancer activities. The constituents responsible for these activities are unknown, pomegranate fractions have shown the potential to prevent UV-B mediated events that could lead to the development of skin cancer. Different pomegranate fractions have shown possible synergistic, interactions against the proliferation and invasiveness of prostate cancer cells. Other areas of possible therapeutic activity include chronic obstructive pulmonary disease, neurological protection, and erectile dysfunction.

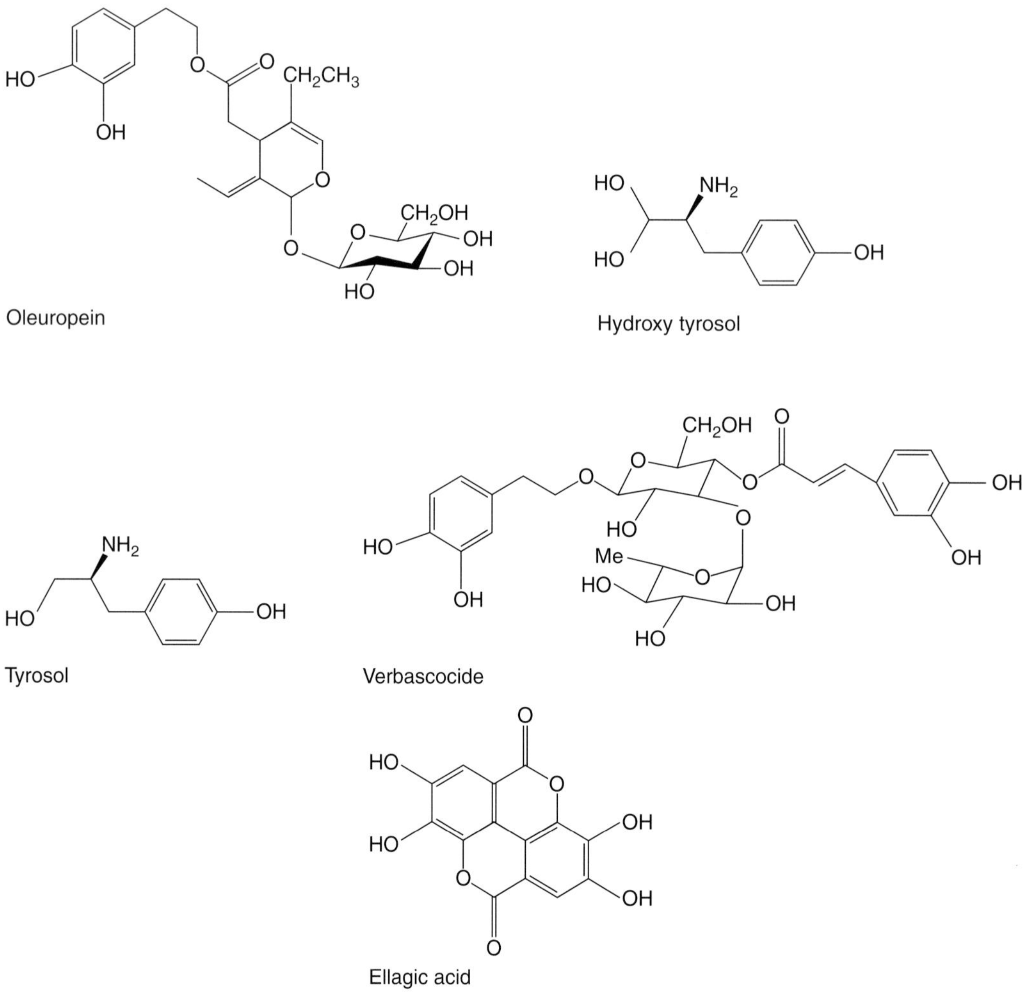

Fig. 32.8
Structures of typical olive and pomegranate phenolics.

Coenzyme Q10

Coenzyme Q10 occurs widely in vegetables, particularly spinach, and it has been estimated that the average level in human plasma is 1 mg/l in human plasma. It is a powerful antioxidant and free-radical scavenger, and is manufactured and used as a medicine in Japan.

Coenzyme Q10 occurs naturally in the body and is mainly located in the mitochondria of myocardium, liver and kidney cells. It acts as an electron carrier in the mitochondrial synthesis of ATP, has membrane-stabilizing effects and has been used for the treatment of cardiovascular diseases, including heart failure, hypertension, angina and arrhythmias, although the evidence to support its use is contradictory. Significantly reduced levels of myocardium coenzyme Q10, of the order of 50% of normal levels, have been reported in heart failure in animals and humans. Contradictory results have been reported in trials using coenzyme Q10 supplementation in heart failure patients.

Deficiency in coenzyme Q10 has been shown to be significantly higher in cancer patients and asthmatics than in healthy people, and supplementation is thought to have beneficial effects in these disease states.

Melatonin

Endogenous levels of melatonin are a result of production by the pineal gland, normally starting as darkness falls, with maximal production between 2 and 4 a.m. Between 5 and 25 µg/day is secreted by juveniles, but levels decrease with age. In extreme diets, the consumption of plant material containing high levels of melatonin could conceivably alter serum concentrations. Melatonin has been identified in bananas, tomatoes, cucumbers and beetroots, but massive amounts of these foods would have to be eaten to achieve pharmacological doses.

Melatonin has been investigated in many different applications, due to its physiological roles. It controls the circadian rhythms, and has been widely researched as an aid to shift work adaptation, jet lag and for insomnia. The 'melatonin replacement' hypothesis states that age-related decline in melatonin production contributes to insomnia, and that replacement with physiological doses improves sleep. Melatonin has also been found to be a powerful free-radical scavenger and its use as an antioxidant in ageing and related problems has been studied.

Trials of melatonin in jet lag have been studied in great detail, and daily doses of melatonin from 0.5 to 5.0 mg are similarly effective when taken close to the target bedtime at the destination, when traversing five or more time zones. However, doses of 5 mg seemed to be no more effective than lower doses. The benefit is also likely to be greater with more time zones crossed, but less for travel in a westerly direction.

It is apparent that light pollution at night increases the risk of breast cancer; and the risk increases with the length of night shifts; night-shift work, including the work of flight attendants, has been shown to increase breast cancer risk by 48%. The reduced risk of breast cancer in blind women, who cannot perceive light and therefore do not have reduced melatonin levels, suggests possible beneficial activity for melatonin in cancer prevention.

The impact of melatonin on various cancers has been studied both alone and with conventional chemotherapy. Melatonin was found to reduce the death risk at 1 year, with similar effects in different cancers.

A rapid decline in melatonin secretion occurs by old age and supplementation has been suggested to be protective against degenerative conditions including osteoporosis. Bone formation/resorption cycles are also thought to follow a circadian pattern, which might in part be modulated by the cyclical secretion of melatonin.

MSM

Methylsulphonyl methane (MSM) has been found in capers and asparagus, amongst a number of food plants, and is one of the compounds responsible for the pungent urinary odour found in individuals after consumption of asparagus. It exists in human plasma at levels of about 4 mg/person, and 4–11 mg are excreted per 24 hours in the urine.

Only two trials of MSM use in patients with osteoarthritis (OA) have been conducted. One trial used 500 mg three times daily and the other 3 g twice daily, both over 2 weeks. Both resulted in statistically significant reduction in the indices for measurement of severity of OA. How MSM acts in joint disease is not known, but its actions might be due to involvement of its sulphur content in the formation of cartilage matrix.

SAMe

S-Adenosylmethionine (SAMe) is found in every living cell, where it acts as a methyl donor in over 100 reactions catalysed by methyltransferases. It acts as a precursor in the aminopropylation pathway leading to the polyamines, e.g. spermidine.

The majority of clinical applications are in the areas of depressive disorders, OA, fibromalgia and liver dysfunction. The benefits of SAMe in reduction of symptoms of OA were accidentally discovered during clinical trials for its use in depression. SAMe (either 400 mg intravenous or 1200 mg/day orally) has been shown to produce similar benefits to non-steroidal anti-inflammatory drugs (NSAIDs) in reduction of pain and functional limitation. SAMe is metaboloically unstable, and enteric formulations and salt derivatives have been used to prolong the activity.

The structures of a number of nutraceuticals obtained from non-plant sources are outlined in Fig. 32.9.

Synergistic effects

Synergistic interactions between a large number of nutraceuticals and conventional medicines have been the subject of numerous patents, although there is often little published research available. Both soy and tea components are widely quoted in these interactions.

The effects of piperine in enhancing bioavailability of a number of nutraceuticals has been reported.

Many combination products are now commercially available, often with no published supporting evidence available.

Adverse effects

The majority of nutraceuticals appear to be remarkably safe when collating data on their LD$_{50}$s from a range of animal species. Interactions with prescription medicines have been reported for a number of them, including melatonin with methamphetamine, policosanol with aspirin, warfarin with cimetidine, SAMe with clomipramine, and coenzyme Q10 with warfarin. Prescription medicines have also been reported to depress levels of nutraceuticals; coenzyme Q10 levels have been adversely affected by a number of these, particularly the statins. Overall, a small range of adverse effects are documented, for the majority these are minor gastrointestinal problems, but caution has been advised with soy products.

Quality of commercially available products

The quality of a number of formulated plant nutraceuticals has been reviewed, but no data are available for resveratrol or pycnogenol products. Poor quality has been reported for a number of these products, based on comparison with levels stated on the labels, and similar great variability in levels of active constituents has been found in flaxseed products, teas, grape products and wines, and soy foods. Similar

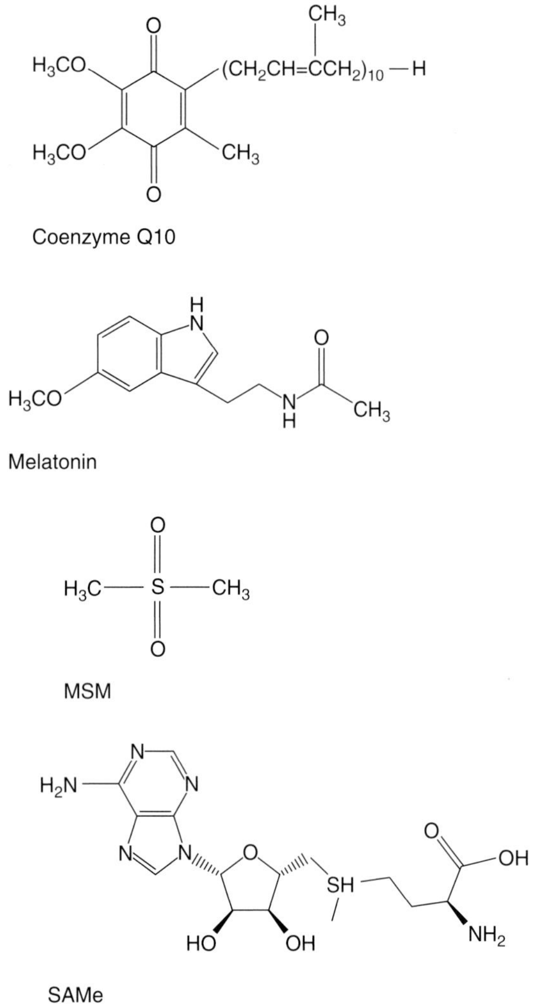

Fig. 32.9
Structures of nutraceuticals commercially obtained from non-plant sources.

variability will undoubtedly occur in other food sources such as the constituents of cocoa and chocolate, cranberry, olives or pomegranate.

Conclusions

There are a number of clearly defined single component nutraceuticals with both *in vitro* and clinical evidence to substantiate their usage. However, others have limited available evidence.

The situation regarding complex supplements, e.g. tea and soy, makes it exceedingly difficult to effectively quantify the evidence, simply because of their complex nature. This fact often makes it difficult to establish which constituent(s) are demonstrating the effects; there is also the associated problem that it is at present unknown whether synergistic effects or the effects of the food matrix are responsible for the reported effects. Similar problems in identification of the precise origin of any effects can occur with grape products containing both resveratrol and GSPE. GSPE, pycnogenol, tea and chocolate all contain catechins and procyanidins, which are most likely the cause of their activity; these components also occur widely in a number of edible plants.

The majority of plant nutraceuticals are antioxidant and, although we have been aware of their claimed benefits for many years, it is apparent that the picture is not clear. It has been proposed that although humans are continually exposed to reactive oxygen species (ROS), we derive most from the oxygen we breathe. Plants are also exposed to high levels of oxidative stress as they produce oxygen via photosynthesis. It is postulated that they synthesize a range of antioxidants to compensate. However, these particular food sources of antioxidants also produce high levels of ROS in the form of H_2O_2. It has been claimed that this situation stimulates a response from human antioxidant systems, but that excessive levels of antioxidant nutraceuticals do not work because they help generate excessive levels of ROS!

Further reading

Davies E, Greenacre D, Lockwood GB 2005 Adverse effects and toxicity of nutraceuticals. Reviews in Food and Nutrition Toxicity 3: 165–195
Eschenauer G, Sweet BV 2006 Pharmacology and therapeutic uses of theanine. American Journal of Health-System Pharmacy 63: 26; 28–30
Lockwood GB 2005 Nutraceutical supplements. Encyclopedia of Pharmaceutical Technology, 1–23
Lockwood GB 2007 Nutraceuticals: a balanced view for healthcare professionals. Pharmaceutical Press, London
Melton S 2006 The antioxidant myth. New Scientist, August 5: 40–43
Payne E, Potts L, Lockwood B 2007 Nutraceuticals for cardiovascular protection. In: Starks TP (ed) Focus on nutrition research. Nova Science Publishers, Haupauge, NY, pp 1–32
Rapport L, Lockwood B 2002 Nutraceuticals. Pharmaceutical Press, London, pp 27–76; 97–136
Soler-Rivas C, Espin JC, Wichers HJ 2000 Oleuropein and related compounds. Journal of the Science of Food and Agriculture 80: 1013–1023

33

Colouring and flavouring agents

In addition to those materials essential to the pharmacological action of medicaments there is a range of others that are present in formulations for either ethical or technical reasons. Included here are colouring matters, flavourings, stabilizers, emulsifiers, thickeners, preservatives, antioxidants and tablet disintegrants and coatings. In the food industry these are classed as additives and for the EU there is a list of permitted substances that may be used in some of the above categories; each substance is given a number prefaced by the letter E. Under EU rules, for appropriate foods, such additives must be included in the labelling. In the UK consumers can obtain further information from the Food Standards Agency and from commercially produced booklets.

For medicinal purposes these additives, which are often identical to those used in foods, are controlled by the Medicines Act and not all manufacturers' data sheets provide information on the nature of the additives present. Thus, if a patient requires a medicament free of gluten or tartrazine it may be necessary for the pharmacist to make enquiries of the manufacturer. In recent years there has been an increasing demand for materials of natural origin and, particularly regarding colouring agents, the toxic nature of many of the synthetic dyes is becoming widely recognized. A considerable number of the additives used in standard medical practice are covered by the monographs of national pharmacopoeias which give standards for purity etc. Others, not so covered, and used in herbal preparations, may be included in the EU list. In some instances e.g. Raspberry Syrup *BP* 1988 and Cherry Syrup the preparation may have the dual role of colourant and flavouring. Also, as in the case of some flavouring and emulsifying agents, there may be an overlap with medicinal action. Thus oils of clove, and peppermint are used as flavours but the former has antibacterial, and the latter, carminative properties. Similarly, natural gums which are widely used as thickening, emulsifying and suspending agents have, in larger doses, a therapeutic action.

COLOURING AGENTS

The essential subsidiary requirements of a medicinal colourant are non-toxicity and stability. Specific factors to be considered are the effect of pH on colour (many natural pigments are pH indicators), solubility in water and oils, and stability to light, heat and sugars. Table 33.1 lists a range of some of the more important natural colourants used in food and medicinals and Fig. 33.1 shows the chemical structures.

For a report covering the legal aspects appropriate to Europe and Japan, see 'Further reading' (Henry 2000).

RED POPPY PETALS

Red poppy petals of the *BP/EP* consist of the dried whole or fragmented petals of *Papaver rhoeas* L. (field poppy, corn poppy) family Papaveraceae. The annual plant is found throughout Europe apart from the far north, N. Africa, temperate Asia and by introduction in N. America, Australia and New Zealand. Once a colourful sight as a weed in cornfields but now, due to the use of selective weed-killers, largely confined in its habit to waste areas and disturbed ground.

When harvested, the petals are a bright scarlet in colour with a dark violet claw and a smooth and shiny upper surface. The dried commercial product is dingy violet, crumpled or broken and often in clumps. Each petal is broadly ovate, about 6 cm long with an entire margin and veins arising from the base and anastomozing just below the margin.

Microscopy of the powder shows sinuously walled epidermal cells, small anomocytic stomata, vascular vibrous tissue, the remains of anthers and pollen grains about 30 μm in diameter with three pores.

The taste is mucilaginous and slightly bitter.

33

Table 33.1   Natural colourants.

Colourant source	Shade	Solubility	Stability	EU No., etc
Anthocyanins: various sources	Red–violet	Water	Colour pH-dependent	E163
Cochineal: *Dactylopius coccus*	Red	Water	Precipitates below pH 3	E120, *BP*
Beetroot powder (betanin); *Beta vulgaris*	Red	Water	Fair stability in acid; poor in alkali	E162
Carmine powder: *D. coccus*	Purplish-red	Alkali	Precipitates below pH 4	E120, *BPC* (1988)
Paprika oleo-resin (capsanthin, capsorubin): *Capsicum annuum*	Orange-red	Oil	Stable	E160(c)
Gardenia yellow: *Gardenia jasminoides, G. augusta*	Yellow (crocetins)	Water	Stable	
Saffron (crocin): *Crocus sativus*	Yellow–orange	Water		
Carotenes: various sources, e.g. carrot root	Orange	Oil/water	Stable	E160(a)
Annatto (bixin): *Bixa orellana*	Yellow–orange	Oil/water	Good in alkali; precipitates in acid	E160 (b)
Curcumin: *Curcuma longa*	Yellow	Water	Good in acid; poor in alkali	E100
Chlorophyll and complexes	Green, olive-green	Water/oil/acid/ alcohol depending on preparation	Fair in alkali; precipitates in acid	E140, E141

The colour of red poppy petals is due to anthocyanidins, including the gentiobioside of cyanidin (mecocyanin; see Table 21.6). On treatment with acid the drug becomes scarlet, whereas alkalis turn it a greenish-blue. The colour and blotching of the petals is variable and the *BP/EP* specifies a colouring capacity of not less than 0.6 when determined by absorbance measurements on an acid ethanolic extract at 525 nm.

Alkaloids with little toxicity (e.g. rhoeadine) and mucilage are also present. For a report on the isolation of two new depsides, (esters composed of two phenolic acids) and other known compounds see M. Hillenbrand *et al.*, *Planta Med.*, 2004, **70**, 380.

Red poppy petals were traditionally employed as an anodyne and expectorant but are now used principally as a colouring for infusions and syrups.

COCHINEAL

Cochineal is the dried female insect *Dactylopius coccus* Costa (*Coccus cacti* Linné) (order Hemiptera), containing eggs and larvae. Cochineal insects are indigenous to Central America. Commercial supplies are derived principally from Peru (85%) amounting in 1998 to 6.99×10^5 kg; other producers are the Canary Islands, Chile, Bolivia and Mexico.

History.   Cochineal was used by the Greeks and Romans and was an important dye in 15th century England. It was derived from the swollen females of two scale insects *Kermes vermilio* and *K. ilicis* close relatives of *D. coccus*. These species use as host the kermes oak, *Quercus coccifera*, a native of the Mediterranean coast (for further details see J. Compton, *The Garden*, 1990, **115**, 385).

Culture and life history.   Each year eggs from the previous crop, which are protected during the rainy season by shelters placed over the plants, are 'sown' on the cacti (usually species of *Opuntia*) on which it is intended to breed. Both male and female insects emerge. The males are about 1 mm long and possess wings, while the females are about 2 mm long and without wings. After fertilization the females attach themselves to the cacti by means of their probosces, which become embedded in the tissues of the plant; the males then die. The females

swell to about twice their former size, owing to the presence of developing larvae, and develop red colouring matter. The larvae mature in about 14 days and escape from the now dead body of the parent. Only a small proportion of the larvae develop into males. For the next fortnight the young females crawl about the plant and the males fly. The sequence of events described above is then repeated. The life cycle thus takes about 6 weeks and three to five generations of the insects may be produced in a season.

Collection and preparation.   The insects are brushed from the plants with small brooms and killed, a certain number being left to provide for subsequent crops. The first crop of the season usually contains the most colouring matter. The insects are killed by plunging in boiling water, by stove heat or by exposure to the fumes of burning sulphur or charcoal. If heat is used, the insects change to a purplish-black colour and are known as 'black grain', while the fume-killed purplish-grey ones are known as 'silver grain'. Small immature insects and larvae which can be separated by sieves are sold as 'granilla' or siftings.

Characters.   Cochineal insects are 3.5–5.5 mm long and somewhat oval in outline. The convex dorsal surface shows from nine to 11 segments, but there are no constrictions between head, thorax and abdomen. The insect has a pair of seven-jointed antennae and three pairs of very inconspicuous legs. The surface bears tubular glands which secrete wax, the melting of which by heat accounts for the difference in colour between the silver grain and black grain varieties.

Cochineal should be examined microscopically after removing the colouring matter by means of solution of ammonia. Within each insect will be found from 60 to 450 eggs and larvae. For illustrations, see previous editions of this book.

Constituents.   Cochineal contains about 10% of carminic acid, (Fig. 33.1), a brilliant purple, water-soluble colouring matter; it is a *C*-glycoside, anthraquinone derivative. The insects also contain about 10% of fat and 2% of wax. Recent research has shown that irradiation, even at the lowest level tested (1 KGy), is effective in eliminating the microbial count and has no significant effect on the stability of the pigment. The *BP* describes a test of absence of salmonellae and

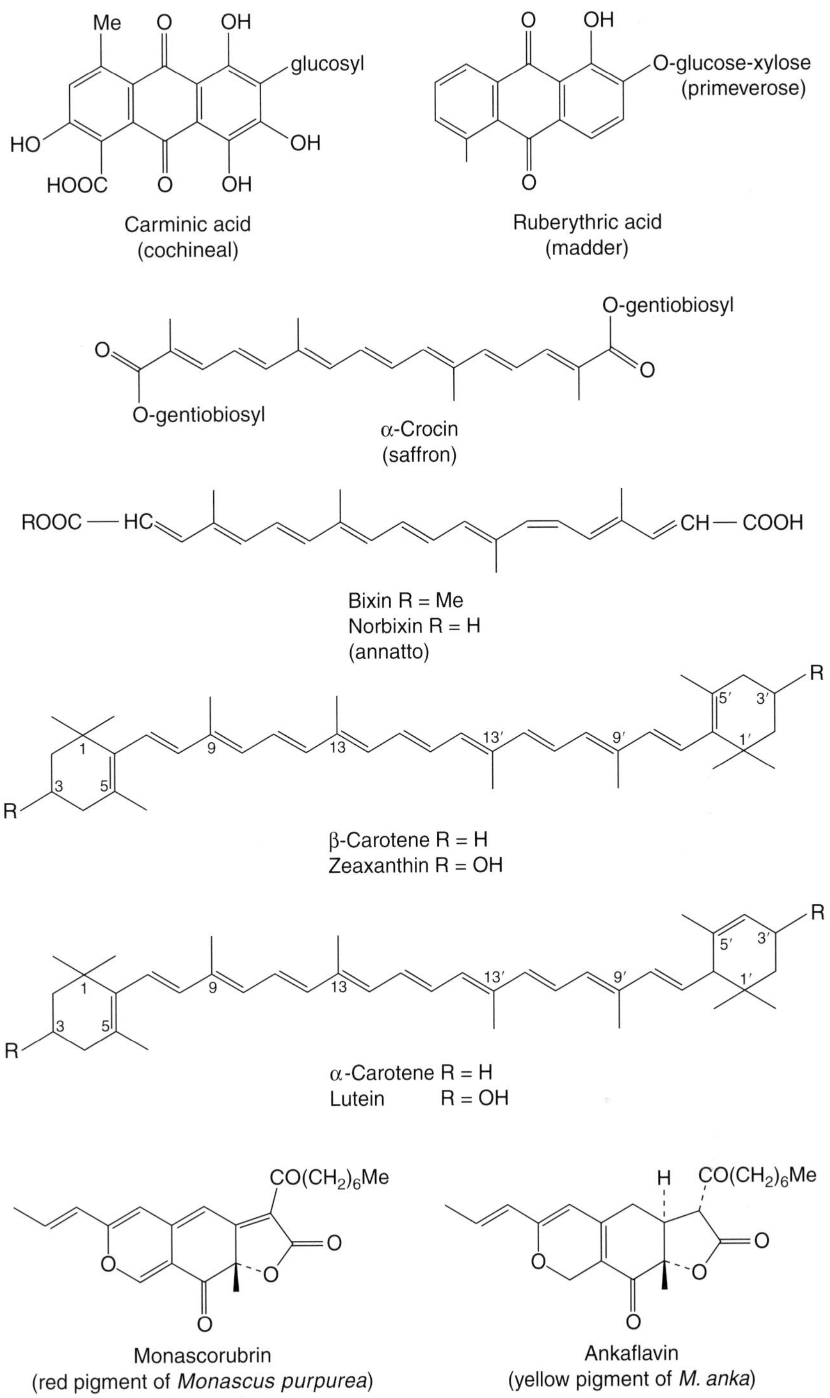

Fig. 33.1
Chemical structures of some natural pigments
of pharmaceutical significance (for anthocyanidins
see Table 21.6).

Escherichia coli and a colour value test in which the extinction of a diluted extract of pH 8.0 is measured at 530 nm.

Carmine, an aluminium lake, is prepared by precipitation by adding aluminium and calcium ions to an extract of cochineal; it contains about 50% of carminic acid. 'Carmines' are produced which vary enormously in shades and tinting strengths.

Adulteration. The weight of cochineal may be increased by 'dressing' it with inorganic matter, the colour of which is chosen so as to blend with the variety of insect being adulterated. If genuine, no insoluble matter should separate when the insects are placed in water and the ash should not exceed 7%.

Uses. Cochineal and carmine are used as colouring agents for liquids and solids and as indicators. No carcinogenic properties have been demonstrated.

Saffron

Saffron consists of the dried stigmas and tops of the styles of *Crocus sativus* (Iridaceae). The drug is prepared in Spain (70% of world supply); other producers are China, Iran and Kashmir. It is included in the *EP*. Saffron was prized by the ancients and was cultivated in Greece, Asia Minor and Persia. Cultivation of the plant in Spain appears to date from the tenth century and in England from the fourteenth century. In 1728 quite large quantities of English saffron were

33

being grown, particularly in the area between Saffron Walden and Cambridge.

The corms are planted in July or August in soil carefully prepared during the previous autumn. The first flowering takes place in September or October of the following year, after which each corm replaces itself by one or more daughter corms. After three harvests of flowers, the corms, which have at least doubled in number, are dug up in May or June. The best of these are reserved for planting in fresh ground in July or August. Saffron culture is labour-intensive. Collection is very much family-orientated. The flowers are gathered in the early morning, placed in baskets or hampers and conveyed to the picking house. The picker takes each flower in turn in the left hand and breaks the style just below the stigmas with the nail of the right thumb. The detached stigmas are dried by artificial heat, usually charcoal stoves, over which they are placed in hair sieves. After about 30–45 min the drug is cooled and stored in a dry place. About 90 000–100 000 flowers give 5000 g of fresh stigmas or about 1000 g of the dried drug.

Saffron or hay-saffron, as it is often called, occurs in loose masses consisting of reddish-brown stigmas among which yellowish pieces, the tops of the styles, can usually be seen. It has a sweetish aromatic odour and a bitter taste. When chewed the saliva is coloured orange–yellow. If the soaked drug is examined under a lens or microscope, the stigmas will be found either separate or united in threes to the apex of the yellowish styles. Each stigma is about 25 mm long and has the shape of a slender funnel, the rim of which is dentate or fimbricate.

Saffron contains a number of carotenoid pigments. A hypothetical protocrocin of the fresh plant is decomposed on drying into one molecule of crocin (a coloured glycoside) (Fig. 33.1) and two molecules of picrocrocin (a colourless bitter glycoside). Crocin on hydrolysis yields gentiobiose and crocetin, while picrocrocin yields glucose and safranal. The latter substance is largely responsible for the characteristic odour and together with picrocrocin the taste of saffron. Other related crocins (crocin-2, -3 and -4) have been described. Five new monoterpenoids, crocusatins A–E, have been obtained from the pollen and a further five, crocusatins F–I, reported from the stigmas (C.-Y. Li and T.-S. Wu, *Chem. Pharm. Bull.*, 2002, **50**, 1305; *J. Nat. Prod.*, 2002, **65**, 1452). Crocusatin H and crocins 1 and 3 were shown to have significant tyrinase inhibitory activity. The same authors (*J. Nat. Prod.*, 2004, **67**, 437) have subsequently described further monoterpenoids, crocusatins J–L, a new naturally occurring acid and 31 known compounds from a methanolic extract of the petals of *C. sativa*. The essential oil from the stigmas and petals contains 34 or more components, mainly terpenes, terpene alcohols and esters.

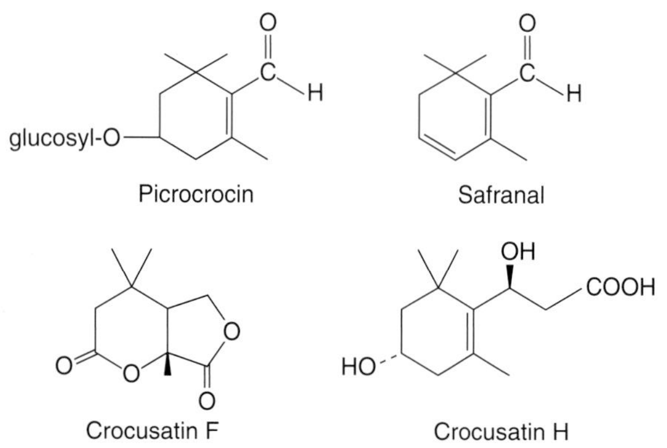

Fig. 33.2
Constituents of saffron (see Fig. 33.1 for formula of crocin).

By the culture of *C. sativus* stigmas on suitable media, stigma-like and style-like tissues which contain crocin, picrocrocin and other pigments have been obtained. Callus cultures at pH 7.0–7.6 with added uridine-diphospho-glucose are able to transform all-*trans*-crocetin into its related glycosides (D. Dufresne *et al.*, *Planta Medica*, 1997, **63**, 150). An antioxidant, 3,8-dihydroxy-1-methylanthraquinone-2-carboxylic, claimed to be superior to Vitamin E in its inhibition of oxidation of linoleic acid, has been isolated from callus stem tissue of saffron.

Although orthodox medicine has generally considered saffron to exert no appreciable therapeutic effects, recent work has demonstrated anticancer, antiarthritic, antihypertensive and other activities which probably arise from the powerful antioxidant properties of the constituents.

Saffron is used in Chinese medicine and in the West it is employed to a limited extent as a colouring and flavouring agent. In Cornwall, UK, it is used for making saffron cakes.

Annatto

Annatto seeds are those of *Bixa orellana* (Bixaceae) and are characterized by having on their surface an edible carotenoid pigment.

The plant is a shrub or small tree, native to northern South America and widely cultivated for the seeds or as an ornamental in the West Indies, tropical Asia and Africa; there are white- and pink-flowered varieties which can be propagated by seeds or cuttings. The estimated world annual production of seeds is 4000 tonnes; Ecuador, India, Kenya and Peru are the principal producers. Annatto usage as a colourant dye is lost in antiquity but with the advent of synthetic dyes at the beginning of the twentieth century its use declined dramatically. However, from the late 1950s, corresponding with the quest for safer food additives, its importance in the food industry has again steadily increased. The solubility of the dye in fixed oil, e.g. castor oil, makes it ideally suitable for use in the dairy industry.

Bixin, a C_{24}-apocarotenoid (Fig. 33.1), is the principal component of the dye and it normally constitutes about 2.5% (dry wt) of the seeds although varieties containing higher proportions are being developed in Ecuador. Isolated for the first time in 1875, it was not until 1961 that its structure was fully established; it belongs to a small group of compounds which also includes crocetin (see Saffron) and abscisic acid (q.v.). Removal of the methyl ester group of bixin yields the dicarboxylic acid norbixin (Fig. 33.1) which forms the basis of the water-soluble annatto dyes. Various semi-synthetic derivatives of bixin also find use as food colourants.

Due largely to the work of A. Z. Mercadante and colleagues (*Phytochemistry*, 1999, **52**, 135 and references cited therein) a considerable number of minor pigments of the seeds have now been characterized. These include C_{30} and C_{32} apocarotenoids; C_{19}, C_{22}, C_{24} and C_{25} diapocarotenoids, three of these being the first examples of geranylgeraniol serving as the esterifying alcohol with a carotenoid carboxylic acid; also isolated were a number of known C_{40} carotenes.

The castor-oil extract of the seeds contains, in addition to the pigments, a small amount of essential oil, the principal component of which is the sesquiterpene hydrocarbon ishwarane.

Chromatographic and spectrophotometric methods are available for the quality control of bixin.

Although used chiefly in the food industry, annatto and bixin have been employed in the production of coloured coating materials for tablets, pills, granules and herbal medicine preparations.

Marigold flowers

Tagetes erecta (Compositae), known commonly as the African marigold, is grown commercially in Mexico, Peru and Ecuador for extraction of xanthophyll pigments from the florets. There is an estimated world area of 7600 ha given over to cultivation; each plant produces on average about 330 mg of xanthophylls. With the exception of flavoxanthin [E161(a)] the xanthophylls have the same carbon skeletons as the carotenes, thus lutein (formerly known as xanthophyll) is 3, 3′-dihydroxy-α-carotene (Fig. 33.1). Lutein finds commercial use as an additive of chicken feed to give colour to egg yolks. The role of lutein in dietary supplements and its pharmacological properties have already been mentioned (Chapter 32).

Note: the common English garden marigold, not to be confused with the above, is *Calendula officinalis*, a well-established herbal remedy.

Red beetroot

Powdered red beetroot, *Beta vulgaris* (Chenopodiaceae), and the isolated red pigment betanin are widely used non-toxic food and pharmaceutical colourants. Betanin is a nitrogen-containing glycoside (Table 33.1) which on hydrolysis gives the aglycone betanidin and glucose. Hairy root cultures of the plant (*Agrobacterium* or *Rhizobium* spp. transformed) release red pigment to the culture medium, which is substantially the same as that contained within the hairy roots and in the original plant cells (M. Taya *et al.*, *J. Ferment Bioeng.*, 1992, **73**, 31).

Additional to its value as a colourant and food, various medicinal activities have been ascribed to red beetroot, including that of a free-radical scavenger; for a report on its potential hepatoprotective value, see M. Agarwal *et al.*, *Fitoterapia*, 2006, **77**, 91.

Monascus

Monascus purpureus is a mould which, when grown on cooked or autoclaved rice and then the whole dried and pulverized, gives a food colourant that has long been used in Chinese cooking. There is now interest in widening the use of this pigment. Strains of mould have been selected to give various shades and that producing the dark red monascorubrin (Fig. 33.1) is particularly important. Considerable work has been carried out on the production of various pigments from chemical and u.v.-mutant strains of the mould using continuous production methods rather than batch processing. With continuous fermentation it is important that the desired product is released to the medium. New chemically defined media have been described which give an increase in the OD_{500} measurements and a reversal of pigment location from predominantly cell-bound to extracellular. It is envisaged that the red pigment will serve as an edible, non-toxic substitute for expensive cochineal.

For recent work on the isolation of alanine or aspartate derivatives of monascorubrin and rubropunctatin see K. Sato *et al.*, *Chem. Pharm. Bull.*, 1997, **45**, 227.

Other species of *Monascus* also produce prigments and Korean workers have described strains of *M. anka*, developed by u.v.-mutation and natural selection, which produce enhanced levels of the pigment ankaflavin (Fig. 33.1). From the same species, a new series of pigments (monankarins A-F) having a conjugated pyrano-coumarin skeleton and exhibiting monoamine oxidase inhibitory activity has been isolated (C. F. Hossain *et al.*, *Chem. Pharm. Bull.*, 1996, **44**, 1535.

Red rose petals

The unexpanded petals of the Provence rose, *Rosa gallica*, were used for preparing the acid infusions of rose of the *BPC* 1949. The drug is mildly astringent and for this reason, and also for the colouring principles, the infusions served as a convenient vehicle for gargles containing alum or tannin. The anthocyanine constituents made the petal extracts unsuitable for prescribing with alkaline salts.

DYESTUFFS

Natural products were at one time of prime importance to the dyeing industry and remain so today in some native societies. Three well-known examples with pharmaceutical links are alkanna, henna and madder. Alkanna and henna contain naphthoquinone derivatives and are described in more detail in Chapter 21. Madder, the root of *Rubia tinctorum* (Rubiaceae) formerly grown in large quantity in the area of Avignon contains anthraquinone derivatives including ruberythric acid (Fig. 33.1). On hydrolysis the latter yields primeverose and alizarin, the pigment responsible for Turkey Red colour. Towards the end of the nineteenth century the use of the natural product was superseded by synthetic material.

For an interesting article on the production of woad, one of the most ancient of dyes known to man, see P. John, 'Further reading,' below.

Further reading

Evans WC 2000 Annatto: a natural choice. Biologist 47(4): 181–184
John P 2006 Indigo reduction in the woad vat: a medieval biotechnology revealed. Biologist 53(1): 31–35
Lauro GL, Francis FJ (eds) 2000 Natural food colorants. Vol 14 of a Basic Symposium Series of the Institute of Food Technologists, Chicago. Marcel Dekker, New York. *This volume includes articles on the following: Carmine, pp 1–9 (J Schul), The betalains, pp 11–30 (JH von Elbe, IL Goldman), Monascus pp 31–85 (RE Mudgett), Paprika pp 97–113 (CL Locey, JA Guzinski), Annatto pp 115–152 (LW Levy, DM Rivadeneira), Lycopene pp 153–192 (ML Nguyen, SJ Schwartz), Turmeric pp 205–226 (R Buescher, L Yang), Chlorophylls pp 227–236 (GAF Hendry), Anthocyanins pp 237–252 (RE Wrolstad), Color measurement pp 273–287 (K Loughrey), Health aspects pp 288–314 (G Mazza), Regulations in Europe and Japan pp 314–327 (BS Henry)*
Negbi M (ed) Hardman R (series ed) 2000 Medicinal and aromatic plants—industrial profiles. Vol. 8. Saffron: *Corcus sativus* L. Harwood Academic, Amsterdam

FLAVOURING AGENTS

Natural flavours are often complex mixtures of compounds such as are found in essential oils and may contain over 100 components, all blending to give a characteristic flavour. Alternatively, a flavouring agent may contain a single compound only, such as vanillin. The design of regulations for flavours for the food industry is obviously a complex task and the EU is currently considering this. Flavours used in medicaments are at present covered by the Medicines Act.

Although food and medicinal flavourings have aspects in common their role in a medicine is different to that in a food. In the former case they are used to disguise an unpleasant taste resulting from the active constituents of the medicine rather than, as in the latter case, to make more attractive an already palatable material. It is questionable whether medicines should be formulated to make them so pleasant to the taste that they are no longer distinguishable as such. Helliwell and Jones discussed this aspect (*Pharm. J.*, 1994, **253**, 181) in an article 'How good should a medicine taste?' mentioning conceptual pharmaceuticals in which a postprandial OTC medicine could be formulated as a liqueur so that the particular brand would become associated with a pleasant after-meal experience.

Certain natural flavours traditionally have been formulated as syrups for addition to the active medicament, a practice now somewhat discouraged on dental health grounds. A number have, in addition to flavour, some medicinal properties. The following, for example, are also, together with their oils, carminatives: citrus peels, ginger, peppermint leaf, fennel fruits, dill fruits, coriander fruits, caraway fruits, cardamom, nutmeg and cinnamon. Liquorice extract is used to disguise the taste of nauseous medicines and Wild Cherry Syrup *BPC* 1988, although employed in cough preparations, is primarily used for flavouring. Raspberry and blackcurrant syrups have no therapeutic value although the juice of the latter is used for its vitamin C content. Similarly saffron (q.v. above) and oil of rose (used to flavour lozenges) have no medicinal effect.

Sweetening agents

There is a need for alternatives to sucrose as a sweetening agent for medical purposes (e.g. for diabetics) and for diet improvement. Although saccharin is the most widely used substitute two natural products are also noteworthy.

Sorbitol. Sorbitol (D-glucitol), *USP/NF* 1995, is a polyhedric alcohol which was first isolated from mountain ash berries (*Sorbus aucuparia*, Rosaceae) and is now known to occur in other members of the family and widely throughout the plant kingdom. It is prepared synthetically by the catalytic hydrogenation of glucose. Sorbitol solution (Sorbitol Liquid) *BPC* 1988 contains 70% of mainly sorbitol and is used as a sweetening agent and vehicle in elixirs, linctuses and mixtures; it has about half the sweetening power of syrup.

Stevioside. A group of ent-kaurane glycosides, derivatives of steviol, have sweetening properties some three hundred times that of sucrose.

Stevioside, the most important, is obtained from *Stevia rebaudiana* (Compositae) a plant native to N.E. Paraguay. Although first isolated in 1931 its structure was not elucidated until 1963 and then some 10 years later it was produced commercially in Japan. New non-glycosidic labdane diterpenoids (sterebins) continued to be isolated (B. D. McGarvey *et al.*, *J. Nat. Prod.*, 2003, **66,** 1395). Now, some 700–1000 tons of plant material are processed annually by Japan, Brazil and other countries. The product is used in the soft drinks and food industries. For a report on the pharmacological and physiological effects of *S. rebaudiana* on animals and humans see M. S. Melis, *J. Ethnopharm.*, 1999, **67,** 157.

Steviol R¹ = R² = H
Stevioside R¹ = Glucose–glucose, R² = Glucose

34

Miscellaneous products

There are a few miscellaneous pharmaceutical materials of natural origin which are not included in the preceding chapters; these are considered below.

KIESELGUHR OR DIATOMITE

Large deposits of diatomite are found in Aberdeenshire in the UK, Virginia and California in the USA, Germany and North Africa. The crude product contains about 65–87% of SiO_2, together with organic matter, clay, iron oxide and about 5–15% of water. The silica is mainly amorphous, being present in the siliceous walls of minute, unicellular plants belonging to a number of families of the Bacillariophyceae. A much smaller percentage of silica occurs in the walls of spicules of siliceous sponges and, in a crystalline form, as sand. Depending on the geographical origin of the diatomite, the diatoms may be either freshwater or marine forms.

The material is dried and crushed, ignited to remove organic matter, boiled with dilute hydrochloric acid to remove impurities such as iron, washed with water and dried. It is then sifted or 'air-blown', the finest grades used in face powders being obtained by the latter method.

Characters. Purified kieselguhr is a fine, white or pale-buff odourless powder. For microscopical examination it may be mounted in cresol or olive oil. In the latter medium the amorphous silica of the diatoms becomes almost invisible, while the crystalline particles of sand remain clear. Only small amounts of sand (Fig. 34.1H) should be present.

The diatoms (Fig. 34.1) consist of two halves or *valves* which fit together like a pill-box. The two positions from which they may be studied are known as the valve-view and the girdle-view. The valves show considerable variation in shape, some samples of kieselguhr showing numerous discoid types resembling that of the *Arachnoidiscus* found in agar, while other samples consist largely of pennate forms. A mixture of both types is usually most suitable for filtration. In many diatoms a median cleft is found in the valves, known as the *raphe*. The valves also show dots and lines, which vary in the different species and are due to minute cavities in the wall.

Kieselguhr is insoluble in all acids except hydrofluoric, but is soluble after fusion with alkalis. It is used for the filtration of oils, fats, syrups, etc., and in the form of the Berkefeld filter for sterilization. Highly purified material is used as an inactive support in column, gas and thin-layer chromatography; the powder will hold up to its own weight of water and still retain its powdery consistency. Diatomite is also employed in face powders, pills, polishing powders and soaps, and to absorb nitroglycerin in the manufacture of dynamite; it is a component of the *BP* (*Vet*) pyrethrum dusting powder.

Extant species of diatoms form an important component of plankton and are involved in the food chains of seas and rivers. (For a wide-ranging illustrated introduction to these single-celled plants see *The Diatoms; Biology and Morphology of the Genera* by F. E. Round *et al.* (1990), Cambridge University Press.)

PREPARED CHALK

Chalk is a whitish or greyish rock which is widely distributed in north-western Europe. It consists mainly of the shells of unicellular animals known as the Foraminifera. Chalk as quarried often contains about 97 or 98% of calcium carbonate, the remainder being largely siliceous and therefore insoluble in acids. The impure chalk is finely ground with water and freed from most of the heavier siliceous impurities by elutriation. The coarser product is sold as 'whiting' and the finer elutriated product is allowed to settle and while still pasty is poured into a funnel-shaped trochiscator. The latter is tapped on a porous chalk slab

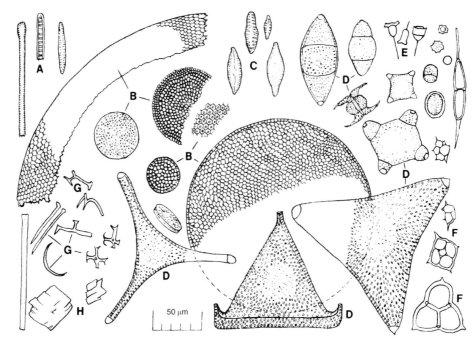

Fig. 34.1
Diatomite (various sources) showing the shells of diatoms and other constituents. A, Diatom skeletons of the Fragilariaceae (e.g. *Synedra*, *Fragilaria*); B, entire or broken portions of *Coscinodiscus* spp.; C, shells of the Naviculaceae (e.g. *Navicula*); D, various forms belonging to the Biddulphioideae (*Biddulphia, Trinacria*, etc.); E, fragments of *Asterionella* spp.?; F, silicoflagellates; G, sponge spicules; H, sand particles.

and ejects the chalk to form 'cones', which are allowed to dry giving Prepared Chalk *BP*. These cones ('crab's eyes') may be powdered.

Characters. For examination chalk should be mounted in cresol, warmed and examined microscopically (Fig. 34.2). Most of the foraminiferous shells have been broken but a number of whole ones usually remain. The whole shells may be concentrated in a small bulk by removing the broken ones by elutriation and examining the residue. Note the following:

Globigerina. In these the shell is of calcite and is perforated by large canals. Each consists of a few lobular chambers arranged in a plane or helicoid spiral. The size varies from about 35 to 80 μm.

Textularia. In these the shell is composed of grains of sand cemented together by calcareous matter. They are usually conical or cuneiform in shape and are composed of numerous chambers in two alternating parallel series. The size varies from about 50 to 180 μm.

Remains of fossil algae. Small rings or discs about 4–9 μm in diameter, termed coccoliths or morpholites.

Prepared chalk is assayed by acid–alkali back-titration; there are pharmacopoeial limits for heavy metals and arsenic; limits for aluminium, iron, phosphate and matter insoluble in hydrochloride acid are determined gravimetrically.

Precipitated chalk. Precipitated chalk (calcium carbonate *BP/EP* is made by the interaction of a soluble calcium salt and a soluble

carbonate. The precipitate varies considerably with the method of preparation. When precipitated at about 0°C, the product is very light and almost entirely amorphous; at about 30°C a denser precipitate of minute rhombohedra is formed, and if boiling solutions are used, the precipitate consists of prismatic rhombohedra with a higher specific gravity than either of the previous forms. The *BP* assay involves a complexometric titration of calcium; there are limits for various metals, etc.

Uses. Chalk is used as an absorbent and antacid.

GELATIN

Gelatin is a mixture of reversible gel-forming proteins derived from certain animal tissues, particularly skin and bones, with hot water. The process converts insoluble collagens into soluble gelatin, the solution of which is then purified and concentrated to a solid form.

The initial stages of the preparation vary with the starting material, bones, for example, being defatted with an organic solvent and sometimes decalcified by treatment with acid. Two types of gelatin are characterized in the *BP/EP*—type A is obtained by partial acid hydrolysis of animal collagen and type B by partial alkaline hydrolysis; mixtures of both types are also permitted.

Characters. Sheet gelatin prepared as above may be cut into strips or made into a granular powder. Gelatin is colourless or pale yellow, is

Fig. 34.2
Shells from prepared chalk. Globigerina in (A) water, (B) cresol (×200). C, *Textularia* in cresol (×200). D, coccoliths (×400).

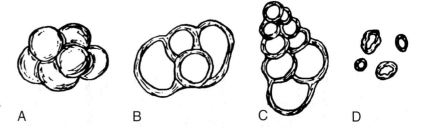

translucent and has little odour or taste. It is insoluble in cold water but absorbs a considerable volume of liquid; it dissolves on heating and a 2% solution forms a jelly on cooling. The gelatinizing power of gelatin is reduced by long boiling. The quality of gelatin is largely judged by its 'jelly strength' or 'Bloom strength' which is determined by a Bloom gelometer. The two types of gelatin (A and B) have isoelectric points in the ranges pH 6.0–9.5 (A) and pH 4.7–5.6 (B). Type B is compatible with anionic substances (e.g. the natural gums), whereas type A is not; for some specific purposes, narrower tolerance limits than above may be required. Note the *BP/EP* limit tests and standards.

Constituents. Gelatin consists mainly of the protein glutin and therefore gives the usual tests for proteins. Thus, it evolves ammonia when heated with soda lime (distinction from agar); with mercuric nitrate solution gives a white precipitate that turns brick-red on warming; it gives a precipitate with a solution of trinitrophenol.

Uses. Gelatin is used in the preparation of pastilles, pastes, suppositories, pessaries, capsules, pill-coatings and gelatin sponge. Specially purified and pyrogen-free gelatins are available for intravenous injection, and a grade with high 'Bloom strength' is used for making gelatin capsules and for bacteriological culture media.

Gelatin sponge

Gelatin sponge can be conveniently mentioned here as an absorbable, water-insoluble haemostatic material. It may be prepared by whisking a warm solution of gelatin to a foam of uniform porosity and drying. After cutting into pieces it is sterilized by dry heat. Note the *BP* standards for this material. It is used in a similar manner to oxidized cellulose.

FISH BODY OILS

The oils expressed from the bodies of a number of 'oily' fish of the families cited on p. 43 contain esters of omega-3 fatty acids. As such, they have become important dietary supplements and two such oils are included in the *BP/EP*. For an explanation of the structural representation of the various acids, as cited below, see Chapter 19, 'Fatty Acids'.

Fish oil, rich in omega-3-acids. The expressed oil is processed in much the same way as for cod-liver oil (q.v.) and involves winterization and deodorization. The esterifying ω-3 acids, as exemplified in the pharmacopoeia, are: α-linolenic acid (C18:3 n-3), moroctic acid (C18:4 n-3), eicosatetraenoic acid (C20:4 n-3), timnodonic (eicosapentaenoic) acid (C20:5 n-3; EPA), heneicosapentaenoic acid (C21:5 n-3), clupanodonic acid (C22:5 n-3) and cervonic (docosahexaenoic) acid (C22:6 n-3; DHA).

It will be noted that up to six double bonds may be involved in these acids; all are ω-3-acids and the positions of the remaining double bonds occur in sequence, separated by one methylene group (see α-linolenic acid, Table 19.3).

The total omega-3-acids, expressed as triglycerides, should be ≮28.0%; that of EPA ≮13.0% and DHA ≮9.0%. Oligomers, determined by size exclusion chromatography (p. 143), should not exceed 1.5%. The maximum permitted anisidine value (p. 180) is 30.0. An antioxidant may be added to the oil.

Farmed Salmon Oil *BP/EP* is obtained from salmon, *Salmo salar*, family Salmonidae, which have been fed in accordance with EU or other applicable regulations. The oil is expressed mechanically at below 100°C either from whole fish or fish from which the fillets have been removed; it is centrifuged and winterized. The pale pink oil

contains the important polyunsaturated acids DHA, EPA and moroctic acid (see above); the two former constitute 10.0–28.0% of the oil, expressed as triglycerides. Chromatography is used to identify the acid components and ^{13}C-NMR for their further evaluation. The anisidine value is maximized at 10.0, considerably less than for the Fish Oil described above; similarly with the peroxide value. These figures indicate the extent of secondary oxidation of the oils.

Preparations derived from fish body oils. The following modifications of fish body oils are included in the pharmacopoeia.

Omega-3-marine triglyceride contains a mixture of the glyceryl esters prepared from the purified concentrated acids or from the omega-3-acid ethyl esters. It contains a minimum 60.0% of total omega-3 acids expressed as triglycerides and a minimum 45% of EPA and DHA, also expressed as triglycerides. The maximum permitted peroxide value is 10.0 and that for the anisidine value 30.0.

Omega-3-acid ethyl esters 60 and *omega-3-acid ethyl esters 90* contain higher minimum concentrations of EPA and DHA than the above, as indicated in their names. They are prepared by transesterification of the body oil of 'oily' fishes with subsequent purification, fractionation and molecular distillation.

These preparations are used to treat such conditions as hypertriglyceridaemia, to reduce the risk of CHD, thrombosis and for other disorders, still under evaluation.

SILK

Silk is the prepared fibre from the cocoons of *Bombyx mori*, the mulberry silkworm, and other species of *Bombyx* and of *Antheraea* (order Lepidoptera). It is produced in China, Japan, India, Asia Minor, Italy, France and many other countries. While the silk of *B. mori* forms the greater part of that used, considerable quantities of the so-called wild silks are produced by *Antheraea mylitta* (India), *A. assama* (India), *A. pernyi* (China) and *A. yama-mai* (Japan).

Before the silkworm passes from the caterpillar to the chrysalis or pupal stage, it secretes around itself an oval cocoon about 2–5 cm long, consisting of a continuous thread up to 1200 m long. This thread consists of two silk or *fibroin* fibres cemented together by a layer of silk glue or *sericin*. Strands of semiliquid fibroin, produced by two glands in the insect, flow into a common exit-tube in the head, where they meet the secretion of silk glue produced by another pair of glands. The double fibre with its coating of sericin emerges from a spinneret in the head of the worm, coagulates and hardens on contact with the air and is spun into the cocoon by figure-of-eight movements of the head. If the chrysalis were allowed to mature, the silk would be damaged by the escaping insect. It is therefore killed by heating at 60–80°C for a few hours or by a short exposure to steam. The cocoons are then graded, placed in hot water and beaten to facilitate removal of the outer layer of fibre, which is only of secondary value, and to soften the silk glue.

The double fibre in the cocoon is known as a *bave* and its constituent fibres are known as *brins*. The reeler takes the loose ends of the fibres of 2–15 cocoons and twists and reels them into a single thread. Most raw silk is reeled from about five cocoons and therefore has 10 brins, fibres containing less than six brins being too fine for commercial purposes. Silk is then usually scoured by treatment with hot soap solution to remove the sericin.

Microscopy. Examine some fibres of raw silk mounted in water. The diameter of these is several times that of a single brin; the individual brins may be seen although difficult to count; and flakes of silk glue may be seen on the surface. If a little of this raw silk is now boiled

34

with soap solution or dilute sodium carbonate solution, the sericin completely dissolves and the constituent brins may be mounted and examined.

The lack of cellular structure and the breadth of the brins are distinguishing characters of mulberry silk. Brins of mulberry silk measure 10–21 μm (mostly about 16 μm), whereas those of wild silks are 30–60 μm. The latter often show well-marked longitudinal striations.

Silk gives the general tests for animal fibres, and the following:

1. Silk is soluble in ammoniacal copper oxide solution. An alkaline solution of copper sulphate and glycerol of a certain strength is used for the separation of silk from wool and cotton.
2. Silk contains little or no sulphur and therefore gives no black precipitate with alkali and lead acetate solution (distinction from wool).
3. Silk rapidly dissolves in concentrated hydrochloric acid (distinction from wool).

Chemical nature.   Natural silk is composed of the protein fibroin. Fibroin on hydrolysis gives mainly glycine (44%) and alanine (27%) together with smaller amounts of serine (11%), tyrosine (5%) and other amino acids. The molecule is a chain-like structure, with a repeating unit 0.7 nm long. This repeating unit, as revealed by radiograph analysis, corresponds in length to that of two fully extended amino acid residues.

Surgically, silk is used as a non-absorbable suture and as such must comply with the *BP* requirements for such materials. (For a general article on silk see M. L. Ryder, *Biologist*, 1995, **42**, 52.)

WOOL, ANIMAL WOOL, SHEEP'S WOOL

Wool is prepared from the fleece of the sheep, *Ovis aries* (order Ungulata), by cleansing and washing. The length and quality of the hair varies not only from animal to animal, but also in different parts of the same fleece. In order to get more or less uniform grades, the wool-sorter spreads each fleece on a frame covered with wire-netting and separates it into wool of different qualities. At the same time he beats much dust and dirt through the netting and picks out burrs, etc. The wool is washed in tanks of warm, soft, soapy water, being squeezed between rollers as it passes from tank to tank.

The approximate composition of raw wool is as follows: wool fibre, 31%; 'wool sweat' or 'suint', consisting mainly of the potassium salts of fatty acids, 32%; earthy matter removable by washing, 26%; and 'wool grease'.

From the washings of the scouring process 'wool grease' may be separated by mechanical means or by the use of organic solvents. When purified it is known as wool fat or anhydrous lanolin (q.v.). Potassium salts may also be recovered. After washing, the wool is dried, and the fibres are mechanically loosened, carded, and spun into yarn.

Microscopical.   The hairs originate in relatively deep pits or hair follicles in the skin and the 'wool grease' is secreted by neighbouring sebaceous glands. If fibres of raw wool are examined under the microscope, they are seen to be covered with irregular masses of grease, the structure of the hair itself being indistinct. If raw wool is to be mounted for microscopical examination, it should be defatted by ether or chloroform, as it will not otherwise wet with water; even with scoured wool, it is advisable to moisten the threads with alcohol before mounting in water, dilute glycerin or solution of picric acid.

Wool hairs are 2–50 cm long and 5–100 μm, usually 13–40 μm, diameter. As the fleeces are removed by shearing, the bases of the hairs are lacking, and tapering ends, known as 'lamb ends' are only found in wool from the first shearing. Three regions of the hair, known as the cuticle, cortex and medulla, are distinguishable.

Cuticle.   This consists of imbricated, flattened, more or less translucent epithelial scales. The shape and arrangement of the scales varies in different breeds of sheep, edges being smooth and straight in some and serrated and wavy in others. The number of scales in a 100 μm length is fairly constant, averaging about 9.7–12.1, in different wools. Such counts may be used to distinguish sheep's wool from angora wool, etc.

Cortex.   The cortex consists of elongated, fusiform cells coalesced into a horny mass in which scattered pigment cells are sometimes found.

Medulla.   The medulla consists of rounded or polyhedral cells containing fatty matter or pigment and is best seen when its cells contain much air or pigment. (For an article on wool describing, among other things, the different fibres found in fleece see M. L. Ryder, *Biologist*, 1994, **41**, 195.)

Tests
1. *Characteristic of animal fibres.* Wool resembles silk in its behaviour with Molisch's test, picric acid, nitric acid and Millon's reagent. It is readily soluble in 5% potash.
2. *Characteristic of wool.*
   (1) Ammoniacal copper oxide solution resembles solution of ammonia in that it causes separation of the scales; it also colours the fibres blue.
   (2) When lead acetate is added to a solution of wool in caustic soda, a black precipitate is formed owing to the high sulphur content (distinction from silk).
   (3) Wool is not appreciably soluble in warm hydrochloric acid (distinction from silk), or in cold concentrated sulphuric acid (distinction from cotton).

Chemical nature of wool.   Wool fibres are composed of the protein keratin. They show elasticity, in contrast to the cellulose and silk fibres. X-ray examination of stretched and unstretched fibre shows that the elasticity arises from a reversible intramolecular transformation of the fibre substance. The radiograph of the stretched fibre closely resembles that given by fibres, such as silk, with fully extended polypeptide chains. In this condition each amino acid residue is 0.34 nm long. This unstable form of keratin is known as β-keratin. The stable form, α-keratin is contracted and the structural unit, corresponding to three amino acid residues, is 0.51 nm long. The chemical relationship between these two forms and its importance in conferring elasticity properties on wool fibres is illustrated in former editions of this work.

Leech

The medicinal leech, *Hirudo medicinalis*, is about 6–10 cm long. The sucker at the anterior end has three radiating jaws provided with 'teeth'. Placed in contact with the skin, the animal produces a triradiate cut and can draw about 4–8 ml of blood. The salivary glands secrete hirudin, an acidic polypeptide of molecular weight around 7000; it retards coagulation of blood and allows bleeding to continue after the leech has been removed. Preparations containing hirudin for the treatment of bruises are manufactured commercially. Other enzymes isolated from the leech include hementin, an antithrombin agent, and orgelase, which degrades hyaluronic acid.

Some 12 000 kg of leeches are used annually in Europe and are exported from France, Italy, Portugal and Central Europe. The animal, classed as a threatened species, is officially protected in some countries including Britain. Future supplies of leech products may need to be met by commercial farms (one currently operates in S. Wales) and by genetically engineered organisms. The cloning and expression of a recombinant gene for hirudin in yeast and bacteria has been reported (1988).

Although used less than formerly, leeches are often the least painful way to reduce inflammation. They have also staged a medical revival by their use in skin grafting for the removal of coagulated blood from beneath the new skin. Unfortunately, the leech is host to *Aeromanas hydrophila*, an organism on which it depends to digest the blood consumed. This is a potential source of infection of wounds and, according to a report in the *British Medical Journal* (11 April 1987), three types of infection, including diarrhoea, have been reported in patients receiving leech treatment. However, the problem can be eliminated by the use of suitable antibiotics.

(For a general review article (20 refs) on the medicinal leech see J. M. Elliot and P. A. Tullett, *Biologist*, 1992, **39**, 153.)

SHELLAC (LAC)

Shellac (lac) is a resinous substance prepared from a secretion that encrusts the bodies of a scale insect *Karria lacca* (*Lucifer lacca*), order Hemiptera. Lac is produced in India, Thailand and to a lesser extent in China (5% of world production). In India the chief plants are members of the Leguminosae (*Acacia* spp., *Butea frondosa*), Euphorbiaceae (*Aleurites laccifera*), Moraceae (*Ficus* spp.), Dipterocarpaceae (*Cajanus indivus, Shorea talura*), Rhamnaceae (*Ziziphus jujuba*) and Sapindaceae (*Schleichera trijuga*). In China the host trees are mainly species of *Ficus* and *Dalbergia* (Leguminosae) (C. Saint-Pierre and O. Binrong, *Econ. Bot.*, 1994, **48**, 21). The insects resemble cochineal insects in structure and life history.

Lac is found most abundantly on the smaller branches and twigs. These are broken off and constitute *stick lac*. Usually, however, the lac is not exported in this form but is scraped from the twigs by means of curved knives. The lac is usually ground in India and the colouring matter extracted with water or dilute soda solution. The solution evaporated to dryness constitutes *lac dye*, and the exhausted lac when dried *seed lac*. From the latter the four types of shellac recognized in the EP/BP are prepared (Table 34.1). Other commercial grades are also utilized. *Button lac* is the molten lac poured into circular moulds and stamped with the maker's name. Flake shellac having a brownish-yellow colour is known in commerce as orange shellac and the darker, reddish-brown varieties are known as ruby or garnet shellac. A number of varieties, required to conform to a table for acid value, loss on drying and wax content, are including in the *USP/NF* 1995. Lac contains about 6% of wax, 6.5% of red water-soluble colouring matter, laccaic acid, 70–85% of resin and a few insect remains, vegetable debris, etc. The resin, composed of two parts, a hard and a soft fraction, is formed from hydroxy fatty acids and sesquiterpenes. An example of the former is aleuritic acid (9,10,16-trihydroxypalmitic acid) and of the latter, a cedrene-type sesquiterpene acid; a water-insoluble yellow pigment is erythrolaccin, a tetrahydroxy-4-methylanthraquinone. The *BP/EP* includes tests for colophony (TLC), arsenic, heavy metals, etc. Shellac is classified as a pharmaceutical aid and is also used in varnishes, polishes, sealing wax, etc.

Isinglass
Russian isinglass or ichthyocolla consists of the dried prepared swimming bladder of the sturgeon, *Acipenser huso*. The fish are caught in South Russian rivers and in the Black and Caspian seas. Isinglass consists chiefly of collagen and resembles gelatin in its properties. Brazilian isinglass is a similar product but derived from fish of different genera.

Ambergris
This very expensive substance used in perfumery is a pathological product found in the intestines of sperm whales or cast by them into the sea. It occurs in streaky grey or brown waxy masses which, exceptionally, may weigh up to 45 kg. It is associated with the beaks of squids on which the whales feed. Ambergris contains about 25% of ambrein. It has a fragrant musk-like odour but its main value lies in the fact that it has a subtle effect on fine perfumes and gives them great tenacity or persistence of odour.

Musk
Musk is the dried secretion from the preputial follicles of the musk deer, *Moschus moschiferus*. This small deer is found in China and

Table 34.1 Pharmacopoeial types of shellac.

Type	Preparation	Characters
Wax-containing shellac	From molten seedlac by filtration through bags or by hot solvent extraction. When sufficiently cool the product is stretched into a large sheet and then broken into flakes	Flakes, brownish-orange or yellow. Almost insoluble in water and partly soluble in ether. With alcohol it gives an opalescent solution
Bleached shellac	Seedlac is dissolved in hot soda solution, bleached with hypochlorite or chlorine and precipitated by acid. It is 'pulled' under water into sticks and dried	A cream to brownish-yellow powder. An opalescent solution is given with alcohol
Dewaxed shellac	From seedlac or wax-containing shellac by treatment with a suitable solvent and removal of the wax by filtration	Flakes as wax-containing shellac. With alcohol it gives a clear solution
Bleached dewaxed shellac	Seedlac or wax-containing shellac is treated with hot soda solution and bleached with hypochlorite; the insoluble wax is removed by filtration, the product precipitated from solution with dilute acid, and dried	Appearance as bleached shellac. With alcohol it gives a clear solution

34

the Himalayas. The musk-containing sacs are known as 'pods'. They are about 5–7 cm diameter, weigh up to 30 g and contain about half their weight of musk. When distilled, musk yields about 1.4% of dark brown volatile oil, the chief odorous constituent of which is muskone. This is a cyclic ketone having a closed chain of 15 carbon atoms. Other constituents of musk are steroidal hormones, muscopyridine and other alkaloids and peptides. A synthetic compound, which differs from muskone only in the absence of a methyl group, is cyclopentadecanone. Most other synthetic musk substitutes have little chemical similarity to the natural product. Musk acts as a fixative and is an important ingredient of many high-class perfumes.

Civet

This product, which resembles musk, is obtained from the perineal follicles of African or Indian civet cats, *Viverra* spp. It contains civetone, a cyclic ketone closely related to muskone but having a closed chain of 17 carbon atoms.

Royal jelly/Queen bee jelly

This hive product of Chinese origin consists of the milky fluid produced by the salivary glands of worker bees and used as essential nourishment for the development of the queen bee larvae. It contains a mixture of amino acids, vitamins (including most of the vitamin B complex and vitamin C), lipids, fatty acids, carbohydrates and minerals. The fresh material is unstable and requires refrigeration. It may also be freeze-dried but more satisfactory preparations are stated to be capsules containing royal jelly stabilized by the addition of honey. Royal jelly is an expensive dietary supplement recommended in health magazines for counteracting the effects of ageing and for the treatment of myalgic encephalomyelitis, depression, dermatitis and other conditions. Its value, which has yet to be clinically proved, may arise from the biologically favourable relative proportions of the many constituents rather than from their quantity.

6 Plants in complementary and traditional systems of medicine

Introduction

The previous chapters have been concerned mainly with those plant drugs that are associated with allopathic medicine, but there are other systems of great significance which also employ plants in the treatment of disease. A number of these, including herbal medicine, homoeopathy, aromatherapy and Bach remedies, are widely practised in the West and are discussed below. A consensus of other alternative systems of medicine which do not involve plants may be obtained from the many publications now available. An indication of the changing conventional attitude towards alternative (complementary) medicine was the establishment in 1987 of a Centre of Complementary Health Studies at the University of Exeter, UK and a Chair in the discipline in 1993. This was the first of its kind in this country and was followed by the introduction of degree courses involving complementary medicine at other universities.

Concerning patients, despite the advances made in orthodox medicine there has been an increasing interest in the complementary systems, particularly by those who have not benefited from previous treatment, by those who have apprehensions concerning the toxicity and safety of modern drugs, and by those who benefit from the holistic approach (rarely achievable in a 5–10 min consultation with a GP). The availability of such treatments under the British NHS, provided referral is made by the patient's general practitioner, has given added status to these treatments and some, such as aromatherapy, are now provided as a hospital service.

In addition to the above there are the traditional systems of medicine widely practised outside Europe. Of these the Asian (Ayurvedic and Unani) and Chinese are two of the most significant, each having a long recorded history. Often disciplines have interacted; thus, traditional Tibetan medicine has been receptive to Ayurvedic, Chinese and Arabian influences and the Japanese is an offshoot of the Chinese (see Chapter 37). In large Asian immigrant populations such as there are in Britain, the Asian and Western types of medicine may have to coexist, sometimes with unforeseeable results.

About 80% of the world's population relies on herbal medicines, and governments of Third World countries, unable to sustain a complete coverage with Western-type drugs, have encouraged the rational development of traditional treatments. At present the World Health Organization is taking an official interest in such developments in order to facilitate its aim of making health care available for all. UNIDO also supports the industrial utilization of medicinal plants which are a source of export earnings for the producers.

Modern research establishments now exist in many countries, e.g. India, Pakistan, Saudi Arabia, China, Japan, South America, etc. and their work is largely devoted to assessing the value of thousands of ethnic remedies along lines acceptable to current medical thinking. Thus the pharmacological effectiveness of many herbal treatments has been vindicated, but unfortunately the side-effects produced are often untenable by modern standards. In some successful instances the drugs have been adopted outside their countries of origin. Another feature is that those plants which have been selected for medicinal use over thousands of years constitute the most obvious choice for examination in the current search for new therapeutically effective drugs.

Except for the well-documented Asian and Chinese drugs it is often a difficult problem to investigate traditional remedies, and researchers in the field need to be skilled in the language, customs, prejudices, etc. of the people and practitioners with whom they are dealing. As religious practices and rituals are often associated with the healing treatment, a multidisciplinary approach is necessary. Abebe (*J. Ethnopharm.*, 1992, **36**, 93) pointed out that researchers all too often report on the alleged therapeutic indications of traditional medicines without recording those adverse effects of which the traditional healers are well aware.

Selection, at this stage, of the crucial botanicals for study is of fundamental importance to the ultimate success of the subsequent lengthy scientific investigation.

For a consideration of the interdisciplinary methods used to record and collect ethnopharmacological field data see F. J. Lipp, *J. Ethnopharm.*, 1989, **25**, 139.

Notices of the numerous symposia and conferences on medicinal plants world-wide are published in the *Newsletter of the International Council for Medicinal and Aromatic Plants* and some journals.

The *Journal of Ethnopharmacology, Fitoterapia*, and *Pharmaceutical Biology* (formerly *International Journal of Pharmacognosy*) have proved particularly valuable for the publication of interdisciplinary research and reviews devoted to indigenous drugs. Many of the reviews cover relatively small regional areas; the following selection of books involve wider geographical regions:

Further reading

Ambasta SP (ed) 1986 Useful plants of India. Publications and Information Directorate, CSIR, New Delhi, India

Appleby JH 1987 A selective index to Siberian, Far Eastern, and Central Asian Russian materia medica. Wellcome Unit for the History of Medicine, Oxford, UK

Duke JA, Ayensu ES 1985 Medicinal plants of China (2 vols). Alegonac Reference Publications Inc, MI, USA

Duke JA, Vasquez R 1994 Amazonian ethnobotanical dictionary. CRC Press, Boca Raton, FL

Ghani A 1998 Medicinal plants of Bangladesh. Asiatic Society of Bangladesh, Dhaka

Hu S-Y, Kong YC, But PPH 1980 An enumeration of Chinese materia medica. Chinese University Press, Hong Kong

Morton JF 1981 Atlas of medicinal plants of Middle America. Chas. C. Thomas, Springfield, IL, USA

Mossa JS, Al-Yahya MA, Al-Meshal IA 1987, 2000 Medicinal plants of Saudi Arabia. King Saud University Libraries, Riyadh, Saudi Arabia, Vols I, II

Oliver-Bever B 1986 Medicinal plants in tropical West Africa. Cambridge University Press, Cambridge, UK

Perry LM 1980 Medicinal plants of East and Southeast Asia. MIT Press, Cambridge, MA, USA

Riley M 1994 Maori healing and herbal. Viking Sevenseas, Paraparaumu, NZ

Sofowora A 1982 Medicinal plants and traditional medicine in Africa. J Wiley & Sons Ltd, Chichester

Van Wyk B-E, Van Oudtshoorn B, Gericke N 1998 Medicinal plants of South Africa. Briza Publications, Pretoria

Watt JM, Breyer-Brandwijk MG 1962 The medicinal and poisonous plants of Southern and Eastern Africa. Churchill Livingstone, London, UK

The wealth of India, raw materials (20 vols). Publications and Information Directorate, CSIR, New Delhi. *A second edition is in the course of publication in stages*

35

Herbal medicine in Britain and Europe: regulation and practice

S. Y. Mills

REGULATORY BACKGROUND

The supply of herbs as healthcare products in Europe is more tightly regulated than other commodities. It is also notoriously complex, covering over-the-counter sales through various outlets, as well provision of 'phytomedicines' by health professionals (i.e. doctors and pharmacists in most of Europe and herbal practitioners in the UK and Ireland). The vague and less regulated 'borderline' area within which many natural products have been supplied direct to the consumer is becoming much more constrained and is intended to disappear altogether after 2010. Essentially, in the case of the direct sale of herbs, there are two regulatory options: food supplements or medicinal products.

Herbal products used for therapeutic purposes are classified as medicines by default under European law. If the UK Medicines and Healthcare products Regulatory Agency (MHRA) determines that a herbal product is a medicinal product then it is a criminal offence to supply it without a licence or registration (or transitional protection until 2011 for products on the market before 2004). In addition, the scope for selling herbs as foods is increasingly limited by 'novel foods' legislation and also by the European Food Standards Agency (see below).

There have been exemptions from requirements of formal licensing in European law for herbal medicinal products provided by professionals. However, this legislation did not envisage exemptions for non-registered practitioners. Herbalists exist in appreciable numbers only in the UK, where, by contrast, there is relatively little interest in herbal medicine by orthodox registered health professionals. There have been exemptions provided in UK law for the provision of herbal remedies on a one-to-one basis but this is not secure in a European framework and the legal status of herbal practitioners is thus undefined. However, with government support, herbal practitioners in the UK are moving towards statutory registration by 2010.

Since the early twentieth century, legislation relating to foods and to medicines has diverged, with natural products gradually falling out of the medicine stream from the 1930s. By the time of the thalidomide tragedy in the early 1960s, and the ensuing new raft of drug laws throughout much of the developed world, natural medicines were largely discounted as a significant force in healthcare. In Europe, the pivotal harmonizing measure, to which all member states of the European Union have subsumed their individual legislations, was passed in 1965. EC Directive 65/65/EEC (now supplanted by Directive 2001/83/EEC) defined medicinal products as any substance or combination of substances:

- presented for treating or preventing disease in human beings or animals;
- which may be administered with a view to making a medical diagnosis or to restoring, correcting or modifying physiological functions in human beings or animals.

These definitions are sweeping. They clearly include any natural materials used for therapeutic ends. In Europe, if one claims for any product an active effect on the human body, one needs by law to have a medicines licence for that product. This means convincing the medicines regulators that any therapeutic effect is warranted, generally by producing controlled clinical trial evidence. It also means that such products have to meet pharmaceutical standards of quality and safety. This default status as medicines is clearly distinct from that applying in the USA, where natural products are in the first instance considered as foods.

In Germany, France and the United Kingdom especially, a large number of herbal medicinal products have obtained marketing authorizations, according to laws within each member state but within the

35

terms of this European legislation. Nevertheless, the governments of Germany, France, the Netherlands and the UK provided exemptions in their own national legislatures to protect herbal medicines from some of the requirements imposed upon synthetic drug manufacturers. These exemptions were highlighted in a report to the European Commission in 1999 and have led to moves for greater harmonization of herbal regulations within new applications of the pivotal 65/65/EEC Directive. The first amendment was enacted quickly and allowed products with 'established use' as medicines to establish their efficacy by reference to this use.

More significantly, and only for 'herbal products with traditional use' registration as a medicine (rather than full licensing) is now possible (Directive 2004/24/EC—an amendment to Directive 2001/83/EC). This will excuse the manufacturer from providing evidence of efficacy, although not from assuring standards of pharmaceutical quality and on-going safety monitoring. Registrations will thus require significant investment by manufacturers and importers. At the time of writing there are concerns that this will be too difficult for many. This option is only available for herbal products where there is evidence of at least 15 years of traditional use somewhere in the European Union, plus at least 15 years elsewhere (i.e. a total of 30 years).

It used to be legal, without a licence, to sell in the UK a simple herbal medicinal product—without claims or brand name (under 'Section 12.2' of the 1968 Medicines Act); this no longer applies. The new traditional use Directive was published on 30 April 2004. Any product that was legally on the UK market under '12:2' on that date has 'transitional protection' and is not required to comply with the Directive until 30 April 2011. After that date, it must have either a traditional herbal registration or a marketing authorization (full licence) or it can no longer be placed on the market. This transitional protection does not apply to any products placed on the UK market at any time after 30 April 2004.

Alone among major industrial countries, the UK has maintained a common law basis to its legal system, in which historical practice provides the default precedent in a court of law. In the delivery of medical care this has meant that there have been very many fewer restrictions than in other developed countries. The statutory rights of doctors, pharmacists and other health professionals have not been monopolies: the common law right of every subject to pursue the health care he or she wishes is still formally protected. Thus unlicensed health professionals and health-food shopkeepers are legally able to provide any service not formally proscribed by Acts of Parliament.

The main statutory control on the supply of medicines is the 1968 Medicines Act. All herbal remedies included on a 'General Sale List' could be freely supplied and under the provisions of section 12.2 for:

2) … the sale, supply, manufacture or assembly of any herbal remedy where the process to which the plant or plants are subjected in producing the remedy consists only of drying, crushing or comminuting, and the remedy is, or is to be, sold or supplied
   a) under a designation which only specifies the plant or plants and the process and does not apply any other name to the remedy, and
   b) without any written recommendation (whether by means of a labelled container or package or a leaflet or in any other way) as to use the remedy.

Although 12.2 has fallen, the General Sale List (GSL) still is referred to as a directory of herbal remedies. Over 300 herbal substances are named for internal use (Schedule 3[A]). Some 30 are listed for external use (Schedule 3[B]). Where maximum doses (MD) or maximum daily doses (MDD) are listed for GSL products it is implied that any dose in excess of that figure cannot be marketed over the counter (OTC) and the medicine becomes prescription only. Herbal remedies on the various schedules are listed in Table 35.1.

Under the terms of the second stage of the Medicines Act (1971) 'Licences of Right' were provided to established medicines already on the market, subject to review before 1990. Around 2000 herbal products obtained these medicines licences. However, the review process was very demanding, with manufacturers having in effect to become modern pharmaceutical companies, ensuring conventional standards of quality medicine production. After 1990, around 600 were successfully reviewed, and now have full medicine licences. However, only a proportion of these are still available on the market and their future in relation to the enactment of the Traditional Use Directive remains uncertain.

INDUSTRY STANDARDS

The British Herbal Medicine Association (BHMA) has, since its founding in 1964, engaged the legislature in productive discussions about the controls of herbal medicines. Its most prominent achievement has been the production of the *British Herbal Pharmacopoeia*, first in 1983 and then, through substantial revisions, to the latest, with 169 monographs published in 1996. The *Pharmacopoeia* has been widely used by regulators in the UK and elsewhere around the world as an effective practical quality standard where official monographs do not exist. The herbal monographs covered in the final 1996 edition are listed in Table 35.2.

The BHMA is also the UK member of a European network of national herbal or phytotherapy associations called the European Scientific Cooperative on Phytotherapy (ESCOP). Since its formation in 1989, ESCOP has been involved in producing harmonized therapeutic monographs for 'plant drugs' as formal submissions to the European medicines regulators. A total of 80 such monographs have been published, listed in Table 35.3. More details of this work can be obtained at the ESCOP website (http://www.escop.com).

THE HERBAL PRACTITIONER

There is another group supplying herbal medicinal products who have clearly been affected by the UK exemptions from European law. Under 12.1 of the 1968 Act no licence is required for:

1) … the sale, supply, manufacture or assembly of any herbal remedy in the course of business where
   a) the remedy is manufactured or assembled on premises of which the person carrying on the business is the occupier and which he is able to close so as to exclude the public, and
   b) the person carrying on the business sells or supplies the remedy for administration to a particular person after being requested by or on behalf of that person and in that person's presence to use his own judgement as to the treatment required.

This exemption for one-to-one supply reflected the fact that herbal medicine in the UK has often been provided by practitioners. As a common folk system, it was first recognized by an Act of Parliament in the reign of Henry VIII in 1533, and its practitioners were in this protected from the hostile intentions of the new physicians and surgeons. With the Industrial Revolution, herbal medicine became an urban phenomenon and the National Association (later Institute) of Medical Herbalists was established in 1864. The NIMH is the oldest professional association of medical herbalists in the developed world. Its members have lately been provided by 4-year BSc programmes at several universities. The NIMH has a full professional constitution, codes of ethics and disciplinary

Table 35.1   General sale list.

Abietis Oil	Caraway	Figwort	Marshmallow
Absinthium	Cardamom	Fir cones	Masterwort
Acacia Powder	Cascara	Fluellin	Maté
Aesculus	Cascarilla	Frangula	Meadow Grass
Agar	Cassia Oil	Fringetree	Meadowsweet
Agrimony	Castor Oil	Frostweed	Melissa
Almond Oil	Catechu	Fucus	Motherwort
Aloes – MD: 100 mg	Catmint	Fumitory	Mountain Flax
Aloin – MD: 20 mg	Caulophyllum	Galangal	Mousear
American Cranesbill Root	Celery Oil	Gamboge	Mugwort
American Liverwort	Celery Seed	Garlic Oil	Muira Puama
Ammoniacum	Centaury	Gentian	Mullein
Angelica Oil	Centella	Germander	Myrrh
Angelica Root	Ceratonia	Ginger	Neroli Oil
Anise	Cetraria	Ginseng	Nettle
Anise Oil	Chamomile	Golden Rod	Nutmeg
Arbutus, Trailing	Chamomile, German	Golden Seal	Oak
Asafoetida	Chestnut	Greater Burnet	Ononis
Asarabacca	Chickweed	Grindelia	Orange Oil
Ash	Chiretta	Ground Ivy	Origanum
Australian	Cimicifuga	Guaiacum	Papaya Leaves
Sandalwood Oil	Cinchona – MD 50 mg	Harts Tongue	Pareira Root
Avocado Oil	Cinnamon Bark	Hay Flower	Parsley Piert
Balm of Gilead Buds	Citrus Bioflavonoids	Heartsease	Parsley Root
Balmony	Clivers	Heather Flowers	Passiflora
Baptisia	Clove	Hemlock Spruce	Peach Leaves
Barberry Bark	Cochlearia	– External 10% max	Pellitory-of-the-wall
Bayberry	Cocillana	Holly	Pennyroyal
Bearberry	Coltsfoot	Holy Thistle	Peony
Bearsfoot	Comfrey	Honeysuckle Flowers	Peppermint
Beech	Condurango	Horehound	Periwinkle
Benzoin	Coriander	Hydrangea	Pichi
Bethroot	Cornflower	Hyssop	Pilewort
Birch, European	Cornsilk	Ipecacuanha	Pimento Oil
Birthwort	Corydalis	Irish Moss	Pimpernel
Bistort	Cotton root	Ispaghula	Pinus Sylvestris
Blackberry Leaf	Couchgrass	Jamaica Dogwood	Pipsissiwa
Blackberry Root Bark	Cowslip	Jambul	Plantain
Black Catechu	Crampbark	Jujube Berries	Pleurisy Root
Black Haw	Cubeb	Juniper	Poke Root
Black Root	Cudweed	Kava	Pollen
Blackthorn	Cynara	Kino	Poplar
Blood Root	Cypripedium	Kola	Potentilla
Blue Flag	Damiana	Krameria	Prickly Ash
Boldo	Dandelion	Lactuca	Prune
Boneset	Dill	Lady's Mantle	Psyllium
Broom	Dogwood	Laminaria	Pulsatilla
Buchu	Echinacea	Larch Bark	Quaking Aspen
Buckbean	Elder	Lavender	Quassia
Buckthorn	Elder, Dwarf	Lemon Grass Oil	Queen's Delight
Bugle	Elecampane	Lemon Oil	Quillaia
Bugleweed	Elm	Leptandrin	Raspberry Leaves
Burdock	Equisetum	Lime Flowers	Red Poppy Petals
Burnet Saxifrage	Eriodictyon	Lime Leaf	Red Sanderswood
Butterbur	Eryngo	Linseed	Rhubarb Rhizome
Butternut	Eucalyptus	Liquorice	Rose Fruit
Calamint	Euonymus	Lobelia – MD 65 mg	Rosemary
Calamus	Eupatorium	Lovage	Rue
Columba	Euphorbia	Lucerne	Rutin
Canella	Eyebright	Lungwort	Safflower
Capsicum	Fennel	Lupulin	Sage Oil
Capsicum Oleoresin	Fenugreek	Lupulus	St John's Wort
– MD 1.2 mg; MDD 1.8 mg;	Feverfew	Maidenhair	Salep
External 2.5% max	Figs	Marigold Flowers	Salicaria

(Continued)

Table 35.1 General sale list. (Cont'd)

Sandalwood Oil	Skunk Cabbage Root	Sumbul	White Pond Lily
Sandarac	Slippery Elm – Powdered Bark	Sundew	Wild Carrot
Sanguinaria	Soya (Protein)	Sunflower	Wild Cherry
Sanicle	Spearmint	Sweet Birch Oil	Wild Oats
Saponaria	Speedwell	Tag Alder	Wild Rose
Sarsaparilla Root	Spigelia	Tansy	Wild Thyme
Sassafras	Squaw Vine	Thyme	Willow, Black
Saw Palmetto	Squill, White	Tolu Balsam	Willow, White
Senega	Star Anise	Tragacanth	Wintergreen Leaves
Senna Fruit	Sterculia – Gum	Unicorn Root, False	Wood Betony
Senna Leaf	Stone Root	Unicorn Root, True	Wood Sage
Serpentary	Storax	Valerian	Yarrow
Shepherd's Purse	Strawberry Leaf	Verbena	Yellow Dock
Skullcap	Sumach	Violet	

General sale (external use only)

Arnica	Coconut Oil	Lycopodium	Pine Oil
Bay Oil	Colophony	Meleleuca Oil	Pyrethrum
Bergamot Oil	Copaiba	Mustard Oil	Rape Oil
Birch Tar Oil	Gall	Neatsfoot Oil	Sassafras Oil
Cade Oil	Geranium Oil	Olibanum	
Cajaput Oil	Hamamelis	Orris	
Camphor Oil	Jaborandi	Palm Kernel Oil	
Cedar Wood Oil	Linseed Oil	Peru Balsam	

Schedule Part I

Areca	Elaterium	Nux Vomica	Slippery Elm Bark (whole)
Canadian Hemp	Embelia	*Podophyllum* spp.	Stavesacre Seeds
Catha edulis	Ergot, prepared	Poison Ivy	*Strophanthus* spp.
Chenopodium ambroisioides	Erysium	Pomegranate Bark	Veratrum, Green
Cocculus indicus	Holarrhena	Poppy Capsule	Veratrum, White
Crotalaria spp.	Ignatius Bean	*Rauwolfia* spp.	Yohimbe
Croton Oil and Seed	Kamala	Sabadilla	
Curcubita maxima	Kousso	Santonica	
Digitalis Leaf	Male Fern	Savin	
Duboisia spp.	Mistletoe Berry	Scopolia	

Schedule Part III Remedies for internal use

False Hellebore	*Adonis vernalis* (100 mg tds)
Quebracho	*Aspidosperma quebracho-blanco* (50 mg tds)
Deadly Nightshade	*Atropa belladonna* (herb:50 mg; root: 30 mg tds)
Greater Celandine	*Chelidonium majus* (2 g tds)
Cinchona Bark	*Cinchona* spp. (250 mg tds)
Meadow Saffron	*Colchicum autumnale* (100 mg tds)
Lily-of-the-valley	*Convallaria majalis* (150 mg tds)
Jimson Weed	*Datura stramonium* (50 mg tds)
Ma-huang	*Ephedra sinica* (600 mg tds)
Yellow Jasmine Root	*Gelsemium sempervirens* (25 mg tds)
Henbane	*Hyoscyamus niger* (100 mg tds)
Lobelia	*Lobelia inflata* (200 mg tds)

Remedies for external use

Aconite	*Aconitum* spp.
Hemlock	*Conium maculatum*
Jaborandi	*Pilocarpus microphyllus*
Poison Oak	*Rhus toxicodendron*
Ragwort	*Senecio jacobaea*

Table 35.2 Monographs in the *British Herbal Pharmacopoeia* 1996.

Monograph name	Botanical name	Action
Agnus Castus	*Vitex agnus-castus* L.	Hormonal modulator
Agrimony	*Agrimonia* spp.	Astringent
Aloes, Barbados	*Aloe barbadensis* Miller.	Stimulant laxative
Aloes, Cape	*Aloe ferox* Miller.	Stimulant laxative
Ammoniacum	*Dorema ammoniacum*	Expectorant
Angelica Root	*Angelica archangelica* L.	Aromatic bitter, spasmolytic
Aniseed	*Pimpinella anisum* L.	Expectorant; carminative
Arnica Flower	*Arnica montana* L.	Topical healing
Artichoke	*Cynara scolymus* L.	Hepatic
Asafoetida	*Ferula assa-foetida* and other *F.* spp.	Spasmolytic
Ascophyllum	*Ascophyllum nodosum* Le Jol.	Thyroactive
Balm Leaf	*Melissa officinalis* L.	Sedative; topical antiviral
Balm of Gilead Bud	*Populus nigra* and other *P.* spp.	Expectorant
Barberry Bark	*Berberis vulgaris* L.	Cholagogue
Bayberry Bark	*Myrica cerifera* L.	Astringent
Bearberry Leaf	*Arctostaphylos uva-ursi* Spreng	Urinary antiseptic
Belladonna Herb	*Atropa belladonna* L.	Antispasmodic
Birch Leaf	*Betula pendula* and other *B.* spp.	Diuretic; antirheumatic
Black Cohosh	*Cimicifuga racemosa* Nutt	Anti-inflammatory
Black Haw Bark	*Viburnum prunifolium* L.	Spasmolytic
Black Horehound	*Ballota nigra* L.	Antiemetic
Bladderwrack	*Fucus vesiculosis* L.	Thyroactive
Blue Flag	*Iris versicolor, I. caroliniana* Watson	Laxative
Bogbean	*Menyanthes trifoliata* L.	Bitter
Boldo	*Peumus boldus* Molina	Cholagogue
Broom Top	*Cytisus scoparius* Link.	Antiarrhythmic, diuretic
Buchu	*Barosma betulina* Bartl. et Wendl.	Urinary antiseptic
Burdock Leaf	*Arctium lappa* L. *A. minus* Bernh.	Dermatological agent
Burdock Root	*Arctium lappa* L. *A. minus* Bernh.	Dermatological agent
Calamus	*Acorus calamus* vars	Carminative
Calumba Root	*Jateorhiza palmata* Miers.	Appetite stimulant
Caraway	*Carum carvi* L.	Carminative
Cardamom Fruit	*Elettaria cardamomum* Maton.	Carminative
Cascara	*Rhamnus purshianus* DC.	Stimulant laxative
Cassia Bark	*Cinnamomum cassia* Blume.	Carminative
Catechu	*Uncaria gambier* (Hunter) Roxb.	Astringent
Cayenne Pepper	*Capsicum frutescens* L.	Rubefacient, vasostimulant
Celery Seed	*Apium graveolens* L.	Diuretic
Centaury	*Centaurium erythraea* Rafn.	Bitter
Cinchona Bark	*Cinchona pubescens* Vahl.	Bitter
Cinnamon	*Cinnamomum zeylanicum* Nees.	Carminative
Clivers	*Galium aparine* L.	Diuretic
Clove	*Syzygium aromaticum* L.	Carminative, topical analgesic
Cocillana	*Guarea rusbyi*	Expectorant
Cola	*Cola nitida, C. acuminata*	Central nervous stimulant
Comfrey Root	*Symphytum officinale* L.	Vulnerary
Coriander	*Coriandrum sativum* L.	Carminative, stimulant
Corn Silk	*Zea mays* L.	Diuretic; urinary demulcent
Couch Grass Rhizome	*Agropyron repens* P. Beauv.	Diuretic
Cranesbill Root	*Geranium maculatum* L.	Astringent
Damiana	*Turnera diffusa* and possibly other spp.	Thymoleptic
Dandelion Leaf	*Taraxacum officinale* Webber.	Diuretic; choleretic
Dandelion Root	*Taraxacum officinale* Webber.	Hepatic
Devil's Claw	*Harpagophytum procumbens* DC.	Antirheumatic
Echinacea Root	*Echinacea angustifolia* DC.	Immunostimulant
Elder Flower	*Sambucus nigra* L.	Diaphoretic
Elecampane	*Inula helenium* L.	Expectorant
Eleutherococcus	*Eleutherococcus senticosus* Maxim.	Adaptogen; tonic
Equisetum	*Equisetum arvense* L.	Diuretic; astringent
Eucalyptus Leaf	*Eucalyptus globulus* Labill.	Antiseptic
Euonymus Bark	*Euonymus atropurpureus* Jacq.	Laxative

(Continued)

Table 35.2 Monographs in the *British Herbal Pharmacopoeia* 1996. (Cont'd)

Monograph name	Botanical	Action
Fennel, Bitter	*Foeniculum vulgare* Miller.	Carminative
Fennel, Sweet	*Foeniculum vulgare* Miller.	Carminative
Fenugreek Seed	*Trigonella foenum-graecum* L.	Demulcent, hypoglycaemic
Feverfew	*Tanacetum parthenium* Schultz Bip.	Migraine prophylactic
Frangula Bark	*Rhamnus frangula* L.	Stimulant laxative
Fumitory	*Fumaria officinalis* L.	Choleretic
Galangal	*Alpinia officinarum* Hance.	Carminative
Garlic	*Allium sativum* L.	Hypolipidaemic; antimicrobial
Gentian	*Gentiana lutea* L.	Bitter
Ginger	*Zingiber officinale* Roscoe.	Carminative; antiemetic
Ginkgo Leaf	*Ginkgo biloba* L.	Vasoactive; platelet aggregation inhibitor
Ginseng	*Panax ginseng* C.A. Meyer.	Adaptogen; tonic
Goldenrod	*Solidago virgaurea* L.	Diuretic; anticatarrhal, diaphoretic
Goldenseal Root	*Hydrastis canadensis* L.	Anti-inflammatory
Grindelia	*Grindelia robusta* Nutt.	Expectorant
Ground Ivy	*Glechoma hederacea* L.	Expectorant
Guaiacum Resin	*Guaiacum officinale* L. *G. Sanctum* L.	Anti-inflammatory
Hamamelis Bark	*Hamamelis virginiana* L.	Astringent
Hamamelis Leaf	*Hamamelis virginiana* L.	Astringent
Hawthorn Berry	*Crataegus monogyna* Jacq.	Cardiotonic
Hawthorn Flowering Top	*Crataegus monogyna* Jacq.	Cardiotonic
Heartsease	*Viola tricolor* L.	Expectorant; dermatological agent
Helonias	*Chamaelirium luteum* A. Gray.	Uterine tonic
Holy Thistle	*Cnicus benedictus* L.	Bitter
Hops	*Humulus lupulus* L.	Sedative; bitter
Horse-chestnut Seed	*Aesculus hippocastanum* L.	Venoactive
Hydrangea	*Hydrangea arborescens* L.	Diuretic
Hyoscyamus Leaf	*Hyoscyamus niger* L.	Antispasmodic
Hyssop	*Hyssopus officinalis* L.	Expectorant
Iceland Moss	*Cetraria islandica* L.	Demulcent
Ipecacuanha	*Cephaelis ipecacuanha, C. acuminata*	Expectorant; emetic
Irish Moss	*Chondrus crispus* Stackh.	Demulcent
Ispaghula Husk	*Plantago ovata* Forssk.	Bulk-forming laxative
Ispaghula Seed	*Plantago ovata* Forssk.	Bulk-forming laxative
Jamaica Dogwood	*Piscidia piscipula* Sarg.	Analgesic
Java Tea	*Orthosiphon aristatus*, (Blume) Miq.	Diuretic
Juniper Berry	*Juniperus communis* L.	Diuretic
Kava-Kava	*Piper methysticum* G. Forst.	Anxiolytic
Lady's Mantle	*Alchemilla xanthochlora*, Rothm. *A. vulgaris* L. S. l.	Astringent
Lily of the Valley Leaf	*Convallaria majalis* L.	Cardioactive
Lime Flower	*Tilia cordata* Mill. and other spp.	Antispasmodic; diaphoretic
Linseed	*Linum usitatissimum* L.	Bulk-forming laxative; demulcent
Liquorice Root	*Glycyrrhiza glabra* L.	Respiratory stimulant
Lobelia	*Lobelia inflata* L.	Respiratory stimulant
Lovage Root	*Levisticum officinale* Koch.	Carminative; mild diuretic
Lucerne	*Medicago sativa* L.	Tonic
Marigold	*Calendula officinalis* L.	Anti-inflammatory, vulnerary
Marshmallow Leaf	*Althaea officinalis* L.	Demulcent
Marshmallow Root	*Althaea officinalis* L.	Demulcent
Maté	*Ilex paraguariensis* A. St.-Hil.	Stimulant
Matricaria Flower	*Matricaria recutita* L.	Anti-inflammatory; antispasmodic
Meadowsweet	*Filipendula ulmaria* Maxim.	Anti-inflammatory
Melilot	*Melilotis officinalis* Pall.	Venotonic, vulnerary
Milk Thistle Fruit	*Silybum marianum* (L.) Gaertn.	Hepatoprotective
Mistletoe Herb	*Viscum album* L.	Hypotensive
Motherwort	*Leonurus cardiaca* L.	Antispasmodic
Mugwort	*Artemisia vulgaris* L.	Emmenogogue
Mullein Leaf	*Verbascum densiflorum* Bertol.	Expectorant
Myrrh	*Commiphora molmol* Engler and other spp. of *C.*	Antiseptic
Nettle Herb	*Urtica dioica* L.	Diuretic
Nettle Root	*Urtica dioica* L.	Prostatic

(Continued)

Table 35.2 **Monographs in the _British Herbal Pharmacopoeia_ 1996. (Cont'd)**

Monograph	Botanical name	Action
Oak Bark	_Quercus robur_ L. and other _Q._ spp.	Astringent
Parsley Herb	_Petroselinum crispum_	Diuretic
Parsley Root	_Petroselinum crispum_	Carminative, diuretic
Passiflora	_Passiflora incarnata_ L.	Sedative
Peppermint Leaf	_Mentha piperata_ L.	Carminative
Pilewort Herb	_Ficaria ranunculoides_ Moench.	Astringent
Poke Root	_Phytolacca americana_ L.	Anti-inflamatory
Prickly Ash Bark	_Zanthoxylum clava-herculis_ L.	Circulatory stimulant
Psyllium Seed	_Plantago afra_ L. _P. indica_ L.	Bulk-forming laxative
Pulsatilla	_Pulsatilla vulgaris_ Miller, _P. pratensis_ (L.) Miller	Sedative
Pumpkin Seed	_Cucurbita pepo_ L.	Prostatic
Quassia	_Picrasma excelsa_	Appetite stimulant
Queen's Delight	_Stillingia sylvatica_ L.	Expectorant
Raspberry Leaf	_Rubus idaeus_ L.	Partus praeparator
Red Clover Flower	_Trifolium pratense_ L.	Anti-inflammatory
Rhatany Root	_Krameria triandra_ Ruiz and Pavon.	Astringent
Rhubarb	_Rheum palmatum_ L., _R. officinale_ Baillon, hybrids	Laxative
Roman Chamomile Flower	_Chamaemelum nobile_ All.	Antispasmodic
Rosemary Leaf	_Rosmarinus officinalis_ L.	Carminative, spasmolytic
Sage Leaf	_Salvia officinalis_ L.	Antiseptic, astringent
Sarsaparilla	_Smilax_ spp.	Anti-inflammatory
Saw Palmetto Fruit	_Serenoa repens_	Prostatic
Senega Root	_Polygala senega_ L. and related spp.	Expectorant
Senna Fruit, Alexandrian	_Cassia senna_ L.	Stimulant laxative
Senna Fruit, Tinnevelly	_Cassia angustifolia_ Vahl.	Stimulant laxative
Senna Leaf	_Cassia senna, C. angustifolia_	Stimulant laxative
Shepherd's Purse	_Capsella bursa-pastoris_ Medik.	Antihaemorrhagic
Skullcap	_Scutellaria lateriflora_ L.	Mild sedative
Slippery Elm Bark	_Ulmnus rubra_ Muhl.	Demulcent
Squill	_Drimia maritima_ Stearn.	Expectorant
Squill, Indian	_Drimia indica_ J.P. Jessop.	Expectorant
St John's Wort	_Hypericum perforatum_ L.	Antidepressant
Stramonium Leaf	_Datura stramonium_ L.	Antispasmodic
Thyme	_Thymus vulgaris, T. zygis_	Expectorant
Valerian Root	_Valeriana officinalis_ L.	Sedative
Vervain	_Verbena officinalis_ L.	Tonic
Violet Leaf	_Viola odorata_ L.	Expectorant
White Deadnettle	_Lamium album_ L.	Astringent
White Horehound	_Marrubium vulgare_ L.	Expectorant
Wild Carrot	_Daucus carota_ L.	Diuretic
Wild Cherry Bark	_Prunus serotina_ Ehrh.	Antitussive
Wild Lettuce	_Lactuca virosa_ L.	Sedative
Wild Thyme	_Thymus serpyllum_ L.	Expectorant
Wild Yam	_Dioscorea villosa_ L.	Spasmolytic, anti-inflammatory
Willow Bark	_Salix alba_ L. and other spp.	Anti-inflammatory
Wormwood	_Artemesia absinthium_ L.	Bitter
Yarrow	_Achillea millefolium_ L.	Diaphoretic

procedures and mandatory professional indemnity cover for its members. Professional members carry the letters MNIMH or FNIMH after their name. A more recent professional association dedicated to a raised professional profile of herbal medicine in the healthcare community in the UK and Europe is the College of Practitioners of Phytotherapy (CPP). Its members carry the letters MCPP or FCPP and often overlap with membership of the NIMH.

There are a number of other practitioner groups in the Western herbal tradition: The Association of Master Herbalists, the International Register of Consultant Herbalists and the Unified Register of Herbal Practitioners. There is also a major practitioner group practising the herbal medicine of China (the Register of Chinese Herbal Medicine) of Tibet (the British Association of Traditional Tibetan Medicine) and three groups practising Ayurvedic medicine from India (the Ayurvedic Medical Association, the Ayurvedic Practitioners Association and the Maharishi Ayurveda Practitioners Assocation).

As the limits of 12.1 exemptions within Europe became more obvious, and herbal practitioner associations faced an uncertain future, the European Herbal and Practitioners Association (now the European Herbal and Traditional Medicine Practitioners Association; EHTPA: http://www.ehpa.eu) was founded in 1993 to represent their interests. The EHTPA has published an agreed core curriculum and developed an accreditation board for educational standards; it has amended its constitution to reflect the standards pertaining for statutory organizations, and constituent organizations of the EHTPA have moved to harmonize with it.

Table 35.3 ESCOP monographs in the medicinal uses of plant drugs.

Monograph name	Common name	Botanical name	Therapeutic indications
Absinthii herba	Wormwood	*Artemesia absinthium* L.	Anorexia, dyspepsia
Agni casti fructus	Agnus castus	*Vitex agnus-castus* L.	Premenstrual syndrome
Allii sativi bulbus	Garlic bulb	*Allium sativum* L.	Prophylaxis of atherosclerosis
Aloe capensis	Cape aloes	*Aloe ferox* Miller.	Short-term use in occasional constipation
Althaeae radix	Marshmallow root	*Althaea officinalis* L.	Dry cough
Anisi fructus	Aniseed	*Pimpinella anisum* L.	Dyspeptic complaints
Arnicae flos	Arnica flower	*Arnica montana*, other *A.* spp.	Treatment of bruises, sprains and inflammation
Betulae folium	Birch leaf	*Betula pendula*, other *B.* spp.	Irrigation of the urinary tract
Boldo folium	Boldo	*Peumus boldus* Mol.	Minor hepatobiliary dysfunction
Calendulae flos	Calendula flower	*Calendula officinalis* L.	Inflammations of the skin and mucosa
Carvi fructus	Caraway	*Carum carvi* L.	Internal use: spasmodic gastrointestinal complaints. External use: flatulent colic of infants
Centaurii herba	Centaury	*Centaurium erythraea* Rafn.	Dyspeptic complaints
Chelidonii herba	Greater celandine	*Chelidonium majus* L.	Mild to moderate spasms of upper gastrointestinal tract; minor gallbladder disorders
Cimicifugae rhizoma	Black cohosh	*Cimicifuga racemosa* (L.) Nutt	Climacteric symptoms
Cinnamomi cortex	Cinnamon	*Cinnamomum zeylanicum* Nees	Dyspeptic complaints
Crataegi folium cum flore	Hawthorn leaf and flower	*Crataegus monogyna* Jacq. Lindm.	Declining cardiac performance
Curcumae longae rhizoma	Turmeric	*Curcuma longa* L.	Mild digestive disturbances and minor biliary dysfunction
Cynarae folium	Artichoke leaf	*Cynara scolymus* L.	Digestive complaints and hepatobiliary disturbances
Echinaceae pallidae radix	Pale coneflower root	*Echinacea pallida* Nutt.	Adjuvant therapy and prophylaxis of recurrent infections of the upper respiratory tract
Echinaceae purpureae herba	Purple coneflower herb	*Echinacea purpurea* Moench.	Adjuvant therapy and prophylaxis of recurrent infections of the upper respiratory tract and also of the urogenital tract
Echinaceae purpureae radix	Purple coneflower root	*Echinacea purpurea* Moench.	Adjuvant therapy and prophylaxis of recurrent infections of the upper respiratory tract
Eleutherococci radix	Eleutherococcus	*Eleutherococcus senticosus* (Rupr. et Maxim) Maxim	Decreased mental and physical capacities
Eucalypti aetheroleum	Eucalyptus oil	*Eucalyptus globulus* and other *E.* spp.	Symptomatic relief of catarrh of the upper respiratory tract
Filipendulae ulmariae herba	Meadowsweet	*Filipendula ulmaria* (L) Maxim	As supportive therapy for the common cold
Foeniculi fructus	Fennel	*Foeniculum vulgare* Miller.	Dyspeptic complaints
Frangulae cortex	Frangula bark	*Rhamnus frangula* L.	Short-term treatment of occasional constipation
Gentianae radix	Gentian root	*Gentiana lutea* L.	Anorexia
Ginkgo folium	Ginkgo leaf	*Ginkgo biloba* L.	Symptomatic treatment of mild to moderate dementia syndromes
Ginseng radix	Ginseng	*Panax ginseng* C.A. Meyer	Decreased mental and physical capacities
Hamamelidis aqua	Hamamelis water	*Hamamelis virginiana* L.	Minor inflammatory conditions of skin and mucosa (topical)
Hamamelidis cortex	Hamamelis bark	*Hamamelis virginiana* L.	Inflammation of the mucous membranes of the oral cavity; short-term symptomatic treatment of diarrhoea
Hamamelidis folium	Hamamelis leaf	*Hamamelis virginiana* L.	Varicose veins and haemorrhoids
Harpagophyti radix	Devil's claw	*Harpagophytum procumbens* DC.	Painful arthrosis
Hederae helicis folium	Ivy leaf	*Hedera helix* L.	Cough, especially associated with hypersecretion of viscid mucus
Hippocastani semen	Horse-chestnut seed	*Aesculus hippocastanum* L.	Chronic venous insufficiency
Hyperici herba	St John's wort	*Hypericum perforatum* L.	Mild to moderate depressive states

(Continued)

Table 35.3 ESCOP monographs in the medicinal uses of plant drugs. (Cont'd)

Monograph name	Common name	Botanical name	Therapeutic indications
Juniperi fructus	Juniper berries	*Juniperus communis* L.	Renal elimination
Lichen islandicus	Iceland moss	*Cetraria islandica* Ach.	Dry cough
Liquiritiae radix	Liquorice root	*Glycyrrhiza glabra* L.	Adjuvant therapy of gastric and duodenal ulcers and gastritis; coughs and bronchial catarrh
Lini semen	Linseed	*Linum usitatissimum*	Constipation
Lupuli flos	Hop strobiles	*Humulus lupulus* L.	Tenseness, restlessness and difficulty in falling asleep
Matricariae flos	Matricaria flower	*Matricaria recutita* L.	Internal use: symptomatic treatment of gastrointestinal complaints External use: minor inflammation and irritations of skin and mucosa
Meliloti herba	Melilotus	*Melilotus officinalis* Desr.	Symptomatic treatment of problems related to varicose veins
Melissae folium	Melissa leaf	*Melissa officinalis* L.	Internal: tenseness, restlessness and irritability External: herpes labialis
Menthae piperitae aetheroleum	Peppermint oil	*Mentha × piperata* L.	Internal use: symptomatic treatment of digestive disorders External use: relief of coughs and colds
Menthae piperitae folium	Peppermint leaf	*Mentha × piperata* L.	Symptomatic treatment of digestive disorders
Myrrha	Myrrh	*Commiphora molmol* and other C. spp.	Topical treatment of gingivitis, stomatitis minor skin inflammations, wounds and abrasions
Myrtilli fructus	Bilberry fruit	*Vaccinium myrtillus* L.	Symptomatic treatment of problems related to varicose veins; topical mild inflammations of mucous membranes of mouth and throat
Ononidis radix	Restharrow root	*Ononis spinosa* L.	Irrigation of the urinary tract
Orthosiphonis folium	Java tea	*Orthosiphon aristatus* and other O. spp	Irrigation of the urinary tract
Passiflorae herba	Passiflora	*Passiflora incarnata* L.	Tenseness, restlessness and irritability
Piperis methystici rhizoma	Kava-kava	*Piper methysticum* G. Forst	Anxiety, tension and restlessness
Plantaginis lanceolatae folium/ herba	Ribwort plantain Leaf/herb	*Plantago lanceolata* L.	Catarrh of the respiratory tract; temporary mild inflammations of the oral and pharyngeal mucosa
Plantaginis ovatae semen	Ispaghula	*Plantago ovata* Forskal.	Habitual constipation
Plantaginis ovatae testa	Ispaghula husk	*Plantago ovata* Forskal.	Relief of constipation
Polygalae radix	Senega root	*Polygala senega* L.	Productive cough
Primulae radix	Primula root	*Primula veris* L.	Productive cough
Psyllii semen	Psyllium seed	*Plantago afra* spp.	Constipation
Rhamni purshiani cortex	Cascara	*Rhamnus purshianus* D.C.	Occasional constipation
Rhei radix	Rhubarb root	*Rheum palmatum* and other R. spp.	Short-term use of occasional constipation
Ribis nigri folium	Blackcurrant leaf	*Ribes nigrum* L.	Adjuvant in the treatment of rheumatic conditions
Rosmarini folium cum flore	Rosemary	*Rosmarinus officinalis* L.	Internal use: hepatic and biliary function External use: adjuvant in rheumatic conditions and peripheral circulatory disorders
Rusci rhizoma	Butcher's broom	*Ruscus aculeatus* L.	Supportive therapy for symptoms of chronic venous insufficiency and haemorrhoids
Salicis cortex	Willow bark	*Salix purpurea* and other S. spp.	Feverish conditions
Salviae folium	Sage leaf	*Salvia officinalis* L.	Inflammations and infections of the mouth and throat
Sennae folium	Senna leaf	*Cassia senna* and other C. spp.	Short-term use for occasional constipation
Sennae fructus acutifoliae	Alexandrian senna pods	*Cassia senna* L.	Short-term use for occasional constipation

(Continued)

Table 35.3 ESCOP monographs in the medicinal uses of plant drugs. (Cont'd)

Monograph name	Common name	Botanical name	Therapeutic indications
Sennae fructus angustifoliae	Tinnevelly senna pods	*Cassia angustifolia* Vahl.	Short-term use for occasional constipation
Serenoae repentis fructus (Sabal fructus)	Saw palmetto fruit	*Serenoa repens* (Bartram) Small	Symptomatic treatment of micturition disorders in mild to moderate benign prostatic hyperplasia
Solidaginis virgaureae herba	Goldenrod	*Solidago virgaurea* L.	Irrigation of the urinary tract
Tanaceti parthenii herba/folium	Feverfew	*Tanacetum parthenium* Sch. Bip.	Prophylaxis of migraine
Taraxaci folium	Dandelion leaf	*Taraxacum officinale* Weber sensu latiore	Adjunct to treatments where enhanced urinary output is desirable
Taraxaci radix	Dandelion root	*Taraxacum officinale* Weber sensu latiore	Restoration of hepatic and biliary function, dyspepsia, loss of appetite
Thymi herba	Thyme	*Thymus vulgaris* and other *T.* spp.	Catarrh of the upper respiratory tract
Trigonellae foenugraeci semen	Fenugreek	*Trigonella foenum-graecum* L.	Adjuvant therapy in diabetes mellitus and adjuvant to diet in mild to moderate hypercholesterolaemia
Urticae folium/herba	Nettle leaf and herb	*Urtica dioica* and other *U.* spp.	Adjuvant treatment of rheumatic conditions
Urticae radix	Nettle root	*Urtica dioica* and other *U.* spp.	Symptomatic treatment of micturition disorders
Uvae ursi folium	Bearberry leaf	*Arctostaphylos uva- ursi* Spreng.	Uncomplicated infections of the lower urinary tract
Valerianae radix	Valerian root	*Valeriana officinalis* L.	Tenseness, restlessness and irritability
Zingiberis rhizoma	Ginger	*Zingiber officinale* L.	Prophylaxis of the nausea and vomiting of motion sickness

In 2000, the House of Lords Select Committee on Science and Technology published its report on Complementary and Alternative medicine and called for the statutory regulation of herbal practice and acupuncture. In its response, the government agreed that this should happen. There is the precedent for such a move in the statutory registration of osteopaths and chiropracters in 1994 and 1996, respectively, although the new regulated profession is most likely to come within the existing Health Professions Council rather than under its own Act of Parliament. Such registration gives the profession the ability to protect its title and thus more effectively control the standard of practice in that discipline (entry into the profession is formally controlled, and a practitioner can be struck off the statutory register and cannot then practice under the title). In the case of the herbal practitioner, there is the additional hope that statutory registration will take over in providing regulatory cover from the increasingly untenable 'section 12.1'. Currently, however, 12.1 does not distinguish between herbal practitioners and anyone else supplying treatment on a one-to-one basis (homoeopaths, naturopaths, aromatherapists, and shop assistants have all become used to supplying herbal products under this cover). It remains unclear how the new statutory regulation will cover these activities.

There are a few doctors practising herbal medicine, usually as members of the NIMH or CPP, but not nearly as many as there are medical phytotherapists in other EU countries.

HERBAL PRACTICE IN THE UK

Unlike the situation pertaining to the use of Chinese herbs (see Chapter 37) and the Ayurvedic traditions of the Indian subcontinent (see Chapter 36), there is no obvious organized therapeutic framework to distinguish Western herbal prescription from that of modern conventional medicine. There are certainly older traditions of practice that certain modern practitioners defer to. In Europe, the historical tradition since Roman times has followed Galenic practices, which are based on making assessments of disturbances of body fluids (or humours), including in particular their temperaments (degrees of heat, cold, dryness and damp) and providing counteracting influences in the herbal materia medica (strictly speaking, this is literally a form of 'allopathic' medicine). Galenic medicine is all but extinct in Europe except as the foundation for classical Islamic medicine. The latter underpins the practice of much ethnic medicine, especially among the Pakinstani and Bangladeshi communities in the UK, but these traditions have not engaged with the legislative initiatives outlined above. Islamic medicine probably informed the practice of Tibetan medicine historically, but this has developed its own blend of Chinese and Indian influences in addition.

Galenic ideas influenced the nineteenth century articulation of European herbalism in North America by Samuel Thomson and his successors, who, ironically, repatriated their ideas, and materia medica, to Britain soon after. The NIMH adopted Thomsonian medicine and its more articulated development, physiomedicalism, soon after its foundation. Right up to the 1980s the NIMH characterized itself as a 'body of physiomedical practitioners' and provided some training in this system that combined some Galenic principles with early insights into the role of the autonomic nervous system. However, these ideas had never been fully developed after the early decades of the twentieth century and they withered as an active tradition.

The prevailing current tradition is to apply herbal medicines empirically to a physiological assessment of the body's needs. The language is most often that of modern Western medicine but the emphasis is different, looking at the underlying disturbances in function, rather than solely at the pathology or symptoms. Herbal remedies are understood by the practitioner as helping the body to do particular things rather than, as in the popular books or media, reducing symptoms. Recent attempts are beginning to better understand this distinction and how it might adapt herbal pharmacology and therapeutics, how medicines of the herbal variety might be suited to supporting self-recuperation that underpins all healing (and as seen in the formidable phenomenon known as the 'placebo effect'). Such modern ruminations will take some years to come to articulation. In the meantime, herbal practice in the UK will be largely pragmatic, imbued by whatever other traditions and practices the individual practitioner finds most helpful.

For the patient, the herbal consultation is usually the start of a remedial path, the timing of which will depend almost entirely on the length of time the illness has been present (the more established the condition, the longer it will take to repair) and could for some conditions be very brief. Typically, a herbal practitioner will take an hour or more at a first visit, with shorter visits thereafter, and much more emphasis than other health professionals on the patient taking a medicine at home. Medicines will often be tinctures or fluid extracts blended into individual mixtures at the end of each consultation in the practitioner's dispensary. Such liquids will most often be provided in bulk by specialist suppliers. It is also likely that solid forms, such as fixed tablets and capsules, will be prescribed as adjuncts; topical creams, ointments and other applications are applied as necessary. Costs often compare favourably with conventional prescription charges, reflecting even today the origins of much herbal medicine among the working class from the time of the Industrial Revolution.

Other current herbal traditions have adapted Chinese and Ayurvedic principles; a few practitioners have applied techniques such as iris diagnosis and other new usually uncharted techniques.

In Europe, there is almost nothing that distinguishes herbal from orthodox medicine. Herbs are simply seen as gentler versions of synthetic medicines, applied by physicians often at the same time and dispensed by pharmacists from the same counters.

36

Asian medicine

Samantha E. Weston

HISTORY OF ASIAN MEDICINE SYSTEMS

Many medical systems have emerged from Asia over the centuries, including Unani, Siddha and Ayurveda. When looking in detail at these systems, obvious similarities exist—the main one being the holistic approach each of them takes in treating patients. However, differences arise when one looks at how the development of each system has been affected by non-Asian medical systems over the centuries.

Unani medicine

Unani can be literally translated from the Arabic language as meaning 'Greek', from the Arabic word for Greece: 'al-Yunaan'. As an alternative medicine, Unani has found favour in Asia, especially India. In India, Unani practitioners can practise as qualified doctors, as the Indian government approves their practice. The principles of Unani medicine are based on the teachings of Hippocrates, Galen and Avicenna, and are based on the four humours (elements: phlegm (*Balgham*), blood (*Dam*), yellow bile (*Safra*) and black bile (*Sauda*). Although the principles of Unani can be traced back to year AD 2 the knowledge and teachings of the medical system were not documented until AD 1025, when Hakim Ibn Sina (known as Avicenna in the West) wrote *The Canon of Medicine* in Persia. The development of Unani medicine, as documented in this medical encyclopaedia, was influenced by Greek and Islamic medicine, and also by the Indian medical teachings of Sushruta and Charaka, the main texts of Ayurvedic medicine; both systems are based on the theory of the presence of elements in the human body, and the balance of these elements determines the state of a person's health. Each person's unique mixture of these substances determines his or her temperament: a predominance of blood gives a sanguine temperament; a predominance of phlegm makes one phlegmatic; yellow bile, bilious (or choleric); and black bile, melancholic. In Unani medicine, many medicines are based on honey, which is considered to have healing properties. Real pearls and metal are also used in the making of Unani medicine based on the kind of ailment it is aimed to heal. In today's modern medical world, honey is often used in wound dressings to kill bacteria because the high sugar content causes movement of water from inside bacterial cells by osmosis, leading to massive dehydration and the eventual death of the infecting organisms.

Ayurveda

Ayurveda is the ancient and sacred (Hindu) system of health care, originating in India over 5000 years ago. It is purely Indian in origin and has not been influenced by other countries or their medical systems. The literal translation of the word 'Ayurveda' from two words in Sanskrit—*āyus*, meaning 'life principle' and *veda*, referring to a 'system of knowledge'—accurately portrays the complexity and depth into which this medical system goes. A more overreaching translation can be taken as 'The knowledge (or science) of life'. The *Charaka Samhita*—an ancient Indian Ayurvedic text on internal medicine defines 'life' as a 'combination of the body, sense organs, mind and soul, the factor responsible for preventing decay and death, which sustains the body over time, and guides the processes of rebirth' and is one of the earliest written texts of Ayurveda, dating back to about 300 BC (see Chattopadhyaya, Further reading). It is believed to be the oldest of three ancient treatises of Ayurveda and is central to the modern-day practice of Ayurvedic medicine. Ayurveda is concerned with measures to protect '*āyus*', which includes healthy living along with therapeutic measures that relate to physical, mental, social and spiritual harmony. It is also one among the few traditional systems of medicine to contain a sophisticated system of surgery (which is referred to as '*salya-chikitsa*'). In today's Western society, the emergence of holistic health systems such as Ayurveda has led to the accommodation of modern science, especially in relation to the testing of medicines, in which research and adaptation are actively encouraged. Indeed, it is perfectly possible to evaluate Ayurvedic medicines using conventional clinical trials, and this is being carried out increasingly. At present, there are only a few Ayurvedic practitioners ('*vaid*') in the West, but the rapidly increasing popularity of more holistic approaches to health—where each patient is considered unique and therefore must be treated individually—has led to the emergence of schools of Ayurveda, Ayurvedic treatment centres and more Ayurvedic medicines being imported. This approach is in contrast to Western medicine where populations are generalized and 'normal' means what is applicable to the majority. Many ethnic populations from India and Pakistan continue to use their own traditional remedies while living in Europe, Australia or the US. Philosophically, Ayurveda has similarities with Traditional Chinese Medicine (TCM). The familiar *yin* and *yang*—the opposing life forces identified in TCM, can be likened to the three 'humours' of Ayurveda—the *tridosha*.

Siddha medicine

Siddha, from the Tamil word for 'achievements', is said to have been developed by eighteen siddhars (beings who have achieved a high degree of physical as well as spiritual perfection or enlightenment), led by the great Siddha Ayastiyar. Some of his works are still standard books of medicine and surgery in daily use among the Siddha medical practitioners of today. Siddha literature is written in Tamil and the medicine is practised largely in Tamil-speaking parts of India and abroad. Like Ayurvedic medicine, this system believes that all objects in the universe, including the human body, are composed of five basic elements: earth, water, fire, air and sky. Siddha medicine is largely therapeutic in nature, and is a form of treatment of disease using substances of all possible origins in a way that balances the possible harmful effects of each substance. The principles and doctrines of this system, both fundamental and applied, have a close similarity to Ayurveda. Additionally, this system also considers the human body as a conglomeration of three humours, seven basic tissues and the waste products of the body. As in both Unani and Ayurvedic medical systems, the equilibrium of humours is considered as a healthy state, and its disturbance or imbalance leads to disease or sickness. Ancient siddhars wrote their recipes on palm-leaves for the use of future generations, and details include preparations that are made mainly out of the parts of the plants and trees, such as leaves, bark, stem, root, etc., but also include mineral and some animal substances. The use of metals like gold, silver and iron powders in some preparations is a special feature of Siddha medicine, which claims it can detoxify metals to enable them to be used for stubborn diseases. The use of mercury in the Siddha medical system is well documented and not uncommon, so patients prescribed medicines containing purified mercury should be treated only by highly qualified practitioners of the art. Over the centuries, the system has developed a rich and unique treasure of drug knowledge in which use of metals and minerals is very much advocated. The depth of knowledge required by practitioners of Siddha medicine is summarized below:

- There are 25 varieties of water-soluble inorganic compounds called '*Uppu*'. These are different types of alkalis and salts.
- There are 64 varieties of mineral drugs that do not dissolve in water but emit vapours when burnt in a naked flame; 32 of these are naturally occurring and the remaining 32 are man-made.
- Seven drugs do not dissolve in water but emit vapour on heating.
- The system has classified separately classes of metals and alloys, which melt when heated and solidify on cooling. These include gold,

silver, copper, tin, lead and iron, which are incinerated according to strict regulations and used in the preparation of medicines.
- There is a group of drugs that exhibit sublimation on heating (including mercury and its salts).
- Sulphur (insoluble in water) is also used in therapeutic diagnosis and in maintenance of health.
- In addition there are drugs obtained from animal sources.

Most medicines and remedies (often common herbs and foods) used in Unani medicine (and Siddha medicine to a lesser extent) are also used in Ayurveda. Whereas Unani was influenced by Islam and Siddha by Alchemy, Ayurveda is associated with Vedic culture, and is generally considered to be the most 'original' form of traditional Asian medicine. The *Materia medica* of all these medical systems consists of many herbs made into pills, syrups, confections and alcoholic extracts, and also some metals. These traditional systems are still practised in rural communities in India and Pakistan—much more so than in cities.

COMMON TERMS AND CONCEPTS USED IN AYURVEDA

Ayurveda is dealt with in more detail because it has influenced the other Asian systems of medicine and remains the philosophical base for them. It is becoming increasingly popular in the West, although the term 'Ayurveda' is often misused. For example, recent newspaper headlines in the US included statements such as:

> *Ayurveda continues to grow rapidly as one of the most important systems of mind–body medicine, natural healing and traditional medicine as the need for natural therapies, disease prevention and a more spiritual approach to life becomes ever more important in this ecological age.*

before going on to calculate the success of this 'eco-friendly science' in material terms—in 2007 the 'global herbal market' was worth US$120 billion, with Ayurvedic treatments and products accounting for 50% of the total (*The Hindu*, 27 October 2007). There can be no argument about the increasing popularity of Ayurveda—clinics and treatment centres exist thousands of miles from India, and the term 'Ayurvedic tourism' is now recognized in many holiday resorts. Unfortunately, the high-class beauty and pampering packages offered in such places are centuries away from the 'real' Ayurveda, and disappoint professional *vaids*, who consider the use of a holistic system of medicine, meant to diagnose and treat a whole person, being reduced to superficial treatments intended to focus on a single part of the body as a travesty.

Prana is known as the 'life energy' and activates both the body and mind in Ayurvedic medicinal systems. It is contained in the head and controls the main functions of the mind, including emotions, memory and thought. Additionally, *prana* kindles the bodily fire '*Agni*' and therefore controls the function of the heart and, via the bloodstream, other vital organs (*dhatus*).

Bhutas are the five basic elements of Ayurveda—ether (or space), air, fire, water and earth. They are seen as manifestations of energy and can be equated to the five senses of hearing, vision, touch, taste and smell. In turn, these senses are associated with a particular sense organ (or organs) of the body, which impact on other 'organs of activity' and result in actions being carried out by the body. Table 36.1 summarizes some of the associations between the bhutas and the activities they govern.

Tridosha are the three humours or basic forces that manifest in the human body. They are formed from the five *bhutas* and are known as *vata*, *pitta* and *kapha*. The *tridosha* govern all functions of the body and mind and, by understanding the relationship between them, a *vaid* may make a diagnosis of the disease affecting a patient. Table 36.2

Table 36.1 The effect of the *Bhutas* on body function.

Bhuta	Body sense	Sense organ	Organs of activity	Action
Ether	Hearing	Ear	Tongue, vocal chords	Speech
Air	Touch	Skin	Muscles, colon, urinary bladder, heart	Movement
Fire	Vision	Eyes	Feet, gastrointestinal system	Walking
Water	Taste	Tongue	Saliva, digestive secretions, blood, muscles	Movement
Earth	Smell	Nose	Tendons, muscles, bones	Stability

Table 36.2 The effect of the *tridosha* on body function.

Dosha	Bhutas	Systems of the body affected	Body activity controlled
Vata	Ether and air	Central nervous system	Breathing, motion, heart beat, nervous impulses
Pitta	Fire and water	Digestion, metabolism, endocrine function	Body temperature, energy levels
Kapha	Water and earth	Immune system, secretions	Wound healing, memory retention, production of secretions

Table 36.3 A summary of constitutional characteristics associated with different *dosha*.

Dosha	Body characteristics
Vata	Lean build, with cool, dry and occasionally rough skin. These types often have small dark eyes and dark, curly hair. They may have a poor appetite, but variable thirst and are often mentally restless. They have a tendency to be emotionally insecure and unpredictable, lots of nervous energy, a fast mode of speech and poor, often interrupted sleep patterns
Pitta	Tend towards a medium build, with soft, warm skin, sharp (often grey or green) eyes and fair, sometimes oily hair. They have a good appetite (sometimes excessive) and are often thirsty. They tend towards sharp, aggressively intelligent mentality, causing a short temper and irritability. They have a strong method of speech, a moderate exercise level, but require little sleep, as it is always very sound
Kapha	Can be overweight, with cool, slightly oily skin. These types often have big blue eyes and thick hair. Often they have a low appetite for food or liquids, and tend to have a calm, considerate mentality. Emotionally they are calm and acquisitive, and tend to think carefully before they speak. They have an aversion to exercise and tend to have deep and lengthy sleep patterns

summarizes how the *bhutas* combine to form each of the *dosha*, and how each *dosha* affects the human body.

It should be noted the *tridosha* govern basic human emotions such as fear, anger and greed, and are involved in more complex emotions such as empathy, compassion and love. It is thought that when the *tridosha* are in equilibrium, the body and mind are healthy and a sense of well-being exists within a person. It is difficult to draw similarities between this philosophy and modern science, but most readers will agree that a sense of well-being exists in most of us when we are rested, well-fed and exercised.

Prakruti is a description of the human constitution—the 'type' of person you are. It is believed the individual's *prakruti* is determined by the parents' *prakruti* at the time of conception. A *vaid* can analyse a patient's constitution by looking at how his or her *tridosha* combine. Most people are a combination of *dosha* elements, and can be described as *vata-pitta* or *pitta-kapha* for instance. Table 36.3 shows the *dosha* characteristics associated with different parts of the human constitution.

As well as the *vata*, *pitta* and *kapha* type of personalities, three attributes provide the basis for distinctions in human temperament, individual differences and psychological and moral dispositions. These basic attributes are *satva*, *rajas* and *tamas*. In brief, *satva* expresses essence, understanding, purity, clarity, compassion and love; *rajas* describes movement, aggressiveness and extroversion; and *tamas* manifests in ignorance, inertia, heaviness and dullness.

Agni is known as the 'digestive fire' and governs metabolic processes. It is essentially *pitta* in nature. *Agni* can become impaired by an imbalance in the *tridosha* and therefore affect metabolism. In these circumstances, food will not be digested or absorbed properly, and toxins will be produced in the intestines and may find their way into the circulation.

Ama are the waste products of the body—faeces, urine and sweat—and are the root cause of disease. Their appearance and properties can give many indications of the state of the *tridosha* and therefore health.

For example, a patient suffering from a *pitta* disorder, such as fever or jaundice, may have dark urine. Additionally, substances such as coffee and tea, which stimulate urination, also aggravate *pitta* and render the urine dark yellow. If a patient has overactive *ama* production, the overcombustion of nutrients may occur, leading to *vata* disorders and emaciation (e.g. overactive thyroid).

Dhatus are the seven tissues or organs of which the human body is composed. Therefore any imbalance in the *tridosha* directly affects the *dhatus*. *Dhatus* are those substances that are retained in the body and always rejuvenated or replenished. The *dhatus* do not correspond to our definition of anatomy, but are more a tissue type than an individual organ. Table 36.4 provides an approximate relationship between *dhatus* and parts of the body.

Gunas Charaka, author of the *Charaka Samhita*, wrote that all material, both organic and inorganic, as well as thought and action, have 'attributes'—qualities that contain potential energy, while the actions with which they are associated express kinetic energy. This is possibly the first reference to the concept of potential and kinetic energy. *Vata*, *pitta* and *kapha* each have their own attributes, and substances having similar attributes will tend to aggravate the related bodily humour. Table 36.5 gives a brief summary of the three *gunas*.

Table 36.4 The Sanskrit name for each of the seven *dhatus* and the tissues or organs with which they are associated.

Dhatu	Associated organ or tissue
Rasa	Nutritional fluid: plasma
Rakta	Blood: life force
Mamsa	Muscles: cover bones
Meda	Adipose tissue: lubrication
Asthi	Bone: help to stand and walk
Majja	Bone marrow: nerve tissue nourishment
Shukra	Testes/ovaries: reproduction

Table 36.5 A summary of the three *Gunas* and their effects upon the body.

Guna	Definition	Effects
Sattva	Essence/subtle	Provision of necessary energy for the body without taxing it
Raja	Activity	Sensuality, sexuality, greed, avarice, fantasies, egotism
Tamas	Inertia/gross	Dullness, drowsiness, pessimism, lack of common sense, laziness, doubt

PRINCIPLES OF AYURVEDA

In addition to the in-depth analysis of a patient's *prakruti* that a *vaid* will undertake to diagnose the patient's ailment, astrological considerations and karma must also be considered. Finally a thorough medical examination, not dissimilar to that undertaken by a TCM practitioner, including the appearance of the tongue, properties of the urine, sweat, sputum and faeces will also be carried out. Once the *vaid* has ascertained the disease and the likely cause of the problem, a complex treatment regimen will be prescribed. As health can be maintained by taking steps to keep *vata-pitta-kapha* in balance through a proper diet, herbal treatment and exercise programme, this is likely to be the first line of action. The concepts governing the pharmacology, therapeutics and food preparation in Ayurveda are based on the action and reaction of the *gunas* to and upon one another. Through understanding of these *gunas*, the balance of the tridosha can be maintained. The diseases and disorders ascribed to *vata, pitta* and *kapha* are treated with the aid of medicines possessing the opposite attribute, to try and correct the deficiency or excess. Many of the medicines prescribed in Ayurvedic medicine are herbs and patients may have to take them as medicines (tinctures, inhalations, pills, capsules or powders) or by combining them into their diet in a prescribed fashion. Table 36.6 provides a brief summary of the herb types used to treat different *dosha*-related illnesses.

Rasayana—widely used herbs

Rasayana (literal translation 'longevity enhancer') are remedies considered to have diverse action and, therefore, affect many systems of the body leading to a positive effect on health—panaceas in other words. The most important are summarized in a Table 36.7 and are included in many recipes to strengthen the tissues of the body. In general, modern research has found them to have antioxidant, immunomodulating and various other activities.

Table 36.6 A summary of herb classes used to treat different *dosha*-related illnesses.

Dosha-related illness	Herbs types used
Vata	Sweet (*madhur*), sour (*amla*) or warm (*lavana*)
Pitta	Sweet (*madhur*), bitter (*katu*) or astringent and cooling (*kashaya*)
Kapha	Pungent (*tikta*), bitter (*katu*) or astringent and dry (*kashaya*)

Preparation of Ayurvedic medicines

In addition to the rasayanas, many other herbs are used in Ayurvedic medicines. Table 36.8 summarizes some of the best documented. Readers should consider that although documented clinical evidence for the activity of some of these herbs can be fairly scarce, practising *vaids* stress the importance of the *combinations* of the herbs—suggesting a synergistic effect between them. Indeed, the main principles that guide Ayurvedic medicinal formulation are: synergy, opposition, enhancement, protection and, as always in holistic systems, balance. Each of these principles is summarized below:

- *Synergy* is the enhancement of the effectiveness of herbs and minerals with similar or complementary action, when combined together.
- *Opposition* is the counterbalancing of an undesirable effect of a herb or mineral by adding another ingredient with the opposite action.
- *Enhancement* is the promotion of the efficacy of the main ingredient, by either increasing its activity or its absorption, by the addition of other ingredients to a formulation.
- *Protection* describes when the potential toxicity of a formula is reduced, by adding mild laxatives or diuretics that promote elimination.
- *Balance* describes when the antagonistic actions of different constituents of a formula are considered to counteract each other.

The preparation of Ayurvedic medicines follows the general Ayurvedic philosophy that emphasizes the whole; that is, substances are combined in such a way that their natural attributes synergistically enhance the action of the whole formula. Traditional formulae are often named, and may denote a specific combination of herbs and other products prepared in a prescribed way, or instead, for their major ingredient(s). In some instances, the name denotes the person who first devised the formula, the therapeutic action of the medicine, or the part of the plant used. For example, *Triphala* powder is a mixture of powders of three fruits—*amla, baheda* and *hirda*—whilst *Chyavanprash* is a semi-solid formulation named after a sage, '*Chyavan*', who first devised the formula.

Preparative methods

As discussed previously, single drugs are rarely used in Ayurvedic practice. The formulations usually contain heterogeneous mixtures of herbs and minerals that have undergone a complex process of purification and preparation. Traditional methods used to prepare Ayurvedic drugs are based on the principles of extraction, concentration and purification, and the choice of preparation method depends on the part of the plant to be used, on its condition (fresh or dried), and on the drug's expected use. For example, cold decoctions are preferred for conditions attributed to an excess of pitta. Table 36.9 gives a summary of some of the most common methods of preparation of herbal material used to produce Ayurvedic medicines. For a more extensive list of herbal ingredients of Asian medicine in general, covering 97 families of plants, see M. Aslam, in the 15th edition of this book, p. 471.

36

Table 36.7 Summarizing the Rasayana herbs most commonly used in Ayurvedic medicinal combinations.

Botanical name	Ayurvedic name	Medicinal use	Clinical evidence
Asparagus racemosa Indian asparagus	*Shatavari*	Tonic, rejuvenative, aphrodisiac, laxative, antispasmodic, antacid, diuretic, antitumor	Constituents isolated from the raw plant, showed increased white cell production in human bone marrow. (Kanitkar et al., J. Res. Ind. Med., 1969; 32)
Emblica officinalis Indian gooseberry	*Amla*	Improves memory and intelligence, tonic, demulcent	*E. officinalis* can heal indomethacin-induced stomach ulceration in rats by their antioxidant action and ability to form mucus. (Bhattacharya et al., J. Clin. Biochem. Nutr., 2007; **41**(2): 106–114)
Piper longum Indian long pepper	*Pimpli*	Antioxidant, digestive stimulant, carminative, expectorant, bronchodilator, anthelmintic, analgesic, circulatory stimulant, aphrodisiac	*In vitro* antioxidant activity of *Piper longum*. (Agbor et al., J. Herb. Pharmacother., 2007; **7**(2): 49–64)
Terminalia chebula Ink nut Black myrobalan	*Haritaki*	Mild laxative, glucose regulator, tonic, alterative, adaptogen, hepatoprotective, antispasmodic, expectorant, antiasthmatic, antiviral and hypoglycaemic, haemorrhoids, dental caries, bleeding gums, ulcerated oral cavity	Chebulagic acid, isolated from *Terminalia chebula*, proved to be a reversible and non-competitive inhibitor of maltase, showing a use for chebulagic acid in managing type-2 diabetes. (Gao et al., Biosci. Biotechnol. Biochem., 2008; **72**: 601–603)
Tinospora cordifolia Heart-leaved moonseed	*Guduchi*	Detoxifier, antioxidant, breaks down exogenous and endogenous toxins, improves comprehension, memory and recollection	Validation of therapeutic claims of *Tinospora cordifolia*: a review promotes regeneration of the liver against CCl$_4$ induced hepatotoxicity. (Panchabhai et al., Phytother. Res., 2007; in press doi:10.1002/ptr.2347)
Withania somnifera Winter cherry	*Ashwagandha*	Analgesic, improves blood glucose control, sedative, rejuvenator, asthma, uterine sedative, relaxant and antispasmodic effects on intestinal, uterine, bronchial, tracheal and blood-vessel muscles	Increases cells capacity to utilise glucose. (Anwer et al., Basic Clin. Pharmacol. Toxicol., 2008; doi:10.1111/j.1742)

Table 36.8 Some important herbs of Ayurveda and their uses.

Botanical name	Ayurvedic name	Effect on dosha	Medical use
Acorus calamus Sweet flag	*Vacha*	Pacifies *vata* and *kapha*	Nerve stimulant, digestive
Adhatoda vasica Malabar nut	*Vasaka*	Pacifies *pitta* and *kapha*	Respiratory disorders, fevers
Aegle marmelos Bengal quince	*Bael, Bel*	Promotes *pitta*	Reduces symptoms of dysentery, digestive, tonic
Andrographis paniculata King of bitters	*Kalmegh*	Pacifies *kapha* and *pitta*	Hepatoprotective properties, jaundice
Eclipta alba Trailing eclipta	*Bhringarajah*	Pacifies *kapha* and *pitta*	Skin and hair disorders
Embelia ribes Embelia	*Viranga*	Pacifies *kapha* and *vata*	Antihelmintic, contraceptive
Nigella sativa Black cumin	*Kalonji*	Pacifies *vata* and *kapha*	Digestive, antiseptic
Ocimum sanctum Sweet basil	*Tulsi*	Pacifies *kapha* and *vata*	Expectorant, febrifuge, immunomodulator
Phyllanthus niruri Stone breaker	*Bhumyamlaki*	Pacifies *kapha* and *pitta*	Diabetes, jaundice, liver protectant

Table 36.8   Some important herbs of Ayurveda and their uses. (Cont'd)

Botanical name	Ayurvedic name	Effect on dosha	Medical use
Picrorrhiza kurroa Kutki, yellow gentian	*Katurohini*	Pacifies *kapha* and *pitta*	Hepatoprotective, immunomodulator
Piper nigrum Black pepper	*Kalmirch*	Pacifies *vata* and *pitta*	Digestive, respiratory disorders
Swertia chirata Chiretta	*Chirayita*	Balances *tridosha*	Appetite stimulant, liver disorders
Terminalia arjuna Arjun myrobalan	*Arjuna*	Pacifies *pitta* and *kapha*	Heart tonic, angina, hypertension
Tribulus terrestris Caltrops	*Gokhru*	Pacifies *vata* and *pitta*	Digestive, diuretic, aphrodisiac

Table 36.9   Methods of preparing Ayurvedic medicines.

Formulation	Method of production
Juice (*Swaras*)	Cold-pressed plant juice
Powder (*Churna*)	Shade-dried, powdered plant material
Cold infusion (*Sita kasaya*)	Herb : water 1 : 6, macerated overnight and filtered
Hot infusion (*Phanta*)	Herb : water 1 : 4, steeped for a few minutes and filtered
Decoction (*Kathva*)	Herb : water 1 : 4 (or 8, 16 then reduced to 1 : 4) boiled
Poultice (*Kalka*)	Plant material pulped
Milk extract (*Ksira paka*)	Plant boiled in milk and filtered

Shodhana (purification) is the process by which toxic substances are purified; that is, rendered less toxic. For example, detoxification of mercury involves a drawn-out process of heating and cooling the mercury salt, grinding it and then suspending and re-suspending the substance in a variety of liquids. Specific products that facilitate the process are added at each stage of preparation and the instructions might call for the use of a specific vessel at different stages of preparation. The instructions can be so detailed, up to the point of stating from which direction the heat is to be applied. It is left to the experience of Ayurvedic practitioners to decide, at the conclusion of an appropriate purification process, that the toxic substances are no longer poisonous but therapeutic. From this brief summary, it can be seen that the classical Ayurvedic methods of preparation are complex and tedious, and that short-cuts in preparation may make a significant difference in the efficacy and safety of the resulting product. Because of this, it may be beyond the scope of the average scientific paper to exactly describe the method by which an herb is prepared, especially if a formula is used, which may go some way as to explaining why such problems exist in replicating the results of other researchers.

Further reading

Chattopadhyaya D (ed) 1982 Case for a critical analysis of the Charaka Samhita. In: Studies in the history of science in India, Vol 1. New Delhi: Editorial Enterprises, pp 209–236
Kapoor LD 1990 Handbook of Ayurvedic medicinal plants. CRC Press, Boca Raton, FL
Lad V 1990 Ayurveda the science of self-healing. Lotus Press, Wisconsin, USA
Puri HS 2003 Rasayana Ayurvedic herbs for longevity and rejuvenation. In: Hardman RH (series ed) Traditional herbal medicine for modern times. Taylor and Francis, London
Rankin-Box D, Williamson EM 2006 Herbal medicine, phytotherapy and nutraceuticals. In: Complementary medicines, a guide for pharmacists. Churchill Livingstone, Edinburgh, pp 52–68
Sairam TV 2000 Home remedies, Vols I, II and III. Penguin, Mumbai, India
Williamson EM (ed) 2002 Major herbs of Ayurveda. The Dabur Foundation, Churchill Livingstone, Edinburgh

37

Chinese herbs in the West

S. Y. Mills

Herbs are used for health care in China more than either Western drugs or acupuncture. If their use in other countries with Chinese influence is taken into account, they form probably the largest tradition of health care in the world.

There is now an increasing use of Chinese herbs outside China and Asia, notably in the USA and the UK. Interest has been expressed within medical circles at cases where the use of Chinese medicine appears to have had dramatic benefits. The following presents a summary of the current status of the use of Chinese herbalism in the West.

HISTORICAL BACKGROUND

Chinese herbal medicine has a strikingly persistent tradition, surviving cultural and dynastic revolutions, with classic texts being preserved as living guides for physicians up to the present day. The earliest known text was unearthed in Hunnan province and dates from the fourth century BC. It lists over 200 herbs, with instructions for 52 pharmaceutical preparations. In around 250 BC, a herbal compendium, the *Pen Tsao Ching* was written in the name of the legendary Emperor Shen Nung, who was said to have lived 5000 years previously. Other still widely used established classics include a commentary on the previous text, the *Shen Nung Pen Tsao Ching Chi Chu* from around the fifth century AD, and the *Hsin Hsiu Pen Tsao* (New Revised *Materia Medica*), written in AD 659. More recent texts include the sixteenth-century *Pen Tsao Kang Mu,* in 52 volumes and containing over 11 000 prescriptions.

In 1977, the Chinese government published a *materia medica* listing almost 6000 herbs and other pharmacological compounds of natural origin. In 1985, in their Drug Administration Law, 8800 patent herbal drugs were identified as requiring re-evaluation. In 1994, an Essential Drug List (of which about 50% would be covered by health insurance) contained almost 1700 herbal drugs.

THERAPEUTIC PRINCIPLES

The approach of traditional Chinese medicine (TCM) is significantly different from that of modern orthodox medicine. Without the modern technology that has allowed isolation of pathogens and pathologies, it developed strategies for understanding and correcting an illness from the broader experience of its impact and associations. There was less opportunity to focus on or directly treat a specific disease entity. Rather, traditional medicine sought to avert adverse influences and to promote normal healthy function so as to help the person eliminate or resist these influences. It was more an interaction with the body's functions than, as in the modern case, with pathologies (that are usually the end-result of dysfunctions).

The underlying principles of Chinese medicine often appear to the Western observer to be wrapped in vague or mystical notions. However, such prejudices arise from the nineteenth-century Western view of the world as clockwork mechanisms. As modern science begins to appreciate the complexities of living systems, it has rediscovered principles that may be consistent with the oriental insights.

The *yin* and *yang* concepts are obvious examples where speculative entities are seen to substitute for empirical data. This disquiet may be diminished, however, if they are instead seen as means of classifying the experience of constant change. The *yang* is the active aspect of any phenomenon, the dispersive, centrifugal, transforming and expansive. Such descriptors are similar to those ascribed to chaotic tendencies in complex dynamic systems. The *yin* is the substantive or nourishing aspect of any phenomenon, the condensing, centripetal, sustaining and preserving. The tendencies to ordered behaviour in dynamic systems have similar qualities.

In the language of complex dynamic systems, life is seen to exist at the edge of chaos, maintaining maximum adaptibility and creativity by balancing static orderliness and turbulent chaos, and avoiding extremes of either. The essential endeavour of the Chinese physician is to restore the balance of the body, the *yin* nourishment and *yang* activity. Obviously this is done in terms of clinical symptoms rather than as an abstract philosophical construct.

The *yin–yang* polarities are imbued with shifting temporal and spatial relationships. At any position or in any event there will always be a blend of the active and the substantial, a blend that is always shifting in time and when viewed from different perspectives. To take a simple example: in the West, a table is an object, fixed and substantial. In the Chinese view that structure is merely in a transitory substantial, *yin*, phase: it also forms a relationship with the people who use it and has an influence on the room in which it stands. Moreover, these active, *yang*, aspects of its existence determine when its *yin* aspect changed from being a tree, and when it changes again to a heap of ash or a children's playhouse! Thus, each table becomes a different entity to each individual human being and at each moment in time, its active aspect always reflecting the position of its substantial and vice versa: it becomes an experience.

Similarly, any symptom of ill health might either be the mark of excessive activity (*yang*) in a system or alternatively relative stasis or congestion (*yin*). In the first case, treatment would concentrate on encouraging the nutritive, assimilative and/or calming influences in the body, mind or spirit; in the second there would need to be a degree of stimulation or mobilization. The art of diagnosis was to distinguish between the two radically different scenarios; the art of medicine to develop appropriate strategies for the particular system defect.

Other polarities would be taken into account (heat versus cold, internal origins versus external, deficient constitutions versus the highly charged, and so on) along with a good number of other qualitative markers of the interior climate. One early view, for example, was that chronic diseases arose when external pathogenic influences drove deeper and deeper into the body. Treatment therefore required that the pathogenic influence was best intercepted at the surface, that is, at its most acute (even alarming, often febrile) stage, to prevent the development of more intractable 'embedded' pathologies. Treatment strategies would be quite different at each stage of penetration.

Another Chinese fundamental is the concept of an underlying energy in all phenomena, as a motive force and determining principle. They did not measure *qi* as calorific or electrical energy. Instead, *qi* is appreciated and judged by ordinary experience, and indeed for this reason is clearly felt as tangible. *Qi* is thus an energetic construct implicit in, and defined by, its outcomes, i.e. by events. It is therefore manifest in all movement and is itself in movement, constantly transforming itself into relatively *yang* and *yin* aspects.

In physiological terms, *qi* was often subdivided into fluids of different densities, some visible and some not. One of the substantial or *yin* aspects of *qi*, for example, is blood or *xue*. Although this was obviously the same fluid as understood anywhere else it also had other qualities. *Xue* can be appreciated as incorporating both what the West knows as blood and the subjective effect of that fluid, warming, pulsing and nourishing. It can also be seen as a deeper, slower, more profound or tangible response to change than other *qi*, a response that is, by definition, also slower to reverse. For example, it may be manifested as long-term physiological responses or the organic change that leads to observable pathologies. Incidentally, in this context herbal medicines were seen to be more effective in moving *xue* (the more substantial shifts in body function) than acupuncture.

The Chinese view of organ function is also quite distinct, derived from induced insights of clinical presentations and the meridianal connections applied in acupuncture. Thus, *gan*, the liver, has the function of distributing energies around the body, governing muscle and sinew activity and eyesight, and is particularly disturbed by emotional distress, particularly anger and frustration. The spleen, *pi*, is responsible for assimilative functions, notably digestion, and for maintaining the integrity of the tissues and circulation, but also includes emotional assimilation as manifested in empathy, maternalism and nurturing. (These notions of concentric repetition of patterns, so that activity at a physical level is manifested also at psychological, emotional, spiritual or even social levels now resonates with one of the mathematical principles of complex system analysis, the fractal, where a pattern is repeated through infinite levels of scale.)

The Chinese herbs were classified according to their perceived ability to affect any of these manifestations of the living body. These classifications are used in Table 37.1, which lists some of the most widely used Chinese herbs in the West. Herbs were also characterized pharmacologically in terms of their taste: bitter, sweet, acrid, salty and sour, this being seen to denote particular properties. Some of the conclusions drawn about such properties can now be supported with modern knowledge of the action of the archetypal plant constituents involved (Mills and Bone, 'Further reading').

It is useful to compare modern and Chinese medical approaches. Faced, for example, with excessive bowel activity, modern physicians would apply diagnostic techniques to eliminate observable pathologies like diverticulitis, dysentery or ulceration, and then lump anything less tangible as 'irritable bowel', with an implicit psychological cause. The traditional Chinese physician would assess the nature of the symptoms, their chronicity, severity and other qualities and correspondences, and might then conclude that the problem was the result of either sluggish digestive metabolism, unwholesome diet, suppressed anger, emotional disruption of assimilative functions, one or more various forms of debility, cold in the stomach or in the bowel, imbalance of heat and cold in the body, damp heat (e.g. hepatic disease), or digestive imbalances. The presence of blood or mucus in the stool, deep persisting pain or wider debility would immediately signify a deep-seated (*xue'*, *yin*) disturbance requiring particularly nurturing treatment (see Porkert, 1983, 'Further reading'). The treatments adopted in each case would be completely different.

Another result of the longevity of Chinese herbal medicine, however, is its reliance on accumulated traditional practices rather than on innovation. Thus, well-established and revered formulae of medicines are more widely used than individual herbs. The mixtures are thought to benefit from interactions between the ingredients that extend the breadth of activities, improve tolerability or potentiate one or more particular effects. These claims have been almost impossible to substantiate in any controlled study. Nevertheless, it is also doubtful whether formulations developed to deal with the diseases of medieval China have the same application to the health priorities of the developed West. Although there is undoubtedly a great deal of favourable human experience of the standard formulations, without controlled clinical scrutiny and the application of clear quality standards for all the many ingredients, it is impossible to verify their value in the modern context.

The adherence to classic texts and precedent rather than assertive enquiry is an essential feature of Chinese medicine, and indeed traditional medicine as a whole. Much that is handed down from Chinese medical history is dogma: there is little sign of a tradition of radical reappraisal, of 'individual seekers after truth'. But this is true of all early traditions. In their struggle for survival, early humans prospered in relation to the fitness of their behaviour to their circumstances. They learned from their elders (who had by definition so prospered) and were justly cautious about reckless questioning.

Table 37.1 Chinese herbs widely used in the West classified by traditional therapeutic activity.

Botanical name	Part used	Action	Constituents
Warming remedies releasing exterior conditions			
Ephedra sinica Stapf	Herb	Diaphoretic, antiasthmatic, diuretic	Ephedrine and related alkaloids
Perilla frutescens L.	Leaves, stem	Diaphoretic, digestive stimulant	Essential oils (including limonene, apinene), perillaidehyde
Angelica dahurica Bentham & Hooker	Root	Diaphoretic, antiseptic, analgesic	Furanocoumarins, angelic acids
Ligusticum sinense Oliver	Root	Diaphoretic, antirheumatic	Essential oil, cnidilide
Zingiber officinale Roscoe	Rhizome	Diaphoretic, antiemetic, expectorant	Zingiberene, shogaol, gingerol, zingiberone, zingiberol
Cooling remedies releasing exterior conditions			
Mentha arvensis L.	Herb	Febrifuge	Essential oil (menthol, menthone, etc.)
Pueraria pseudohirsuta Tang & Weng	Root	Diaphoretic, analgesic, febrifuge, vasodilator	Isoflavones (including daidzein), puerarin
Bupleurum falcatum L.	Root, herb	Febrifuge, digestive tonic, relaxant	Saponins (including saikosaponin, daikogenin)
Cimicifuga foetida L.	Rhizome	Diaphoretic, detoxifier	Triterpenoid (including dahurinol), cimicifugoside, cimicifugin, visnagin
Purgatives			
Rheum palmatum L.	Root	Laxative, choleretic, detoxifier	Anthraquinones (including rhein, emodin)
Cooling remedies			
Anemarrhena asphodeloides Bunge	Rhizome	Febrifuge, anti-inflammatory, antiasthmatic	Steroidal saponins (including timosaponin, sarsapogenin)
Gardenia jasminoides Ellis	Fruit	Febrifuge, sedative, detoxifier, choleretic	Iridoid glycosides (including gardenin, genipin, gardenoside, crocetin)
Trichosanthes kirilowii Maximowicz	Root	Anti-inflammatory, detoxifier, increasing mucosal secretions	Saponins
Camellia sinensis Kuntze	Leaves	Anti-inflammatory, choleretic	Xanthines
Remedies cooling gan (liver function)			
Cassia tora L.	Seeds	Laxative, sedative, ophthalmic remedy	Anthraquinones (including emodin, chrysophanol, rhein), mucilage
Remedies cooling xue (blood)			
Paeonia suffruticosa Andrews	Bark	Antipyrexic, vasostimulant, antitoxaemic	Paeonolide, paeonoside, paeonoflorin, tannins
Cooling and drying remedies			
Scutellaria baicalensis Georgi	Root	Bitter digestive, choleretic, detoxifier, haemostatic	Flavonoid glycosides (including balcalein, baicalin, woogonin)
Coptis chinensis Franchet	Rhizome	Bitter digestive, choleretic, sedative	Alkaloids (including herberine, columbamine, coptisine, palmatine)
Phellodendron amurensei Ruprecht	Bark	Bitter digestive, choleretic, detoxifier, febrifuge, tonic	Alkaloids (including berberine, palmatine, phellodendrine), triterpenoids, sterols
Sophora flavescens Aiton	Root	Bitter digestive, choleretic, diuretic, antipruritic	Alkaloids (including matrine, sophoranol), flavonoids
Gentiana scabra Bunge	Root	Bitter digestive, choleretic, urinary antiseptic, anxiolytic	Gentianine, gentiopicrin, gentisin
Cooling and disinfecting remedies			
Lonicera japonica Thunberg	Flowers	Antipyretic, detoxifier	Luteolin, tannin
Forsythia suspensa Vahl	Fruit	Anti-infective, antipyretic, urinary antiseptic, anti-inflammatory	Saponins, flavonoids
Taraxacum mongolicum Handel-Mazetti	Whole plant	Anti-infective, antipyretic, choleretic	Bitter principles, taraxasterol
Aromatic remedies transforming damp			
Agastache rugosa Fischer & Meyer	Herb	Digestive stimulant, antiemetic	Essential oil (including anethole, methyichavicol, limonene, pinene)
Atracyloides lancea Thunberg	Rhizome	Digestive stimulant, antirheumatic	Essential oil (including atracylol, atracylone, atracylin)
Magnolia officinalisi Rehder & Wilson	Bark	Digestive stimulant, expectorant	Magnolol, essential oil (including eudesmol) alkaloids (including magnocurarine, magnoflorine)
Amomum cardomomum L.	Fruit	Antiemetic, digestive stimulant, expectorant, antinausea	Essential oil (including camphor, borneol)
Inula britannica L.	Root	Expectorant, antinausea	Essential oil (including camphor, alantol, alantoic acid), bitter principles (including lactones), triterpenes

Diuretic remedies			
Poria cocos Wolff	Fungus sclerotium	Diuretic, sedative	Triterpenes, polysaccharides
Alisma plantago aquatica L.	Rhizome	Diuretic	Alisol, triterpenes, resin
Artemisia capillaris Thunberg	Herb	Diuretic, choleretic	Essential oil (including pinene, capillene), esculetin, scoparone
Coix lachryma jobi L.	Seed	Diuretic, antidiarrhoeal, antirheumatic	Coixol, starches
Remedies expelling wind and damp			
Chaenomeles sinensis (Thouin) Koehne	Fruit	Spasmolytic, anticramping, diuretic	Saponins, flavonoids, tannins
Acanthopanax gracilistylus W.W. Smith	Root bark	Antirheumatic, diuretic	Salicylates
Remedies warming the interior			
Cinnamomum cassia Blume	Bark	Diaphoretic, circulatory stimulant	Essential oil (including cinnamic aldehyde), resin
Eugenia caryophyllata Thunberg	Flowers	Antiemetic, digestive stimulant, circulatory stimulant	Essential oil (including eugenol, caryophylene)
Sedative remedies			
Biota orientalis (L.) Enlicher	Seeds	Sedative, aperient	Essential oil, fatty oil
Sedative remedies calming gan (liver function)			
Gastrodia elata Blume	Rhizome	Spasmolytic, sedative, antirheumatic	Vanillyl alcohol, vanillin
Uncaria rynchophyllai (Miguel) Jackson	Stems with hooks	Spasmolytic, antipyretic	Alkaloids (including rhynchophylline, hirsutine)
Remedies regulating qi			
Citrus tangerina Hort & Tanaka	Peel	Carminative, expectorant	Essential oil (including limonene, linalool), carotene
Lindera strychnifolium Villars	Root	Carminative, reducing urinary irritation, antidysmenorrhoeic	Essential oil (including borneol, linderane, linderalactone)
Remedies moving xue (blood)			
Ligusticum wallachii Franchet	Rhizome	Circulatory stimulant, analgesic, menstrual regulator	Essential oil (including cnidium lactone)
Carthamus tinctorius L.	Flowers	Circulatory stimulant, analgesic, menstrual regulator	Carthamin
Achyranthes bidentata Blume	Root	Circulatory stimulant, tonic	Saponins, insect-moulting hormone (ecdysterone, inokosterone)
Prunus persica (L.) Batsch.	Seed	Circulatory stimulant, aperient, antitussive	Cyanogenic glycosides (including amygdalin)
Remedies transforming phlegm and stopping coughs			
Platycodon grandiflorum (Jacqain) de Candolle	Root	Expectorant, antiseptic	Saponins, sterols
Cooling remedies transforming hot phlegm			
Peucedanum praeruptorum Dunn	Root	Expectorant, antiasthmatic	Coumarins
Antitussives			
Eriobotryajaponica Lindley	Flowers	Expectorant, antitussive, antiemetic	Essential oil, cyanogenic glycosides (including amygdalin)
Remedies tonifying qi			
Panax ginseng C. A. Meyer	Root	Tonic, sedative	Saponins (including ginsenosides), panax acid, glycosides (including panaxin, panaquilin, ginsenin) sterols
Astragalus membranaceus (Fischer) Bunge	Root	Tonic, immune stimulant, diuretic	Sterols, betaine, astragalin
Atractyloides macrocephala Koidzumi	Rhizome	Tonic, digestive stimulant, diuretic	Atractylone
Zizyphus jujuba Muller	Seed	Tonic, sedative, digestive stimulant	Triterpenes
Glycyrrhiza uralensis Fischer	Root	Tonic, spasmolytic, expectorant, pharmaceutical moderator	Saponins (including glycyrrhizin), flavonoids (including liquiritin)

(Continued)

Table 37.1 Chinese herbs widely used in the West classified by traditional therapeutic activity. (Cont'd)

Botanical name	Part used	Action	Constituents
Remedies tonifying yang			
Trigonella foenum-graecum L.	Seed	Tonic, spasmolytic, warming	Alkaloids (including trigonelline), steroidal saponins (including diosgenin), mucilage
Eucommia ulmoides Oliver	Bark	Tonic	Resin, gutta-percha
Remedies tonifying xue			
Rehmannia glutinosa (Gaertner) Liboschitz	Prepared root, rhizome	Tonic	Iridoid glycosides (including catalpol), rehmannin, mannitol, sterols
Angelica sinensis (Oliver) Diels	Root	Tonic, menstrual regulator, aperient	Essential oil (including carvacrol, safrol), furanocoumarins
Paeonia lactiflora Pallas	Root	Tonic, analgesic, spasmolytic	Paeoniflorin, paeonol
Remedies tonifying yin			
Lycium chinense Miller	Bark	Tonic, antiasthmatic, antitubercular	Solanaceous alkaloids, betaine, physaline, carotene
Asparagus cochinensis (Loureiro) Merrill	Root	Tonic, expectorant, aperient	Asparagin, mucilage, sterols
Ophiopogon japonicus (Thunberg) Ker-Gawler	Root	Tonic, sedative, antitussive	Saponins, mucilage
Codonopsis pilosula Franch	Root	Tonic	Saponin, alkaloids, mucilage

Such survival imperatives, however, no longer apply in the a modern Western context. It is now necessary for the potential of Chinese herbal remedies to be assessed more rigorously and with reference to the undoubted benefits of modern Western medical techniques. It is otherwise too easy to characterize the new Western interest in Chinese herbal medicine as a romantic retreat.

CHINESE HERBAL MEDICINE IN WESTERN PRACTICE

The use of Chinese herbs has continued in traditional manner by physicians and pharmacists serving Chinese communities around the world. In many major Western cities, the Chinatown districts support many herb shops and practices, with remedies imported diectly from Asia and practitioners trained by the old system of apprenticeship. Much of this activity has remained closed to Westerners, although this has changed in recent years as the remedies have become better known and demand for treatment has increased. In recent years, there has been a proliferation of Chinese herb shops in towns and shopping precincts across the UK. Concerns have been raised about their promotional and labelling activities, given the current state of the law in the UK, and nor have these businesses been involved in steps to statutorily register herbal practitioners (see Herbal Medicine in Britain and Europe: regulation and practice). The traditional separation between Chinese and western cultures within western countries is in this case challenging the legislature.

Chinese herbal medicine is also among the most rapidly growing in popularity of the complementary therapies in the English-speaking Western world. It is particularly applied as a second tier of treatment by Western acupuncturists who, having started with the most accessible Chinese therapy, discover how closely herbs and acupuncture are integrated into clinical practice in China itself. Thus, many of the colleges of acupuncture in the USA and UK have introduced courses in herbalism. At least some of these new courses are rather brief, despite the fact that their graduates face different legislative and professional responsibilities as prescribers of pharmacologically active medicines.

The leading professional group of practitioners of Chinese herbal medicine in the UK is the Register of Traditional Chinese Medicine, which has around 400 members. It provides a 2-year course covering around 300 herbs and 150 classical formulae, a course often taken up by Western acupuncturists, the majority of whom will have received several years of training in that discipline in one of the main acupuncture colleges in the UK. Further postgraduate seminars are available on an occasional basis. Very few Western physicians have been persuaded to prescribe Chinese herbs.

Consultations with practitioners of Chinese herbal medicine average around an hour in the first instance. Treatment will often be combined with acupuncture and advice on diet and exercises (these often based on the Chinese Qi Gong routine). The average cost of a prescription is between £5–8 in a consultation that might cost £40–50 (in 2008). Herbs are traditionally provided as mixtures of individual dried plant parts that patients have to cook or steep themselves at home. This is an involved process in which taste and smell contribute fully to the experience of taking the medicine. For those who are ill-suited to this labour, there is a wide range of patented preparations in coated pill, tablet and recently tincture or capsule form. The diagnostic and therapeutic principles applied are of the 'Eight Principle' approach based on classifications derived from the eight polarities alluded to above: yin–yang, 'cold–hot', 'internal–external', 'full–empty'), which has also been applied as the basis of the TCM acupuncture treatment most widely used in the West.

STATE RECOGNITION: EVIDENCE OF EFFICACY

There is a considerable and growing literature of clinical and other experimental evidence published from China with, however, very much less from Western countries. Much of the evidence cited from China has been of uncontrolled studies, although this is now improving, and the regulatory agencies in North America, Australasia and Europe will not accept Chinese data in support of applications for licensing as medicines. The attitude of such agencies is generally sceptical of the case for such remedies, although there is also widespread acceptance of their pharmacological potential in pharmaceutical development.

In part, the view of the medical establishment is affected by a general unease about the lack of pharmaceutical precision in all herbal remedies. Regulators in the West have been persuaded (reluctantly) that remedies that have been traditionally used among the population have a continuing place in healthcare. What they resist is the prospect of recognizing the claims of 'new' herbal remedies from abroad. In almost all Western countries, therefore, Chinese herbalism is practised without endorsement or recognition from the state. The one notable exception is the state of California, which registers OMDs (Doctors of Oriental Medicine) as practitioners who can legally prescribe herbal remedies, and conducts State examinations with a standard syllabus of around 300 herbs.

Conventionally conducted clinical trials in the West are relatively rare and have not been sufficient to change this climate of scepticism. The case for such a radical challenge to conventional pharmacology is unlikely to be swung without consistent clinical trial evidence showing significant effect over and above the effect of placebo. Unfortunately, for many of the less clinically severe conditions for which Chinese herbalism is now applied in the West, the placebo effect is likely to be considerable. This means that studies have to be larger and particularly well-conducted, and adds another to the many difficulties (like lack of patentability, low retums on investment and the scepticism of ethics committees and potential collaborating physicians) faced in providing such evidence.

Questions of efficacy also raise issues of safety in the conventional view. A substance with pharmacological effect has, by definition, the possibility of a toxicological effect. The claim of proponents of herbal medicine is that in plant remedies the pharmacological effect is a balanced complex of interactions: in those that have stood the test of time this complex has demonstrated a lack of risk, possibly by the synergism of low-level constituents or by the buffering of one constituent with another. There is little evidence of at least acute adverse effects in clinical experience. However, the pharmacotoxicological case is still circumstantial.

Chinese remedies that establish clinical efficacy in clinical trials will suffer the default implication that they will manifest concordant risks until they demonstrate otherwise. Even those who report with enthusiasm the results of a controlled clinical study of the use of a mixture of Chinese herbs in the treatment of persistent atopic eczema of children (M. P. Sheehan et al., Lancet, 1992, 340: 13–17) advised that such herbs should only be prescribed with 6-monthly monitoring of liver and kidney function, and not supplied to women of child-bearing age without contraception and to those with histories of jaundice or alcohol misuse. It is important to note that there has been no follow-up to these important studies, not least because it proved impractical to generate a licensable medicine out of the formalation.

QUALITY OF CHINESE HERBS IN WESTERN MARKETS

All herbal remedies suffer the complications of being crude natural products grown or collected from a wide range of sources. The consumer is protected only by sound industrial practices informed by effective pharmacognostic disciplines. With the rapid increase in demand of Chinese herbs in the West there is undoubtedly greater temptation for suppliers to test the market with whatever they can sell. The faking of Chinese pharmaceuticals in some Asian countries is now suspected to be widespread. There have been serious incidents where adulteration has led to adverse effects, notably in a case in Belgium where adulteration with an *Aristolochia* species (especially *Aristolochia fang-chi*) for *Stephania tetranda* (mandarin name *hang fang ji*) was implicated in an outbreak of kidney failure among patients at a slimming clinic. Over 30 patients sustained terminal kidney failure and a number have since developed kidney cancer. Although the prospect of interaction with the concurrent prescription of diuretics is high, aristolochic acid in *Aristolochia* is known to be moderately nephrotoxic. Unfortunately, this form of substitution has been found to be common and ongoing, and regulators in the UK, Europe and North America have banned not only *Aristolochia* but a number of other remedies, such as *Stephania tetandra* and species of *Clematis* and *Akebia* (either of which may be sold as *mu tong*), as well as some formulae containing the above, because the risk of substitution could not reasonably be ruled out.

The whole incident has cast a serious cloud in the minds of Western regulators over the reliability of herbal medicines imported from China and Asia, and it is likely that there will be other developments. For the practitioner or user of Chinese herbs, problems are most likely in those buying from unfamiliar or small suppliers, especially those providing 'patented' formulations. Fortunately, there are a number of responsible importers in the West, some of whom use Chinese pharmacognostic expertise through their production process, and who favour dealing with State pharmaceutical houses on mainland China where quality regulation is applied. The *Chinese Pharmacopoeia* (Guangdong Science and Technology Fress, Guangzhou) provides quality standards for most of the herbal products available in the West. The best samples of Chinese herbs are among the highest-quality products available on the market. It behoves a potential user to ensure that they seek out such sources.

Further reading

Bensky D, Gamble A 1986 Chinese herbal medicine: materia medica. Eastland Press, Seattle, WA

Bensoussan A, Myers SP 1996 Towards a safer choice: the practice of traditional Chinese medicine in Australia. University of Western Sydney, Campbelltown, New South Wales

Chang H-M, But PP-H 1986 Pharmacology and applications of Chinese materia medica, Vol I and Vol II. World Scientific Publishing, Singapore

Kaptchuk T 1983 The web that has no weaver. Congdon and Weed, New York

Larre Fr.C, Schats J, Rochat de la Vailee E 1986 Survey of traditional Chinese medicine. Institut Ricci, Paris

Mills S 1991 Out of the earth. Viking, London

Mills SY, Bone K 2000 Principles and practice of phytotherapy. Churchill Livingstone, London

Needham J 1956 Science and civilisation in China, Vol 2. Cambridge University Press, Cambridge, UK

Perry LM 1980 Medicinal plants of east and southeast Asia: attributed properties and uses. MIT Press, Cambridge, MA

Porkert M 1974 The theoretical foundations of Chinese medicine. MIT Press, Cambridge, MA

Porkert M 1983 The essentials of Chinese diagnostics. Acta Medicinae Sinensis, Zurich, Switzerland

Unschuld PU 1985 Medicine in China: a history of ideas. University of California Press, CA

Yen K-Y 1992 The illustrated Chinese materia medica: crude and prepared. SMC Publishing Inc, Taipei, Taiwan

38

Plants in African traditional medicine—some perspectives

A. Sofowora

In 1991, the World Health Organization (WHO) redefined traditional medicine (TM) as comprising 'therapeutic practices that have been in existence, often for hundreds of years, before the development and spread of modern scientific medicine and are still in use today. These practices vary widely, in keeping with the social and cultural heritage of different countries'. The practice of TM in Africa, even today, contains considerable mysticism and secrecy. Therefore, the WHO's original definition of TM, coined in the African region in 1976, and which took cognisance of the importance of 'the concept of nature which includes the material world, the sociological environment whether living or dead and the metaphysical forces of the universe' is still valid in Africa.

TRADITIONAL MEDICINE PRACTITIONERS AND THEIR TECHNIQUES

The practitioners of TM in Africa include herbalists, herb sellers, traditional birth attendants, bone setters, diviners, faith healers, traditional surgeons, spiritualists and others. The training of these practitioners is still by an apprenticeship of about 7 years minimum. The content of such training is not standardized. The techniques used in African TM derive from the basic understanding of the aetiology of disease, as conceived by traditional medical practitioners (TMPs), who believe that diseases arise not only from physical ailments and psychological causes (as in Western medicine) but also from astral influences, spiritual causes (due to evil thoughts and machination by enemies), esoteric causes (i.e. originating from the soul or caused by deeds of an individual before reincarnation). Because TMPs in Africa place so much emphasis on supernatural forces, they are consulted not only for sickness but also when misfortunes occur in the family or to an individual, as many such evil omens are ascribed in Africa to supernatural forces. TMPs observe their patients for symptoms and signs but do not perform any pathological examination because they lack training in such techniques. Diagnosis of the disease is made through anamnesis—observation of the patient for signs and symptoms, including visual examination, clinical examination, biological examinations (such as tasting of urine for the presence of sugar in the case of diabetics, or allowing the patient to urinate on the ground and watching for infestation by ants, smelling of sores for putrefaction etc.), divination, which can be by throwing of seeds (Sofowora, 2008) or bones, use of mind-changing plant drugs, use of astronomical signs and analysis of dreams. Although many of these methods can be utilized by TMPs, specializations do occur. The practitioners also refer patients to one another in appropriate cases.

Treatment types in African traditional medicine

African TM provides holistic treatment. The type of treatment varies and is sometimes indicative of the specialization of the practitioner.

Medicaments intended for internal and external application involve the use of vegetable organs (leaves, barks, roots, etc.), latex, resin, etc. Whole or parts of animals (snail, bone, etc.) and mineral substances (alum, kaolin, etc.) are also used. Although the medicine prescribed may contain only a single active item, it is often a multi-component mixture, some of the components of which act as preservatives, flavours or colouring agents. The multi-component preparation also contains ingredients for all the ailments (or symptoms) that need to be removed to restore the patient's balance. In this way, African TM differs from Western medicine, where a patient can receive a prescription of various tablets, capsules, mixtures along with other dosage forms to eradicate a reported case of illness. The medicaments used in African TM can be administered in the form of a liquid (decoctions, oily mixtures, etc.), solid (powders, ointments), semi-solid (balsams, etc.) or gas (steam inhalation, incense, etc.). The only route of drug administration that is absent in TM in Africa is the intravenous (i.v.) route. The other routes are employed though in rather crude forms.

Other types of treatment used in African TM include therapeutic fasting and dieting, hydrotherapy, treatment of burns, dry heat therapy, blood letting (cupping or venesection), bone setting, spinal manipulation, massage, psychotherapy, faith healing (spiritual healing), therapeutic occultism and also obstetric and gynaecological practice.

Surgical operations carried out in African TM include male and female circumcision, tribal marks, whitlow operation, cutting of the umbilical cord, piercing ear-lobes, uvulectomy, tooth abstraction, trephination (or trepanation) and abdominal surgery. Common complications from the various surgical operations include tetanus, meningitis and septicaemia. No anaesthesia or X-ray diagnosis is used for these operative procedures. After each of the operations, the patient is treated with herbs to heal the wound.

Preventive medicine in African TM takes the form of simple hygiene in some cases, or the performance of regular sacrifices against the wrath of those gods, which, it is believed, leads to periodic epidemic diseases like smallpox and plague. However, health education is helping to modify these beliefs. Armlets, medicated rings, waist leather bands or special necklaces or charms are often worn as a preventive measure or talisman. Some charms are also used to prevent car crashes or to ward off evil spells from witchcraft; the efficacy of such preventive care has yet to be proven. Again, education by road safety corps personnel helps to dispel beliefs in charms for preventing road accidents.

Although there are minor differences all over Africa in TM practice, there is considerable similarity because of the closeness of the cultures of the African peoples, especially between neighbouring countries as the geographical barriers are artificial. For example, the sale of herbs is usually in the markets where food items (vegetables, etc.) can be purchased. This is so all over Africa, although a section of a big market may be set aside for herb sellers' stalls.

In divination, bone throwing is done in southern Africa but seed throwing is done in Western and Central Africa. Seven seeds are used in Central Africa, whereas seed throwing of sixteen or eight seeds is used in Western Africa. The divination process involves, in all cases, the interpretation of the arrangement of the elements (seeds or bones) after being thrown on the ground by the TMP in order to predict or divine on a particular complaint or situation for the patient. These practices continue despite education, and diviners are consulted both by the educated elite as well as by the illiterate.

Ethnopharmacological themes, as illustrated by sub-Saharan art objects and utensils, have been discussed in an illustrated article by De Smet (1998).

Scientific evidence supporting some practices and remedies in African traditional medicine

Attempts have been made by scientists to justify or rationalize, on a scientific basis, many aspects of the practice of the African TMP. Some of these practices are inexplicable, whereas others, like the use of many of the herbs, can be rationalized.

Plants of *Ageratum conyzoides* L. collected at night are used to treat children who cry too often for no known cause, especially at night. Night collection of this herb is particularly indicated when the frequent crying is suspected to be due to the influence of witchcraft, or to persistent disturbance from the spirits of the child's playmates (dead or alive), thus requiring the use of the 'occult' power of the herb. The following procedure is followed: A suitable location of *A. conyzoides* is found during the day. Very late at night, the collector approaches the plant and chews nine or seven seeds (for male or female, respectively) of melegueta pepper (*Aframomum melegueta* K. Schum.). The chewed grains are spat on the plant while the appropriate incantations are recited. The plant is then plucked and warmed over a fire at home before the juice is expressed. Palm oil (expressed from the mesocarp of *Elais guiniensis* family, Palmaceae) is added to the pressed juice and the mixture used to rub the whole body of the patient. *Ageratum conyzoides* is commonly used in TM for dressing wounds and ulcers, for scabies and as an eyewash. It is used as a styptic in East Africa (Kokwaro, 1993). These common uses result from its antimicrobial properties, which have been demonstrated scientifically but the special effect (occult power) it is claimed to possess when collected at night cannot easily be rationalized on a scientific basis, especially when there is no precise diagnosis of the disease. There are, however, other practices in African TM that are justifiable scientifically. Some examples are given below.

In many African homes, teeth are cleaned in the morning by chewing the root or slim stem of certain plants until they acquire brush-like ends. The fibrous end is then used to brush the teeth thoroughly. These chewing sticks impart varying taste sensations: a tingling, peppery taste and numbness is provided by *Zanthoxylum zanthoxyloides* Waterman (*Fagara zanthoxyloides* Lam.) root, a strong bitter taste and frothing by *Masularia acuminata* (G. Don.) Bullock ex Hoyle stem, and an initial bitterness becoming sweet later by *Vernonia amygdalina* Del. root. The root of *Terminalia glaucescens* Planch. produces a discoloration of the mouth. The most popular chewing sticks are those with a good flavour and texture, and a recognized effect on the teeth and supporting tissues. Freshly cut specimens are always desirable because they are more easily chewed into a brush. Some of them, however, possess such tough fibres that they penetrate the gums during use, thus causing some discomfort (Sofowora, 2008).

Buffered extracts of the common chewing sticks show antimicrobial activity against oral microbial flora but to varying degrees (Sote and Wilson, 1995; Taiwo *et al.*, 1999; Almas, 2002; Ndukwe *et al.*, 2005). Some African chewing sticks are also reported to contain fluoride ions, silicon, tannic acid, sodium bicarbonate and other natural plaque-inhibiting substances that can reduce bacterial colonization and plaque formation. The antimicrobial activity of the most effective (*Z. zanthoxyloides*) was shown to be due to berberine, chelerythrine and canthine-6-one (Fig. 38.1), which are most active at pH 7.5 (or during tooth decay) and simple benzoic acid derivatives, which are most active around pH 5 (or after an acid drink like lime juice). These data indicate that the chewing sticks, in addition to providing mechanical stimulation of the gums and removing food particles from the teeth crevices, also destroy oral microbes. Some African chewing sticks have been reported to contain fluoride ions, although their fluoride content was considered insufficient to produce a significant increase in the fluoride content of the dental enamel. Plant parts used as chewing sticks also have been shown to contain not only fluoride but also silicon, tannic acid, sodium bicarbonate and other natural plaque-inhibiting substances that could reduce bacterial colonization and plaque formation (Ogunmodede, 1991; Sote and Wilson, 1995; Taiwo *et al.*, 1999; Almas, 2002; Ndukwe *et al.*, 2005).

Other practices used in African TM, such as collecting certain plants only at certain seasons, using cold extraction instead of hot for some herbs, using young instead of old leaves of certain plants, using fallen dead leaves of certain plants rather than fresh ones, etc. have been rationalized as being due to seasonal, diurnal or age variations in active constituents of plants or the thermolability of the active ingredients of certain plants.

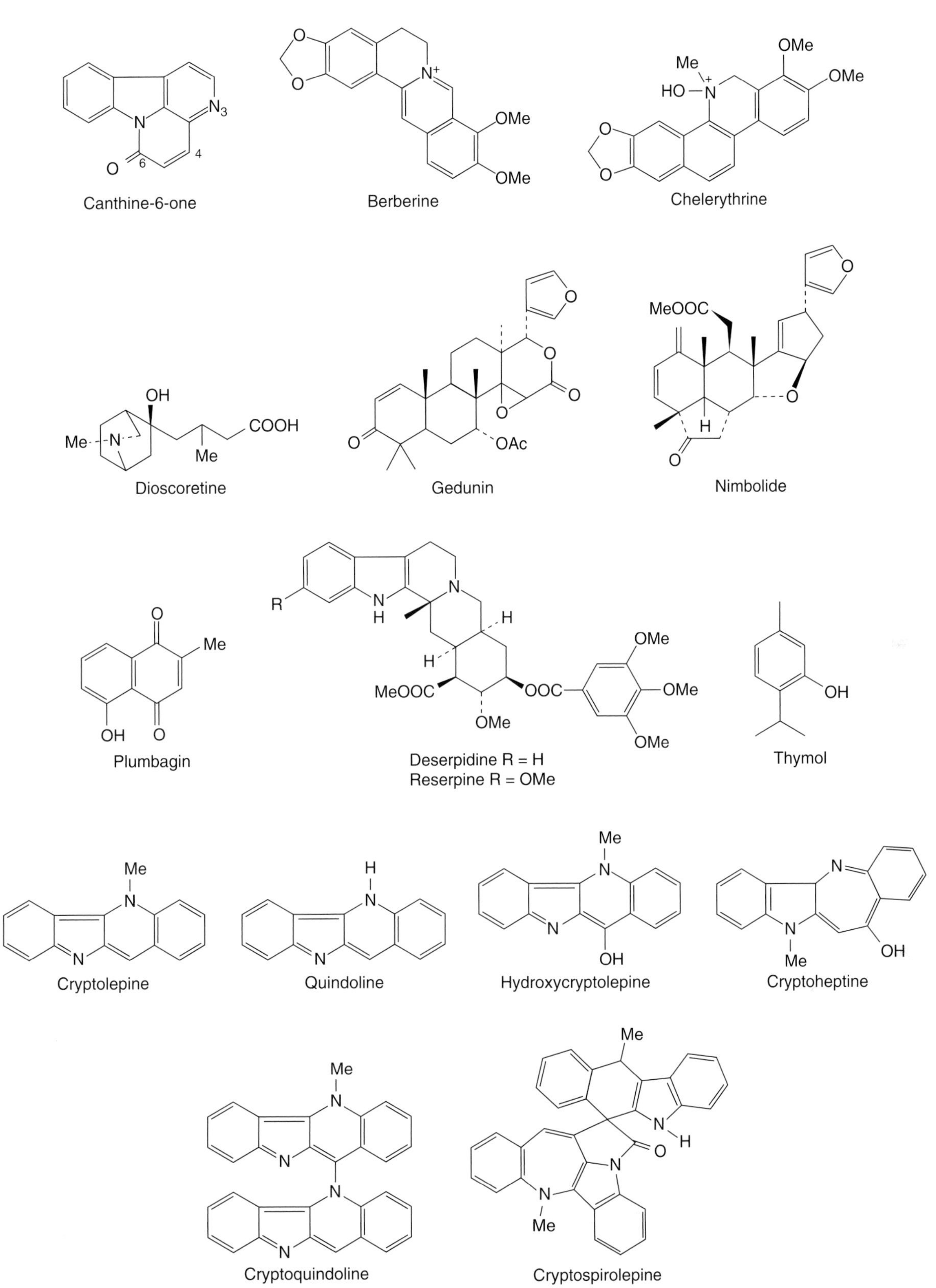

Fig. 38.1
Some chemical structures associated with African medicinal plants (see text).

(Continued)

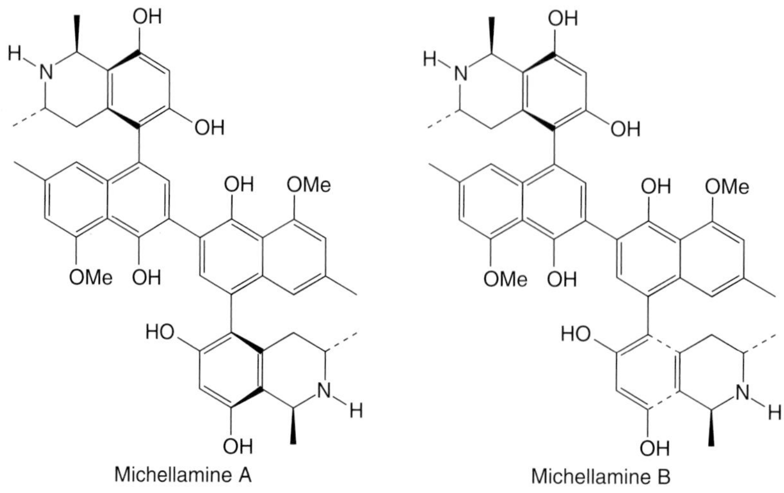

Michellamine A

Michellamine B

Fig. 38.1—Cont'd

The following are the summarized results from a few examples of the investigations carried out to prove the efficacy claimed for medicinal plants used in African TM.

Dioscorea dumetorum (Kunth) Pax tubers are used in African TM, in carefully regulated doses, for the management of diabetes mellitus (Iwu, 1993). Crude extracts of the tuber were shown to possess a hypoglycaemic effect in normal rats and rabbits and were checked for hypoglycaemia produced by alloxan. From the active aqueous fraction, dioscoretine (Fig. 38.1) was characterized as the hypoglycaemic agent by using bioassay-guided fractionation of the extract. Of the solvent fractions tested for toxicity, the aqueous fraction used in TM was the least toxic $LD_{50} = 1400$ mg kg^{-1}. Further work has been recommended by the researchers before dioscoretine or the extract of the tuber can be exploited commercially as careful control of the dosage was found necessary even by TMPs.

Polygala nyikensis is used by the highlanders of Malawi and bordering countries to treat various skin problems of fungal origin. The root of the plant was recently shown to exert its antifungal activity owing to the presence of xanthones (Marston *et al.*, 1993).

Azadirachta indica leaves and stem bark are used in treating malaria and have been shown to be effective *in vitro* and *in vivo*. Rochanankij *et al.* (1985) associated the antimalarial activity with nimbolide while Khalid and Duddeck (1989), using a bioassay-directed purification procedure, named another limonoid, gedunin (Fig. 38.1), as the active principle. The possibility that the extract of neem acts by causing a redox perturbation by imposing substantial oxidant stress during malarial infection has been postulated. The antiplasmodial and larvicidal activity of neem has been confirmed by others (Dhar *et al.*, 1998; Isah *et al.*, 2003; Nathan *et al.*, 2005; Udeinya *et al.*, 2006; Okumu *et al.*, 2007; Soh and Benoit-Vical, 2007).

The published scientific proof for the efficacy of other African plants was reviewed by Sofowora (1993) while the efficacy of others can be readily deduced from their active constituents. For example, the use of *Rauwolfia vomitoria* roots (containing reserpine) in treating some mentally ill patients; *Plumbago zeylanica* root (containing the naphthoquinone, plumbagin) for treating various fungal skin diseases; *Ocimum gratissimum* leaves (containing essential oils rich in thymol) for treating diarrhoea are all clearly justifiable (Sofowora, 2008). Other plants whose active constituents have not been characterized have also been demonstrated experimentally in the laboratory to be efficacious. Examples of these include remedies used in treating skin diseases and the use of *Combretum mucronatum* and *Mitragyna stipulosa* as anthelminthics (Sofowora, 2008).

Theories on the origin of herbal medicine in Africa

Although it is not known exactly when the humans first practised herbalism in Africa, a number of theories have been advanced by scholars and TMPs alike to explain the acquisition of this knowledge by early Africans. One such theory states that early man in Africa deliberately selected specific plant materials for the treatment of his ailments as man had the ability to rationalize rather than to rely on instinct as do lower animals. The choice was certainly not based on the knowledge of the plant constituents. Some anthropologists state that early man lived in fear, and that, to allay this, he indulged in mystical and religious rituals. Thus, it could well be that the initial selection of plant materials for medicinal purposes was influenced by religious thoughts and collections were accompanied by magical rituals. Some plants are still used in the rituals of traditional religion in many parts of Africa today.

It has been proposed that the knowledge of medicinal plants in Africa was gained by accident, although this theory has been refuted by a number of African TMPs, who claim that information on such plants was communicated to their ancestors in various ways. However, early Africans could have gained some specific knowledge by watching the effects produced by various plants when eaten by domestic animals. Even today, some herbalists try out remedies, in the presence of their patients, on domestic animals, especially when testing for toxicity, and on themselves or their relations. Such tests prove to the patient that the preparation is harmless and sometimes also confirm that the dosage prescribed is also justifiable. Such information on African medicinal and toxic plants has been passed on orally from generation to generation and even today there are many herbal cures in Africa that have not been written down (Sofowora, 2008).

According to some TMPs another possibility is that knowledge of traditional cures came from wizards and witches. It is believed that some witches, whether living or dead, attend village markets in strange forms—as goats, sheep or birds. If their presence in this disguise is detected by someone very shrewd or gifted, such as a TMP, the practitioner is promised some useful herbal cures in return for not exposing the witch in disguise. The same reward would be offered if a real-life witch was caught in the process of performing an evil act.

Hunters, especially in African countries, have been reported as the original custodians of some effective traditional herbal recipes. Such knowledge could have been acquired when, for example, a hunter shot an elephant. If the elephant ran away, chewed leaves from a specific plant and did not die, it is believed the hunter noted the plant as a possible antidote for wounds or for relieving pain. Similar observations were made in villages where, for example, a domestic animal chewed the leaf of a specific plant when that animal was ill and recovered later or when another animal accidentally chewed a leaf and died (Sofowora, 2008). Similar observations by scientists have confirmed that chimpanzees use medicinal plants in Africa for self-medication (Huffman and Wrangham, 1993).

TMPs also claim that, when in a trance, it is possible to be taught the properties of herbs by the spirit of an ancestor who practised herbalism. Spirits are said sometimes to assume various forms, e.g. an alligator, or a human being with one leg and one arm using a walking stick. If one encounters such a creature very late at night it can be a useful source of original information of herbal cures. In whatever manner the early Africans gained their knowledge of the curative powers of herbs, one must assume that they were able, thereafter, to recognize the plant, as the detailed flora available today describing medicinal plants were then non-existent.

RESEARCH INTO AFRICAN MEDICINAL PLANTS

Information on the use of medicinal plants has been obtained from herbalists, herb sellers and indigenous people in Africa over many years (Baba et al., 1992). Under the umbrella of Agence de Coopération Culturelle et Technique (ACCT) in Paris, ethnobotanical surveys with international teams had been carried out by 1988 in the following African countries: Central African Republic, Rwanda, Mali, Niger, Federal Islamic Republic of Comoros, Mauritius, Seychelles, Gabon, Dominica, Tunisia, Madagascar, Togo, Congo and Benin Republic. The African Union's Scientific Technical and Research Commission (AU/STRC) carried out similar surveys in Western Nigeria, Uganda, Cameroon, Ghana, Swaziland and Mozambique as at 2004 (Adjanohoun et al., 1989, 1993, 1996; Mshana et al., 2000; Adeniji et al., 2001, 2004). All these ethnobotanical surveys have been published. Other ethnobotanical surveys on the region have also been published (Samuelsson et al., 1991).

As early as 1968, it was decided at a conference organized in Dakar by the AU/STRC that the efficacy of herbs used by TMPs should be tested, particularly in the following areas: anticancer, antimalarial, antihelminthic, antimicrobial, antihypertensive, cardiac activity, antisickling and antiviral. The following is a summary of the research to date, as indicated by publications on African medicinal plants collated by NAPRALERT database for natural products. Only 36% of all publications dealt with bioassay-guided isolation of plant constituents along with their pharmacological and toxicological testing. The remainder dealt with purely phytochemical research (including quantitative analysis). Biological screening work resulted in publications on antimicrobial activity (16%), molluscicidal (11%), antimalarial (7%), toxicity testing (7%) and antitumour related (4%), while other minor biological testing amounted to 55% of the total publications relating to bioassay-guided research on African medicinal plants to 1993 (Sofowora, 1993, 2008). In molluscicidal testing, three plants came out as having potential commercial exploitation, namely *Phytolacca dodecandra*, *Swartzia madagascariensis* and *Tetrapleura tetraptera*. The field trials on these and toxicity studies against non-target organisms have been carried out successfully in ponds where the intermediate host snail of schistosomiasis is prevalent (Hostettmann, 1991).

Cryptolepis sanguinolenta, which is used for treating urinary infections in TM, has been shown to be strongly antimicrobial. Cryptolepine was identified as the active alkaloid. The extract of this root has been formulated for therapeutic use by the Centre for Research into Plant Medicine in Ghana. A new alkaloid, named cryptospirolepine (Fig. 38.1), was characterized from this root by Tackie et al. (1993) whereas hydroxycryptolepine, cryptoheptine and cryptoquindoline (three new alkaloids) were reported from a specimen of the same root collected

in Guinea Bisau by Houghton et al. (1993). Paulo et al. (1993) have examined the alkaloids characterized by Houghton et al. (1993) from this root for antibiotic activity. All the alkaloids showed activity but to varying degrees against the test organisms used. According to Cimanga et al. (1996, 1997), this plant showed potent antibacterial, anticomplementary and moderate antiviral activities, but no antifungal effect. The results obtained by Paulo et al. (1994a, 1994b) after testing the root extracts and its alkaloids against diarrhoeal and other bacteria suggested that the roots could be a therapeutic alternative for bacterial etiologic diarrhoea in West Africa. See Sofowora (2008) for more research on *Cryptolepis sanguinolenta*.

Garcinia kola seeds are chewed for protection against liver disease and were shown to contain biflavonoids (Iwu, 1993; Tarashima et al., 2002). The biflavonoids and the crude extracts of the seed have been shown to be effective in protecting against liver damage (Farombi et al., 2004, 2005; Odunola et al., 2005; Adaramoye and Adeyemi, 2006a) and they ameliorate di-*n*-butylphthalate-induced testicular damage in rats (Farombi et al., 2007). The mechanisms involved in the hepatoprotection were explained by Farombi in 2000. 'Kolaviron' has been patented for commercial exploitation and the methods for its isolation and quantification have been enunciated. Other activities reported for 'Kolaviron' and the extract of *Garcinia kola* include: Attenuation of indomethacin- and HCl/ethanol-induced oxidative gastric mucosa damage in rats, and hypoglycaemic and hypolipidaemic effects (Adaramoye and Adeyemi, 2006b), whereas toxicological investigations include on erythrocytes (Esomonu et al., 2005), alteration of oestrous cycle in rats (Akpantah et al., 2005) as well as the brine shrimp lethality and mutagenicity tests (Sowemimo et al., 2007). The amino acid composition of the seeds has been reported by Adeyeye et al. (2007).

Thaumatococcus danielli produces a red fruit, the aril of the seed of which contains the polypeptide thaumatin. Thaumatin is almost 5000 times as sweet as sucrose on molar basis. It is a low-calorie, high-intensity sweetener suitable for sweetening pharmaceuticals for diabetics. The plant grows readily in the moist areas of Africa and the early researches on its development were carried out jointly by researchers in Ife (Nigeria) and Tate and Lyle Ltd in UK. It is used in soft drinks in Japan (Sofowora, 2008). Thaumatin I and Thaumatin II have been cloned and synthesized through recombinant DNA. The cloning experiments showed that the N- and C-terminal regions of both of the thaumatin molecules do not play any important role in eliciting the sweet taste of thaumatin (Masuda et al., 2004; Zemanek and Wassermann, 2005; Ide et al., 2007).

Cassia podocarpa, which is used as a laxative in TM, has been shown to contain anthraquinone derivatives similar to those found in official senna of the *British Pharmacopoeia*. The leaves and pods were also compared for their biological efficacy with official senna and shown to be just as effective on a weight basis. *C. podocarpa* was also shown to be less toxic than official senna. This leaf has been formulated into tablets and recommended as a substitute for official senna in Africa through the work of African researchers (Abo and Adeyemi, 2002; Akomolafe et al., 2004). Danafco (Ghana) Ltd. produces standardized tea bags of this leaf on a commercial scale. Similar work on *C. italica* has led to the development of laxatives based on this plant, now commercially available in Mali and other African countries.

Euphorbia hirta is used traditionally in treating diarrhoea and dysentery in African TM. Although it contains phorbol derivatives this plant has been shown to be effective *in vitro* and *in vivo* against *Entamoeba*, which causes amoebic dysentry. The plant has been formulated into mixtures and a preparation of the whole plant is also available commercially in Mali for use against amoebic dysentery (Keita, 1994; see also Sofowora, 2008).

Zanthoxylum zanthoxyloides (Lam.) Waterm. The 'antisickling' property of the root of *Z. zanthoxyloides* was discovered when it was observed that the aqueous extract preserved the red colour of blood in blood-agar plates during a screen for its antimicrobial activity. The extract was later shown to revert sickled HbAS, HbSS and crenated HbAA red blood cells to normal *in vitro*. The activity was also demonstrated in the root of other *Zanthoxylum* species, and *Z. gilletti* was found to be just as active as *Z. zanthoxyloides*. This, and previous observations, led to postulation of a membrane-based activity earlier reported for the extracts. Activity-directed fractionation of the aqueous extract located the ether fraction as the active fraction. GC-MS analysis of the ether fraction indicated the presence of phenolic and fatty acids. These acids are 2-hydroxymethyl-benzoic acid, *p*-hydroxybenzoic acid, vanillic acid, *m*-hydroxybenzoic acid, 2-hydroxy-3-phenylpropionic acid, traces of stearic acid, linoleic and palmitic acids. Further analysis of the fraction confirmed the presence of these acids and identified additional ones: *p*-coumaric, caffeic and ferulic acids. Xanthoxylol [2-dimethylallyl-4-(3-hydroxypropyl)phenol] was also isolated from the root. *p*-Hydroxybenzoic acid, 2-hydroxymethylbenzoic acid, vanillic acid, 2,2-dimethyl-2H-1-benzopyran-6-butyric acid (DBA; which is a chemical modification of xanthoxylol) and two uncharacterized non-acidic isomers of butyric acid isolated from the root have all been shown to possess antisickling activity. DBA also causes a slight increase in the pO_2 of the HbSS. Although the extract from the root (*Z. zanthoxyloides*) and DBA have been reported as generally non-toxic to (whole) animals and intracellular enzymes of the red blood cell, such as glucose-6-phosphate and 6-phosphogluconate dehydrogenases, the extract was observed to revert sickled cells to round rather than discoid shapes in some experiments. DBA, however, has been shown to increase the activity of Ca^{2+}-activated Mg^{2+}-dependent ATPase in both normal HbAA and sickle HbSS cell membranes, suggesting an antisickling activity based on Ca^{2+} mobilization in the HbSS red cell membrane for the root extractives. Other synthetic benzoic acid derivatives known to possess antisickling activities are *p*-methoxybenzoic acid, 3,4-dihydroxybenzoic acid, 3,4-dimethylbenzoic acid and *p*-fluorobenzoic acid. Relating the observed antisickling activity to physicochemical parameters of substituted benzoic acids showed that increased lipophilicity enhances sickle-cell reversal activity and that electron-donating substituents play an important role in antisickling activity. Although the attempted preliminary clinical trial on sickle cell anaemia (SCA) patients was plagued with a high default rate, the results obtained appear to indicate significant diminution of painful episodes in treated individuals (Adesanya and Sofowora, 1994). A product developed from the extract of 'Fagara' is being marketed under the name DREPANOSTAT® in Togo and Benin Republics. In Burkina Faso and surrounding countries the herbal product FACA® which is a mixture of 'Fagara' and *Calotropis procera* is marketed for SCA (Sofowora 2008). The use of a leaf extract of *Terminalia catappa* as having antisickling potential has been supported by recent research involving human blood samples (Mgbemene and Ohiri, 1999). Research on other plants used in the management of SCA have been discussed by Adesanya and Sofowora (2008).

The development of bioassay techniques (Hostettmann, 1991) for antiviral activity in plants and the importance of finding a cure for HIV/AIDS has brought some African medicinal plants into prominence. About 120 plants have been reported to show antiviral activity (many of these grow in Africa, e.g. *Diospyros, Spondias, Terminalia* spp.), whereas others are reported to have immunomodulating properties, such as *Aloe* and *Zingiber* spp. etc. A new plant species, *Ancistrocladus korupensis* (Ancistrocladaceae), was discovered in Cameroon and found to contain new alkaloids: michellamines A and B, which have a wide spectrum of antiviral activity, including anti-HIV cytopathic activity. Efforts were made to develop michellamine B for use in HIV/AIDS treatment. It was characterized by collaborative effort of some Cameroon scientists and the National Cancer Institute in the USA. The plant is rare. Efforts are in progress to germinate the seeds in its natural habitat at Korup National Park, in glass houses and through tissue culture in collaboration with J. B. Johnson Biotech Laboratories (Manfredi *et al.*, 1991; Jato *et al.*, 1993). Readers should consult the review by Elujoba (2008) on plants used for the management of HIV/AIDS in Africa.

Nwosu (1999) has reported on 30 plants from 21 families which are used traditionally for the treatment of mental disorders in southern Nigeria.

In a review of over 240 higher plants that are used in Africa as arrow poisons, Neuwinger (1996) cites many as having medicinal properties.

TRADE IN MEDICINAL PLANTS IN AFRICA

The amount of trade in the area of medicinal plants in some African countries is well documented (see Table 38.1). It is known, for example,

Table 38.1 African medicinal plants exported for their active ingredients.

Species	Part used	Ingredient	Source area
Allanblackia floribunda	Fruit	Fat	Côte d'Ivoire
Ancistrocladus abbreviatus	Plant	Michelamine A and B(Alk) (Fig. 38.1)	Cameroon, Ghana
Corynanthe pachyceras	Bark	Yohimbine, corynanthine, corynanthidine	Ghana
Dennetia tripetala	Fruit	Essential oil	Ghana
Griffonia simplicifolia	Seed	BS11 lectin	Ghana, Côte d'Ivoire, Cameroon
Harpagophytum procumbens	Root	Glucoiridoids	Namibia
H. zeyheri	Root	Glucoiridoids	Namibia
Hunteria eburnea	Bark	Eburine, etc.	Ghana
Jateorhiza palmata	Root	Palmatine, jateorhizine, colombamine	Tanzania
Pausinystalia yohimbe	Bark	Yohimbine	Cameroon
Pentadesma butryacea	Fruit	Fat	Côte d'Ivoire
Physostigma venenosum	Fruit	Physostigmine (eserine)	Ghana, Côte d'Ivoire
Prunus africana	Bark	Sterols, triterpenes, n-decosanol	Cameroon, Kenya, Madagascar
Rauwolfia vomitoria	Root	Reserpine (Fig. 38.1), yohimbine, etc.	Zaire, Rwanda, Mozambique
Strophanthus spp.	Fruit	Ouabain	West Africa
Voacanga africana	Seed	Voacamine	Côte d'Ivoire, Cameroon, Ghana
V. thouarsii	Seed	Voacamnie	Cameroon

After Cunningham (1993a & b)

that the government of Cameroon is the major source for the world market of *Prunus africana* bark, where it has been harvested since 1972. Over a 6-year period (1986–1991), 11 537 metric tons of the bark (reaching an average of 700 tons) were processed by Plantecam Medicam, a French-owned company based in south-west Cameroon. *P. africana* bark represents 86% of the medicinal plants exported by this company between 1985 and 1991 (Cunningham and Mbenkum, 1993). The bark is used in treating prostate gland hypertrophy and benign prostate hyperplasia (Shenouda *et al.*, 2007; Dedhia *et al.*, 2008). Another major plant material exported by Cameroon is the seed of *Voacanga africana* (Apocynaceae), which is used for the production of the alkaloid tabersonine, used as a CNS depressant in geriatric patients. Cameroon exported US$40 million worth of *V. africana* in 1993 alone. Cameroon also exports *Tabernanthe iboga* and *Myrianthus arboreus*, but in small quantities (Cunningham and Mbenkum, 1993).

Capsules containing the extract of *P. africana* bark are marketed in Europe, where the market value of this trade is estimated at US$150 million per year. In addition to Cameroon, Kenya (1923 tons per year), Uganda (193 tons per year), Zaire (300 tons per year) and Madagascar (78–800 tons per year) export this bark to various pharmaceutical companies in Europe, mainly to Madaus in Germany and Spain, Laboratoires Debat in France, Prosynthèse in France, Inverni Della Beffa and Indena Spa in Italy (Cunningham and Mbenkum, 1993).

Three plants out of the 24 000 indigenous species of the Republic of South Africa have been developed as export products. These are Rooibos tea (*Asplathusa linearis*), Marula (*Sclerocarya birrea*) and *Aloe ferox*. About 500 million South African Rands per annum are spent on traditional remedies in the Republic of South Africa.

Namibia exports 200 tons of *Harpagophytum procumbens* and *H. zeyheri* tubers annually to Germany (80.4%), France (12.8%), Italy (1.9%), USA (1.5%), Belgium (1%) and South Africa (1.2%) (Cunningham *et al.*, 1992).

In Madagascar, the export sale of *Catharanthus roseus* and other plants represents a major export earner.

The roots of *Swartzia madagascariensis* and *Entada africana* are traded 500–800 kilometres from Burkina Faso and Mali to Abidjan in Côte d'Ivoire. Similarly, most of the common chewing sticks are sold across the borders of neighbouring countries in West Africa; 75–80 tons of *Griffonia simplicifolia* seeds are exported each year to Germany from Ghana; commercial gatherers in Côte d'Ivoire chop down *Griffonia simplicifolia* vines and *Voacanga africana* and *Voacanga thouarsii* trees in order to obtain the fruits for export (Cunningham, 1993a, 1993b). Large quantities of various medicinal plants are also exported to France by SETEXFARM in Senegal. These plants are collected from the wild and there is currently no evidence of any replanting. The harvesting of such large quantities of medicinal plants from the wild will eventually result in serious social or environmental consequences. To ensure the sustainable use of the medicinal plant resources of Africa, uncontrolled exportation of plants collected from the wild should give way to large-scale cultivation of the desired plants. Table 38.2 shows African medicinal plants whose demand exceeds supply.

Office National de Développement des Forêts (ONADEF) in Cameroon has applied its experience of indigenous (e.g. *Terminalia superba*) and exotic timber to species with medicinal values. Three species cultivated for bark production (*Prunus africana* and two exotic *Cinchona* species) and *Voacanga africana* cultivated for its seed have been propagated on a large scale. The foresight of ONADEF in implementing medicinal tree cultivation in plantations and through enrichment planting is exceptional in Africa and is encouraging (Cunningham and Mbenkum, 1993).

Table 38.2 African medicinal plants whose demand exceeds supply.

Species	Families
Alepidea amatymbica	Apiaceae
Asclepias cucullata	Asclepiadaceae
Begonia homonymma	Begoniaceae
Bowiea volubilis	Liliaceae
Cassia abbreviata	Fabaceae
Cassia sp.	(unidentified species known as muwawani)
Dianthus zeyheri	Illecebraceae
Garcinia afzellii	Clusiaceae*
Garcinia mannii	Clusiaceae*
Howorthia limifolia	Liliaceae
Monanthotaxis capea	Annonaceae
Pimpinella caffra	Apiaceae
Plectranthus grallatus	Lamiaceae
Siphonochilus aethiopicus	Zingiberaceae
Warburgia salutaris	Canellaceae*

*Trees/shrubs with agroforestry potential
Compiled from Cunningham (1993a, b)

Conservation of medicinal plants in Africa

More than 200 000 out of about 300 000 plants species identified in the whole of our planet are in the tropical countries of Africa and elsewhere. Among the potential uses of these African plants, those involving traditional medicines and pharmacopoeial drugs are foremost; 80% of the population of Africa living in rural areas relies on TM.

Approximately 1.8 million km^2 of the world's tropical rain forest (totalling roughly 9 million km^2) are in Africa, the rest being in America, Asia and few patches in the Indian Ocean and Pacific Islands. One-fifth of the total 120 000 (including 30 000 undescribed species) seed plants present in the tropical moist forest has been estimated to be present in Africa (Farnsworth and Soejarto, 1991). All over the world, and especially in Africa, factors that cause forest depletion include direct human pressure as well as indirect factors: commercial logging in the forest, fuel wood consumption, cattle ranching (where either excessive grazing causes depletion or selective grazing by cattle results in prolific growth of poisonous species), forest farming and forest fires. Environmental factors such as desert encroachment, pollution, acid rain, the greenhouse effect and erosion are other factors causing loss of forests.

The collection of medicinal plants by herbalists and herb sellers (herb traders) for local use and export also has had a noticeable depletion effect on this important forest resource in Africa, where collectors now have to travel farther afield to obtain the herbs to be used in their practice, as few of these are cultivated. According to Cunningham (1993a, 1993b), indigenous forests cover only 0.3% of South Africa but are a source of over 130 commercially exploited traditional plants; over 400 indigenous species and 70 exotic species are commercially sold to Zulu people as herbal medicines. These indigenous species are causing concern because of the depletion of wild stocks when demand exceeds supply. Scarce, slow-growing forest species are particularly vulnerable to this over-exploitation.

Mauritius and Rodriguez have two of the most threatened flora in the world. Over 150 species of plants on these African islands are threatened with extinction, out of which at least 30 species are known from less than 10 collections (Owadally *et al.*, 1991). According to Kokwaro (1991), high- and medium-potential land in Kenya constitutes about 17% of the country and supports 90%

of the population, which is mostly rural. The plant communities in such areas are usually the most threatened by over-utilization. The depletion rates of the forest resources, which include medicinal plants, are very high. For example, Kakamega, North and South Mandi forests, which occur in high-potential areas, are being cleared at the rate of 245, 295 and 490 ha per year, respectively (Kokwaro, 1991).

The sustainable management of the forest resources and the medicinal plants in them is important, so that while the benefits to present generations are satisfied the potential to meet the needs and aspirations of future generations is not jeopardized. Conservation activities involving medicinal plant gardens maintained by herbalists, herbaria and various arboreta are scattered all over Africa. Some countries have also started special programmes to conserve the genetic resources of their medicinal plants. Although there is a need to utilize all the conventional methods of conservation (*in situ* and *ex situ* conservation, gene banks, biotechnology, etc.), the education of rural dwellers, particularly the herbalists and the herb sellers, in conservation awareness is important for an effective approach to the sustainable utilization of the medicinal plant resources in Africa. One group of TMPs in South Africa collaborates with the conservation of Traditional Healing Practices and Plants Project (CTHPPP) at Bulwer, in South Africa, for the conservation of medicinal plants. The project successfully cultivated more than 30 indigenous plant species. This young ethnobotanical reserve is currently being used to train TMPs in the Bulwer area in the identification of medicinal plants. This kind of approach, rather than merely relying on legislation, is to be encouraged. Attempts to stop the exploitation of *Prunus africana* in Cameroon by banning merely led to a rise in its exportation through illegal channels from 700 tons per year to over 1000 tons per year (Mbenkum and Thomas, 1993). Since 1995, *P. africana* has been included in CITES Appendix II as an endangered species. In 2000, Plantecam, the largest bark exporter in Africa, closed its extraction factory in Cameroon, due to complex ecological, social and economic factors. Wild collection is no longer sustainable (and probably never was) where harvest seriously affects morbidity and mortality rates of harvested populations (Stewart, 2003). Alternatives to wild collection to meet future market demand—including conservation practices, enrichment plantings, small- and large-scale production and protection of genetic resources—have been proposed by Stewart (2003). *P. africana* is at the beginning of a transition from an exclusively wild-collected species to that of a cultivated medicinal tree.

THE AFRICAN PHARMACOPOEIA

Reports of the uncontrolled dosage of herbal remedies used by TMPs necessitated a research programme to carry out quantitative pharmacognostical analysis on some common African medicinal plants. Data accumulated from such research were used to compile the first *African Pharmacopoeia* (*AP*) published by AU/STRC (1985, 1986). The *AP* specifies quality control standards to be met by the plants when used in commerce and in manufacturing pharmaceutical preparations. Volume 1 of the *AP* contains monographs on 100 medicinal plants, whereas volume 2 describes the methods to be used in their quality control. Some of the old reliable methods of plant analysis are still retained (along with the most modern techniques) as alternatives in this volume as many African countries cannot afford the sophisticated spectroscopic instruments used in quality control today. The *AP* is available in English, French and Arabic. Some African countries have produced their own national herbal pharmacopoeiae, e.g. Ghana and Nigeria.

CONCLUSION

With the development of simpler, inexpensive bench-top bioassays (Hostettmann, 1991), it is expected that in future many hitherto untested natural products isolated from African plants will be put through a variety of biological tests.

The current awareness of HIV/AIDS in Africa and the development of screening programmes for anti-HIV activity in plants will herald the screening of more African plants claimed by TMPs to be used in treating HIV/AIDS-related symptoms. This is of increasing importance because, in addition to being a sexually transmitted disease, HIV/AIDS is also contracted through blood transfusion when adequate care is not taken to use only HIV-free blood. Some patients with diseases like sickle-cell anaemia who require blood transfusion because of lack of an available cure (this disease kills 120 000 or more children annually in Africa) need to be considered especially in HIV/AIDS and primary health care programmes. More attention should also be given to the possibility of cures, from plant sources, for HIV/AIDS. However, it will be necessary to determine what indications in the treatment or diagnostic mode of the TMP should be looked for in identifying candidate plants for HIV/AIDS cure (see Elujoba, 2008).

Tissue and suspension cultures of some African medicinal plants have also been developed in various laboratories, but mainly outside Africa, for the future biotechnological production of the secondary plant metabolites of these plants for drugs needed world-wide. Examples include *Catharanthus roseus*, *Ammi majus* and *A. visnaga*, and *Tribulus terrestris* (see also *Thaumatococcus danielli*, above). This trend will probably be intensified to prepare for the future demand for drugs in relation to conservation efforts.

While national *materia medica* of herbs are being compiled, it is expected that efforts will continue to eliminate toxic plants from the recipes of the TMPs, and to encourage the use of the harmless ones, which will be made available on a large scale in standardized dosage forms not only for home use but also for export.

Many countries in Africa (for example, Rwanda, Egypt, Mali) now cultivate medicinal plants on a large scale for local processing into galenicals, teas, various dosage forms and other standardized preparations for use in health care. It is expected that activity in this direction will increase in Africa with assistance from UNIDO as more can be derived economically by making simple extracts of medicinal plants rather than exporting them as raw materials. Drug production from medicinal plants in Africa should be further intensified in African countries through public/private/partnership (PPP) arrangements, so that Africa can contribute more to the global trade in medicinal plant products.

The formation of networks of laboratories to bring African countries together for collaborative research and development work on natural products generally and medicinal plants in particular is expected to increase. The creation of the Natural Products of East and Central Africa (NAPRECA) network by UNESCO has given a boost to inter-African collaborative research efforts on medicinal plants in that subregion of Africa. This led to the creation of the West African network, also with UNESCO support. The International Organization for Chemistry in Development (IOCD) has encouraged the creation of a Network of Analytical and Bioassay Services in Africa (NABSA), with headquarters in Addis Ababa University, Ethiopia. This network was created to encourage the bioassay of natural products from phytochemical research by pooling existing analytical facilities in African laboratories. All these efforts are expected to boost output in research and development work in this field. With institutional strengthening of African laboratories taking place, it is hoped that more and more of the collaborative research with developed countries can take place in Africa where labour is relatively cheap.

The old methods and practices of traditional medicine in Africa are being transformed with the awareness of the TMPs for the need for more precise dosage in the use of their herbal remedies. Retraining programmes are going on in several countries, with a view to improving the competence of the TMPs and the quality of health care that they deliver on a continent where 80% of the people have only TM available to them. Research has provided evidence for the rationalization of some of the practices of the TMPs and the efficacy of some of the herbs they use while new natural products with potential for drug development for management of diseases rampant world-wide are emerging from African plants. It is hoped that increased inter-African and international collaborative research and sustainable use of biodiversity resources in Africa will help to develop new drugs from the rich untapped forests of Africa for the betterment of mankind.

Further reading

Abo KA, Adeyemi AA 2002 Seasonal accumulation of anthraquinones in leaves of cultivated *Cassia podocarpa* Guill et Perr. African Journal of Medicine and Medical Science 31(2): 171–173

Adaramoye OA, Adeyemi EO 2006a Hepatoprotection of D-galactosamine-induced toxicity in mice by purified fractions from *Garcinia kola* seeds. Basic Clinical Pharmacology and Toxicology 98(2): 135–141

Adaramoye OA, Adeyemi EO 2006b Hypoglycaemic and hypolipidaemic effects of fractions from kolaviron, a biflavonoid complex from Garcinia Kola in streptozotocin-induced diabetes mellitus rats. Journal of Pharmacy and Pharmacology 58(1): 121–128

Adesanya SA, Sofowora A 1994 Phytochemical investigation of plants for the management of sickle cell anaemia. In: Hostettmann K (ed) Phytochemistry of plants used in traditional medicine. Oxford University Press Oxford, UK

Adesanya SA, Sofowora A 2008 Medicinal plants and management of sickle cell anaemia. In: Sofowora A (ed) Medicinal plants and traditional medicine in Africa. Spectrum Books, Ibadan, Nigeria

Adeyeye EI, Asaolu SS, Aluko AO 2007 Amino acid composition of two masticatory nuts (*Cola acuminata* and *Garcinia kola*) and a snack nut (*Anacardium occidentale*). International Journal of Food Science and Nutrition 58(4): 241–249

Adjanohoun EJ, Adjakidje V, Ahyi MRA *et al* 1989 Contribution aux études ethnobotaniques et floristiques en République du Benin. ACCT, Paris, France

Adjanohoun E, Ahyi MRA, Ake-Assi L *et al* 1991 Contribution to ethnobotanic and floristic studies in Western Nigeria. AU/STRC, Lagos, Nigeria

Adjanohoun E, Ahyi MRA, Ake-Assi L *et al* 1993 Contribution to ethnobotanic and floristic studies in Uganda. OAU/STRC, Lagos, Nigeria

Adjanohoun JE, Aboubakar N, Dramane K *et al* 1996 Contribution to ethnobotanic and floristic studies in Cameroon. AU/STRC, Lagos, Nigeria

Adeniji, KO, Amusan OOG, Dlamini PS *et al* 2001 Contribution to the ethnobotanic and floristic studies in Swaziland. AU/STRC, Lagos, Nigeria

Adeniji K, Agostinho AB, Amusan OOG *et al* 2004 Contribution to the ethnobotanic and floristic studies in Mozambique. AU/STRC, Lagos, Nigeria

Akomolafe RO, Adeoshun IO, Ayoka AO *et al* 2004 An in vitro study of the effects of *Cassia podocarpa* fruit on the intestinal motility of rats. Phytomedicine 11(2–3): 249–254

Akpantah AO, Oremosu AA, Noronha CC *et al* 2005 Effects of garcinia kola seed extract on ovulation, oestrous cycle and foetal development in cyclic female sprague-dawley rats. Nigerian Journal of Physiological Science 20(1–2): 58–62

Almas K 2002 The effect of *Salvadora persica* extract (miswak) and chlorhexidine gluconate on human dentin: a SEM study. Journal of Contemporary Dental Practice 3(3): 27–35

AU/STRC 1985 African Pharmacopoeia, Vol 1. OAU/STRC, Lagos, Nigeria

AU/STRC 1986 African Pharmacopoeia, Vol 2. OAU/STRC, Lagos, Nigeria

Baba S, Akerele O, Kawaguchi Y (eds) 1992 Natural resources and human health. Elsevier, Tokyo, Japan

Cimanga K, De Bruyne T, Lasure A *et al* 1996 *In vitro* biological activities of alkaloids from *Cryptolepis sanguinolenta*. Planta Medica 62(1): 22–27

Cimanga K, De Bruyne T, Pieters L *et al* 1997 *In vitro* and *in vivo* antiplasmodial activity of cryptolepine and related alkaloids from *Cryptolepis sanguinolenta*. Journal of Natural Products 60(7): 688–691

Cunningham AB 1993a Ethics, ethnobiological research and biodiversity. WWF, Gland

Cunningham AB 1993b African medicinal plants. Setting priorities at the interface between conservation and primary healthcare. People and Plants Working Paper I. UNESCO, Paris, France

Cunningham AB, Mbenkum FT 1993 Sustainability of harvesting *Prunus africana* bark in Cameroon. People and Plants Working Paper 2. UNESCO, Paris, France

Cunningham AB, Jasper PJ, Hansen LCB 1992 The indigenous plant use programme. Foundation for Research Development, Paris, France

De Smet PAGM 1998 Journal of Ethnopharmacology 63: 1–179

Dedhia RC, Calhoun E, McVary KT 2008 Impact of phytotherapy on utility scores for five benign prostatic hyperplasia/lower urinary tract symptoms health states. Journal of Urology 179(1): 220–225

Dhar R, Zhang K, Talwar GP *et al* 1998 Inhibition of the growth and development of asexual and sexual stages of drug-sensitive and resistant strains of the human malaria parasite *Plasmodium falciparum* by neem (*Azadirachta indica*) fractions. Journal of Ethnopharmacology 61(1): 31–39

Elujoba AA 2008 Traditional medicine and HIV/AIDS in Africa. In: Sofowora A (ed) Medicinal plants and traditional medicine in Africa. Spectrum Books, Ibadan, Nigeria

Esomonu UG, El-Taalu AB, Anuka JA et al 2005 Effect of ingestion of ethanol extract of Garcinia Kola seed on erythrocytes in Wistar rats. Nigerian Journal of Physiological Science 20(1–2): 30–32

Farnsworth NR, Soejarto DD 1991 Global importance of medicinal plants. In: Akerele O, Heywood N, Synge H (eds) Conservation of medicinal plants. Cambridge University Press, Cambridge, UK

Farombi EO 2000 Mechanisms for the hepatoprotective action of kolaviron: studies on hepatic enzymes, microsomal lipids and lipid peroxidation in carbontetrachloride-treated rats. Pharmacological Research 42(1): 75–80.

Farombi EO, Møller P, Dragsted LO 2004 Ex-vivo and in vitro protective effects of kolaviron against oxygen-derived radical-induced DNA damage and oxidative stress in human lymphocytes and rat liver cells. Cell Biology and Toxicology 20(2): 71–82

Farombi EO, Adepoju BF, Ola-Davies OE, Emerole GO 2005 Chemoprevention of aflatoxin B1-induced genotoxicity and hepatic oxidative damage in rats by kolaviron, a natural bioflavonoid of *Garcinia kola* seeds. European Journal of Cancer Prevention 14(3): 207–214

Farombi EO, Abarikwu SO, Adedara IA, Oyeyemi MO 2007 Curcumin and kolaviron ameliorate di-n-butylphthalate-induced testicular damage in rats. Basic Clinical Pharmacology and Toxicology 100(1): 43–48

Hostettmann K 1991 Assays for bioactivity. In: Methods in plant biochemistry, Vol 6. Academic Press, London

Houghton PJ, Paulo MA, Gomez ET 1993 New alkaloids of *Cryptolepis sanguinolenta*. In: Phytochemistry of plants used in traditional medicine—an international symposium of the Phytochemical Society of Europe, Lausanne September/October 1993. Book of Abstracts, Number P73

Huffman MA, Wrangham RW 1993 Diversity of medicinal plant use by wild chimpanzees. In: Heltne PG, Marquardt LA (eds) Chimpanzee behavioural diversity. Harvard University Press, Cambridge, MA, pp 1–14

Ide N, Kaneko R, Wada R *et al* 2007 Cloning of the thaumatin I cDNA and characterization of recombinant thaumatin I secreted by Pichia pastoris. Biotechnology Progress 23(5): 1023–1030

Isah AB, Ibrahim YK, Iwalewa EO 2003 Evaluation of the antimalarial properties and standardization of tablets of *Azadirachta indica* (Meliaceae) in mice. Phytotherapy Research 17(7): 807–810

Iwu MM 1993 A handbook of African medicinal plants. CRC Press, Boca Raton, FL

Jato J, Symonds P, Thomas D *et al* 1993 Conserving a rare medicinal plant: the case of *Ancistroclaudus korupensis* (Ancistrocladaceae). Proceedings of the 5th OAU/STRC Symposium on African Traditional Medicine and Medicinal Plants. OAU/STRC, Lagos, Nigeria

Keita A 1994 Activities of the traditional medicine department in Mali. International workshop by the GIFTS of Health, Mbarara, Uganda, December 6–9, 1994

Khalid SA, Duddeck H 1989 Isolation and characterization of an antimalarial agent of the neem tree *Azadirachta indica*. Journal of Natural Products 52(5): 922–927

Kokwaro JO 1991 Conservation of medicinal plants in Kenya. In: Akerele O, Heywood V, Synge H (eds) Conservation of medicinal plants. Cambridge University Press, Cambridge, pp 315–319

38

Kokwaro JO 1993 Medicinal plants of East Africa, 2nd edn. Kenya Literary Bureau, Nairobi, Kenya

Manfredi KP, Blunt JW, Cardelina II JH *et al* 1991 Journal of Medicinal Chemistry 34: 3402–3405

Marston A, Maillard M, Hostettmann K 1993 Search for antifungal, molluscicidal and larvicidal compounds from African medicinal plants. Journal of Ethnopharmacology 38: 215–223

Masuda T, Tamaki S, Kaneko R *et al* 2004 Cloning, expression and characterization of recombinant sweet-protein thaumatin II using the methylotrophic yeast *Pichia pastoris*. Biotechnology and Bioengineering 85(7): 761–769

Mbenkum FT, Thomas DN 1993 Sustainable use of secondary products from Cameroon's forests: a survey of medicinal, insecticidal and molluscicidal plants. In: Proceedings of the 5th OAU/STRC Symposium on African Traditional Medicine and Medicinal Plants. OAU/STRC, Lagos, Nigeria

Mgbemene CN, Ohiri FC 1999 Pharmaceutical Biology 37: 152

Mshana NR, Abbiw DK, Addae-Mensah I *et al* 2000 Contribution to the ethnobotanic and floristic studies in Ghana. AU/STRC, Lagos, Nigeria

Nathan SS, Kalaivani K, Murugan K 2005 Effects of neem limonoids on the malaria vector *Anopheles stephensi* Liston (Diptera: Culicidae). Acta Tropica 96(1): 47–55

Ndukwe KC, Okeke IN, Lamikanra A *et al* 2005 Antibacterial activity of aqueous extracts of selected chewing sticks. Journal of Contemporary Dental Practice 6(3): 86–94

Neuwinger JD (translated from the German by Aileen Porter) 1996 African ethnobotany—poisons and drugs. Chapman and Hall, Weinheim

Nwosu MO 1999 Fitoterapia 70: 58

Odunola OA, Adetutu A, Olorunnisola OS, Ola-Davis O 2005 Protection against 2-acetyl aminofluorene-induced toxicity in mice by garlic (*Allium sativum*), bitter kola (*Garcina kola* seed) and honey. African Journal of Medicine and Medical Science 34(2): 167–172

Odusanya SA, Songonuga OO, Folayan JO 1979 Fluoride ion distribution in some African chewing sticks. IRCS Medical Science, 7, 580

Ogunmodede E 1991 Dental care: the role of traditional healers. World Health Forum 12(4): 443–444

Okumu FO, Knols BG, Fillinger U 2007 Larvicidal effects of a neem (*Azadirachta indica*) oil formulation on the malaria vector *Anopheles gambiae*. Malaria Journal 6: 63

Owadally AW, Dulloo ME, Straham W 1991 Measures that are required to help conserve the flora of Mauritius and Rodriquez in *ex situ* collections. In: Heywood VH, Wyse-Jackson PS (eds) Tropical botanic gardens. Their role in conservation and development. Head Press, London

Paulo A, Duarte A, Gomes ET 1993 Antibiotic activity of some alkaloids isolated from *Cryptolepis sanginolenta*. International Symposium Phytochemistry of Plants used in Traditional Medicine, Book of Abstracts, Poster No. 108. Lausanne, September, 1993

Paulo A, Pimentel M, Viegas S *et al* 1994a *Cryptolepis sanguinolenta* activity against diarrhoeal bacteria. Journal of Ethnopharmacology 44(2): 73–77

Paulo A, Duarte A, Gomes ET 1994b *In vitro* antibacterial screening of *in vitro Cryptolepis sanguinolenta* alkaloids. Journal of Ethnopharmacology 44(2): 127–130

Rochanankij S, Tebttearanonth Y, Yenjai Ch, Yuthavong Y 1985 Journal of Tropical Medicine and S.E. Asian Public Health 16: 66

Samuelsson G, Farah MH, Claeson P *et al* 1991 Inventory of plants used in traditional medicine in Somalia. I. Plants of the families Acanthaceae—Chenopodiaceae. Journal of Ethnopharmacology 35: 25–63

Shenouda NS, Sakla MS, Newton LG *et al* 2007 Phytosterol *Pygeum africanum* regulates prostate cancer *in vitro* and *in vivo*. Endocrine 31(1): 72–81

Sofowora A 1993 Recent trends in research into African medicinal plants. Journal of Ethnopharmacology 38: 209–214

Sofowora A 2008 Medicinal plants and traditional medicine in Africa, 3rd edn. Spectrum Books Ltd, Ibadan, Nigeria

Soh PN, Benoit-Vical F 2007 Are West African plants a source of future antimalarial drugs? Journal of Ethnopharmacology 114(2): 130–140

Sote EO, Wilson M 1995 In-vitro antibacterial effects of extracts of Nigerian tooth-cleaning sticks on periodontopathic bacteria. African Dental Journal 9: 15–19

Sowemimo AA, Fakoya FA, Awopetu I *et al* 2007 Toxicity and mutagenic activity of some selected Nigerian plants. Journal of Ethnopharmacology 113(3): 427–432

Stewart KM 2003 The African cherry (*Prunus africana*): can lessons be learned from an over-exploited medicinal tree? Journal of Ethnopharmacology 89(1): 3–13

Tackie AN, Boye GI, Sharaff MHM *et al* 1993 Journal of Natural Products 56: 653–670

Taiwo O, Xu HX, Lee SF 1999 Antibacterial activities of extracts from Nigerian chewing sticks. Phytotherapy Research 13(8): 675–679

Terashima K, Takaya Y, Niwa M 2002 Powerful antioxidative agents based on garcinoic acid from *Garcinia kola*. Bioorganism and Medicinal Chemistry 10(5): 1619–1625

Udeinya IJ, Brown N, Shu EN *et al* 2006 Fractions of an antimalarial neem-leaf extract have activities superior to chloroquine, and are gametocytocidal. Annals of Tropical Medicine and Parasitology 100(1): 17–22

WHO 1976 African traditional medicine. Report of the African Regional Expert Committee. WHO Afro's Technical Report Series, No 1

WHO 1991 Traditional medicine and modern health care: Progress Report by the Director General. World Health Organization, Geneva, Switzerland, Document No A44/10 22 March 1991

Zemanek EC, Wasserman BP 2005 Issues and advances in the use of transgenic organisms for the production of thaumatin, the intensely sweet protein from *Thaumatococcus danielli*. Critical Reviews of Food Science and Nutrition 35(5): 455–466

PART

7 | Non-medicinal toxic plants and pesticides

39

Hallucinogenic, allergenic, teratogenic and other toxic plants

The plants included in this chapter are toxic species which, although finding little use in modern medicine, are, because of the pharmacological effects which they produce, of considerable interest to pharmacognosists.

HALLUCINOGENS

Most cultures of man, from earliest times, have had recourse to some form of narcotic, often hallucinogenic, drug. These hallucinogens, often derived from plants, have frequently been used within a religious context. In recent years peyote, Indian hemp and lysergic acid derivatives have received much attention, but there are many other similar drugs used by local populations whose existence and use are still being investigated by ethnobotanists. In this respect, Professor R. E. Schultes (1915–2001) made extensive studies of such plants in South America and has emphasized the great need for recording the wealth of knowledge possessed by native tribes on narcotic plants before the activities of these peoples are overcome by 'civilization'.

With the exception of cannabis, the principal known hallucinogenic plants contain alkaloids related to the neurophysiological transmitters noradrenaline and 5-hydroxytryptamine (serotonin).

FUNGI

Some of the poisonous fungi when taken orally produce hallucinations; these include toadstools of the genera *Amanita, Psilocybe* and *Conocybe*.

The Amanitas. A number of *Amanita* species, in addition to promoting hallucinogenic effects, are extremely toxic. The appearance of the serious symptoms is considerably delayed (particularly with amatoxins, formula Fig. 39.1) after ingestion, by which time effective treatment becomes difficult. Three classes of toxins are recognized in the genus—tryptamines (e.g. bufotenine), cyclic peptides (phallotoxins and amatoxins) and isoxazole alkaloids (e.g. ibotenic acid, formula Fig. 39.1). The three classes of compound appear to be restricted to certain specific sections of the genus.

The fly agaric. The fly agaric (*Amanita muscaria*) is readily distinguished by its red or orange cap, often covered with white flecks. It contains a mixture of isoxazole alkaloids ibotenic acid and muscimol. Polysaccharides and a carboxymethylated derivative of the fungus have been shown to possess antitumour activity (T. Kiho *et al.*, *Biol. Pharm. Bull.*, 1994, **17**, 1460). The pigments (betalains) of the fungus, also found in the Caryophyllales, are formed from tyrosine and the rapid development of pigment formation in *A. muscaria* has given an ideal system for isolating the enzymes involved (L. A. Mueller *et al.*, *Phytochemistry*, 1996, **42**, 1511; 1997, **44**, 567).

The pharmacological effects appear within an hour or so of ingestion, with an initial period of excitation followed by muscular twitches, a slowed pulse rate, impaired breathing, delirium and coma; however, ingestion of the fungus is rarely fatal. The mushroom has a traditional use as an inebriant in regions of Siberia; one hypothesis suggests it to be the *soma* of the Rig Veda. The panther cap, *A. pantherina*, contains similar principles including pantherine (5-aminomethyl-3-hydroxyisoxazole), a flycidal alkaloid. A branched $(1{\rightarrow}3)$-β-D-glucose isolated from an alkaline extract of the fungus exhibited significant activity in mice.

Hallucinogenic Mexican mushrooms. A number of small toadstools—particularly species of *Psilocybe* (*P. mexicana*), *Conocybe*

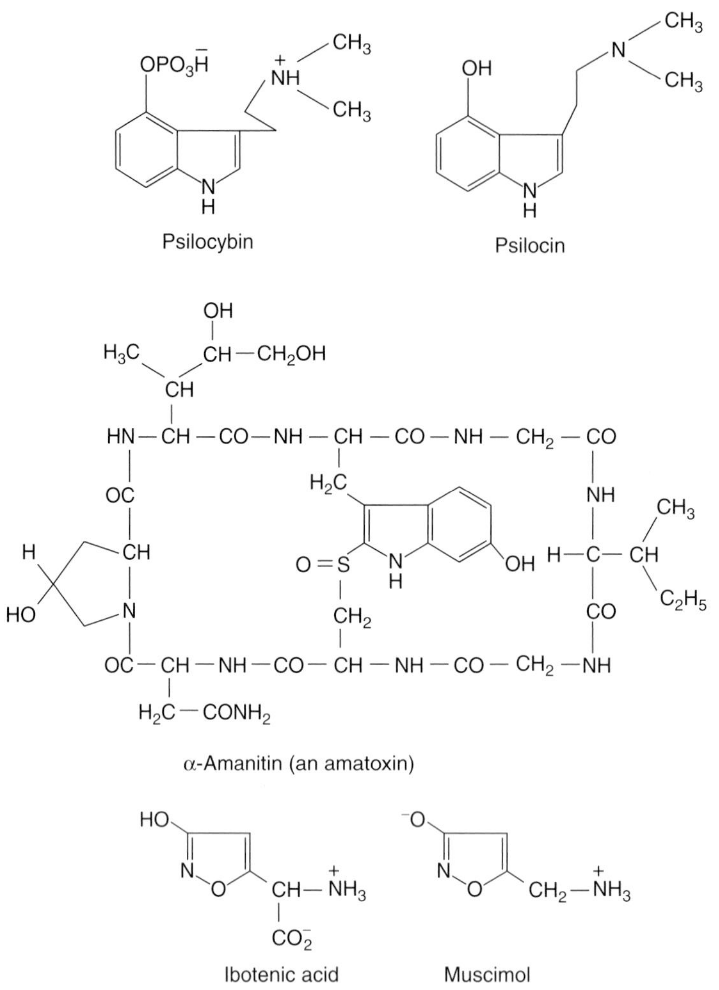

Fig. 39.1
Toxic and hallucinogenic constituents of fungi.

(*C. cyanopus*) and *Stropharia*—constitute the Mexican hallucinogenic mushrooms (*teonanacatl*, 'flesh of the gods', much revered by the Aztecs). The onset of symptoms after ingestion of the fungi is rapid, and includes inability to concentrate and the occurrence of hallucinations. The active constituents are the tryptamine derivatives psilocybin and psilocin, compounds related to serotonin. These compounds are also found in similar toadstools (e.g. *Psilocybe* and *Paneolus, Copelandia, Gymnopilus, Inocybe, Panneolina, Pluteus* and *Stropharia* spp.) which are found in temperate regions. In Britain the 'liberty cap', *Psilocybe semilanceata*, a small toadstool common on lawns and parkland, and in Australia *P. subaeruginosa* both contain psilocybin. What is claimed to be the highest proportion of psilocin contained in any mushroom (3.3%, dry weight) was reported in *Psilocybe cubensis*; for a review of the mushroom alkaloids (567 refs), see R. Autkowiak *et al.*, *Alkaloids*, 1991, **40**, 189); for the concise large-scale synthesis of psilocin and psilocybin, see O. Shirota *et al.*, *J. Nat. Prod.*, 2003, **66**, 885.

Puffballs. Species of *Lycoperda* contain constituents which produce auditory hallucinations and a state of half-sleep about half an hour after consumption. The effects are distinct from those caused by the mushrooms. Puffballs are used by the Mixtecs of Southern Oaxaca in Mexico.

LYSERGIC ACID DERIVATIVES

The hallucinogenic properties of lysergic acid, and, in particular, the diethylamide derivative (LSD), are well-known. This acid forms the non-peptide portion of a number of ergot alkaloids (q.v.) and can also be produced by suitable cultivation of the fungus in liquid culture. It was with some surprise that lysergic acid was also found as a component of some convolvulaceous seeds (species of *Ipomoea, Rivea* and *Argyreia*), and as far as is known at present they constitute the only higher plants containing ergot-type alkaloids.

Morning Glory seeds. In the sixteenth century the Spaniards in Mexico reported the use of sacred hallucinogenic seeds known as 'ololiuqui'. The climbing plant from which they were obtained was subsequently identified as *Rivea corymbosa*. Closely related in constituents and action are the seeds of *Ipomoea tricolor* (*I. violacea*) and those of various species of *Argyreia*. The name 'Morning Glory' is applied to *Ipomoea tricolor* but also to a number of other species (e.g. to *I. purpurea* and to the Japanese Morning Glory, *I. hederacea*). The trade names of species of *Ipomoea* are endlessly mixed. The seeds of the above-mentioned *Ipomoea hederacea* have long been used in the East as a purgative and were formerly official in the *British Pharmacopoeia* under the name 'kaladana' or 'pharbitis seeds'.

PEYOTE

Certain cacti are of pharmaceutical and pharmacological interest, as they contain protoalkaloids, some of which have marked hallucinogenic properties. One of these is the cactus *Lophophora williamsii* which has long been used by Mexican Indians. It is known as peyotl, anhalonium or mescal buttons. The latter name is derived from the cactus stems, which are cut into slices about 20–50 mm in diameter. An interesting report (H. R. El-Seedi *et al.*, *J. Ethnopharm.*, 2005, **101**, 238) sheds more light on its possible use by native N. Americans some 5700 years ago: two specimens from the Witte Museum in San Antonio were radiocarbon-dated to 3780–3600 BCE and, on analysis (TLC and GC-MS), gave alkaloids (2%) in which mescaline was identified, making these the oldest examples of a plant drug to yield a major bioactive compound. The chief active constituent is the alkaloid mescaline. The chemistry dates back to 1888, in which year Lewin isolated anhalonine, a crystalline tetrahydroisoquinoline alkaloid. By 1973 some 56 alkaloids had been characterized from the cactus and these could be classified as (1) mono-, di- and trioxygenated phenethylamines and their amides; (2) tetrahydroisoquinoline alkaloids and their amides; (3) phenethylamine conjugates with Kreb's cycle acids; (4) pyrrole derivates. Examples of these groups are given in Fig. 39.2. The alkaloids can arise in the plant from dopamine, and grafting experiments involving *Trichocereus pachanoi* ('San Pedro') (a mescaline-producing species) and *T. spachianus* (no mescaline) have indicated that biosynthesis of the hallucinogen is confined to the aerial parts.

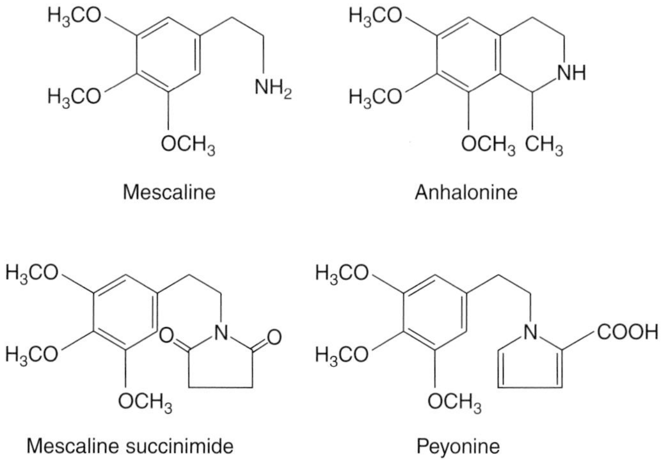

Fig. 39.2
Representative alkaloids of peyote.

INDIAN HEMP

The Indian hemp plant was originally considered as a distinct species but came to be regarded as a variety of *Cannabis sativa*, the common European hemp, which thus exhibited a variety of ecotypes giving rise to differing cannabinoid mixtures. Subsequently (in 1974), a case was presented by American taxonomists for the recognition of three distinct species. *C. sativa, C. indica* and *C. ruderalis*. Other botanists have proposed sub-species of *C. sativa*.

The plant is found wild in India, Bangladesh and Pakistan. The drug consists of the dried flowering and fruiting tops of the pistillate plants from which no resin has been removed. Limited cultivation is permitted in some countries. The drug has been produced in East Africa, South Africa, Tripoli, Asia Minor and USA. Large confiscations of illicit cannabis and its preparations continue to be made in most countries.

In temperate climates large quantities of hemp are grown for the stem fibre and for the seeds, which yield 30–35% of a drying oil.

History. Hemp has been cultivated for its seeds and fibres from a very remote period, but the narcotic properties are usually not marked in plants grown in temperate regions, and even in India an active drug can only be grown in certain districts. The drug is mentioned in early Hindu and Chinese works on medicine, and its use slowly spread through Persia to the Arabs. It was used by the Mohammedan sect known as the Hashishin or Assassins, who came into contact with the Crusaders in the eleventh and twelfth centuries. The drug attracted the attention of Europeans at the time of Napoleon's Egyptian expedition.

Hemp products

Three main type of narcotic product are produced.

1. The Indian hemp or *ganja* of the *Indian Pharmacopoeia* (1955) is required to contain 'not more than 10% of its fruits, large foliage leaves and stems over 3 mm'. This is the *flat-* or *Bombay-ganja*, which was formerly official in many pharmacopoeias. Round- or *Bengal-ganja* is prepared by rolling the wilted tops between the hands.
2. *Bhang* (Hindustani) or *Hashish* (Arabic) consists of the larger leaves and twigs of both male and female plants. It is used in India for smoking, either with or without tobacco and drugs such as opium or datura, or is taken in the form of an electuary made by digestion with melted butter.
3. *Charas* or *churrus* is the crude resin. This is obtained by rubbing the tops between the hands, beating them on cloths or carpets, or by natives who wear leather aprons walking among the growing plants. The resin is scraped off and forms an ingredient of numerous smoking mixtures. Like *bhang*, it is also used with butter.

In America and Europe the product used by addicts is known as *marihuana*, in north Africa as *kief*, in South Africa as *dagga*, and in Arabia and Egypt as *hashish*.

Production of ganja. This is legally only produced by a few licensed growers in Bengal, Mysore and Madras. The seed is sown in rows about 1.3 m apart and male plants are eliminated as soon as they can be recognized. The resinous tops, largely of unfertilized female plants, are cut about 5 months after sowing and pressed into cakes. The yield is about 120 kg per acre.

Macroscopical characters. The flat- or Bombay-ganja occurs in agglutinated flattened masses of a dull green or greenish-brown colour. The resin is no longer sticky but hard and brittle; the odour, which is very marked in the fresh drug, is faint. The drug has a slightly bitter taste. Here and there ovoid hemp seeds may be picked out. Before further examination the drug should be soaked in successive quantities of alcohol to remove the resin and then softened in water.

The lower digitate leaves of the plant are seldom found in the drug. The thin, longitudinally furrowed stems bear simple or lobed, stipulate bracts. These subtend the bracteoles, enclosing the pistillate flowers. The bracts are stipulate and the lamina may be simple or three-lobed. The bracteole enclosing each flower is simple. The perigone enveloping the lower part of the ovary and the two reddish-brown stigmas can be seen with a lens.

Microscopical characters. The resin is secreted by numerous glandular hairs, 130–250 µm long (see Figs 39.3; 42.5). The head is usually eight-celled and the pedicel multiseriate or unicellular. To differentiate these from similar trichomes (e.g. those of the Labiatae) specific

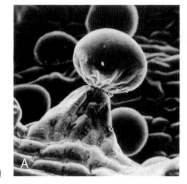
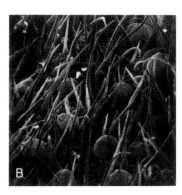

Fig. 39.3
A, typical stalked glandular trichome from bracteole ×270. B, sessile glandular trichomes and covering trichomes, ×130. (J. W. Fairbairn.)

stains can be used. These include Fast Blue Salt B and, as described by Corrigan and Lynch in 1978, a reagent consisting of vanillin in ethanolic sulphuric acid which stains the cannabis glands a deep reddish-purple. It is possible to analyse individual trichomes by GLC by which means it has been shown that the glands represent a dynamic system in the cannabinoid synthetic activity of the plant. In addition, sessile glands (Fig. 39.3), abundant conical, curved, unicellular hairs, are also found, many having cystoliths of calcium carbonate in their enlarged bases (see Figs 39.3; 42.3); however, these cystolith hairs are not confined solely to the genus *Cannabis*. Cluster crystals of calcium oxalate are abundant, particularly in the bracteoles.

Constituents.   The narcotic resin is a brown, amorphous semisolid; soluble in alcohol, ether and carbon disulphide. It contains over 60 compounds (cannabinoids) all composed of an aromatic portion (C_{11} or C_{12}), theoretically derivable from six acetate units, and an isoprenoid component (C_{10}). They appear to form a natural group of C_{21} terpeno-phenolics of unique occurrence. Some principal components are cannabinol, tetrahydrocannabinol (THC), cannabidiol (CBD), cannabidiol-carboxylic acid, cannabigerol and cannabichromene (Fig. 39.4). Cannabinodiol is the aromatic analogue of cannabidiol. Cannabigerol precedes Δ^9-THC in the biosynthetic pathway and is incorporated, by the plant, into the latter and other neutral cannabinoids. The identification

Mevalonate derived | Acetate derived

Cannabidiol-carboxylic acid

$-CO_2 \rightarrow$

Cannabidiol

Δ^9-Tetrahydrocannabinol

Δ^8-Tetrahydrocannabinol

Cannabinol

Cannabichromene

Nabilone
A synthetic THC analogue

Fig. 39.4
Principal cannabinoids of *Cannabis sativa* and synthetic analogue.

of phloroglucinol β-D-glucoside in the shoot laticifer exudate of *C. sativa*, and phloroglucinol as a prominent component, and the only phenol, in the glandular trichomes suggests that it may have an important role in the *in vivo* enzymatically regulated biosynthesis of the cannabinoids (C. T. Hammond and P. G. Mahlberg, *Phytochemistry*, 1994, **37**, 755).

Cannabipinol, isolated in 1967, contains a bicyclic monoterpene moiety in addition to the acetate-derived portion. Cannabidivarin, described in 1969, is a cannabidiol homologue with a 5-propyl-resorcinol moiety. In view of the importance of the detection of Indian hemp, a number of gas and thin-layer chromatographic techniques coupled with mass spectrometry have been developed for the separation of these substances.

Δ^9-THC is the principal psychoactive constituent; Δ^8-THC is almost as active but is only present in the plant in small amounts; cannabinol is less potent; although lacking psychotropic properties cannabidiol has anticonvulsant and possible analgesic effects. Cannabichromene may enhance THC activity and has antifungal, antimicrobial and anti-inflammatory activity; for enzyme studies related to its formation see S. Morimoto *et al.*, *Phytochemistry*, 1998, **49**, 1525.

The plant also contains a small quantity of laevorotatory volatile oil (about 30 components) containing terpenes and a sesquiterpene (cannibene); the bases choline, trigonelline, spermidine and an alkaloid cannabisativine; flavonoid *O*-glycosides of both vitexin and orientin; and calcium carbonate. It yields about 15% of ash and 10–18% of alcoholic extract.

Resin production.   The study of resin production in cannabis continues to attract considerable attention. In practice, two varieties of *Cannabis sativa* are recognized: one produces fibre and the other resin. However, there is still no unanimity of opinion on the generic status of resin production, a situation which makes difficult a realistic legal definition of the narcotic drug. Cannabinoid production does not appear to be directly dependent on the presence of chlorophyll, and both green shoots and completely white shoots (as from a sport) will continue synthesis in the dark. Some evidence indicates that the plant's ability to produce resin is governed mainly by the environment; thus, progeny of seeds of European fibre-producing plants when grown in Egypt reverted to resin-producing plants in a matter of a few years and, conversely, seeds from resin-producing plants of the Middle East failed to produce abundant narcotic resin when grown in temperate Europe. These observations have been supported by work at the phytotron near Paris, which suggests that cannabis has, from its early growth stages, the chemical capacity to become either fibrous or resinous, depending on the climate. Nevertheless, it is possible to raise resin-containing plants in temperate regions and plants raised in the UK from overseas seed-stock (Morocco, Sri Lanka, Zambia) for a number of generations broadly retained the cannabinoid content typical of the source countries but tetrahydro-cannabinolic acid (THCA) consistently predominated over THC, the ratio THCA/THC being 17 compared with 2 in plants from the original areas (J. E. Pitts *et al.*, *J. Pharm. Pharmacol.*, 1992, **44**, 947).

Apart from ability to produce resin *per se*, it appears certain that resin-producing plants do exist as chemical races. The principal chemotypes recognized are those involving a preponderance of Δ^9-THC, CBD or cannabigerol together with others having various ratios of THC/CBD. There may also be a variation in resin content between male and female plants; again, this may be an inherited feature or may be differing climatic responses of the male and female. A study of wild-growing plants of cannabis collected in northern India at different altitudes and locations showed that these, too, showed great variations in the proportions of cannabinoids present. Possibly, a complete range of genetic types covering the transition from the fibrous form to the various resin types will emerge, with climatic factors also influencing the chemical products of any one type.

All the above factors obviously contribute to the very variable narcotic action of different samples of the drug.

Cannabis evaluation.   The many factors above which determine the cannabinoid composition mean that care must be taken in ascertaining the chemical phenotype of a plant. The general view that cannabis preparations can be evaluated on their Δ^9-THC content neglects other active components, and in attempts to classify cannabis on the basis of its narcotic/fibre content a number of systems, some very complex, have been devised. A relatively simple relationship introduced by Waller is based on the combined Δ^9-THC and cannabinol (CBN) in relation to cannabidiol (CBD).

The phenotype is expressed as

$$= \frac{\Delta^9\text{-}THC + CBN}{CBD}$$

A sample with a value greater than 1 = a drug type of cannabis; a sample with a value less than 1 = a fibre type.

High potency grades of marihuana (>20% Δ^9-THC dry wt.) are reportedly available on the illicit drug market and from one such sample S. A. Ahmed *et al.* have characterized eleven new cannabinoid esters (*J. Nat. Prod.*, 2008, **71**, 536).

Uses.   Medicinal properties of cannabis were recognized some 5000 years ago. In the mid-nineteenth century it was used in Europe as a hypnotic, anticonvulsant, analgesic, antianxiety and antitussive agent and was still official in the *BPC* 1949, together with the extract and tincture. Over many years it fell into disuse in human and veterinary medicine, and because of its narcotic properties importation into many countries became illegal. Promising results on the use of Δ^9-THC (dronabinol) for the relief of nausea and vomiting caused by cancer chemotherapy led to its use in the USA as an antiemetic. It is also employed to stimulate the appetite of AIDS patients. It can be prescribed in the UK under licence on a named-patient basis. Sativex is a relatively new Canadian product containing a mixture of THC and CBD. It is a spray not licensed for production in the UK but can be prescribed under Home Office licence for specific patients. Nabilone (Fig. 39.4), a synthetic cannabinoid antiemetic, is described in the *British National Formulary*; it is recommended to be administered in a hospital setting under close observation.

Cannabis also appears to have value in the relief of the symptoms of multiple sclerosis and other neurological disorders. The debate on its clinical usefulness continues. Subject to Medicines Control Agency approval, Phase II trials by GW Pharmaceuticals involving MS sufferers and patients with other neurological disorders were proposed (Report, *Pharm. J.*, 1999, **263**, 811).

Addiction has been common in many parts of Asia for more than 1000 years but only in recent years has the problem become world-wide.

Further reading

Amar BA 2006 Cannabinoids in medicine. A review of their therapeutic potential. J Ethnopharmacology 105 (1–2): 1–25. *A review with over 170 refs*
British Medical Association 1997 Therapeutic uses of cannabis. Harwood Academic Publishers, Amsterdam, The Netherlands
Brown DT (ed), Hardman R (series ed) 1998 Medicinal and aromatic plants – industrial profiles, Vol 4. Cannabis the genus *Cannabis*. CRC Press, Taylor and Francis Group, Boca Raton, FL. *904 references*
Mechoulam R (ed) 2005 Cannabinoids as therapeutics – milestones in drug therapy. Birkhauser Verlag, Basel. *282 references*

OTHER HIGHER PLANTS

Apocynaceae. Iboga root (*Tabernanthe iboga*), an African narcotic, contains alkaloids of the indole group. The alkaloid ibogaine has received attention as a possible antiaddictive drug (P. Popik and P. Skolnick, *The Alkaloids*, 1999, **52**, 197).

Compositae. *Calea zacatechichi*; in Mexico taken first as an infusion and then smoked.

Labiatae. *Salvia divinorum*: the leaves have long been used in Mazatec shamanistic divination ceremonies in the region of Oaxaca, Mexico. R. G. Wasson, working in the 1950s and 1960s, reported and identified this unusual intoxicant plant, which he believed to represent the sacred Aztec narcotic called pipilzintzintli. He stated that the hallucinogenic effects were similar to, but shorter and less striking than, those of the Mexican narcotic mushrooms (q.v.). Later, the ethnobotanist Daniel Siebert described the hallucinogenic effects of a minute amount of the active constituent, salvinorin A, as 'awesome and frightening'.

The active constituents comprise a considerable number of neoclerodane diterpenes, including salvinorins A–I, salvinicins A and B and others. Salvinorin A is a κ-opioid selective agonist and salvinicin A is a partial κ-opioid agonist; salvinicin B is the first known neoclerodane μ-opioid antagonist (T. A. Munro and M. A. Rizzacasa, *J. Nat. Prod.*, 2003, **66**, 703; A. K. Bigham *et al.*, *J. Nat. Prod.*, **66**, 1242; O. Shirota *et al.*, *J. Nat. Prod.*, 2006, **69**, 1782).

The use of *S. divinorum* ('magic mint', 'Sally D') as an hallucinogen has now spread globally and its possession in Australia, Italy, Sweden and four American States is illegal. For a current overview, see G. Vince, *New Scientist*, 2006, Sept. 30, 44; and for a review update on the pharmacology and analytical methodology of the plant and salvinorin, A. O. Grundmann *et al.*, *Planta Medica*, 2007, **73**, 1039.

Leguminosae. The beans of *Anadenanthera peregrina* are used in northern South America for the preparation of snuff. A root decoction of *Mimosa hostilis* is used in east Brazil. Both contain tryptamines. *M. ophthalmocentra* root is used similarly and contains *N,N*-dimethyltryptamine, *N*-methyltryptamine and hordenine (L. M. Batista *et al.*, *Pharm. Biol.*, 1999, **37**, 50).

Malpighiaceae. A number of *Banisteriopsis* species, e.g. *B. caapi*, a forest liana, are used as a snuff or beverage in the Amazon basin. Such species are reportedly psychoactive and contain tryptamine derivatives and the simple β-carboline alkaloids harmine, harmaline and tetrahydroharmine (Fig. 39.5).

Ayahuasca (hoasca) is an Amazonian ritual decoction made by boiling together a mixture of *B. caapi* and *Psychotria viridis* (Rubiaceae) the latter containing the psychedelic compound *N,N*-dimethyltryptamine (DMT) (Fig. 39.5). Modern research involving human volunteers has demonstrated the subtlety of this shamanistic preparation in which DMT consumed orally exerts its full effect by the build-up of 5-hydroxytryptamine made possible by the monoamine oxidase inhibitory properties of the *Banisteriopsis* alkaloids. It would appear that the combination of these two drugs produces a pharmacological response equivalent to that observed in acute psychotic unmedicated patients. For details of the above research see A. B. Pomilio *et al.*, *J. Ethnopharmacology*, 1999, **65**, 29; J. C. Callaway *et al.*, *ibid.*, 1999, **65**, 243.

Ayahuasca is banned in the USA but in 2006 the Supreme Court unanimously ruled that a small religious sect could continue to import and utilize a hallucinogenic tea central to its ritual ceremonies (see report by C. Cavaliere and M. Blumenthal, *HerbalGram*, 2006, **17**, 62).

Myristicaceae. Nutmeg has received attention as a psychotropic agent and this action may possibly arise from the myristicin and elemicin components; the formal relationship of these compounds to the amphetamines (some of which exert hallucinogenic effects) is of interest. Dimeric phenylpropanoids are also found in the seeds.

Virola spp. are also of the family Myristicaceae. They yield a blood-red, bark resin which is used by Indian tribes of the Amazon region for the preparation of hallucinogenic snuffs. They contain various tryptamines. *Virola sebifera*, used in Venezuela, contains the well-known psychotomimetic *N,N*-dimethyltryptamine (DMT) and also 5-hydroxy-DMT, 5-methoxy-DMT and 2-methyl-1,2,3,4-tetrahydro-β-carboline. *V. multinerva* also contains diarylpropanoids similar to those found in nutmeg.

Besides nutmeg, other essential oils that contain elemicin are those of parsley (*Petroselinum sativum*) and elemi-tree (*Canarium commune*) (M. DeVincenzi *et al.*, *Fitoterapia*, 2004, **75**, 615).

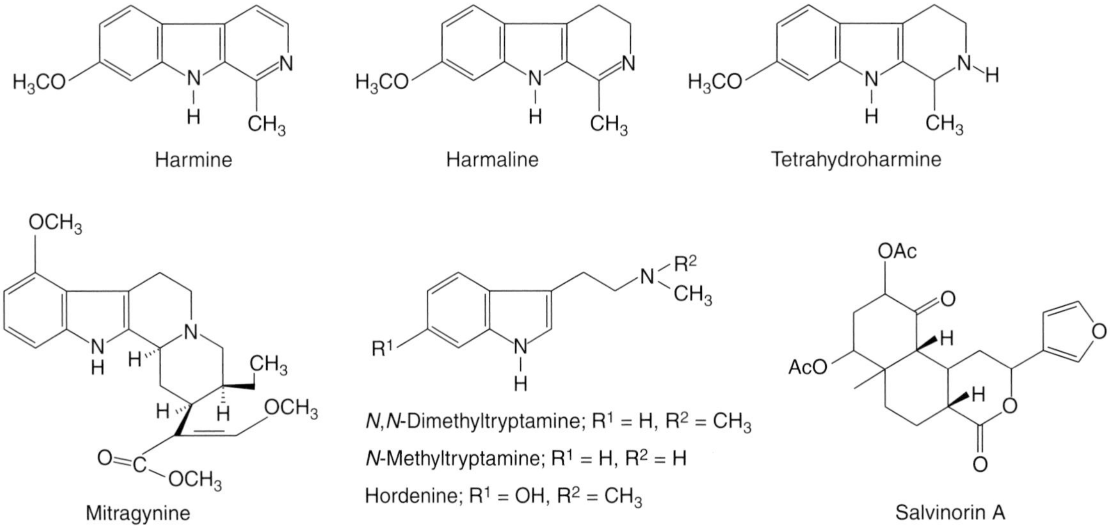

Harmine

Harmaline

Tetrahydroharmine

Mitragynine

N,N-Dimethyltryptamine; R¹ = H, R² = CH₃
N-Methyltryptamine; R¹ = H, R² = H
Hordenine; R¹ = OH, R² = CH₃

Salvinorin A

Fig. 39.5
Constituents of various hallucinogenic plants (see text).

Myristicin | Elemicin | Amphetamine corresponding to elemicin

Rubiaceae. *Mitragyna speciosa* leaves (q.v.) contain the alkaloid mitragynine, which binds to the same opioid receptor in the brain as morphine, codeine and diamorphine. The leaves (kraton) are widely available in the US, where it is used for its energizing and euphoric effects. It is an illegal substance in some S.E. Asian countries and in Australia. For a survey, see G. Vince under *Salvia divinorum* above.

Solanaceae. A number of genera containing tropane alkaloids feature in native rituals.

Zygophyllaceae. *Peganum harmala* produces a range of harmine alkaloids and the seeds are recognized in India for their psychoactive properties.

African hallucinogens. For ethnopharmacological notes on genera including *Alchornea*, *Monadenium*, *Mostuea* and *Voacanga* see P. A. G. M. De Smet, *J. Ethnopharm.*, 1996, **50**, 141.

The so-called Iboga alkaloids, which possess a catharanthine-type structure, are found in a number of African plants and are used locally as a stimulant. Apparently, a global medical subculture has arisen in which the alkaloid ibogaine is used principally to alleviate the symptoms of opioid withdrawal (K. R. Alper *et al.*, *J. Ethnopharm.*, 2008, **115**(1), 9–24).

Further reading
Dobkin de Rios M 1996 Hallucinogens. Cross-cultural perspectives. Waveland Press Inc., IL, USA

NATURAL ALLERGENS

A large number of plant and animal materials give rise to allergic reactions in certain individuals. The allergenic material is transmitted by direct skin contact, by airborne pollens, smoke and dried plant particles, and on the coats of domestic animals. Once a person has been sensitized to a particular allergen, subsequent exposure to the materials produces an antigen–antibody reaction which results in the liberation of histamine or histamine-like compounds which in turn cause the allergic symptoms. Allergies are commonly manifested as hay fever, asthma and dermatitis. Desensitization is often possible once the specific cause has been established, and a considerable number of allergenic extracts are now available for diagnostic and prophylactic treatments. As fatal anaphylactic reactions are possible, desensitization using allergenic extracts should be carried out only in situations where full cardiorespiratory resuscitation facilities are available. The following allergens are well-known.

Pollens. Responsible for seasonal hay fever, which may progress to chronic asthma. Pollen counts of the atmosphere are regularly recorded and published. Grass pollens form the highest proportion of the total count and may constitute 62% of the total count during June and July. In London, for these months, daily counts of 200 m^{-3} are not uncommon. Pollen counts of 50, and as low as 10, will produce discomfort in susceptible individuals. Common grasses involved include timothy (*Phleum pratensis*), cocksfoot (*Dactylis glomerata*) and perennial rye (*Lolium perenne*). The pollen of nettle (*Urtica dioica*) is second in importance to the grasses in this connection in the UK. It occurs in the air throughout the summer, reaching a peak in late June to July. Other relevant pollens are those of the plantain (*Plantago* spp.) and mugwort (*Artemesia vulgaris*). In the USA pollens of the ragweeds (*Ambrosia* spp.) are important. Tree pollens are contained in the atmosphere in the spring; they are not as common as allergens as those of grasses, the ones of most clinical importance being from the birch and plane trees.

Spores. A number of common moulds produce spores which cause rhinitis and asthma in sensitive individuals. They are often responsible for those conditions which extend beyond the normal pollen season and up to the beginning of frosts. Moulds flourish in damp conditions where organic decay is progressing, and peak sporulation occurs during hot, dry conditions when the atmosphere may become heavily contaminated. In the UK the spores of *Cladosporium herbarum* and *Sporobolomyces roseus* cause the most trouble. Exposure to lycopodium spores (q.v.) has caused allergic reactions varying from dermatitis to severe asthma attacks. There are also reports of spores causing adhesions on serous surfaces and foreign-body granulomas in soft tissues. This could have implications for the use of lycopodium powder as a dusting powder for non-lubricated condoms.

***Rhus* (Toxicodendron) spp.** *Rhus radicans* (poison ivy), *R. toxicodendron* (poison oak), *R. diversiloba* (Pacific poison oak) and *R. vernix* (poison sumach, poison elder) (Anacardiaceae) contain contactant allergens which produce severe dermatitis associated with watery blisters which burst and quickly spread across the skin. The allergens are contained in the plant sap and are easily transmitted (on clothing, hands, animal fur and even as the result of bush fires). These compounds are known as urushiols and belong to a class of alkenyl polyphenols found in the Anacardiaceae. They constitute an interesting chemotaxonomic group and are an example of the use of a starter other than acetyl-CoA in fatty-acid synthesis by which C$_2$ units derived from malonate are added to an unsaturated fatty acid; subsequent cyclization forms, as one example, the urushiols. With the exception of the cultivated sumach, which does not appear to be troublesome, these plants are not found in Britain, but they constitute a consider-

Urushiol phenols
For poison ivy:
R = C$_{15}$ aliphatic side-chain
For poison oak:
R = C$_{17}$ aliphatic side chain
R may possess 0, 1, 2 or 3 double bonds

Parthenin

able hazard in the USA, where poison ivy, in particular, is particularly widespread as a woody vine. Lacquer, used in the sixteenth and seventeenth centuries for producing an oriental-type finish on furniture, was derived from *R. vernicifera*, and its use constituted an industrial hazard for the craftsmen. Similar compounds to the above have been isolated from the fruit pulp of *Ginkgo biloba* and from the glandular trichomes of annual *Phacelia* spp. (Hydrophyllaceae) of the Californian Mojave desert. The dermatitic action of these compounds is consistent with oxidation of the allergen to a quinone which then binds covalently to a protein nucleophile giving an antigenic complex.

Sesquiterpene lactones.   These compounds (see Chapter 24), obtained from members of the Compositae, Lauraceae and Magnoliaceae and from the liverwort *Frullania* (Jubulaceae), are a major class of substances causing allergic contact dermatitis in man. The presence of an α-methylene group, exocyclic to the γ-lactone, appears to be the principal immunochemical requisite for activity. The compounds are illustrated, from the many, by the pseudoguaianolide parthenin, obtained from the plant *Parthenium hysterophorus*, an aggressive weed causing public health problems in parts of India. Some individuals are sensitive to feverfew and others to chrysanthemums. Two other plant species which can give rise to allergic reactions are the common rue (*Ruta graveolens*) and the indoor ornamental 'dumb cane' (*Dieffenbachia seguine*, Araceae). In the latter instance it would appear that the irritant substances are introduced into the body tissues by abrasion, through punctures caused by acicular crystals of calcium oxalate contained in idioblasts.

Miscellaneous.   Hair, feathers and house dust can all act as allergenic material; house dust often includes mites. Numerous other materials, not of natural origin (e.g. detergents, dyes, cosmetics), may also act as contact allergens.

TERATOGENS OF HIGHER PLANTS

Teratogenic substances, when ingested by the mother, can cause abnormalities in the developing fetus; thalidomide represents the tragic example of a synthetic drug having such undetected properties at the time of its use. Such substances undoubtedly occur also in plants, but no species has been shown as having been responsible for malformations in humans. That the possibility exists is demonstrated by the teratogenic effects of certain plants when incorporated into animal fodder.

Teratogens usually, but not invariably, act during a short, relatively early period of the gestation cycle, so that when the abnormalities become apparent in the offspring the causative plant may have disappeared from the fodder source. The range of plant constituents known to have teratogenic effects, albeit often demonstrated using only laboratory animals and large doses not normally experienced by humans, includes 14 different groups of alkaloids, coumarins, lignans, macrolides, nitriles, terpenoids, toxic amino acids and unidentified

compounds of many plants. As with the hallucinogens, the majority of teratogens contain nitrogen; for some examples see Table 39.1.

OTHER TOXIC PLANTS

In addition to those plants mentioned in this chapter and those of medicinal significance considered in Chapters 19–26, there remain many others with poisonous properties. Such plants are generally of local importance, and it is desirable that the pharmacist should have some knowledge of those found in his own locality, be familiar with those characters by which the plant can be identified and be aware of the antidotes required for the treatment of poisoning.

Cases of poisoning of humans by higher plants are most likely to occur with children and to involve those plants that produce attractive berries (e.g. belladonna, cotoneaster), seeds (e.g. laburnum) eaten for green peas, and those which may be introduced into the mouth for other reasons (e.g. the hollow stems of hemlock used as pea-shooters). Mistaken identity occasionally leads to fatalities and this is particularly so in the case of members of the Umbelliferae. Cases include a fatality in Maine, USA from consumption of *Cicuta maculata* (spotted cowbane) in mistake for ginseng. The poisonous principle present in *Cicuta* spp. is a C$_{17}$-polyunsaturated alcohol named cicutoxin. Some eleven such polyacetylenes have been isolated from *C. virosa* (water-hemlock) and using a model neurone, U. Wittstock *et al.* have suggested that the toxic property of cicutoxin could be due to a prolonged neuronal action potential (*Planta Medica*, 1997, **63**, 120). In Holland, four people were poisoned by *Oenanthe crocata* (hemlock water dropwort) consumed in mistake for celery (these people probably survived because the roots were boiled before eating). This plant its widespread in marshy and damp woodland areas of Europe; its roots have an odour and taste resembling parsnips or celery and the poisonous principle is oenanthetoxin, isomeric with cicutoxin.

The poisoning of livestock by plants is relatively common, particularly in extensive grazing areas where there is no attempt to control weeds. Poisonous plants may be consumed by animals because the plants happen to be growing among the fodder or were collected and dried with hay. In the latter case some unstable poisonous constituents may disappear with drying and storage. In poor seasons animals may forage and consume plants which they would not normally eat. During the dry summer of 1976 numerous cows died near Crediton, UK after eating *O. crocata*.

Some widespread poisonous plants owe their properties to the presence of hepatotoxic pyrrolizidine alkaloids (see Fig. 26.10). These include the *Senecio* spp. (ragworts) and members of the tribe Eupatorieae of the Compositae. Several commonly used herbs containing small quantities of these alkaloids include comfrey, Russian comfrey, coltsfoot and petasites. Human fatalities have been reported in relation to the herbal use of *Senecio longibobus* in the USA. In the UK, a voluntary agreement by herbal medicine suppliers not to supply senecio products is now being followed with proposed legislation by the Medicines and Healthcare products Regulatory Agency to implement a ban (*Pharm. J.*, 2007, **278**, 448).

Another group of compounds which has been shown to promote liver cancer in rats is that containing safrole and other alkenylbenzene derivatives. Although these are weak carcinogens and concentrations in products for human consumption never approach the toxic levels observed in laboratory tests, the desirability of their use has been questioned. Oils in which they occur include sassafras, Brazilian sassafras, star-anise, nutmeg, cinnamon, camphor (natural), calamus, tarragon, basil and ylang-ylang. M. De Vincenzi *et al.* have consid-

Table 39.1   Teratogens of higher plants.

Plant source	Constituents	Notes
Senecio spp. (Compositae)	Pyrrolizidine alkaloids: lasiocarpine, retrorsine	Possible teratogenic effects in rats and *in utero* deaths of calves
Indigofera spicata (Leguminosae)	$H_2N-C-(CH_2)_4-CH-COOH$, with NH and NH_2 groups — Indospicine	Cleft palate and embryo lethality in rats. Possible malformations in domestic livestock. Indospicine teratogenesis
Nicotiana spp. (Solanaceae), *Lobelia* spp. (Campanulaceae)	Pyridine alkaloids	Probably responsible for some skeletal deformations in pigs but effect not positively attributable to alkaloids
Blighia sapida (Akee) fruits and seeds (Sapindaceae)	$H_2C=$ ... $CH_2-CH-COOH$ with NH_2 — Hypoglycin A	Hypoglycin A is known to be hypoglycaemic in humans and teratogenic in rats; it is twice as toxic as its peptide derivative hypoglycin B
Leucaena leucocephala; *Mimosa* spp. (Leguminosae)	Mimosine	Large quantities toxic to livestock. Teratogenic effects demonstrated in pigs and rats
Locoplants e.g. *Astragalus lentiginosus* (Leguminosae)	Unknown	Contains osteolathyrogens (substances ingested by young through mother's milk), and teratogens characterized by causing excessive flexure of carpal joints or contracted tendons
Lupins e.g. *Lupinus sericeus* (Leguminosae)	Quinolizidine alkaloids, e.g. cytisine, anagyrine — Anagyrine, Cytisine	Teratogenic effect results in crooked calf disease
Conium maculatum (Umbelliferae)	Coniine	Alkaloid teratogenic, shown to produce crooked calf disease
Veratrum californicum (Liliaceae)	Many steroidal alkaloids — Cyclopamine	Teratogenic effect causes cyclopian and related cephalic malformations in lambs. The three active alkaloids have a fused furanopiperidine ring E/F arrangement as in cyclopamine

ered the specific occurrence of methyleugenol as a component of aromatic plants (*Fitoterapia*, 2000, **71**, 216).

Other carcinogens or cocarcinogens discussed elsewhere are the betel quid and tigliane and daphnane derivatives and related diterpenes.

The fruits of *Blighia sapida* have been mentioned elsewhere in connection with teratogenesis (Table 39.1) and hypoglycaemia (Chapter 29). The unripe fruits present an exceptional hazard for young children in the areas in which the trees grow. In 1998 an epidemic of fatal encephalopathy involved 29 preschool children in Burkina Faso, W. Africa (H. A. Meda *et al.*, *Lancet*, 1999, **353**, 536) and a similar explanation was suggested for an epidemic involving more than 100 children in the Ivory Coast in 1984 and for poisonings in Jamaica. The unripe fruits contain the highest hypoglycin A content but nevertheless the ripe fruits also need to be par-boiled before consumption. As in all cases of poisoning, rapid identification of the poison is essential if the most effective treatment is to be given. Often, the material available for identification is scant and rarely sufficient to enable identification by means of standard methods based on a flora; this reinforces a need for knowledge of the local poisonous plants and the characters of their various morphological parts.

Fungi have a geographically universal potential as toxic agents, and the significance of their active constituents, mycotoxins, is only now coming to be fully appreciated. Well-established are the poisonous principles of various Basidiomycetes which may be confused with the edible mushroom and toadstools. Also, the infection of rye with the ergot fungus resulting in the disease St Anthony's Fire, which, although now rare, still occasionally occurs in rye-eating countries. The polyketide patulin is produced by species of *Penicillium* and is often present in mouldy apples; it was originally studied for its antibiotic properties but proved also to be a potent carcinogen.

The more widespread danger of mycotoxins became apparent in World War II, when the consumption of mouldy grain in Russia led to thousands of fatalities. The mycotoxins produced by various *Aspergillus* spp. (e.g. *A. flavus, A. parasiticus*) are termed aflatoxins, all having a coumarin nucleus fused to a bifuran unit and possessing in addition a pentenone ring (B series) or a six-membered lactone (G series). Examples are given in Fig. 39.6.

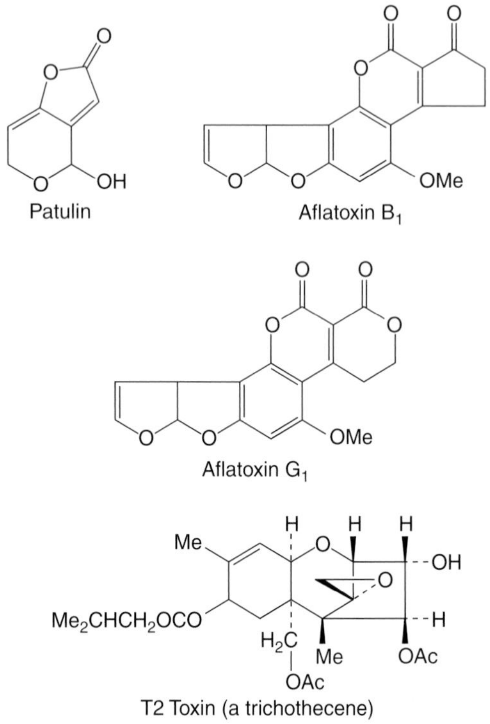

The above moulds are particularly likely to occur in oil-seed meals and in cereals; they have been circumstantially implicated in the deaths of children in a number of countries. Animal tests have shown the aflatoxins to be potentially harmful in a number of respects—as potent toxins, as carcinogens, as teratogens and as mutagens. In Britain these compounds came to prominence in 1959 when great numbers of turkeys and chickens in East Anglia rapidly succumbed to their toxicity after being fed contaminated groundnut meal imported from S. America. The recognition of the serious health hazards to humans and animals of aflatoxins in foods has led to the legal imposition in the UK of a limit of 10 µg kg^{-1} aflatoxin B$_1$ in nuts and nut products for human consumption, and an EU guideline for a limit of 20 µg kg^{-1} aflatoxin B$_1$ for animal feedstuffs. Methods of assay for these compounds have been developed in recent years and include HPLC and TLC (slow and cumbersome) and various RIA and EIA techniques.

Another condition arising from consumption of overwintered mouldy cereals, and reported to occur principally in Russia, is alimentary toxic aleukia; other manifestations include weight loss, skin inflammation and death. The responsible organisms (largely *Fusarium* and *Trichothecium* spp.) produce active constituents termed trichothecenes of which about 172 had been reported by 1981 (see J. F. Grove, *Nat. Prod. Rep.*, 1993, **10**, 429). These compounds are tricyclic sesquiterpenes and the majority are exemplified by the structure of T2 toxin (Fig. 39.6). However, some 67 compounds are macrocyclic in structure and it is interesting that they also occur in two toxic Brazilian species of *Baccharis* (Compositae), a finding which was originally incorrectly attributed to fungal infection (B. B. Jarvis *et al.*, *J. Nat. Prod.*, 1988, **51**, 736; *Phytochemistry*, 1991, **30**, 789). Matossian of the University of Maryland considers that *F. tricinctum* was the probable fungal food contaminant causing 'putrid malignant fever', a great child-killer of the early eighteenth century. These compounds also achieved notoriety as alleged agents of chemical warfare ('yellow rain').

Crude drugs, unless sterilized, are often grossly contaminated with mould spores, and if such drugs are to be consumed as such (as distinct from use for the isolation of active constituents), then it is important that they are free of dangerous mycotoxins. A Polish survey of 246 crude drug samples found only two (salvia leaves and tormentilla rhizome) which contained *Aspergillus* spp. producing aflatoxin B$_1$. Nevertheless, it is a situation that requires monitoring.

Fig. 39.6
Structures of some mycotoxins.

Further reading

Frohn D, Pfander HJ, Alford I (translator) 2005 Poisonous plants: a handbook for doctors, pharmacists, toxicologists, biologists and veterinarians, 2nd edn. Timber Press, Portland, OR. *An appendix includes information concerning N. American plants*

Harborne J B, Baxter H, Moss G P (eds) 1996 Dictionary of plant toxins. John Wiley, Chichester, UK. *A number of books on poisonous plants, now mostly out of print but useful if accessible, are given in the 14th edition of this book, p. 532*

40

Pesticides of natural origin

Pesticides may be classified according to the type of organism against which they are effective, namely, fungicides, herbicides, insecticides, molluscicides, nematocides, rodenticides. The origin of the use of natural products in these respects is lost in antiquity (see Further Reading) and a large number of such materials, of local use, still remain to be chemically investigated and evaluated. Although the majority of pesticides used in modern agriculture are synthetic, plant products still contribute to the insecticides and rodenticides. Phytochemicals can also serve as lead compounds from which others, exhibiting, for example, a greater toxicity towards the pest, a wide spectrum of activity such as the inclusion of mites, a lowered mammalian toxicity and a decrease in photodecomposition, can be developed.

ACARICIDES

Mites and ticks are small arachnids of the order Acarina (Acari). Specific mites infest crude drugs and food (Chapter 13) and the house-dust mite, *Dermatophagoides pteronyssinus*, is well known for its possible association with asthma. Ticks are the largest members of the order and economically the most important. They are all blood-sucking parasites responsible for microbial infections, e.g the spirochaete infection causing Lyme disease, and protozoal diseases in animals.

The control of mites by plant products has centred largely on essential oils. In a report (*Pharm. J.*, 1998, **261**, 406) on the laboratory testing of three oils by I. Burgess and colleagues, tea tree oil was the most effective, giving 100% immobilization of house-dust mites at 30 min, and 100% mortality at 2 h; for the same exposure times lavender oil gave figures of 87% and 87% and lemon oil 63% and 80% respectively. Australian workers have demonstrated that for laundering purposes several essential oils are effective acaricides when emulsified in low concentrations of the laboratory detergent Tween and that a simple washing procedure with eucalyptus oil, without the use of very hot water, controlled house-dust mites and their allergens in clothing and bedding (E. R. Tovey and L. G. McDonald, *J. Allergy Clin. Immunol.*, 1997, **100**, 464).

For Third World countries where synthetic acaricides are relatively expensive the exploitation of suitable local plants is important. The essential oils of some members of the Capparidaceae have been shown to be effective antitick agents and the situation is outlined by W. Lwande *et al.* (*Phytochemistry*, 1999, **50**, 40) in their studies on the tick-repellent properties of the essential oil of *Gynandropsis gynandron*. This East African annual species has been proposed as an antitick pasture plant as it disrupts the free-living stages of *Rhipicephalus appendiculatus*, the vector of the pathogen causing East Coast fever in animals. Twenty-eight compounds were identified in the essential oil, carvacrol, phytol and linalool being the major constituents, although greatest repellency towards the tick was shown by a number of minor constituents. Methyl isothiocyanate was also identified in the oil (2.1%) and could contribute towards the activity. It may be noted here that *G. gynandron* is also employed in traditional medicine for a number of conditions and its essential oil is used as a repellant for head-lice.

INSECTICIDES

PYRETHRUM FLOWER

Pyrethrum flowers (Insect flowers, Dalmatian insect flowers) are the dried flower-heads of *Chrysanthemum cinerariifolium* (Trev.) Vis. [*Tanacetum cinerariifolium* (Trev.) Sch. Bip., *Pyrethrum cinerariifolium* Trev.] (Compositae). The plant is perennial, about 1 m high, and indigenous to the Balkans. Principal cultivated sources are Kenya, Tasmania, Tanzania and Rwanda. Smaller amounts are grown in Japan, Eastern Europe, Brazil and India.

History. The insecticidal properties of Persian or Caucasian insect flowers (*Chrysanthemum coccineum* Willd. and *C. marshallii* Aschers) have long been known in their country of origin, but the use of the Yugoslavian species dates from the middle of the last century. Persian insect flowers are now rarely seen in British commerce, and Kenya, the largest exporter, produces flowers of the Dalmatian type, the original Dalmatian seed being introduced by Gilbert Walker in 1928.

Collection. Conditions for pyrethrum cultivation are particularly favourable in Kenya; the producing areas have an altitude of 1900–2700 m and an annual rainfall of 76–180 cm. The altitude is important, giving a low night temperature (5–15°C), which stimulates maximum bud production. Collection takes place for about 9 months of the year. As about 90% of the insecticidal activity of the plant is present in the flowers, only these are collected. Before drying they are not toxic to insects. In Kenya all the flowers are delivered to the Pyrethrum Marketing Board at Nakuru. Here all samples are analysed and the growers paid on the pyrethrin content of their deliveries. The thousands of African smallholders are organized on cooperative lines and all the profits of the Board are returned to the growers. At the factory of the Board some of the flowers are baled for export but the majority are made either into powder or into standardized liquid extract. Current developments may be followed in the biannual journal *Pyrethrum Post*.

Characters. The closed flower-heads are about 6–9 mm in diameter and the open ones about 9–12 mm in diameter. They bear a short peduncle which is striated longitudinally. The involucre consists of two or three rows of yellowish or greenish-yellow, lanceolate, hairy bracts. The receptable is nearly flat and devoid of palae. It bears numerous, yellow tubular florets and a single row of cream or straw-coloured ligulate florets. The ligulate corollas are 10–20 mm in length and have about 17 veins and three rounded teeth, the central one very small (distinction from ox-eye daisies, *C. leucanthemum*, in which the ligulate corollas have seven veins and three teeth, the centre one being the largest). The achenes are five-ribbed (achenes of Persian flowers usually 10-ribbed). The flowers have a slightly aromatic odour and a bitter, acrid taste.

Characters of powders. The species used as insecticides are *C. cinerariifolium*, *C. coccineum* and *C. marshallii*, the powders from which show the following elements: parenchyma often containing aggregate crystals, T-shaped hairs, numerous spherical pollen grains, sclerenchymatous cells (particularly from Persian flowers), tracheids and epidermal cells having a striated, papillose cuticle. Kenya flowers are guaranteed to contain not less than 1.3% of pyrethrin; Japanese usually contain 0.9–1.0% and Dalmatian about 0.7–0.8%.

Constituents. Pyrethrum owes its insecticidal properties to esters which are reportedly produced by a number of different cell types (oil glands, resin ducts and mesophyll cells). Pyrethrin I, jasmolin I and cinerin I are esters of chrysanthemic acid (chrysanthemum monocarboxylic acid), while pyrethrin II, jasmolin II and cinerin II are esters of pyrethric acid (monomethyl ester of chrysanthemum dicarboxylic acid). The alcohol component of the pyrethrins is the keto-alcohol pyrethrolone and of the cinerins the keto-alcohol cinerolone. Pyrethrum flowers also contain sesquiterpene lactones and the triterpenoid pyrethrol. The biosynthesis of pyrethrin I in seedlings of *C. cinerariifolium* has been studied using [1-^{13}C]-D-glucose as a precursor; the acid portion of the molecule is derived from D-glucose and the alcohol

moiety possibly from linoleic acid (K. Matsuda *et al.*, *Phytochemistry*, 2005, **66**, 1529).

Pyrethrum Extract of the *BP* (*Vet.*) contains 24.5–25.5% of pyrethrins; it may be prepared extemporaneously from the flower-heads and is used for the preparation of the *BP* (*Vet.*) dusting powder and spray. The dusting powder (pyrethrum extract, diatomite, talc) has a pyrethrin content of 0.36–0.44%, of which not less than half consists of pyrethrin I. It is assayed by titrimetry for both pyrethrin I and II. Extracts containing 50% more active material compared with commercial extracts can be obtained by extraction of the plant material with liquified carbon dioxide (100 bar). The extract is usually diluted on farms with kerosene to a pyrethrin strength of about 0.2%. For work on *Pyrethrum* hybrids, see Chapter 14.

The popularity of pyrethrum derived from its rapid knock-down action (largely due to pyrethrin II), lethality to insects (pyrethrin I) and low mammalian toxicity. However, synthetic analogues of natural pyrethrins with higher insecticidal activity (over 1000 times that of pyrethrin I), more photostability and a similar low toxicity have virtually displaced pyrethrin from the market, particularly in the area of domestic insecticidal sprays. There continues, however, to be a market for natural pyrethrins in special areas such as food processing plants and insecticidal spraying of edible fruits and vegetables shortly before harvest.

	R	R^1
Pyrethrin I	CH$_3$	CH=CH$_2$
Jasmolin I	CH$_3$	CH$_2$–CH$_3$
Cinerin I	CH$_3$	CH$_3$
Pyrethrin II	COOCH$_3$	CH=CH$_2$
Jasmolin II	COOCH$_3$	CH$_2$–CH$_3$
Cinerin I	COOCH$_3$	CH$_3$

Uses. Insect flowers are a contact poison for insects. They are largely used in the form of powder, but sprays in which the active principles are dissolved in kerosene or other organic solvent are more efficient. For recent developments, see above.

Derris and lonchocarpus

The roots of many species of *Derris* and *Lonchocarpus* (Leguminosae) have insecticidal properties which are usually, but not invariably, due to the presence of rotenone. The former *British Veterinary Codex* included monographs on 'Derris', the dried rhizome and roots of *Derris elliptica*, *D. malaccensis* and possibly other species, and on 'Lonchocarpus', the dried roots of *Lonchocarpus utilis*, *L. urucu* and possibly other species. Other genera of the same family with rotenoid-producing species are *Millettia*, *Neorautanenia* and *Tephrosia*.

Derris is indigenous to Malaya and is cultivated there and in Burma, Thailand and tropical Africa. Lonchocarpus is indigenous to Peru and Brazil and it is the usual source of material on the UK and USA markets, frequently being sold as a black resinous extract containing about 30% of isolatable rotenone and about 20% of the structurally related deguelin.

Characters. Derris roots are up to 2 m long and 1 cm or more diameter. They are sometimes attached to short pieces of rhizome. The outer surface is greyish-brown to reddish-brown and bears fine longitudinal furrows and, in the larger pieces, elongated lenticles. The drug is flexible and breaks with a fibrous fracture. It has a slight aromatic odour; and when chewed, gradually produces a feeling of numbness in the tongue and throat. Prolonged grinding of the drug is necessary on account of its fibrous nature, and special precautions are necessary, owing to the objectionable properties of the dust. A transverse section shows a thin brown bark and a cream to pale-brown wood which in the larger pieces show three or four concentric rings.

Lonchocarpus usually occurs in pieces 4–30 cm long and 1.5–2.5 cm in diameter. The outer surface is brownish-grey, with wrinkles and scars and, in the larger pieces, transverse lenticles.

Constituents. Derris and lonchocarpus contain about 3–10% of rotenone, a colourless crystalline substance which is insoluble in water but soluble in many organic solvents. However, rotenone is not the only constituent with insecticidal properties, and the evaluation of the drug depends both on rotenone content and on the amount of chloroform extractive it contains.

Rotenone is an isoflavone derivative and is biosynthesized from acetate, mevalonate and phenylalanine with an extra carbon arising from a C-1 pool. Its toxicity to mammals limits its usefulness.

Rotenone (a rotenoid)

The roots also contain deguelin which is similar to rotenone but possesses a *gem*-dimethylpyran moiety. Flavonoids and stilbenes with the same moiety are minor components.

Rotenoid derivatives, having a larvicidal property, have been isolated from *Derris trifoliata*; activity is due mainly to rotenone (A. Yenesew *et al.*, *Phytochemistry*, 2006, **67**, 988).

Nicotinoids

As early as 1763 nicotine, in the form of a tea prepared from tobacco, was recommended for the destruction of aphids.

The genus *Nicotiana* (Solanaceae) comprises about 100 species. Tobacco for smoking, chewing and snuffing is prepared by a curing process, largely of the cultivated Virginian tobacco, *N. tabacum*, and the Turkish tobacco, *N. rustica*. Tobacco is believed to be a native of tropical America, and was cultivated and used by the native inhabitants before the discovery of the American continent by Europeans. *N. tabacum* is of hybrid origin, and various 'synthetic tobaccos', somewhat resembling it, have been raised by crossing and breeding wild, possibly ancestral, species. Nicotine (structure and biogenetic origin, Fig. 26.2) is the characteristic alkaloid of the genus and is prepared commercially from waste material of the tobacco industry; it has long been used as an effective insecticide but is gradually being replaced by safer products. Other species (e.g. *N. glutinosa*) produce nornicotine by demethylation of nicotine in the leaves, whereas some (e.g. *N. glauca*) contain, in addition to the nicotine alkaloids, the homologous anabasine (structure and biogenetic origin, Fig. 26.11). Nornicotine and anabasine are also insecticidal. An interesting report (J. E. Huesing and D. Jones, *Phytochemistry*, 1987, **26**, 1381) indicated that extracts of species of *Nicotiana*, section Repandae, caused high levels of mortality in *Manduca sexta*, the tobacco hornworm, a tobacco-associated insect which is not susceptible to the toxic effects of nicotine. The insecticidal component is an *N*-acylnornicotine which is found only in this section of the genus and is absent from the other 65 spp.

The nicotinoids are also found in some other members of the Solanaceae (spp. of *Duboisia*, *Anthocercis*, *Cyphanthera* and *Crenidium*), a few *Erythroxylum* spp., *Asclepias syriaca* and *Anabasis aphylla*.

Cevadilla seed. Cevadilla or sabadilla consists of the seeds of *Schoenocaulon officinale* (Liliaceae), a plant found from Mexico to Venezuela. The seeds are dark brown to black, sharply pointed and about 6 mm long. They contain about 2–4% of mixed alkaloids known as 'veratrine'. The chief alkaloids, cevadine and veratridine, are closely related to the ester alkaloids of veratrum (q.v.). The powdered seeds and preparations of 'veratrine' are used as a dust or spray to control thrips and various true bugs which attack vegetables.

Ryania. The roots and stems of *Ryania speciosa* (Flacourtiaceae), a plant native to South America, contain 0.16%–0.2% of alkaloids having insecticidal properties. Ryanodine, the principal alkaloid, is a complex ester involving 1-pyrrole-carboxylic acid. The plant is used in the control of various lepidopterous larvae which attack fruits, and particularly the European corn borer.

Miscellaneous

A number of other plants containing insecticidal compounds with scope for synthetic improvement include *Mammea* spp., Guttiferae (coumarins); Ebenaceous spp., containing the naphthoquinone plumbagin (q.v.) and *Phryma leptostachya*, Verbenaceae (a highly active lignan, haedoxan A). *Melia azedarach* (Meliaceae), native to N.W. India, has been long recognized for its insecticidal properties and is still the subject of considerable research. Three diacylated meliacarpin derivatives with strong insecticidal activity against the larvae of *Spodoptera littoralis* have been isolated from the leaves (F. I. Bohnenstengel *et al.*, *Phytochemistry*, 1999, **50**, 977); two insecticidal tetranortriterpenoids have potential for further development (B. S. Siddiqui *et al.*, *Phytochemistry*, 2000, **53**, 371) and positive antifeedant properties have been demonstrated with extracts of unripe fruits and green or senescent leaves against mature adults of the elm leaf beetle, *Xanthogaleruca luteola* (M. Defagó *et al.*, *Fitoterapia*, 2006, **77**, 500).

RODENTICIDES

Red squill. Red squill and white squill (see 'Cardioactive Drugs', Chapter 23) are both varieties of *Urginea maritima* (Liliaceae). The red squill may be distinguished in either the whole or powdered state by the reddish-brown outer scales and the white to deep purple inner ones. In addition to other cardioactive glycosides, the bulb of the red squill also contains the glucosides scilliroside and scillirubroside. Strains selected for high scilliroside content have been developed from plants introduced to southern California in 1946. Unlike other mammals, rodents do not regurgitate the squill bulb, and death follows convulsions and respiratory failure.

Strychnine. The occurrence of strychnine in *Strychnos* species (Loganiaceae) has already been discussed. This alkaloid has been used traditionally for the extermination of moles, but its toxicity to other animals and its painful poisonous action do not make it a poison of choice.

MOLLUSCICIDES

Pharmaceutical interest in molluscicides is concerned primarily with the control of schistosomiasis (bilharzia), a parasitic disease of humans in which certain freshwater snails act as intermediate hosts for the blood flukes, *Schistosoma haemotobium, S. mansoni* and *S. japonicum*. The disease, which causes intestinal and bladder damage, is prevalent in S. America, Africa and the Far East and is increasing as a result of the construction of dams and irrigation systems which provide enlarged breeding areas for snails. Eggs are eliminated in the faeces or urine of infected humans and, in water, hatch as miracidia which enter the host snails (*Biomphalaria pfeiffer* (S. America), *B. glabrata, Bulinus globosus*, etc.) where numerous cercaria are produced. The cercaria emerge into the water and infect humans by passing through the skin into the bloodstream. Synthetic drugs are available to combat the infection but for the general control of the disease the eradication of the intermediate stages of the life-cycle of the fluke is necessary together with improved sanitary arrangements. In 1998 it was estimated that there were over 20 million severely diseased individuals in the tropics and some ten times that number infected to some degree.

During the last two decades it has been shown that a wide range of phytochemicals exhibit molluscicidal activity. Prominent families in this connection are the Leguminosae, Araliaceae, Compositae and Liliaceae. However, before a plant, shown to possess molluscicidal activity in laboratory tests, can be utilized on a large scale a number of other, fairly obvious, criteria need to be satisfied. Thus, the plant material must be available in sufficient quantity and, if necessary, capable of easy propagation in the region where required; the active constituents should be water-soluble and easily extractable from the plant source; the molluscicidal activity should be high and the toxicity towards other organisms, including humans, low. Few plants as yet examined appear to have satisfied all of these requirements.

The berries of the Ethiopian plant *Phytolacca dodecandra* (Phytolaccaceae) have proved effective in clearing stretches of waterways of snails, but cultivation in areas outside of the natural habitat has produced disappointingly low yields of fruits. The most active components of this plant are triterpenoid saponins composed of oleanolic acid (Fig. 23.10) with a branched sugar side-chain at C-3; they are liberated by the enzymatic cleavage of the ester-bound saccharide chains of non-molluscicidal bidesmodic saponins (S. T. Thiilborg *et al., Phytochemistry*, 1993, **32**, 1167). A plant the pods of which contain similar saponins is *Swartzia madagascariensis* (Leguminosae), a tree widespread throughout Africa; it has local medicinal, insecticidal and piscicidal uses. The leaves of the S. America species *S. simplex* have a similar activity to those of the African plant and glycosides of oleanolic acid, gypsogenin (Fig. 23.10) and gypsogenic acid have been isolated as active constituents. Saponins are also present in *Tetrapleura tetraptera* (Leguminosae), a promising Nigerian molluscicide. A number of these plants containing effective saponins are also well established piscicides.

Spirostanol saponins, as found in *Balanites aegyptica* (Zygophyllaceae), are potent molluscicides. This plant contains balanitin-1, -2 and -3; balanitin-1, for example, possesses a yamogenin aglycone (q.v.) with a branched glucose and rhamnose side-chain. In the same family, saponins from the pericarps of *Guaiacum officinale* have molluscicidal activity. In an evaluation of plant molluscicides against the freshwater snail *Lymnaea luteola*, the vector of animal schistosomiasis in India, *Sapindus trifoliatus* (Sapindaceae) was the most effective of the species tested (D. Sukumaran *et al., Pharm. Biol.*, 2002, **40**, 450). The aqueous extracts of three other Indian-grown plants (*Thevetia peruviana, Alstonia scholaris* and *Euphorbia pulcherrina*) have also been shown to possess considerable molluscicidal activity (A. Singh and S. K. Singh, *Fitoterapia*, 2005, **76**, 747).

Tannins constitute the active principles of some Leguminosae e.g. *Acacia* spp., and napthoquinones of the juglone and plumbagin type (p. 251) constitute those of the Malawi Ebenaceous species *Diospyros usambarensis*. The disadvantage of the latter source, investigated by Hostettman *et al.*, is that the naphthoquinones are at their highest concentration in the root-bark.

Other phytochemical groups of compounds having recognized molluscicidal activity are isobutylamides of the Asteraceae, Rutaceae and Piperaceae, steroidal glycoalkaloids (*Solanum mammosum*), anthraquinones (*Morinda lucida*, Rubiaceae) and flavonoids of various families. Two N.E. Brazilian species of *Solanum* (*S. jabrense* and *S. stipulaceum*) have shown promising activity (T. M. S. Silva *et al., Fitoterapia*, 2006, **77**, 449).

Some of the most active substances known are the unsaturated anacardic acids of cashew nut shells (*Anacardium occidentale*), but unfortunately field trials carried out in Mozambique showed the treated water to give rise to dermatitis.

Continued progress in this area is to be expected; other plants tested and shown to possess molluscicidal activity include *Ambrosia maritima, Ammi majus, Azolla pinnata, Calendula micrantha officinalis, Croton campestris, Cucumis prophetarum, Euphorbia splendens, Millettia thonningii* and *Rhynchosia minimum*.

Further reading

Casida JE, Quistad GB (eds) 1995 Pyrethrum flowers, production, chemistry, toxicology and uses. Oxford University Press, New York
Dales MJ 1996 A review of plant materials used for controlling insect pests of stored products. Bulletin 65, Natural Resources Institute, Chatham, UK
Regnault-Roger C, Philogène BJR 2008 Past and current prospects for the use of botanicals and plant allelochemicals in integrated pest management. Pharmaceutical Biology 46(1–2): 41–52. *A review with 90 references*

PART

8

Morphological and microscopical examination of drugs

Introduction

In standard works such as the *European Pharmacopoeia*, the *British Pharmacopoeia*, the *British Herbal Pharmacopoeia* and similar publications of other countries one will find detailed morphological and anatomical descriptions of those plant drugs that are included as monographs. Microscopical characteristics of the powdered drugs are also given. Such descriptions form the basis for the identification of drugs and from this the detection of adulterated and poor quality material.

Of recent significance concerning the above is the introduction of EU directives governing the quality control of licensed herbal medicinal products. These regulations require manufacturers of such medicinals to have available personnel with the particular expertise to carry out identification tests and to recognize adulterants, the presence of fungal growth, infestation and non-uniformity within a delivery of crude drugs, etc.

To understand, and to make practical use of, the pharmacopoeial and other descriptions requires a knowledge of the botanical terminology used and an acquired skill in recognizing the structures cited for both the whole and powdered plant. It is also necessary to appreciate the function of, and to select the most appropriate, mounting reagents for the microscopical examination of drugs. Formerly, a student's practical training in pharmacognosy was largely devoted to developing such skills but now, particularly in the UK, USA and Australia these studies have been reduced to a minimum with greatest emphasis being placed on the theoretical aspects, and practical applications, of the more recent developments of the subject. Nevertheless as readers will have perceived from Part 5 of this book, such morphological and anatomical studies still form a very necessary core of the subject and are a prerequisite to the use, for medicinal purposes, of any plant consignment.

For the UK, further explanation of the EU regulatory requirements is given in 'Rules and Guidance for Pharmaceutical Manufacturers and Distributors 2007, Annex 7—Manufacture of Herbal Medicinal Products' compiled by the Inspection and Standards Division of the Medicines and Healthcare products Regulatory Agency, published by the Pharmaceutical Press.

41

Plant description, morphology and anatomy

Plant form ranges from unicellular plants—for example, yeasts and some green algae—to the strongly differentiated higher plants. Examples of pharmaceutical interest may be found in most of the larger groups and a quick perusal of the families involved in Chapter 5 of this textbook illustrates this point.

Characteristically the higher plants consist in the vegetative phase of roots, stems and leaves with flowers, fruits and seeds forming stages in the reproductive cycle. Modifications of the above structures are frequently present—rhizomes (underground stems), stolons (runners with a stem structure), stipules, bracts (modified leaves), tendrils (modified stems), etc. Certain organs may appear to be missing or much reduced—for example, the reduction of leaves in some xerophytic plants.

It is most important that students acquire the ability to interpret morphological and anatomical descriptions of crude drugs as found in pharmacopoeias and allied works and also to record adequately the features of whole or powdered drugs and adulterants of commercial significance.

As indicated in Chapter 2, for convenience of study, drugs may be arranged not only according to families and chemical constituents, but also into such morphological groups as barks, roots, leaves, seeds, etc. Some drugs constitute more than one morphological part—for example, whole herbs and commercial 'roots', which may consist of both rhizomes and roots.

LEAVES AND TOPS ('HERBS')

These consist of stems (often limited in their girth by 'official' requirements) and leaves often associated with flowers and young fruits. All portions of such drugs need to be described.

Aerial stem. Note dimensions, shape, colour, whether herbaceous or woody, upright or creeping, smooth or ridged, hairs present or not and if so whether of the glandular or covering form. Note arrangement of tissues as seen in transverse section.

Position and arrangement of leaves. *Radical* (arising from the crown of the root) or *cauline* (arising from the aerial stem). In the Solanaceae note *adnation* (the fusion of part of the leaf with the stem). The arrangement may be *alternate* (e.g. lobelia), *opposite, decussate* (in pairs alternately at right angles; e.g. peppermint) or *whorled*.

Leaves, flowers and fruits. These can be described according to the schedules given below.

Structure of the aerial stem. The primary stem (Fig 41.1A) shows the following structure: epidermis, cortex, medullary rays, medulla and a vascular system taking the form of a dictyostele. The epidermis is composed of a single layer of compactly arranged cells and bears stomata. The cortex is usually parenchymatous, the outer layers of cells in aerial stems containing chloroplasts. The layers of cortex cells immediately underlying the epidermis may be collenchymatous, constituting a hypodermis. The endodermis is usually not well-differentiated in aerial stems, although a layer of cells containing starch (starch sheath) and corresponding in position to the endodermis may be defined. Underground stems often resemble roots in showing a more or less well-differentiated endodermis with characteristic Casparian strips (thickenings).

The pericycle may take the form of a complete or a discontinuous ring of fibres or may be parenchymatous and ill-defined. Pericycle fibres may form a cap outside each primary phloem group.

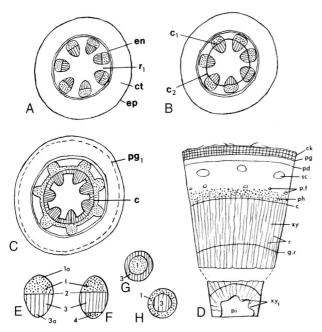

Fig. 41.1
Stem structure of dicotyledons (transverse section). A, primary structure
showing seven vascular bundles; B, development of a complete cambial ring
by formation of the interfascicular cambium; C, beginning of a secondary
growth; D, stem after a number of seasons of growth, outer cork now
present. E–H, types of vascular bundle: E, collateral; F, bicollateral;
G, amphivasal; H, amphicribral. c, Cambium; c_1, fascicular cambium;
c_2, interfascicular cambium; ck, cork; ct, cortex; en, endodermis; ep,
epidermis; g.r, growth ring; pd, phelloderm; p.f, pericyclic fibres; pg,
phellogen; pg_1, developing phellogen; pi, pith; r, rays; r_1, primary
medullary ray; sc, sclerenchyma; xy, xylem; xy_1, primary xylem; 1,
phloem; 1a, protophloem; 2, fascicular cambium; 3, xylem; 3a,
protoxylem.

The vascular bundles of the dictyostele are usually collateral, but are
in some cases bicollateral (Cucurbitaceae, Solanaceae, Convolvulaceae)
(Fig. 41.1E–H). The xylem is differentiated centrifugally and the protoxylem is endarch; the phloem is differentiated centripetally and the
protophloem is exarch (cf. the root). The differentiation, in dicotyledons, is usually incomplete, so that a zone of meristematic cells (the
intrafascicular cambium) separates the primary vascular tissues. Such
a bundle is described as open, in contrast to the closed bundle typical
of monocotyledons. In the bicollateral bundle the intrafascicular
cambium occurs between the xylem and the outer phloem group.

Secondary thickening is initiated by tangential divisions in the
intrafascicular cambium. The daughter cells cut off on the inner side
differentiate into xylem and those cut off to the outside into phloem.
The amount of secondary xylem produced in both stems and roots, in
general, exceeds the amount of secondary phloem. As the process of
secondary thickening of the stem proceeds, its dictyostele is converted
into a solid cylinder of secondary tissues. The intrafascicular cambia
become linked to form a continuous cambial cylinder by the development of interfascicular cambia in the ray tissue (Fig. 41.1B, C). The
cambial activity may spread out from the intrafascicular cambia across
the rays, or in other cases cambial activity may originate at a median
point in the ray and then by lateral extension from both intrafascicular
and interfascicular cambia the cambial cylinder may be completed.

In woody perennials the cambial divisions are arrested during the
winter but are renewed each spring. The xylem produced at different
seasons varies in texture. The spring wood is characterized by abundance

of relatively thin-walled large conducting elements; the autumn wood,
by a high proportion of thick-walled mechanical elements such as wood
fibres. A similar alteration between sieve tissue and phloem fibres may
occur in the secondary phloem. With increase in girth the central core
of xylem may become non-functional, dark in colour and packed with
metabolic byproducts forming a heartwood or duramen. Sandalwood is
the heartwood of *Santalum album* and is packed with volatile oil. The
blocking of the vessels in the formation of heartwood occurs by the
development of tyloses (see Fig. 42.6P).

The secondary increase in diameter of the vascular cylinder is
accompanied by changes in the outer tissues. The epidermis and part
or all of the primary cortex may be shed. A phellogen may arise in
the epidermis, cortex or pericycle and give rise externally to cork and
internally to a variable amount of phelloderm (Fig. 41.1D).

For the investigation of the anatomy of stems, transverse sections
and radial and tangential longitudinal sections should be prepared from
the drug previously moistened or soaked. For a study of the individual
elements, disintegrated material should be used (see Chapter 43).

The following structures are constantly present in powdered stems:
cork and vascular tissues in varying amount; abundant parenchyma
often containing starch. Calcium oxalate and other cell inclusions may
be present. Aleurone grains are absent.

The relative amounts, size, shape and form of the structural elements are of first importance in identification. The xylem elements,
which are well-preserved in dry drugs, are of particular importance.

BARKS

As understood in commerce, barks consist of all tissues outside the
cambium. In botany the term 'bark' is sometimes restricted to the
'outer bark'—that is, the periderm and all tissues lying outside it.

A young bark (Fig. 41.1) is composed of the following tissues.

1. Epidermis: a layer of closely fitting cuticularized cells with occasional stomata.
2. Primary cortex: a zone usually consisting of chlorophyll-containing
   collenchyma and parenchyma.
3. Endodermis: or inner layer of the cortex, which frequently contains
   starch.
4. Pericycle: which may be composed of parenchyma or of fibres.
   Groups of fibres often occur opposite each group of phloem.
5. Phloem: which consists of sieve tubes, companion cells and phloem
   parenchyma separated by radially arranged medullary rays.

In commercial barks the above structures have been modified by the
activity of the cambium and the cork cambium or *phellogen*. Growth of
the new tissues produced by the cambium causes the tissues of the
primary bark to be tangentially stretched, compressed or torn. As these
cells are stretched tangentially they may be divided by radial walls—
for example, in the medullary rays. During this dilatation groups of
parenchymatous cells in the cortex and phloem may be thickened into
sclerenchymatous cells. The cambium produces secondary phloem,
which often consists of alternating zones of sieve elements and phloem
fibres. The pericycle is frequently ruptured, and parenchymatous cells
which grow into the spaces may develop into sclerenchyma.

The cork cambium or *phellogen* may arise in the epidermis (e.g. willow), primary cortex or pericycle. The phellogen produces on its outer
side *cork*, and on its inner side chlorophyll containing suberized cells
which form the *secondary cortex* or *phelloderm*. These three layers are
known as the *periderm*. If the cork cambium develops in or near the
pericycle, a part of the whole of the primary cortex will lie outside
the cork and will be gradually thrown off. *Lenticels* replace stomata for

purposes of gaseous exchange; and as the cork increases, the amount of chlorophyll-containing tissue decreases.

The natural curvature of the bark increases when the bark is removed from the tree and dried. Large pieces of trunk bark, especially if subjected to pressure, may be nearly flat. Terms used to describe the curvature are illustrated in Fig. 41.2. Some commercial barks (e.g. cinnamon and quillaia) consist of the inner bark only. In quillaia the dark patches often found on the outer surface are known as *rhytidome* (literally, 'a wrinkle'). This term is applied to plates of tissue formed in the inner bark by successive development of cork cambia.

Barks may be described under the following headings.

Origin and preparation. From trunk branches or roots. Whole or inner bark.

Size and shape

Outer surface. Lichens, mosses, lenticels, cracks or furrows, colour before and after scraping.

Inner surface. Colour, striations, furrows.

Fracture. Short, fibrous, splintery, granular, etc. The fracture depends largely on the number and distribution of sclereids and fibres. A bark frequently breaks with a short fracture in the outer part and a fibrous fracture in the phloem.

Transverse surface. A smoothed transverse surface, especially if stained with phloroglucinol and hydrochloric acid, will usually show the general arrangement of the lignified elements, medullary rays and cork. Sections, however, are more satisfactory and can be used for a microscopical examination of calcium oxalate.

Anatomy

The cork cells in transverse section are often tangentially elongated and arranged in regular radial rows. In surface view they are frequently polygonal. The cell walls give a suberin reaction; the cell contents frequently give a positive tannin reaction. The cortex is usually composed of a ground mass of parenchyma. An outer band of collenchyma often occurs. Secretion cells, sclereids and pericyclic fibres may occur scattered or in groups in the cortex. The cortical cells often contain starch or other typical cell inclusions such as calcium oxalate.

Sieve tubes, companion cells, phloem parenchyma and medullary ray cells are always present in the phloem, but these soft tissues may not be well-preserved in medicinal barks. The sieve tubes, unless well-developed, are observed only after special treatment. Secretion cells, phloem fibres and sclereids may or may not be present in the phloem.

Xylem tissue is usually absent but may be present in small amounts on the inner surface of the bark.

The following should all be carefully noted in the anatomical examination of barks: the presence or absence of outer bark (cork, phellogen, phelloderm); the structure, amount and site of origin of the cork; the extent, cell structure and cell contents of the cortex; the presence or absence and, if present, the distribution, size and form of sclereids, phloem fibres and secretion cells; and the width, height, distribution and cell structure and contents of the medullary rays. When calcium oxalate is present, its crystalline forms and their distribution should be studied.

Transverse and longitudinal sections should be prepared. The size and form of sclereids and phloem fibres are best studied in disintegrated material. Preparations treated with cellulose, lignin, starch, callus, oil, suberin and tannin stains should be examined.

The cell types mentioned above are discussed in Chapter 42.

Powdered barks. Powdered barks always possess sieve tubes and cellulose parenchyma. Cork, fibres, sclereids, starch, calcium oxalate and secretory tissues are frequently present. Xylem tissues are absent or only present in very small amount. Chlorophyll and aleurone grains are absent.

WOODS

Although few drugs consist solely of wood, no description of a stem or root is complete without an account of its wood. Wood consists of the secondary tissues produced by the cambium on its inner surface. The cells composing these tissues—the vessels, tracheids, wood fibres

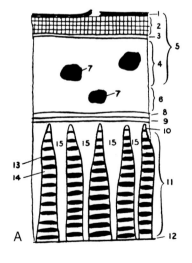
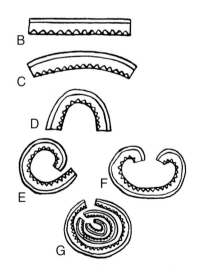

Fig. 41.2

Barks. A, diagram showing a typical arrangement of the tissues: 1, outer surface frequently showing lichens, lenticels and remains of primary tissues cut off by the cork; 2, cork; 3, cork cambium or phellogen; 4, phelloderm or secondary cortex; 5, periderm; 6, inner part of primary cortex; 7, groups of cortical sclerenchyma; 8, endodermis; 9, pericycle; 10, primary phloem; 11, secondary phloem; 12, cambium; 13, band of lignified fibres; 14, sieve elements; 15, medullary rays. B–G, shapes of barks: B, flat; C, curved; D, channelled; E, single quill; F, double quill; G, compound quill.

and parenchyma—are not necessarily all lignified. In some cases (e.g. the wood of belladonna root) non-lignified elements predominate. The distribution of the lignified elements may be ascertained by treating smoothed transverse, radial and tangential surfaces or sections with phloroglucinol and hydrochloric acid. In trees, the cells of the old wood frequently become coloured as they fill with waste products such as resins, tannins and colouring matters. This central region is called the *heartwood*, while the outer wood, which still retains its normal appearance and functions, is called the *sapwood*. Commercial guaiacum wood and logwood consist of heartwood.

In transverse section woods usually show annual rings each of which normally represents a season's growth. In some tropical species the annual rings are not well-marked, owing to the absence of a seasonal interruption in growth. The so-called *false annual rings* found in, for example, quassia are irregular rings formed by alternating zones of wood parenchyma and fibres. The width and height of *medullary rays* are of diagnostic importance in the case of Jamaica and Surinam quassias and rhubarbs. The *grain* of wood primarily results from the arrangement of the annual rings and medullary rays, but is modified by the wavy course of the wood elements which causes the wood to split irregularly. Irregular splitting is largely dependent on the number of lateral branches which cause knots in the wood.

Woods may be described under the following headings.

Size and colour. Note any differentiation into sapwood and heartwood. The latter may not be coloured uniformly (e.g. logwood).

Relative density. Woods vary considerably in this respect (e.g. guaiacum has a relative density of 1.33 and poplar one of 0.38).

Hardness and behaviour when split

Transverse surface. The lignified elements may show a markedly radiate arrangement or they may be irregularly scattered. Note distribution of wood fibres and wood parenchyma and of true and false annual rings. Measure the distances between medullary rays and between annual rings.

Longitudinal surfaces. Measure height of medullary rays.

LEAVES OR LEAFLETS

The following features can be used to describe leaves.

Duration. *Deciduous* or *evergreen*.

Leaf base. *Stipulate* or *exstipulate*; if stipulate, describe shape, etc; if sheath is present, describe it (e.g. *amplexicaul*—stem-clasping).

Petiole. *Petiolate* or *sessile*. If present, describe size, shape, colour, hairs, etc.

Lamina
1. Composition. If simple, whether *pinnate* or *palmate*. If compound, whether *paripinnate* (with an equal number of leaflets) or *imparipinnate* (Fig. 41.3).
2. Incision. The leaf may be more or less cleft, the amount being indicated by adding *-fid*, *-partite* or *-sect* to a prefix denoting whether the leaf is of a pinnate or a palmate type.
3. Shape. If the shape is obscured by drying, soak the leaf in warm water and spread it on a tile. The appropriate terms connected with leaf-shapes are given in Fig. 41.3.
4. Venation. *Parallel, pinnate* (feather-like), *palmate, reticulate* (net-veined).
5. Margin. See Fig. 41.3 for terminology.
6. Apex. See Fig. 41.3 for terminology.
7. Base. Symmetrical or asymmetrical; cordate, reniform, etc.

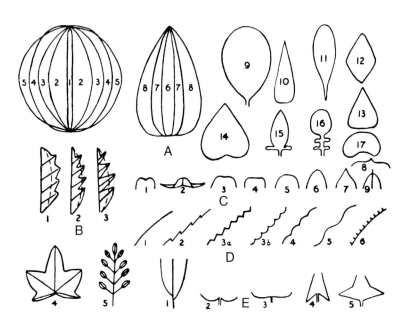

Fig. 41.3
Terms applied to leaves. A, Shape: 1, acicular; 2, elliptical; 3, oval; 4, oblong; 5, round; 6, linear; 7, lanceolate; 8, ovate; 9, obovate; 10, subulate; 11, spatulate; 12, diamond-shaped; 13, cuneate; 14, cordate; 15, auriculate; 16, lyrate; 17, reniform. B, Composition and incision: 1, pinnatifid; 2, pinnatipartite; 3, pinnatisect; 4, palmatifid; 5, imparipinnate. C, Apex: 1, emarginate; 2, recurved; 3, retuse; 4, truncate; 5, obtuse; 6, acute; 7, acuminate; 8, mucronate; 9, apiculate. D, Margin: 1, entire; 2, serrate; 3a and 3b, dentate; 4, crenate; 5, sinuate; 6, ciliate; E, Base: 1, asymmetric; 2, cordate; 3, reniform; 4, sagittate; 5, hastate.

8. Surface. Colour; glabrous (free from hairs) or pubescent (hairy); if the latter, whether hispid (with rough hairs), hirsute (with long distinct hairs) or with glandular hairs; punctate (dotted with oil glands). Note lines on surface of coca leaves, raised points on belladonna, press marks on Tinnevelly senna, etc. Note any differences between the upper and the lower surfaces.

9. Texture. Brittle, coriaceous, papery, fleshy, etc.

Anatomy

A study of the anatomy of the leaf reveals that there is a basic structural pattern yielding characters that enable the presence of a leaf to be detected in a powder. Other less general characters will make possible such distinctions as that between monocotyledonous and dicotyledonous leaves, and between xerophytic and mesophytic leaves. The more detailed anatomical characters will, when taken together, allow of the identification of the genus and ultimately of the species of leaf. A knowledge of the diagnostic characters of any leaf permits of the detection of contaminants and substitutes.

The leaf (Fig. 41.4) is built up of a protective epidermis, a parenchymatous mesophyll and a vascular system. The shape, size and wall structure of the epidermal cells; the form, distribution and relation to the epidermal cells of the stomata; the form, distribution and abundance of epidermal trichomes are all of diagnostic importance.

The mesophyll may or may not be differentiated into spongy mesophyll and palisade tissue. Palisade tissue may be present below both surfaces or occur only below the upper epidermis. In all green leaves the mesophyll cells are rich in chloroplasts. The mesophyll, although typically parenchymatous, may contain groups of collenchyma or sclerenchyma, secretion ducts or latex tissue, oil or mucilage cells, or

hydathodes (water pores). Cells may contain inclusions such as crystals or calcium oxalate, the form, size and distribution of which may have importance.

The vascular systems of leaves fall into two main classes: the reticulate venation typical of dicotyledons and the parallel venation of monocotyledons. The structure of the individual veins is subject to considerable variation. The midrib bundle of the dicotyledonous leaf may be poorly or markedly differentiated. In leaves with a well-differentiated midrib the palisade tissue is usually interrupted in the midrib region and collenchyma frequently occurs above and below the midrib bundle. The main veins, in dicotyledonous leaves, are open and usually collateral (Fig. 41.4); less commonly they are bicollateral. The xylem faces towards the upper surface. Various degrees of secondary thickening of the midrib bundle are seen. The lateral veins are almost entirely collateral even in cases where the midrib bundle is bicollateral. The smallest veins often consist of xylem only. The veins of monocotyledonous leaves are closed bundles.

The midrib bundle is often, as in the Solanaceae, enclosed in an endodermis which may take the form of a starch sheath. The development of the pericycle is variable, in some cases being parenchymatous and containing secretion cells, in some cases consisting of a sheath of pericyclic fibres with their long axes parallel to the vein.

For the investigation of the structure of a leaf it is necessary to examine transverse sections of the lamina and midrib; portions of the whole leaf, including leaf margin, cleared in chloral hydrate; and surface preparations of both epidermi. Sections should be cleared, if necessary, and stained for cellulose and lignin. In individual cases it may be necessary to apply microchemical tests for mucilage, tannin, cutin, volatile oil, calcium oxalate or carbonate.

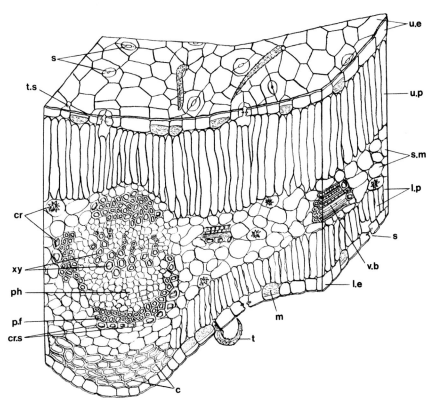

Fig. 41.4
Transverse section of senna leaflet: c, collenchyma; cr, calcium oxalate crystals; cr.s, crystal sheath; l.e, lower epidermis; l.p, lower palisade; m, mucilage cell; ph, phloem; p.f, pericyclic fibre; s, stomata; s.m, spongy mesophyll; t, trichome; t.s, trichome scar; u.e, upper epidermis; u.p, upper palisade; v.b, vascular bundle; xy, xylem vessels.

Powdered leaves. The following are consistently present: epidermis with stomata; cellulose parenchyma; not very abundant small-sized vascular elements and chlorophyll (except in bulb leaves). Structures frequently present are epidermal trichomes, glands, palisade cells, crystals of calcium oxalate, collenchyma and pericyclic fibres (see also Chapter 42).

For the differentiations of closely allied leaves it may be necessary to make determinations of such differential characters as vein-islet number, stomatal number, stomatal index and palisade ratio (q.v.).

INFLORESCENCES AND FLOWERS

The following features serve to describe the complex structure of flowers.

Type of inflorescence. *Racemose, cymose* or mixed (e.g. racemes of cymes in clove).

Axis or receptacle of inflorescence. The main axis of an inflorescence is called the *rachis*, while the branches bearing flower clusters and individual flowers are termed *peduncles* and *pedicels*, respectively. The term *receptacle of the inflorescence* must not be confused with the receptacle of the flower (see below). In the Roman chamomile the receptacle of the inflorescence is conical and solid, a membranous palea subtends each floret and the capitulum is surrounded by an involucre of bracts.

Type of flower. Monocotyledon or dicotyledon. Unisexual or hermaphrodite. Regular or zygomorphic. Hypogynous, perigynous or epigynous (Fig. 41.5).

Receptacle of the flower (thalamus or torus) is the extremity of the peduncle on which the calyx, corolla, etc. are inserted. When the receptacle is elongated below the calyx, it is called a *hypanthium*, or if below the ovary, a *gynophore* or stalk of the ovary (cf. clove).

Calyx. Note number of sepals if *polysepalous* or divisions if *gamosepalous*. *Caducous* (e.g. poppy) or *persistent* (e.g. belladonna). Describe colour, shape, hairs, etc., as for a leaf.

Corolla. Note number of petals if *polypetalous* or divisions if *gamopetalous*. Observe any special characteristics such as venation (henbane) and oil glands (clove petals).

Androecium. Note number of stamens; whether free or joined (*monadelphous, diadelphous*, etc.), *didynamous* or *tetradynamous, epipetalous*, etc. Dehiscence of anthers (valves, pores or slits).

Gynaecium. Note number of carpels; apocarpous or syncarpous; superior or inferior. Sizes and shapes of stigma, style and ovary. The enlarged base of the styles in the Umbelliferae is called a *stylopod*. Number of loculi, placentation (parietal, axile, free-central, etc.).

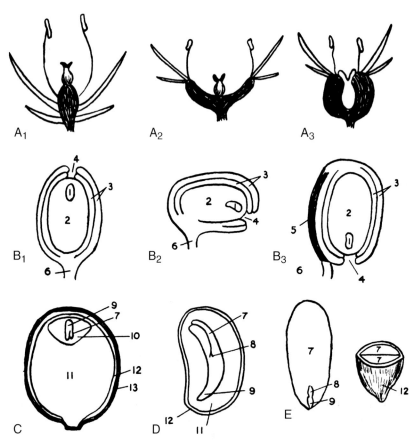

Fig 41.5
A₁, A₂ and A₃, hypogynous, perigynous and epigynous flowers; B₁, B₂ and B₃, orthotropous, campylotropous, and anatropous ovules; C, fruit of *Piper* with single albuminous seed; D, albuminous seed of *Papaver*, E, exalbuminous seed of almond. 1, embryo sac; 2, nucellus; 3, integuments; 4, micropyle; 5, raphe; 6, funicle; 7, cotyledon; 8, plumule; 9, radicle; 10, endosperm; 11, perisperm; 12, testa; 13, pericarp.

Ovules. Note number in each loculus; *orthotropous, campylotropous, anatropous* (Fig. 41.5).

Anatomy

The flower stalk or pedicel has a stem structure and in the powdered form exhibits the appropriate elements. The bracts, calyx and, to a lesser extent, corolla have a leaf structure and will yield such elements as epidermis with stomata, glandular and covering hairs, mesophyll cells, oil glands and crystals. The epidermal cells of the corolla often have a papillose or striated cuticle. Delicate coloured fragments of the corolla can often be distinguished in coarsely powdered drugs. A characteristic papillose epidermis may sometimes be present on the stigmas of the gynaecium. Characteristic fragments of the anther wall are diagnostic of the presence of flowers. Of first importance is the occurrence, size, shape and wall structure of pollen grains.

With powdered flowers the pollen grains, portions of the fibrous layer of the anther wall and the papillose epidermis of the stigmas are obvious features.

FRUITS

The following classification shows the principal types of fruit met with in pharmacognosy.

  A. *Simple* (i.e. formed from a gynaecium with one pistil).
  B. *Aggregate* (i.e. formed from more than one pistil, e.g. aconite).
  C. *Collective* (i.e. formed not from one flower but from an inflorescence, e.g. fig).

1. Simple, dry, indehiscent fruits

(1) *Achene.* A small hard indehiscent fruit. The term is strictly only applied to those formed from one carpel, but is sometimes used for those formed from two carpels (e.g. the fruit of the Compositae). The latter is better termed a *cypsela*.
(2) *Nut.* This is similar to an achene, but is typically formed from two or three carpels (e.g. dock fruit).
(3) *Caryopis.* This is the type of fruit in which the testa and pericarp are fused (found in the cereals).

2. Simple, dry, dehiscent fruits

(1) *Legume.* A fruit formed from one carpel which splits along both dorsal and ventral sutures (e.g. senna).
(2) *Follicle.* A fruit from one carpel which dehisces by the inner suture only. Follicles are usually found in aggregates or etaerios (e.g. aconite and strophanthus).
(3) *Capsules.* Capsules are dry dehiscent fruits formed from two or more carpels. Some bear special names (e.g. the *siliqua* and *silicula* of the Cruciferae, and the *pyxis* or *pyxidium* found in henbane). The latter is a capsule which opens by means of a lid.

3. Schizocarpic or splitting fruits

A familiar example of this group is the *cremocarp*, the bicarpellary fruit of the Umbelliferae, which splits into two *mericarps*.

4. Succulent fruits

(1) *Drupe.* This is typically formed from one superior carpel (e.g. almond and prune). The inner part of the pericarp, which is called the endocarp, is hard and woody and encloses one seed.
(2) *Berry.* This fruit is formed from one or more carpels and the pericarp is entirely fleshy. It is usually many-seeded. Examples: nux vomica, colocynth, orange, lemon, capsicum. Special terms which

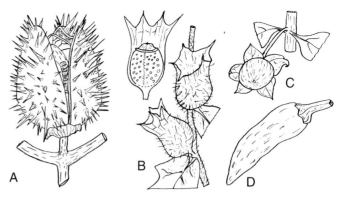

Fig. 41.6
Fruits of the Solanaceae. A and B, capsules: A, ripe fruit of *Datura stramonium*; B, pyxidia of *Hyoscyamus niger* with upper fruit showing calyx partly removed. C and D, berries of *Atropa belladonna* and *Capsicum* sp., respectively. All four fruits are basically bilocular but stramonium fruit becomes almost completely four-celled by the development of a false septum.

are sometimes used are *pepo* for the berry of the Cucurbitaceae and *hesperidium* for that of the orange and similar rutaceous fruits.

Examples of fruits of the Solanaceae are shown in Fig. 41.6. The description of a fruit may be arranged as follows.

Class

See above.

Shape and dimensions

Adhesion. Superior or inferior. Fruits from inferior ovaries usually show floral remains at the apex (e.g. cardamom, fennel, unpeeled colocynth and lobelia).

Dehiscence. Dehiscent or indehiscent. Different types of dehiscence are shown by the legume, follicle, siliqua and the pyxidium and other capsules. Most capsules split longitudinally into valves which are usually equal in number to or double those of the loculi or placentae. Dehiscence is termed *septicidal* if the valves separate at the line of junction of the carpels or *loculicidal* if the valves separate between the placentae or dissepiment. In the latter case the placentae or dissepiment may remain attached either to the axis or to the valves.

Pericarp. Colour, texture, markings, number of sutures. Note whether uniform throughout or modified into epicarp, mesocarp and endocarp.

Placentation (e.g. marginal in senna, parietal in poppy, axile in cardamom, etc.).

Seeds. Number. Describe in detail (see under 'Seeds' below).

Other characters. Odour, taste, food reserves.

Anatomy

The pericarp is bounded by inner and outer epidermi which, in general, resemble those of leaves. The outer epidermis may bear stomata and hairs. In fleshy fruits the internal tissue is mainly parenchymatous, resembling the mesophyll of leaves. In dry fruits and fleshy dry fruits it usually contains fibres or sclereids. Secretory tissues such as vittae, oil ducts or cells, and latex tissue are commonly present in the pericarp of medicinal fruits. Husk of cardamoms can be detected by the presence

41

of pitted fibres, spiral vessels and abundant empty parenchymatous cells. The endocarp of almond, sometimes used as an adulterant, consists mainly of sclereids.

Portions of receptacle (e.g. the rind of colocynth), persistent sepals and flower stalk may be present.

SEEDS

Seeds may be produced from orthotropous, campylotropous or anatropous ovules (Fig. 41.5). Care must be taken to distinguish seeds from fruits or parts of fruits containing a single seed (e.g. cereals and the mericarps of the Umbelliferae). The seed consists of a kernel surrounded by one, two or three seed coats. Most seeds have two seed coats, an outer *testa* and an inner *tegmen*. The seed is attached to the placenta by a stalk or *funicle*. The *hilum* is the scar left on the seed where it separates from the funicle. The *raphe* is a ridge of fibrovascular tissue formed in more or less anatropous ovules by the adhesion of funicle and testa. The *micropyle* is the opening in the seed coats which usually marks the position of the radicle. An expansion of the funicle or placenta extending over the surface of the seed like a bag is known as an *aril* or *arillus*. A false aril or *arillode* resembles an aril, but is a seed coat. A *caruncle* or *strophiole* is a protuberance arising from the testa near the hilum.

The kernel may consist of the embryo plant only (*exalbuminous seeds*), or of the embryo surrounded by *endosperm* or *perisperm* or both (*albuminous seeds*) (Fig. 41.5). Endosperm and perisperm are tissues containing food reserves and are formed, respectively, inside and outside the embryo sac.

The description of a seed may be arranged as follows.

Size, shape and colour

Funicle, etc. Describe funicle and, if present, raphe and aril.

Hilum and micropyle. Size and positions.

Seed coats. Number. If present, describe arillode, caruncle or strophiole. Thickness and texture of testa; whether uniform in colour or not; smooth, pitted or reticulate. If hairs are present, describe their length, texture and arrangement. Mechanism for dispersal (e.g. awn of strophanthus).

Perisperm. Present or absent. Nature of food reserves.

Endosperm. Present or absent. Nature of food reserves.

Embryo. Size and position (e.g. straight in *Strophanthus*, curved in stramonium, folded in mustard). Size, shape, number and venation of cotyledons. Size and shape of radicle.

Anatomy

The testas of seeds often yield highly diagnostic characters. A highly diagnostic sclerenchymatous layer is often present (Fig. 41.7K, I). The number of cell layers, and their structure, arrangement, colour and cell contents are subject to characteristic variations. The epidermis of the testa is often composed of highly characteristic, thick-walled cells (Fig. 41.7A, B, E, J, L). It may bear characteristic hairs (Fig. 41.7M).

The storage tissues perisperm and endosperm, and in other cases cotyledons, are composed of uniform cells often containing characteristic cell contents (e.g. aleurone, starch, calcium oxalate, fixed oil, volatile oil). The cell walls are often considerably thickened (e.g. nux vomica).

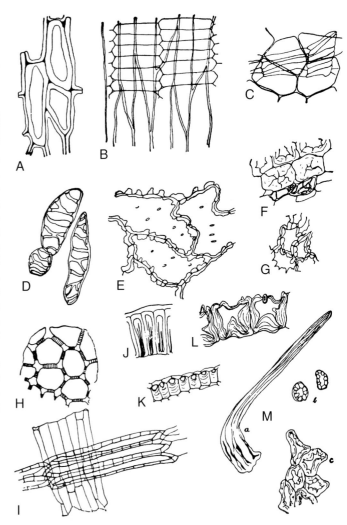

Fig. 41.7
Some diagnostic structures of fruits and seeds. A, lignified epidermal cells of testa of seed of *Lobelia inflata*; B, epidermis of testa of cardamom seed, with fragment of the underlying parenchymatous layer attached; K, sclerenchymatous layer of testa of cardamom seed in transverse section; C, 'parqueting cells' of inner epidermis of the pericarp of fennel, with parenchyma of mesocarp attached; D, lignified reticulate 'parenchyma' cells of the mesocarp of fennel. E, epidermis of capsicum seed in surface view; F, sclereids and reticulate cells of testa of colocynth seed; G, sclereids of same in surface view; J, epidermis of testa of colocynth seed in transverse section; H, pigment layer of testa of linseed in surface view; I, sclerenchymatous layer of testa of linseed seen in surface view and with hyaline layer adherent; L, epidermis of testa of stramonium seed in transverse section; M, lignified hair of nux vomica: a, whole hair; b, transverse sections of limb of hair; c, periclinal section through the bases of several hairs.

The radicle, plumule and leaf-like cotyledons yield little of diagnostic significance to the powdered drug.

Transverse and longitudinal sections of fruit and seeds should be prepared. Disintegration makes possible a study of the structure of the individual layers and elements and of structures such as vittae.

The variation in structure between different fruits and seeds is considerable. Aleurone grains, carbohydrate reserves and a little vascular tissue are constantly present in seeds. Fruits yield similar characters, except that the amount of vascular tissue is greater and lignified elements of the pericarp are often present.

SUBTERRANEAN ORGANS

Under this heading it is convenient to discuss: (1) stem structures such as corms, bulbs, stem-tubers and rhizomes and (2) root structures such as true and adventitious roots and root-tubers. Many drugs which are commonly spoken of as roots consist wholly or partly of rhizomes (e.g. rhubarb and gentian) and in many cases the gradual transition from stem to root makes an accurate differentiation of the two parts impossible.

Monocotyledonous rhizomes can be distinguished from dicotyledonous rhizomes by the scattered arrangement of their vascular bundles. Stem structures may usually be distinguished from roots by the fact that they bear buds and possess a well-marked pith. In underground organs chlorophyll is absent, and starch, when present, is usually abundant and in the form of large grains of reserve starch.

The following scheme may be used with suitable modifications for the description of most subterranean organs.

Morphological nature.   Rhizome, root, etc.

Condition.   Fresh or dry; whole or sliced; peeled or unpeeled.

Subaerial stems.   Remains of subaerial stems occur in aconite, serpentary, etc. Note whether present in sufficient amount to constitute an adulteration.

Subterranean stems
1. **Size and shape**.
2. **Direction of growth and branching**.
3. **Surface characters**. Colour, stem scars, buds, cataphyllary leaves, roots or root scars, lenticels, cracks, wrinkles, surface crystals, evidence of insect attack, peeling, etc.

4. **Fracture and texture**. Flexible, brittle, hard, horny, mealy, splintery, etc.
5. **Transverse section**. Colour (cf. male fern); distribution of lignified and secretory elements (e.g. in ginger); relative sizes of bark, wood and pith. Note any abnormalities such as the star spots and absence of a lignin reaction in rhubarb.

Roots
1. **Kind**. True (i.e. developed from the radicle or its branches) or adventitious.
2. **Size and shape**. Tuberous, conical, cylindrical, etc.
3. **Surface characters**. Colour; cracks, wrinkles, annulations, lenticels, etc.
4. **Fracture and texture**.
5. **Transverse section**. Note absence of pith, whether the wood is markedly radiate or not, and any abnormalities such as are found in jalap and senega.

Food reserves and chemical tests
Odour and taste
Anatomy
Most of the important drugs derived from roots are those of dicotyledons and the following brief description of their fundamental structural pattern is restricted to that of the typical dicotyledonous type.

The primary root (Fig. 41.8A) shows the following structures: a piliferous layer composed of a single layer of thin-walled cells, devoid of cuticle and bearing root hairs formed as lateral outgrowths of the cells; a parenchymatous cortex, the innermost layer of which is differentiated into an endodermis; and a vascular cylinder or stele taking the form of a radial protostele or less frequently of a medullated protostele. The vascular tissues of the stele are enclosed in a single

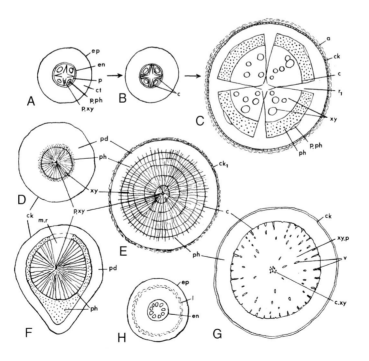

Fig. 41.8
Root structures in transverse section. A–C, initiation of secondary growth in liquorice root: A, primary structure; B, development of cambium; C, formation of secondary phloem and xylem and of the cork cambium. D–G, variations in root structure: D, ipecacuanha; E, *Rauwolfia serpentina*; F, senega; G, belladonna; H, veratrum, a monocotyledon with no secondary thickening. a, Degenerative cortex; c, cambium; ck, cork; ck_1, stratified cork; ct, cortex; c.xy, central xylem; en, endodermis; ep, epidermis; l, lacuna; m.r, medullary ray; p, pericycle; pd, phelloderm; ph, phloem; p.ph, primary phloem, p.xy, primary xylem; r_1, primary medullary ray; v, xylem vessels, xy, xylem; xy.p. xylem parenchyma.

or many-layered pericycle. The protostele is composed of a central mass of xylem tissue with two or more radiating arms and of phloem groups located between the xylem arms. The xylem is differentiated in a centripetal direction, so that the protoxylem groups occupy the ends of the xylem arms and the metaxylem makes up the inner xylem mass. The number of protoxylem groups is usually fairly constant for a given species, but some variation is not uncommon (e.g. valerian). The xylem is described as diarch (*Solanum* spp.), triarch (alfalfa), tetrarch (liquorice, *Ipomoea* spp.) or polyarch, according to the number of protoxylem groups present. The central xylem cylinder is medullated in some cases (e.g. valerian). The phloem groups are usually separated from the xylem cylinder by a narrow zone of parenchyma ('fundamental parenchyma').

In many roots increase in diameter of the axis is accomplished by secondary thickening. Secondary thickening is initiated in the zone of 'fundamental parenchyma', the whole or part of which becomes meristematic. The derived cells mature as secondary phloem centrifugally and as secondary xylem centripetally. From the point of initial cambial activity there is a progressive tangential development, the cambia extending laterally until they reach the points where the protoxylem groups abut on to the pericycle. The pericycle opposite the protoxylem groups becomes meristematic and thus a continuous cambial cylinder is formed (Fig. 41.8B). The activity of the cambium opposite the protoxylem groups gives rise to the broad primary rays (Fig. 41.8C).

The cylinder of secondary tissues is composed of xylem and phloem elements which at first tend to be arranged in regular radial rows. This arrangement often becomes less regular, owing to irregular growth of the individual elements and further division and growth of the xylem and phloem parenchyma cells. The structure of the secondary xylem and phloem is described in Chapter 42.

Coincident with the development of the secondary vascular tissues other changes take place (Fig. 41.8C). The primary phloem groups are forced outwards and gradually obliterated. Divisions take place in the pericycle, so that it increases in diameter with the expansion of the vascular cylinder. Often the pericycle also increases in thickness, becoming many layers, and forms a 'secondary cortex'. The piliferous layer, cortex and endodermis become fractured and are cut off by the formation of a phellogen in the outermost layer of cells derived from

the pericycle. At a still later stage a new phellogen may arise in the secondary phloem, with a consequent disintegration of the pericycle.

The structures of the primary and secondary roots of dicotyledons show many deviations from the general plan described above. Figure 41.8D–G indicates variations in root structure arising from the preferential development of certain tissues. Monocotyledons characteristically exhibit no secondary thickening (Fig. 41.8H). Jalap shows anomalous secondary thickening.

UNORGANIZED DRUGS

Many types of unorganized drugs are discussed in Part 5, namely: fixed oils, fats and waxes; volatile oils; resins, oleoresins, oleo-gum-resins, balsams and gums. To these must be added dried juices (e.g. aloes), latices (e.g. opium) and extracts (e.g. agar and catechu).

The following scheme may be used in their examination.

Physical state

Solid, semi-solid or liquid.

1. **If solid.** (a) Size and form: Tears, lumps, etc., and their approximate size and weight. (b) Packing: Paper, skins, leaves, plastic, etc. (c) External appearance: Colour, shiny or dusty; opaque or translucent; presence of vegetable fragments. (d) Hardness and fracture: Conchoidal, porous, etc. (e) Solubility in water and organic solvents. (f) Vegetable debris, if any, remaining insoluble (e.g. in myrrh and asafoetida). (g) Effect of heat: Does substance melt, char, sublime or burn without leaving appreciable ash? (h) Microscopical appearance of powder, sublimate (e.g. balsams) or insoluble matter (e.g. opium and catechu).

2. **If liquid.** (a) Colour and fluorescence. (b) Viscosity. (c) Density. (d) Solubility (e.g. of balsam of Peru in a solution of chloral hydrate).

Odour and taste

Chemical tests, chromatographic and spectroscopic characteristics

42

Cell differentiation and ergastic cell contents

Modifications to the basic structure of the living plant cell involving composition of the cell wall, cell shape and cell contents, are found in the various plant tissues and furnish those microscopical characters of drug plants which are of value in identification and in the detection of adulteration.

THE CELL WALL

The original cell wall may, during the differentiation of the cell, undergo various chemical modifications that profoundly change its physical properties. Principal among these are the deposition of further cellulose or hemicellulose and incrustation of the wall by lignin, cutin or suberin. Algal cell walls, which commonly contain pectin mixed with cellulose, xylose, mannose or silica, may contain also hemicellulose, alginic acid, fucoidin and fucin (Phaeophyta), geloses (Rhodophyta) and chitin.

Cellulose walls. Certain colour reactions can be applied for the recognition of cellulose cell walls. The colour reactions vary with differences in the relative proportions of cellulose, hemicellulose and pectin present.

1. Chlor-zinc-iodine gives a blue colour with true celluloses and a yellow with pectic substances. Walls containing these in different proportions stain blue, violet, brownish-violet or brown. Similar colours are obtained with iodine followed by concentrated acids.
2. Iodine, when used alone, gives no colour with true celluloses but may give a blue if hemicelluloses are present (e.g. in the cotyledons of tamarind seeds).
3. Ammoniacal solution of copper oxide dissolves true celluloses, and on pouring the alkaline liquid into dilute sulphuric acid the cellulose is precipitated. Walls containing hemicelluloses, etc., are incompletely soluble in this reagent.
4. Phloroglucinol and hydrochloric acid gives no pink or red colour with cellulose walls.

Lignified walls. Lignin is a strengthening material which impregnates the cell walls of tracheids, vessels, fibres and sclereids of vascular plants; it constitutes 22–34% of woods. Chemically, it is a complex phenylpropanoid (C_6–C_3) polymer which differs according to its source, lignin from dicotyledons being different from that of the conifers (Fig. 21.1). In the wall, it appears to occur chemically combined with hemicellulose and is built up in greatest concentration in the middle lamellae and in the primary walls. Lignified cell walls after treatment with Schultze's macerating fluid will show cellulose reactions.

For the identification of lignified walls the following tests are available:

1. On treatment with 'acid aniline sulphate' the walls become bright yellow.
2. Phloroglucinol and hydrochloric acid stains lignified walls pink or red. A similar colour is obtained when pentose sugars are warmed with this reagent.
3. Chlor-zinc-iodine stains lignified walls yellow.

Suberized and cutinized walls. Suberin and cutin consist of mixtures of substances, chiefly highly polymerized fatty acids such as suberic acid, $COOH[CH_2]_6COOH$, although the acids present in the two substances are not identical. These materials waterproof cells in which they occur. Suberin thickenings, such as are found in cork cells and endodermal cells, usually consist of carbohydrate-free suberin lamellae. Cutin forms a secondary deposit on or in a cellulose wall. Leaves are frequently covered with a deposit of cutin which may show characteristic

42

papillae, ridges or striations. Beneath the cuticle, the cellulose wall may also be impregnated with cutin (cutinized), so that these walls may show a gradation from pure cellulose on the inside, through layers of cellulose impregnated with pectin compounds and fatty substances, to the outer cuticle, which is free of cellulose. Waxes (largely esters of higher monohydric alcohols and fatty acids) occur with suberin and cutin. Unlike the latter, they readily melt on warming and are extractable with fat solvents. Such waxes in the form of minute rods or particles give a glaucous effect to the structures which they cover and are responsible for the 'bloom' of many fruits, stems, etc. Wax is found in larger amounts on the leaves of *Myrica*, and in the wax palms, *Copernicia*, it coats the leaves heavily (Carnauba wax).

The reactions of suberin and cutin are almost identical.

1. Chlor-zinc-iodine gives a yellow to brown colour.
2. Sudan-glycerin colours both suberin and cutin red, especially on warming. The reagent is made by dissolving 0.01 g of Sudan III in 5 ml of alcohol and adding 5 ml of glycerin.
3. Strong solution of potash stains suberin and cutin yellow. On warming suberin with a 20% solution of potash, yellowish droplets exude, but cutin is more resistant.
4. Diluted tincture of alkanna stains the walls red.
5. Concentrated sulphuric acid does not dissolve suberin or cutin.
6. Oxidizing agents. At ordinary temperatures concentrated chromic acid solution has little effect. When heated with potassium chlorate and nitric acid, the walls change into droplets, which are soluble in organic solvents or in dilute potash.

Mucilaginous cell walls. Certain cell walls may be converted into gums and mucilages. This gummosis (gummous degeneration) may be observed in the stems of species of *Prunus, Citrus* and *Astragalus*, in testas of many seeds (e.g. linseed and mustard) and in the outer layers of many aquatic plants. In the case of gum-yielding species of *Astragalus*, gummosis commences near the centre of the pith and spreads outwards through the primary medullary rays. The polysaccharide walls, excepting the primary membranes, swell and are converted into gum, the lumen, which frequently contains starch, becoming very small. When the stem is incised, whole tissues are pushed out by the pressure set up by the swelling of the gum. The commercial gum has a definite cell structure. The reaction of gums and mucilages is described below under 'Cell Contents'.

Chitinous walls. Chitin $(C_8H_{13}O_5N)_n$, a polyacetylamino-hexose, forms the major part of the cell walls of crustaceans, insects and many fungi (e.g. ergot). It gives no reactions for cellulose or lignin. When heated with 50% potash at 160–170°C for 1 h, it is converted into chitosan, $C_{14}H_{26}O_{16}N_2$, ammonia and acids such as acetic and oxalic. The mass may be dissolved in 3% acetic acid and the chitosan reprecipitated by the addition of a slight excess of alkali. Chitosan gives a violet colour when treated first with a 0.5% solution of iodine in potassium iodide, and then with 1% sulphuric acid. The test may be applied to shrimp scales, first freed from carbonate by means of 5% hydrochloric acid, to the elytra of beetles or to defatted ergot.

PARENCHYMATOUS TISSUE

Meristematic tissue is usually composed of cells characterized by isodiametric form (except in the case of the provascular tissues), by possessing a protoplast capable of division and a primary cell wall composed of cellulose. The fundamental parenchyma occurring in various parts of the plant is potentially meristematic, and such cells achieve maturity without further differentiation except for an increase in cell size and wall thickness and a restricted change of form. The pith, cortex and rays of the plant axis and the mesophyll of the leaves are composed, at least in part, of such parenchyma. The mesophyll cells often contain abundant chloroplasts, and may be differentiated into palisade and spongy mesophyll. An early stage of differentiation may be seen in the lignified pitted parenchyma constituting the pith of the stems of *Lobelia inflata* and *Cephaelis ipecacuanha*, and the pitted cellulose parenchyma of the pulp of *Citrullus colocynthis*.

THE EPIDERMIS

The epidermis consists of a single layer of cells covering the whole plant. The epidermis of the root constitutes the piliferous layer and that of the shoot is a highly differentiated and compact layer of cells. The epidermal cells, in contrast to the stomatal guard cells, are often devoid of chloroplasts. Epidermal cells show great variety in form, giving characteristic patterns when seen in surface view. In transection they are often flattened parallel to the surface, and square or rectangular in shape. The outer walls are often convex and the most markedly thickened.

The epidermis of the stems of trees and shrubs is usually obliterated early by the development of a cork cambium, but on the stems of herbaceous plants and in leaves, fruits and seeds the epidermis persists and often yields highly diagnostic characters.

For leaves in particular, the shape of the epidermal cells in surface view and in section (Fig. 42.1A–D), the nature and distribution of the wall thickening, the presence or absence of cuticle and its form, the distribution and structure of the stomata, the presence or absence of well-differentiated subsidiary cells to the stomata, the presence of characteristic cell inclusions such as cystoliths, the presence or absence and form, size and distribution of epidermal trichomes and the presence and distribution of water-pores should all be carefully noted in describing the characters of an epidermis.

The structures of the epidermis and stomata are of first importance in the microscopical identification of leaves (see Fig. 42.2). Straight-walled epidermal cells are seen in, for example, jaborandi, coca and senna leaves; wavy-walled epidermal cells in stramonium, hyoscyamus and belladonna; beaded walls in *Lobelia inflata* and *Digitalis lanata*; a papillose epidermis in coca leaf. A thick cuticle is developed in *Aloe* leaf and bearberry leaf; a striated cuticle in belladonna, jaborandi, *Digitalis lutea* and *D. thapsi*. Mucilage is present in the epidermis of senna and buchu leaves. Cystoliths of calcium carbonate occur in the epidermal cells of Urticaceae and Cannabinaceae; sphaero-crystals of diosmin occur in buchu epidermis (Fig. 42.1B).

The stomata may be surrounded by cells resembling the other epidermal cells (anomocytic, formerly ranunculaceous, type), but in other cases definite subsidiary cells may be distinguished. Three main types are distinguishable: the anisocytic (formerly cruciferous) type, with the stoma surrounded by three or four subsidiary cells, one of which is markedly smaller than the others; the paracytic (formerly rubiaceous) type, with two subsidiary cells with their long axes parallel to the pore; and the diacytic (formerly caryophyllaceous) type with two subsidiary cells, with their long axis at right angles to the pore of the stomata (Fig. 42.2). There are variations among these types (e.g. the actinocytic type, in which the subsidiary cells are arranged along the radii of a circle) and altogether some 31 types have been recognized. (For a survey of the classification of morphological types of stomata see M. Baranova, *Bot. Rev.*, 1992, **58**, 49).

Often, when viewed under the light microscope as cleared preparations, the outlines of the epidermal cells and stomata do not appear as definite as the line drawings (Fig. 42.2) might suggest. This is due to

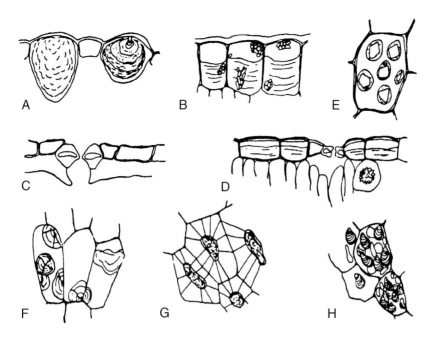

Fig. 42.1
A, Epidermal cells of *Urtica dioica* containing cystoliths of calcium carbonate. B, Epidermal cells of the leaf of *Barosma betulina* showing sphaero-crystalline masses of diosmin and a thick deposit of mucilage on the inner tangential walls. C, Cells of the lower epidermis of *Arctostaphylos uva-ursi* showing thick cuticle and sunken stomata. D, Upper epidermis of *Cassia angustifolia* showing mucilage cells and stomata; a cell of the underlying mesophyll contains a cluster crystal of calcium oxalate. E, Aleurone grains showing crystalloid and globoid, from the endosperm of the seed of *Ricinus communis*. F, Sphaerocrystalline masses of inulin in dahlia tuber. G, Cells of the endosperm of the seed of *Strychnos nux-vomica* showing walls of reserve cellulose, traversed by plasmodesmata. H, Parenchymatous cells from the rhizome of *Zingiber officinale* containing starch grains.

the convoluted arrangements of cells on the leaf surface and is illustrated by the scanning electron micrographs included in the digitalis and Solanaceae descriptions in Part 5.

The distribution of stomata between the upper and lower epidermis shows great variation. The stomata may be entirely confined to the lower epidermis, as in *Ficus* species, bearberry, boldo, buchu, coca, jaborandi and maté leaves. The leaves of savin show stomata confined to two localized areas of the lower surface. The floating leaves of aquatics have stomata confined to the upper epidermis. Sometimes they are evenly distributed on both surfaces; most commonly they are more numerous on the lower surface. For 'stomatal number' and 'stomatal index' see Chapter 43.

The epidermis of fruits and seeds may yield characters of diagnostic value (see Fig. 41.7). The outer and inner epidermi of the pericarp of the umbelliferous fruits are highly characteristic structures. Characteristic cells with thickened pitted walls form the outer epidermis of the pericarp in vanilla, juniper and capsicum. The outer epidermi of the pericarp of coriander and vanilla contain prisms of calcium oxalate. A striated cuticle is seen in aniseed, caraway and star anise fruits. Thickened palisade-like cells form the epidermis of the testa of colocynth and fenugreek seeds. Characteristic elongated tapering cells form the epidermis of cardamoms. Thickened lignified cells form the epidermis of lobelia seed, and mucilage cells that of linseed and of white and black mustard.

EPIDERMAL TRICHOMES

Most leaves and many herbaceous stems, flowers, fruits and seeds possess hairs or trichomes of one kind or another. Many show hairs of more than one type. Hairs may be grouped into non-glandular or clothing hairs, and glandular hairs. Clothing hairs may be unicellular or

multicellular. Unicellular hairs vary from small papillose outgrowths to large robust structures (Figs 42.3, 42.4). Multicellular hairs may be uniseriate, biseriate or multiseriate or complicated branched structures (Fig. 42.4). The chemical nature of the cell wall, and the presence of pits or protuberances or of cell inclusions, such as cystoliths, should be noted.

Glandular hairs may have a unicellular or a multiseriate stalk; the glandular head may be unicellular or multicellular (Fig. 42.5). The cuticle of the gland may be raised by the secretion (Fig. 42.5E and F). In peppermint the oil secretion beneath the cuticle contains crystals of menthol. A particular type of hair is often characteristic of a plant family or genus—for example, biseriate hairs of the form shown in Fig. 42.4J are common in the Compositae, while glandular hairs such as Fig. 42.5A, B and C are found in the Solanaceae, and such as Fig. 42.5E in the Labiatae. For types of hairs found on seeds, see sections on cotton, strophanthus seeds and nux vomica seeds.

Trichomes serve a number of functions, which include physical and chemical protection for the leaf against microbial organisms, aphids and insects, and the maintenance of a layer of still air on the leaf surface, thus combating excess water loss by transpiration. The secretions of glandular trichomes of certain genera constitute important materials for the perfumery, food and pharmaceutical industries; some secretions contain narcotic resins and others give rise to skin allergies. The sesquiterpenes of the capitate and non-capitate glandular trichomes of *Helianthus annuus* are antimicrobial and the glandular trichomes of some *Solanum* species contain sucrose esters of carboxylic acids such as 2-methyl-propanoic and 2-methylbutyric acid, which are aphid deterrents. The isolated secretory cells of the pellate glandular trichomes of *Mentha piperita* can carry out the *de novo* synthesis of monoterpenes. These studies have been facilitated by improved methods of trichome microsampling.

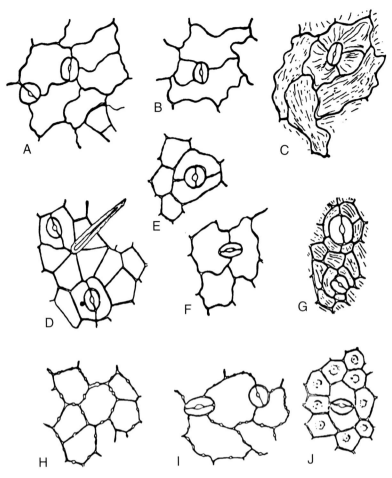

Fig. 42.2
Epidermis of leaves: A, lower epidermis of *Digitalis purpurea*; B, lower epidermis of *Hyoscyamus niger*, C, upper epidermis of *Atropa belladonna*; D, lower epidermis of *Cassia angustifolia*; E, lower epidermis of *Rosmarinus officinalis*; F, lower epidermis of *Mentha piperita*; G, lower epidermis of *Pilocarpus jaborandi*; H, upper epidermis of *Lobelia inflata*; I, lower epidermis of *Digitalis lanata*; J, lower epidermis of *Erythroxylum coca*. A, Anomocytic type of stomata; B and C, anisocytic type of stomata; D, paracytic type of stomata; E and F, diacytic type of stomata; G, actinocytic type of stomata.

THE ENDODERMIS

The endodermis is a specialized layer of cells marking the inner limit of the cortex. A typical endodermis is usually present in roots, in aquatic and subterranean stems and in the aerial stems of certain families (e.g. Labiatae and Cucurbitaceae). Leaves and aerial stems often show a starch sheath, probably representing a modified endodermis.

The cells of the endodermis appear in transverse section four-sided, oval or elliptical and often extended in the tangential direction. The cells are longitudinally elongated, with the end walls often transverse. A primary endodermis, such as can be studied in lobelia stem, is characterized by the deposition, in the radial walls, of special modified material (resembling cutin) in the form of a Casparian strip. Subsequently, a suberin lamella may be laid down within the primary wall, giving a secondary endodermis. This may be followed by the deposition of a secondary wall of lignocellulose, giving a tertiary endodermis, as in *Aletris* and *Smilax*. The structure of the endodermis is of value in differentiating between the commercial species of *Smilax*.

CORK TISSUE

As the plant axis increases in diameter, a cork cambium or phellogen usually arises which, by its activity, produces new protective tissues, known collectively as periderm, which replace the epidermis and part or all of the primary cortex. The cells of the cork cambium undergo tangential divisions giving rise externally to phellem or cork tissue and internally to phelloderm or secondary cortex. Usually, only a limited production of phelloderm occurs, so that the number of cork layers greatly exceeds the number of phelloderm layers. However, wide secondary cortex is seen in ipecacuanha root (Fig. 41.8) and taraxacum.

In roots the cork cambium arises in the pericycle; in stems it may arise in the epidermis or the subepidermal layer or be deep-seated. The first-formed cork cambium may be functional throughout the life of the plant and may itself keep pace with the increase in girth, giving rise to an even smooth bark. A persistent cork cambium, failing to increase in diameter, gives rise to the fissured bark of the cork oak and cork elm. Often, however, the first-formed cork cambium has only a limited period of activity and is replaced by secondary cambia of more deep-seated origin; this process may be repeated again and again.

Cork tissue is built up of a compact mass of cells, usually rectangular in transverse sections (Fig. 21.13C) five- or six-sided in surface view (see Fig. 21.13E) and often arranged in regular radial rows. The cell wall is composed of inner and outer cellulose layers and a median suberin lamella, or of a suberin lamella laid down upon the primary cellulose wall. The cellulose layers may be lignified, as in cassia bark. The mature cork cell is dead, impermeable to water and often filled with dark reddish-brown contents rich in tannins and related substances.

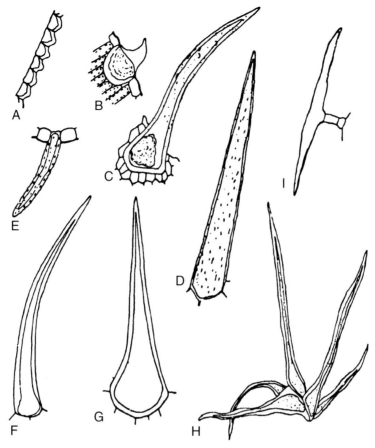

Fig. 42.3
Epidermal trichomes. A, Papillae of lower epidermis of *Coca* leaf. B–G, Unicellular hairs; B, papillose epidermal cell with cystolith from leaf of *Cannabis*; C, cystolith clothing hair from floral bract of *Cannabis*; D, *Lobelia inflata* leaf; E, senna leaf; F, lignified hair of *Ailanthus*; G, comfrey. H, Group of unicellular hairs from *Hamamelis* leaf. I, T-shaped hair of *Artemisia absinthium*.

The presence of cork cells in powdered drugs may show adulteration or use of low-quality or improperly peeled drug (e.g. cinnamon, ginger and liquorice).

The formation of cork puts out of action the stomatal apparatus, and involves the formation of special breathing pores or lenticels. The lenticels are larger in size and smaller in number than the stomata they replace. The simplest form of lenticel consists of a mass of unsuberized thin-walled cells which become rounded off and are known as complementary tissue. Often, however, in the lenticel area, the cork cambium gives rise not only to complementary tissue, but also, alternating with it, to diaphragms of suberized cells, with well-marked intercellular air spaces.

COLLENCHYMA

Collenchyma is a living tissue, directly derived from parenchyma, but having greater mechanical strength. The walls are thickened, the thickening being composed of cellulose and being laid down in longitudinal strips commonly located at the angles of the cells. The cells are usually four- to six-sided in transverse section, axially elongated when seen in longitudinal section. Their walls, being composed of cellulose, have considerable plasticity, and, hence, collenchyma constitutes the typical mechanical tissue of herbaceous stems and of the petioles and midribs of leaves. Collenchyma is present above and below the midrib bundle in many leaves (e.g. senna, stramonium, hyoscyamus, belladonna, digitalis and lobelia); in the wings of lobelia

stem; in the cortex of cascara bark; and in the pericarp of colocynth and capsicum.

SCLEREIDS

Sclereids or stone cells are sclerenchymatous cells approximately isodiametrical in shape. The walls of the typical sclereid are thick, lignified, often showing well-marked stratification and traversed by pit-canals which are often funnel-shaped or branched. The cell lumen is usually small, sometimes almost completely obliterated. Cell contents of diagnostic significance may be present (e.g. prisms of calcium oxalate in calumba, starch grains in cinnamon).

Sclereids commonly occur in the hard outer coats of seeds and fruits and in the bark and pericyclic regions of woody stems. They occur isolated or in small groups in quillaia and calumba, in larger groups in cascara (Fig. 21.13) and wild cherry bark (Fig. 25.3) or in definite sclereid layers, as in cinnamon (Fig. 22.10) and cassia bark. The absence of sclereids from frangula and cinchona barks aids in their microscopical identification. The presence of elongated sclereids in powdered ipecacuanha is diagnostic of the presence of stem; lignified sclereids, which are present in clove stalk (Fig. 22.12), should be almost absent from powdered cloves. Characteristic sclereids are present in the rind and seed coat of colocynth (Fig. 41.7F and G).

Attention can appropriately be called, in this section, to the sclerenchymatous layer of the testas of linseed (Fig. 41.7I) and cardamoms (Fig. 41.7K); to the pitted fusiform sclerenchymatous cells of

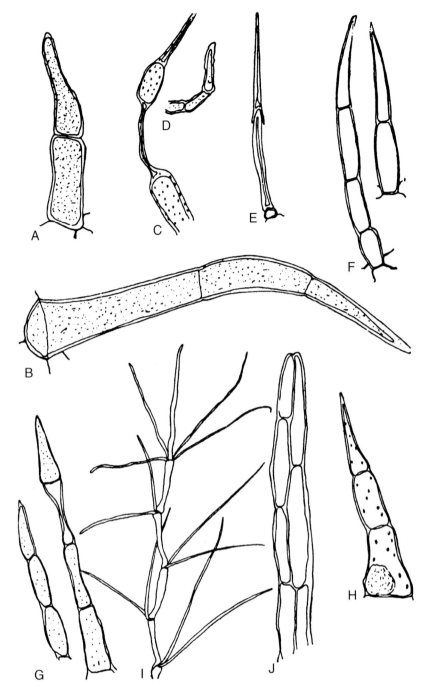

Fig. 42.4
Epidermal trichomes. A–H, Uniseriate clothing hairs; I, multicellular branched hair; J, biseriate hair. A, *Datura metel*; B, *Datura stramonium*; C, *Mentha piperita*; D, *Thymus vulgaris*; E, *Plantago lanceolata*; F, *Hyoscyamus niger*; G, *Digitalis purpurea*; H, *Xanthium strumarium*; I, *Verbascum thapsus*; J, *Calendula officinalis*.

the mesocarp of coriander (Fig. 22.6); to the lignified reticulate cells occurring in the mesocarp of fennel (Fig. 41.7D) and dill, and in the inner part of the testa of colocynth (Fig. 41.7F); and to the lignified idioblasts seen in the lamina of hamamelis leaf.

FIBRES

Tissue composed of spindle-shaped or elongated cells with pointed ends is known as prosenchyma. When cells of this kind are thick-walled, they are known as fibres. The cell wall may be composed of almost pure cellulose or may show various degrees of lignification in the form of sclerotic or sclerenchymatous fibres.

Fibres are developed from a single cell, the fibre initial, which during its development grows rapidly in the axial direction. During this period of growth the tips of the elongating cells may push past one another, a process known as 'gliding growth' and made possible by a modification in the state of the middle lamella. Most mature fibres are unicellular, but occasionally transverse septa develop (e.g. ginger). Fibres are best differentiated on the basis of the tissue in which they occur (i.e. as cortical fibres, pericyclic fibres, xylem fibres or phloem fibres).

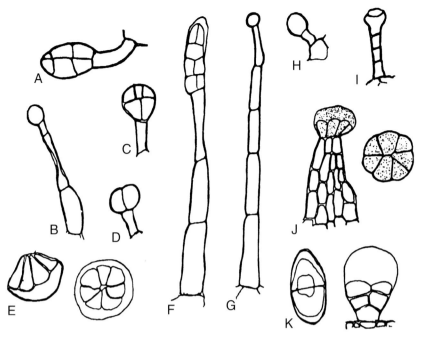

Fig. 42.5
Glandular hairs: A and B, *Atropa belladonna*; C, *Datura stramonium*; D, *Digitalis purpurea*; E, multicellular labiate glandular hair; F, *Hyoscyamus niger*; G and H, *Primula vulgaris*; I, *Digitalis lutea*; J, *Cannabis sativa*; K, *Artemisia maritima*.

Frequently, fibres are differentiated in the pericycle; thus flax consists of the *pericyclic fibres* of *Linum usitatissimum* and hemp of the pericyclic fibres of *Cannabis sativa*. The cell wall of the flax fibre is composed of almost pure cellulose; in hemp some lignification has taken place.

Isolated groups of pericyclic fibres occur in lobelia stem and in cinnamon bark. The meristeles of clove hypanthium are enclosed in an incomplete sheath of pericyclic fibres. The lignified, moderately thick-walled pericyclic fibres, accompanied by a parenchymatous sheath of cells containing prisms of calcium oxalate, constitute an important diagnostic character of senna leaf (Fig. 21.10). The presence of pericyclic fibres in the midrib of the leaves of *Digitalis lutea* and *D. thapsi* contrasts with their absence in *D. purpurea* and *D. lanata*.

Xylem fibres may be regarded as being directly derived from tracheids, and intermediate forms, having a limited conducting function and known as fibre-tracheids occur (Fig. 42.6A–C). The fibre-tracheid has smaller pits, thicker walls and usually more tapering ends than the typical tracheid. Wood fibres have thicker walls and pits reduced to minute canals. Occasionally, wood fibres are septate (Fig. 42.6D). Cells having a fibre-like form with living contents and simple pits but which are really fusiform xylem parenchyma cells are termed 'substitute fibres'. The mature wood fibre is a dead lignified element. The autumn wood is usually characterized by containing a higher proportion of wood fibres than the spring wood. The ground mass of secondary xylem of *Picroena excelsa* is built up of compactly arranged thick-walled wood fibres and the secondary xylem of liquorice (Fig. 23.11) contains wood fibres arranged in bundles, which alternate with the small groups of vessels and are enclosed in a sheath of xylem parenchyma containing prisms of calcium oxalate. The secondary xylem in gentian, rhubarb and jalap is free from fibres.

Phloem fibres may occur in both primary and secondary phloem; they may or may not be lignified. Their thickened walls are traversed by simple pits, in contrast to the fine-bordered pits of the wood fibres. Phloem fibres constitute the 'hard bast' of earlier writers. Jute consists of the phloem fibres from the stems of various species of *Corchorus*.

The phloem fibres of liquorice resemble those of the xylem in being enclosed in a crystal sheath. The distribution, abundance, size and shape of the phloem fibres constitute important characters for the differentiation of medicinal barks. Phloem fibres occur isolated or in irregular rows in the barks of cinnamon (Fig. 22.10), cassia and cinchona (Fig. 26.33). The phloem fibres of cinnamon can be differentiated from those of cassia by their smaller diameter. In barks, in which fibres occur isolated or in rows, the area of fibres per gram of powdered bark can be made a criterion for determining the amount present in mixtures. The phloem fibres of cinchona constitute a prominent feature of the powder; they are large (80–90 μm in diameter), are fusiform in shape and have very thick walls, conspicuously striated and traversed by funnel-shaped pits (Fig. 26.33). The secondary phloem of cascara, frangula and quillaia is composed of alternating zones of hard and soft phloem. The phloem fibres of cascara are accompanied by a crystal sheath (Fig. 21.13); those of quillaia are characterized by their tortuous, irregular outline and often exhibit enlarged and forked apices. Fibres are absent from the phloem of gentian and ipecacuanha.

XYLEM

The primary xylem is composed of protoxylem and metaxylem. Secondary growth in thickness of the stem and root of gymnosperms and dicotyledons is accompanied by the formation of secondary xylem. The structural elements of xylem are tracheids, vessels or tracheae, xylem fibres, xylem parenchyma and rays.

The *tracheid* is derived from a single cell and can be regarded as the basic cell type of xylem tissue. It takes the form of an elongated water-conducting cell, with a lignified and variously thickened and pitted cell wall (Fig. 42.6A). At maturity it is a dead element. The pits are bordered (Fig. 42.6L–N), although in some cases the borders are so narrow that the pits appear simple. In gymnosperms the pits are confined to the radial walls.

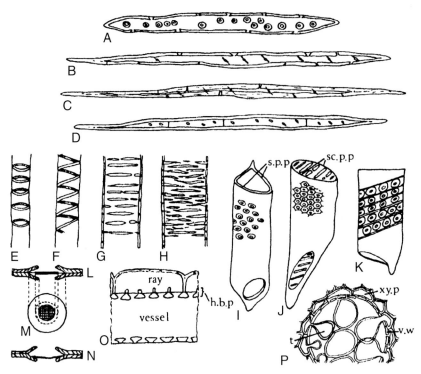

Fig. 42.6
Xylem components. A, Tracheid; B, fibre-tracheid; C, xylem fibre; D, septate fibre; E, annular vessel; F, spiral vessel; G, scalariform vessel; H, reticulate vessel; I, vessel segment with round bordered pits and simple perforation plate (s.p.p.) at either end; J, vessel segment with hexagonal pits caused by crowding, and scalariform perforation plate (sc.p.p) at either end; K, vessel segment with bordered pits and band of tertiary thickening. L, M, N, structure of the bordered pit; L and N, sections show overarched secondary wall, pit membrane and central torus, the latter, in N, closing the pit mouth; M, surface view of same; O, half-bordered pit pairs (h.b.p.) connecting a vessel and ray cells; P, vessel in transverse section showing development of tyloses. t, Tylosis; v.w, vessel wall; xy.p, xylem parenchyma.

The character of the secondary wall thickening enables us to distinguish annular, spiral, scalariform and reticulate tracheids. Transition forms between these types are not uncommon. Annular and spiral tracheids occur most frequently in protoxylem; scalariform and reticulate tracheids most frequently in metaxylem and secondary xylem. True vessels are absent in gymnosperms, in which the secondary xylem consists of a homogeneous tracheidal system only broken by narrow medullary rays and in some cases by a slight development of xylem parenchyma. Cellulose wadding is made from high grade sulphite pulp usually prepared from coniferous wood, and when examined microscopically shows typical coniferous tracheids, with bordered pits and a small amount of wood parenchyma. The tissues are completely delignified in the preparation of the pulp. Tracheids occur in the secondary xylem of some angiosperms (e.g. ipecacuanha).

Vessels or *tracheae* constitute the fundamental conducting elements of the xylem of the angiosperms. The vessel is derived from a vertical series of cells, in which increase in diameter and dissolution of the end-walls occurs so that a continuous tube is formed. The most primitive type of vessel consists of a vertical series of tracheid-like segments in which some of the scalariform pits of the adjacent end-walls have broken down to give slit-like openings; the most advanced type of vessel shows complete dissolution of the end-walls of the constituent segments (see Fig. 42.6I–K). The vessels of the protoxylem show annular or spiral thickening, those of the later-formed xylem scalariform and reticulate thickening (Fig. 42.6E–H). The secondary wall thickening is composed of lignocellulose. Larger vessels may have a complete secondary wall perforated only by pits. These pits are subject to considerable variation in size, form and crowding and

sometimes bands of tertiary thickening are laid down within the secondary wall (Fig. 42.6K).

Spiral and annular vessels are typical of protoxylem, and usually occur in the protoxylem of stems and roots, in small vascular bundles and in the veins of leaves. Thus, small amounts of such vessels are seen in gentian, clove, squill and most leaves (e.g. senna, belladonna, hyoscyamus and stramonium). Spiral and scalariform vessels occur in lobelia stem. Reticulate vessels occur in gentian, ginger and rhubarb, those of the last two drugs being almost non-lignified. Vessels showing numerous bordered pits occur in quassia, jalap, sandalwood, hydrastis and the stems of belladonna and aconite.

The living meshwork of the secondary xylem is made up of *rays* and *xylem parenchyma* which permeate the dead mass of mature vessels, tracheids and wood fibres. The xylem parenchyma cells are often axially elongated, sometimes thin-walled but often with walls showing thickening and lignification. The walls are traversed by simple pits or, where the cells abut on vessels or tracheids, by half-bordered pits. Xylem parenchyma may function as a storage tissue, the cells becoming blocked with starch (as in ipecacuanha). The xylem parenchyma cells may grow into the vessel cavities and form tyloses which block up the vessel and render it non-functional, a process which occurs in the development of heartwood (Fig. 42.6P). The distribution of xylem parenchyma may be diffuse, vasicentric when it forms sheaths around the larger vessels, or terminal when a zone of xylem parenchyma is formed towards the end of each year's growth. The formation of concentric zones of xylem parenchyma may give rise to 'false annual rings', as in quassia. In transverse sections the medullary rays appear radially arranged and where the ray cells about on to vessels they may possess half-bordered pits (Fig. 42.6O).

PHLOEM

The structural elements of phloem include sieve tubes, companion cells, phloem parenchyma and secretory cells. The sieve tube is the conducting element of the phloem. It is formed from a vertical series of elongated cells, interconnected by perforations in their walls in areas known as sieve plates. The perforations may be restricted to smaller areas, sieve fields, several of which are contained in each sieve plate. The sieve plates may occur in the end-walls or lateral walls of the sieve tube (Fig. 42.7). The mature sieve plate is coated with a film of callus, which may increase in amount and form a callus pad completely blocking the sieve plate (Fig. 42.7D). The development of the callus pad may render the sieve tube permanently functionless; in other cases the callus pad formed in the autumn is redissolved in the spring. The mature sieve tube lacks a nucleus, but while functional contains cytoplasm. Sieve tubes may often be detected by recognition of the callus pads, which show typical staining reactions.

1. Alkaline solution of corallin: stains callose red.
2. Aniline Blue: stains callose blue.
3. Chlor-zinc-iodine: stains callose a reddish-brown.
4. Solution of Ammoniacal Copper Nitrate *BP*: does not dissolve callose.
5. Solution of potash: as even a cold 1% solution of potash dissolves callose, this should not be used as a clearing agent if it is afterwards desired to test the section for callose.

In view of their delicate structure and lack of lignification, sieve tubes are difficult to observe in commercial drugs. The sieve tubes of cascara bark can often be detected, even in the powdered drug, when stained with corallin soda. They are sometimes also to be observed in powdered gentian.

The companion cells are intimately associated with the sieve tubes both structurally and functionally. The sieve tube and the companion cells are derived from a common mother cell of the procambial strand in primary phloem or from a phloem mother cell derived from the cambium in secondary phloem. The phloem mother cell undergoes longitudinal division into two daughter cells of unequal size, the smaller of which becomes the companion cell. The companion cell is characterized by its dense protoplast and well-developed nucleus, and by possessing a thin cellulose wall.

The cells of the phloem parenchyma are usually axially elongated, although they may remain isodiametric and be arranged in linear series. They remain typically thin-walled.

The phloem often contains secretory cells (e.g. ginger, cinnamon, cassia and jalap). Laticiferous tissue may also occur in the phloem (e.g. lobelia and taraxacum) (Fig. 42.7E).

SECRETORY TISSUES

Secretory tissues include secretory cells, secretory cavities or sacs, secretory ducts or canals and latex tissue.

Oil cells occur in ginger (Fig. 48.8D), pepper, mace, cardamoms, cinnamon (Fig. 42.8G) and cassia. Large oil cells form an important diagnostic character of powdered sassafras root bark. Cells containing resins (Fig. 42.8H), oleoresins and mucilage are common. Enzyme storage cells occur in many endospermic seeds (e.g. the myrosin cells of the Cruciferae). Storage cells, crystal cells and tannin cells may also be considered under this heading.

Secretory cavities or *sacs* may arise by separation of the cells and subsequent formation of a secretory epithelium (schizogenously) or by breakdown of the cells forming a cavity not bounded by a definite epithelium (lysigenously). Schizogenous oil cavities occur in eucalyptus, lysigenous oil cavities in *Gossypium* species. Secretory products may appear in cells before the latter break down to give a lysigenous cavity. Schizolysigenous oil cavities occur in the Rutaceae and the Burseraceae. The oil cavity develops from a mother cell, which undergoes division to give daughter cells which separate, leaving a schizogenous central cavity. The walls of the cells surrounding this central cavity then break down, forming an oily secretion, and the cavity continues to increase in size lysigenously (Fig. 42.8E, F).

The vittae of the Umbelliferae are schizogenous oleoresin canals (Fig. 42.8A–C) and they occur in the stem, roots and leaves.

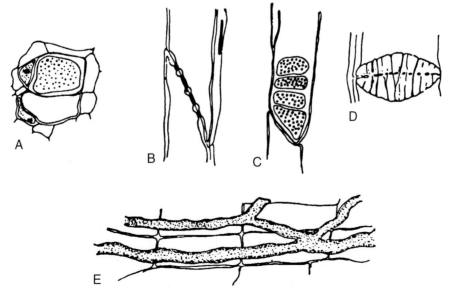

Fig. 42.7
Phloem elements. A, Sieve tubes and companion cells in transverse section, one of the sieve tubes showing a transverse sieve plate in surface view; B and C, respectively, tangential and radial longitudinal views of a sieve tube, showing an oblique sieve plate with four sieve fields; D, sieve plate in winter condition, showing deposit of callus; E, radial longitudinal view of laticifers in the root of *Taraxacum officinale*.

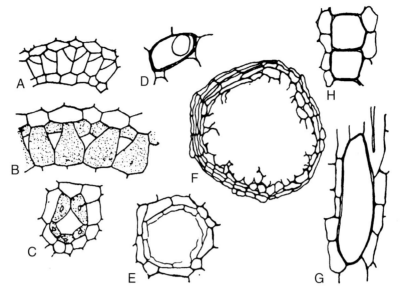

Fig. 42.8
Secretory cells and ducts. A, B, C, Stages in development of a typical schizogenous oil duct in the Umbelliferae (after Hayward); D, oil cell of ginger; E and F, schizolysigenous oil glands in *Barosma* and *Citrus*; G, oil cell of cinnamon seen in longitudinal section; H, resin cells of jalap.

The oleoresin ducts of *Pinus* species are also of schizogenous origin. Schizogenous oleoresin ducts which enlarge lysigenously occur in some members of the Leguminosae (e.g. *Copaifera*).

Latex (Laticiferous) tissue consists of either cells or tubes which contain a fluid with a milky appearance arising from the suspension of small particles in a liquid dispersion medium with a very different refractive index. The suspended particles vary in nature, and may be hydrocarbons composed of essential oils, resins and rubber. Alkaloids are present in the latex of Papaveraceae, the proteolytic enzyme papain in the latex of *Carica* (pawpaw) and vitamin B_1 in that of *Euphorbia*. Latex cells are typical of the Euphorbiaceae, Moraceae, Cannabinaceae, Apocynaceae and Asclepiadaceae. In the Euphorbiaceae the cells destined to form the latex systems are differentiated in the embryo. From these embryonic initials the branched tubular latex cells of the mature plant are developed. The latex cells have thickened walls and numerous nuclei, and contain latex in which characteristic dumb-bell-shaped starch grains may be present. The long, sinuous latex cells of *Cannabis sativa* are unbranched.

Laticifers are also formed by the partial or complete fusion of a longitudinal series of cells. They occur in Convolvulaceae, Campanulaceae and the suborder Liguliflorae of the Compositae. The Papaveraceae possess latex elements intermediate in structure between latex cells and vessels. The laticifers of *Ipomoea* consist of longitudinal rows of cells which retain their transverse walls. A similar condition is seen in *Sanguinaria*. In *Chelidonium* the marginal parts of the transverse walls persist; in *Papaver* and *Argemone* there is only slight evidence of the original transverse walls. The laticifers in the Liguliflorae take the form of a continuous non-septate series of passages usually occurring in the primary and secondary phloem. *Taraxacum officinale* (Fig. 42.7E) shows concentric zones of anastomosing latex vessels in the phloem of both rhizome and root.

It is often difficult or impossible to determine the mode of origin of the laticifers except by following their development from the embryonic or seedling stages. A further difficulty in delimiting elements of a laticiferous nature arises from their association in some plants with idioblasts containing tannins, mucilage, etc., and from the fact that latex material may also occur in schizogenous canals.

ERGASTIC CELL CONTENTS

The cell contents with which we are concerned in pharmacognosy are those which can be identified in vegetable drugs by microscopical examination or by chemical and physical tests. These cell contents represent either food-storage products or by-products of metabolism, and include carbohydrates, proteins, fixed oils and fats, alkaloids and purines, glycosides, volatile oils, gums and mucilages, resins, tannins, calcium oxalate, calcium carbonate and silica; being non-living, they are referred to as *ergastic*.

Starch

Starch occurs in granules of varying sizes in almost all organs of plants; it is found most abundantly in roots, rhizomes, fruits and seeds, where it usually occurs in larger grains than are to be found in the chlorophyll-containing tissues of the same plant. The small granules formed in chloroplasts by the condensation of sugars are afterwards hydrolysed into sugars so that they may pass in solution to storage organs where, under the influence of leucoplasts, large grains of reserve starch are formed. Starch is of considerable pharmaceutical importance and is fully discussed in Chapter 20.

Proteins

Storage protein occurs in the form of aleurone grains which are particularly well seen in oily seeds (e.g. castor seed (see Fig. 42.1E) and linseed). The simplest aleurone grain consists of a mass of protein surrounded by a thin membrane. Often, however, the ground mass of protein encloses one or more rounded bodies or globoids and an angular body known as the crystalloid. Aleurone grains are best observed after defatting and removal of starch, if these are present in large amount. Sections being examined for aleurone should be treated with the following reagents:

1. Millon's reagent stains the protein red on warming.
2. Iodine solution stains the ground substance and crystalloid yellowish-brown but leaves the globoids unstained.
3. Picric acid stains the ground substance and crystalloid yellow.

The endosperm cells of nutmeg each contain one large and several smaller aleurone grains. The large aleurone grains are 12–20 μm in diameter, and contain a large well-defined crystalloid. Aleurone grains, containing globoids, are present in the endosperm and cotyledons of linseed. Some of the aleurone grains of the endosperm of fennel contain a minute cluster crystal of calcium oxalate; others contain one or more globoids.

Fixed oils and fats

Fixed oils and fats are widely distributed and occur in both vegetative and reproductive structures. They often occur in seeds, where they may replace the carbohydrates as a reserve food material, and are not uncommonly associated with protein reserves. As lipids, fats form an essential component of biological membranes.

Reserve fats occur in solid, frequently coloured or crystalline masses which melt on warming. Feathery crystalline masses of fat occur in the endosperm of nutmeg. Fixed oils occur as small highly refractive drops. Oil globules, associated with aleurone grains, can be well seen in the cotyledons of linseed and colocynth and in the endosperm of nux vomica and umbelliferous fruits. Oils and fats are soluble in ether-alcohol, but, with a few exceptions, such as castor oil, are sparingly soluble in alcohol. They are coloured brown or black with a 1% solution of osmic acid, and red with a diluted tincture of alkanna. The latter stains rather slowly and should be allowed to act for at least 30 min. A cold mixture of equal parts of a saturated solution of potash and strong solution of ammonia slowly saponifies fixed oils and fats. After some hours, characteristic soap crystals may be observed. For a full discussion of fixed oils and fats, see Chapter 19.

Gums and mucilages

Gums, mucilages and pectins are polysaccharide complexes formed from sugar and uronic acid units. They are insoluble in alcohol but dissolve or swell in water. They are usually formed from the cell wall (e.g. tragacanth) or deposited on it in successive layers. When such cells are mounted in alcohol and irrigated with water, the stratification may often be seen (e.g. mustard and linseed).

Specific tests for these substances are at present lacking, but the following are useful. The official Solution of Ruthenium Red stains the mucilage of senna and buchu leaves, althaea, linseed and mustard. It also stains sterculia gum but has less action on tragacanth. A lead acetate medium can be used to prevent undue swelling or solution of the substance being tested. Some forms of mucilage are stained by the *BP* Alkaline Solution of Corallin, e.g. that found in squill. Others are stained by chlor-zinc-iodine or methylene blue dissolved in alcohol and glycerin.

The pharmaceutical gums are described in Chapter 20.

Volatile oils and resins

Volatile oils occur as droplets in the cell. They are sparingly soluble in water but dissolve in alcohol (cf. fixed oils). They resemble fixed oils (q.v.) in their behaviour towards osmic acid and tincture of alkanna, but they are not saponified when treated with ammoniacal potash.

Resins may be associated with volatile oil or gum, or may be found in irregular masses which are insoluble in water but soluble in alcohol. Resins, oleoresins and gum resins are usually secreted into secretory cavities or ducts. They stain slowly with diluted tincture of alkanna. For details of volatile oil and resin-containing drugs see Chapter 22.

Tannins

Tannins are widely distributed in plants and occur in solution in the cell sap, often in distinct vacuoles. If it is desired to study the distribution of the tannins in the plant, the sections must be cut dry, since tannins are soluble in water and alcohol. If sections of galls are so cut and mounted in clove oil, plates of tannin may be observed. Sections containing tannins acquire a bluish-black or greenish colour when mounted in a dilute solution of ferric chloride. For tannin-containing drugs see Chapter 21.

Alkaloids and glycosides

These important secondary metabolites are rarely visible in plant cells without the application of specific chemical tests.

Crystals

Various crystalline deposits may occur in plant cells.

Calcium oxalate. Oxalic acid rarely occurs in the free state in plants but is extremely common as its calcium salt in the form of crystals. It is dimorphous and is found either as the trihydrate, belonging to the tetragonal system of crystals, or as the monohydrate, belonging to the monoclinic system.

Crystals of the tetragonal system form as a result of supersaturation of the cell sap with calcium oxalate. They have all three axes at right angles to one another; two of the axes are equal in length and the third, or principal axis, may be either shorter or longer. They are illustrated in Fig. 42.9A–D; and in addition to these forms, the tiny sandy crystals or microcrystals found in the Solanaceae (Fig. 26.8) and other families probably belong to this system. In the monoclinic system the crystals have such forms as shown in Fig. 42.9E–I, and result from an excess of oxalic acid in the cell sap. They have three unequal axes with the two lateral axes at right angles to one another, but one only of these is at right angles to the third axis. These crystals shine more brightly when viewed in polarized light than do the trihydrate crystals.

Usually it is sufficient to describe the general form and size of the crystals, without reference to a crystallographical class. The most common forms encountered are prisms (senna, hyoscyamus, quassia, liquorice, cascara, quillaia, rauwolfia, calumba); rosettes (rhubarb, stramonium, cascara, senna, clove, jalap); single acicular crystals (ipecacuanha, gentian, cinnamon); bundles of acicular crystals (squill); microsphenoidal or sandy crystals (belladonna).

When calcium oxalate is present, it is important that the types of crystal, their size and distribution be recorded. Cascara shows cluster crystals generally distributed in the ground mass of parenchyma and prisms confined to the rows of parenchymatous cells forming a sheath round the fibres (Fig. 21.13). The prisms of calcium oxalate in calumba are contained in the sclereids.

The cells containing calcium oxalate may differ from those surrounding them in size, form or contents, and are often referred to as idioblasts.

Calcium oxalate is usually present to the extent of about 1% in plants but in some structures such as the rhizome of rhubarb it may exceed 20% of the dry weight. It often forms a character of considerable diagnostic importance. The solanaceous leaves may be distinguished from one another, belladonna by its sandy crystals, stramonium by its cluster crystals, and henbane by its single and twin prisms. Similarly, phytolacca leaves and roots, which both possess acicular crystals, are distinguished from belladonna leaves and roots, which have sandy crystals. Other instances of the diagnostic importance of calcium oxalate are given under the individual drugs and no attempt is made to give here more than a few selected examples, which will be extended by the student in further reading.

Sections to be examined for calcium oxalate may be cleared with chloral hydrate or caustic alkali, as these reagents only very slowly dissolve the crystals. The polarizing microscope will often assist in the detection of small crystals. Crystals may be identified as

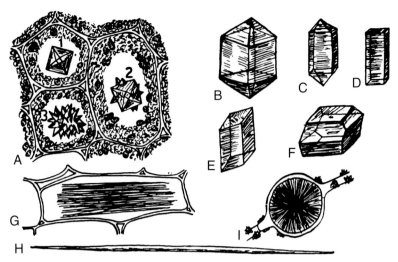

Fig. 42.9
Calcium oxalate. A–D, Crystals of the tetragonal system; E–I, crystals of the monoclinic system. A3, A rosette crystal formed of tetragonal crystals as seen in A1 and A2; D, a tetragonal prism; E, a monoclinic prism; G, raphides; H, a single needle crystal; I, a sphaerocrystal. (After Thoms' *Handbuch der Pharmazie*.)

calcium oxalate if they are insoluble in acetic acid and caustic alkali, soluble in hydrochloric and sulphuric acids without effervescence and show, after solution in 50% sulphuric acid, a gradual separation of needle-like crystals of calcium sulphate at the site of the original crystals.

Calcium carbonate. This may be found embedded in or incrusted in the cell walls. Concretions of calcium carbonate formed on outgrowths of the cell wall are termed cystoliths. They occur in the orders Urticaceae, Moraceae, Cannabinaceae and Acanthaceae, and in some of the Combretaceae and Boraginaceae. Well-formed cystoliths are seen in the enlarged upper epidermal cells and in the clothing hairs of the lower epidermis of the leaf of *Cannabis sativa* (Fig. 42.3). When the mineral substance of the cystolith is dissolved out in dilute acid, there remains a small, often stratified, basis composed of cellulose. Calcium carbonate can be identified by the fact that it dissolves with effervescence in acetic, hydrochloric or sulphuric acid. If 50% sulphuric acid is used, needle-shaped crystals of calcium sulphate gradually separate.

Hesperidin and diosmin. These occur as feathery-like aggregates or sphaerocrystalline masses in the cells of many of the Rutaceae and in isolated plants of other families. Crystalline masses of diosmin are present in the upper epidermal cells of buchu leaves (Fig. 42.1B). These crystals are insoluble in organic solvents but soluble in potassium hydroxide.

Silica. This substance forms the skeletons of diatoms (see 'agar' and 'kieselguhr'), and occurs as an incrustation on cell walls or as masses in the interior of cells (e.g. in the cells of the sclerenchymatous layer of cardamom seeds). Silica is insoluble in all acids except hydrofluoric. It may be examined by igniting the material and treating the ash with hydrochloric acid, the silica remaining unaltered.

43

Techniques in microscopy

The microscopical characters of many drugs have already been described, but it will be realized that microscopical techniques require considerable skill; years of experience are necessary to acquire a really good knowledge of the microscopy of drugs, foodstuffs and other plant materials. It is first necessary to learn how to use a microscope properly and to understand the purpose of the different reagents used in the examination of crude drugs. The preparation of systematic and illustrated reports is also important.

Mountants for specimens

Definition, particularly of colourless structures, is increased by choice of a mountant of refractive index different from that of the object. A mountant of lower refractive index is to be preferred so that the outline shadow is on the side away from the object. The ratio refractive index of object to refractive index of mountant should be of the order of 1.06. The value of this relative refractive index for cellulose (cotton) to water is 1.17, to chloral hydrate solution (5:2) 1.08 and to glycerin 1.06. This serves to emphasize the value of chloral hydrate and glycerin as mountants for plant structures.

THE MICROSCOPE

Magnification and field of view

For work in pharmacognosy, microscopes are usually fitted with two objectives, 16 mm and 4 mm, two or three eyepieces and a condenser. The procedure for making microscopical measurements is described below. Different combinations of eyepiece and objective give different magnifications and fields of view, as indicated in the table below.

When using the microscope, it is useful to know the size of the fields of view. For instance, if we know that using a 4 mm objective and a ×6 eyepiece our field of view is approximately 0.5 mm, or 500 µm, the size of objects such as the *Arachnoidiscus* diatom in agar (100–300 µm) or the large rosette crystals of calcium oxalate in rhubarb (up to 200 µm) may be roughly estimated. For accurate measurement, however, an eyepiece micrometer or camera lucida is used.

Apparatus for making microscopical measurements and drawings to scale

Microscopical measurements can be made using a stage micrometer in conjunction with an eyepiece micrometer, camera lucida or microprojector.

Micrometers

Two scales are required, known, respectively, as a *stage micrometer* and an *eyepiece micrometer*. The stage micrometer is a glass slide 7.6 × 2.5 cm (3 × 1 inch) with a scale engraved on it. The scale is usually 1 or 1.1 mm long and is divided into 0.1 and 0.01 parts of a millimetre. The eyepiece micrometer may be a linear scale (Fig. 43.1A and the scale 0–10 in Fig. 43.1B) or it may be ruled in squares. The value of one eyepiece division is determined for every optical combination to be used, a note being made in each case of the objective eyepiece and length of draw-tube.

To do this, unscrew the upper lens of the eyepiece, place the eyepiece micrometer on the ridge inside, and replace the lens. Put the stage micrometer on the stage and focus it in the ordinary way. The two micrometer scales now appear as in Fig. 43.1B, when the 4 mm objective is in use. In the example figured, it will be seen that when the 7 line of the stage micrometer coincides with the 0 of the eyepiece, the 10 of the stage coincides with 7.7 of the eyepiece. As the distance between 7 and 10 on the stage scale is 0.3 mm, 77 of the small eyepiece divisions equal 0.3 mm or 300 µm; therefore, 1 eyepiece division equals 300/77 or 3.9 µm.

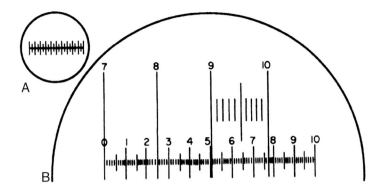

Fig. 43.1
A, Eyepiece micrometer; B, eyepiece micrometer superimposed on portion of stage micrometer scale.

Focal length of objective	Initial magnifying power	Approximate magnification (field of view in brackets) with eyepiece		
		×6	×10	×15
16 mm (2/3 inch)	10	62 (2.0 mm)	110 (1.1 mm)	155 (0.89 mm)
4 mm (1/6 inch)	45	285 (0.5 mm)	490 (0.25 mm)	690 (0.21 mm)

Camera lucida

Various forms of apparatus have been designed so that a magnified image of the object under the microscope may be traced on paper. The Swift-Ives camera lucida and the Abbé drawing apparatus are examples. The former fits over the eyepiece, and when in use light from the object passes direct to the observer's eye through an opening in the silvered surface of a prism. At the same time, light from the drawing paper and pencil is reflected by a second prism and by the silvered surface, so that the pencil appears superimposed on the object, which may thus be traced.

When the instrument is in use, the illumination of both object and paper must be suitably adjusted and the paper must be tilted at the correct angle to avoid distortion. The Abbé drawing apparatus utilizes, instead of the adjustable prism, a plane mirror carried on a side-arm; with the mirror at 45° to the bench surface, no inclined board is necessary.

To make measurements or scale drawings, the divisions of a stage micrometer are first traced on paper and then, using the same objective, eyepiece and length of draw-tube, the object to be recorded is traced.

The above camera lucidas which have served pharmacognosists well in the past do not now appear to be available commercially. This seems apparent from some of the line illustrations now submitted for publication!

Microprojection

With a suitable apparatus objects beneath a microscope can be transmitted to a screen or on to paper. Suitable particles can then be traced at the desired magnification.

Photomicrography

Modern research microscopes have built-in facilities for photomicrography; with less expensive or with older microscopes it is necessary to fit a suitable camera to the equipment. The photographic record may seem, at first sight, to dispense with the older tracing techniques discussed above. However, although the photographic record is suitable for thin sections of plant material, rarely is it completely so for powdered drugs. A photograph contains everything visible in a particular field of view and much of this is usually uninformative; rarely does a single field of view show all the diagnostic features of the powdered drug to best advantage, and also, owing to limitations on depth of focus, structures such as large fibres, vessels, trichomes, etc. are seldom seen with all details completely in focus. Fragments of disintegrated material adhering to, or partly covering, the element photographed are also confusing to the inexperienced observer.

Polarization

The apparatus consists of a polarizer, or Nicol prism, fitting below the microscope stage, and a similar prism forming the analyser fitting above the objective. As in the case of the polarimeter, with which students will be familiar, one Nicol is kept stationary while the other is rotated. With geological microscopes, polarizers are usually permanently fitted, but for botanical work the analyser is usually fitted when required, either between the objective and nosepiece or over the eyepiece. Less cumbersome are discs cut from polaroid sheets; one of these can be of a size to fit into the filter holder of the microscope and the other to rest on the eyepiece.

When both the polarizer and analyser have their diagonal surfaces parallel, the ray of plane polarized light is transmitted by the analyser. If now the polarizer is revolved, the light diminishes in intensity until at a position 90° from the first it is entirely extinguished, the polarized light being now totally reflected by the analyser. This position, when the diagonal surfaces of the two Nicols are at right angles, is termed 'crossed Nicols'.

Isotropic substances are characterized by having the same physical properties in all directions (e.g. gases, liquids and isometric crystals). Such substances are monorefringent (i.e. they have only one refractive index). Isotropic substances are not visible, however they be oriented, when examined between crossed Nicols. They in no way affect the polarized light passing through them from the polarizer.

Anisotropic substances exhibit different physical properties according to the direction along which they are examined. Such substances show more than one refractive index. The great majority of crystalline materials show birefringence. When a uniaxial crystal is placed with its optical axis horizontal to the stage and examined between crossed Nicols, then as the stage is rotated it will alternately shine bright (or coloured) and disappear. Through the 360° it becomes invisible (i.e. shows extinction) four times. The examination of crystals between crossed Nicols enables us to determine their crystal system (see 'Calcium oxalate' Chapter 42). The crystal is placed with its axis parallel to the longer diagonal of the polarizing Nicol. If the crystal belongs to the tetragonal system, the polarized light passes unchanged and on reaching the analyser is completely absorbed, the field appearing dark (i.e. extinction takes place). Conversely, monoclinic crystals show extinction only when the vertical axis makes an angle with the diagonal of the Nicol known as the extinction angle.

Many crystalline substances show brilliant colours when examined in polarized light (e.g. asbestos, sucrose, cinnamic acid). Starch grains often show a black cross, a phenomenon due to the crystalline refraction of the material. Polarized light is useful for the detection of calcium oxalate, especially when only small quantities are present in the tissues under examination. It appears bright on a black background.

Phase-contrast microscopy

This has proved particularly useful for the examination of living cells, the constituents of which normally show little differentiation. Monochromatic light is employed; light directly transmitted through the sample is reduced in intensity and the deflected light is brought half a wavelength out of phase with the transmitted light. Strong contrasts in the material under examination are thereby obtained without reduction in the resolving power of the microscope.

Ultraviolet microscopy

The limit of resolution of any microscope is governed by the wavelength of the beam employed; the shorter the wavelength, the smaller the object which can be resolved. The ultraviolet microscope with lenses of fused quartz will transmit radiation down to the wavelength of 240 nm. The images produced are recorded photographically. The instrument has been valuable in the study of cell division and differentiation.

Electron microscopy

Just as a beam of light can be focused by an optical lens, so a stream of electrons can be focused by an electromagnet acting as a lens. Objects placed in the path of the electrons produce an image which can be recorded either on a fluorescent screen or on a photographic plate. Both the focal length and the magnification can be varied by regulation of the field strength, which is controlled by the current passing through the lens. Good stabilization of the lens current is essential for the best lens performance. Because gas molecules will cause a scattering of electrons, electron images are formed only in a high vacuum (less than 10^{-4} mmHg). Although commercial electron microscopes were available in 1939, it was not until the 1950s that their potential could be fully exploited for biological work. The breakthrough in this field centred on the preparation of ultra-thin sections of biological tissue by the use of glass knives and on the development of suitable staining, fixation and embedding materials. To prevent complete scattering of the electrons by the tissue, sections of the order of 20–200 nm are used and a buffered solution of osmium tetroxide is commonly employed for fixation and staining. Unstained cell components of a tissue have a fairly uniform electron scattering power, similar to that of the embedding medium, so that little contrast of the image is obtainable. However, the incorporation of electron-dense atoms (osmium) into the cell organelles enables a good degree of contrast to be obtained on the electron micrographs of the sections. There is, at present, no objective way of determining how much the fine structure of cells is altered by the fixation methods employed, but indirect correlation of the results obtained with those from other techniques is reassuring.

The light microscope gives magnifications of the order of ×1000 with a resolution, set by the wavelength of the light employed, down to about 0.2 μm for visible light; no further magnification of the image can increase the detail. The theoretical limit of resolution of the electron microscope is similarly governed by the wavelength of the electrons (about 0.003 nm) and in practice electron microscopes give resolutions to about 0.4 nm. Magnifications of ×10 000 to ×24000 are commonly employed and to show all the available detail on high-quality

electron micrographs, prints at magnifications of around ×500 000 may be required.

Much knowledge of the detailed structure of the living cell has only been made possible by the advent of the electron microscope. For the routine examination of vegetable drugs the light microscope with polarizing attachment is generally fully adequate, but scanning electron micrographs at a much lower magnification than the above can be extremely useful for depicting structural details not obvious with the light microscope, for example, maize starch and digitalis (Fig. 23.17).

Drawings for publication and thesis work

For the detailed steps involved in the preparation of these line drawings, see earlier editions of this book.

PREPARATION OF DRUGS FOR MICROSCOPICAL EXAMINATION AND GENERAL USE OF REAGENTS

The following aims should be kept in mind for the microscopical examination of crude drugs.

1. The determination of the size, shape and relative positions of the different cells and tissues.
2. The determination of the chemical nature of the cell walls.
3. The determination of the form and chemical nature of the cell contents.

Dried material often requires softening by exposing it to a moist atmosphere (leaves) or by boiling in water (roots and barks). Botanical sections of the plant material may need to be made (cut either by hand or with a freezing microtome). Sections of the dry material may be necessary for the examination of mucilage or water-soluble cell components. Disintegration serves for the isolation of specific tissues and bleaching and defatting techniques for observing deeply coloured materials and fatty seeds respectively. Almost certainly, clearing reagents will be required together with a range of suitable stains for cell walls and cell contents.

Any report should state what characters appear to be of the greatest diagnostic importance and these should be illustrated by suitable sketches.

Distribution of tissues

A general idea of the distribution of tissues can be obtained by the examination of transverse and radial and tangential longitudinal sections. Such sections should first be mounted in water or dilute glycerin. Subsequently sections should be cleared by means of chloral hydrate or other clearing agents (see below) and some stained as follows.

Phloroglucinol and hydrochloric acid. Mount the section in a 1% solution of phloroglucinol in ethanol (90%) and allow to stand for about 2 min; remove any alcohol which has not evaporated with a piece of filter paper; add concentrated hydrochloric acid, cover and examine. All lignified walls stain pink or red.

Hydrochloric acid is a powerful clearing agent and it must be remembered that it will dissolve many cell contents, including calcium oxalate. The vegetable debris of catechu contains phloroglucinol and in this case the wood stains on the simple application of hydrochloric acid.

To prevent damage to the microscope either by liquid contact or by vapours, preparations mounted in concentrated hydrochloric acid should be free of excess acid and must be removed from the microscope stage as soon as possible.

Chlor-zinc-iodine solution. The reagent, often somewhat slowly, stains cellulose walls blue or violet, lignified or suberized walls yellow or brown, and starch grains blue.

43

Clearing, defatting and bleaching

Structures are frequently obscured by the abundance of cell contents, the presence of colouring matters and the shrinkage or collapse of the cell walls. Therefore, reagents are used for the removal of cell contents, for bleaching and for restoring as far as possible the original shape of the cell wall. If the microscopical examination is to be made from the section mounted in the clearing agent, the refractive index of the latter is important. It may be advisable to wash the section and mount in a different medium. The commonly used mountants glycerin, alcohol, carbolic acid, lactophenol, clove oil and Canada balsam all have some clearing effect. The following clearing and bleaching agents are particularly useful.

Solution of chloral hydrate. This dissolves starch, proteins, chlorophyll, resins and volatile oils, and causes shrunken cells to expand. Chloral hydrate may be used, not only for sections but also for whole leaves, flowers, pollen grains, etc. It does not dissolve calcium oxalate and is therefore a good reagent for detection of these crystals.

Solution of potash. Solutions of potassium hydroxide, both aqueous and alcoholic, up to a strength of 50% are used for different purposes, but for use as a clearing agent a 5% aqueous solution is most generally useful. A 0.3% solution of potash may be used to dissolve aleurone grains. A 5% solution is much more powerful, and rapidly dissolves starch, protein, etc., causing the swelling of cell walls. Potash should be washed out as soon as clearing is completed, as more prolonged action is liable to cause disintegration (see below).

Ether–ethanol. A mixture of equal parts of ether and ethanol (96%) is useful for the removal of fixed oils, fats, resins, volatile oils, tannins or chlorophyll. Defatting is particularly necessary in the case of oily seeds such as linseed and strophanthus.

Solution of sodium hypochlorite. This solution is useful for bleaching dark-coloured sections such as those of many barks and for removing chlorophyll from leaves. When bleaching is complete, the sections should not be left in the reagent but should be removed and washed with water. Prolonged contact with solution of chlorinated soda causes the removal of starch and lignin, which may not be desirable.

Disintegration and isolation of tissues

The use of reagents for purposes of disintegration is based on their action on the cell wall, particularly the middle lamella. Woody tissues are usually disintegrated by means of oxidizing agents, as these oxidize away the middle lamella, which is composed mainly of lignin. Thus, dilute nitric acid has a marked disintegrating effect on wood, whereas dilute sulphuric acid has not. The middle lamella of cellulose cells is composed of pectic substances which are made soluble by dilute acids or dilute alkalis, which thus effect disintegration. Pure celluloses, however, are resistant to hydrolysing and oxidizing agents, and the stability of cellulose in boiling 5% potash is made use of for the separation of cotton from wool. Other materials such as mannans, galactans, pectin, hemicelluloses, gums and lichenin, which may occur in the cell wall, are much more readily attacked by hydrolysing agents. It will thus be seen that the composition of the 'crude fibres' (i.e. those tissues which remain after the material has been subjected to the action of hydrolysing agents under controlled conditions) is likely to vary in both amount and chemical nature in different drugs. However, quantitative comparisons of the crude fibres of different samples of the same drug are useful.

Potassium chlorate and nitric acid. The strength of the reagent and the time it is allowed to act must be varied according to the nature of the material. For woods (e.g. quassia) the material, in small pieces or thick sections, is immersed in 50% nitric acid. *Minute* quantities of potassium chlorate are added at intervals to maintain an evolution of gas. From time to time a fragment of the wood should be removed and teased with needles. When it breaks up readily, it should be washed free from acid and examined. The process should not be continued longer than is necessary, since prolonged bleaching causes more or less complete destruction of the lignin.

Chromic acid and nitric or sulphuric acid. The reagent usually consists of a mixture of equal parts of 10% chromic acid and 10% nitric or sulphuric acid. It is frequently used for the disintegration of sclerenchymatous tissues such as the testas of capsicum and colocynth seeds or for the separation of lignified hairs such as those of nux vomica and strophanthus.

Solution of potash or soda. As mentioned above, alkalis are used both for clearing and disintegrating. The material is usually digested with 5% potash on a water-bath until the more resistant cells can be teased out of the more or less completely disintegrated parenchyma. The method is useful for the separation of the heavy cuticularized epidermis of leaves and for the isolation of secretory tissue such as the vittae of umbelliferous fruits and the latex vessels of lobelia. Suberized and cutinized tissues are very resistant to the potash. Potash is also useful for the isolation of lignified elements such as are found in the veins of leaves, in senna stalks and in many barks.

Preparation of a crude fibre

For qualitative work the following procedure may be adopted. Mix about 2 g of the drug, in No. 60 powder, with 50 ml of 10% nitric acid in a casserole. Bring to the boil and maintain at the boiling point for 30 s. Dilute with water and strain through a fine filter cloth held over the mouth of a filter funnel. Transfer the washed residue to the casserole and boil for a further 30 s with 50 ml of a 2.5% solution of sodium hydroxide. Collect and wash the residue as before, mount and examine. It will be found that the tissues disintegrate readily and are in a condition well suited to microscopical examination.

Reagents

Directions for making the following reagents, if not given below, will be found in the appendices of the *BP*. Some of the uses of each are mentioned, but further details will be found elsewhere.

Ethanol. Different strengths are used for preserving material and for hardening. Alcohol acts as a clearing agent by dissolving oils, resins, chlorophyll, etc. It does not dissolve gums and mucilages (therefore a useful mountant for drugs containing them).

Alkanna tincture. A supply sufficient for a few months only should be made by macerating 1 part of alkanet root and 5 parts of alcohol 90% for 1 week, afterwards filtering. Stains oils and fats and suberized and cuticularized walls.

Chloral hydrate and glycerin combines the properties of chloral hydrate and glycerin and is therefore useful for slow clearing without heat. Preparations mounted in it may be left for some days without undue evaporation.

Chloral hydrate solution BP (chloral 80 g, water 20 ml). A valuable and widely used clearing agent. See above.

Chromic acid solution. 25% Chromic acid in water. See 'Disintegration and isolation of tissues'.

Chromic and nitric acids solution. 10% Chromic acid and 10% nitric acid. See 'Disintegration and isolation of tissues'.

Clove oil. A useful clearing agent for powders containing much oil.

Cresol. A suitable mountant for chalks, kieselguhr, etc.

Chlor-zinc-iodine solution (syn. Schulze's solution). Prepared by adding a solution of zinc chloride (zinc chloride 20 g; water 8.5 ml) dropwise to a solution of potassium iodide (1.0 g) and iodine (0.5 g) in water (20 ml) until a precipitate of iodine forms which does not disappear on cooling. This requires about 1.5 ml. Used as test for walls containing celluloses. Iodine solution followed by sulphuric acid gives similar results.

Copper oxide, ammoniacal solution of, BP. This solution must be freshly prepared. It causes swelling and solution of cellulose walls. The balloon-like swellings produced in raw cotton are best observed if the reagent be diluted with an equal volume of distilled water. This solution is commonly known as cuoxam.

Corallin, alkaline solution of, BP (syn. Corallin-soda). Stains the callose of sieve-plates and some gums and mucilages.

Ether–ethanol. A defatting agent.

Ferric chloride solution; iron (III) chloride solution BP. See 'Tannins'.

Glycerin, dilute. One volume of glycerin is mixed with two volumes of distilled water. A useful mountant for preparations which may be left for some time, as it does not dry up. It has some clearing action, but is much inferior in this respect to chloral hydrate. It can usefully be added to a mount cleared with chloral hydrate solution to prevent the formation of crystals. It is not a good mountant for starch, as the grains tend to become transparent and striations, etc. are difficult to see; water is preferable.

Hydrochloric acid. This (density *c.* 1.18; *c.* 11.5 M) is used in testing silk and preparations containing colchicine, and with phloroglucinol as a test for lignin.

Iodine water, BP (see BP Iodine Solutions R1 and R2). This gives a blue colour with starch and hemicelluloses. Iodine Tincture *BP*, followed by sulphuric acid, resembles chlor-zinc-iodine (q.v.).

Lactophenol BP. See 'Clearing'.

Mercury–nitric acid solution BP (syn. Millon's Reagent). Test for protein-containing materials e.g. aleurone grains, wool and silk.

Nitric acid 10%. See 'Crude fibre'.

Phloroglucinol solution. A 1% solution in 90% ethanol with hydrochloric acid as a test for lignin.

Picric acid solution. A saturated solution in water which is used to stain aleurone grains and animal fibres.

Potash solution. A 5% solution is commonly used for clearing and disintegrating (q.v.) and for the separation of cotton from wool. A 50% solution is used in testing for chitin in ergot and for eugenol in clove. A 2.5% solution is used for preparing crude fibre (q.v.).

Potassium cupri-tartrate, solution of (syn. Fehling's Solution). Used in testing for reducing sugars such as glucose.

Potassium iodobismuthate R1. Precipitates with alkaloids.

Potassium tetraiodomercurate solution BP (syn. Mayer's Reagent). A precipitant for most alkaloids.

Potassium chlorate and nitric acid (syn. Schultze's macerating fluid). Produces bleaching, disintegration and delignification.

Ruthenium red, solution of, BP. Stains many gums and mucilages. It must be freshly prepared.

Sodium carbonate solution BP. This is useful for the disintegration of fibres such as flax, where the use of an oxidizing agent is not required.

Sodium hypochlorite solution. The *BP* includes a strong and weak solution; for use see 'Clearing, defatting and bleaching'.

Sudan III (Sudan red) solution. A solution in equal parts of glycerin and alcohol, stains oils and suberized walls, and is useful in the examination of secretory cells and ducts.

Sulphuric acid 80%. Concentrated sulphuric acid causes rapid charring, but dilutions containing 80% or less form useful reagents. The behaviour of cotton, wool, chalks, calcium oxalate and sections of strophanthus seeds should be noted. The acid dissolves cellulose and lignified walls, but has little action on suberin.

Water, distilled. A useful mountant for starches. Sections which have been bleached with solution of chlorinated soda or similar reagent may be freed from the bubbles of gas which they frequently contain by placing them in freshly boiled distilled water.

POWDERED DRUGS

The systematic approach to the identification of powdered drugs can proceed in a number of ways; for organized drugs, however, all methods depend on the microscopical recognition of characteristic cell types and cell contents. Identification can then be made by reference to tables and appropriate illustrations, by the use of punched cards, and by employing a suitable computer program. For dealing with mixtures of drugs, greater skills and practice are required and only the first of the above approaches is applicable. When a tentative identification has been made, further confirmatory observations and chemical tests can be performed; most pharmacopoeial drugs now have TLC tests for identity.

Preliminary tests

1. Note the colour. *White*: acacia, tragacanth; *light yellow*: colocynth, peeled liquorice, ginger, quassia, squill; *light brown*: ipecacuanha, unpeeled liquorice, nux vomica, opium, fennel, gentian, cascara, coriander, cardamoms, jalap, linseed, aloes; *cinnamon brown*: cinnamon, catechu; *dark brown*: clove, Curaçao aloes; *dark reddish-brown*: nutmegs; *violet*: ergot; *red*: cinchona; *orange*: rhubarb; *pale green*: lobelia; *green*: henbane, belladonna, stramonium, senna, digitalis.
2. Note odour. The following are particularly characterized: ginger, fennel, gentian, opium, coriander, cardamoms, cinnamon, clove, nutmegs.
3. Taste (NB: Students should *not* taste powdered drugs without the consent of their supervisor. Adulterated or spoiled drugs may be harmful, others such as capsicum too pungent to taste, and alkaloid-containing drugs poisonous). *Aromatic*: coriander, cardamoms, cinnamon, clove, nutmegs; *aromatic and pungent*: ginger;

43

bitter: colocynth, quassia, nux vomica, gentian, aloes, squill, cinchona, rauwolfia; *sweet*: liquorice; *astringent*: catechu; *mucilaginous*: marshmallow root, slippery elm bark, ispaghula husk.

4. Mix a small quantity of the powder with a few drops of water and allow to stand. Aqueous extracts and inspissated juices such as catechu and aloes dissolve almost completely, while the gummy or mucilaginous nature of drugs such as acacia, tragacanth and linseed becomes apparent.

   Mix a small quantity of the powder with dilute sulphuric acid. Effervescence followed by solution occurs with chalk.

5. Press a small quantity of the powder between filter paper. An oily stain, spreading but persisting when the paper is heated in an oven, occurs with powders containing fixed oil. Volatile oil will give a stain, disappearing on heating in an oven.

6. Shake a little powder in half a test-tube-full of water, and if any marked frothing occurs, suspect saponin-containing drugs; boil gently and note the odour of any volatile oil evolved. Filter and divide into two portions which may be tested for tannins and for anthraquinone derivatives as follows.

   (1) Test for tannin (see Chapter 21, 'Tannins'). *Tannins absent* from quassia, squill, strophanthus, capsicum and ginger; *gallitannins present* in cloves and rhubarb; *phlobatannins present* in catechu, krameria, prunus serotina, cinnamon and cinchona.

   (2) Test for anthraquinones by shaking the aqueous extractive with ether, separating and adding to the ethereal solution about one-third of its volume of ammonia. After shaking, a pink colour is obtained in the aqueous layer with rhubarb, cascara and senna.

Microscopical examination

If the preliminary tests have shown that the drug dissolves or becomes mucilaginous in water, trials should be made with other liquids such as alcohol, olive oil or lactophenol until one is found in which the drug is insoluble. In most cases, however, the following procedure may be adopted.

Examination for starch. Mount in water, examine and sketch any granules observed and prove whether they are starch or not by irrigation with iodine water. Do not waste time trying to find other structures that are best seen in the following mountants.

Examination for epidermal trichomes and calcium oxalate solution. Mount in chloral hydrate solution, boil gently until clear, and examine. To ensure that calcium oxalate, if present in small quantity, is not overlooked, polarized light may be used.

Examination for lignin. Moisten the powder with an alcoholic solution of phloroglucinol and allow to stand until nearly dry; add concentrated hydrochloric acid, apply a cover-glass, and examine. Note the presence or absence of lignified vessels, fibres, parenchyma, sclereids or hairs (e.g. nux vomica). If vessels or fibres do not stain pink, suspect rhubarb or ginger.

A considerable amount of information should have been derived from the preliminary tests and the above three mounts, and the examination may be continued by the application of further microchemical tests (chlor-zinc-iodine, tincture of alkanet, ruthenium red, corallin soda, etc.). It is often advisable to defat oily powders, to bleach highly coloured ones and to prepare a crude fibre of those powders containing much starch.

Microscopical measurements of cells and cell contents should be made whenever possible and compared with those published in the literature.

The application of a knowledge of the anatomy of those plant organs occurring in drugs should make possible a recognition of the organs represented. This should be followed by reference to an atlas of vegetable powders or tables of the diagnostic characters of powdered drugs. The identity of a powder should not be regarded as established until it has been compared with one of known authenticity.

A series of tables to assist with the identification of powdered drugs, based on the presence or absence of starch, epidermal trichomes and calcium oxalate, will be found in earlier editions of this book (up to and including the 13th edition). Tables of histological characters of drugs are also given in Wallis's *Textbook of Pharmacognosy* (1967); in these a morphological arrangement is employed so that in order to commence the identification process the student must first decide to which group his unknown powder belongs. For the appropriate illustrations of the elements present in powdered drugs see Jackson and Snowdon (1990) in the literature cited in Chapter 2.

Computer-assisted identification of powdered drugs

In 1976 Jolliffe and Jolliffee published details of a computer program for the identification of 174 powdered drugs of organized structure (*Analyst*, **101**, 622). Further elaboration of the method followed as indicated in the literature quoted below. The procedure involves the examination of a single unknown powder in four different mountants for the presence or absence of eleven histological characters, namely, calcium oxalate (if present, type of crystal), aleurone, cork, lignified parenchyma, stomata (if present, which of six types), trichomes (if present, type and structure), vessels/tracheids (if present, lignified or non-lignified), sclereids, fibres, starch and pollen. The information is coded as a string of characters comprising six blocks of five digits, each of which indicates the absence or presence of the microscopical characters being examined. Processing involves a validity check of the input data and a comparison of the observed characters for the unknown with those of the 174 powdered drugs stored in the data bank. The output then gives those drugs having zero errors compared with the input followed by those having 1, 2, etc., errors. Allowance is made in the program for the fact that a particular feature of the drug might be present in such small amount that it could be missed by the inexperienced microscopist. For drugs where the computer cannot give a unique identification, simple distinguishing tests are suggested e.g. the measurement of starch grains and fibres for cassia and cinnamon. Contamination of the drug with moulds, mites, etc. does not affect the identification and the presence of additional material in the powder affording one characteristic only, e.g. starch, is accommodated.

In addition to organized single powders it should be noted that computer-aided identification programs have also been described for unorganized drugs, homoeopathic tinctures, textile and surgical dressing fibres, and food materials (see below).

Further reading

Bannerman HJ, Cox BJ, Musset JH 1982 Computer-assisted identification of unorganised drugs. Pharmaceutical Journal 228: 716–717 [CAIDUD]

Jolliffe GH, Jolliffe GO 1978 Microcomputer-aided identification of powdered vegetable drugs. Pharmaceutical Journal 221: 385–386 [POWDERS]

Jolliffe GH, Jolliffe GO 1979 'MICROAID'. Practical Computing 2: 120–132

Jolliffe GH, Jolliffe GO 1989 The microcomputer as an analytical aid in drug microscopy. In: Trease and Evans' Pharmacognosy (13th edition). Baillière Tindall, London, UK, pp 784–798

Stevens RG 1980 Computer-aided identification of textile and surgical dressing fibres. Pharmaceutical Journal 223: 293–294 [FIBRES/BAS]

QUANTITATIVE MICROSCOPY

In addition to the simple measurement of the sizes of tissues, cells and cell contents by means of the micrometer eyepiece or camera lucida, it is possible to estimate the percentage of foreign organic matter in many powdered drugs by a lycopodium spore method which was developed by T. E. Wallis (Analytical Microscopy, 3rd ed., 1965) and subsequently adopted by the *Pharmacopoeia*. Although the method appears now to be little used, the principles involved, as cited below, are of interest. Other microscopical determinations which may usefully be made in certain cases are vein-islet numbers, palisade ratios, stomatal numbers and stomatal indices.

Lycopodium spore methods

Wallis showed that lycopodium spores are exceptionally uniform in size (about 25 μm) and that 1 mg of lycopodium contains an average of 94 000 spores. The number of spores mg^{-1} was determined by direct counting and by calculation based on specific gravity and dimensions of the spores. The methods gave values in good agreement. These facts make it possible to evaluate many powdered drugs, provided that they contain one of: (1) well-defined particles which may be *counted* (e.g. pollen grains or starch grains); or (2) single-layered tissues or cells the *area* of which may be traced at a definite magnification and the actual area calculated; or (3) characteristic particles of uniform thickness, the length of which can be measured at a definite magnification and the actual length calculated. Whichever method is adopted, mounts containing a definite proportion of the powder and lycopodium are used and the lycopodium spores are counted in each of the fields in which the number or area of the particles in the powder is determined. The method is somewhat laborious and has not been subjected to statistical assessment. For powdered pharmacopoeial drugs reliance is now placed on other methods. Details can, however, be found in the *BP* 1973 and earlier editions of this book. Classical examples of drugs to which it was applied are senna and linseed (area measurements), nux vomica (trichome-rib lengths) and pypethrum and ginger (counts).

Leaf measurements

A number of leaf measurements are used to distinguish between some closely related species not easily characterized by general microscopy.

Palisade ratio.   The average number of palisade cells beneath each upper epidermal cell is termed the *palisade ratio*. Quite fine powders can be used for the determination.

Pieces of leaf about 2 mm square, or powder, are cleared by boiling with chloral hydrate solution, mounted and examined with a 4 mm objective. A camera lucida or other projection apparatus is arranged so that the epidermal cells and the palisade cells lying below them may be traced. First a number of groups each of four epidermal cells are traced and their outlines inked in to make them more conspicuous. The palisade cells lying beneath each group are then focused and traced. The palisade cells in each group are counted, those being included in the count which are more than half-covered by the epidermal cells; the figure obtained divided by 4 gives the palisade ratio of that group. The range of a number of groups from different particles should be recorded.

Drugs for which palisade ratios have been utilized include belladonna, stramonium, buchu, senna, digitalis and, for recognition as adulterants, xanthium and phytolacca.

Stomatal number.   The average number of stomata per square millimetre of epidermis is termed the *stomatal number*. In recording results the range as well as the average value should be recorded for each surface of the leaf and the ratio of values for the two surfaces.

Fragments of leaf from the middle of the lamina are cleared with chloral hydrate solution or chlorinated soda. Timmerman counted the number of stomata in 12–30 fields and from a knowledge of the area of the field was able to calculate the stomatal number; the camera lucida method described for vein-islet numbers may also be used, the position of each stoma being indicated on the paper by a small cross.

Using fresh leaves, replicas of leaf surface may be made which are satisfactory for the determination of stomatal number and stomatal index. An approximate 50% gelatin and water gel is liquefied on a water-bath and smeared on a hot slide. The fresh leaf is added, the slide is inverted and cooled under a tap and after about 15–30 min the specimen is stripped off. The imprint on the gelatin gives a clear outline of epidermal cells, stomata and trichomes.

The early investigations by Timmerman (1927) indicated that stomatal numbers are usually useless for distinguishing between closely allied species, but that in certain cases the ratio between the number of stomata on the two surfaces may be of diagnostic importance. It is possible, for example, to distinguish *Datura innoxia* from other species of *Datura* by this means.

Stomatal index.   The percentage proportion of the ultimate divisions of the epidermis of a leaf which have been converted into stomata is termed the *stomatal index*:

$$I = \frac{S \times 100}{E + S} \times 100$$

where S = number of stomata per unit area and E = number of ordinary epidermal cells in the same unit area. While stomatal number varies considerably with the age of the leaf, stomatal index is highly constant for a given species and may be determined on either entire or powdered samples. It is employed in the *BP* and *EP* to distinguish leaflets of Indian and Alexandrian sennas.

Pieces of leaf other than extreme margin or midrib are suitably cleared and mounted, and the lower surface examined by means of a microscope with a 4 mm objective and an eyepiece containing a 5 mm square micrometer disc. Counts are made of the numbers of epidermal cells and of stomata (the two guard cells and ostiole being considered as one unit) within the square grid, a cell being counted if at least half of its area lies within the grid. Successive adjacent fields are examined until about 400 cells have been counted and the stomatal index value calculated from these figures. The stomatal index may be determined for both leaf surfaces.

Rowson (1943 and 1946) found that stomatal index values may be used to distinguish between leaves of co-generic species (Table 43.1).

Vein-islet number.   The term 'vein-islet' is used to denote the minute area of photosynthetic tissue encircled by the ultimate divisions of the conducting strands. The number of vein-islets mm^{-2} calculated from four contiguous square millimetres in the central part of the lamina, midway between the midrib and the margin, is termed the *vein-islet number*. When determined on whole leaves, the area examined should be from the central part of the lamina, midway between the margin and midrib.

Many leaves may be cleared by boiling in chloral hydrate solution in a test-tube placed in a boiling water-bath. Those which are difficult to clear in this way may, after soaking in water, be treated successively with sodium hypochlorite to bleach, 10% hydrochloric acid to remove calcium oxalate, and finally chloral hydrate.

A camera lucida or projection apparatus is set up and by means of a stage micrometer the paper is divided into squares of 1 mm^2 using a 16 mm objective. The stage micrometer is then replaced by the cleared preparation and the veins are traced in four contiguous squares, either in a square 2 mm × 2 mm or a rectangle 1 mm × 4 mm (Fig. 43.2). When counting, it is convenient to number each vein-islet on the tracing. Each numbered area must be completely enclosed by veins, and

Table 43.1 Stomatal index values.

| | Stomatal index | |
Species	Upper surface	Lower surface
Atropa acuminata	1.7 to **4.8** to 12.2	16.2 to **17.5** to 1.83
Atropa belladonna	2.3 to **3.9** to 10.5	20.2 to **21.7** to 23.0
Cassia senna	11.4 to **12.4** to 13.3	10.8 to **11.8** to 12.6
Cassia angustifolia	17.1 to **19.0** to 20.7	17.0 to **18.3** to 19.3
Datura inermis	18.1 to **18.3** to 18.7	24.5 to **24.9** to 25.3
Datura metel	12.7 to **17.4** to 19.4	21.2 to **22.3** to 23.9
Datura stramonium	16.4 to **18.1** to 20.4	24.1 to **24.9** to 26.3
Datura tatula	15.6 to **20.2** to 22.3	28.3 to **29.8** to 31.0
Digitalis lanata	13.9 to **14.4** to 14.7	14.9 to **16.1** to 17.6
Digitalis lutea	2.5 to **5.5** to 8.4	21.6 to **22.9** to 25.2
Digitalis purpurea	1.6 to **2.7** to 4.0	17.9 to **19.2** to 19.5
Digitalis thapsi	5.9 to **7.0** to 7.8	11.9 to **12.4** to 13.5
Erythroxylum coca	Nil	12.2 to **13.2** to 14.0
Erythroxylum truxillense	Nil	8.9 to **10.1** to 10.7
Phytolacca acinosa	Nil	**15.0**
Phytolacca americana	2.9 to **4.2** to 5.7	13.0 to **13.2** to 13.4

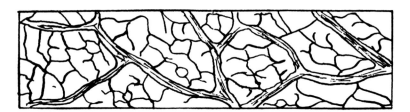

Fig. 43.2
The vein-islets of 4 mm² of the leaf of *Erythroxylum truxillense*. (After Levin.)

Table 43.2 Vein-islet numbers.

	Species	Range of vein-islet numbers	Average
Senna	Cassia senna	15–29.5	26
	Cassia angustifolia	19.5–22.5	21
Coca	Erythroxylum coca	8–12	11
	Erythroxylum truxillense	15–26	20
Digitalis	Digitalis purpurea	2–5.5	3.5
	Digitalis lanata	2–3.5	2.7
		3–8	4.4
	Digitalis lutea	1–1.5	1.2
	Digitalis thapsi	8.5–16	

Table 43.3 Veinlet termination numbers.

Atropa acuminata	1.4–3.5
Atropa belladonna	6.3–10.3
Cassia angustifolia	25.9–32.8
Cassia senna	32.7–40.2
Datura stramonium	12.6–20.1
Digitalis purpurea	2.5–4.2
Erythroxylum coca	16.8–21.0
Erythroxylum truxillense	23.1–32.3
Hyoscyamus niger	12.4–19.0

those which are incomplete are excluded from the count if cut by the top and left-hand sides of the square or rectangle but included if cut by the other two sides. For example, the vein-islets in Fig. 43.2 total 62 and the vein-islet number is therefore 15.5.

The vein-islet number frequently serves to distinguish closely related plants (Table 43.2).

Veinlet termination number. Hall and Melville (1951) determined veinlet termination number, which they define as 'the number of veinlet terminations per mm² of leaf surface. A vein termination is the ultimate free termination of a veinlet or branch of a veinlet'. By this character they distinguished between Peruvian and Bolivian coca leaves and between Alexandrian and Tinnevelly senna leaflets. The values are recorded in Table 43.3.

One practical difficulty in the measurement of vein-islet and veinlet-termination numbers is deciding exactly where, and if, a veinlet terminates. This may appear to vary according to the preliminary treatment a leaf has received.

At present, of the above leaf measurements, only stomatal index is employed officially. With the increasing number of whole herbs and leaves now being introduced into the *European* and *British Pharmacopoeias* and the need for standardization of the many herbal products of interest world-wide, a further investigation of the possible usefulness of these leaf measurements might prove rewarding. For acceptance, the results from any future measurements would necessitate a more sophisticated statistical analysis than was probably afforded the examples quoted above.

Index

Page numbers in **bold** refer to principal references, those in *italics* refer to figures, tables and chemical formulae.

T